Evidence-Based Obstetrics and Gynecology

Evidence-Based Obstetrics and Gynecology

EDITED BY

Errol R. Norwitz, MD, PhD, MBA

Louis E. Phaneuf Professor of Obstetrics & Gynecology
Tufts University School of Medicine
Chief Scientific Officer
Chair, Department of Obstetrics & Gynecology
Tufts Medical Center
Boston, MA, USA

Carolyn M. Zelop, MD

Director of Ultrasound and Perinatal Research
Division of MFM and Department of Obstetrics and Gynecology
The Valley Hospital, Ridgewood, NJ, USA
Clinical Professor of Obstetrics and Gynecology
NYU School of Medicine, New York, NY, USA

David A. Miller, MD

Division of Maternal-Fetal Medicine
Department of Obstetrics and Gynecology
Keck School of Medicine
University of Southern California
Los Angeles, CA, USA

David L. Keefe, MD

Stanley H. Kaplan Professor
Department of Obstetrics and Gynecology
NYU Langone Medical Center
New York, NY, USA

WILEY Blackwell

This edition first published 2019

Registered Office(s)
John Wiley & Sons, Inc., 111 River Street, Hoboken, NJ 07030, USA
John Wiley & Sons Ltd, The Atrium, Southern Gate, Chichester, West Sussex, PO19 8SQ, UK

Editorial Office
9600 Garsington Road, Oxford, OX4 2DQ, UK

For details of our global editorial offices, customer services, and more information about Wiley products visit us at www.wiley.com.

Wiley also publishes its books in a variety of electronic formats and by print-on-demand. Some content that appears in standard print versions of this book may not be available in other formats.

Library of Congress Cataloging-in-Publication Data

Names: Norwitz, Errol R., editor. | Zelop, Carolyn M., editor. | Miller, David A. (David Arthur), 1961- editor. | Keefe, David (David L.), editor.
Title: Evidence-based obstetrics and gynecology / edited by Errol R. Norwitz, Carolyn M. Zelop, David A. Miller, David L. Keefe.
Other titles: Evidence-based obstetrics and gynecology (Norwitz)
Description: Hoboken, NJ : Wiley, 2019. | Includes bibliographical references and index. |
Identifiers: LCCN 2018041057 (print) | LCCN 2018041689 (ebook) | ISBN 9781119072928 (Adobe PDF) | ISBN 9781119072959 (ePub) | ISBN 9781444334333 (hardback)
Subjects: | MESH: Genital Diseases, Female | Pregnancy Complications | Evidence-Based Medicine
Classification: LCC RG101 (ebook) | LCC RG101 (print) | NLM WP 140 | DDC 618.1–dc23
LC record available at https://lccn.loc.gov/2018041057

Cover Design: Wiley
Cover Images: © monkeybusinessimages/Getty Images
© John Fedele/Getty Images, © Bohbeh/Shutterstock
© Doro Guzenda/Shutterstock

Set in 9/12pt and MeridienLTStd by SPi Global, Chennai, India
Printed in Singapore by C.O.S. Printers Pte Ltd

10 9 8 7 6 5 4 3 2 1

Contents

List of contributors

Veronica Ades
Department of Obstetrics and Gynecology
NYU Langone Medical Center
New York, NY, USA

Jennifer Amorosa
Department of Obstetrics, Gynecology and Reproductive Sciences
Icahn School of Medicine, Mt Sinai Hospital
New York, NY, USA

Karen Archabald
Legacy Health
Portland, OR, USA

Stephanie Bakaysa
Department of Maternal-Fetal Medicine
Tufts Medical Center
Boston, MA, USA

Oren Barak
Rehovot, affiliated with the Hadassah-Hebrew University School of Medicine, Department of Obstetrics and Gynecology
Kaplan Medical Center
Jerusalem, Israel

Marie Beall
Obstetrics and Gynecology
Harbor UCLA Medical Center
Torrance, CA, USA

Mila de Moura Behar Pontremoli Salcedo
Department of Gynecology and Obstetrics
Federal University of Health Sciences (UFCSPA)/Santa Casa de Porto Alegre
Porto Alegre, RS, Brazil

Rana Snipe Berry
Department of Obstetrics and Gynecology
Indiana University School of Medicine
Indianapolis, IN, USA

Stephanie V. Blank
Division of Gynecologic Oncology, Department of Obstetrics and Gynecology
NYU Langone Medical Center
New York, NY, USA

Isaac Blickstein
Obstetrics and Gynecology, Kaplan Medical Center, Rehovot,
The Hadassah-Hebrew University School of Medicine, Jerusalem, Israel

Anne-Sophie Boes
Leuven University Fertility Centre (LUFC)
UZ Leuven, Leuven, Belgium

Ware Branch
Division of Maternal-Fetal Medicine, Department of Obstetrics and Gynecology, Medical Director of Women and Newborns Clinical Program for Intermountain Healthcare, Intermountain Medical Center
University of Utah
Murray, UT, USA

Haywood Brown
Morsani College of Medicine
University of South Florida Health Center
Tampa, FL, USA

Julie Brown
Department of Obstetrics and Gynecology
University of Auckland
New Zealand

Steve N. Caritis
Division of Maternal-Fetal Medicine, Department of Obstetrics, Gynecology and Reproductive Sciences
Magee Women's Hospital of UPMC
Pittsburgh, PA, USA

H. J. A. Carp
Department Obstetrics and Gynecology
Sheba Medical Center
Tel HaShomer, Israel

Steven L. Clark
Department of Obstetrics and Gynecology
Baylor College of Medicine Obstetrics and Gynecology, Service Chief
MFM, Texas Children's Hospital, TCH Pavilion for Women
Houston, TX, USA

Joshua Copel
Department Obstetrics, Gynecology & Reproductive Sciences,
Division of Maternal-Fetal Medicine
Yale School of Medicine
New Haven, CT, USA

Sabrina D. Craigo
Division of Maternal-Fetal Medicine, Department of Obstetrics and Gynecology
Tufts Medical Center
Boston, MA, USA

John P. Curtin
Division of Gynecologic Oncology, Department of Obstetrics and Gynecology
NYU Langone Medical Center
New York, NY, USA

Thomas D'Hooghe
Division of Reproductive Medicine and Biology, Department of Obstetrics and Gynecology
University of Leuven
Leuven, Belgium

Gary A. Dildy
Department of Obstetrics and Gynecology
Baylor College of Medicine Obstetrics and Gynecology, Service Chief
MFM, Texas Children's Hospital, TCH Pavilion for Women
Houston, TX , USA

Margaret Dziadosz
Department of Obstetrics and Gynecology, NYU School of Medicine
New York University
New York, NY, USA

Britt K. Erickson
Division of Gynecologic Oncology
University of Alabama at Birmingham
Birmingham, AL, USA

Christine Farinelli
Obstetrix Medical Group
Tucson Medical Center
Tucson, AZ, USA

Cynthia Farquhar
Department of Obstetrics and Gynecology
University of Auckland
New Zealand

Maisa N. Feghali
Division of Maternal-Fetal Medicine, Department of Obstetrics, Gynecology and Reproductive Sciences
Magee Women's Hospital of UPMC
Pittsburgh, PA, USA

Kimberley Ferrante
Division of Female Pelvic Medicine and Reconstructive Pelvic Surgery,
Department of Obstetrics and Gynecology
NYU Langone Medical Center
New York, NY, USA

Michael R. Foley
Banner University Medical Center Phoenix, Obstetrics and Gynecology
University of Arizona College of Medicine Phoenix
Phoenix, AZ, USA

Karin Fox
Maternal-Fetal Medicine, Baylor College of Medicine
Texas Children's Hospital, Pavilion for Women
Houston, TX, USA

Jenna Friedenthal
Department of Obstetrics and Gynecology
New York University
New York, NY, USA

Joanna Gibson
Obstetrics and Gynecology
Yorkshire and Humber, UK

Veronica Gillispie
Ochsner Health System
New Orleans, LA, USA

Dianne Glass
Division of Female Pelvic Medicine and Reconstructive Pelvic Surgery,
Department of Obstetrics and Gynecology
NYU Langone Medical Center
New York, NY, USA
Division of Female Pelvic Medicine and Reconstructive Pelvic Surgery,
Department of Urology
NYU Langone Medical Center
New York, NY, USA

Katherine R. Goetzinger
Department of Obstetrics, Gynecology and Reproductive Sciences
University of Maryland School of Medicine
Baltimore, MD, USA

Jane Goldman
Division of Maternal-Fetal Medicine, Department of Obstetrics and Gynecology
The Valley Hospital
Ridgewood, NJ, USA

Steven Goldstein
Department of Obstetrics and Gynecology
NYU Langone Medical Center
New York, NY, USA

George Graham
Department of Maternal-Fetal Medicine
Tufts Medical Center
Boston, MA, USA

Jeanne-Marie Guise
Division of Maternal-Fetal Medicine, Departments of Obstetrics and Gynecology, Medical Informatics and Clinical Epidemiology, Public Health and Preventive Medicine, and Emergency Medicine
Oregon Health and Science University
Portland, OR, USA

Cynthia Gyamfi-Bannerman
Columbia University Medical Center
New York, NY, USA

Cara Heuser
Division of Maternal-Fetal Medicine, Department of Obstetrics and Gynecology
University of Utah and Intermountain Medical Center
Murray, UT, USA

Alexandria J. Hill
High Risk Pregnancy Center
Las Vegas, NV, USA

Texas A&M College of Medicine
College Station, TX, USA

University of Arizona
Phoenix, AZ, USA

Kathy Huang
Department of Obstetrics and Gynecology
NYU Langone Medical Center
New York, NY, USA

Warner K. Huh
Division of Gynecologic Oncology
University of Alabama at Birmingham
Birmingham, AL, USA

Joses A. Jain
Columbia University Medical Center
New York, NY, USA

Arun Jeyabalan
Division of Maternal-Fetal Medicine, Department of Obstetrics, Gynecology and Reproductive Sciences
University of Pittsburgh School of Medicine, Magee-Women's Hospital
Pittsburgh, PA, USA

Carrie Lynn Johnson
Department of Obstetrics and Gynecology
University of Miami, Miller School of Medicine
Miami, FL, USA

Emily L. Johnson
Johns Hopkins Bayview Medical Center, Department of Neurology
Johns Hopkins University School of Medicine
Baltimore, MD, USA

Megan L. Jones
The University of Ohio Wexner Medical Center
Columbus, OH, USA

Peter W. Kaplan
Johns Hopkins Bayview Medical Center, Department of Neurology
Johns Hopkins University School of Medicine
Baltimore, MD, USA

David L. Keefe
Department of Obstetrics and Gynecology
NYU Langone Medical Center
New York, NY, USA

Rasha S. Khoury
Division of Family Planning and Global Women's Health
Department of Obstetrics, Gynecology & Reproductive Biology
Brigham and Women's Hospital, Harvard Medical School
Boston, MA, USA

Sarah J. Kilpatrick
Department of Obstetrics and Gynecology
Cedars-Sinai Medical Center
Los Angeles, CA, USA

David L. Kulak
Department of Obstetrics and Gynecology
Johns Hopkins Medical Center
Baltimore, MD, USA

Jessica Lee
Division of Gynecologic Oncology, Department of Obstetrics and Gynecology
NYU Langone Medical Center
New York, NY, USA

Richard H. Lee
Division of Maternal-Fetal Medicine, Department of Obstetrics and Gynecology, University of Southern California, Keck School of Medicine
Los Angeles, CA, USA

Patricia A. Lohr
bpas (British Pregnancy Advisory Service)
Stratford Upon Avon, UK

Sherri Longo
Ochsner Health System
New Orleans, LA, USA

Richard Lyus
bpas (British Pregnancy Advisory Service) Richmond
East Twickenham, UK

Dominique Malacarne
Division of Female Pelvic Medicine and Reconstructive Pelvic Surgery,
Department of Obstetrics and Gynecology
NYU Langone Medical Center
New York, NY, USA

Division of Female Pelvic Medicine and Reconstructive Pelvic Surgery,
Department of Urology
NYU Langone Medical Center
New York, NY, USA

Peter W. Marks
Center for Biologics Evaluation and Research, U.S. Food and Drug Administration
Silver Spring, MD, USA

Jovana Y. Martin
Department of Obstetrics and Gynecology
University of Alabama at Birmingham
Birmingham, AL, USA

Stephanie R. Martin
Clinical Concepts in Obstetrics
Scottsdale, AZ, USA

Christel Meuleman
Leuven University Fertility Centre (LUFC)
UZ Leuven, Leuven, Belgium

David A. Miller
Division of Maternal-Fetal Medicine, Department of Obstetrics and Gynecology, Keck School of Medicine
University of Southern California
Los Angeles, CA, USA

Payam Mohassel
Johns Hopkins Bayview Medical Center, Department of Neurology
Johns Hopkins University School of Medicine
Baltimore, MD, USA

Jane Moore
Nuffield Department of Obstetrics and Gynecology
University of Oxford
Oxford, UK

Lila Nachtigall
Department of Obstetrics and Gynecology
NYU Langone Medical Center
New York, NY, USA

Frederick Naftolin
Department of Obstetrics and Gynecology
New York University
New York, NY, USA

Jennifer A. Namazy
Scripps Clinic
San Diego, CA, USA

James Neilson
Obstetrics and Gynecology
University of Liverpool
Liverpool, UK

Diane De Neubourg
Leuven University Fertility Centre (LUFC)
UZ Leuven, Leuven, Belgium

Errol R. Norwitz
Louis E. Phaneuf Professor of Obstetrics & Gynecology
Tufts University School of Medicine
Chief Scientific Officer Chair, Department of Obstetrics & Gynecology
Tufts Medical Center
Boston, USA

Anthony O. Odibo
Department of Obstetrics and Gynecology
University of South Florida
Tampa, FL, USA

Joseph G. Ouzounian
Division of Maternal-Fetal Medicine, Department of Obstetrics and Gynecology
University of Southern California, Keck School of Medicine
Los Angeles, CA, USA

Michael J. Paidas
Department of Obstetrics, Gynecology and Reproductive Sciences, Yale School of Medicine
Section of Maternal-Fetal Medicine
New Haven, CN, USA

Lubna Pal
Department of Obstetrics, Gynecology and Reproductive Sciences
Yale University School of Medicine
New Haven, CT, USA

Joong Shin Park
Department of Obstetrics and Gynecology
Seoul National University College of Medicine
Seoul National University Hospital
Seoul, Korea

Anita Patel
University of Central Florida
Center for Reproductive Medicine
Orlando, FL, USA

Shivani R. Patel
Division of Maternal-Fetal Medicine, Department of Obstetrics and Gynecology
University of Southern California, Keck School of Medicine
Los Angeles, CA, USA

Shefali Pathy
Department of Obstetrics, Gynecology and Reproductive Sciences
Yale University School of Medicine
New Haven, CT, USA

Karen Peeraer
Leuven University Fertility Centre (LUFC)
UZ Leuven, Leuven, Belgium

Ashley T. Peterson
Division of Maternal-Fetal Medicine, Department of Obstetrics and Gynecology
Tufts Medical Center
Boston, MA, USA

Joanne Quinones
Department of Obstetrics and Gynecology, Maternal Fetal Medicine, Lehigh Valley Health Network
The Center for Advanced Perinatal Care, Allentown, PA, USA

University of South Florida-Morsani College of Medicine
Tampa, FL, USA

Diana A. Racusin
Department of Obstetrics and Gynecology, Division of Maternal-Fetal Medicine
Baylor College of Medicine, Texas Children's Hospital Pavilion for Women
Houston, TX, USA

A. Reza Radjabi
Department of Obstetrics and Gynecology
NYU Langone Medical Center
New York, NY, USA

Andrei Rebarber
Mount Sinai St. Luke's and Mount Sinai West, Mount Sinai Beth Israel, The Mount Sinai Hospital
Obstetrics, Gynecology and Reproductive Sciences
New York, NY, USA

Danielle M. Roncari
Division of Family Planning, Department of Obstetrics and Gynecology
Tufts University School of Medicine
Boston, MA, USA

Ashley S. Roman
Department of Obstetrics and Gynecology, NYU School of Medicine
New York University
New York, NY, USA

Michael Ross
Obstetrics and Gynecology
Harbor UCLA Medical Center
Torrance, CA, USA

B. Ryan Ball
Department of Obstetrics, Gynecology and Reproductive Sciences,
Yale School of Medicine
Section of Maternal-Fetal Medicine
New Haven, CN, USA

Nada Sabir
Obstetrics and Gynecology/Maternal Medicine,
Bradford Teaching Hospitals NHS Foundation Trust
Bradford, UK

Michael Schatz
Kaiser Permanente
San Diego, CA, USA

Kathleen M. Schmeler
Department of Gynecologic Oncology and Reproductive Medicine
The University of Texas, MD Anderson Cancer Center
Houston, TX, USA

Zachary P. Schwartz
Division of Gynecologic Oncology, Department of Obstetrics and Gynecology
NYU Langone Medical Center
New York, NY, USA

James H. Segars
National Institute of Child Health and Human Development
National Institutes of Health
Bethesda, MD, USA

Lili Sheibani
Maternal-Fetal Medicine, Department of Obstetrics and Gynecology
University of California
Irvine, Orange, CA, USA

Celso Silva
University of Central Florida, Center for Reproductive Medicine
Orlando, FL, USA

Michael K. Simoni
Department of Psychiatry
Yale School of Medicine
Yale, New Haven, CN, USA

Scott W. Smilen
Division of Female Pelvic Medicine and Reconstructive Pelvic Surgery,
Department of Obstetrics and Gynecology
NYU Langone Medical Center
New York, NY, USA

Division of Female Pelvic Medicine and Reconstructive Pelvic Surgery,
Department of Urology
NYU Langone Medical Center
New York, NY, USA

John Smulian
Department of Obstetrics and Gynecology, Maternal Fetal Medicine,
Lehigh Valley Health Network
The Center for Advanced Perinatal Care, Allentown, PA, USA

University of South Florida-Morsani College of Medicine
Tampa, FL, USA

Rhoda Sperling
Department of Obstetrics, Gynecology and Reproductive Sciences
Icahn School of Medicine, Mt Sinai Hospital
New York, NY, USA

Medicine, Infectious Diseases
Icahn School of Medicine, Mt Sinai Hospital
New York, NY, USA

Carla Tomassetti
Leuven University Fertility Centre (LUFC)
UZ Leuven, Leuven, Belgium

Maria Victoria Vargas
Department of Obstetrics and Gynecology
George Washington University Medical Center
USA

Alex C. Vidaeff
Department of Obstetrics and Gynecology, Division of Maternal-Fetal Medicine
Baylor College of Medicine, Texas Children's Hospital Pavilion for Women
Houston, TX, USA

Deborah Wing
Maternal-Fetal Medicine, Department of Obstetrics and Gynecology
University of California
Irvine, Orange, CA, USA

Kimberly Yonkers
Department of Psychiatry
Yale School of Medicine
Yale, New Haven, CN, USA

Carolyn M. Zelop
Ultrasound and Perinatal Research, Division of MFM and
Department of Obstetrics and Gynecology, The Valley Hospital,
Ridgewood, NJ, USA

Department of Obstetrics and Gynecology
NYU School of Medicine, New York, NY, USA

Lisa C. Zuckerwise
Department of Obstetrics, Gynecology & Reproductive Sciences,
Division of Maternal-Fetal Medicine
Yale School of Medicine
New Haven, CT, USA

1

CHAPTER 1

Evidence-based medicine in obstetrics and gynecology

Jeanne-Marie Guise
Division of Maternal-Fetal Medicine, Departments of Obstetrics and Gynecology, Medical Informatics and Clinical Epidemiology, Public Health and Preventive Medicine, and Emergency Medicine, Oregon Health and Science University, Portland, OR, USA

> ... decisions about the care of individual patients should be based on the conscientious, explicit, and judicious use of the current best evidence on the effectiveness of clinical services.
>
> *IOM Knowing What Works in Health Care 2008 [1]*

While all clinicians want to use the best evidence to make health care decisions, with 37 reviews, 47 randomized control trials (RCTs), and two guidelines published every day, it is impossible for practicing clinicians to keep up with all the new evidence and decide whether it is sufficient to suggest that they should change their practice. This book provides a summary of evidence for the major clinical areas of practice within the specialty of Obstetrics and Gynecology (OB/GYN), and this chapter (i) provides an overview and context, discussing the history of evidence based medicine (EBM) in OB/GYN; (ii) describes the importance and conduct of a systematic evidence review, a hallmark of EBM and contemporary evidence-based decision-making; and (iii) provides additional EBM resources and references for interested readers.

History of obstetrics and evidence-based medicine

OB/GYN has played a long and important role in shaping what is known today as EBM, although it did not always embrace evidence. The beginnings of OB/GYNs relationship with EBM may have started in the 1800s when women went to Lying-in Hospitals to stay for days or months in preparation for and recovery from childbirth. Lying-in hospitals were often crowded, and rates of maternal and child death from childbed fever (puerperal sepsis) were high. Some women were said to prefer giving birth in the streets, pretending to have given birth *en route* to the hospital. Ignac Semmelweiss, perplexed by the lower rates of maternal mortality for women delivering outside the hospital said: "To me, it appeared logical that patients who experienced street births would become ill at least as frequently as those who delivered in the clinic ... What protected those who delivered outside the clinic from these destructive unknown endemic influences?" [2]. He also observed that there were higher rates of maternal mortality from childbed fever in the First Division Hospital, which was staffed by physicians, compared with the Second which was staffed by midwives. Both units had trainees, performed examinations, and saw roughly similar populations. He realized that unlike the midwives, physicians all performed autopsies on women who died the night before prior to beginning their clinical duties on the maternity ward. In 1847, Semmelweiss figured out what might be occurring when a forensic medical professor, Jakob Kolletschka, died of sepsis after sustaining an accidental finger stick during an autopsy. He concluded that, "In Kolletschka, the specific causal factor was the cadaverous particles that were introduced into his vascular system. I was compelled to ask whether cadaverous particles had been introduced into the vascular systems of those patients whom I had seen die of this identical disease. I was forced to answer affirmatively" [2]. He required physicians wash their hands with chlorinated lime before examining patients. The mortality rate in District 1 fell from 11.4% prior to handwashing to 1.27% (rates were 2.7% and 1.33% in District 2). The medical community did not embrace this new evidence. Semmelweiss was ridiculed by physicians who were offended by the suggestion they were unclean, and his theory was rejected because it was contrary to the accepted belief that childbed fever was caused by miasmas or "bad air." In response, Semmelweiss could only figuratively shake his head: "One would believe that the clarity of things would have made the truth apparent to everyone and that

Evidence-Based Obstetrics and Gynecology, First Edition. Edited by Errol R. Norwitz, Carolyn M. Zelop, David A. Miller, and David L. Keefe.

they would have behaved accordingly. Experience teaches otherwise. Most medical lecture halls continue to resound with lectures on epidemic childbed fever and with discourses against my theories" [2].

Fast forward to the 1950s and 1960s and two stories demonstrate how difficult it is for new evidence to change clinical practice even when that evidence is strong – and how profound the consequences for this failure.

In the 1950s, diethylstilboestrol (DES) therapy was used to prevent miscarriage. Its use was established through uncontrolled studies. Even though randomized controlled trials were published in the mid-1950s that found no significant prevention offered by DES, its use had become so commonplace that it continued despite the evidence. It was not until 1971 that the food and drug administration (FDA) brought national attention to the harms of DES exposure (associated with vaginal clear cell carcinoma) and banned its use in pregnancy. Total exposure to DES for mothers and daughters has been estimated to exceed 10 million worldwide.

The story of antenatal corticosteroids is not only a major discovery in obstetrics but is also emblematic of the importance of EBM. In the 1960s, Graham "Mont" Liggins, an Australian obstetrician, had a sheep farmer neighbor and wondered why ewes delivered prematurely when worried by dogs [3]. Liggins suspected it may have something to do with the stress-response in the mother and the release of cortisol. He conducted an experiment where he administered corticosteroids to pregnant ewes and found they delivered prematurely. Unexpectedly, he also found that the lambs delivered by ewes that received corticosteroids survived in far greater numbers than he would have expected given the severe degree of their prematurity [4]. In the 1970s, Liggins and a pediatrician colleague, Ross Howie, conducted the first randomized trial in humans to test their theory that corticosteroids reduced the occurrence of respiratory distress syndrome (RDS). RDS and mortality rates were significantly reduced in the treated group (6.4%) as opposed to 18% in placebo treated mothers. Within a decade of this first RCT additional studies supported the conclusion that corticosteroids significantly reduced infant mortality for prematurely born children. However it was not until the mid-1990s that antenatal steroids became part of routine practice for women at risk of premature delivery (after a meta-analysis was published in 1989). The forest plot from a meta-analysis of antenatal corticosteroids represents this delay, demonstrates the potential power of systematic reviews and meta-analyses of a body of evidence, and has become the symbol for the Cochrane Collaboration, the most recognized source for evidence-based systematic reviews in medicine. It has been estimated that tens of thousands of babies would have been saved by earlier implementation of steroids.

It is perhaps not a surprise that Archie Cochrane, for whom the Cochrane Collaboration is named awarded the field of OB/GYN the first wooden spoon award for failing to evaluate the care they provide with RCTs and failing to apply results of RCTs in practice [5]. He went further stating that GO in Gynecology and Obstetrics should stand for "go ahead without evidence" [6].

What is evidence-based medicine?

EBM, refers to a process of turning clinical problems into questions and systematically locating, appraising, and synthesizing research findings as a basis for clinical decision-making. Gordon Guyatt [7] first used the term "EBM" in the 1980s to describe an approach to residency training at McMaster University School of Medicine where residents were taught how to identify, interpret, and use the literature in their clinical decision-making. At first he wanted to call it "Scientific Medicine" but reconsidered when others argued that the title would imply all other medicine was non-scientific [8]. Further refined by David Sackett, "EBM requires a bottom-up approach that integrates the best external evidence with individual clinical expertise and patient choice" [9].

The systematic review is a hallmark of EBM. Systematic reviews apply a scientific review strategy that limits bias by the systematic assembly, critical appraisal, and synthesis of all relevant studies on a specific topic. As shown in Figure 1.1, systematic reviews are at the top of the evidence hierarchy pyramid. Clinicians in pursuit of the best evidence, should first search for high-quality systematic reviews. Since systematic reviews are such an important part of EBM and are instrumental to clinical decision-making, this chapter provides a brief description of the systematic review process.

Systematic review processes

If, as is sometimes supposed, science consisted in nothing but the laborious accumulation of facts, it would soon come to a standstill, crushed, as it were, under its own weight... Two processes are thus at work side by side, the reception of new material and the digestion and assimilation of the old [10]

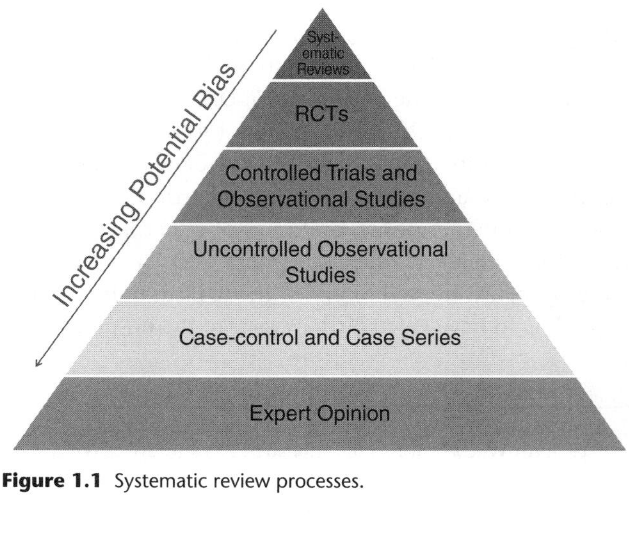

Figure 1.1 Systematic review processes.

Table 1.1 Steps for evidence-based obstetrics

1. Formulate a clear clinical question
2. Search the literature and identify relevant reviews and studies
3. Critically appraise individual studies and the overall body of evidence
4. Synthesize results given context and patient factors
5. Implement
6. Evaluate the application into clinical practice

A systematic review is a scientific review strategy that limits bias by the systematic assembly, critical appraisal, and synthesis of all relevant studies on a specific topic. Table 1.1 presents the six steps for Evidence-based Obstetrics. The first four of these are covered by, and critical to, systematic review. Therefore, busy clinicians can shortcut these steps if they are able to find a high-quality systematic review that answers their clinical question.

Each of these steps is covered briefly below.

Formulating the question

A prudent question is one-half of wisdom [11]
Sir Francis Bacon

Questions arise every day a clinician cares for patients: some they can answer easily, others they know where to find the answers quickly, and many require investigation. The ability to take an everyday dilemma and turn it into an answerable and searchable question is important not only for systematic reviews, but also for good clinical care. Questions often fall into specific categories: incidence/ prevalence, causation/etiology, screening, diagnostic, therapeutic/treatment, prevention, outcomes (benefits and/or harms), prognostic, and they can be expressed as, "In patients with … how effective is … compared with … for the outcome[s] of … ". Formulating an answerable and relevant question is a critical foundational step to determining the relevant scope of a review; too big and the review may not be feasible, too narrow and the results may not be relevant. Systematic review questions are often formulated according to a PICOTS format, that is, **P**opulation, **I**ntervention, **C**omparator, **O**utcome, **T**iming, and **S**etting (Table 1.2).

Table 1.2 PICOTS

Population – Who does the review topic pertain to
Intervention – What is the intervention or treatment that is being evaluated?
Comparator – What is the intervention being compared with?
Outcome – What are the benefits and harms?
Timing – What is the timing of outcomes or follow-up?
Setting – What settings are relevant to this topic?

Population – Understanding the population of reviews and research studies is often one of the clearest ways clinicians can determine whether the scope of a review or study is pertinent to their clinical population. Factors often considered include age (e.g. child, teen, young adult, elderly), sex, medical conditions, pregnancy status, and social factors (education required, skill-level, access to care). A description of such factors helps clinicians understand whether the review will be applicable to their patient population.

Intervention – The intervention is often the main subject of reviews. Interventions can involve medical, surgical, health systems, social, or behavioral interventions and can have one or many components.

Comparator – The comparator group is often overlooked, yet is critical to understanding the relative effectiveness of an intervention. Comparators include no treatment, placebo, "standard of care," active alternative treatment. It is important to describe the underlying condition considered "standard of care" as what is considered standard might be an intervention in other settings.

Outcomes – Outcomes include health outcomes, intermediate outcomes, and harms.

Timing – Timing is increasingly recognized as an important consideration. Timing refers to the timing of the intervention or parts of the intervention and also may describe the time of patient eligibility, intervention, and follow-up for a target trial.

Setting – Setting or context factors such as organizational characteristics, financial setting (fee-for- service, capitated, uninsured; geographic and clinical settings (solo or group practice, public or private, for profit or non-profit, etc.) are often critical to interventional effectiveness and should be described in systematic reviews.

Often the S in PICOTS is used to refer to study design. While that use is not usually an element in the question, it can be helpful to consider the types of studies that are most likely to inform particular types of questions. Table 1.3 aligns common types of questions with study designs.

Descriptions of these PICOTS elements enables the reader of a systematic review to understand whether the question is

Table 1.3 Studies applicable to particular review questions

Question type	Study design
Incidence	Cohort
Prevalence	Cohort, cross-sectional
Treatment/therapy	Randomized controlled trial (RCT)
Screening	RCT, cohort
Diagnostic accuracy	RCT, case series
Prognosis	RCT, cohort
Harms	RCT, cohort, case–control, case report
Etiology	Cohort, case–control
Prevention	RCT, cohort

relevant to their clinical dilemma and setting. The questions also specify search terms and the inclusion and exclusion criteria for studies.

Searching the literature and identifying relevant studies

A comprehensive search and a systematic, unbiased approach to finding, selecting, and interpreting evidence are distinguishing features of systematic reviews. Searches of systematic reviews are meant to include all of the evidence and not just published articles. In general, bibliographic searches for systematic reviews in health care should always include MEDLINE® and the Cochrane Central Register of Controlled Trials. Additional databases that are often useful include Embase, CINAHL, Scopus, and PsychINFO. In addition to searching bibliographic databases, systematic reviews search reference lists of relevant reviews and articles and conduct searches for unpublished literature from registries, government or industry documents, Websites, and other sources. Once you have conducted a comprehensive search, the next critical ingredient of a systematic review is applying an unbiased approach to including and excluding articles. This process involves a priori decision-making about issues such as date range, study design, language, key subject matter issues etc. A PRISMA [12] or QUORUM [13] figure is often used to detail finding and selecting pertinent literature for a review.

Critically appraising studies and assessing the strength of a body of literature

Critically appraising the literature involves two major stages: (i) evaluating the risk of bias for individual studies based upon study design; and (ii) grading the overall strength of evidence for a body of literature. Problems with an individual study's design or conduct have the potential to introduce bias or inferential error, and raise questions about the validity of their findings. Numerous tools exist to evaluate the risk of bias for controlled trials [14–16] and observational studies [16–25]. In general risk of bias tools evaluate participant selection; outcome, exposure, and process measures; study processes such as blinding; and appropriate analytic methods including intent to treat and considerations for confounding. This stage of individual study evaluation is critically important. One element in assessing the strength of the body of literature, it can inform quantitative syntheses such as meta-analyses, and provide insights on how to strengthen future research studies in design and conduct. Because raters may vary in their interpretation, reviewers will usually pilot test the application of the tool prior to wide-scale use across studies.

Understanding the reliability of the overall body of evidence is critical for guideline groups, policymakers, and clinicians. Methods for evaluating the overall strength of evidence have evolved over the past several decades. Organizations such as the US Preventive Services Task Force (USPSTF) [19] the US Evidence-based Practice Centers (EPCs) Program [20], and the Oxford Center for Evidence-based Medicine [21] have all developed criteria. The USPSTF risk of bias/quality rating scale has been adapted for easy use by relative novices and is available at www.storc.org) In 2000, a collaboration of international experts formed the Grading of Recommendations Assessment, Development, and Evaluation (GRADE) Working Group to establish common and transparent criteria to grade the literature. The group has grown tremendously over the years and experts in the field continue to refine the application of GRADE criteria by examining and debating their experiences and exemplars (www.gradeworkinggroup.org). According to GRADE, evidence from randomized controlled trials starts as high quality and that from observational studies starts as low quality based on the assumption that randomization controls for systematic bias in effect estimates. The body of evidence is evaluated using five main criteria: (i) risk of bias; (ii) inconsistency of results across studies; (iii) indirectness; (iv) imprecision; and (v) publication bias [22]. Risk of bias was discussed above. Consistency involves determining the degree to which studies were similar in direction and range of effect sizes. Directness involves assessing whether the evidence reflects a single direct link to the outcome or whether it involves several indirect links in a chain of evidence or surrogate outcomes. Precision has to do with the certainty of the effect which is often judged by the narrowness of the confidence interval. Publication bias is the last major GRADE criterion. It has long been recognized that studies with positive findings are more likely to be published. (Several factors can contribute to this, including journal bias toward positive results and author awareness of those journal preferences.) This alone can bias the overall body of literature. Published studies can show an intervention's effect while there could be a large body of unpublished evidence suggesting no effect. Because of this, GRADE recommends conducting an evaluation for publication bias. After considering GRADE elements, the entire body of literature for a given outcome is rated as high, moderate, low, or very low. Table 1.4 presents the summary grades and their meaning.

Knowing that guideline groups, policymakers, and clinicians have limited time, the GRADE working group also recommends use of a summary of evidence table to summarize: (i) key outcomes; (ii) effect sizes (magnitude and confidence interval); (iii) numbers of studies and participants; (iv) overall GRADE of evidence by outcome; and (v) important notes or comments. Ultimately, the GRADE approach provides a system for evaluating the strength of the literature as a whole and determining the strength of recommendation that can be made. For example a strong

Table 1.4 GRADING the quality of a body of literature [22]

High – Further research is very unlikely to change our confidence in the estimate of effect. (e.g. High confidence that the evidence reflects the true effect).
Moderate – Further research may change our confidence in the estimate of effect and may change the estimate. (e.g. Moderate confidence that the evidence reflects the true effect).
Low – Further research is very likely to have an important impact on our confidence in the estimate of effect and is likely to change the estimate. (e.g. Low confidence that the evidence reflects the true effect).
Very low – any estimate of effect is very uncertain (e.g. very low confidence that the evidence reflects a true effect)

recommendation could be made when the effect size is large and overall evidence quality is high, meaning that it is unlikely to have occurred in the absence of a true effect of the intervention. However, a weak recommendation would be made for low or very low evidence where any effect could have occurred solely as a result of bias from confounding factors. The GRADE system or adaptations of the GRADE system are used by numerous guideline groups including since 2015 the International Consensus on cerebroplacental ratio (CPR) and endocervical curettage (ECC), Science with Treatment Recommendations provided by the International Liaison Committee for Resuscitation (ILCOR) which are used in this book [23]. Ultimately these processes and products are tools to promote transparency, understanding, and dialogue around the totality of evidence, our certainty in that evidence, and a rationale for practice.

Evidence-based resources

Table 1.5 provides the interested reader with additional resources to find evidence-based reviews and guidance and/or to learn more about evidence-based practices. Some of the major resources are discussed in some detail.

The Cochrane Collaboration

Realizing that it is a daunting if not impossible challenge for the individual practicing clinician to keep abreast and synthesize the medical literature, Sir Ian Chalmers, motivated by Archie Cochrane's wooden spoon challenge to obstetrics, developed a database of all existing and relevant randomized controlled clinical trials for interventions in OB/GYN and a repository of systematic reviews the Cochrane library. The Cochrane Collaboration (http://www.cochrane.org) is now one of the largest networks of global scientists, with more than 37 000 volunteers who synthesize the world's evidence and produce high-quality systematic reviews. The Collaboration is organized into review groups that are responsible for conducting and updating systematic reviews for specific topic areas. Several review groups are pertinent to OB/GYN including:

Pregnancy and Childbirth
The Cochrane Menstrual Disorders and Subfertility Group
The Cochrane Fertility Regulation Group
The Cochrane Gynecological Cancer Group

The Cochrane Library (http://www.cochranelibrary.com) has become one of the world's most recognized sources of high-quality systematic reviews in medicine. The origins and symbol of the Cochrane are connected to obstetrics, and as mentioned earlier, the very symbol for the Cochrane reflects the story of antenatal corticosteroid therapy.

Table 1.5 List of evidence-based organizations and resources

Agency for Healthcare Research and Quality (AHRQ) – http://www.ahrq.gov
AHRQ Evidence-based Practice Centers Program (EPC) – http://www.ahrq.gov/research/findings/evidence-based-reports/index.html
Bandolier – http://www.medicine.ox.ac.uk/bandolier
Centre for Reviews and Dissemination (CRD) – www.york.ac.uk/crd
Cochrane Collaboration – http://www.cochrane.org
Cochrane Pregnancy and Childbirth – http://pregnancy.cochrane.org
Cochrane Gynecology and Fertility Group – http://cgf.cochrane.org
Cochrane Fertility Regulation Group – http://fertility-regulation.cochrane.org
Cochrane Gynecological Cancer Group – http://gnoc.cochrane.org
GRADE Working Group – http://www.gradeworkinggroup.org
JAMA Evidence – http://jamaevidence.mhmedical.com
James Lind – http://www.jameslindlibrary.org
National Institute for Health and Clinical Excellence (NICE) – www.nice.org.uk
Oxford Centre for Evidence-based Medicine – http://www.cebm.net
PRISMA – http://www.prisma-statement.org
US Preventive Services Task Force (USPSTF) – http://www.uspreventiveservicestaskforce.org

The US preventive services task force and the US evidence-based practice centers program

The USPSTF (www.uspreventiveservicestaskforce.org) is an excellent resource for evidence and recommendations in primary care and prevention. The USPSTF was established in 1984 as an independent, volunteer panel of national experts in prevention and EBM who issue recommendations on clinical preventive services such as screenings, counseling services, and preventive medications. Topics relating to OB/GYN and women's health include cervical cancer screening; screening for bacterial vaginosis in pregnancy to prevent preterm birth; mammography; breastfeeding; screening for BRCA-related cancer, chlamydia, and gonorrhea, depression, genital herpes; counseling for gynecologic cancers; immunizations, and many more. It is an excellent resource for primary care issues and is considered by the US government when making coverage decisions. All USPSTF recommendations are paired with systematic evidence reviews conducted by EPCs. In 1997, Agency for Healthcare Research and Quality (AHRQ) (then known as the Agency for Health Care Policy and Research) established the EPC program to develop evidence reports to inform health policy, guidelines, coverage decisions, patient decision-making, and clinical practice for clinical professional societies, insurers, employers, healthcare organizations, and policymakers. Examples of reports that are relevant to OB/GYN include comparative effectiveness of therapies to treat menopausal symptoms, antidepressant treatment of depression during pregnancy and postpartum, smoking cessation interventions in pregnancy and postpartum care, oral contraception use for the prevention of ovarian cancer, progestogens for the prevention of preterm birth, and nitrous oxide for the management of labor pain (a full list can be found at http://www.ahrq.gov/research/findings/evidence-based-reports/search.html?f[0]=field_evidence_based_reports%3A13971).

Rationale for this book

Clinicians have more access to evidence than ever before; this is both a cure and a curse. While the process of finding, appraising, and synthesizing evidence is possible for practitioners, studies suggest that the process is too time consuming for most [24, 25]. Inadequate time (74%), limited searching skills (41%), and limited access to evidence (43%) have been cited by physicians as barriers to implementing evidence-based care [25]. This book is written to provide a central resource for evidence in OB/GYN for the busy clinician. The chapters that follow provide an overview of the evidence across major clinical topics faced on a daily bases by Obstetricians and Gynecologists.

References

1 Eden, J., Levit, L., Berg, A. et al. (eds.) (2011). *Finding What Works in Health Care: Standards for Systematic Reviewers*. The National Academies Press.

2 Semmelweis, I. and Carter, K.C.T. (1983). *Etiology, Concept and Prophylaxis of Childbed Fever*. University of Wisconsin Press.

3 Norwitz, E. and Greeberg, J. (2010). Beyond antenatal corticosteroids: what did mont liggins teach us? *Reviews in Obstetrics and Gynecology* **3** (**3**): 79.

4 Gluckman, P. and Buklijas, T. (2013). Sir Graham Collingwood (Mont) Liggins. *Biographical Memoirs of Fellows of the Royal Society* **59**: 193–214.

5 Ohlsson, A. and Clark, K. (2002). Evidence-based perinatal and paediatric health care: the contribution of the Cochrane collaboration and tte Canadian Cochrane network and Centre. *Paediatrics & Child Health* **7**: 319–322.

6 The Cochrane Pregnancy and Childbirth Database. (1989). Effective Care in Pregnancy and Childbirth. http://journals.sagepub.com/doi/abs/10.1177/016327879501800406.

7 Guyatt, G. and Voelker, R. (2012). Everything you ever wanted to know about evidence-based medicine. *JAMA* **313** (**18**): 1783–1785.

8 Smith, R. and Rennie, D. (2014). Evidence-based medicine—an oral history. *JAMA* **311** (**4**): 365–367.

9 Sackett, D., Rosenberg, W., and Gray, J. (1996). Evidence based medicine: what it is and what it isn't. *BMJ* **312**: 71–72.

10 Raleigh, L. (1884). Address by the Rt. Hon. Lord Rayleigh. In: *Report of the Fifty-Fifty-Fourth Meeting of the British Association for the Advancement of Science*, 3–23. John Murray.

11 Bacon S.F. http://www.azquotes.com/quotes/topics/prudent.html

12 Moher, D., Liberati, A., Tetzlaff, J., and Altman, D. (2009). Preferred reporting items for systematic reviews and meta-analyses: the PRISMA statement. *Annals of Internal Medicine* **151** (**4**): 264–269.

13 Clarke, M. (2000). The QUORUM statement. *Lancet* **355**: 756–757.

14 Collaboration TC (2011; 5.1.0). *Cochrane Handbook for Systematic Reviews of Interventions* (ed. H. JPT and S. Green). Wiley.

15 Higgins, J. and Altman, D. (2011). The Cochrane Collaboration's tool for assessing risk of bias in randomised trials. *BMJ* **343**: d5928.

16 Viswanathan M., Ansari M., Berkman N., et al. (2012) Assessing the Risk of Bias of Individual Studies in Systematic Reviews of Health Care Interventions Agency for Healthcare Research and Quality; Methods Guide for Comparative Effectiveness Reviews (AHRQ Publication No. 12-EHC047-EF).

17 Harris, R., Helfand, M., Woolf, S. et al. (2001). Methods work group, third US preventative services task force. Current methods of the US preventative services task force: a review of the process. *American Journal of Preventative Medicine* **20** (**3**): 21–35.

18 Wells G., Shea B., O'Connell D., et al. The Newcastle-Ottawa Scale (NOS) for Assessing the Quality of Nonrandomised Studies in Meta-Analyses https://www.ncbi.nlm.nih.gov/books/NBK99082/bin/appb-fm4.pdf.

19 Force USPST. Grade Definitions. 2015. https://www.uspreventiveservicestaskforce.org/Page/Name/grade-definitions.

20 Berkman, N.D.L.K., Ansari, M., McDonagh, M. et al. (2013). Grading the strength of a body of evidence when assessing health care interventions for the effective health care program of the Agency for Healthcare Research and Quality: an update. *Methods Guide for Comparative Effectiveness Reviews AHRQ* Publication No. 13(14)-EHC130-EF.

21 Howick, J., Chalmers, I., Glasziou, P. et al. (2011). The 2011 Oxford CEBM levels of evidence (introductory document). *Oxford Centre for Evidence-Based Medicine*.

22 Guyatt, G., Oxman, A., Vist, G. et al. (2008). Rating quality of evidence and strength of recommendations GRADE: an emerging consensus on rating quality of evidence and strength of recommendations. *British Medical Journal* **336**: 92.

23 Morrison, L., Chair, L., Gent, E. et al. (2015). Part 2: evidence evaluation and Management of Conflicts of interest 2015 American Heart Association guidelines update for cardiopulmonary resuscitation and emergency cardiovascular care. *Circulation* **132**: S368–S382.

24 Cumbers, B. (1999). Evidence-based practice data day. *Health Services Journal* **109** (**5650**): 30–31.

25 Craig, J., Irwig, L., and Stockler, M. (2001). Evidence-based tools: useful tools for decision making. *The Medical Journal of Australia* **174**: 248–253.

SECTION 1
Gynecology

David L. Keefe

General Gynecology

2

CHAPTER 2

Abnormal menstrual bleeding

Cynthia Farquhar and Julie Brown

Department of Obstetrics and Gynecology, University of Auckland, Auckland, New Zealand

CLINICAL SCENARIO

A 42-year-old mother of four children presents to her general practitioner on the eighth day of her menstrual period. She fainted at home when she got up that morning and her husband has brought her to the clinic. She recovered completely from the faint and walks into the clinic. She usually has regular periods and the typical duration is six days. The first four days are heavy and she changes pads and tampons hourly during the day and twice during the night. They are not painful. She has no other health problems except that she is 90 kg and 159 cm tall. The body mass index (BMI) is 35.6 $kg\,m^{-2}$.

On examination she looked very pale. She has a pulse rate of 88b m^{-1} and her blood pressure is 125/80. The rest of the findings are normal. A vaginal examination is not done but there are no abdominal masses.

The general practitioner arranges an urgent hemoglobin test and later that day the result is reported as 60 $g\,l^{-1}$.

Background

The International Federation of Gynecology and Obstetrics (FIGO) defines chronic abnormal uterine bleeding (AUB) as "bleeding from the uterine corpus that is abnormal in duration, volume, and/or frequency and has been present for the majority of the last 6 months" [1, 2]. The prevalence of AUB in the general population is predicted to range between 11% and 13% rising to 24% for those women aged 36–45 years [3]. The extent of the menstrual bleeding has been linked to the likelihood of anemia [4, 5].

Heavy menstrual bleeding (HMB) without underlying pathology (also known as menorrhagia or dysfunctional uterine bleeding) can be a major health problem for many women, frequently resulting in referral for hysterectomy (National Health Committee, 1998) [6]. The National Institute for Health and Clinical Excellence defines HMB as "as excessive menstrual blood loss which interferes with the woman's physical, emotional, social, and material quality of life, and which can occur alone or in combination with other symptoms." (p8) [7]. Table 2.1 indicates that menstrual blood loss per month in excess of 80 ml is considered to be "heavy" [8]. Unfortunately, measurement of the volume of monthly menstrual blood loss is not possible outside the research setting, and clinicians are dependent on self-report by women about the heaviness of their menstrual loss.

Table 2.1 Suggested "normal" limits for menstrual parameters in the mid-reproductive years

Clinical dimensions of menstruation and menstrual cycle	Descriptive term	Normal limits (5th–95th centile)
Volume of monthly blood loss (ml)	Heavy	>80
	Normal	5–80
	Light	<5

Source: Fraser et al. 2007 [8].

HMB may occur at any time between puberty and the menopause and is typically described as either ovulatory or anovulatory. A history of HMB with regular menstrual cycles is usually associated with ovulation whereas an anovulatory pattern of bleeding with erratic intervals between menstrual periods, is common in puberty and as women near the menopause. Anovulatory menorrhagia may also be present in women with polycystic ovaries who often have irregular and heavy menses. This "dysfunctional uterine bleeding" is defined in the NICE guidelines as "Abnormal vaginal bleeding that occurs during a menstrual cycle that produced no egg (ovulation did not take place). The occurrence of irregular or excessive uterine bleeding in the absence of pregnancy, infection, trauma, new growth or hormone treatment" (p. xiii) [7].

Vannella et al. (2008) reported iron deficiency anemia (serum ferritin <30 $\mu g\,dl^{-1}$) in two-thirds (67%) of women

Evidence-Based Obstetrics and Gynecology, First Edition. Edited by Errol R. Norwitz, Carolyn M. Zelop, David A. Miller, and David L. Keefe.

(aged 20–56 years) who had a diagnosis of menorrhagia [9]. As HMB is the most common presentation of abnormal menstrual bleeding this chapter will focus on HMB.

Differential diagnoses of HMB that should be considered include uterine pathology such as fibroids and hyperplastic endometrium, complications of early pregnancy such as miscarriage, carcinoma of the cervix and endometrium (rarely), and exogenous hormones taken for menopausal symptoms. Fibroids are present in about 40% of women with menorrhagia [7] although they are probably only responsible for menorrhagia when they result in an enlargement of the endometrial cavity or when they are submucous fibroids. Rarely, disorders of coagulation may be present. Approximately 5% of women with menorrhagia have endometrial hyperplasia, a premalignant condition of the endometrium, which is more likely to occur in women who weigh 90 kg or more and women who are 45 years old. In the majority of women no obvious cause is found for their HMB [6, 7].

Scope: This chapter is limited to women with HMB without pathology and does not cover the management of women with known pathology such as endometrial hyperplasia and uterine fibroids.

Clinical questions

1. Are there tests to establish the severity of HMB?
2. In women with HMB, what initial investigations should be undertaken?
3. Which women with HMB should have investigations to exclude serious pathology?
4. In a woman with HMB, what is the management of acute anemia?
5. In women with HMB, what is the effectiveness and safety of oral progestogens?
6. What is the effectiveness and safety of antifibrinolytics for women with HMB?
7. What is the effectiveness and safety of non-steroidal anti-inflammatory drugs for women with HMB?
8. What is the effectiveness and safety of combined oral contraceptives for women with HMB?
9. What is the effectiveness and safety of progesterone containing intrauterine devices for women with HMB?
10. What is the effectiveness and safety of injected/depot progestogens for women with HMB?
11. What is the effectiveness and safety of surgery, e.g. endometrial ablation/resection or hysterectomy for women with HMB?

Search strategy

The following search strategy was used to identify potential studies to answer the clinical questions. The databases that were searched included MEDLINE, Embase, and the Cochrane Database of Systematic Reviews from inception until January 2012. The following search terms were used: uterine hemorrhage/or menorrhagia/or metrorrhagia, dysfunctional uterine bleeding, AUB, metrorrhagia, menometrorrhagia, HMB, hypermenorrhagia, and systematic review and meta-analysis.

Critical appraisal of literature for each clinical question

1. Are there tests to establish the extent of HMB?

The clinical symptoms that women with HMB experience is variable with some women only presenting after severe anemia has been diagnosed and others presenting with no derangement in their hematology results. The NICE guidelines for HMB recommend that history taking should cover the nature of the bleeding (frequency, heaviness, and length) and seek to identify any potential pathology (pain or pressure symptoms) and also to identify the woman's concerns and expectations [7]. Although it is possible to objectively measure menstrual blood, the tests involve the collection of menstrual pads and tampons and are rarely undertaken except in the research setting. Subjective measures such as pictorial bleeding charts are reported to have highly variable sensitivity and sensitivity and are not recommended. [7] (p35). There is no simple and reliable way of identifying women who have severe HMB and the question of whether menstrual blood loss is a problem can only truly be determined by the woman herself [7] (p35).

Women with anemia have been found to be more likely to have excessive menstrual blood loss and therefore anemia can be used as an indicator of the severity of HMB providing other factors such as diet are taken into account. Ferritin levels have been reported to be the most sensitive test for diagnosing Fe deficiency anemia [10].

2. In women with HMB, what initial investigations should be undertaken?

A full history should be obtained including the nature of bleeding and symptomology that may indicate structural or histological abnormalities. A physical examination (observation, abdominal palpation, visualization of the cervix, and bi-manual examination) is recommended prior to investigations for structural or histological abnormalities, and prior to levonorgestrel intrauterine system (LNG-IUS) fitting [7].

The preceding paragraph has described that anemia is common and testing is recommended.

There are other conditions that may be present such as hormonal, thyroid, and coagulation disorders. Studies have reported on the association between hormonal conditions and HMB and no link has been reported [11, 12]. There is only one case-control study that considered thyroid disorders and there was no evidence of a link between thyroid disorders and menstrual disorders [13]. With regard to coagulation disorders such as von Willebrand disease, two systematic reviews suggested a prevalence between 5% and

20% [14, 15]. No case-control studies were available to establish the prevalence in the general population.

The NICE guidelines 2007 made the following recommendations for laboratory testing for women with HMB:

- A full blood count test should be carried out on all women with HMB. This should be done in parallel with any HMB treatment offered. [C]
- Testing for coagulation disorders (for example, von Willebrand disease) should be considered in women who have had HMB since menarche and have personal or family history suggesting a coagulation disorder. [C]
- A serum ferritin test should not routinely be carried out on women with HMB. [B]
- Female hormone testing should not be carried out on women with HMB. [C]

Thyroid testing should only be carried out when other signs and symptoms of thyroid disease are present. [C] National Institute for Health and Clinical Excellence, 2007 [7].

3. Which women with HMB should have investigations to exclude serious pathology?

The question of which women should be further investigated for pathology such as fibroids and endometrial pathology is an important one as some serious underlying conditions may be present (for example, endometrial hyperplasia) and some conditions are not amenable to medical treatments (e.g. use of tranexamic acid in women with HMB in association with uterine bleeding has been shown not be effective).

Therefore, women at risk of endometrial hyperplasia and carcinoma should have an assessment of their endometrium by either ultrasound or by endometrial biopsy. For women in the premenopausal age group the threshold for endometrial biopsy is ≥12 mm [6, 16]. Risk factors for endometrial pathology include high body mass indices (≥90 kg), age > 45 years, persistent intermenstrual bleeding and treatment failure [3, 6, 16–18].

Women with a clinical examination that suggests a structural or histological abnormality further investigations such as pelvic ultrasound is recommended [3, 7]. If there is uncertainty about the location of a centrally located fibroid, then saline infusion sonography is a useful second line investigation. There is no role for magnetic resonance imaging in the investigation of AUB as a first line test [6, 16].

4. In a woman with HMB, what is the management of acute anemia?

The NICE guideline 2007 notes the common association between anemia and women with HMB with iron deficiency anemia emerging as a clinical problem with a menstrual blood loss of 60–80 ml [7]. Serum ferritin is the most accurate test for iron deficiency anemia (likelihood ratio (LR) 51.85 at a level of $<15\,ng\,ml^{-1}$) [7]. Marret et al. (2010) recommended that iron must be administered to women with iron deficiency anemia [3]. There are a number of options for administration including daily and intermittent doses via oral or intravenous routes.

The evidence for the management of women with iron deficiency anemia in women with HMB is limited. A meta-analysis of daily versus intermittent treatment with iron supplements in menstruating women found that intermittent iron supplementation resulted in more frequent presentations with anemia compared with daily supplementation (Risk Ratio (RR) 1.26, 95%CI 1.04–1.51). Intermittent iron supplementation did reduce the risk of anemia (RR 0.73, 95%CI 0.56–0.95) and improve hemoglobin concentration (MD $4.58\,g\,l^{-1}$, 95%CI 2.56–6.59) and ferritin (MD 8.32, 95%CI 4.97–11.66) compared with no treatment or placebo [19].

In a randomized trial, intravenous administration of ferric carboxymaltose (≤1 g over 15 minutes, administered weekly to achieve a total calculated replacement dose) has also been shown to be safe and more effective than oral ferrous sulfate (325 mg, three times daily for six weeks) in women with iron deficiency anemia associated with heavy uterine bleeding [20].

5. In women with HMB, what is the effectiveness and safety of oral progestogens?

Progestogen therapy given in the luteal phase has been widely used in the treatment of dysfunctional uterine bleeding for many years. However, randomized controlled trials have shown it to be repeatedly ineffective in ovulatory menorrhagia. It can be used to manage irregular anovulatory cycles as it will induce a regular withdrawal bleed when given for seven days of each calendar month. Once menstruation commences other therapies may be given such as non-steroidal anti-inflammatory drugs (NSAIDs) or tranexamic acid.

Although progesterone therapy no longer has a place in the maintenance therapy of regular heavy periods it still has an important role in emergency suppression of a heavy extended menstrual bleeding episode. This is achieved by giving Norethisterone (15 mg per day) or medroxyprogesterone acetate (30 mg per day) for three to four weeks. The dosage can be decreased once bleeding has ceased. Bleeding should stop in the first week, but if it does not the dosage can be increased. Once the patient has been free of bleeding for three to four weeks progestogen can be stopped and a withdrawal bleed should occur. Maintenance therapy can then be instituted. Another regime is to give medroxyprogesterone acetate 10 mg per day initially and increase the dosage each day until the bleeding has stopped.

6. What is the effectiveness and safety of antifibrinolytics for women with HMB?

The mode of action of tranexamic acid is to depress the fibrinolytic activity of peripheral blood through the inhibition of plasminogen activation [18]. The dosage is 1 g three or four times a day on the days of heavy bleeding.

A Cochrane systematic review reported that antifibrinolytic therapy (tranexamic acid) resulted in a significant reduction in menstrual blood loss (weighted mean difference (WMD) −94, 95%CI (CI) −151.4 to −36.5) and significant change in mean reduction of blood loss (WMD −110.2, 95%CI −146.5 to −73.8) compared with placebo [21]. This was supported in another systematic review that found that tranexamic acid resulted in a reduction of menstrual blood loss of 34–54% in women with idiopathic menorrhagia [22].

Antifibrinolytics have also been reported to result in a significant reduction in mean blood loss when compared with other medical therapies, including mefenamic acid, norethisterone (administered in the luteal phase) and ethamsylate [21].

Non-specific side effects are reported in approximately one-third of women and include nausea and leg cramps [18]. There is no overall benefit in reduction in dysmenorrhea with antifibrinolytic agents [23] and no effect on duration of menses compared with control [22]. There is also thought to be an increased risk of thromboembolism. No differences in adverse effects between tranexamic acid and placebo were reported by Naoulou (2012) [22]. Longitudinal Swedish studies have also shown no difference in the occurrence of thrombosis in women treated with tranexamic acid compared with spontaneous thrombosis in women [21, 22].

The available evidence suggests that tranexamic acid is safe and effective at reducing menstrual blood loss and may also improve quality of life, including reduced flooding/leakage and improved sex life [22].

7. What is the effectiveness and safety of non-steroidal anti-inflammatories for women with HMB?

Endometrial prostaglandins are elevated when menstruation is excessive. NSAIDs reduce prostaglandin levels by inhibiting the enzyme cyclo-oxygenase [7, 18]. Randomized controlled trials have consistently shown that NSAIDs decrease menstrual blood loss by between 20 and 50% [7]. Mefenamic acid, Ibuprofen, Naproxen, and Diclofenac have all been shown to be effective. NSAIDs are also helpful for women who have dysmenorrhea and up to 70% of women experience significant relief of pain [6]. NSAIDS were not as effective as danazol or tranexamic acid but had fewer side effects than danazol. The common side effects associated with NSAIDs are headaches and gastrointestinal disturbances, including dyspepsia, nausea, vomiting, and diarrhea. These disturbances can be avoided by taking the medication with food and are unlikely to occur if taken for a short time or intermittently. Women with a previous history of gastrointestinal ulceration or a history of bronchospasm with aspirin, should not be given NSAIDS. Non-steroidal anti-inflammatories should be taken regularly from the onset of menses, or just before, until heavy bleeding has subsided [7].

8. What is the effectiveness and safety of the combined oral contraceptive pill for women with HMB?

The combined oral contraceptive pill is useful in reducing menstrual blood loss and establishing regular cycles but the reduction in menstrual blood loss is less certain. Use of the combined oral contraceptive pill has the additional advantage of reducing dysmenorrhea and providing contraception [18].

A Cochrane systematic review identified only one randomized trial. There was no evidence of a significant difference in menstrual blood loss between those women treated with the oral contraceptive pill and those treated with danazol, or mefenemic acid, or naproxen [24]. A 2011 placebo controlled randomized trial comparing estradiol (E2) valerate and dienogest with placebo found that the oral contraceptive pill was effective in the treatment of women with idiopathic heavy and/or prolonged menstrual bleeding when compared with placebo with a mean reduction of −64.2% in the oral contraceptive group compared with −7.8% in the placebo group [25].

9. What is the effectiveness and safety of progesterone containing intrauterine devices for women with HMB?

Medicated intrauterine devices which release levonorgestrel (LNG-IUS; Mirena™) in a controlled manner have been shown to reduce menstrual blood loss by up to 90% in women with menorrhagia [7, 26] with increasing effectiveness after approximately six months of use [26]. Patient satisfaction has also been shown to be high over 3–24 months of use, ranging from 63% to 87% [26]. The side effects reported are minor and include irregular bleeding, breast tenderness, and expulsion of the device [26].

The evidence currently suggests that LNG-IUS is more effective at reducing menstrual blood loss that other medical interventions (combined oral contraceptive, oral progestogens, tranexamic acid, mefenamic acid, and fluriprofen). Reductions in mean blood loss volume ranging from 62% to 96% have been reported for LNG-IUS compared with 11–44% for other pharmacological interventions [26] (Table 2.2).

A recent review reported similar outcomes of pictorial blood loss between LNG-IUS and endometrial ablation after 24 months follow-up [26], whereas the NICE guideline favored surgical ablation compared with LNG-IUS at 12 months follow-up (WMD 33.2 ml; 95%CI 27.2–39.2 ml) [7]. The NICE guideline indicated that when LNG-IUS was compared with endometrial ablation the odds ratio for amenorrhea at up to one year follow-up was 0.75 (95%CI 0.36–1.54) in favor of surgical ablation [7]. A recent individual patient data meta-analysis has also shown similar rates of dissatisfaction between LNG-IUS (18%) and endometrial destruction techniques (17%). After six months follow-up, more women reported heavy bleeding following endometrial destruction compared with LNG-IUS (OR 4.3, 95%CI

Table 2.2 Pharmacological treatment options for heavy menstrual bleeding

Pharmacological therapy	Mechanism	Dosage	Reduction in menstrual blood loss	Benefits	Potential unwanted effects
Levonorgestrel releasing intrauterine system (LNG-IUS)	Prevents proliferation of the endometrium	20 μg/24 h	Up to 95% after 6 months	No impact on future fertility, Minimal side effects (systemic) Effective for up to 3 years Cost effective	Irregular bleeding for up to 6 months, minor and transient breast tenderness, acne or headaches. Less common – amenorrhea and rarely perforation of the uterus at the time of insertion of the device.
Tranexamic acid	Antifibrinolytic agent	1 g tds – QID	58%	No impact on future fertility, taken only during heavy menstrual bleeding, effective within 3 hours, useful where hormonal treatments are not acceptable	Common side effects include gastrointestinal disturbances and headaches. Less common are allergic skin responses.
Non-steroidal anti-inflammatory drugs (NSAIDS) Includes mefenamic acid, naproxen, and diclofenac	Reduce production of prostaglandin	Oral medication taken just prior to heavy bleeding or from day 1 until heavy bleeding ceases	Up to 49%	No impact on future fertility, only taken for 3 to 5 days, useful where hormonal treatments are not acceptable, inexpensive	Common side effects are gastrointestinal disturbances. Rarely there is worsening of asthma in sensitive people, peptic ulcers with possible bleeding and peritonitis
Combined Oral Contraceptives pill	Prevents proliferation of the endometrium	30 μg EE + desogestrol taken daily for 21 days followed by 7-day break	Up to 45%	No impact on future fertility, effective contraceptive	Common side effects include mood changes, headaches, nausea, fluid retention, and breast tenderness. Rarely there may be thromboembolic event or heart attack
Oral progestogen includes norethisterone	Prevents proliferation of the endometrium	10–15 mg daily	Up to 83% in the long term	No impact on future fertility, can be used where estrogen use is contra-indicated	Common side effects are usually minor and transient and include weight gain, bloating, breast tenderness, headaches and acne. Rarely there may be depression
Injected or implanted progestogen	Prevents proliferation of the endometrium	Depot intramuscular injections given 3-monthly	Bleeding likely to stop completely	No impact on future fertility, Long lasting, and effective, can be used where estrogen use is contra-indicated	Common side effects can include irregular bleeding, weight gain, amenorrhea, pre-menstrual like syndrome. Less common effects include revisable loss of bone mineral density
Gonadotrophin releasing hormone analogue (GnRHa)	Stops production of estrogen and progesterone	Monthly injection given for 3 to 6 months. Use of "Add-back" therapy recommended if therapy exceeds 6 months	Bleeding likely to stop completely in 89%	No impact on future fertility, reduces pain associated with endometriosis	Common side effects include menopause-like symptoms. Less common there may be osteoporosis with use over 6 months

Source: Adapted from National Institute for Health and Clinical Excellence (2007) and Lumsden and Wedisinghe (2011) [7, 23].

Table 2.3 Benefits and harms of the two surgical approaches

	Endometrial ablation/resection	Hysterectomy
Benefits	• Short surgical time • Short recovery time • Less likely to need pelvic floor repair	• Complete cure of abnormal bleeding • May assist other problems such as pelvic pain
Harms	• Need symptoms such as pain may occur • Only 80% of women have improved outcomes	• Intraoperative and postoperative side effects more common such as injury, infection, need for blood transfusion, pelvic floor repair and stress incontinence • Longer surgical time • Slower recovery

Sources: Middleton et al., 2010; Lethaby et al., 2009; Cooper et al., 2011 [27, 29, 30].

1.8–10.6, p = 0.001); this difference was still apparent at two years follow -up (OR 13, 95%CI 2.0–84.2, p = 0.007) [27] (Table 2.3).

LNG-IUS also appears to be more cost-effective than pharmacological therapies [7]. Based on an individual patient data meta-analysis, hysterectomy was identified as the overall preferred strategy for the treatment of HMB based on an incremental cost ratio [28]. This is based on the assumption that in LNG-IUS failures, women will proceed to second generation endometrial ablation and then hysterectomy if required [28].

LNG-IUS appears to be an effective means of reducing menstrual blood loss in women with HMB compared with pharmacological therapies and is also an effective contraceptive. In the long term it may not be as cost-effective as hysterectomy, but there is no compromise to future fertility and may be the first choice of preference for women.

10. What is the effectiveness and safety of injected/depot progestogens for women with HMB?

Depot medroxyprogesterone acetate (DMPA) is usually used as an injectable contraceptive administered every three months. One of the side effects is amenorrhea. Randomized controlled trial evidence suggested that amenorrhea was achieved in more women using DMPA than norethisterone at one year (12% versus 7%) and two years (24% versus 15%) [7]. Another trial reported in the NICE guideline indicated that up to 47% of women receiving DMPA (100–150 mg) had amenorrhea at one year follow-up.

11. What is the effectiveness and safety of surgery, e.g. endometrial ablation/resection or hysterectomy for women with HMB?

There are two main surgical options for women with menorrhagia:

(i) endometrial destruction by either laser or resectoscope, roller ball ablation, or thermal balloon ablation, microwave endometrial ablation; or

(ii) hysterectomy.

Endometrial destruction

The hysteroscopic methods of laser, resectoscope, or rollerball have become well established over the past five years as methods of removing endometrium. The thermal balloon ablation system is relatively new in New Zealand and has some advantages in being simple to use and avoids major complications that accompany other techniques. It can also be performed under local anesthetic. Microwave endometrial ablation has the advantages of short operating time and being suitable for women with fibroids up to 5 cm in diameter, regardless of position.

Hysterectomy

There are three major techniques for performing a hysterectomy. Providing the uterus is not larger than 12 weeks then the majority of hysterectomies should be performed through the vaginal route. The abdominal route is restricted to those women with severe pelvic disease such as endometriosis or large fibroids. The laparoscopic route is particularly suited to those women who have no descent of the cervix such as nulliparous women and women with moderate endometriosis. The cervix is usually removed at hysterectomy, although some women may choose to conserve it.

A Cochrane systematic review reported that hysterectomy was significantly better at improving HMB compared with endometrial ablation or resection techniques at one year follow-up (OR0.04, 95%CI 0.01–0.2). A greater percentage of women were more dissatisfied following first generation endometrial ablation than hysterectomy after 12 months (13% versus 5%) [27] and another systematic review reported greater satisfaction with hysterectomy at two years follow-up (OR 0.5, 95%CI 0.3–0.8) [29].

Despite the initial benefits of endometrial ablation/resection such as reduced surgical and recovery times and reduced complications, hysterectomy was identified as the more cost effective option in the long term due to the costs of repeated endometrial ablation interventions as a results of treatment failure [28, 29].

Conclusion

Although hysterectomy is undoubtedly effective for the cessation of HMB, and cost-effective in the long term compared to all other treatments, it is not recommended as a first line treatment [7]. Pharmacological treatments including LNG-IUS are useful initial treatments for women to be offered prior to surgical interventions.

Acknowledgements

We are grateful to Marian Showell of the Cochrane Menstrual Disorders and Subfertility Group for assisting with the electronic searches for studies.

References

1 Munro, M. et al. (2011). The FIGO classification system ("PALM-COEIN") for causes of abnormal uterine bleeding in non-gravid women in the reproductive years, including guidelines for clinical investigation. *International Journal of Gynaecology and Obstetrics* **113**: 3–14.

2 Fraser, I. et al. (2011). The FIGO recommendations on terminology and definitions for normal and abnormal uterine bleeding. *Seminars in Reproductive Medicine* **29**: 383–390.

3 Marret, H. et al. (2010). Clinical practice guidelines on menorrhagia: management of abnormal uterine bleeding before menopause. *European Journal of Obstetrics and Gynaecology and Reproductive Biology* **152**: 133–137.

4 Janssen, C.A., Scholten, P.C., and Heintz, A.P. (1995). A simple visual assessment technique to distinguish between menorrhagia and normal menstrual blood loss. *Obstetrics and Gynecology* **85**: 977–982.

5 Palacios, S. (2011). The management of iron deficiency in menometrorrhagia. *Gynecological Endocrinology* **27** (**S1**): 1126–1130.

6 National Health Committee (1998). *Guidelines for the Management of Heavy Menstrual Bleeding*. Christchurch, New Zealand: National Health Committee.

7 National Institute for Health and Clinical Excellence (2007). *Heavy Menstrual Bleeding*. London: National Collaborating Centre for Women's and Children's Health, RCOG Press.

8 Fraser, I. et al. (2007). A process designed to lead to international agreement on terminologies and definitions used to describe abnormalities of menstrual bleeding. *Fertility and Sterility* **87** (**3**): 466–476.

9 Vannella, L. et al. (2008). Benefit of concomittant gastrointestinal and gynaecological evaluation in premenopausal women with iron deficiency anaemia. *Alimentary Pharmacology & Therapeutics* **28**: 422–430.

10 Guyatt, G. et al. (1992). Laboratory diagnosis of iron-deficiency anemia: an overview. *Journal of General Internal Medicine* **7** (**2**): 145–153.

11 Eldred, J. and Thomas, E. (1994). Pituitary and ovarian hormone levels in unexplained menorrhagia. *Obstetrics and Gynecology* **84** (**5**): 775–778.

12 Haynes, P., Anderson, A., and Turnbull, A. (1979). Patterns of menstrual blood loss in menorrhagia. *Research and Clinical Forums* **1** (**2**): 73–78.

13 Krassas, G. et al. (1994). Menstrual disturbances in thyrotoxicosis. *Clinical Endocrinology* **40** (**5**): 641–644.

14 James, A., Matchar, D., and Myers, E. (2004). Testing for von Willebrand disease in women with menorrhagia: a systematic review. *Obstetrics and Gynecology* **104** (**2**): 381–388.

15 Claessens, E. and Cowell, C. (1981). Acute adolescent menorrhagia. *American Journal of Obstetrics and Gynecology* **139** (**3**): 277–280.

16 Farquhar, C. et al. (2003). A systematic review of transvaginal ultrasonography, sonohysterography and hysteroscopy for the investigation of abnormal uterine bleeding in premenopausal women. *Acta Obstetricia et Gynecologica Scandinavica* **82**: 493–504.

17 Farquhar, C. et al. (1999). An evaluation of risk factors for endometrial hyperplasia in premenopausal women with abnormal menstrual bleeding. *American Journal of Obstetrics and Gynecology* **181**: 525–529.

18 Vilos, G., Lefebvre, G., and Graves, G. (2001). Guidelines for the management of abnormal uterine bleeding. *Journal of Obstetrics and Gynaecology Canada* **106**: 1–6.

19 Fernández-Gaxiola, A.C. and De-Regil, L.M. (2011). Intermittent iron supplementation for reducing anaemia and its associated impairments in menstruating women. *Cochrane Database of Systematic Reviews*. 12 (Art. No.: CD009218) doi: 10.1002/1405651858.CD009218.pub2.

20 Van Wyck, D. et al. (2009). Large-dose intravenous ferric carboxymaltose injection for iron deficiency anaemia in heavy uterine bleeding: a randomized controlled trial. *Transfusion* **49** (**12**): 2719–2728.

21 Lethaby, A., Farquhar, C., and Cooke, I. (2000). Antifibrinolytics for heavy menstrual bleeding. *Cochrane Database of Systematic Reviews*. 4 (Art. No.: CD000249) doi: 10.1002/14651858.CD000249.

22 Naoulou, B. and Tsai, M. (2012). Efficacy of tranexamic acid in the treatment of idiopathic and non-functional heavy menstrual bleeding: a systematic review. *Acta Obstetrica et Gynecologica Scandinavica* **91**: 529–537.

23 Lumsden, M. and Wedisinghe, L. (2011). Tranexamic acid therapy for heavy menstrual bleeding. *Expert Opinion on Pharmacotherapy* **12** (**13**): 2089–2095.

24 Farquhar, C. and Brown, J. (2009). Oral contraceptive pill for heavy menstrual bleeding. *Cochrane Database of Systematic Reviews*. 4 (Art. No.: CD000154) doi: 10.1002/14651858.CD000154.

25 Jensen, J. et al. (2011). Effective treatment of heavy menstrual bleeding with estradiol valerate and dienogest. *Obstetrics and Gynecology* **117** (**4**): 777–787.

26 Kaunitz, A. and Inki, P. (2012). The levonorgestrel-releasing intrauterine system in heavy menstrual bleeding. *Drugs* **72** (**2**): 193–215.

27 Middleton, L. et al. (2010). Hysterectomy, endometrial destruction, and levonorgestrel releasing intrauterine system (Mirena) for heavy menstrual bleeding: systematic review and meta-analysis of data from individual patients. *British Medical Journal* **341**: c3929.

28 Roberts, T. et al. (2011). Hysterectomy, endometrial ablation, and levonorgesterel releasing intrauterine system (Mirena) for treatment of heavy menstrual bleeding: cost effectiveness analysis. *British Medical Journal* **342**: b2202.

29 Lethaby, A. et al. (2009). Endometrial resection and ablation versus hysterectomy for heavy menstrual bleeding. *Cochrane Database of Systematic Reviews*. 2 (Art. No.: CD000329) doi: 10.1002/14651858.CD000329.pub2.

30 Cooper, K. et al. (2011). Outcomes following hysterectomy or endometrial ablation for heavy menstrual bleeding: retrospective analysis of hospital episode statistics in Scotland. *British Journal of Obstetrics and Gynaecology*.

3

CHAPTER 3

Termination of pregnancy

Richard Lyus[1] and Patricia A. Lohr[2]
[1]*bpas (British Pregnancy Advisory Service) Richmond, East Twickenham, UK*
[2]*bpas (British Pregnancy Advisory Service), Stratford Upon Avon, UK*

> **CASE SCENARIO**
>
> A 24-year-old woman, gravida 1, presents to her primary care physician stating that she performed a pregnancy test at home which was positive. She believes that she is approximately eight weeks from her last menstrual period. She has been in a relationship with her partner for seven months and using condoms for birth control. Her past medical, surgical, family, and social histories are otherwise unremarkable. She would like to have an abortion and to discuss how she can prevent unintended pregnancy in the future.

Background

Induced abortion is one option for managing unintended or unwanted pregnancy. An estimated 43 million abortions are undertaken each year worldwide making it the most commonly performed gynecological procedure [1]. While some intended pregnancies become unwanted, most women who have abortions did not intend to become pregnant. Data on pregnancy intention are not collected in every country, but those from the United States illustrate its relationship with the incidence of abortion. Exclusive of miscarriages, 22% of pregnancies in the US end in abortion. However, of the nearly one half that are unintended, 40% end in abortion [2, 3].

Unintended pregnancy is the result of contraceptive method failures in some cases, but most occur either because no contraception was used or because the method was used inconsistently or incorrectly [4–6]. Ambivalence about contraception or pregnancy and a perceived low risk of pregnancy have also been associated with non-use or inconsistent use of contraception, and use of less effective methods [7]. That a pregnancy is unintended is only a first level explanation of the decision to terminate a pregnancy however [8]. Underlying that decision is typically a complex set of reasons such as interference with education, economic resources, health concerns, or relationship difficulties [9, 10].

Induced abortion using modern methods is very safe. When performed by trained clinicians with the appropriate resources, the chance of a woman dying from an induced abortion is considerably lower than chance of dying from childbirth [11, 12]. In the most recent Confidential Enquiry into Maternal Deaths in the United Kingdom, only two direct deaths related to induced abortion were recorded in the period 2006–2008 [13]. During this time, approximately 600 000 abortions would have been performed in England and Wales [14]. In contrast, when abortion is performed in unsafe conditions it is the cause of almost 70 000 deaths per year worldwide [15].

This chapter focuses on elective, induced abortion to 24 weeks gestation; termination of pregnancy for fetal or maternal indications is not considered in detail. Abortion at these gestations may be performed surgically or with medications. The choice of method is determined by multiple factors including patient preference, medical eligibility, and service availability.

Clinical questions

1. What counseling is needed for a woman who is considering ending a pregnancy by abortion?
2. What medical assessments are necessary before an abortion is performed?
3. What are the methods of abortion in the first trimester of pregnancy and which is optimal?
4. What are the methods of abortion in the second trimester of pregnancy and which is optimal?
5. What are the risks associated with surgical and medical abortion? What can be done to mitigate abortion-related risks?
6. Does abortion affect future reproductive outcomes?

Evidence-Based Obstetrics and Gynecology, First Edition. Edited by Errol R. Norwitz, Carolyn M. Zelop, David A. Miller, and David L. Keefe.

7. What contraceptive methods can be initiated immediately following an abortion?
8. What follow-up is required after an abortion?

1. What counseling is needed for a woman who is considering ending a pregnancy by abortion?

A woman with an unwanted pregnancy may choose to have an abortion, continue the pregnancy and arrange for adoption, or continue the pregnancy and undertake parenting. Most women requesting abortion will have decided to have a termination of pregnancy before coming to a healthcare provider for assistance. While the decision may not be easy and some women may find the experience stressful, most will not require further counseling [16, 17]. Requirements for counseling may also be viewed as intrusive when a woman is certain of her decision and can result in unnecessary delays to treatment [18, 19]. An explanation of treatment options and their associated risks provided in an a supportive non-judgmental manner and prompt referral for treatment summarizes the expectations and needs of most women once the decision to have an abortion has been made [18].

For some women, the decision to end or continue a pregnancy may not be straightforward. Feelings about whether a pregnancy is wanted are not always clear or may change over time, affected by factors such as a change in personal circumstances or antenatal screening results. Healthcare providers can help a woman consider her pregnancy options with non-directive decision-making support. A small proportion of women may anticipate that they will not cope well after an abortion [20]. Thus the option of supportive counseling before and after an abortion should be available if needed [21].

Importantly, whether a woman continues an unintended pregnancy or chooses to have an abortion, the mental health outcomes will be the same [22, 23]. Adverse mental health outcomes after an abortion or birth are most reliably predicted by a history of mental health problems. Referral pathways to therapeutic counseling should be in place [21]. Women who continue unintended pregnancies or are denied an abortion may also need additional support during and after their pregnancy [24–27].

For women considering abortion due to fetal abnormality or a maternal medical condition, discussion with an obstetrician, fetal medicine specialist, or pediatrician may be necessary to facilitate informed decision-making.

Conclusions

• Non-judgmental decision making support and prompt referral characterizes the needs of most women requesting induced abortion.
• Counseling should be available for the small proportion of women who require it whether ending or continuing an unintended or unwanted pregnancy.
• Providers should be reassured that abortion is not a cause of adverse mental health outcomes.

2. What medical assessments are necessary before an abortion?

If a woman has presented to her clinician without having performed a home pregnancy test, urine beta-hCG testing should be undertaken [17]. Once pregnancy has been confirmed, determination of gestational age is important because the methods used for medical and surgical abortion are gestational age dependent. In addition, gestational age limits are integral to abortion law in most countries. Gestational age may be determined by ultrasound or by clinical assessment (bimanual pelvic examination and/or last menstrual period). Where ultrasound is readily available, it is often used to verify gestational age and exclude ectopic or non-viable pregnancies or uterine anomalies. One systematic review has highlighted the lack of comparative data justifying the routine use of ultrasound prior to abortion with regard to safety and effectiveness [28]. Therefore ultrasound should not be considered a requirement.

The pre-abortion medical evaluation is not intended to assess whether a woman may safely have an abortion or not. Rather, it is focused on determining if any contraindications to choice of method or anesthesia exist, and whether the abortion needs to be performed in a hospital setting. A brief, targeted physical examination is usually sufficient and can be tailored to the anticipated treatment and the woman's medical history. This may include height and weight (to determine body mass index), observations, cardiac, pulmonary, abdominal, and pelvic examinations. Blood testing is typically limited to determination of Rhesus (D) antigen status [21]. Administration of anti-D immunoglobulin is recommended for Rh negative women, unless the father of the pregnancy is known to be Rh negative [29]. Hemoglobin determination is often undertaken where there is a concern for anemia or if significant blood loss anticipated although data to support this practice are limited [30]. Opportunistic screening for sexually transmitted infections or abnormal cervical cytology is also a frequent recommendation [21, 31].

Conclusions

• The medical assessment prior to abortion should be focused on a determination of gestational age, eligibility for a choice of treatment options including anesthetic, and Rhesus (D) antigen status.
• Ultrasound is often used as a means of determining gestational age and excluding pregnancy-related or uterine anomalies before abortion but is not a requirement.
• Opportunistic screening for sexually transmitted infections and abnormal cervical cytology may be incorporated into pre-abortion care.

3. What are the methods of abortion in the first trimester of pregnancy and which is optimal?

In both the first and second trimesters, abortion may be performed surgically or achieved by the administration of abortifacient medications. In the first trimester, the main surgical techniques are vacuum aspiration and dilation and sharp curettage (D&C). Cochrane meta-analyses have found few statistically significant differences between these methods. However, vacuum aspiration was shown to be faster than D&C when used for abortion and to be faster and associated with less pain and bleeding when used for miscarriage management [32, 33]. An additional advantage of vacuum aspiration is that it may be undertaken in an office setting under local anesthetic. Dilation and curettage is conducted in an operating theater with general anesthetic requiring greater resources [21, 34].

Vacuum aspiration may be performed using a manual or electrical suction device. Randomized comparisons have found no differences between electric and manual vacuum aspiration in terms of complications or patient preference, but more clinicians report difficulty with manual vacuum aspiration after nine weeks gestation [35]. One study found that significantly more women are bothered by the noise associated with electric vacuum aspiration [36].

Medical abortion allows a woman to have a safe, effective termination of pregnancy without a surgical procedure. Early medical abortion refers to the use of abortifacient medications up to 63 days gestation, although some regimens are effective beyond 63 days.

In the past, medical abortions were performed only in the second trimester using intra-amniotic instillation of hyper-osmolar agents or prostaglandins [35]. The development of prostaglandin analogues that could be administered vaginally or by injection made medical abortion possible earlier in pregnancy [37]. However the need to administer the medication in a hospital setting and a high incidence of gastrointestinal side effects and pain limited their use. The introduction of the anti-progestogerone mifepristone in the late 1980s led to a transformation in early medical abortion care.

Mifepristone causes cervical softening, decidual necrosis, and increased myometrial sensitivity to prostaglandins [38]. Initially studied for use alone in very early pregnancy, mifepristone was found to be only 60–80% effective [38]. When administered 36–48 hours before a prostaglandin analogue, however, the efficacy increased to nearly 100%. Multiple randomized trials have since demonstrated that the combination of mifepristone and a prostaglandin analogue is the most effective regimen for early medical abortion [39]. Defined as a complete abortion without resort to surgical intervention, success is upwards of 95% in most studies [39].

The most widely used and recommended prostaglandin analogue for medical abortion is misoprostol [21, 40]. Gemeprost (16, 16-dimethyl-trans-delta^2 PGE1 methyl ester) is a vaginally administered prostaglandin analogue that was initially approved for use with mifepristone in Europe. Although effective to 63 days gestation, it is expensive and requires refrigeration. Misoprostol, in contrast, is inexpensive, stable at room temperature, and can be administered by a variety of routes including oral, vaginal, sublingual, and buccal. Compared to Gemeprost, misoprostol administered vaginally has a similar side effect profile and is more effective to 63 days gestation [41].

Initial studies of medical abortion with 600 mg mifepristone and 400 mcg oral misoprostol were limited to gestations up to and including 49 days. When evaluated beyond 49 days gestation, oral misoprostol was shown to be associated with an unacceptably high failure rate [42]. A dose of 800 mcg misoprostol administered vaginally was, however, shown to be as effective at all gestations up to and including 63 days with a faster onset of action and fewer side effects [43, 44]. Vaginal administration was also shown to allow for a flexible dosing interval between mifepristone and misoprostol of anywhere from 6 to 72 hours without a decrement in effectiveness [45]. More recent studies have investigated misoprostol administered sublingually and buccally, which are also effective and acceptable routes of administration [42]. Reducing the dose of mifepristone from 600 to 200 mg is as effective in inducing a complete abortion [42].

Most early medical abortions are undertaken outside of a medical facility. Women are given tablets of misoprostol to take home and use within a specified interval, followed by abortion at home. A large body of evidence demonstrates that this is safe, effective, and acceptable to women [46].

Where mifepristone is not available, misoprostol may be used alone for early medical abortion. However multiple doses are often required and the success rate is lower, ranging from 85% to 90% in most studies [42]. The anti-dihydrofolate reductase agent methotrexate can also be used in combination with misoprostol up to 56 days gestation. Rather than acting as an abortifacient, the main effect of methotrexate is to cause embryonic demise. Methotrexate-based regimens have a less reassuring safety profile than those with mifepristone, require a longer interval before administration of the prostaglandin, and are about as effective as misoprostol alone [42].

A Cochrane review of six studies comparing medical and surgical methods in the first trimester found the rate of abortions not completed with the intended method to be significantly higher in the medical abortion group (OR 2.7, 95% CI 1.1, 6.8) [47]. There was no difference between the groups for ongoing pregnancies or pelvic infections, but one major complication, a uterine perforation, was reported in the surgical group. Duration of bleeding was longer with medical as compared to surgical abortion, but only rarely does this result in anemia requiring transfusion. In one large retrospective review of approximately 80 000 women undergoing early medical abortion, only 13 patients required blood transfusions [48]. Data on acceptability, side effects, or women's satisfaction with the procedure were not available for inclusion in the Cochrane review.

One randomized trial comparing early medical abortion with mifepristone and misoprostol to vacuum aspiration under general anesthetic up to 14 weeks gestation was published following the Cochrane review [49]. This study validated the finding of a longer duration of bleeding with early medical abortion. It also found while most women having an early medical abortion were satisfied with their care, acceptability was lower than with vacuum aspiration particularly as gestational age increased. Cohort studies have shown that acceptability and satisfaction with both medical and surgical abortion is greatest when women are able to receive the method of their choosing [50].

Conclusions

- Vacuum aspiration is the preferred method for first trimester surgical abortion.
- A combined regimen of mifepristone and misoprostol is the most effective method of early medical abortion.
- Both medical and surgical methods of first trimester abortion have very low complication rates and are acceptable to patients.
- In the absence of medical contraindications, the choice of method should be determined by the patient after discussion of both options.

4. What are the methods of abortion in the second trimester and which is optimal?

Surgical abortion can be performed with electric vacuum aspiration up to 16 weeks gestation using large-bore suction cannula and tubing [51]. However, the most commonly used method of surgical abortion in the second trimester is dilatation and evacuation (D&E). This procedure is characterized by the attainment of wide cervical dilation and the use of crushing forceps remove the fetus and placenta. Cervical dilation is usually achieved by inserting slowly expanding synthetic or natural cervical tents several hours before the procedure or with the use of medications such as mifepristone or misoprostol that soften the cervix making manual dilation easier. Following extraction of the fetus and placenta, a vacuum aspiration is performed to remove any remaining blood and tissue. Outdated surgical abortion methods include hysterotomy and hysterectomy. These are only used in modern abortion care when a transcervical approach is not possible [52]. Obstruction by a large, distorting cervical or uterine tumor is one example of when these methods might be employed.

Medical abortion in the second trimester also necessitates the passage of a larger fetus through a more dilated cervix and usually requires repeated administration of medications. The process is sometimes referred to as medical "induction" abortion as it mimics induction of labor. Older methods include intra- and extra-amniotic instillation of hypertonic solutions or prostaglandin, trans-cervical insertion and insufflation of a Foley balloon, and intravenous or intramuscular prostaglandins or oxytocics. Randomized trial data support the use of modern prostaglandin analogues with mifepristone as the most efficacious with the shortest induction to abortion interval [53]. The induction to abortion interval is usually defined as the time between the administration of medications and the passage of the fetus. In some studies, the time is extended to include the passage of the placenta which can occur several hours later.

As with early medical abortion, second trimester medical abortion involves the administration of mifepristone followed by a waiting period, typically of 24–48 hours. Women are then given repeated doses of a prostaglandin analogue to induce labor. Misoprostol is most commonly recommended but Gemeprost is an alternative [21, 54]. The median induction to abortion interval with a combined regimen is 6–8 hours in most studies. Prostaglandin analogues, like misoprostol, may also be used alone; however the median induction to abortion interval is increased significantly to 12–16 hours [53].

A Cochrane review comparing medical and surgical methods in the second trimester identified two randomized trials only one of which compared D&E to medical abortion with mifepristone and misoprostol [55]. Due to difficulties in recruitment, this study was underpowered to detect a difference in individual complications between the methods. Nevertheless, this study found a lower overall rate of adverse events in the D&E group (OR 0.06, 95% CI 0.01, 0.76). These adverse events were limited to presumed infection and retained placental tissue. Fewer subjects randomized to D&E required overnight hospitalization. Although women treated with mifepristone and misoprostol reported significantly more pain than those undergoing D&E, efficacy and acceptability were the same in both groups.

A more recent trial randomized 122 women at 13–20 weeks gestation to medical induction with mifepristone and misoprostol or surgical evacuation [56]. In this study, vacuum aspiration was performed up to 15 weeks gestation and D&E beyond. There were several statistically significant findings favoring surgical abortion. Women found surgery more acceptable and compared with medical induction and more women would opt for the same procedure again (100% versus 53%). Fewer women in the surgical arm found the experience worse than expected (0% versus 53%). Women who had medical induction also experienced more bleeding and pain. Similar to previously published randomized trials of medical and surgical abortion in the second trimester, a large proportion of women eligible to participate declined enrolment because they had a strong preference for a surgical abortion method.

A systematic review of the available cohort studies and case-series concluded that, given trained providers and where otherwise feasible, D&E is preferable to medical abortion in the second trimester, based on an overall lower rate of complications and patient preference [57]. In addition, D&E is quicker and less costly than medical abortion in the second trimester [58].

Traditionally, abortion for fetal abnormality or death has been accomplished by medical induction, as this practice allows pathological examination of the intact fetus. However, retrospective studies have demonstrated that there is a role for D&E in this setting based on greater safety and effectiveness [59, 60]. Genetic abnormalities are able to be confirmed without an intact fetus as are most structural anomalies [60–62]. Importantly, where women are given a choice of methods, grief resolution is the same with either a medical or surgical abortion for fetal anomaly [63].

Conclusions

- D&E is the preferred method of surgical abortion in the second trimester.
- Mifepristone and misoprostol is the most effective regimen for second trimester medical abortion and has the shortest induction to abortion interval.
- In the second trimester, D&E is preferred by women, associated with a lower rate of adverse events, faster, and more cost-effective than medical induction abortion.
- Patient preference should guide choice of method for elective abortion as well for abortion in cases of fetal anomaly.

5. What are the risks associated with surgical and medical abortion? What can be done to mitigate abortion-related risks?

Complications with surgical abortion are very low at any gestational age. Among 170 000 first trimester vacuum aspirations performed in low-risk women, minor complications occurred in 8.5 per 1000 cases and complications requiring hospitalization in 0.7 per 1000 cases [64]. D&E has a similar low rate of complications although the risk of a major complication increases with gestational age [65, 66]. A history of two or more Cesarean deliveries has been shown to be the strongest predictor for having a major complication with D&E (OR 7.4, 95% CI 3.4, 15.8) [66]. Mortality from surgical abortion is extremely rare but increases as gestational age advances. The lowest case fatality rate for abortion is at eight weeks gestation or less (0.1 per 100 000 procedures) and the risk of death increases by 38% with each successive gestational week [12].

Serious complications with medical abortion are also rare. However the overall rate of complications with medical abortion is higher than with surgical abortion [47, 49, 55, 57]. Two per 1000 women having an early medical abortion experience a complication requiring treatment in a hospital, most commonly due to heavy bleeding [67]. Surgical intervention for any reason, most commonly evacuation of retained products of conception, occurs in 2 in 100 procedures [68]. Mortality from early medical abortions with mifepristone is estimated to be 1 per 100 000 procedures [67, 69]. In the mid-trimester, complications with medical abortion increase, mainly due to retained placental tissue which is an indication for surgical intervention in 8 in 100 procedures [70].

An understanding that the overall rate of complications with any modern abortion method at any gestational age should provide reassurance to patients and providers. Women should also be informed of the relevant risks of the methods of termination she is considering as part of an informed decision-making process.

Cervical injury and uterine perforation

The rate of recognized uterine perforation during vacuum aspiration ranges from 0.1 to 4 per 1000 procedures [21, 71]. The rate of cervical injury ranges from 0.1 to 10 per 1000 procedures but is higher in adolescents [67]. Other risk factors for immediate complications of surgical abortion are performance by an inexperienced provider and increasing gestational age. With D&E, perforation of the uterus occurs in 2–3 per 1000 procedures and cervical laceration in up to 1 in 100 procedures [72].

Pharmacologic and mechanical methods of cervical preparation reduce the need for and facilitate rigid dilation of the cervix making procedures less difficult to perform and faster. Cervical preparation can also reduce the risk of cervical and uterine injury [73–75]. Mifepristone and misoprostol are the most effective pharmacologic methods of cervical preparation before first trimester surgical abortion [76]. Although mifepristone achieves greater baseline cervical dilation than misoprostol, it requires administration at least 24 hours pre-operatively compared to 2–3 hours with misoprostol. Mifepristone is also significantly more expensive than misoprostol.

Misoprostol may also be used for cervical preparation before D&E but osmotic dilators provide superior cervical dilatation [77]. Osmotic dilators are also effective for cervical preparation before first trimester surgical abortion.

Intra-operative ultrasound is widely used during second trimester surgical abortion to locate fetal parts and monitor the position of instruments. Continuous ultrasound guidance has also been shown in one retrospective cohort study to reduce the risk of uterine perforation during D&E [78]. Continuous ultrasound can also be used to monitor the placement of instruments at first trimester surgical abortion, although the evidence supporting this practice, is less-compelling [79].

Procedures to cause fetal demise before D&E are widely used in an effort to make the procedure safer, but lack an evidence base. Their posited benefit is the softening of fetal tissues to facilitate removal of fetal parts. The only randomized controlled trial available found that intra-amniotic digoxin administered 24-hours prior to D&E did not reduce the duration of the procedure or subjective difficulty compared to placebo [80]. However, a retrospective cohort study of 128 D&Es also found no difference in operating time when intra-cardiac potassium chloride was used to induce fetal demise prior to the procedure [81].

Cervical and uterine injury is largely obviated by avoiding instrumentation of the uterus with a medical abortion. However, uterine rupture can occur with second trimester medical abortion and is associated with a prior history of Cesarean delivery. A systematic review found the risk of uterine rupture in women with prior Cesarean delivery is estimated to be 0.28% (95% CI 0.08, 1%). The risk of uterine rupture in women without prior Cesarean delivery is estimated to be 0.04% (95% CI 0.01, 0.20%) [82].

Hemorrhage

Following first trimester vacuum aspiration, 0.007% of procedures are complicated by vaginal bleeding of a severity requiring hospitalization [64]. In a large cohort study of 11,747 D&Es up to 26 weeks gestation, blood loss greater than 500 ml was encountered in 0.9% of cases [66]. However, only 0.08% of cases had bleeding severe enough to warrant hospitalization and either observation or blood transfusion.

Significant bleeding after surgical abortion may be due to uterine atony, trauma to the reproductive tract, retained tissue or, less commonly, coagulopathy. Atony is the most common cause and while uterotonics such as oxytocin or ergot alkaloids are effective treatments, their prophylactic use in the context of first trimester surgical abortion is not supported by the available evidence [83–85]. One randomized controlled trial has demonstrated a statistically significant reduction in blood loss with D&E when vasopressin was added to a paracervical block [86].

Surgical intervention to achieve hemostasis is required in 2 of 1000 early medical abortions [67]. However the necessity for a blood transfusion is lower at 0.5–2 per 1000 procedures [12, 67]. Heavy bleeding is more common after later medical abortions with blood transfusions being required in 5– 7 in 1000 procedures [69, 87].

Infection

The rate of upper genital tract infection after abortion is influenced by the diagnostic criteria used [31]. When objective measures are employed, the rate after first trimester vacuum aspiration ranges from 0.01% to 2.4% [64, 88, 89]. Prior to the introduction of routine antibiotic prophylaxis, 0.8% of D&Es in one large cohort study were associated with febrile complications [81]. Infection after early medical abortion is infrequently reported. The best estimate based on prospective studies appears to be approximately 0.3% [86]. Rates with medical "induction" abortion in the second trimester are more difficult to estimate as fever is a common side effect of prostaglandin analogues, but reported ranges are from 1% to 3% [86].

Upper genital tract infection following surgical abortion is reduced by approximately 40% with antibiotic prophylaxis [90]. Although *Chlamydia* cervicitis is one of the strongest risk factors for post-abortion infection, universal prophylaxis leads to a greater reduction in the diagnosis of post-abortion infections and is more and cost-effective than a screen-and-treat approach [91, 92]. Bacterial vaginosis may also be a risk factor for post-abortion infection however the benefit of a screen and treat strategy has not been consistently demonstrated [86]. Short courses of doxycycline, tetracycline, metronidazole, and tinidazole administered pre-operatively are all effective for prophylaxis [86, 88].

The benefit of prophylactic antibiotics in medical abortion is less clear, as the risk of infection with this method is extremely low. However, the very small percentage of serious infections were shown to be further reduced with administration of treatment doses of doxycycline in one large cohort study (0.025% to 0.006%) [93]. Based on this study, some guidelines recommend routine prophylaxis for medical abortion.

Retained products of conception

Incomplete evacuation of the products of conception is one of the more common complications of medical and surgical abortion. Clinically it leads to prolonged bleeding and uterine cramping and is usually treated by vacuum aspiration. The frequency of re-aspiration following first trimester surgical abortion ranges from 0.3% to 2% and from 0.4% to 3% following second trimester surgical abortion [94]. One randomized trial found its incidence to be reduced with routine intra-operative ultrasound [74]. Cervical preparation with misoprostol is also associated with a risk reduction following vacuum aspiration [79].

Approximately 2% of early medical abortions require surgical intervention for incomplete evacuation including retention of a non-viable pregnancy [68]. Although clinicians frequently use routine repeat doses of misoprostol to increase the effectiveness of early medical abortion regimens there is limited evidence to support this practice [95]. Retained placenta requiring surgical intervention is reported in 2.5–10% of medical "induction" abortions in the second trimester [96]. Many studies have reported routine operative removal of placental tissue after a specified time period elevated operative intervention rates. In the absence of bleeding, however, waiting for spontaneous expulsion is safe and preferred [54, 97].

Failed abortion

Continuing pregnancy after surgical abortion occurs in 2 of 1000 procedures performed at 12 weeks gestation or less [98]. Procedures in women with one or more prior pregnancies and those conducted at less than or equal to six weeks gestation, particularly when small suction cannulae are used, are at higher risk for failure. Failures are also more likely when abortions were performed by inexperienced surgeons and in women with uterine anomalies. The risks of failed abortion with very early pregnancies can be reduced by application of a strict protocol that employs transvaginal ultrasound to confirm gestational age, inspection of the aspiration for the gestational sac, and serial beta-hCG measurements when evacuation cannot be confirmed visually [99].

Continuing pregnancy occurs in less than 1% of early medical abortions with most combined regimens. Vacuum aspiration is the treatment of choice as another dose of misoprostol is effective in less than 40% of cases [100]. One non-randomized trial found a reduced risk of continuing pregnancy at 50–63 days gestation when a second dose of misoprostol was routinely administered four hours following the initial dose but other studies have not demonstrated a clear benefit to routine repeat dosing of misoprostol.

Conclusions

- Risks of medical and surgical abortion are rare at any gestation.
- Complications should be discussed with women intending to terminate a pregnancy so that she can make an informed decision as to her choice of method.
- Interventions shown to reduce the risks of surgical abortion include the use of cervical preparation, ultrasound guidance, and prophylactic antibiotics.
- Induced fetal demise is not recommended before D&E to reduce risks based on a lack of objective evidence that it improves safety or effectiveness.

6. Does abortion affect subsequent reproductive outcomes?

A number of epidemiologic studies of have examined whether abortion negatively impacts on future pregnancies. These studies vary widely in their quality and conclusions, which can make interpretation difficult. None have been designed to determine causal relationships. There are no proven associations between induced abortion and subsequent ectopic pregnancy or infertility [101]. One systematic review reported that abortion may be linked with an increased risk of low birth weight, miscarriage, and placenta previa, but may also be protective for pre-eclampsia [102]. A 2009 meta-analysis identified 37 studies at "low to moderate risk of bias" and found an increased odds ratio for preterm delivery in women with a history of one abortion (OR 1.36, 95% CI 1.24, 1.50); a history of more than one abortion increased the odds-ratio (OR 1.93, 95% CI 1.28, 2.71) [103]. However, the authors advised caution against interpreting results to mean that a causal relationship had been established as the confounding effects of socioeconomic factors were considered in very few studies and abortion is often underreported. Further reassurance regarding the safety of surgical abortion is provided by a Danish population-based study of 11 814 pregnancies ended either by medical or surgical abortion in the first trimester [104]. This study found no difference in subsequent pregnancy outcomes between the groups.

Conclusion

- The current evidence is inadequate to implicate abortion as a causative factor of subsequent pregnancy morbidity.

7. What contraceptive methods can be initiated immediately following an abortion?

Ovulation can resume within 10–14 days following an abortion [105, 106]. All methods of contraception can be initiated at the time of an uncomplicated surgical abortion of any gestation, including hormonal methods and insertion of intrauterine devices (IUDs) [21]. Hormonal methods may be started on the day of misoprostol for a medical abortion and IUD insertion can occur at the time of follow-up [21].

Insertion of an IUD immediately after an early first trimester surgical abortion is not associated with an increased risk of procedural complications compared to interval insertion [107, 108]. Older randomized trials demonstrated significantly higher expulsion rates when an IUD was inserted after second trimester abortion compared to insertion after first trimester abortion [108]. However, more recent prospective studies have demonstrated only slightly higher or similar expulsion rates, possibly due to the use of ultrasound guidance during insertion [109, 110]. One randomized trial comparing insertion at the time of D&E at 15–23 weeks gestation with insertion three to six weeks post-procedure also found no difference in expulsion rates (6.8% versus 5% respectively, $p = 1.0$) [111]. Importantly, all of the women randomized to immediate insertion received their IUD as planned, however only 46% returned to the clinic to have the IUD placed at a later time [111]. In a similar randomized trial of immediate versus delayed insertion after first trimester abortion, only 71% of women in the delayed group returned to have the IUD inserted [112].

Recent studies have examined the insertion of IUDs at the time of follow-up after early medical abortion. An observational study of 118 women who had either a levonorgestrel IUS or copper IUD placed the time of confirmation of a complete first trimester medical abortion found an expulsion rate of 4.1% [113]. One randomized trial compared copper IUD insertion at one week after mifepristone with delayed insertion at four to six weeks after mifepristone. It found relatively high expulsion rates but no significant difference between the groups (11% in immediate group vs. 12% in delayed group, $p = 0.88$) [114]. Rates of IUD insertion were higher in the immediate group and duration of bleeding was not affected by timing of insertion.

Conclusion

- All methods of contraception can be started at the time of a surgical abortion.

- IUD insertion at the time of surgical abortion is safe in both the first and second trimester.
- The risk of expulsion with IUD insertion at second trimester surgical abortion is low, but is slightly higher that with delayed insertion, or insertion at the time of first trimester surgical abortion.
- After a medical abortion, an IUD can be inserted as soon as the procedure is felt to be complete.
- Starting contraception immediately after an abortion increases uptake rates and reduces the risk of subsequent unplanned pregnancy.

8. What follow-up is required after an abortion?

A 2004 literature review concluded that, when a first trimester surgical abortion is uncomplicated and the success of the procedure is immediately verified, routine follow-up is not necessary [115]. In complicated cases, or where the success of the abortion is not verified at the time of treatment, follow-up should be considered. Patients should be able to attend a follow-up visit if they request one [21].

When early medical abortion was first studied, protocols required women to be observed until the pregnancy had passed. Most early medical abortion now take place outside of a medical facility and some form of follow-up is used to ensure the procedure is complete. The best protocol for follow-up after early medical abortion is the subject of ongoing research. A follow-up visit for an ultrasound examination is often recommended and is and efficient and accurate means of confirming expulsion of the gestational sac [116]. Alternative protocols under investigation involve the use of standardized questionnaires that can be administered by phone, home pregnancy tests, and quantitative serum b-HCG testing [117].

Conclusions

- Routine follow-up after early surgical abortion is not required.
- Follow-up after early medical abortion conducted outside of a medical facility is recommended to ensure the abortion is complete.
- All women should be able to access a follow-up visit if they want one.

After a pregnancy options discussion and medical history, the patient was offered a surgical abortion with various anesthetic options, or an early medical abortion at home. She chose to have an early medical abortion and returned to the clinic two weeks later for an ultrasound scan which confirmed expulsion of the gestational sac. She chose to have a progestogen-releasing IUD inserted at this time.

Abortion is an integral part of women's healthcare. All obstetricians, gynecologists, and general practitioners should be familiar with the standards of care relevant to this common procedure. Counseling before treatment should be supportive, non-directive, and focused on the patient's needs. Both surgical and medical abortion are safe and effective and both methods should be available to women throughout the first and second trimesters of pregnancy, regardless of the reason for the abortion. For those women wishing to use it, contraception can be easily integrated into abortion care.

References

1 Sedgh, G., Singh, S., Shah, I. et al. (2012). Induced abortion: incidence and trends worldwide from 1995 to 2008. *Lancet* **379** (**9816**): 625–632.

2 Finer, L.B. and Henshaw, S.K. (2006). Disparities in rates of unintended pregnancy in the United States, 1994 and 2001. *Perspect. Sex. Reprod. Health* **38**: 90–96.

3 Jones, R.K. and Kooistra, K. (2011). Abortion incidence and access to services in the United States, 2008. *Perspect. Sex. Reprod. Health* **43**: 41–50.

4 Jones, R.K., Darroch, J.E., and Henshaw, S.K. (2002). Contraceptive use among US women having abortions in 2000–2001. *Perspect. Sex. Reprod. Health* **34**: 294–303.

5 Rasch, V. (2002). Contraceptive failure: results from a study conducted with accepted and unaccepted pregnancies in Denmark. *Contraception* **66**: 109–116.

6 Schünmann, C. and Glasier, A. (2006). Measuring pregnancy intention and its relationship with contraceptive use among women undergoing therapeutic abortion. *Contraception* **73**: 520–524.

7 Bruckner, H., Martin, A., and Bearman, P.S. (2004). Ambivalence and pregnancy: adolescents' attitudes, contraceptive use and pregnancy. *Perspect. Sex. Reprod. Health* **36**: 248–257.

8 Bankole, A., Singh, S., and Haas, T. (1998). Reasons why women have induced abortions: evidence from 27 countries. *Int. Fam. Plan. Perspect.* **24**: 117–127.

9 Kirkman, M., Rowe, H., Hardiman, A. et al. (2009). Reasons women give for abortion: a review of the literature. *Arch. Womens Ment. Health* **12**: 365–378.

10 Larsson, M., Aneblom, G., Odlind, V., and Tydén, T. (2002). Reasons for pregnancy termination, contraceptive habits and contraceptive failure among Swedish women requesting an early pregnancy termination. *Acta Obstet. Gynecol. Scand.* **81**: 64–71.

11 Raymond, E.G. and Grimes, D.A. (2012). The comparative safety of legal induced abortion and childbirth in the United States. *Obstet. Gynecol.* **119** (**2 Pt 1**): 215–219.

12 Bartlett, L.A., Berg, C.J., Shulman, H.B. et al. (2004). Risk factors for legal induced abortion-related mortality in the United States. *Obstet. Gynecol.* **103**: 729–737.

13 Cantwell, R., Clutton-Brock, T., Cooper, G. et al. (2011). Saving Mothers' Lives: reviewing maternal deaths to make motherhood safer: 2006–2008. *BJOG* **118**: 1–203.

14 Department of Health. (2011). Abortion Statistics for England Wales, 2010. www.dh.gov.uk/prod_consum_dh/groups/dh_digitalassets/documents/digitalasset/dh_127202.pdf (accessed 22 June 2018).

15 Haddad, L.B. and Nour, N.M. (2009). Unsafe abortion: unnecessary maternal mortality. *Rev. Obstet. Gynecol.* **2**: 122–126.

16 Rowlands, S. (2008). The decision to opt for abortion. *J. Fam. Plan. Reprod. Health Care* **34**: 175–180.

17 Moore, A.M., Frohwirth, L., and Blades, N. (2011). What women want from abortion counseling in the United States: a qualitative study of abortion patients in 2008. *Soc. Work Health Care* **50**: 424–442.

18 Kumar, U., Baraitser, P., Morton, S., and Massil, H. (2004). Decision making and referral prior to abortion: a qualitative study of women's experiences. *J. Fam. Plan. Reprod. Health Care* **30**: 51–54.

19 Henshaw, S.K. (1994). Abortion services under national health insurance: the examples of England and France. *Fam. Plan. Perspect.* **26**: 87–89.

20 Foster, D.G., Gould, H., and Kimport, K. (2012). How women anticipate coping after an abortion. *Contraception* **86** (**1**): 84–90.

21 The Royal College of Obstetricians and Gynaecologists (2011). *The Care of Women Requesting Induced Abortion. Evidence-Based Clinical Guideline Number* 7. London: RCOG.

22 American Psycological Association (2008). *Task Force on Mental Health and Abortion. Report of the Task Force on Mental Health and Abortion*. Washington DC: APA.

23 National Collaborating Centre for Mental Health (2011). *Induced Abortion and Mental Health. A Systematic Review of the Mental Health Outcomes of Induced Abortion, Including their Prevalence and Associated Factors*. London: Academy of Medical Royal Colleges.

24 Russo, N.F. (1992). Psychological aspects of unwanted pregnancy and its resolution. In: *Abortion, Medicine, and the Law*, 4e (ed. J.D. Butler and D.F. Walbert), 593–626. New york, NY: Facts on File.

25 David, H.P. (2011). Born unwanted: mental health costs and consequences. *Am. J. Orthopsychiatry* **81**: 184–192.

26 Dagg, P.K. (1991). The psychological sequelae of therapeutic abortion – denied and completed. *Am. J. Psychiatry* **148**: 578–585.

27 Gipson, J.D., Hindin, M.J., and Koenig, M.A. (2008). The effects of unintended pregnancy on infant, child, and parental health: a review of the literature. *Stud. Fam. Plan.* **39**: 18–38.

28 Kulier, R. and Kapp, N. (2011). Comprehensive analysis of the use of pre-procedure ultrasound for first- and second-trimester abortion. *Contraception* **83**: 30–33.

29 National Institute for Health and Clinical Excellence (2008). *Routine Antenatal Anti-D Prophylaxis for Women Who Are Rhesus D Negative: Review of NICE Technology Appraisal Guidance 41 (NICE Technology Appraisal Guidance 156)*. London: NICE.

30 Munro, J., Booth, A., and Nicholl, J. (1997). Routine pre-operative testing: a systematic review. *Health Technol. Assess.* **1** (**2**): 1–62.

31 Achilles, S.L., Reeves, M.F., and Society of Family Planning (2011). Prevention of infection after induced abortion: release date October 2010: SFP guideline 20102. *Contraception* **83**: 295–309.

32 Kulier, R., Fekih, A., Hofmeyr, G.J., and Campana, A. (2001). Surgical methods for first trimester termination of pregnancy. *Cochrane Database Syst. Rev.* (**4**): CD002900. doi: 10.1002/14651858.CD002900.

33 Tunçalp, O., Gülmezoglu, A.M., and Souza, J.P. (2010). Surgical procedures for evacuating incomplete miscarriage. *Cochrane Database Syst. Rev.* (**9**): CD001993. doi: 10.1002/14651858.CD001993.pub2.

34 World Health Organization (2011). *Safe Abortion: Technical and Policy Guidance for Health Systems*, 2e. Geneva: WHO.

35 Fiala, C. and Gemzel-Danielsson, K. (2006). Review of medical abortion using mifepristone in combination with a prostaglandin analogue. *Contraception* **74**: 66–86.

36 Dean, G., Cardenas, L., Darney, P., and Goldberg, A. (2003). Acceptability of manual versus electric aspiration for first trimester abortion: a randomized trial. *Contraception* **67**: 201–206.

37 Bygdeman, M., Bremme, K., Christensen, N. et al. (1980). A comparison of two stable prostaglandin E analogues for termination of early pregnancy and for cervical dilatation. *Contraception* **22**: 471–483.

38 Bygdeman, M. and Swahn, M.L. (1985). Progesterone receptor blockage. Effect on uterine contractility and early pregnancy. *Contraception* **32**: 45–51.

39 Kulier, R., Kapp, N., Gülmezoglu, A.M. et al. (2011). Medical methods for first trimester abortion. *Cochrane Database Syst. Rev.* (**11**): CD002855. doi: 10.1002/14651858.CD002855.pub4.

40 American College of Obstetricians and Gynecologists (ACOG) (2005). *Medical Management of Abortion*, 12. Washington (DC): American College of Obstetricians and Gynecologists (ACOG). (ACOG practice bulletin; no. 67).

41 Bartley, J., Brown, A., Elton, R., and Baird, D.T. (2001). Double-blind randomized trial of mifepristone in combination with vaginal gemeprost or misoprostol for induction of abortion up to 63 days gestation. *Hum. Reprod.* **16**: 2098–2102.

42 Spitz, I.M., Bardin, C.W., Benton, L., and Robbins, A. (1998). Early pregnancy termination with mifepristone and misoprostol in the United States. *N. Engl. J. Med.* **338**: 1241–1247.

43 el-Refaey, H., Rajasekar, D., Abdalla, M. et al. (1995). Induction of abortion with mifepristone (RU 486) and oral or vaginal misoprostol. *N. Engl. J. Med.* **332**: 983–987.

44 Schaff, E.A., Fielding, S.L., and Westhoff, C. (2001). Randomized trial of oral versus vaginal misoprostol at one day after mifepristone for early medical abortion. *Contraception* **64**: 81–85.

45 Wedisinghe, L. and Elsandabesee, D. (2010). Flexible mifepristone and misoprostol administration interval for first-trimester medical termination. *Contraception* **81**: 269–274.

46 Ngo, T.D., Park, M.H., Shakur, H., and Free, C. (2011). Comparative effectiveness, safety and acceptability of medical abortion at home and in a clinic: a systematic review. *Bull. World Health Organ.* **89**: 360–370.

47 Say, L., Kulier, R., Gülmezoglu, M., and Campana, A. (2005). Medical versus surgical methods for first trimester termination

of pregnancy. *Cochrane Database Syst. Rev.* (**1**): CD003037. doi: 10.1002/14651858.CD003037.

48 Hausknecht, R. (2003). Mifepristone and misoprostol for early medical abortion: 18 months experience in the United States. *Contraception* **67**: 463–465.

49 Robson, S.C., Kelly, T., Howel, D. et al. (2009). Randomised preference trial of medical versus surgical termination of pregnancy less than 14 weeks' gestation (TOPS). *Health Technol. Assess.* **13**: 1–124, iii–iv.

50 Henshaw, R.C., Naji, S.A., Russell, I.T., and Templeton, A.A. (1993). Comparison of medical abortion with surgical vacuum aspiration: women's preferences and acceptability of treatment. *BMJ* **307**: 714–717.

51 Stubblefield, P.G., Albrecht, B.H., Koos, B. et al. (1978). A randomized study of 12-mm and 15.9 mm cannulas in midtrimester abortion by laminaria and vacuum curettage. *Fertil. Steril.* **29**: 512–517.

52 Stubblefield, P.G., Carr-Ellis, S., and Borgatta, L. (2004). Methods for induced abortion. *Obstet. Gynecol.* **104**: 174–185.

53 Wildschut, H., Both, M.I., Medema, S. et al. (2011). Medical methods for mid-trimester termination of pregnancy. *Cochrane Database Syst. Rev.* (**1**): CD005216. doi: 10.1002/14651858.CD005216.pub2.

54 Borgatta, L., Kapp, N., and Society of Family Planning (2011). Clinical guidelines. Labor induction abortion in the second trimester. *Contraception* **84**: 4–18.

55 Lohr, P.A., Hayes, J.L., and Gemzell-Danielsson, K. (2008). Surgical versus medical methods for second trimester induced abortion. *Cochrane Database Syst. Rev.* (**1**): CD006714. doi: 10.1002/14651858.CD006714.pub2.

56 Kelly, T., Suddes, J., Howel, D. et al. (2010). Comparing medical versus surgical termination of pregnancy at 13–20 weeks of gestation: a randomised controlled trial. *BJOG* **117**: 1512–1520.

57 Grossman, D., Blanchard, K., and Blumenthal, P. (2008). Complications after second trimester surgical and medical abortion. *Reprod. Health Matters* **16** (**31 Suppl**): 173–182.

58 Cowett, A.A., Golub, R.M., and Grobman, W.A. (2006). Cost-effectiveness of dilation and evacuation versus the induction of labor for second-trimester pregnancy termination. *Am. J. Obstet. Gynecol.* **194**: 768–773.

59 Bryant, A.G., Grimes, D.A., Garrett, J.M., and Stuart, G.S. (2011). Second-trimester abortion for fetal anomalies or fetal death: labor induction compared with dilation and evacuation. *Obstet. Gynecol.* **117**: 788–792.

60 Edlow, A.G., Hou, M.Y., Maurer, R. et al. (2011). Uterine evacuation for second-trimester fetal death and maternal morbidity. *Obstet. Gynecol.* **117** (**2 Pt 1**): 307–316.

61 Bernick, B.A., Ufberg, D.D., Nemiroff, R. et al. (1998). Success rate of cytogenetic analysis at the time of second-trimester dilation and evacuation. *Am. J. Obstet. Gynecol.* **179**: 957–961.

62 Shulman, L.P., Ling, F.W., Meyers, C.M. et al. (1990). Dilation and evacuation for second-trimester genetic pregnancy termination. *Obstet. Gynecol.* **75**: 1037–1040.

63 Burgoine, G.A., Van Kirk, S.D., Romm, J. et al. (2005). Comparison of perinatal grief after dilation and evacuation or labor induction in second trimester terminations for fetal anomalies. *Am. J. Obstet. Gynecol.* **192**: 1928–1932.

64 Hakim-Elahi, E., Tovell, H.M., and Burnhill, M.S. (1990). Complications of first-trimester abortion: a report of 170,000 cases. *Obstet. Gynecol.* **76**: 129–135.

65 Cates, W. Jr., Schulz, K.F., Grimes, D.A. et al. (1982). Dilatation and evacuation procedures and second-trimester abortions. The role of physician skill and hospital setting. *JAMA* **248**: 559–563.

66 Peterson, W.F., Berry, F.N., Grace, M.R., and Gulbranson, C.L. (1983). Second-trimester abortion by dilatation and evacuation: an analysis of 11,747 cases. *Obstet. Gynecol.* **62**: 185–190.

67 Henderson, J.T., Hwang, A.C., Harper, C.C., and Stewart, F.H. (2005). Safety of mifepristone abortions in clinical use. *Contraception* **72**: 175–178.

68 Ashok, P.W., Templeton, A., Wagaarachchi, P.T., and Flett, G.M. (2002). Factors affecting the outcome of early medical abortion: a review of 4132 consecutive cases. *BJOG* **109**: 1281–1289.

69 Meites, E., Zane, S., and Gould, C.; C. sordellii Investigators(2010). Fatal *Clostridium sordellii* infections after medical abortions. *N. Engl. J. Med.* **363**: 1382–1383.

70 Ashok, P.W., Templeton, A., Wagaarachchi, P.T., and Flett, G.M. (2004). Midtrimester medical termination of pregnancy: a review of 1002 consecutive cases. *Contraception* **69**: 51–58.

71 Allen, R.H., Goldberg, A.B., and Board of Society of Family Planning (2007). Cervical dilation before first-trimester surgical abortion (<14 weeks' gestation). SFP guideline 2007. *Contraception* **76**: 139–156.

72 Fox, M.C., Hayes, J.L., and Society of Family Planning (2007). Cervical preparation for second-trimester surgical abortion prior to 20 weeks of gestation. *Contraception* **76**: 486–495.

73 Grimes, D.A., Schulz, K.F., and Cates, W.J. Jr. (1984). Prevention of uterine perforation during curettage abortion. *JAMA* **251**: 2108–2111.

74 Schulz, K.F., Grimes, D.A., and Cates, W. Jr. (1983). Measures to prevent cervical injury during suction curettage abortion. *Lancet* **1**: 1182–1185.

75 Meirik, O., Huong, N.T., Piaggio, G. et al. (2012). Complications of first-trimester abortion by vacuum aspiration after cervical preparation with and without misoprostol: a multicentre randomised trial. *Lancet* **379** (**9828**): 1817–1824.

76 Kapp, N., Lohr, P.A., Ngo, T.D., and Hayes, J.L. (2010). Cervical preparation for first trimester surgical abortion. *Cochrane Database Syst. Rev.* (**2**): CD007207. doi: 10.1002/14651858.CD007207.pub2.

77 Newmann, S.J., Dalve-Endres, A., Diedrich, J.T. et al. (2010). Cervical preparation for second trimester dilation and evacuation. *Cochrane Database Syst. Rev.* (**8**): CD007310. doi: 10.1002/14651858.CD007310.pub2.

78 Darney, P.D. and Sweet, R.L. (1989). Routine intraoperative ultrasonography for second trimester abortion reduces incidence of uterine perforation. *J. Ultrasound Med.* **8**: 71–75.

79 Acharya, G., Morgan, H., Paramanantham, L., and Fernando, R. (2004). A randomized controlled trial comparing surgical termination of pregnancy with and without continuous ultrasound guidance. *Eur. J. Obstet. Gynecol. Reprod. Biol.* **114**: 69–74.

80 Jackson, R.A., Teplin, V.L., Drey, E.A. et al. (2001). Digoxin to facilitate late second-trimester abortion: a randomized, masked, placebo-controlled trial. *Obstet. Gynecol.* **97**: 471–476.

81 Singh, S., Seligman, N.S., Jackson, B., and Berghella, V. (2012). Fetal intracardiac potassium chloride injection to expedite second-trimester dilation and evacuation. *Fetal Diagn. Ther.* (**1**): 31, 63–38.

82 Goyal, V. (2009). Uterine rupture in second-trimester misoprostol-induced abortion after cesarean delivery: a systematic review. *Obstet. Gynecol.* **113**: 1117–1123.

83 Nygaard, I.H., Valbø, A., Heide, H.C., and Kresovic, M. (2011). Is oxytocin given during surgical termination of first trimester pregnancy useful? A randomized controlled trial. *Acta Obstet. Gynecol. Scand.* **90**: 174–178.

84 Ali, P.B. and Smith, G. (1996). The effect of syntocinon on blood loss during first trimester suction curettage. *Anaesthesia* **51**: 483–485.

85 Beeby, D. and Morgan Hughes, J.O. (1984). Oxytocic drugs and anaesthesia. A controlled clinical trial of ergometrine, syntocinon and normal saline during evacuation of the uterus after spontaneous abortion. *Anaesthesia* **39**: 764–767.

86 Schulz, K.F., Grimes, D.A., and Christensen, D.D. (1985). Vasopressin reduces blood loss from second-trimester dilatation and evacuation abortion. *Lancet* **2**: 353–356.

87 Hamoda, H., Ashok, P.W., Flett, G.M., and Templeton, A. (2005). Medical abortion at 9–13 weeks' gestation: a review of 1076 consecutive cases. *Contraception* **71**: 327–332.

88 Heisterberg, L. and Kringelbach, M. (1987). Early complications after induced first-trimester abortion. *Acta Obstet. Gynecol. Scand.* **66**: 201–204.

89 Fried, G., Ostlund, E., Ullberg, C. et al. (1989). Somatic complications and contraceptive techniques following legal abortion. *Acta Obstet. Gynecol. Scand.* **68**: 515–521.

90 Sawaya, G.F., Grady, D., Kerlikowske, K., and Grimes, D.A. (1996). Antibiotics at the time of induced abortion: the case for universal prophylaxis based on a meta-analysis. *Obstet. Gynecol.* **87**: 884–890.

91 Penney, G.C., Thomson, M., Norman, J. et al. (1998). A randomised comparison of strategies for reducing infective complications of induced abortion. *Br. J. Obstet. Gynaecol.* **105**: 599–604.

92 Cameron, S.T. and Sutherland, S. (2002). Universal prophylaxis compared with screen-and-treat for Chlamydia trachomatis prior to termination of pregnancy. *BJOG* **109**: 606–609.

93 Fjerstad, M., Trussell, J., Sivin, I. et al. (2009). Rates of serious infection after changes in regimens for medical abortion. *N. Engl. J. Med.* **361**: 145–151.

94 Lichtenberg, E.S. and Grimes, D.A. (2009). Surgical complications: prevention and management. In: *Management of Unintended and Abnormal Pregnancy: Comprehensive Abortion Care*. Oxford: Wiley-Blackwell.

95 Gallo, M.F., Cahill, S., Castleman, L., and Mitchell, E.M. (2006). A systematic review of more than one dose of misoprostol after mifepristone for abortion up to 10 weeks of gestation. *Contraception* **74**: 36–41.

96 Kapp, N. and Von Herten, H. (2009). Medical methods to induce abortion in the second trimester. In: *Management of Unintended and Abnormal Pregnancies: Comprehensive Abortion Care*. Oxford: Wiley-Blackwell.

97 Green, J., Borgatta, L., Sia, M. et al. (2007). Intervention rates for placental removal following induction abortion with misoprostol. *Contraception* **76**: 310–313.

98 Kaunitz, A.M., Rovira, E.Z., Grimes, D.A., and Schulz, K.F. (1985). Abortions that fail. *Obstet. Gynecol.* **66**: 533–537.

99 Edwards, J. and Carson, S.A. (1997). New technologies permit safe abortion at less than six weeks' gestation and provide timely detection of ectopic gestation. *Am. J. Obstet. Gynecol.* **176**: 1101–1106.

100 Reeves, M.F., Kudva, A., and Creinin, M.D. (2008). Medical abortion outcomes after a second dose of misoprostol for persistent gestational sac. *Contraception* **78**: 332–335.

101 Royal College of Obstetricians and Gynaecologists. (2009). Induced Termination of Pregnancy and Future Reproductive Outcomes – Current Evidence. RCOG Opinion issued 16th September 2009. Accessed 22 June 2018 from: www.rcog.org.uk/induced-termination-pregnancy-and-future-reproductive-outcomes-%E2%80%93-current-evidence.

102 Lowit, A., Bhattacharya, S., and Bhattacharya, S. (2010). Obstetric performance following an induced abortion. *Best Pract. Res. Clin. Obstet. Gynaecol.* **24**: 667–682.

103 Shah, P., Zao, J., and on behalf of Knowledge Synthesis Group of Determinants of Preterm/LBW Births (2009). Induced termination of pregnancy and low birthweight and preterm birth: a systematic review and meta-analyses. *BJOG* **116**: 1425–1442.

104 Virk, J., Zhang, J., and Olsen, J. (2007). Medical abortion and the risk of subsequent adverse pregnancy outcomes. *N. Engl. J. Med.* **357**: 648–653.

105 Marrs, R.P., Kletzky, O.A., Howard, W.F., and Mishell, D.R. Jr. (1979). Disappearance of human chorionic gonadotropin and resumption of ovulation following abortion. *Am. J. Obstet. Gynecol.* **135** (**6**): 731–736.

106 Schreiber, C.A., Sober, S., Ratcliffe, S., and Creinin, M.D. (2011). Ovulation resumption after medical abortion with mifepristone and misoprostol. *Contraception* **84**: 230–233.

107 Grimes, D.A., Lopez, L.M., Schulz, K.F., and Stanwood, N.L. (2010). Immediate postabortal insertion of intrauterine devices. *Cochrane Database Syst. Rev.* (**6**): CD001777. doi: 10.1002/14651858.CD001777.pub3.

108 Steenland, M.W., Tepper, N.K., Curtis, K.M., and Kapp, N. (2011). Intrauterine contraceptive insertion postabortion: a systematic review. *Contraception* **84**: 447–464.

109 Fox, M.C., Oat-Judge, J., Severson, K. et al. (2011). Immediate placement of intrauterine devices after first and second trimester pregnancy termination. *Contraception* **83** (**1**): 34–40.

110 Drey, E., Reeves, M.F., Ogawa, D.D. et al. (2009). Insertion of intrauterine contraceptive immediately following first- and second-trimester abortions. *Contraception* **79** (**5**): 397–402.

111 Hohmann, H.L., Reeves, M.F., Chen, B.A. et al. Immediate versus delayed insertion of the levonorgestrel-releasing intrauterine device following dilatation and evacuation: a randomised controlled trial. *Contraception* **85** (**3**): 240–245.

112 Bednarek, P.H., Creinin, M.D., Reeves, M.F. et al.; Post-Aspiration IUD Randomization (PAIR) Study Trial Group(2011). Immediate versus delayed IUD insertion after uterine aspiration. *N. Engl. J. Med.* **364**: 2208–2217.

113 Betstadt, S.J., Turok, D.K., Kapp, N. et al. (2011). Intrauterine device insertion after medical abortion. *Contraception* **83**: 517–521.

114 Shimoni, N., Davis, A., Ramos, M.E. et al. (2011). Timing of copper intrauterine device insertion after medical abortion: a randomized controlled trial. *Obstet. Gynecol.* **118**: 623–628.

115 Grossman, D., Ellertson, C., Grimes, D.A., and Walker, D. (2004). Routine follow-up visits after first-trimester induced abortion. *Obstet. Gynecol.* **103**: 738–745.

116 Rørbye, C., Nørgaard, M., and Nilas, L. (2004). Prediction of late failure after medical abortion from serial beta-hCG measurements and ultrasonography. *Hum. Reprod.* **19**: 85–89.

117 Clark, W., Bracken, H., Tanenhaus, J. et al. (2010). Alternatives to a routine follow-up visit for early medical abortion. *Obstet. Gynecol.* **115**: 264–272.

4

CHAPTER 4
Miscarriage and ectopic pregnancy

Celso Silva and Anita Patel
University of Central Florida, Center for Reproductive Medicine, Orlando, FL, USA

> **CASE SCENARIO**
>
> A 25-year-old now G1Po, last menstrual period (LMP) six weeks ago, presents with vaginal spotting. She also reports vague, intermittent, left lower quadrant achey pain. She had a remote history of chlamydial infection and recently engaged in unprotected intercourse. Home pregnancy test was positive.

Background

Vaginal bleeding during the first trimester of the pregnancy is one of the most common clinical scenarios encountered in Obstetrics and Gynecology, occurring in approximately one fourth of all pregnancies [1]. The differential diagnosis of first trimester bleeding classically includes not only ectopic pregnancy (EP), but also miscarriage (threatened, inevitable, incomplete, missed, septic, and complete), and gestational trophoblastic disease. Recurrent pregnancy loss and gestational trophoblastic disease are outside of the scope of this chapter.

Miscarriage or spontaneous abortion is one of the most common complications of the pregnancy. The incidence is approximately 20–25% when the pregnancy is clinically recognized and may be higher if very early pregnancy losses or biochemical pregnancies are included [2]. In many cases, a spontaneous abortion will occur before a woman recognizes that she is pregnant, and the presenting symptoms are mistaken for late menses.

The rate of EP is approximately 19.7 cases per 1000 pregnancies. In the presence of first trimester vaginal bleeding, the risk increases above the normal population rate [3]. Emergency Room series have reported that 7–24% of women presenting with first trimester pain or bleeding are ultimately diagnosed with ectopic pregnancies [4].

When evaluating a pregnant patient with first trimester vaginal bleeding it is important to use an evidence-based approach of the steps of history, physical examination, laboratory and imaging studies, and treatment. Fortunately, the incorporation of improved transvaginal ultrasound (TVS) technology and serial measurements of the beta subunit of human chorionic gonadotropin (β-hCG) into routine clinical practice has resulted in an increased rate of correct diagnosis and introduction of early therapy.

During the assessment of patients with first trimester vaginal bleeding it is important to correctly identify those women with viable intra-uterine pregnancies (IUP) versus those with ectopic pregnancies or non-viable intrauterine pregnancies. When this is done correctly, appropriate intervention is possible, and the appropriate treatment course can be instituted, be it observation, pharmacologic intervention, or surgical intervention. It is also important to provide patients with counseling about possible implications for future reproductive prognosis, and emotional support.

Ectopic pregnancy

Ectopic pregnancy is defined as any pregnancy implanted outside of the endometrial cavity. It is considered the main cause of maternal death in the first trimester of the pregnancy [5], and the attention of the clinician must be on early diagnosis and institution of therapy before tubal rupture. EPs comprise 1–2% of all first trimester pregnancies in the United States, however this small portion accounts for nearly 6% of all pregnancy-related deaths [5, 6]. Up to 73.9% of women with an EP may be diagnosed on an initial TVS assessment and 94% are diagnosed prior to the need for emergency surgical intervention [7, 8].

Heterotopic pregnancy is another rare condition that occurs when EP is found in conjunction with an intrauterine pregnancy. The incidence of heterotopic pregnancy is higher when the pregnancy is achieved through Assisted Reproductive Technologies (ART), and it estimated to be 1–3 in every 100 ART pregnancies [9, 10] in contrast to 1 in every 7000–30 000 spontaneous pregnancies [11]. The risk is

Evidence-Based Obstetrics and Gynecology, First Edition. Edited by Errol R. Norwitz, Carolyn M. Zelop, David A. Miller, and David L. Keefe.

directly correlated with the number of embryos transferred during the *In Vitro* Fertilization (IVF) process. When four or more embryos are transferred, it is estimated that the risk for an heterotopic pregnancy is as high as 1 in 45 pregnancies [12]. Thus, in clinical practice it is important to remember that a visualized IUP does not exclude the risk of EP in women undergoing IVF treatment. Ovulation induction also is associated with an incidence of heterotopic pregnancy of nearly 0.5–1% [13]. Rare cases of twin tubal pregnancies, with both embryos in the same fallopian tube or one embryo is each fallopian tube have also been reported [14, 15].

Historical perspective

The first known report describing an ectopic pregnancy is from Abulcasis in 963 CE [16]. Duverney, in 1708, was probably the first to describe a heterotopic pregnancy in an autopsy case. Parvey, in 1876, described 22 cases of ruptured tubal pregnancies. Until the end of the nineteenth century, the therapy of ectopic pregnancies was not surgical, and the mortality rates was as high as 60% [17]. In 1884, the British surgeon, Robert Lawson Tait (1845–1899) reported the first salpingectomy for the treatment of an ectopic pregnancy. In 1888, Tait reported only two deaths out of 42 operated cases, a marked improvement for a condition that had been almost always fatal [18].

In 1891, Whitcomb described a case of a ruptured tubal ectopic pregnancy associated with an intra-uterine pregnancy in a bicornuate uterus. In 1894, Bussieri described a case of an intact ectopic pregnancy in an autopsy of a prisoner after her execution. Interestingly, at the time, it was felt that ectopic pregnancies were the result of an embryo passing through the tube and implanting there secondary to an interrupted coitus. In subsequent years, the number of described cases increased. In 1902, Zinke described 88 cases and in 1904 Simpson reported 113 cases [19].

In 1941, Caffier described 10 cases of salpingostomia rather than salpingectomy for the treatment of ectopic pregnancy. Of these patients, four proceeded to have subsequent IUP.

It was not until the mid-twentieth century that technological advancements, including the advent of laparoscopy and ultrasound, the radioimmunoassay for the determination of (β-hCG), and more recently the introduction of IVF have made it possible the early diagnosis of an unruptured ectopic pregnancy and better prognosis for patients at risk for ectopic pregnancy [20].

Today, we have an improved understanding of the natural history of ectopic pregnancies, including the fact that some patients with this condition may indeed experience spontaneous resolution. The therapeutic armamentarium has expanded and now includes the use of conservative surgery, when indicated, and the use of medical therapy with methotrexate (MTX).

Clinical questions

1. How common is ectopic pregnancy?

Ectopic pregnancy remains a frequency condition during a woman's reproductive life. In the developed world, the incidence of EP is 11–20 per 1000 live births [21–23]. In the developing world, the incidence is thought to be higher, but the data is not clear. Epidemiological studies have consistently reported a sixfold increase in the incidence of ectopic pregnancies between 1970 and 1992 [24]. This increase is thought to be secondary to a higher incidence of pelvic inflammatory disease (PID), more women of reproductive age with the habit of smoking, increased use of ART, and increased awareness of the conditions. In assisted conception populations the incidence is as high as 4% [10].

The epidemiology of ectopic pregnancy is easier to understand when divided in two distinct entities: ectopic pregnancies due to contraceptive methods failure, which have a low incidence as the modern contraceptive methods have a low failure rate; and ectopic pregnancies due to reproductive failure rate, with a higher incidence [25]. The estimated failure rate of tubal sterilization ranges from 0.1–0.8%, and a third of these pregnancies are ectopic [26].

2. What effects does ectopic pregnancy have on morbidity and mortality?

Improved methods for early diagnosis and treatment have reduced the fatality rate in developed countries [23]. Nonetheless, ectopic pregnancy remains the leading cause of first trimester pregnancy-related maternal death, with a rate of 0.35 cases per 1000 ectopic pregnancies [16, 27]. However, in countries in development, the maternal death rate is much higher [28].

Ectopic pregnancy is also considered a frequent cause of maternal morbidity. Acute symptoms, including pelvic pain and vaginal bleeding are common. In the long term, chronic pelvic pain, infertility, and psychological issues are frequently present in women with a previous history of ectopic pregnancy [29].

3. What are the risk factors for ectopic pregnancy?

Though many risk factors have been found in association with EP, up to one-third of cases occur in women without any apparent risk factors [30].

Of the risk factors associated with EP, the highest risk is attributed to tubal pathology that results from PID, especially those caused by *Chlamydia trachomatis* and *Neisseria gonorrheae* [31–33]. The exact mechanism is not determined, but in addition to compromise of the tubal architecture, it may be due to a disruption of the tubal microenvironment. The tubal lumen or ostia may be partially obstructed due to the formation of synechiae or tubal torsion due to pelvic adhesions, obstructing the passage of the embryo, although allowing the passage of the sperm due to its smaller size.

Tubal pathology due to previous pelvic surgery is another important risk factor for ectopic pregnancies. This is especially true in women who have undergone surgical procedures for sterilization or fertility restoration, including fimbrioplasty, salpingoplasty, and neosalpigostomy.

A history of multiple sexual partners is also associated with EP, but this correlation is likely due to the higher incidence of PID in women with multiple sexual partners.

It is important to note that the use of contraceptive methods including tubal sterilization, copper and progestin releasing intrauterine devices (IUDs), and progestin-only contraceptives is associated with an overall lower rate of ectopic pregnancies due to the efficacy of these contraceptive methods. While IUD use lowers EP rate by 10% when compared to women not using contraception, when the IUD fails women are at a higher risk of EP, perhaps due to the higher risk of PID in these patients. In a multicenter study, the World Health Organization concluded that in low risk populations, the risk for PID due to the use of an IUD is temporary and limited to the insertion period [34–37]. Congenital anomalies of the fallopian tubes, including diverticulums, septums, hypoplasia, and accessory ostia may be involved in the cause of an ectopic pregnancy. In addition, when the lumen of the tube is narrowed, for example due to extrinsic compression caused by uterine fibroids, there could be an increased risk for ectopic pregnancies. Other conditions can also predispose to EP including salpingitis isthmica nodosa (SIN) and congenital fallopian tube anomalies secondary to in utero diethylstilbestrol exposure (DES) [37, 38]. DES exposure increases the rate of EP by ninefold [39]. The etiology of SIN is unknown, and occurs when tubal mucosa penetrates the myosalpinx in the isthmic segment of the tube resulting in muscular hypertrophy.

A previous EP increases the risk of subsequent EP by more than 10%, and approximately 9% of women with a single episode of salpingitis have a subsequent EP [33, 40, 41]. This risk may be attributable to the predisposing tubal disorder that led to the first EP.

One-third of all cases of ectopic pregnancies are associated with smoking [33], and smoking has been found to be an independent risk factor for EP. There is a dose–effect relationship present, and the risk is higher when a woman uses more than 20 cigarettes a day [42]. Though the mechanism is unknown, several mechanisms have been proposed, including delayed ovulation, altered tubal and uterine motility, impaired tubal ciliary motility, and impaired immunity [31].

Ectopic pregnancy is more common in women with infertility, even in the absence of tubal disease [43]. Assisted reproductive technologies are particularly associated with EP, with a risk of 2–5%, and it may be higher when tubal disease is present [31]. One study found that women taking clomiphene citrate doubled their risk of ectopic pregnancy from 3–6% [44]. Similarly, controlled ovarian stimulation with gonadotropins has been associated with an increased risk of ectopic pregnancy [45, 46].

4. What causes ectopic pregnancy?

Ectopic pregnancies occur when there is a disruption to the blastocyst migration through the fallopian tube or when there are conditions that promote early implantation. The exact mechanisms are not well-established. Of note, ectopic pregnancies are unique to the human species, and perhaps to higher primates. Because of this species-specificity, there is no good animal model to study this condition.

Approximately 93–98% of EPs occur within the fallopian tube. Of these, 70% implant in the ampulla, followed by the isthmus, fimbria, and cornual/interstitial locations. [47]. Up to 7% of EPs are located outside the fallopian tube [47]. These sites include the ovary, cervix, peritoneal cavity, and prior cesarean scar. The fallopian tube lacks a submucosal layer; thus a zygote is able to quickly invade the epithelium and the rapidly proliferating trophoblast often invades as far as within the muscularis, and may even reach the tubal serosa. Commonly, the developing embryo in an EP is absent or poorly developed.

The patognomonical finding is an ectopic gestation is the presence of chorionic villi in the lumen or in the wall of the fallopian tube or another extra-uterine site. The pathology evaluation of these villi revealed it to be normal or with hyaline degeneration. However chromosomal abnormality is not likely an important etiology of ectopic pregnancy [48, 49]. In one study in which chorionic villi were karyotyped from 30 viable surgically excised ectopic gestations, the rate of karyotype abnormality was no different from that of controls with intrauterine pregnancies [49].

Chronic salpingitis is observed in up to 90% of ectopic pregnancies [50]. Infection produces an inflammatory response that damages the tubal ciliary epithelium, potentially disrupting the embryonic transport through the fallopian tube or may result in the formation of intra-tubal synechiae, thus contributing to closure of fallopian tube. PID can promote adhesion formation with adjacent pelvic organs, disrupting the anatomy of the fallopian tube, and potentially also resulting in altered tubal transport.

We previously discussed the higher incidence of EP in patients undergoing ART. One theory for this higher rate is that the medications used to stimulate ovarian follicle development result in high levels of progesterone and estradiol that may slow tubal peristalsis and promote uterine relaxation, thus promoting early embryo implantation. Women with tubal infertility undergoing IVF are at even higher risk of EP. This is one of the reasons physicians may recommend removal of diseased tubes before undergoing IVF treatment [51].

Oocyte or embryonic anomalies may also participate in the pathogenesis of ectopic pregnancy. An abnormal embryo may have sub-optimal transport through the fallopian tube. Although not necessarily related to chromosome abnormalities, it could be speculated that this could also be associated with the fact that women older than 35 years of age have a higher rate of EP [52].

In relation to the uterus, the endometrium undergoes decidualization and the endometrial mucosa may present an atypical aspect. This has been called the Arias–Stella reaction, and it is characterized by increased cellular volume, hyperchromatosis, pleomorphism, and increased mitotic activity [53]. In 5–10% of ectopic pregnancies a decidual cast may be passed and often mistaken for products of conception. This occurs because the abnormal pregnancy does not produce enough progesterone to maintain the decidua. Notably, on pathologic examination only decidua will be seen and chorionic villi will be absent. This may often be confused with a miscarriage.

EP rupture is usually spontaneous. Early rupture, 6–8 weeks, occurs with isthmic implantations due to the small diameter size of the fallopian tube at this location. Ampullar ruptures occur later around 8–12 weeks because it is more easily distensible compared to the isthmus. Interstitial ruptures occur even later at 12–16 weeks as the myometrium provides more room for the embryo to develop. Interstitial rupture is the most dangerous because proximity to uterine and ovarian vessels can result in massive hemorrhage.

5. How is the diagnosis of ectopic pregnancy made?

The early diagnosis of an ectopic pregnancy is important as it decreases the risk of tubal rupture and ameliorates the success rates of conservative therapy. Special attention must be given to patients at risk for ectopic pregnancy, including patients with previous history of ectopic pregnancy, tubal surgery (including tubal ligations), infertility, use of assisted reproductive technologies therapy, history of PID, presence of endometriosis, use of IUD, and history of smoking.

In patients with delayed menses, vaginal bleeding, and/or pelvic pain are possible indicators of an ectopic pregnancy. In these cases, it is important to maintain close follow-up until a final diagnosis is confirmed.

In patients that are hemodynamically stable, it is possible to proceed with non-invasive diagnostic steps, including transvaginal ultrasound and β-hCG measurements. Conversely, in hemodynamic unstable patients, it may be necessary to resort to surgical diagnosis, either with a laparoscopy or laparotomy. In certain cases, a uterine curettage may be employed with the goal to verify the presence of intra-uterine villi, confirm a non-viable intra-uterine pregnancy. Culdocentesis, to verify the presence of intra-pelvic blood, is rarely performed in today's clinical practice.

Historically the triad of pain, vaginal bleeding or spotting, and delayed or missed menstruation raised suspicion of EP in women of child bearing age [54]. Decades ago women often presented with symptoms of acute abdomen and/or hypovolemic shock secondary to ectopic rupture. Today, with the advent of commercially available urine pregnancy tests in combination with early utilization of TVS and serial measurements of plasma β-hCG, women are diagnosed earlier in the course of the disease. In fact, most patients with EP deny symptoms of abdominal pain or this is a late finding [55]. Up to 10% are asymptomatic and one in three women have no clinical signs [55].

Information regarding date of LMP, date of first positive home pregnancy test, dates of positive urine and/or blood pregnancy tests, date of HCG administration for ovulation triggering or date of oocyte retrieval if the pregnancy resulted from infertility treatment are all important information in the evaluation of patient at risk for ectopic pregnancy.

The patient's history must include information regarding the onset, volume, and duration of vaginal bleeding as well as nature, intensity, and location of the pelvic pain. Early presentation symptoms of EP are subtle or may even be absent. It is common for patients to believe they are carrying a normal pregnancy or having a miscarriage. Up to 30% of patients with ectopic pregnancies have no vaginal bleeding [56].

Because the symptoms of EP are non-specific, it may be misdiagnosed as other gynecological, gastrointestinal, or urological disorders. Common conditions that may present similarly to EPs include appendicitis, salpingitis, ovarian cyst rupture, miscarriage, adnexal torsion, urolithiasis, and urinary tract infection [57].

Other symptoms that are not specific for EP include nausea, vomiting, and diarrhea. Symptoms of ruptured EP are the same as those of an acute abdomen: abdominal distension, tenderness, peritoneal signs, and shock. Therefore the diagnosis of EP should be considered for all reproductive age women who present with acute abdominal pain or GI symptoms [23].

The overall likelihood of ectopic pregnancy is 39% in a patient with abdominal pain and vaginal bleeding, but no other risk factors. The probability increases to 54% if the patient has other risk factors [58]. It is important to note that 30–50% of patients with ectopic pregnancies may not bleed [59]. Conversely, only 29% of pregnant patients presenting to a hospital emergency room with bleeding or pain, findings of peritoneal irritation, and cervical motion tenderness turned out to have ectopic pregnancies in one series. Even though this was fourfold higher than the 7.7% prevalence of ectopic pregnancies among the entire cohort of pregnant patients presenting with pain and bleeding, the majority of pregnancies in the high-risk group were still intrauterine [59].

Physical examination in patients at risk for ectopic pregnancy should include an assessment of the volume of vaginal bleeding, presence of abdominal/pelvic tenderness, presence of adnexal mass and cervical motion tenderness, uterine size, and hemodynamic status. Tenderness to palpation may be elicited on abdominal and bimanual examination. EPs of older gestational age may produce mass effect and push the uterus to one side.

Symptoms of dizziness, lightheadedness, and syncope should raise suspicion for intra-abdominal bleeding from a ruptured EP. Blood accumulation in the rectouterine cul-de-sac may present as posterior vaginal fornix bulging. Women with hemoperitoneum may complain of symptoms of diaphragmatic irritation characterized by referred pain to the neck, shoulder or scapula which worsens with maximal inspiration.

Only 10% of patients with an ectopic pregnancy have a palpable adnexal mass, and up to 10% have negative pelvic examinations [60].

There are significant limitations in using medical history and physical examination in the diagnosis of ectopic pregnancy. Therefore, decision–analysis studies have determined that diagnostic algorithms using a combination of pelvic transvaginal ultrasound and β-hCG offered the most accurate means of diagnosing ectopic pregnancy [59].

The presence of an intrauterine gestation on ultrasound almost always rules out an ectopic pregnancy, since the incidence of heterotopic pregnancies has been reported as 1/30 000 spontaneous conceptions. In pregnancies achieved through assisted reproductive technologies, heterotopic gestation must always be a consideration as reported incidence is much higher, approaching 1/100–1/1000 pregnancies [59].

Unless the patient is hemodynamically unstable as in cases of ruptured ectopic pregnancies, or the diagnosis is definite as when products of conception are seen at the external os or in the vagina during pelvic examination, an initial ultrasound evaluation should be undertaken. Transvaginal sonography provides an accurate diagnosis of pregnancy status for most intrauterine pregnancies [61].

A transvaginal ultrasound can visualize an intra-uterine gestational sac when the gestational age is approximately five to six weeks [62]. When the gestational age is unknown, the β-hCG values may help determine the gestational age and improve the interpretation of the transvaginal ultrasound findings [63–65]. The discriminatory value (also called the "discriminatory zone") of the β-hCG is defined as the value above which a gestational sac must be identified by the ultrasound, when the pregnancy is intra-uterine and normal. The discriminatory values for transvaginal ultrasounds are usually between 1500 and 2000 $\mathrm{mIU\,ml^{-1}}$. The discriminatory value for abdominal ultrasound is usually around 6500 $\mathrm{mIU\,ml^{-1}}$ [66].

However, these values are also largely dependent on ultrasound equipment resolution and examiner experience. Moreover, inter-assay variability also contributes to made it very difficult to establish a universally reproducible discriminatory β-hCG value [67], and therefore these values are often defined by each institution.

When the β-hCG value is above the discriminatory zone, an intra-uterine pregnancy (gestational sac) must be seen by an ultrasound. The absence of an intra-uterine pregnancy when the β-hCG is above the discriminatory zone indicates an unviable pregnancy, but it cannot distinguish between an ectopic pregnancy or a miscarriage [68]. The presumptive diagnosis of an ectopic pregnancy in these cases can be incorrect in more than 50% of the cases [69]. However, it is also important to take into consideration the cases of multiple gestation, in which the β-hCG values are higher than when compared to singleton gestations [70].

Care must be taken to confirm the presence of a true gestational sac, rather than a pseudosac. A true gestational sac is eccentrically placed and adjacent to the central echogenic endometrial stripe, reflecting implantation of the conceptus in the endometrial tissue rather than in the endometrial cavity. A pseudosac is a collection of fluid within the endometrial cavity and can be seen in ectopic pregnancies [71].

The sensitivity and specificity of a transvaginal ultrasound to accurately diagnose an ectopic pregnancy depends upon the criteria used to establish the diagnosis. If stringent criteria are used, like for example the extra-uterine presence of embryonic heart activity or a gestational sac containing a yolk sac or embryo, the sensitivity is low, ranging from 20.1% to 64.6%, and the negative predictive value of the test is also low. Alternatively, if less stringent criteria are used, like for example any adnexal mass other than a simple cyst, with or without cul-de-sac fluid, the sensitivity of ultrasound improves to 69–84.4%, and the negative predictive value improves to 95%, at the expense of minimal losses in specificity and positive predictive value [72, 73]. If ultrasound demonstrates neither an intrauterine pregnancy nor an adnexal mass in early pregnancy, further evaluation is required and an ectopic gestation must be considered. The presence of an intrauterine gestation on ultrasound almost always rules out an ectopic pregnancy, since the incidence of heterotopic pregnancies has been reported as 1/30 000 spontaneous conceptions [11].

Knowledge of the temporal appearance of embryonic structures as visualized by transvaginal ultrasound is essential to the correct diagnosis of a viable intra-uterine pregnancy. For example, an intrauterine gestational sac can often be imaged by a transvaginal ultrasound approximately 4.5 – 5 weeks after the first day of the LMP, and should almost always be detectable by 5 ½ weeks gestation [73]. Failure to image an intrauterine gestation should be interpreted with caution when LMP is the reference, since dating can be incorrect due to recall bias and delayed ovulation. Initially, the diameter of the gestational sac may only be 2–3 mm, and will increase by 1 $\mathrm{mm\,d^{-1}}$ in early pregnancy, and a yolk sac should be imaged at a gestational sac diameter of 8–10 mm, or approximately one week after the appearance of the gestational sac. This correlates to 5.5–6.5 weeks gestation [74]. Embryonic cardiac activity adjacent to the yolk sac is detected next. Fetal cardiac activity can be detected prior to six weeks gestation in some instances, and should be confirmed by 46 days gestational age and a mean sac diameter of 16 mm in almost all viable gestations [67].

In reproductive aged patients, the symptoms of vaginal bleeding and/or pelvic pain should always raise suspicion for a possible pregnancy, and β-hCG measurements in blood or urine should be obtained to confirm or rule-out a pregnancy. In conjunction with transvaginal ultrasound, quantitative β-hCG assays are integral in the diagnosis of ectopic pregnancy. Serial quantitative β-hCG measurements are an integral part of the clinical follow-up of a pregnant patient with an early pregnancy and trimester vaginal bleeding and/or pain until it is determined if the pregnancy is viable, or if the presenting symptoms are due to a miscarriage or an ectopic pregnancy. Similarly, serial β-hCG measurements following a diagnosis of a miscarriage or an ectopic pregnancy are essential to confirm resolution of these problems.

When the gestational age is unknown, β-hCG values may help in the determination of the gestational age. Moreover, quantitative β-hCG values serve as a reference when interpreting the results of the transvaginal ultrasound. The trophoblast begins to secrete hCG into maternal blood upon implantation. For this reason β-hCG can be detected in maternal serum even prior to the anticipated menses, and 2½ weeks prior to the ability of ultrasound to consistently image a gestational sac [67]. As already mentioned, the "discriminatory zone" of the β-hCG values, is the β-hCG level above which an intrauterine gestational sac, if the pregnancy is normal and intrauterine, will always be detected by ultrasound.

6. What if the location of the pregnancy remains unknown following ultrasound?

Although initially there was confusion in the literature regarding the definition for a "Pregnancy of Unknown Location" (PUL), today the term is generally applied to describe women with a positive pregnancy test who have no evidence of either an intra-uterine pregnancy or an ectopic pregnancy on transvaginal ultrasound [72, 75].

At presentation, a pregnant woman with first trimester vaginal bleeding or pain can be classified as being in one of five categories based on ultrasound findings: definite ectopic pregnancy (extra-uterine gestational sac with yolk sac and/or embryo with or without cardiac activity), probable ectopic pregnancy (adnexal mass or extra-uterine sac-like structure), PUL (no signs of either ectopic pregnancy or intra-uterine pregnancy), probable intra-uterine pregnancy (intrauterine sac-like structure), and definite intrauterine pregnancy (intrauterine gestational sac with yolk sac and/or embryo with or without cardiac activity) [72, 75].

As many as 5–42% of women presenting for an early pregnancy ultrasound assessment will be classified as having a PUL [7, 76–78]. It is important to note that PUL is a classification and not a final diagnosis, and as such, when a PUL is present, women must be followed until a final diagnosis is confirmed. Balance must be achieved in evaluating the risk of morbidity due to an ectopic pregnancy and the risk of interventions used to reach a final diagnosis and treatment.

Once diagnosed with a PUL, the following final outcomes are possible: a visualized ectopic pregnancy; a visualized intra-uterine pregnancy; a spontaneously resolved PUL (women who start as having a PUL, with spontaneous resolution of β-hCG to undetectable levels without surgical or medical therapy); a persisting PUL; a non-visualized ectopic pregnancy (rising β-hCG levels after uterine evacuation); or histological intra-uterine pregnancy (identification of chorionic villi after uterine evacuation) [72, 75].

When the values of β-hCG are below the discriminatory zone or the transvaginal ultrasound does not detect a definite intra-uterine pregnancy or a definite ectopic pregnancy, the rate of change of β-hCG has been used to assist in final diagnosis of a PUL [79].

It is common in clinical practice to expect that the β-hCG values should double every 48 hours when the pregnancy is viable. However, a recent retrospective analysis of a large database of women presenting with first trimester bleeding or pain found that viable intrauterine pregnancies occurred when the rate of increase was as low as 53% in 48 hours [68]. Importantly, based on this new data, if former criteria considering a pregnancy to be unviable when the β-hCG rise was inferior to 66% in 48 hours [64] were to be used, this could result in the interruption of viable pregnancies.

The majority of ectopic pregnancies have slower rates of increase, but a significant percentage of these ectopic pregnancies have β-hCG that mimic those of a viable intra-uterine pregnancy [80].

When the values of the β-hCG are above the discriminatory zone, a transvaginal ultrasound should be performed to document the presence or absence of an intra-uterine pregnancy. The absence of a definite intra-uterine pregnancy with the β-hCG levels above the discriminatory zone, or with levels rising inappropriately or declining suggest the presence of an unviable pregnancy, but cannot distinguish between an ectopic pregnancy or a miscarriage. A presumptive diagnosis of an ectopic pregnancy in these situations may be incorrect in more than 50% of the cases [69].

Progesterone levels may also be used to complement the diagnostic armamentarium of a PUL, although this is an ancillary test with limited value in diagnosing the status of a pregnancy. Levels greater than 20–25 $ng\,ml^{-1}$ are reassuring for a normal intrauterine pregnancy. However, levels below 5 $ng\,ml^{-1}$ are highly suggestive of a non-viable pregnancy, either an ectopic pregnancy or a non-viable intrauterine pregnancy. A total of 31% of viable pregnancies, 52% of ectopic pregnancies, and 23% of spontaneous miscarriages have intermediate values between 10 and 20 $ng\,ml^{-1}$, an overlap which limits the ability of progesterone measurements to discriminate between viable and non-viable pregnancies. When the pregnancy is non-viable, a progesterone level cannot discern an intrauterine pregnancy from an ectopic pregnancy [81].

Uterine curettage and anatomo-pathological examination of the obtained tissue may help to determine the differential diagnosis between an ectopic pregnancy and a miscarriage. In situations where β-hCG curves have confirmed an abnormal gestation, but the location of the pregnancy is unknown and ectopic pregnancy remains in the differential, a uterine curettage may be performed. If the obtained tissue is confirmed to be chorionic villi, then an abnormal intra-uterine pregnancy is confirmed, except in cases of heterotopic pregnancies (although this is a rare clinical circumstance). If chorionic villi are not present, then the suspicion for ectopic pregnancy is high. Some clinicians choose to offer empiric treatment with MTX, without the need for curettage, and do so based on the fact that chorionic villi are not detected in 20% of curettage specimens from elective terminations [82]. A Pipelle curette, traditionally used to perform endometrial biopsies can also be used to obtain intrauterine tissue in these scenarios, but with a sensitivity of only 30% compared with curettage in identifying intrauterine villi [83].

Other clinicians advocate curettage, and reserve MTX therapy only for those patients in whom no intrauterine villi was found to be present. Proponents of this option argue that up to 40% of pregnancies in this clinical scenario turn out to be intrauterine pregnancies [84], and therefore MTX would be used unnecessarily in a large proportions of patients.

When the transvaginal ultrasound and serial measurements of β-hCG levels do not diagnose a definite ectopic pregnancy, the likelihood of detecting an ectopic pregnancy at laparoscopy is only 7% [85].

7. How is ectopic pregnancy managed?

The incorporation of improved diagnostic methods and work-up protocols into routine clinical practice have allowed for a progressive earlier detection of ectopic pregnancy. As a result, patients with this condition rarely present with a life-threatening situation, requiring emergency surgery. It is not uncommon that patients are diagnosed with an ectopic pregnancy when they are not yet symptomatic. As a result of this paradigm shift, the therapeutic approach y for an ectopic pregnancy has also changed, with more options available to the modern clinician.

Treatment options for ectopic pregnancies include expectant management, medical management with MTX, and surgical. MTX can be administered parenterally as a single dose, parenterally in a multi-dose protocol, or by direct injection into the ectopic under ultrasound or laparoscopic guidance. Surgical options include laparotomy or laparoscopic approaches. Surgical interventions can include conservation of the affected tube with a salpingostomy, segmental salpingectomy with the option to re-anastomose the affected tube at a later date, or total salpingectomy. The clinical presentation often dictates the treatment approach [86].

Surgical treatment

Surgery is the definitive treatment of an ectopic pregnancy. Laparotomy should be performed in cases where the patient is hemodynamically unstable with tubal rupture. In the other clinical situations, laparoscopy should be performed. The laparoscopic route has several advantages, including less blood loss, shorter operative time, hospital stay, faster recovery, and lower costs [87].

Laparoscopic and laparotomy surgery have similarly high rates of post-operative tubal patency, and similar rates of subsequent intrauterine pregnancies [88].

When tubal conservation is undertaken, the likelihood of residual trophoblastic tissue and the need for further treatment is significantly higher after laparoscopy than after laparotomy. Post-laparoscopic residual trophoblastic tissue has been reported in 15% after salpingostomy by laparoscopy and 5% after salpingostomy by laparotomy [89].

Most ectopic gestations implant in the ampulla of the fallopian tube, and as such are potentially amenable to either salpingostomy or salpingectomy. The patient and the clinician must weigh the benefits of a conservative surgery (salpingostomy) as a means of optimizing reproductive potential in the future but with the risks of residual trophoblastic tissue and recurrent ectopic pregnancy against the risks and benefits of the radical surgery (salpingectomy).

Salpingectomy is the treatment of choice in patients who have no future reproductive desire, who have a recurrent ectopic pregnancy in the same tube, in patients with tubal rupture or tubal damage that is irreparable, and in patients with bleeding that cannot be controlled with attempted salpingostomy. When the β-hCG level is above $5000\,\text{mIU ml}^{-1}$, tubal damage is likely to be more extensive, and therefore tubal conservation may be contra-indicated [90, 91].

Although salpingostomy is indicated in patients who want to maintain their reproductive capacity, it is not clear if this procedure indeed result in a higher rate of future IUP when compared to the radical salpingectomy. Some studies have demonstrated a higher rate of a future intrauterine pregnancy but also a higher risk for a future ectopic pregnancy salpingostomy compared with salpingectomy (IUP: 61% vs 38%; EP: 15% vs 10% [89] . Other studies have not shown that salpingostomy results in a higher chance for a future intra-uterine pregnancy or another ectopic pregnancy [92, 93]. An important contributor to future reproductive prognosis is the status of the contralateral fallopian tube. Even after salpingectomy, high intrauterine pregnancy rates have been reported when the remaining fallopian tube is patent and appears healthy. When the contralateral tube is damaged, there may be an advantage in terms of a future intra-uterine pregnancy when the salpingostomy is performed [94].

Salpingostomy should be limited to patients desiring to preserve fertility. When tubal conservation with salpingostomy is performed there is a 3–20% risk of persistent trophoblastic tissue, and therefore follow-up with serial β-hCG levels is mandatory [95]. When the β-hCG levels after surgery increase or plateau, there is indication to proceed with subsequent treatment with MTX [96]. When the ectopic pregnancy is diagnosed early and the adnexal mass is less than 2 cm in size or when the initial β-hCG levels are high, the risk for persistent trophoblast tissue is increased [97].

Those patients unwilling to accept the risk of residual ectopic tissue and perhaps a higher risk of recurrent ectopic pregnancy should choose salpingectomy. Such patients can be counseled that their reproductive potential remains high, as long as the remaining tube is healthy.

When surgery is being performed for isthmic or interstitial ectopic pregnancies, conservative surgery is rarely possible.

Medical management

Medical management of ectopic pregnancy, primarily with MTX (MTX), is a non-invasive alternative to surgery. MTX is a folic acid antagonist. Folic acid is converted into tetrahydrofolate by the enzyme dihydrofolate reductase. Tetrahydrofolate is an essential cofactor in the de novo synthesis of purines and pyrimidines, which are the "building blocks" of DNA and RNA. MTX inhibit the dihydrofolate reductase, resulting in nucleic acid synthesis inhibition [98].

Post MTX abdominal pain, presumably from tubal abortion or distention, occurs in 20–25% of patients, and can often be difficult to differentiate from tubal rupture. Hospitalization for observation is occasionally required, but surgical intervention is rarely required [99]. Folinic acid (Leucovorin) is a MTX antagonist and reduces the side effects and complications rates, particularly when high MTX doses are used [98].

The American College of Obstetrics and Gynecology lists the following criteria for the use of MTX [100]: **Absolute indications** include: (i) hemodynamic stability without active bleeding or signs of hemoperitoneum; (ii) non-laparoscopic diagnosis of ectopic pregnancy; (iii) patient desires future fertility; (iv) general anesthesia poses significant risk; (v) patient is able to return for follow-up care; (vi) informed consent. **Absolute contraindications** include: (i) breastfeeding; (ii) overt or laboratory evidence of immunodeficiency; (iii) alcoholism, alcoholic liver disease, other chronic liver disease; (iv) pre-existing blood dyscrasias and/or marrow hypoplasia; (v) leucopenia (leukocytes <2000 cells mm^{-3}; thrombocytopenia (platelets <100 000) or significant anemia; (vi) known sensitivity to MTX; (vii) active pulmonary disease; (viii) peptic ulcer disease; (ix) hepatic, renal, or hematologic dysfunction. **Relative contraindications** include: (i) adnexal mass ≥ 3.5 cm; (ii) presence of embryonic cardiac activity; (iii) initial β-hCG > 5000 mIU ml^{-1}.

Before therapy with MTX, it is important to obtain a complete blood count (CBC), liver enzymes (Alanine aminotransferase (ALT), aspartate transaminase (AST), renal function (creatinine, Biochemistry, Ultrasound, Nuchal Translucency (BUN)), blood type, coagulation panel.

In properly selected patients, MTX therapy is as effective as laparoscopic conservative surgery [101, 102]. MTX results in successful non-surgical treatment in 78–96% of patients. Tubal patency by follow-up hysterosalpingography is present in 78–84% of the cases. The rate of subsequent intra-uterine pregnancy is 65% and the risk for a recurrent ectopic pregnancy is 13% [102–104]. MTX can also be used to treat cervical, abdominal, or cornual ectopic gestations as surgical options in these cases are dangerous and could result in loss of reproductive potential. In these rare instances, MTX treatment may be chosen, after adequate counseling, even in the presence of relative contraindications to its use such as high β-hCG values or the presence of cardiac activity.

Two systemic MTX protocols have been described: single dose and multiple dose protocol.

In the single dose protocol, MTX is administered intramuscularly at a dose of 50 mg m^{-2} of body surface. Follow-up with serial β-hCG levels is initiated. β-hCG is measured at baseline (day 0), day 4 and day 7. Those patients with a β-hCG decline higher than 15% between day 4 and day 7 have good prognosis, and must be followed with serial β-hCG until the levels are negative. If the hCG decline is less than 15% between day 4 and 7, a repeat dose is given, with similar hCG follow-up. Approximately 15–20% of patients require a second dose. Subsequent MTX dose can be given in selected cases [105–107].

The single dose MTX protocol, with a repeat dose as dictated by protocol, is as effective as laparoscopic salpingostomy. Subsequent pregnancy rates and tubal patency are comparable. Avoidance of surgery and hospitalization render single dose MTX more cost-effective than surgery, as long as surgery is not required to diagnose the ectopic pregnancy.

The multi-dose protocol employs MTX at a dose of 1 mg kg^{-1}, followed by Leucovorin in a dose of 0.1 mg kg^{-1} 24 hours later. One injection is given daily. This regimen is continued until the β-hCG decreases by at least 15% on two consecutive days and up to four doses can be given. β-hCG is measured at baseline (day 0), day 1, day 3, day 5 and day 7, until the necessary decline in hCG is seen. After this initial decline, hCG is followed weekly until it is not detectable. If treatment is unsuccessful after four doses, additional MTX is unlikely to be effective. Approximately 50% of the patients do not need the complete eight days treatment protocol [104, 107].

As mentioned, when the β-hCG is in decline, in both protocols, the levels should be followed with weekly measurements until it is negative. For most patients, the levels become negative within three weeks. However, when the initial levels are very high, it may take up to eight weeks for the levels to become negative. When the levels plateau or start to rise again, it is an indication of persistent trophoblastic tissue [101, 104, 107].

Systematic literature reviews have concluded that the multi-dose protocol may be slightly more effective than the single dose protocol, but at the expense of a greater risk of medical complications. Single dose treatment was successful in treating 88.1% of ectopic gestations, and multiple dose treatment successful in 92.7%. However, if the initial β-hCG levels and the presence of embryonic cardiac activity are taken into consideration, both protocols appear to be similar in terms of result [107]. Due to study design differences, it is difficult to draw definite conclusions regarding direct comparisons between the single versus double dose MTX protocols.

Most clinicians prefer the single dose regimen, which is easier to administer and has fewer side effects [108]. Multiple dose therapy may be preferred by some, particularly when medical therapy is being considered in patients with relative contraindications such as high initial β-hCG levels or presence of cardiac activity, or for atypical ectopic pregnancies, such as cervical, interstitial or cesarean section scar ectopic gestations.

More recently, a new MTX protocol has been described, where two doses of MTX 50 mg m^{-2} are given on days 1 and 4, without the use of Leucovorin. The follow-up is the same as done for the single dose protocol. If the β-hCG level decline between the 4th and the 7th day is less than 15%, two extra doses of MTX are given [109, 110].

Independently of the MTX protocol utilized, patients should be instructed to have serial follow-up until the β-hCG levels are negative. It is important to observe that commonly the β-hCG levels will increase between day 1 and day 4 of therapy, and this is not a sign of treatment failure. Routine physical exam and transvaginal ultrasound are indicated when there is pain exacerbation. In approximately 40% of the patients there is pelvic pain when the MTX is used, usually between the 3rd and 7th day of therapy, most likely due to destruction and separation of the trophoblast and tubal abortion [111]. It is also important to avoid the use of non-steroidal anti-inflammatory drugs and aspirin as well as folic acid. If the pain is persistent or is worsening, treatment failure, or tubal rupture are possible, particularly when associated with hemodynamic instability and/or increase in β-hCG levels.

MTX is usually well tolerated. Rarely there are complications, but unfortunately serious side effects including alteration of liver function and bone marrow suppression as well as maternal death have been described [112, 113]. The most common side effects are abdominal distension, vaginal bleeding, pelvic pain, nausea and vomiting, stomatitis, gastritis, enteritis, dermatitis, pleuritis, alopecia, and neutropenia. Most side effects are mild and self-limited.

Several studies have evaluated the predictive factors for the success of MTX therapy. Gestational age, presence of vaginal bleeding and/or pelvic pain, initial β-hCG levels, progression of β-hCG levels, progesterone levels, the size of the adnexal mass, presence of embryonic cardiac activity, presence of free intra-peritoneal fluid, and vascularization of the adnexal mass have all been evaluated.

Of all of these parameters, it appears that the initial β-hCG levels has the highest predictive value. When this level is above 5000 mIU ml^{-1}, the risk for therapy failure is high [86]. When the adnexam mass is greater than 4 cm, there is free intra-peritoneal fluid; the β-hCG levels increase dramatically in the first 48 hours, or the ratio of β-hCG values between day 4 and day 7 are inappropriate; the risk of treatment failure is also higher [114–118].

There is controversy in the literature regarding the best therapy in terms of future reproductive status. The reproductive future can be evaluated indirectly by a hysterosalpingogram or directly if a future intrauterine pregnancy indeed occurs. It appears that conservative surgery and medical management offer the best chance for a successful future intrauterine pregnancy [119–121].

Local therapy

Ultrasound-guided intra-ectopic injection of MTX or other substances, including prostaglandins, potassium chloride, and hyperosmolar glucose have been described, usually with concurrent aspiration of the gestational sac, for the treatment of an ectopic pregnancy. The dose of MTX is 1 mg kg^{-2}. Although the systemic administration of MTX is easier, local injection has been described in an effort to minimize the risk of systemic side effects [122–124].

The technique appears to be as efficacious as systemic MTX and it is specially indicated when there is embryonic cardiac activity present and in cases of ectopic pregnancy in atypical locations. Although these ectopic pregnancies are rare, they have increased morbidity [125].

Other techniques employed to treat ectopic pregnancies in unusual locations include local injections of potassium chloride and uterine artery embolization [126].

Interstitial ectopic pregnancy

Approximately 5% of the ectopic pregnancies are in the interstitial location, and are associated with high morbidity. If there is embryonic cardiac activity present, local potassium chloride to interrupt cardiac activity and local MTX to interrupt trophoblast proliferation are indicated. When there is no cardiac activity present, systemic MTX may be used. Multiple doses may be necessary, but successful therapy with a single dose has been described. When the treatment fails or if there is evidence of rupture, cornual resection of the uterus may be necessary, either via laparotomy, laparoscopy, or robotic [127–131].

Cervical ectopic pregnancy

Approximately 0.5% of ectopic pregnancies are in this location. As the cervix is highly vascularized, these ectopic pregnancies may be accompanied by extensive hemorrhage and significant morbidity.

As early diagnosis is now possible, the need for radical therapy with hysterectomy has decreased. Conservative therapy options include local injection of MTX, potassium chloride, or prostaglandins; systemic therapy with MTX; cervical curettage; or hysteroscopic resection of the ectopic pregnancy with placement of an intra-cervical balloon for bleeding control; uterine artery embolization with selective catheterization of cervical branches of the uterine artery; or traquelectomy [132–135].

Ovarian ectopic pregnancy

The incidence of ovarian ectopic pregnancy ranges from 1 : 2000 to 1 : 60 000 deliveries, accounting for approximately 3% of all ectopic pregnancies [136, 137]. They are usually difficult to differentiate from a corpus luteum or a tubal pregnancy, and are associated with poor clinical outcomes secondary to rupture and intense hemoperitoneum due to the increased vascularity of the ovary. *In Vitro* fertilization and use of IUD have been shown to be risk factors for ovarian ectopic pregnancies [138]. Treatment options include local or systemic MTX, resection of the ectopic pregnancy or oophorectomy [139, 140].

Cesarean section Scar Ectopic Pregnancy

This form of ectopic pregnancies is very rare, however its incidence is increasing as there are more cesarean section being performed [141].

Heterotopic ectopic pregnancy

The incidence of this condition is 1: 30 000 spontaneous pregnancies. However, the incidence increases dramatically when ART are performed. As ART is more and more common, heterotopic pregnancies are now present in approximately 1% of the ectopic pregnancies. The diagnosis is deceiving, and in 50% of the cases, it is only diagnosed after tubal rupture. If the intra-uterine pregnancy is viable, the indicated treatment is the laparoscopy with salpingectomy as MTX cannot be utilized. Alternatively, ultrasound guided potassium chloride injection directly into the gestational sac when there is embryonic cardiac activity present. When the intrauterine pregnancy is not viable, MTX is an alternative [10].

Expectant management

With a better understanding of the natural history of ectopic pregnancies, it is now well know that a large percentage of these pregnancies may resolve spontaneously at a rate of approximately 40–60% of the cases [142, 143]. When the ectopic pregnancy resolves spontaneously, there is a high degree of post-resolution tubal patency [144].

Several criteria have been utilized to determine if an ectopic pregnancy could be followed expectantly. Expectant management should only be contemplated if the β-hCG levels are declining, there is no embryonic cardiac activity present, and the patient is hemodynamically stable. A recent β-hCG curve characterization in patients undergoing spontaneous miscarriages revealed that β-hCG declines of <21% in two days or < 60% in seven days implied the ongoing presence of trophoblast, regardless of location [145]. American College of Obstetricians and Gynecologists (ACOG) criteria allow for ongoing observation after a single dose of MTX when a 15% decline in β-hCG level has occurred from the value three days post-MTX to six days post-MTX [146]. In patients with known ectopic pregnancies being managed expectantly because of a downward trend in β-hCG levels, they have a higher chance of failure if the initial β-hCG values are excess of 1500–2000 mIU ml^{-1} [147].

Although there is no evidence for a size threshold beyond which expectant management is contraindicated, ACOG recommends that expectant management only be considered when the ectopic is early and small [146]. It is important to note that there are reports of ruptured ectopic pregnancies with very low β-hCG levels [148, 149].

When expectant management is adopted, close patient surveillance is mandatory.

Rh status and antibody screen

Rh immunoglobulin should be considered to non-sensitized Rh negative women who have an ectopic pregnancy or a spontaneous miscarriage. An embryo at six to seven weeks gestation already has red blood cells in sufficient volume to sensitize the mother, and fetal-maternal hemorrhage has been documented at the time of a first trimester threatened miscarriage. There is controversy in the literature regarding the cost-benefit of Rh immunoglobulin in these clinical scenarios [150].

References

1 Hasan, R. et al. (2010). Patterns and predictors of vaginal bleeding in the first trimester of pregnancy. *Ann. Epidemiol.* **20** (**7**): 524–531.

2 Wilcox, A.J. et al. (1988). Incidence of early loss of pregnancy. *N. Engl. J. Med.* **319** (**4**): 189–194.

3 Centers for Disease Control and Prevention (1995). Ectopic pregnancy – United States, 1990–1992. *MMWR Morb. Mortal. Wkly. Rep.* **44** (**3**): 46–48.

4 McRae, A., Murray, H., and Edmonds, M. (2009). Diagnostic accuracy and clinical utility of emergency department targeted ultrasonography in the evaluation of first-trimester pelvic pain and bleeding: a systematic review. *CJEM* **11** (**4**): 355–364.

5 Berg, C.J. et al. (2010). Pregnancy-related mortality in the United States, 1998 to 2005. *Obstet. Gynecol.* **116** (**6**): 1302–1309.

6 Stulberg, D.B. et al. (2013). Ectopic pregnancy rates in the Medicaid population. *Am. J. Obstet. Gynecol.* **208** (**4**): 274.e1–274.e7.

7 Kirk, E. et al. (2008). Why are some ectopic pregnancies characterized as pregnancies of unknown location at the initial transvaginal ultrasound examination? *Acta Obstet. Gynecol. Scand.* **87** (**11**): 1150–1154.

8 Condous, G. et al. (2005). The accuracy of transvaginal ultrasonography for the diagnosis of ectopic pregnancy prior to surgery. *Hum. Reprod.* **20** (**5**): 1404–1409.

9 Molloy, D. et al. (1990). Multiple-sited (heterotopic) pregnancy after in vitro fertilization and gamete intrafallopian transfer. *Fertil. Steril.* **53** (**6**): 1068–1071.

10 Fernandez, H. and Gervaise, A. (2004). Ectopic pregnancies after infertility treatment: modern diagnosis and therapeutic strategy. *Hum. Reprod. Update* **10** (**6**): 503–513.

11 Noor, N., Bano, I., and Parveen, S. (2012). Heterotopic pregnancy with successful pregnancy outcome. *J. Hum. Reprod. Sci.* **5** (**2**): 213–214.

12 Dor, J. et al. (1991). The incidence of combined intrauterine and extrauterine pregnancy after in vitro fertilization and embryo transfer. *Fertil. Steril.* **55** (**4**): 833–834.

13 Mukul, L.V. and Teal, S.B. (2007). Current management of ectopic pregnancy. *Obstet. Gynecol. Clin. North Am.* **34** (**3**): 403–419. x.

14 Eze, J.N., Obuna, J.A., and Ejikeme, B.N. (2012). Bilateral tubal ectopic pregnancies: a report of two cases. *Ann. Afr. Med.* **11** (**2**): 112–115.

15 Svirsky, R. et al. (2010). Twin tubal pregnancy: a rising complication? *Fertil. Steril.* **94** (**5**): 1910.e13–1910.e16.

16 Nama, V. and Manyonda, I. (2009). Tubal ectopic pregnancy: diagnosis and management. *Arch. Gynecol. Obstet.* **279** (**4**): 443–453.

17 Golden, A. (1950). Ovarian pregnancy. *Am. J. Surg.* **80** (**4**): 482–484.

18 Golditch, I.M. (2002). Lawson Tait: the forgotten gynecologist. *Obstet. Gynecol.* **99** (**1**): 152–156.

19 Lurie, S. (1992). The history of the diagnosis and treatment of ectopic pregnancy: a medical adventure. *Eur. J. Obstet. Gynecol. Reprod. Biol.* **43** (**1**): 1–7.

20 Thorburn, J.E., Janson, P.O., and Lindstedt, G. (1983). Early diagnosis of ectopic pregnancy. A review of 328 cases of a five-year period. *Acta Obstet. Gynecol. Scand.* **62** (**6**): 543–547.

21 Boufous, S. et al. (2001). Trends in the incidence of ectopic pregnancy in new South Wales between 1990-1998. *Aust. N. Z. J. Obstet. Gynaecol.* **41** (**4**): 436–438.

22 Bakken, I.J. and Skjeldestad, F.E. (2003). Reduced number of extrauterine pregnancies – increased fertility of women during the 1990s? *Tidsskr. Nor. Laegeforen.* **123** (**21**): 3011–3014.

23 Lewis, G. (2007). *The Confidential Enquiry into Maternal and Child Health (CEMACH). Saving Mothers' Lives: Reviewing maternal deaths to make motherhood safer: 2003–2005*. London: CEMACH.

24 Chang, J. et al. (2003). Pregnancy-related mortality surveillance – United States, 1991–1999. *MMWR Surveill. Summ.* **52** (**2**): 1–8.

25 Coste, J. et al. (2000). Recent declining trend in ectopic pregnancy in France: evidence of two clinicoepidemiologic entities. *Fertil. Steril.* **74** (**5**): 881–886.

26 Peterson, H.B. et al. (1997). The risk of ectopic pregnancy after tubal sterilization. U.S. collaborative review of sterilization working group. *N. Engl. J. Med.* **336** (**11**): 762–767.

27 Farquhar, C.M. (2005). Ectopic pregnancy. *Lancet* **366** (**9485**): 583–591.

28 Leke, R.J. et al. (2004). Ectopic pregnancy in Africa: a population-based study. *Obstet. Gynecol.* **103** (**4**): 692–697.

29 Varma, R. and Gupta, J. (2009). Tubal ectopic pregnancy. *BMJ Clin. Evid.* **2009**.

30 Karaer, A., Avsar, F.A., and Batioglu, S. (2006). Risk factors for ectopic pregnancy: a case-control study. *Aust. N. Z. J. Obstet. Gynaecol.* **46** (**6**): 521–527.

31 Waylen, A.L. et al. (2009). Effects of cigarette smoking upon clinical outcomes of assisted reproduction: a meta-analysis. *Hum. Reprod. Update* **15** (**1**): 31–44.

32 Hillis, S.D. et al. (1997). Recurrent chlamydial infections increase the risks of hospitalization for ectopic pregnancy and pelvic inflammatory disease. *Am. J. Obstet. Gynecol.* **176** (**1 Pt 1**): 103–107.

33 Ankum, W.M. et al. (1996). Risk factors for ectopic pregnancy: a meta-analysis. *Fertil. Steril.* **65** (**6**): 1093–1099.

34 Arias, R.D. (2002). Compelling reasons for recommending IUDs to any woman of reproductive age. *Int. J. Fertil. Womens Med.* **47** (**2**): 87–95.

35 Steen, R. and Shapiro, K. (2004). Intrauterine contraceptive devices and risk of pelvic inflammatory disease: standard of care in high STI prevalence settings. *Reprod. Health Matters* **12** (**23**): 136–143.

36 Furlong, L.A. (2002). Ectopic pregnancy risk when contraception fails. A review. *J. Reprod. Med.* **47** (**11**): 881–885.

37 Schippert, C. et al. (2012). The risk of ectopic pregnancy following tubal reconstructive microsurgery and assisted reproductive technology procedures. *Arch. Gynecol. Obstet.* **285** (**3**): 863–871.

38 Hoover, R.N. et al. (2011). Adverse health outcomes in women exposed in utero to diethylstilbestrol. *N. Engl. J. Med.* **365** (**14**): 1304–1314.

39 Goldberg, J.M. and Falcone, T. (1999). Effect of diethylstilbestrol on reproductive function. *Fertil. Steril.* **72** (**1**): 1–7.

40 Skjeldestad, F.E., Hadgu, A., and Eriksson, N. (1998). Epidemiology of repeat ectopic pregnancy: a population-based prospective cohort study. *Obstet. Gynecol.* **91** (**1**): 129–135.

41 Westrom, L. et al. (1992). Pelvic inflammatory disease and fertility. A cohort study of 1, 844 women with laparoscopically verified disease and 657 control women with normal laparoscopic results. *Sex. Transm. Dis.* **19** (**4**): 185–192.

42 Bouyer, J. et al. (2003). Risk factors for ectopic pregnancy: a comprehensive analysis based on a large case-control, population-based study in France. *Am. J. Epidemiol.* **157** (**3**): 185–194.

43 Clayton, H.B. et al. (2006). Ectopic pregnancy risk with assisted reproductive technology procedures. *Obstet. Gynecol.* **107** (**3**): 595–604.

44 Cohen, J. et al. (1986). In-vitro fertilization and embryo transfer: a collaborative study of 1163 pregnancies on the incidence and risk factors of ectopic pregnancies. *Hum. Reprod.* **1** (**4**): 255–258.

45 Gemzell, C., Guillome, J., and Wang, C.F. (1982). Ectopic pregnancy following treatment with human gonadotropins. *Am. J. Obstet. Gynecol.* **143** (**7**): 761–765.

46 McBain, J.C. et al. (1980). An unexpectedly high rate of ectopic pregnancy following the induction of ovulation with human pituitary and chorionic gonadotrophin. *Br. J. Obstet. Gynaecol.* **87** (**1**): 5–9.

47 Bouyer, J. et al. (2002). Sites of ectopic pregnancy: a 10 year population-based study of 1800 cases. *Hum. Reprod.* **17** (**12**): 3224–3230.

48 Coste, J. et al. (2000). Role of chromosome abnormalities in ectopic pregnancy. *Fertil. Steril.* **74** (**6**): 1259–1260.

49 Goddijn, M. et al. (1996). Cytogenetic characteristics of ectopic pregnancy. *Hum. Reprod.* **11** (**12**): 2769–2771.

50 Kutluay, L. et al. (1994). Tubal histopathology in ectopic pregnancies. *Eur. J. Obstet. Gynecol. Reprod. Biol.* **57** (**2**): 91–94.

51 Chang, H.J. and Suh, C.S. (2010). Ectopic pregnancy after assisted reproductive technology: what are the risk factors? *Curr. Opin. Obstet. Gynecol.* **22** (**3**): 202–207.

52 Bouyer, J. et al. (1996). Ectopic pregnancy: factors related to ovum anomalies? *Rev. Epidemiol. Sante Publique* **44** (**2**): 101–110.

53 Arias-Stella, J. (2002). The Arias–Stella reaction: facts and fancies four decades after. *Adv. Anat. Pathol.* **9** (**1**): 12–23.

54 Weckstein, L.N. et al. (1985). Accurate diagnosis of early ectopic pregnancy. *Obstet. Gynecol.* **65** (**3**): 393–397.

55 Bottomley, C. et al. (2009). The optimal timing of an ultrasound scan to assess the location and viability of an early pregnancy. *Hum. Reprod.* **24** (**8**): 1811–1817.

56 Buckley, R.G. et al. (1999). History and physical examination to estimate the risk of ectopic pregnancy: validation of a clinical prediction model. *Ann. Emerg. Med.* **34** (**5**): 589–594.

57 Birkhahn, R.H. et al. (2003). The ability of traditional vital signs and shock index to identify ruptured ectopic pregnancy. *Am. J. Obstet. Gynecol.* **189** (**5**): 1293–1296.

58 Mol, B.W., van Der Veen, F., and Bossuyt, P.M. (1999). Implementation of probabilistic decision rules improves the predictive values of algorithms in the diagnostic management of ectopic pregnancy. *Hum. Reprod.* **14** (**11**): 2855–2862.

59 Wieringa-de Waard, M. et al. (2002). Threatened miscarriage in general practice: diagnostic value of history taking and physical examination. *Br. J. Gen. Pract.* **52** (**483**): 825–829.

60 Della-Giustina, D. and Denny, M. (2003). Ectopic pregnancy. *Emerg. Med. Clin. North Am.* **21** (**3**): 565–584.

61 Polena, V. et al. (2015). Non-invasive tools for the diagnosis of potentially life-threatening gynaecological emergencies: a systematic review. *PLoS One* **10** (**2**): e0114189.

62 Timor-Tritsch, I.E. et al. (1989). The use of transvaginal ultrasonography in the diagnosis of ectopic pregnancy. *Am. J. Obstet. Gynecol.* **161** (**1**): 157–161.

63 Kadar, N. and Romero, R. (1987). hCG determinations in early pregnancy. *Fertil. Steril.* **47** (**4**): 722–724.

64 Kadar, N. and Romero, R. (1987). Observations on the log human chorionic gonadotropin-time relationship in early pregnancy and its practical implications. *Am. J. Obstet. Gynecol.* **157** (**1**): 73–78.

65 Romero, R. et al. (1986). The value of serial human chorionic gonadotropin testing as a diagnostic tool in ectopic pregnancy. *Am. J. Obstet. Gynecol.* **155** (**2**): 392–394.

66 Tenore, J.L. (2000). Ectopic pregnancy. *Am. Fam. Physician* **61** (**4**): 1080–1088.

67 Butt, K. and Lim, K. (2014). Determination of gestational age by ultrasound. *J. Obstet. Gynaecol. Can.* **36** (**2**): 171–183.

68 Barnhart, K.T. et al. (2004). Symptomatic patients with an early viable intrauterine pregnancy: HCG curves redefined. *Obstet. Gynecol.* **104** (**1**): 50–55.

69 Barnhart, K.T. et al. (2002). Presumed diagnosis of ectopic pregnancy. *Obstet. Gynecol.* **100** (**3**): 505–510.

70 Chung, K. et al. (2006). Defining the rise of serum HCG in viable pregnancies achieved through use of IVF. *Hum. Reprod.* **21** (**3**): 823–828.

71 Ahmed, A.A., Tom, B.D., and Calabrese, P. (2004). Ectopic pregnancy diagnosis and the pseudo-sac. *Fertil. Steril.* **81** (**5**): 1225–1228.

72 Barnhart, K. et al. (2011). Pregnancy of unknown location: a consensus statement of nomenclature, definitions, and outcome. *Fertil. Steril.* **95** (**3**): 857–866.

73 Perriera, L. and Reeves, M.F. (2008). Ultrasound criteria for diagnosis of early pregnancy failure and ectopic pregnancy. *Semin. Reprod. Med.* **26** (**5**): 373–382.

74 Blaas, H.G. (2014). Detection of structural abnormalities in the first trimester using ultrasound. *Best Pract. Res. Clin. Obstet. Gynaecol.* **28** (**3**): 341–353.

75 Condous, G. et al. (2006). Pregnancies of unknown location: consensus statement. *Ultrasound Obstet. Gynecol.* **28** (**2**): 121–122.

76 Hahlin, M., Thorburn, J., and Bryman, I. (1995). The expectant management of early pregnancies of uncertain site. *Hum. Reprod.* **10** (**5**): 1223–1227.

77 Cacciatore, B., Stenman, U.H., and Ylostalo, P. (1989). Comparison of abdominal and vaginal sonography in suspected ectopic pregnancy. *Obstet. Gynecol.* **73** (**5 Pt 1**): 770–774.

78 Banerjee, S. et al. (1999). The expectant management of women with early pregnancy of unknown location. *Ultrasound Obstet. Gynecol.* **14** (**4**): 231–236.

79 Schuneman, M., Von Wald, T., and Hansen, K. (2015). Pregnancy of unknown location. *S. D. Med.* **68** (**4**): 163–167.

80 Silva, C. et al. (2006). Human chorionic gonadotropin profile for women with ectopic pregnancy. *Obstet. Gynecol.* **107** (**3**): 605–610.

81 Lu, Q. et al. (2015). The value of ratio of hCG, progesterone in local blood of pregnancy location versus venous blood in the diagnosis of ectopic pregnancy. *Int. J. Clin. Exp. Med.* **8** (**6**): 9477–9483.

82 Lindahl, B. and Ahlgren, M. (1986). Identification of chorion villi in abortion specimens. *Obstet. Gynecol.* **67** (**1**): 79–81.

83 Barnhart, K.T. et al. (2003). Usefulness of pipelle endometrial biopsy in the diagnosis of women at risk for ectopic pregnancy. *Am. J. Obstet. Gynecol.* **188** (**4**): 906–909.

84 Chung, K. et al. (2011). Reevaluating the role of dilation and curettage in the diagnosis of pregnancy of unknown location. *Fertil. Steril.* **96** (**3**): 659–662.

85 Ankum, W.M. et al. (1993). Laparoscopy: a dispensable tool in the diagnosis of ectopic pregnancy? *Hum. Reprod.* **8** (**8**): 1301–1306.

86 Hajenius, P.J. et al. (2007). Interventions for tubal ectopic pregnancy. *Cochrane Database Syst. Rev.* (**1**): CD000324. doi: 10.1002/14651858.CD000324.pub2.

87 Lundorff, P. et al. (1991). Laparoscopic surgery in ectopic pregnancy. A randomized trial versus laparotomy. *Acta Obstet. Gynecol. Scand.* **70** (**4–5**): 343–348.

88 Wang, Y.L. et al. (2014). Laparoscopic management of ectopic pregnancies in unusual locations. *Taiwan J. Obstet. Gynecol.* **53** (**4**): 466–470.

89 Seifer, D.B. et al. (1993). Comparison of persistent ectopic pregnancy after laparoscopic salpingostomy versus salpingostomy at laparotomy for ectopic pregnancy. *Obstet. Gynecol.* **81** (**3**): 378–382.

90 Natale, A. et al. (2003). Human chorionic gonadotropin level as a predictor of trophoblastic infiltration into the tubal wall in ectopic pregnancy: a blinded study. *Fertil. Steril.* **79** (**4**): 981–986.

91 Cabar, F.R. et al. (2006). Predictive factors of trophoblastic invasion into the ampullary region of the tubal wall in ectopic pregnancy. *Hum. Reprod.* **21** (**9**): 2426–2431.

92 Clausen, I. (1996). Conservative versus radical surgery for tubal pregnancy. A review. *Acta Obstet. Gynecol. Scand.* **75** (**1**): 8–12.

93 Mol, B.W. et al. (1996). Conservative versus radical surgery for tubal pregnancy. *Acta Obstet. Gynecol. Scand.* **75** (**9**): 866–867.

94 Mol, B.W. et al. (1998). Fertility after conservative and radical surgery for tubal pregnancy. *Hum. Reprod.* **13** (**7**): 1804–1809.

95 Lund, C.O. et al. (2002). Persistent ectopic pregnancy after linear salpingotomy: a non-predictable complication to conservative surgery for tubal gestation. *Acta Obstet. Gynecol. Scand.* **81** (**11**): 1053–1059.

96 Graczykowski, J.W. and Mishell, D.R. Jr. (1997). Methotrexate prophylaxis for persistent ectopic pregnancy after conservative treatment by salpingostomy. *Obstet. Gynecol.* **89** (**1**): 118–122.

97 Gracia, C.R., Brown, H.A., and Barnhart, K.T. (2001). Prophylactic methotrexate after linear salpingostomy: a decision analysis. *Fertil. Steril.* **76** (**6**): 1191–1195.

98 Barnhart, K., Coutifaris, C., and Esposito, M. (2001). The pharmacology of methotrexate. *Expert Opin. Pharmacother.* **2** (**3**): 409–417.

99 Lipscomb, G.H. (2012). Medical management of ectopic pregnancy. *Clin. Obstet. Gynecol.* **55** (**2**): 424–432.

100 American College of Obstetricians and Gynecologists (2014). Practice bulletin no. 143: medical management of first-trimester abortion. *Obstet. Gynecol.* **123** (**3**): 676–692.

101 Pisarska, M.D., Carson, S.A., and Buster, J.E. (1998). Ectopic pregnancy. *Lancet* **351** (**9109**): 1115–1120.

102 Lipscomb, G.H., Stovall, T.G., and Ling, F.W. (2000). Nonsurgical treatment of ectopic pregnancy. *N. Engl. J. Med.* **343** (**18**): 1325–1329.

103 Silva, P.M. et al. (2015). Effectiveness of expectant management versus methotrexate in tubal ectopic pregnancy: a double-blind randomized trial. *Arch. Gynecol. Obstet.* **291** (**4**): 939–943.

104 Stovall, T.G., Ling, F.W., and Buster, J.E. (1989). Outpatient chemotherapy of unruptured ectopic pregnancy. *Fertil. Steril.* **51** (**3**): 435–438.

105 Stovall, T.G., Ling, F.W., and Gray, L.A. (1991). Single-dose methotrexate for treatment of ectopic pregnancy. *Obstet. Gynecol.* **77** (**5**): 754–757.

106 Lipscomb, G.H. et al. (1998). Analysis of three hundred fifteen ectopic pregnancies treated with single-dose methotrexate. *Am. J. Obstet. Gynecol.* **178** (**6**): 1354–1358.

107 Barnhart, K.T. et al. (2003). The medical management of ectopic pregnancy: a meta-analysis comparing "single dose" and "multidose" regimens. *Obstet. Gynecol.* **101** (**4**): 778–784.

108 Tabatabaii Bafghi, A. et al. (2012). Fertility outcome after treatment of unruptured ectopic pregnancy with two different methotrexate protocols. *Int. J. Fertil. Steril.* **6** (**3**): 189–194.

109 McLaren, J.F. et al. (2014). Success of the two-dose methotrexate protocol for treatment of ectopic pregnancy in women with a history of prior ectopic pregnancy. *J. Reprod. Med.* **59** (**7–8**): 379–384.

110 Hamed, H.O., Ahmed, S.R., and Alghasham, A.A. (2012). Comparison of double- and single-dose methotrexate protocols for treatment of ectopic pregnancy. *Int. J. Gynaecol. Obstet.* **116** (**1**): 67–71.

111 Lipscomb, G.H. et al. (1999). Management of separation pain after single-dose methotrexate therapy for ectopic pregnancy. *Obstet. Gynecol.* **93** (**4**): 590–593.

112 Isaacs, J.D. Jr., McGehee, R.P., and Cowan, B.D. (1996). Life-threatening neutropenia following methotrexate treatment of ectopic pregnancy: a report of two cases. *Obstet. Gynecol.* **88** (**4 Pt 2**): 694–696.

113 Schoenfeld, A. et al. (1992). Methotrexate pneumonitis in nonsurgical treatment of ectopic pregnancy. *Obstet. Gynecol.* **80** (**3 Pt 2**): 520–521.

114 Dudley, P.S. et al. (2004). Characterizing ectopic pregnancies that rupture despite treatment with methotrexate. *Fertil. Steril.* **82** (**5**): 1374–1378.

115 Tawfiq, A., Agameya, A.F., and Claman, P. (2000). Predictors of treatment failure for ectopic pregnancy treated with single-dose methotrexate. *Fertil. Steril.* **74** (**5**): 877–880.

116 Potter, M.B., Lepine, L.A., and Jamieson, D.J. (2003). Predictors of success with methotrexate treatment of tubal ectopic pregnancy at Grady memorial hospital. *Am. J. Obstet. Gynecol.* **188** (**5**): 1192–1194.

117 Lipscomb, G.H. et al. (1999). Predictors of success of methotrexate treatment in women with tubal ectopic pregnancies. *N. Engl. J. Med.* **341** (**26**): 1974–1978.

118 Nguyen, Q. et al. (2010). Are early human chorionic gonadotropin levels after methotrexate therapy a predictor of response in ectopic pregnancy? *Am. J. Obstet. Gynecol.* **202** (**6**): 630 e1–630 e5.

119 Seror, V. et al. (2007). Care pathways for ectopic pregnancy: a population-based cost-effectiveness analysis. *Fertil. Steril.* **87** (**4**): 737–748.

120 Juneau, C. and Bates, G.W. (2012). Reproductive outcomes after medical and surgical management of ectopic pregnancy. *Clin. Obstet. Gynecol.* **55** (**2**): 455–460.

121 de Bennetot, M. et al. (2012). Fertility after tubal ectopic pregnancy: results of a population-based study. *Fertil. Steril.* **98** (**5**): 1271–1276.

122 Jeng, C.J., Ko, M.L., and Shen, J. (2007). Transvaginal ultrasound-guided treatment of cervical pregnancy. *Obstet. Gynecol.* **109** (**5**): 1076–1082.

123 Dadhwal, V. et al. (2009). Successful management of live ectopic pregnancy with high beta-hCG titres by ultrasound-guided potassium chloride injection and systemic methotrexate. *Arch. Gynecol. Obstet.* **280** (**5**): 799–801.

124 Hung, T.H. et al. (1996). Treatment of cervical pregnancy with methotrexate. *Int. J. Gynaecol. Obstet.* **53** (**3**): 243–247.

125 Jourdain, O. et al. (2003). Management of other ectopic pregnancies (cornual, interstitial, angular, ovarian). *J. Gynecol. Obstet. Biol. Reprod. (Paris)* **32** (**7 Suppl**): S93–S100.

126 Krissi, H. et al. (2014). Outcome, complications and future fertility in women treated with uterine artery embolization and methotrexate for non-tubal ectopic pregnancy. *Eur. J. Obstet. Gynecol. Reprod. Biol.* **182**: 172–176.

127 Barnhart, K., Spandorfer, S., and Coutifaris, C. (1997). Medical treatment of interstitial pregnancy. A report of three unsuccessful cases. *J. Reprod. Med.* **42** (**8**): 521–524.

128 Tulandi, T. and Al-Jaroudi, D. (2004). Interstitial pregnancy: results generated from the Society of Reproductive Surgeons Registry. *Obstet. Gynecol.* **103** (**1**): 47–50.

129 Corioni, S. et al. (2015). Interstitial pregnancy treated with a single-dose of systemic methotrexate: a successful management. *J. Res. Med. Sci.* **20** (**3**): 312–316.

130 Ansari, A. et al. (2015). Robotic-assisted laparoscopic resection of cornual ectopic pregnancy. A case report. *J. Reprod. Med.* **60** (**1–2**): 58–64.

131 Watanabe, T. et al. (2014). Laparoscopic cornuotomy for interstitial pregnancy and postoperative course. *J. Obstet. Gynaecol. Res.* **40** (**8**): 1983–1988.

132 Ushakov, F.B. et al. (1997). Cervical pregnancy: past and future. *Obstet. Gynecol. Surv.* **52** (**1**): 45–59.

133 Asante, A. et al. (2015). Single-dose intramuscular methotrexate treatment of cervical ectopic pregnancy. A case report. *J. Reprod. Med.* **60** (**1–2**): 78–82.

134 Hosni, M.M., Herath, R.P., and Mumtaz, R. (2014). Diagnostic and therapeutic dilemmas of cervical ectopic pregnancy. *Obstet. Gynecol. Surv.* **69** (**5**): 261–276.

135 Mangino, F.P. et al. (2014). Successful rescue hysteroscopic resection of a cervical ectopic pregnancy previously treated with methotrexate with no combined safety precautions. *Clin. Exp. Obstet. Gynecol.* **41** (**2**): 214–216.

136 Grimes, H.G., Nosal, R.A., and Gallagher, J.C. (1983). Ovarian pregnancy: a series of 24 cases. *Obstet. Gynecol.* **61** (**2**): 174–180.

137 Seinera, P. et al. (1997). Ovarian pregnancy and operative laparoscopy: report of eight cases. *Hum. Reprod.* **12** (**3**): 608–610.

138 Zhu, Q. et al. (2014). Risk factors and clinical features of ovarian pregnancy: a case-control study. *BMJ Open* **4** (**12**): e006447.

139 Pagidas, K. and Frishman, G.N. (2013). Nonsurgical management of primary ovarian pregnancy with transvaginal ultrasound-guided local administration of methotrexate. *J. Minim. Invasive Gynecol.* **20** (**2**): 252–254.

140 Scutiero, G. et al. (2012). Primary ovarian pregnancy and its management. *JSLS* **16** (**3**): 492–494.

141 Ash, A., Smith, A., and Maxwell, D. (2007). Caesarean scar pregnancy. *BJOG* **114** (**3**): 253–263.

142 Lund, J. (1955). Early ectopic pregnancy; comments on conservative treatment. *J. Obstet. Gynaecol. Br. Emp.* **62** (**1**): 70–76.

143 Shalev, E. et al. (1995). Spontaneous resolution of ectopic tubal pregnancy: natural history. *Fertil. Steril.* **63** (**1**): 15–19.

144 Rantala, M. and Makinen, J. (1997). Tubal patency and fertility outcome after expectant management of ectopic pregnancy. *Fertil. Steril.* **68** (**6**): 1043–1046.

145 Seeber, B.E. et al. (2006). Application of redefined human chorionic gonadotropin curves for the diagnosis of women at risk for ectopic pregnancy. *Fertil. Steril.* **86** (**2**): 454–459.

146 American College of Obstetricians and Gynecologists (2001). ACOG practice bulletin. Clinical management guidelines for obstetrician-gynecologists. Medical management of abortion. *Obstet. Gynecol.* **97** (**4**): 1–13.

147 Elson, J. et al. (2004). Expectant management of tubal ectopic pregnancy: prediction of successful outcome using decision tree analysis. *Ultrasound Obstet. Gynecol.* **23** (**6**): 552–556.

148 Resta, S. et al. (2012). Rupture of ovarian pregnancy in a woman with low beta-hCG levels. *Case Rep. Obstet. Gynecol.* 213169.

149 Fu, J. et al. (2007). Rupture of ectopic pregnancy with minimally detectable beta-human chorionic gonadotropin levels: a report of 2 cases. *J. Reprod. Med.* **52** (**6**): 541–542.

150 ACOG practice bulletin. Prevention of Rh D alloimmunization. Number 4 May 1999 (replaces educational bulletin Number 147, October 1990). American College of Obstetrics and Gynecology (1999). Clinical management guidelines for obstetrician-gynecologists. *Int. J. Gynaecol. Obstet.* **66** (**1**): 63–70.

5

CHAPTER 5
Pelvic pain

Jane Moore
Nuffield Department of Obstetrics and Gynecology, University of Oxford, Oxford, UK

> **CASE SCENARIO**
>
> A 27-year-old woman, para 2, attends the gynecology clinic complaining of pelvic pain. She has been suffering daily pain since the birth of her second child two years ago. She was previously fit and well apart from period pain since her teens which she controlled with either ibuprofen or paracetamol or sometimes both. Her first pregnancy and delivery were straightforward five years ago, but during her second pregnancy she developed pelvic girdle pain (PGP) and needed crutches in the last six weeks. She went into labor at 36 weeks and although the delivery was normal in the end, she delivered with her legs in stirrups. She does not really know why but it left her feeling out of control and frightened. Her partner was not there because he is in the military and couldn't get home in time. She has managed over the last two years but is now afraid that she won't be able to cope with the pain when her partner goes overseas again. She wants an operation to sort it out.

Background

Chronic pelvic pain (CPP) can be defined as intermittent or constant pain in the lower abdomen or pelvis present for at least six months, not associated exclusively with menstruation or intercourse. It is common affecting about one in six of the adult female population [1]. Not all of these women will seek health care or indeed be limited by pain in their working or personal lives, but the reality of living with chronic pain can be grueling. In the absence of adequate diagnosis and treatment women can become frustrated and may alter their patterns of behavior to cope with the situation, perhaps choosing a less demanding job or becoming isolated from friends.

Women with CPP present as frequently to primary care physicians as people with asthma and back pain [2], and yet there is a striking lack of evidence regarding the best way to manage this complex symptom. In part, the difficulty lies in the fact that CPP is a symptom and not a diagnosis in itself. Women with CPP may have a range of factors contributing to their pain and although some approaches and therapeutic interventions may be helpful for many women with pelvic pain, it is important to try to identify the various contributory factors and tailor treatments for each component.

The management of pelvic pain has been greatly advanced by the developing appreciation of the role of the central nervous system (CNS) in the genesis of pain. As will be explored later in the chapter, it is clear that although pathology such as endometriosis can create inflammatory changes in the pelvis which stimulate peripheral pain fibers, the response of the CNS is crucial to the development of symptoms. Pre-existing influences on the CNS such as previous pain experience or depression may alter the pattern of symptoms which develop.

Consensus on an approach to the management of CPP

Evidence-based approaches to the initial management of CPP have been developed by a number of professional organizations including RCOG, EAU, and ACOG. A brief summation of this general approach is given here.

Given that there are likely to be a number of factors contributing to the pain experience, it is important to take a broad approach to diagnosis from the start. The *history* should include discussion of the nature of the pain as well as the factors which provoke or relieve the pain including movement or posture. Enquiry should be made regarding menstrual symptoms, dyspareunia, urinary and bowel symptoms including dyschezia (rectal pain on opening bowels) and rectal bleeding. A diagnosis of irritable bowel syndrome (IBS), can be made on the basis of the history alone using the Rome Criteria (see Box 5.1). Time spent discussing the patient's own ideas about the cause of the pain, her concerns perhaps regarding fertility or past experiences,

Evidence-Based Obstetrics and Gynecology, First Edition. Edited by Errol R. Norwitz, Carolyn M. Zelop, David A. Miller, and David L. Keefe.

and her expectations of investigation or treatment is always rewarded either with useful diagnostic information or with a more effective working partnership.

The *examination* can also be revealing. Evidence of pelvic abnormality can help to make a diagnosis such as endometriosis. Palpation of the lower spine, sacro-iliac joints, and symphysis pubis may reveal a musculoskeletal component and pain which is highly localized and exacerbated by contraction of the underlying muscle, may indicate a "trigger point" in the abdominal wall or pelvic floor. Importantly the examination may offer a psychodynamic opportunity, through the patient's response to examination, to explore her feelings about the pain and perhaps other aspects of her life or history.

General search strategy

The evidence base for the diagnosis and management of CPP is poor. This arises partly from the variety of conditions which can present with pelvic pain and partly from the limited understanding of the genesis of pain. This makes it difficult to identify relevant literature and challenging to perform adequate trials. However, to try to answer the clinical questions posed, reference is made to consensus guidelines as well as Medline (using the Medical Subject Headings (MeSH) term pelvic pain) and the Cochrane library.

Clinical questions

1. What is the role of the CNS in the experience of CPP?
2. In women with CPP how does the initial consultation influence outcome?
3. What is the prevalence of musculo-skeletal abnormalities in women of reproductive age with CPP?
4. What is the sensitivity and specificity of laparoscopy in identifying the cause of CPP in women?
5. Which methods of pain relief are safe and effective in reducing CPP?

Discussion of the evidence

1. What is the role of the CNS in the experience of CPP?

Search Strategy: Pelvic pain (MeSH) AND CNS.

Since early pain studies of the hypothalamic pituitary axis in the late 1990s [3], interest has grown in the notion that the key to understanding CPP lies in the CNS rather than the pelvis. More recently studies have focused on the structure and function of the brain itself comparing pain patients to controls.

Two studies have examined changes in gray matter volume in women with CPP. As-Sanie et al. used voxel-based morphometry to demonstrate that a similar reduction in gray matter volume in brain regions associated with pain processing was seen in women with CPP, whether or not endometriosis had been demonstrated in the pelvis. Pain-free women with and without endometriosis did not show any such reduction [4]. Tu et al. used a similar methodology to compare 32 women with primary dysmenorrhea and 32 pain-free controls. Again, alterations in gray matter volume were observed in areas of the brain known to be involved in pain processing and these persisted throughout the menstrual cycle i.e. beyond the duration of pain [5]. The same group identified altered cerebral metabolism in pain associated regions in women with menstrual pain compared to pain-free menstruating women [6].

Vincent et al. used functional magnetic resonance imaging (MRI) (which detects alterations in blood flow identifying activation and deactivation of specific regions within the brain) to examine responses to experimental pain in women with dysmenorrhea but no ongoing pelvic pain compared to controls. Again changes in response to experimental pain were observed in pain subjects throughout the menstrual cycle, not just during the painful period. Mean serum cortisol levels were lower in women with dysmenorrhea compared to controls and levels correlated with duration of symptoms. Physical but not mental quality of life was also lower for women with dysmenorrhea [7].

Stratton and Berkley reviewed the existing literature to explore what is known of the link between endometriosis (as a potential association with pelvic pain) and the CNS. It is clear that endometriotic lesions can establish their own nerve supply and that this could provide a two-way interaction between the disease and the CNS. It seems clear therefore that in addition to treating pathologies known to be associated with CPP, a focus on the CNS may also open potential conceptual and therapeutic options in the understanding and management of CPP [8].

Two helpful reviews summarize the clinical situation well. Baranowksi describes the potential genesis of pelvic pain starting from a relatively benign initial trigger which in a predisposed individual may progress to involve multiple layers of dysfunction including alteration in the perception of physiological sensation, associated musculo-skeletal tension particularly in the pelvic floor, autonomic dysfunction, and difficulty in functioning both physically and socially. This has been termed a complex regional pain syndrome [9]. Aslam et al. explores the concept of visceral hyperalgesia a condition which describes the hypersensitivity of other organs in the same region which can develop in response to pain arising from the pelvis, and can lead to dysfunction in those organs [10].

In clinical discussions with patients suffering from CPP, the notion that the CNS may be involved in the genesis of pelvic pain seems to resonate with sufferers. Women are often aware of the way in which their symptoms are affected by psychological factors or their menstrual cycle and are glad of a template for this discussion which avoids the dichotomy between an organic and a psychological cause for their pain, but rather promotes a conversation about influences and factors which could be amended.

The recognition of the impact that primary dysmenorrhea has on women's lives as well as these primary research data which demonstrate its effect on the CNS, has led to the inclusion of dysmenorrhea as a CPP syndrome in the most recent IASP taxonomy [11].

2. In women with CPP how does the initial consultation influence outcome?

Search Strategy: Pelvic pain (MeSH) AND consultation AND outcome.

In addition to the information included in the existing evidence-based guidelines, this search identified two additional papers of interest. In a study by Verheul et al., 30 healthy women with menstrual pain participated in a study in which they were asked to imagine having severe symptoms and take part in a scripted consultation with a general practitioner. Subjects completed questionnaires to measure their anxiety and expectations of success following the General Practitioner (GP) consultation. They were randomized to receive a scripted communication style from their GP which was either warm and empathic or cold and formal. In addition the GP adopted an outlook with either a positive expectation of the future or an uncertain outlook. In this highly controlled study which involved simulated patients and female GPs only, results suggested that only a warm empathic style associated with a positive outlook was likely to reduce anxiety and help the patient anticipate benefit from treatment [12].

In a second paper which provides a helpful synthesis of existing qualitative studies and an exploration of the potential and limitations of combining qualitative data, Souza et al. describe the emerging themes in studies of the doctor–patient interaction concerning CPP. Using clear methodology they include seven studies in a metasynthesis and draw out key themes. First they examine the considerable impact of CPP on women's lives and the extent to which it disrupts their ability to fulfill their roles, with consequent effects on employment and on their families as well as their own sense of fulfillment. They explore the concept of secondary gain demonstrating how the focus of care should be on quality of life as a whole rather than on the pain itself. Second, they highlight the importance placed by patients on finding an explanation for the pain and the strain placed on the doctor–patient relationship if a pathological cause cannot be identified. It is clear that the doctor has an important role in validating pain and needs to understand how the pain is impacting on the patient's life and what her expectations are with regard to investigation and treatment. They discuss the limitations of the biomechanical model of disease to understand a symptom of this kind and provide very helpful food for thought for clinicians seeking to treat women with CPP [13].

3. What is the prevalence of musculo-skeletal abnormalities in women of reproductive age with CPP?

Search Strategy: Pelvic pain: etiology (MeSH) AND musculoskeletal pain (MeSH).

Somatic (body wall) pain is poorly taught and understood among medical practitioners. Routine assessment of women with pelvic pain would not traditionally include assessment of the musculo-skeletal system. Assessment even by those with an interest in the field is hampered by a lack of standardized tests. However, prevalence studies suggest that musculo-skeletal dysfunction either as a primary cause of pain or secondary to chronic pain is common among patients with CPP. In a retrospective study of 987 women attending a CPP clinic, 22% of women were recorded as having pelvic floor tenderness [14]. In a prospective study of 19 women with CPP by the same author, subjects were significantly more likely than healthy controls to have abnormal musculo-skeletal findings such as asymmetric iliac crests (61% vs 25%) [15]. In a blinded study of 48 women, abnormal musculo-skeletal findings and pelvic floor tenderness were found significantly more commonly in the 19 women with CPP than in the 29 pain-free women [16, 17].

Although the evidence base in this field is poor, clinicians should consider the involvement of a physiotherapist in their initial assessment particularly where the pain is movement or posture related or examination reveals focal tenderness.

4. What is the sensitivity and specificity of laparoscopy in identifying the cause of CPP in women?

Search Strategy: pelvic pain (MeSH) AND diagnostic laparoscopy AND specificity and sensitivity.

No trials have been performed which adequately answer this question, because of the challenge of identifying an objective measure against which to judge the sensitivity and specificity of diagnostic laparoscopy which has traditionally been seen as the gold standard in the diagnosis of CPP. Although endometriosis can be identified at laparoscopy, it can also be asymptomatic and it is therefore not always clear whether the endometriosis is indeed the cause of the CPP. Some variants of endometriosis such as deep infiltrating disease and adenomyosis, may not be visible at laparoscopy and therefore the correct diagnosis may be missed.

Given the uncertain value of diagnostic laparoscopy several recently published guidelines advocate the use of a therapeutic trial of hormonal treatment to test the possible diagnosis of endometriosis rather than the first line use of diagnostic laparoscopy. MRI and transvaginal ultrasonography also have a useful role in the diagnosis of adenomyosis, endometriomas, and nodular (particularly bowel related) endometriosis http://www.eshre.eu/Guidelines-and-Legal/Guidelines/Endometriosis-guideline.aspx.

Adhesions can also be identified reliably at laparoscopy but again, it is not always clear that adhesions cause pain. Certainly it is far from clear that dividing adhesions reduces pain [18]. Other conditions such as hernia may be visible at laparoscopy but their relevance is yet to be established.

It is important to remember that diagnostic laparoscopy is not without risk, with an incidence of injury to bladder, bowel, or blood vessel of approximately 2.4 per 1000 of which two-thirds will need laparotomy [19]. Before undergoing diagnostic laparoscopy women should understand not only that these risks exist but also that a cause of their pain may not be found. It is vital that when this happens it is clear to both clinician and patient that the failure to identify pathology does not mean that the pain does not exist.

In managing women with CPP, screening for sexually transmitted infections (STIs) should always be offered to sexually active women even if the STI is not ultimately thought to be the cause of the pain. Failure to detect and treat an STI may lead to future sub-fertility and increased risk of ectopic pregnancy, and increases the risk of onward transmission.

5. Which methods of pain relief are safe and effective in reducing CPP?

Search Strategy: pelvic pain (MeSH) AND analgesia (MeSH).

The literature regarding effective treatment for CPP is hampered by the difficulties of defining the condition which is being treated. Clearly, if a treatable component of the pain is identified, then drugs or interventions specific to that condition should be considered. The search described above yielded no high quality studies of analgesia for CPP. What *is* known is that laparoscopic utero-sacral nerve ablation (LUNA) is ineffective in the management of CPP [20].

In line with the WHO pain ladder, patients with CPP should be offered paracetamol with or without non-steroidal anti-inflammatory drugs (NSAIDs) in combination, taken regularly unless contraindicated. Although there is no evidence concerning CPP directly, Cochrane reviews concerning the use of NSAIDs for dysmenorrhea, suggest that no particular NSAID is better than another and patient or clinician experience should lead the choice [21]. The addition of opiate based drugs such as codeine or tramadol can be helpful particularly if taken only occasionally for peaks of pain but care should be taken to avoid constipation and addiction.

Little evidence exists to support the use of complementary therapies in CPP, although if the patient finds them helpful and wishes to explore their use, this seems reasonable, provided the patient is aware of potential interactions with other drugs.

It can be difficult to know whether there is a neuropathic element to a patient's pain although the description of pain as burning, aching, or stabbing may be suggestive of nerve involvement. If pain is not well controlled with conventional analgesia, it may be worth trying an adjuvant analgesic such as amitriptyline (particularly helpful if sleep disturbance is an issue), pregabalin, gabapentin, or duloxetine. Some clinicians have identified innovative methods to diagnose and treat neuropathic pain including nerve blocks and surgery, but as summarized in a useful review article, more evidence is needed before these can be recommended unanimously [22].

A recent systematic review attempted to determine the value of psychological treatments in the management of CPP, emphasizing the need to adopt a biopsychosocial model in understanding and treating pain. Only four studies of adequate quality were identified and the heterogeneity in their design and small size made it difficult to draw conclusions. However two of the papers reported three-month [23] and 12-month follow-up [24] in a study using Mensendieck somatocognitive therapy which can be seen as a hybrid of physiotherapy and psychotherapy. Results were encouraging with a significant improvement in pain scores 12 months after treatment. Further research is needed to explore its use in other settings.

Several helpful evidence-based guidelines on the use of adjuvant analgesics have been published in recent years (Box 5.2). The reader is referred to the NICE guidelines: Neuropathic Pain – Pharmacological Management [25]. This gives a simple algorithm for treatment and includes the important advice to avoid starting opiates for benign pain without the advice of a specialist pain team.

Summary

The mechanistic paradigm of seeking to identify a single unifying pathology to explain and treat a patient's symptoms, leaving the woman a passive recipient of medical care, is inadequate to explain the principles underlying the management of CPP. The origin of CPP is complex including a person's emotional, physical, and sexual persona as well as her own sense of her future and her past. Resolution of this pain must therefore be a process which she can direct albeit with the skilled advice of a clinician. Whilst a detailed history can often identify treatable components of pain and new understanding of the role of the CNS can explain symptom patterns and offer new therapeutic options, it could be argued that the most important advance relevant to the management of pelvic pain is a new paradigm for the doctor–patient relationship in which patients experience their doctor as listening to their problems, validating their symptoms, taking them seriously as agents in their own recovery, and working with them to improve their quality of life.

Case resolution

The 27-year-old woman presented initially found the approach of her new gynecologist refreshing and for the first time she felt listened to and taken seriously and felt that she no longer needed to demand anything, in particular an operation, possibly hysterectomy, in order to get people to take her seriously. During the initial conversation with the gynecologist she realized that her periods were actually quite a strain and that as a result she had been functioning at less than her best for years. Recognizing that she also needed effective contraception, she opted for a Mirena coil with which she was delighted since she no longer menstruated. They discussed endometriosis as a possible cause and the gynecologist's opinion was that it probably was a contributory factor, but they agreed that it didn't need to be established either way at present provided they could control the pain adequately with appropriate treatment.

The gynecologist had examined her at the initial consultation and she was surprised and pleased that he had actually been able to recreate the pain by pressing on her symphysis pubis and then the left sacroiliac joint. No one else had been able to demonstrate her pain before. This reassured her that he did believe that her pain was real. Thinking back she realized that this same pain had been present during her second pregnancy but had gone away immediately after the birth. She could therefore readily accept that it might be linked to the pelvic girdle pain (PGP) of pregnancy and was happy to see the physiotherapist again before proceeding to the laparoscopy. The doctor also pointed out that if this pain was PGP it might actually be made worse by a diagnostic laparoscopy with her legs placed in lithotomy under general anesthetic.

In the short term she found a low dose of amitriptyline helpful in reducing the pain and helping her sleep well for the first time in months since the pain no longer woke her up and worried her when she turned over in bed. She also used diclofenac with paracetamol regularly in the initial two or three weeks of treatment and reduced it gradually at her own pace. Once she was pain-free, she decided to stop the amitriptyline after about four months of treatment including hydrotherapy with the physio and she found she could maintain strength and pain-free mobility with regular attendance at a local Pilates class.

Finally through having the space to consider her fears and concerns, she realized just how confused and frightened she still felt about what had happened during the birth and decided to access the "After thoughts" service through the community midwife. They looked at the obstetric notes together and she now understood that the baby's heart beat had suddenly dropped and that is why her legs had been put in stirrups so that delivery could be achieved quickly (which may have exacerbated her pelvic girdle problem). She could now process her fears from that the time that something had gone wrong and been covered up and see that the baby had recovered completely and there was no ongoing cause for concern.

Six months after the first appointment, she saw the gynecologist for the second time. They had spent 45 minutes together the first time but this time the appointment took just eight minutes. She said that she was now functioning very well, her husband was overseas as planned but she was as fine with that strain as any other military wife, accessing the support of other women effectively now that she was no longer isolated by her pain. She could handle the normal stress of life with young children because she was pain-free provided she made time for her exercise class. He asked her if she still wanted the laparoscopy but she said no because she now understood her pain and knew how to keep it at bay.

Box 5.1 Diagnosis of irritable bowel syndrome

Rome III criteria http://romecriteria.org/assets/pdf/19_RomeIII_apA_885-898.pdf.

Continuous or recurrent abdominal pain or discomfort on at least three days a month in the last three months, with the onset at least six months previously, associated with at least two of the following:

- Improvement with defecation
- Onset associated with a change in frequency of stool
- Onset associated with a change in form of stool

Symptoms such as abdominal bloating and the passage of mucus are commonly present and are suggestive of IBS. Extra-intestinal symptoms such as lethargy, backache, urinary frequency, and dyspareunia may occur in association with IBS.

Box 5.2 Adjuvant analgesics [25]

Drug	Starting dose	Maximum dose	possible alternative
amitriptyline	10 mg at night	75 mg at night	nortriptyline, imipramine
pregabalin	75 mg twice daily	300 mg twice daily	gabapentin
duloxetine	60 mg once daily	120 mg once daily	

Further reading

Guidelines

Royal College of Obstetricians and Gynecologists. *RCOG Guidelines for the Initial Management of Chronic Pelvic Pain* (2012). www.rcog.org.uk/womens-health/clinical-guidance/initial-management-chronic-pelvic-pain-green-top-41, accessed 25 June 2018.

Fall, M., Baranowski, A.P., Elneil, S. et al. (2010). EAU guidelines on chronic pelvic pain. *Eur. Urol.* **57** (**1**): 35–48.

American College of Obstetricians and Gynecologists (2004). ACOG Practice Bulletin No. 51. Chronic pelvic pain. *Obstet. Gynecol.* **103** (**3**): 589–605.

Patient education brochure

Available at: http://www.pelvicpain.org/docs/patients/Patient-Education-Brochure.aspx, accessed 25 June 2018.

References

1 Zondervan, K.T., Yudkin, P.L., Vessey, M.P. et al. (2001). The community prevalence of chronic pelvic pain in women and associated illness behaviour. *Br. J. Gen. Pract.* **51** (**468**): 541–547.

2 Zondervan, K.T., Yudkin, P.L., Vessey, M.P. et al. (1999). Prevalence and incidence of chronic pelvic pain in primary care: evidence from a national general practice database. *Br. J. Obstet. Gynaecol.* **106** (**11**): 1149–1155.

3 Heim, C., Ehlert, U., Hanker, J.P., and Hellhammer, D.H. (1998). Abuse-related posttraumatic stress disorder and alterations of the hypothalamic-pituitary-adrenal axis in women with chronic pelvic pain. *Psychosom. Med.* **60** (**3**): 309–318.

4 As-Sanie, S., Harris, R.E., Napadow, V. et al. (2012). Changes in regional gray matter volume in women with chronic pelvic pain: a voxel-based morphometry study. *Pain* **153** (**5**): 1006–1014.

5 Tu, C.H., Niddam, D.M., Chao, H.T. et al. (2010). Brain morphological changes associated with cyclic menstrual pain. *Pain* **150** (**3**): 462–468.

6 Tu, C.H., Niddam, D.M., Chao, H.T. et al. (2009). Abnormal cerebral metabolism during menstrual pain in primary dysmenorrhea. *Neuroimage* **47** (**1**): 28–35.

7 Vincent, K., Warnaby, C., Stagg, C.J. et al. (2011). Dysmenorrhoea is associated with central changes in otherwise healthy women. *Pain* **152** (**9**): 1966–1975.

8 Stratton, P. and Berkley, K.J. (2011). Chronic pelvic pain and endometriosis: translational evidence of the relationship and implications. *Hum. Reprod. Update* **17** (**3**): 327–346.

9 Baranowski, A.P. (2009). Chronic pelvic pain. *Best Pract. Res. Clin. Gastroenterol.* **23** (**4**): 593–610.

10 Aslam, N., Harrison, G., Khan, K., and Patwardhan, S. (2009). Visceral hyperalgesia in chronic pelvic pain. *BJOG* **116** (**12**): 1551–1555.

11 IASP Task Force on Taxonomy (ed. H. Merskey and N. Bogduk) *Classification of Chronic Pain*, 2e. Seattle: IASP Press http://www.iasp-pain.org.

12 Verheul, W., Sanders, A., and Bensing, J. (2010). The effects of physicians' affect-oriented communication style and raising expectations on analogue patients' anxiety, affect and expectancies. *Patient Educ. Couns.* **80** (**3**): 300–306.

13 Souza, P.P., Romão, A.S., Rosa-e-Silva, J.C. et al. (2011). Qualitative research as the basis for a biopsychosocial approach to women with chronic pelvic pain. *J. Psychosom. Obstet. Gynaecol.* **32** (**4**): 165–172.

14 Tu, F.F., As-Sanie, S., and Steege, J.F. (2006). Prevalence of pelvic musculoskeletal disorders in a female chronic pelvic pain clinic. *J. Reprod. Med.* **51** (**3**): 185–189.

15 Tu, F.F., Holt, J., Gonzales, J., and Fitzgerald, C.M. (2008). Physical therapy evaluation of patients with chronic pelvic pain: a controlled study. *Am. J. Obstet. Gynecol.* **198** (**3**): 272.e1–272.e7.

16 Neville, C.E., Fitzgerald, C.M., Mallinson, T. et al. (2012). A preliminary report of musculoskeletal dysfunction in female chronic pelvic pain: a blinded study of examination findings. *J. Bodyw. Mov. Ther.* **16** (**1**): 50–56.

17 Fitzgerald, C.M., Neville, C.E., Mallinson, T. et al. (2011). Pelvic floor muscle examination in female chronic pelvic pain. *J. Reprod. Med.* **56** (**3–4**): 117–122.

18 Swank, D.J., Swank-Bordewijk, S.C., Hop, W.C. et al. (2003). Laparoscopic adhesiolysis in patients with chronic abdominal pain: a blinded randomised controlled multi-Centre trial. *Lancet* **361**: 1247–1251.

19 Jansen, F.W., Kapiteyn, K., Trimbos-Kemper, T. et al. (1997). Complications of laparoscopy: a prospective multicentre observational study. *Br. J. Obstet. Gynaecol.* **104** (**5**): 595–600.

20 Daniels, J.P., Middleton, L., Xiong, T. et al. (2010). International LUNA IPD meta-analysis collaborative group. Individual patient data meta-analysis of randomized evidence to assess the effectiveness of laparoscopic uterosacral nerve ablation in chronic pelvic pain. *Hum. Reprod. Update* **16** (**6**): 568–576.

21 Marjoribanks, J., Proctor, M., Farquhar, C., and Derks, R.S. (2010). Nonsteroidal anti-inflammatory drugs for dysmenorrhoea. *Cochrane Database Syst. Rev.* (**1**): CD001751. doi: 10.1002/14651858.CD001751.pub2.

22 Tu, F.F., Hellman, K.M., and Backonja, M.M. (2011). Gynecologic management of neuropathic pain. *Am. J. Obstet. Gynecol.* **205** (**5**): 435–443.

23 Haugstad, G.K., Haugstad, T.S., Kirste, U.M. et al. (2006). Mensendieck somatocognitive therapy as treatment approach to chronic pelvic pain: results of a randomized controlled intervention study. *Am. J. Obstet. Gynecol.* **194** (**5**): 1303–1310.

24 Haugstad, G.K., Haugstad, T.S., Kirste, U.M. et al. (2008). Continuing improvement of chronic pelvic pain in women after short-term Mensendieck somatocognitive therapy: results of a 1-year follow-up study. *Am. J. Obstet. Gynecol.* **199** (**6**): 615.

25 NICE CG173 (2013, updated 2018). *Neuropathic Pain – Pharmacological Management*. London: National Institute for Clinical Excellence. www.nice.org.uk/guidance/CG96.

CHAPTER 6
Genital tract infections

Veronica Ades
Department of Obstetrics and Gynecology, NYU Langone Medical Center, New York, NY, USA

> **CASE SCENARIO**
> A 23-year-old Go presents with new onset mucopurulent vaginal discharge. She recently initiated a sexual relationship with a new partner. She takes oral contraceptive pills, but does not use barrier contraception.

Background

Genital tract infections affect millions of people worldwide, and clinicians may encounter a variety of clinical presentations in both men and women. Diagnostic modalities have advanced rapidly with the development of polymerase chain reaction (PCR) and other highly sensitive techniques, and it is essential for clinicians to quickly and accurately recognize presenting symptoms of the various infections and select the appropriate diagnostic tests. In addition, antibiotic resistance has made treatment selection more challenging, and recent recommendations have changed. Pregnancy further complicates the picture of genital tract infections, both for diagnosis and management. This chapter will review the most up to date literature regarding the presentation, diagnosis, and management of genital tract infections in men and women, and how these differ in pregnancy.

Search strategy

Resources: Cochrane library, Pubmed, CDC Guidelines and Recommendations.
Search Terms
Question 1: [Disease name], Epidemiology Clinical manifestations symptoms.
Question 2: [Disease name], Diagnosis, screening, culture, NAAT.
Question 3: [Disease name], Management, treatment.

Clinical questions

1. What are the most common clinical presentations for gonorrhea, chlamydia, herpes simplex virus (HSV), trichomonas, *Mycoplasma genitalium*, and genital warts?
2. What is the optimal diagnostic method for gonorrhea, chlamydia, HSV, trichomonas, *mycoplasma genitalium*, and genital warts?
3. What is the recommended treatment of gonorrhea, chlamydia, HSV, trichomonas, *mycoplasma genitalium*, and genital warts?
4. How does the presentation or management of these infections differ in pregnancy?

Discussion of the evidence

1. What are the most common clinical presentations for gonorrhea, chlamydia, HSV, trichomonas, *Mycoplasma genitalium*, and genital warts?

Gonorrhea is more common in men that in women, and is more likely to be asymptomatic in women [1]. Men who have sex with men and HIV-infected individuals are at especially high risk of gonorrhea infection [1]. In women who are symptomatic, vaginal discharge, and abdominal pain are the most common presenting symptoms, with arthralgia, skin lesions, and bartholin gland abscess occurring less commonly [2]. When symptomatic in men, gonorrhea often presents as pyuria or dysuria, and less commonly as epididymitis [3–6].

The vast majority (>95%) of individuals infected with **chlamydia** are asymptomatic [5, 7, 8]. When symptoms are present, the most common among women is mucopurulent cervicitis or urethritis, and less common is pelvic inflammatory disease [9–11]. Among men, presenting symptoms, when present, can include urethritis and epididymitis [12, 13]. *Chlamydia trachomatis* has also been identified as the single most common cause of non-gonococcal reactive arthritis, or Reiter's syndrome, which typically presents as

Evidence-Based Obstetrics and Gynecology, First Edition. Edited by Errol R. Norwitz, Carolyn M. Zelop, David A. Miller, and David L. Keefe.

a single-site, lower limb arthritis approximately four weeks after genital tract infection occurs [14].

Genital herpes simplex presents with painful ulcers, vesicles, papules, pustules, crusts, fissures along the skin and mucous membranes of the genitals, thighs, or buttocks. However, it can also present with less typical symptoms, such as cystitis, urethritis, cervicitis, and even meningitis [15, 16]. Dysuria can lead to urinary retention, and constitutional symptoms such as headache, fever, malaise, and lymphadenopathy can also be present [16]. These symptoms can be preceded by a prodrome of tingling, burning, or pain in the area where the lesions will appear [16]. While 60% of new HSV-2 infections are symptomatic, 40% are asymptomatic [15]. In addition, while HSV-2 is commonly thought to be a genital infection and HSV-1 an orolabial infection, in fact, new genital HSV-1 infections are as common as new orolabial HSV-1 infections, and the incidence of HSV-1 genital infections appears to be increasing [15, 17]. Primary outbreaks, usually the first outbreak that occurs after acquisition of the virus, are usually significantly more painful and incapacitating, with multiple lesions, while subsequent outbreaks are less painful and demonstrate fewer, more localized lesions or only a single lesion [16, 18].

Trichomonas infections can be asymptomatic in up to 50% of cases and symptoms, when present, can be sufficiently mild that they can be mistaken for normal vaginal discharge, and infections can last for long durations untreated [19, 20]. The most common presenting symptom in women is vaginal discharge and in men, urethral discharge [19, 21]. The vaginal discharge can be yellow or malodorous ("musty"), and a pruritic or irritated sensation can be described [20]. Other symptoms include dyspareunia, dysuria, vulvar erythema, vulvar pruritis, and abdominal pain [20, 22]. Colpitis macularis or "strawberry cervix" is an appearance of the cervix created by punctate hemorrhages on the cervix; however it is difficult to see with the naked eye and is more visible with colposcopy (90%) than with the naked eye (2%) [20, 22]. Mucopurulent discharge is uncommon unless coinfection with chlamydia or gonorrhea is present [20].

The pathological nature of *Mycoplasma genitalium* is still under investigation. While it is a common cause of non-gonococcal urethritis in men, it has not been shown to cause them long-term sequelae, such as infertility [23]. And while mycoplasma has been associated with adverse outcomes in women such as preterm birth, mycoplasma can also be asymptomatic, with over half of women testing positive reporting no symptoms [24]. Among women who do report symptoms, cervicitis and postcoital bleeding are common, and urethritis can also be seen occasionally [23–25]. While a cervicitis may be seen on presentation, this cervicitis is often asymptomatic [26, 27]. Other pelvic inflammatory disease symptoms are not usually seen with mycoplasma, such as vaginal discharge, pelvic pain, or dyspareunia, though it has been suggested that mycoplasma may increase the risk of developing pelvic inflammatory disease [24].

Genital warts appear as multiple polymorphic lesions, potentially appearing as cauliflower-like, papular, or keratotic, that can coalesce into larger masses [28, 29]. In men, common locations include the frenum, corona, coronal sulcus, inner surface of the prepuce, and urethra or urinary meatus [28]. In women, warts can appear at the fourchette and adjacent labia, but also other part of the vulva, perineum, groin, and anus [28, 29]. Warts can also be seen inside the vagina and on the cervix, but are rarely seen on the thighs or trunk [28]. Warts usually do not have additional symptoms other than their presence, but may occasionally be accompanied by pruritis, irritation, or pain [29].

2. What is the optimal diagnostic method for gonorrhea, chlamydia, HSV, trichomonas, *Mycoplasma genitalium*, and genital warts?

The optimal diagnostic test for both *N. gonorrhea* and *C. trachomatis* is nucleic acid amplification testing (NAAT) [30]. Previously the gold standard test was culture; however, this method required invasive testing (urethral swabs for men or cervical swabs for women), expedited transportation and maintenance of a cold chain for adequate specimen handling [30]. Additionally, testing required 48–72 hours for bacterial growth in order to provide results [30]. NAAT testing does not require viable organisms; instead detecting infection based on as little as a single copy of DNA or RNA, greatly increases sensitivity [30]. It is estimated that the use of NAAT improves detection of chlamydia by 20–50% over culture or earlier nonculture tests [30]. Sensitivity of NAAT testing for both *N. gonorrhea* and *C. trachomatis* is over 90% while specificity is greater than 99% [30]. The improved sensitivity of NAAT testing also permits less invasive methods of testing for gonorrhea and chlamydia, including urine specimens for both men and women, and self-collected vaginal swabs for women [30]. Self-collected vaginal swabs have equal sensitivity and specificity when compared with provider-collected endocervical swabs [31, 32]. While *N. gonorrhea* and *C. trachomatis* can be detected in the first void urine for women, the organism load is substantially lower than at other detection sites (cervix, vagina), and evidence indicates that up to 10% of chlamydia or gonorrhea infections may be missed [30, 33, 34]. However, urine testing is a highly convenient and useful diagnostic modality and need not be eliminated as an option for women in the appropriate clinical scenario, especially in patients who are apprehensive about having a pelvic exam or performing a vaginal self-swab, or who prefer the convenience of a urine sample. NAAT is not FDA-cleared for rectal, oropharyngeal, or conjunctival diagnosis of gonorrhea or chlamydia, and the specificity may not be as high as with urinary and endocervical samples [23]. When antimicrobial resistance is suspected, such as in cases of treatment failure, culture may still be a useful diagnostic modality despite the logistical challenges [23]. For point-of-care testing of symptomatic men, Gram or methylene blue or gentian violet (MB/GV) stain of urethral secretions showing polymorphonuclear leukocytes with intracellular Gram-negative diplococci can provide high specificity, but does not rule out infection due to low sensitivity [23].

Diagnosis of **genital herpes simplex** virus can be made clinically, with the appearance of typical lesions as described above. While laboratory diagnosis is not required, it can help confirm the diagnosis and establish the timing of acquisition. If lesions are present, a viral culture can be taken by swabbing the base of an active lesion [16]. Sensitivity of herpes viral culture can be reduced by poor specimen handling, swabbing of healing lesions, or recurrent rather than primary infections; therefore a negative viral culture does not rule out herpes infection [16]. Because of the low sensitivity of viral culture, NAAT tests are becoming more widely available, and are the test of choice for central nervous system and systemic infections [23]. Cytologic detection of herpes cellular changes (Tzanck preparation) and monoclonal antibody detection are insufficiently sensitive [23]. Serum antibodies to herpes rise within a few weeks of exposure, with IgM antibodies rising first, followed by IgG antibodies; the latter remain permanently detectable in the serum [16]. Therefore, serum antibodies may be negative in the setting of an acute primary outbreak, and should be repeated after several weeks [16]. Additionally, presence of HSV-1 antibodies does not differentiate between oral and genital transmission; HSV-2 is still rare in the oral cavity and therefore infection is still presumed to occur in the genital tract [23]. While screening with serology in the general population is not recommended, serologic testing may be useful for patients without symptoms whose partners have genital herpes in order to determine immunity status [23].

The mainstay of **trichomonas** diagnosis is light microscopy with wet mount because it is low cost and widely accessible. *T. vaginalis* has a classic appearance on wet mount of motile flagellated protozoa [35]. However, sensitivity of light microscopy can be as low as 51–65% [23, 35]. *T. vaginalis* organisms can be detected on Pap smear, but specificity is low, and therefore clinical correlation is recommended; confirmation via alternative diagnostic method is recommended in patients in whom trichomonas infection is unlikely [36]. NAAT tests are also now available and FDA-approved for *T. vaginalis*, and offer the benefit of increased sensitivity and specificity, with the disadvantage of increased cost and precluding immediate diagnosis and treatment [37, 38]. NAAT testing can detect trichomonas three to five times more often than wet mount, and are equally sensitive (95–100%) from urethral swabs or urine in men and from vaginal swabs, endocervical swabs, and urine in women [23]. Rapid tests have been developed, but are not yet FDA approved, and while specificity is high, they have lower sensitivity than NAAT tests. Prior to the widespread availability of NAAT tests, culture offered the highest sensitivity and specificity (75–96% and 100%, respectively) but is less useful now in the era of widespread NAAT availability [23].

Mycoplasma genitalium has only recently been recognized as a sexually transmitted infection, and therefore testing for mycoplasma is not widely commercially available [26, 39, 40]. Culture is not a useful diagnostic tool for mycoplasma because of its slow growth, and the ability to isolate it is limited to few laboratories [23]. Studies of mycoplasma have found that NAAT and PCR-based detection offers the best sensitivity and specificity, but none have been FDA-approved [23, 39, 40]. The optimal specimen collection in men is from urine and in women is from cervical or vaginal swabs [39, 40]. While the clinical implications of mycoplasma are still being elucidated [27, 41, 42] development of a commercially available test would further both clinical testing and research into mycoplasma.

Genital warts can be adequately diagnosed by visual inspection of typical lesions as described above [23]. Biopsy is not required unless lesions are atypical or unresponsive to treatment [29]. Atypical appearance can include hyperpigmentation, induration, fixation to underlying tissue, friability, or ulceration [23].

3. What is the recommended treatment of gonorrhea, chlamydia, HSV, trichomonas, *Mycoplasma genitalium*, and genital warts?

Treatment of **gonorrhea** is becoming an increasing challenge as the prevalence of antimicrobial resistance rises [23, 43]. Fluoroquinolones are no longer effective against *N. gonorrhea*, and combination therapy is currently recommended in order to improve treatment efficacy and slow the spread of antimicrobial resistance [23, 43]. Additionally, as part of the 2015 CDC Guidelines, oral cephalosporins are no longer recommended as a first line as part of the combination therapy for *N. gonorrhea* [23]. While both doxycycline and azithromycin are effective against *N. gonorrhea*, azithromycin is preferred due to its ease of use and low side effect profile. Therefore the recommended regimen to treat cervical, urethral, or rectal gonorrhea is ceftriaxone 250 mg IM single dose + azithromycin 1 g orally single dose [23]. If ceftriaxone is not available, then it may be replaced with a single dose of oral cefixime 400 mg, but this is not optimal as the serum levels are lower and shorter-lasting, and efficacy for pharyngeal gonorrhea is lower [23]. Given that treatments are single dose and antimicrobial resistance is high, directly observed therapy is recommended for gonorrhea [23]. Expedited partner therapy (EPT), in which a prescription is given to the patient for oral combination single-dose therapy (cefixime and azithromycin) to be given to her or his partner along with educational materials about gonorrhea in order to prevent reinfection of the patient, is a helpful public health approach that can be considered [44].

The recommended treatment of **chlamydia** is azithromycin 1 g orally in a single dose or doxycycline 100 mg orally twice a day for seven days [23]. Treatment with azithromycin offers the obvious advantage of immediate effectiveness without concerns about adherence, but a meta-analysis of 12 randomized controlled trials comparing azithromycin and doxycycline found no difference between the two, with 97–98% cure rates [45]. Erythromycin is less effective than azithromycin or doxycycline, while levofloxacin and ofloxacin are effective but more expensive than the standard treatments [23]. In order to prevent reinfection, EPT can be considered, with either azithromycin or doxycycline, and the patient should abstain from sex for seven days from the start of treatment regardless of regimen [23]. If EPT is being given and the partner is female, the teratogenicity of doxycycline should be considered in choosing an EPT regimen, given that the physician will not be able to assess for pregnancy in the partner prior to medication administration. Test of cure is not necessary in asymptomatic patients unless reinfection or poor adherence is suspected, and NAAT may be falsely positive up to three weeks after treatment, thereby limiting the utility of repeat testing [23].

Treatment of **genital herpes** is aimed at shortening the duration and severity of outbreaks, as well as reducing the frequency of outbreaks. The primary genital herpes outbreak can be severe and prolonged, and therefore warrants treatment in most patients [23]. This can be accomplished with acyclovir 400 mg three times a day for 7–10 days, valacyclovir 1 g orally twice a day for 7–10 days, or famciclovir 250 mg orally three times a day for 7–10 days [23]. If outbreaks last longer than 10 days, therapy duration can be extended [23]. Recurrent outbreaks are shorter and less painful, and therefore some patients may decline treatment while others may want treatment to mitigate and shorten the duration of symptoms. Acyclovir, valacyclovir, and famciclovir are all appropriate for treatment of recurrent outbreaks; the dose and frequency can vary, but listed here is the lowest frequency of dosing for increased convenience (see Table 6.1) [23]. A Cochrane review found that antiviral medications prevent recurrent outbreaks in individuals suffering four outbreaks or more per year, but found no difference in effectiveness between acyclovir, valacyclovir, and famciclovir [46]. Treatment of primary disease does not seem to reduce the likelihood or frequency of subsequent outbreaks [47]. Oral acyclovir can reduce asymptomatic viral shedding of HSV-2 by over 90%, though it is unclear whether this translates into a reduction in viral transmission [48].

Table 6.1 Dosing and frequency options for medications to treat recurrent HSV infection [23]

Medication	Dose options	Frequency	Duration
Acyclovir	400 mg	QID	5 d
	800 mg	BID	5 d
	800 mg	TID	2 d
Valacyclovir	500 mg	BID	3 d
	1 g	QD	5 d
Famciclovir	125 mg	BID	5 d
	1 g	BID	1 d
	500 mg once, then 250 mg	BID	2 d

The recommended treatment for **trichomoniasis** is single-dose oral metronidazole 2 g or tinidazole 2 g [23]. Tinidazole is better tolerated and reaches higher levels in serum and genitourinary tract, but is more expensive than metronidazole [23]. However, a Cochrane review found that a treatment of longer duration may have a lower frequency of gastrointestinal side effects (7% compared with 15% with single dose) [49]. The same review found that while vaginal preparation is inferior to oral treatment, combined vaginal and oral treatment is more effective than oral treatment alone [49]. While oral single dose, oral longer dose, and combination treatment all have cure rates of over 90%, vaginal treatment has a cure rate of under 50% [49]. Individuals testing positive for trichomonas are at high risk of acquiring chlamydia, gonorrhea, or trichomonas in the near future, and therefore it is recommended that they be retested for infections three months after treatment [50].

Many basic antibiotics, such as beta-lactams and penicillins, are ineffective against *Mycoplasma genitalium* because it lacks a cell wall. The most effective treatment is a single dose of azithromycin, with a median cure rate of 85%; however, a resistant strain appears to be emerging, reducing the cure rate to 40% [23, 51]. The seven-day doxycycline treatment used for chlamydia treatment is ineffective against mycoplasma [23]. While a longer period of administration of azithromycin (500 mg dose followed by 250 mg daily for four days) may reduce the development of resistance, it does not improve treatment efficacy when an organism is already resistant [23, 52]. There have been reports of success with moxifloxacin 400 mg daily for 7, 10, or 14 days for treatment failures, but it has not been evaluated in a clinical trial, and moxifloxacin resistance has also been reported [23]. Current regimens for pelvic inflammatory disease treatment are not effective against mycoplasma; therefore if a patient does not respond to antibiotic therapy, NAAT testing for mycoplasma could be considered, and if positive, adding moxifloxacin to the antibiotic regimen may improve the clinical response [23].

Genital warts may be treated or left alone to resolve spontaneously; 30% will resolve within four months [23]. There are several options for treatment of warts, and none have been shown to be more effective than any other, therefore treatment can be guided based on patient and clinician preference and circumstances [23]. Imiquimod is topical and patient-applied, used for up to 16 weeks. It works by stimulating production of interferon and other cytokines at the site of the wart [23]. Success rates of 77% in women and 40% in men have been cited, with 13% recurrence [53]. Common side effects include local inflammatory reactions or irritation, hypopigmentation, ulcerations, or worsening of preexisting dermatoses [23, 54]. Podophyllotoxin is also a patient-applied topical agent that causes wart necrosis through antimitotic activity. It can be used for up to four weeks [23]. The area of treatment should be limited in size (less than 10 cm^2) [23]. Success rates can be as high as 45–77% with recurrence rates of approximately 38% [53]. Side effects are common and include mild to moderate pain or local irritation [23, 53]. Sinecatechins are a third topical option that are extracted from green tea and can be used for up to 16 weeks; side effects are similar to those of imiquimod [23, 55]. Success rates of 58% have been found, with short-term recurrence estimated at 6–9% [53]. Safety in immunocompromised individuals and those with genital herpes has not been evaluated [23]. Topical agents administered by the clinician include trichloroacetic acid (TCA) and bichloroacetic acid, with clearance rates of 70–80% but recurrence rates of 36% [53]. Side effects can include pain, ulceration and crusting, as well as damage to healthy surrounding tissue if misapplied [23, 53]. Cryotherapy, or freezing of tissue with nitrous oxide or liquid nitrogen, may be used by appropriately trained providers; side effects include pain during and after the procedure, as well as necrosis and blistering of warts. Success rates are high, approximately 79–88% after the first three treatments, though recurrence rates may be higher, at 25–40%, because treatment does not affect subclinical underlying infection [53]. Local anesthesia can be helpful for pain control [23, 53]. Surgical removal can be useful, especially for larger lesions, and can be accomplished with a scalpel, carbon dioxide laser, or curettage [23]. Suturing is usually not required as hemostasis can be achieved with pressure and electrocautery or a chemical hemostatic agent [23]. In order to prevent transmission to healthcare workers, appropriate precautions should be taken, including masks and ventilation [56]. While surgical removal has a high success rate, at approximately 72% clearance, it tends to be reserved for larger lesions because it is more painful and causes significant bleeding, and therefore topical agents are usually preferable [53]. Laser treatment is more costly and has lower success rates, 23–52%, with recurrence as high as 77% [53].

4. How does the presentation or management of these infections differ in pregnancy?

The regimen for treating gonorrhea in pregnancy is unchanged; pregnant women should be treated with IM ceftriaxone and oral azithromycin [23]. For treatment of chlamydia in pregnancy, only the single dose azithromycin treatment is an option because it is both safe and effective; doxycycline is teratogenic, and therefore is contraindicated [23]. Among the alternative regimens, ofloxacin, and levofloxacin do not have any known teratogenic effects from human studies, but animal studies raise a concern for cartilage damage in neonates, and therefore it is recommended that they be avoided [23]. Should alternatives to azithromycin be required, amoxicillin or erythromycin can be used, though these are not ideal regimens due to resistance and poor tolerance, respectively [23]. Due to the concern for serious sequelae from persistent infection or reinfection, test of cure is recommended three to four weeks after treatment, as well as three months after treatment [23]. Women who tested positive for chlamydia in early pregnancy should be rescreened in the third trimester to prevent complications of vertical transmission [23].

The incidence of neonatal acquisition of genital HSV is extremely low, and therefore a Cochrane review of antiviral prophylaxis was unable to determine whether suppression prevents transmission because no cases occurred [57, 58]. Nonetheless, antiviral prophylaxis did reduce the risk of having an HSV outbreak at delivery, having a cesarean delivery for genital herpes, and having HSV detected at delivery [57]. Therefore, suppressive therapy with acyclovir or valacyclovir can be beneficial in order to prevent cesarean delivery associated with genital HSV outbreak [23]. Suppression is not helpful in women who have serology showing antibodies to HSV but who do not report a history of HSV outbreaks [23]. The highest risk of neonatal HSV is in women without a history of HSV who acquire HSV late in pregnancy as maternal antibodies appear to be protective [59]; therefore women whose partners have known genital HSV but who themselves do not have a history of HSV should be counseled to abstain from sex late in pregnancy [23].

The treatment of trichomonas in pregnancy is unchanged; a single dose of metronidazole is recommended. However, a Cochrane review also found that while metronidazole was more effective than placebo or no treatment at clearing the infection, treatment increased the risk of preterm birth by 78%, though later, larger studies showed no association [23, 60].

Mycoplasma may be a cause of preterm birth, given that it has been detected both in the amniotic cavity and in cord cultures from preterm infants [42]. It has been suggested that treatment of mycoplasma colonization may reduce rates of preterm birth and neonatal complications, but the precise utility and magnitude of impact are unclear, and further research is needed [61, 62]. For overt mycoplasma infections in pregnancy, the first line of treatment, azithromycin, is safe and effective in pregnancy [23]. In the case of treatment failures, moxifloxacin is generally avoided in pregnancy due to the concerns about cartilage damage cited above with quinolone antibiotics in infants, and therefore treatment should be individualized with input from a specialist [23].

For treatment of genital warts, podophyllin is contraindicated due to its antimitotic activity, and imiquimod and sinecatechins have not been evaluated and therefore are better avoided [23]. TCA is non-systemically absorbed, and therefore can be used in pregnancy [53]. Cryotherapy and surgical removal are both local procedures and therefore can be performed in pregnancy [53]. However, given that most genital warts are otherwise asymptomatic and nonpathologic, it is acceptable and often preferable to defer treatment until after the pregnancy in order to use a patient-applied topical agent, which is often the most convenient option.

References

1 Delpech, V., Martin, I.M.C., Hughes, G. et al. (2009). Epidemiology and clinical presentation of gonorrhoea in England and Wales: findings from the Gonococcal resistance to antimicrobials surveillance programme 2001–2006. *Sex. Transm. Infect.* **85** (**5**): 317–321. doi: 10.1136/sti.2008.034843.

2 McCormack, W.M., Johnson, K., Stumacher, R.J., and Donner, A. (1977). Clinical spectrum of gonococcal infection in women. *The Lancet* **309** (**8023**): 1182–1185. doi: 10.1016/s0140-6736(77)92720-9.

3 Klouman, E., Masenga, E.J., Sam, N.E., and Klepp, K.I. (2000). Asymptomatic gonorrhoea and chlamydial infection in a population-based and work-site based sample of men in Kilimanjaro, Tanzania. *Int. J. STD AIDS* **11** (**10**): 666–674.

4 Holmes, K.K., Berger, R.E., and Alexander, E.R. (1979). Acute epididymitis: Etiology and therapy. *Syst. Biol. Reprod. Med.* **3** (**4**): 309–316. doi: 10.3109/01485017908988421.

5 Miller, W.C., Ford, C.A., Morris, M. et al. (2004). Prevalence of chlamydial and Gonococcal infections among young adults in the United States. *JAMA* **291** (**18**): 2229–2236. doi: 10.1001/jama.291.18.2229.

6 Watson, R.A. (1979). Gonorrhea and acute epididymitis. *Mil. Med.* **144** (**12**).

7 Cecil, J.A., Howell, M.R., Tawes, J.J. et al. (2001). Features of chlamydia trachomatis and Neisseria gonorrhoeae infection in male Army recruits. *J. Infect. Dis.* **184** (**9**): 1216–1219. doi: 10.1086/323662.

8 Detels, R., Green, A.M., Klausner, J.D. et al. (2011). The incidence and correlates of symptomatic and asymptomatic chlamydia trachomatis and Neisseria Gonorrhoeae infections in selected populations in five countries. *Sex. Transm. Dis.* 1–7. doi: 10.1097/OLQ.0b013e318206c288.

9 Marrazzo, J.M. (2005). Mucopurulent cervicitis: no longer ignored, but still misunderstood. *Infect. Dis. Clin. North Am.* **19** (**2**):333–49–viii): doi: 10.1016/j.idc.2005.03.009.

10 Geisler, W.M., Wang, C., Morrison, S.G. et al. (2008). The natural history of untreated chlamydia trachomatis infection in the interval between screening and returning for treatment. *Sex. Transm. Dis.* **35** (**2**): 119–123. doi: 10.1097/OLQ.0b013e318151497d.

11 Frej-Mądrzak, M., Teryks-Wołyniec, D., Jama-Kmiecik, A. et al. (2015). Diagnosing chlamydia trachomatis urinary tract infections – preliminary report. *Adv. Clin. Exp. Med.* **24** (**3**): 441–445.

12 Takahashi, S., Takeyama, K., Kunishima, Y. et al. (2006). Analysis of clinical manifestations of male patients with urethritis. *J. Infect. Chemother.* **12** (**5**): 283–286. doi: 10.1007/s10156-006-0466-7.

13 Berger, R.E., Alexander, E.R., Monda, G.D. et al. (1978). Chlamydia trachomatisas: a cause of acute idiopathic epididymitis. *N. Engl. J. Med.* **298** (**6**): 301–304. doi: 10.1056/NEJM197802092980603.

14 Keat, A., Dixey, J., Sonnex, C. et al. (1987). Chlamydia trachomatis and reactive arthritis: the missing link. *The Lancet* **329** (**8524**): 72–74. doi: 10.1016/S0140-6736(87)91910-6.

15 Langenberg, A.G.M., Corey, L., Ashley, R.L. et al. (1999). A prospective study of new infections with herpes simplex virus type 1 and type 2. *N. Engl. J. Med.* **341** (**19**): 1432–1438. doi: 10.1056/NEJM199911043411904.

16 Fatahzadeh, M. and Schwartz, R.A. (2007). Human herpes simplex virus infections: epidemiology, pathogenesis, symptomatology, diagnosis, and management. *J. Am. Acad. Dermatol.* **57** (**5**): 737–763. doi: 10.1016/j.jaad.2007.06.027.

17 Xu, F., Sternberg, M.R., Kottiri, B.J. et al. (2006). Trends in herpes simplex virus type 1 and type 2 Seroprevalence in the United States. *JAMA* **296** (**8**): 964–973. doi: 10.1001/jama.296.8.964.

18 Steben, M. (2005). Genital herpes simplex virus infection. *Clin. Obstet. Gynecol.* **48** (**4**): 838–844.

19 Van Der Pol, B., Williams, J.A., Orr, D.P. et al. (2005). Prevalence, incidence, natural history, and response to treatment of Trichomonas vaginalis infection among adolescent women. *J. Infect. Dis.* **192** (**12**): 2039–2044. doi: 10.1086/498217.

20 Heine, P. and McGregor, J.A. (1993). Trichomonas vaginalis: a reemerging pathogen. *Clin. Obstet. Gynecol.* **36** (**1**): 137–144.

21 Krieger, J.N., Jenny, C., Verdon, M. et al. (1993). Clinical manifestations of trichomoniasis in men. *Ann. Intern. Med.* **118** (**11**): 844–849.

22 Wølner-Hanssen, P., Krieger, J.N., Stevens, C.E. et al. (1989). Clinical manifestations of vaginal Trichomoniasis. *JAMA* **261** (**4**): 571–576. doi: 10.1001/jama.1989.03420040109029.

23 Workowski, K.A., Bolan, G.A., and Centers for Disease Control and Prevention (2015). Sexually transmitted diseases treatment guidelines, 2015. *MMWR Recomm. Rep.* **64** (**RR-03**): 1–137.

24 Sonnenberg, P., Ison, C.A., Clifton, S. et al. (2015). Epidemiology of mycoplasma genitalium in British men and women aged 16-44 years: evidence from the third National Survey of sexual attitudes and lifestyles (Natsal-3). *Int. J. Epidemiol.* doi: 10.1093/ije/dyv194.

25 Moi, H., Reinton, N., and Moghaddam, A. (2009). Mycoplasma genitalium in women with lower genital tract inflammation. *Sex. Transm. Infect.* **85** (**1**): 10–14. doi: 10.1136/sti.2008.032748.

26 Lis, R., Rowhani-Rahbar, A., and Manhart, L.E. (2015). Mycoplasma genitalium infection and female reproductive tract disease: a meta-analysis. *Clin. Infect. Dis.* **61** (**3**): 418–426. doi: 10.1093/cid/civ312.

27 Huppert, J.S., Mortensen, J.E., Reed, J.L. et al. (2008). Mycoplasma genitalium detected by transcription-mediated amplification is associated with Chlamydia trachomatis in adolescent women. *Sex. Transm. Dis.* **35** (**3**): 250–254. doi: 10.1097/OLQ.0b013e31815abac6.

28 Oriel, J.D. (1977). Genital warts. *Sex. Transm. Dis.* **4** (**4**): 153–159.

29 Lynde, C., Vender, R., Bourcier, M., and Bhatia, N. (2013). Clinical features of external genital warts. *J. Cutan. Med. Surg.* **17** (**Suppl 2**): S55–S60.

30 Centers for Disease Control and Prevention (2014). Recommendations for the laboratory-based detection of chlamydia trachomatis and Neisseria gonorrhoeae – 2014. *MMWR Recomm. Rep.* **63** (**RR-02**): 1–19.

31 Knox, J., Tabrizi, S.N., Miller, P. et al. (2002). Evaluation of self-collected samples in contrast to practitioner-collected samples for detection of Chlamydia trachomatis, Neisseria gonorrhoeae, and Trichomonas vaginalis by polymerase chain reaction among women living in remote areas. *Sex. Transm. Dis.* **29** (**11**): 647–654.

32 Masek, B.J., Arora, N., Quinn, N. et al. (2009). Performance of three nucleic acid amplification tests for detection of Chlamydia trachomatis and Neisseria gonorrhoeae by use of self-collected vaginal swabs obtained via an internet-based screening program. *J. Clin. Microbiol.* **47** (**6**): 1663–1667. doi: 10.1128/JCM.02387-08.

33 Michel, C.-E.C., Sonnex, C., Carne, C.A. et al. (2007). Chlamydia trachomatis load at matched anatomic sites: implications for screening strategies. *J. Clin. Microbiol.* **45** (**5**): 1395–1402. doi: 10.1128/JCM.00100-07.

34 Schachter, J., Chernesky, M.A., Willis, D.E. et al. (2005). Vaginal swabs are the specimens of choice when screening for Chlamydia trachomatis and Neisseria gonorrhoeae: results from a Multicenter evaluation of the APTIMA assays for both infections. *Sex. Transm. Dis.* **32** (**12**): 725.

35 Krieger, J.N., Tam, M.R., Stevens, C.E. et al. (1988). Diagnosis of Trichomoniasis: comparison of conventional wet-mount examination with Cytologic studies, cultures, and monoclonal antibody staining of direct specimens. *JAMA* **259** (**8**): 1223–1227. doi: 10.1001/jama.1988.03720080057028.

36 Wiese, W., Patel, S.R., Patel, S.C. et al. (2000). A meta-analysis of the Papanicolaou smear and wet mount for the diagnosis of vaginal trichomoniasis. *Am. J. Med.* **108** (**4**): 301–308. doi: 10.1016/S0002-9343 (99)00466-0.

37 Nye, M.B., Schwebke, J.R., and Body, B.A. (2009). Comparison of APTIMA Trichomonas vaginalis transcription-mediated amplification to wet mount microscopy, culture, and polymerase chain reaction for diagnosis of trichomoniasis in men and women. *Am. J. Obstet. Gynecol.* **200** (**2**): 188.e1–188.e7. doi: 10.1016/j.ajog.2008.10.005.

38 Hobbs, M.M. and Seña, A.C. (2013). Modern diagnosis of Trichomonas vaginalis infection. *Sex. Transm. Infect.* **89** (**6**): 434–438. doi: 10.1136/sextrans-2013-051057.

39 Mobley, V.L., Hobbs, M.M., Lau, K. et al. (2012). Mycoplasma genitalium infection in women attending a sexually transmitted infection clinic: diagnostic specimen type, coinfections, and predictors. *Sex. Transm. Dis.* **39** (**9**): 706–709. doi: 10.1097/OLQ.0b013e318255de03.

40 Jensen, J.S., Björnelius, E., Dohn, B., and Lidbrink, P. (2004). Comparison of first void urine and urogenital swab specimens for detection of mycoplasma genitalium and chlamydia trachomatis by polymerase chain reaction in patients attending a sexually transmitted disease clinic. *Sex. Transm. Dis.* **31** (**8**): 499–507.

41 Casin, I., Vexiau-Robert, D., La Salmonière De, P. et al. (2002). High prevalence of mycoplasma genitalium in the lower genitourinary tract of women attending a sexually transmitted disease clinic in Paris, France. *Sex. Transm. Dis.* **29** (**6**): 353–359.

42 Goldenberg, R.L., Culhane, J.F., Iams, J.D., and Romero, R. (2008). Epidemiology and causes of preterm birth. *The Lancet* **371** (**9606**): 75–84. doi: 10.1016/S0140-6736(08)60074-4.

43 FDCAP, C.D.C. (2012). Update to CDC's sexually transmitted diseases treatment guidelines, 2010: oral cephalosporins no longer a recommended treatment for gonococcal infections. *MMWR Morb. Mortal. Wkly. Rep.* **61** (**31**): 590–594.

44 Handsfield, H.H., Hogben, M., and Schillinger, J. (2006). *Expedited Partner Therapy in the Management of Sexually Transmitted Diseases*. Atlanta, GA: Centers for Disease Control and Prevention. US Department of Health and Human Services.

45 Lau, C.Y. and Qureshi, A.K. (2002). Azithromycin versus doxycycline for genital chlamydial infections: a meta-analysis of randomized clinical trials. *Sex. Transm. Dis.* **29** (**9**): 497–502. doi: 10.1097/00007435-200209000-00001.

46 Le Cleach, L., Trinquart, L., and Do, G. (2014). Oral antiviral therapy for prevention of genital herpes outbreaks in immunocompetent and nonpregnant patients. *Cochrane Database Syst. Rev.* CD009036. doi: 10.1002/14651858.CD009036.pub2/pdf/standard.

47 Koelle, D.M. and Wald, A. (2000). Herpes simplex virus: the importance of asymptomatic shedding. *J. Antimicrob. Chemoth.* **45** (**suppl 4**): 1–8. doi: 10.1093/jac/45.suppl_4.1.

48 Wald, A., Zeh, J., Barnum, G. et al. (1996). Suppression of subclinical shedding of herpes simplex virus type 2 with acyclovir. *Ann. Intern. Med.* **124** (**1_Part_1**): 8–15. doi: 10.7326/0003-4819-124-1_Part_1-199601010-00002.

49 Forna, F. and Gülmezoglu, A.M. (1996). *Interventions for Treating Trichomoniasis in Women* (ed. F. Forna). Chichester, UK: Wiley. doi: 10.1002/14651858.cd000218.

50 Peterman, T.A., Tian, L.H., Metcalf, C.A. et al. (2006). High incidence of new sexually transmitted infections in the year following a sexually transmitted infection: a case for rescreening. *Ann. Intern. Med.* **145** (**8**): 564–572. doi: 10.7326/0003-4819-145-8-200610170-00005.

51 Bissessor, M., Tabrizi, S.N., Twin, J. et al. (2015). Macrolide resistance and azithromycin failure in a mycoplasma genitalium-infected cohort and response of azithromycin failures to alternative antibiotic regimens. *Clin. Infect. Dis.* **60** (**8**): 1228–1236. doi: 10.1093/cid/ciu1162.

52 Jensen, J.S., Bradshaw, C.S., Tabrizi, S.N. et al. (2008). Azithromycin treatment failure in mycoplasma genitalium-positive patients with nongonococcal urethritis is associated with induced macrolide resistance. *Clin. Infect. Dis.* **47** (**12**): 1546–1553. doi: 10.1086/593188.

53 Yanofsky, V.R., Patel, R.V., and Goldenberg, G. (2012). Genital warts: a comprehensive review. *J. Clin. Aesthet. Dermatol.* **5** (**6**): 25–36.

54 Kumar, B. and Narang, T. (2011). Local and systemic adverse effects to topical imiquimod due to systemic immune stimulation. *Sex. Transm. Infect.* doi: 10.1136/sextrans-2011-050025.

55 Tatti, S., Swinehart, J.M., Thielert, C. et al. (2008). Sinecatechins,

a defined green tea extract, in the treatment of external Anogenital warts: a randomized controlled trial. *Obstet. Gynecol.* **111** (**6**): 1371. doi: 10.1097/AOG.0b013e3181719b60.

56 Siegel, J.D., Rhinehart, E., Jackson, M., and Chiarello, L. (2007). Guideline for isolation precautions: preventing transmission of infectious agents in health care settings. *Am. J. Infect. Control* doi: 10.1016/j.ajic.2007.10.007.

57 Hollier, L.M. and Wendel, G.D. (2008). *Third Trimester Antiviral Prophylaxis for Preventing Maternal Genital Herpes Simplex Virus (HSV) Recurrences and Neonatal Infection* (ed. L.M. Hollier). Chichester, UK: John Wiley & Sons, Ltd. doi: 10.1002/14651858.CD004946.pub2.

58 Whitley, R., Davis, E.A., and Suppapanya, N. (2007). Incidence of neonatal herpes simplex virus infections in a managed-care population. *Sex. Transm. Dis.* **34** (**9**): 704. doi: 10.1097/01.olq.0000258432.33412.e2.

59 Brown, Z.A., Benedetti, J., and Ashley, R. (1991). Neonatal herpes simplex virus infection in relation to asymptomatic maternal infection at the time of labor. *N. Engl. J. Med.* **324**: 1247–1252.

60 Gulmezoglu, A.M. (2013). Interventions for trichomoniasis in pregnancy (review). *Cochrane Database Syst. Rev.* 1–18. doi: 10.1002/14651858.CD000220.pub2.

61 Vouga, M., Greub, G., Prod'hom, G. et al. (2014). Treatment of genital mycoplasma in colonized pregnant women in late pregnancy is associated with a lower rate of premature labour and neonatal complications. *Clin. Microbiol. Infect.* **20** (**10**): 1074–1079. doi: 10.1111/1469-0691.12686.

62 Larsen, B. and Hwang, J. (2010). Mycoplasma, Ureaplasma, and adverse pregnancy outcomes: a fresh look. *Infect. Dis. Obstet. Gynecol.* **2010**: doi: 10.1155/2010/521921.

7

CHAPTER 7
Uterine fibroids

David L. Kulak[1] and James H. Segars[2]
[1]*Department of Obstetrics and Gynecology, Johns Hopkins Medical Center, Baltimore, MD, USA*
[2]*National Institute of Child Health and Human Development, National Institutes of Health, Bethesda, MD, USA*

Introduction

Fibroids have been documented in medical literature for over 2500 years. Causes were often ascribed to melancholy and other female-associated diseases. Treatments were limited to medical herbs and expectant management. As medical advancements and science have progressed, so has the understanding and treatment of fibroids, and that change is now occurring at a rapid pace. Currently, fibroids are one of the most common diseases an obstetrician/gynecologist will encounter in his or her career. The disease can present with a wide variety of clinical symptoms from vaginal bleeding, pelvic pain, infertility, to poor obstetric outcomes. Yet, because of this variability in the fibroids and their presentation, the evidence guiding a provider can be overwhelming, confusing, or conflicting. It is often difficult to find clear and significant evidence for the care of women with fibroids. In this chapter we have summarized the current evidence-based medical and scientific knowledge on the causes, risks, sequelae, and treatments of fibroids with a focus on the Level I evidence behind that knowledge.

Epidemiology

Uterine leiomyomas, also known as fibroids, are benign smooth muscle monoclonal growths that are believed to originate from the uterine myometrium [1]. They are the most common benign neoplasm in reproductive age women, and are found in 70–80% of women by the age of menopause [2, 3]. Fibroids are significantly more common and more severe in blacks when compared to whites, and affect up to 80% of black women [4]. Black women are more likely to be diagnosed at a young age, have multiple fibroids, and undergo surgery for their fibroids compared to white women [5, 6]. Asians and Hispanics in the US have similar rates to whites [7, 8]. European studies have reported a lower disease incidence in these populations; however there too 50% of effected women are asymptomatic [9–11]. Fibroids become more common with increasing age, however as they are hormonally-sensitive their symptomatology, in white women specifically, drops off sharply with menopause [12, 13]. It is estimated that the direct cost of treating fibroids is \$4.1–9.4 billion in the US annually [14]; the total cost including lost work and obstetric sequelae may approach \$5.9–34.4 billion annually [15].

Classification

Leiomyomas are a heterogeneous disease process. Multiple methods have been proposed to classify fibroids that would account for both clinical significance and epidemiologic uniformity. The most commonly used system of classification, classifies fibroids in comparison to the uterine layers: submucosal, intramural, and subserosal [16]. Submucosal, refers to the region that is below the endothelium, the term is actually a misnomer as the uterus does not contain any mucosal tissue, the term "subendothelial" would be more accurate [17]. Intramural fibroids are those that do not distort the endometrial cavity and <50% protrusion into the serosal surface. Subserosal are then defined as those with >50% protrusion into the serosal surface [18]. Classification for submucosal fibroids has been further subdivided to allow for greater clinical significance. The ESHRE/ESGE classification system further subdivides submucosal fibroids into three categories. Type 0 are >90% within the uterine cavity and are also called pedunculated or intra-cavitary. Type I are sessile submucosal fibroids that are >50% in the cavity, and type II are <50% in the cavity [19]. A more detailed classification system known as the STEP W system, that includes fibroid size, location, and depth of invasion has been proposed with the goal of more accurately predicting the success of treatment [20, 21]. This new system has not gained widespread acceptance. There is currently no widely used or universally accepted classification system that takes into account location, size, and number of fibroids.

Evidence-Based Obstetrics and Gynecology, First Edition. Edited by Errol R. Norwitz, Carolyn M. Zelop, David A. Miller, and David L. Keefe.

Etiology

The etiology of fibroids is not well understood, and rather than a single disease process, there appear to be at least two types of fibroids: genetic or common (sporadic) fibroids. The best characterized cause of genetic fibroids in both North America and Europe, are those due to hereditary leiomyomatosis and renal cell carcinoma (HLRCC). These cellular fibroids are associated with fumarate hydratase gene mutations and more severe disease [22–24]. For fibroids not related to HLRCC, a genetic predisposition seems likely, as there is high racial correlation and first degree relatives of women with fibroids have a 2.5 times greater risk of developing fibroids themselves [25]. Genetic studies of fibroid tissue have shown mutations that increase the HOX gene, catechol-o-methyltransferase (COMT) expression, and lower retinoic acid [26–28]. Karyotype studies of the tumors themselves show that up to 40% of fibroids have at least one anomaly [29]. It should also be noted that as fibroids are monoclonal neoplasms, and within one uterus, each may have a different genotype.

Fibroids are hormonally responsive, sensitive to both estrogen and progesterone, and thus different physiologic states that effect or change the hormonal milieu may affect fibroid growth [12]. Early menarche, nulliparity, and elevated BMI are associated with higher levels of estrogen and are also associated with increased risk of fibroid disease [5, 30]. Fibroids express much higher levels of aromatase within them, creating a microenvironment with supra-physiologic estrogen levels; the levels of fibroid aromatase compared to normal myometrium are 38-fold higher in white women and 83-fold higher in black women [31]. Estrogen has traditionally been viewed as the primary cause of fibroid proliferation and growth, however it is now clear that without progesterone, estrogens do not cause fibroid growth or even maintenance of fibroid size [32]. Furthermore, lack of estrogen in the presence of progesterone does not lead to fibroid regression. Progesterone antagonists cause shrinkage of fibroid tissue [33–35].

The inciting event for fibroid development may be related to inflammatory and hyperplastic processes. It appears that seedling fibroids develop in areas of myometrial hyperplasia (MMH) and disordered collagen, and afterword become neoplastic [36, 37]. Myometrial smooth muscle cells (MSMCs) can react in different ways to inflammation, and fibroids cells, which communicate via autocrine and paracrine pathways, contain all markers of inflammation including cyclo-oxygenase and lipo-oxygenase [38]. Fibroids have fewer progenitor/stem cells [39] and lower levels of anti-fibrotic factors such as vitamin D3 [40]. It has been suggested that certain risk factors for fibroids may be the source of the inciting inflammation or irritation of MSMC. Hypertension, more specifically diastolic hypertension increases the risk by 24% of symptomatic fibroids, this correlation was also incremental or graded in that for every 10 mmHg increase in BP there was an 8–10% increase in risk of fibroids [41]. It is postulated that this relationship arises from myometrial injury or cytokine release due to hypertension. Studies have linked fibroids to infections of smooth muscle such as Chagas' disease [42].

Fibroids are very dynamic and it has become apparent that every fibroid behaves differently. A recent longitudinal study that followed fibroid growth with serial MRIs reported there was an overall growth of 9% over a six month period for fibroids. However fibroid growth patterns could be further classified: 34% were rapidly growing (>20% increase in size over 6 m) and 7% were spontaneously regressing (> decrease in size over 6 m). Interestingly, even individual fibroids in the same patient behaved independently, showing that factors other than circulating hormone levels drive fibroid growth. Additionally, the study found that in white women over age 45, growth slowed to 2%; however this was not the case for black women at the same age, had an average fibroid growth rate of 15% in six months [13]. Studies assessing fibroid growth and regression relating to pregnancy found that pregnancy eliminated 36% of fibroids and 72% had >50% fibroid regression [34]. In summary, while fibroids tend to grow over time, within one uterus each may behave differently, and some will shrink, especially post-partum.

Diagnosis

While clinical history and physical exam are always crucial to the assessment of fibroids, imaging studies are key for proper diagnosis and treatment. Fibroids can be evaluated with many different imaging modalities, each with its own sensitivity, convenience, and cost. The most widely used and generally readily accessible method is ultrasound. This method is limited by its inability to fully assess a fibroids relationship to endometrium, distinguish adenomyosis from myometrial contractions from fibroids, and ovarian or adnexal masses from pedunculated fibroids. Saline infusion sonograms, with or without 3D technology, are able to articulate the endometrial surfaces and more clearly define the nature of submucosal fibroids. Hysterosalpingograms are only able to indirectly characterize the endometrial cavity, but have the advantage of showing tubal status or patency, which may be effected by fibroids or other sources. MRI is now the method of choice as it is able to delineate a fibroid's proximity to other tissues including endometrium, bowel, and bladder. MRI is also able to distinguish adenomyosis, atypical cellular fibroids, sarcoma, and degenerating fibroids [43]. Historically, CT scans were used to assess the relationship of fibroids to surrounding organs or vessels; this modality is rarely used if MRI ultrasound is available. Surgical pathology remains the only method to definitively diagnose fibroids (see Figure 7.1, which shows ultrasound).

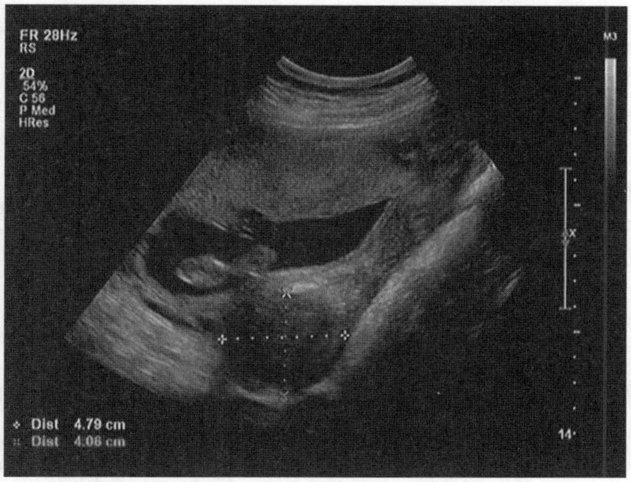

Figure 7.1 Sonographic image showing a single 4.8 × 4.1 cm posterior submucosal/intramural fibroid in early pregnancy. The fetus and placenta can be seen anterior to the fibroid.

Evidence-based approach to clinical management

Uterine fibroids can present with a multitude of clinical scenarios that stem from their differences in size, location, and number. The management of fibroids is thus based on the clinical signs and symptoms with which they present.

Vaginal bleeding is the most common complaint associated with fibroids. It is clear that fibroids are the source of abnormal uterine bleeding for many women, however no study has been able to correlate with it specific fibroid characteristics and predict with accuracy which fibroids will cause bleeding [10]. Submucosal and large fibroids >5 cm both increase the risk for abnormal bleeding [44]. The major cause of this bleeding is abnormal endometrium in the area around the fibroid. Other potential sources include the increased endometrial surface area [45], local endometrial atrophy [46], and global changes in the endometrium related to altered expression of the HOX gene [47]. Consistent with these findings is the increasing likelihood of global endometrial changes and glandular atrophy observed with large fibroids beginning at 4 cm, with 100% correlation by 8 cm [48]. Even those fibroids that do not physically distort the endometrial cavity but are within 5 mm of the cavity are likely to cause endometrial changes [46].

Pressure or pain from the fibroids is also a common presenting complaint. It is not uncommon for fibroids to grow to well over 20 cm in height or 10 cm in width. Additionally they can be found abutting the bladder anteriorly and the rectum posteriorly. Fibroids can cause urinary frequency, incontinence, and even renal failure by compressing the ureters. Posterior fibroids can cause constipation, obstruction, and diarrhea. As fibroids age, they may become calcified and hard, exhibiting greater pressure on their surrounding tissue. A degenerating or twisting pedunculated fibroid can cause sudden onset and severe pain [49]. Women with fibroids were twice as likely to report severe non-cyclic pelvic pain (95% CI 0.9–7.6), although only a trend as the difference detected was not statistically significant [50, 51]. Of women undergoing hysterectomy for fibroid disease, black women are more likely to have severe pelvic pain, 59% vs. 40% for white women [52]. Cyclic pain or dysmenorrhea is not associated with fibroids [50, 51].

Dyspareunia is strongly associated with fibroids as patients with known fibroids were 40% more likely to have mild and 80% more likely to have severe dyspareunia when compared to their non-fibroid counterparts (95% CI 0.9–8.3), although again, only a trend but not statistically significant [50]. Anterior fibroids were more likely to cause deep dyspareunia than those in other locations [53].

Evidence-based pregnancy outcomes related to fibroids

Fibroids can affect pregnancy from preconception to the post-partum period (see Tables 7.1 and 7.2). They can cause infertility by obstructing fallopian tubes and impaired gamete transport [54]. As stated above fibroids cause both focal and global changes in the endometrium, altering its physiologic receptivity and its physical shape. Besides being hormonally sensitive, fibroids are also hormone generating. They can change the local hormone milieu and create a hyper-estrogenic environment, which can be inhospitable to an embryo; this is aside from the changes in HOX gene expression [55]. The clinical role of fibroids, and the characteristics of those fibroids that effect pregnancy rates and outcomes has been extensively studied. However, many studies lacked appropriate control groups or uniform study methods and thus the results are often contradictory [55]. Recently there have been a series of meta-analyses that summarize the evidence. In 2001, a meta-analysis concluded that women with fibroids had a relative risk (RR) of 1.7 for a

Table 7.1 Fibroid effect on fertility compared to age matched control

	Submucosal	Intramural	Large (>4–5 cm)	Small (<4–5 cm)	Subserosal
Pregnancy rate	↓↓[a]	↓[b]	↓↓	Depends on location	–
Live birth rate	↓↓[a]	↓[b]	–	–	–

↓ Decreased risk.
↓↓ Decreased risk, by more than 50%.
– No significant difference.
[a]Risk is removed if the fibroid is removed and returns are not significantly different from counterparts without fibroids.
[b]Risk does not change with removal of these fibroids.

Table 7.2 Fibroid effect on pregnancy compared to age matched control

	Submucosal	Intramural	Large(>4–5 cm)	Small(<4–5 cm)
Preterm labor	No clear evidence[a]	No clear evidence[a]	↑/↑↑	–
Cesarean section	↑↑	No clear evidence[a]	Evidence contradict: No dif vs. ↑↑	–
Post-partum hemorrhage	No clear evidence[a]	No clear evidence[a]	OR 1.8	–

↑ Increased risk.
↑↑ Increased risk, more than 200%.
– No significant difference.
[a]Studies are small, inconclusive, or contradictory.

spontaneous abortion after clinical pregnancy, the study also showed these patients had decreased RR, 0.7, for live births. These risks could have been secondary to the significantly worse prognosis for submucosal fibroids that had a RR of 0.36 for clinical pregnancy and 0.32 for live birth when compared to their normal counterparts [56]. To elucidate and further classify the risk, a more recent meta-analysis was performed that showed intramural fibroids decreased pregnancy rates, RR 0.8, and increased spontaneous abortion rates, RR 1.7 [57]. Both of these meta-analyses contained data from assisted reproductive technology (ART) cycles and spontaneous pregnancies. An Italian study focusing on women undergoing ART reported that the odds ratio for women with submucosal fibroids was 0.3 for both clinical pregnancy and live birth. For women with intramural fibroids the odds ratios were 0.8 for clinical pregnancy and 0.7 for live birth, respectively, when compared to the unaffected controls. The study also confirmed earlier evidence that subserosal fibroids were not correlated with decreased ART success rates [58]. The reduced pregnancy rates of women with intramural fibroids can be further divided by size. Those women with intramural fibroids that are greater than 4 cm had pregnancy rates of 12%, while those with smaller fibroids had pregnancy rates of 30%, similar to the general population [59].

After clinical pregnancy is established there are further risks associated with fibroids (see Table 7.2). Although it was commonly believed that fibroids were risk factors for many adverse obstetrical outcomes, there were few data to confirm these suspicions. As high-quality obstetric ultrasound became more frequently used, the data have consistently shown adverse outcomes associated with fibroids. Early studies showed that women with even one fibroid were about twice as likely to have cesarean section, 23% vs. 12% [60]. The study did not mention the indication for the cesarean sections, but it could have been impacted by an almost fourfold increased risk of malpresentation associated with submucosal fibroids [61]. More recent studies have confirmed a similarly increased risk of cesarean section in women with fibroids, but have also found a 1.5–2.5 fold increased risk of preterm delivery, almost sevenfold increase risk of preterm premature rupture of membranes (PPROM), 4.5 fold increased risk of short cervix, and increased risk of post-partum hemorrhage with a greater than 10-fold increased risk of receiving a blood transfusion [62–64]. Early evidence showed that the location of the fibroid with relation to the placenta was paramount in determining risk in pregnancy, while overall size played a less significant role [65]. More recent studies have confirmed that the risk of preterm labor is increased when the placenta is directly overlying the fibroid, or if there are multiple fibroids evident [61]. During pregnancy as many as 20% of women with known fibroids will have clinical evidence of fibroid degeneration, 50% of which will be confirmed with ultrasound [66]. Fortunately, for those women with fibroids that are able to conceive, carry the fetus to term and deliver, there is a high rate of fibroid resolution or shrinkage post-partum secondary to myometrial remodeling, hormonal flux, and uterine involution [12, 34].

Quantitative measures of fibroid disease

The ability to accurately qualify and quantify in an objective, replicable, and analytical system the symptoms of fibroid disease is crucial to any accurate and therefore meaningful epidemiologic, diagnostic, or therapeutic analysis or study. Many systems have been used and most focus on just one aspect of the disease.

For vaginal bleeding alkaline hematin (AH) is the gold standard. Alkaline hematin has been used as marker or quantitative correlate of hemoglobin since the 1940s. A method of extracting the substance from sanitary napkins for measuring menstrual blood loss has been in use in the US since the 1970s. This method is limited by the use of only specific sanitary napkins from which the alkaline hematin can be removed and specific labs with the capabilities of measuring the alkaline hematin. This method is prohibitively laborious and expensive. Thus, the pictorial blood loss assessment chart (PBAC) was created to simplify, using pictures, the assessment of menstrual blood loss. The PBAC system takes into account the degree to which each item of a sanitary napkin is soiled with blood as well as the total number of pads or tampons used. The system has an 80% sensitivity and specificity as a diagnostic test for menorrhagia, using alkaline hematin as the control. Since its advent in 1990, it has been used frequently as a qualitative and quantitative marker of menorrhagia, however alkaline hematin remains the gold standard [67].

To assess the bulk symptoms of fibroids The Medical Outcomes Study Short-Form 36 (SF-36) Health Survey was often applied. This 36-item self-administered questionnaire assesses eight categories of pain: physical function, physical role limitations, vitality, general health perceptions, bodily pain, social function, emotional role limitations, and mental health. The SF-36 has been used extensively as an indicator of health-related quality of life, and its reliability and validity are well documented [68]. Although the SF-36 had been well validated and extensively used in many disciplines including gynecology, it was not designed to assess for the specific somatic complaints and pain that can be related to fibroids.

To more accurately gauge fibroid related physical, psychological, social, and emotional pain from the patient's perspective, The Uterine Fibroid Symptom and Quality of Life Scale (UFSQOL) was created [51, 69]. The questionnaire succeeded in not only being internally valid, meaning that the same women would have similar scores within a relatively short time period, but also correlated well on the physical pain with the SF-36. It did not correlate well with the SF-36 on its other components bolstering the claim that it was a necessary tool for accurately assessing overall disease burden for women with fibroids, as their specific complaints and lifestyle modifications are different than people afflicted with other diseases [51, 69].

Evidence-based treatment of fibroids

It should be emphasized that treatment choices for fibroids are variable and cross a wide spectrum based on the patient's symptoms, age, parity, comorbidities, goals of care, and type of fibroid. Within the first year of care 94% of women with fibroids will have either a diagnostic or therapeutic procedure [15]. Treatment is generally recommended for symptomatic patients, as 77% of patients followed with expectant management will not improve over a 1-year period [70]. While hysterectomy is the definitive treatment for fibroids, it removes the possibility of a woman ever having her own biological children in the future without the use of a gestational surrogate. Although myomectomy, surgical removal of a fibroid, is fertility sparing, myomectomy carries significant comorbidities which will be discussed below. However, the spectrum of treatment choices for fibroids is rapidly changing and growing with the advent of new medical agents and the proliferation and development of new minimally invasive surgeries and procedures. While, medical treatments are only FDA approved to temporize symptoms pre-operatively or decrease surgical morbidity for those undergoing procedures, some medical strategies are used as long-term therapy, and in those instances adjunct add-back hormonal therapy is given.

Evidence-based medical treatment

Medical treatments act on different aspects of the hormone pathway, as fibroids are hormonally responsive as stated above. Leuprolide, a GnRH agonist which acts in-vivo as an antagonist when given continuously, is the only FDA-approved medical treatment for fibroids. GnRH agonists are generally used for between three and six months preoperatively, with their major benefits peaking at about three months. In that time, they are able to reduce fibroid size about 30% and overall uterine volume by as much as 65% [71, 72]. The reduction in size is likely secondary to vascular changes, alterations in osmotic regulation, and altered signaling pathways [73, 74]. In combination with supplemental iron, GnRH agonists have also been shown to improve hemoglobin levels by at least $2\,g\,dl^{-1}$ in 74% of women with fibroids and menorrhagia, as opposed to iron alone, which only caused that improvement in 46% of women [75]. Because GnRH agonists have such a significant effect on overall uterine volume, when given preoperatively, many women will be able to have a vaginal hysterectomy, a less morbid procedure, when otherwise they would have a needed a laparotomic hysterectomy [76]. If hysterectomy was performed by laparotomy there was no difference in blood loss for patients that were treated with GnRH agonists. For patients that undergo myomectomy after GnRH agonist use there may be a higher risk of recurrence: 8.8% for women treated with GnRH-a vs. 2.3% for those not treated ($P = 0.34$) [77]. The risks associated with GnRH agonists are related to its hypoestrogenic effects. As many as 95% of women undergoing treatment will complain of hot flushes, vaginal dryness or frontal headaches within the first eight weeks of use [78]. Additionally, if continued for six months, there was significant bone loss associated with its use [79]. To avoid these symptoms, add back hormonal therapy has been used. After cessation of therapy, uterine volume returns to its pretreatment size by four to six months, however 64% of women will remain asymptomatic for as long as one year [78].

Letrozole, an aromatase inhibitor, inhibits local estrogen biosynthesis, thus decreasing estrogen levels in the tissue. Since fibroids have extremely high levels of local aromatase [31] and consequently the ability to synthesize their own estrogen, fibroids are very sensitive to letrozole. Clinically, letrozole 2.5 mg has been shown to decrease fibroid size by over 40% in three months, with the greatest rate of shrinkage in the first month. It also has a significantly lower side effect profile than GnRH agonists with few patients complaining of hot flushes, and no measurable bone mineral density changes in three months [80, 81].

Letrozole treatment of fibroids, while effective, is currently an off-label use of the drug.

Newer research has focused on progesterone antagonists and selective progesterone receptor modulators (SPRMs), their effects on fibroids, and potential treatment modalities. The most basic treatment in this category is a direct progesterone antagonist, Mifepristone. A meta-analysis of mifepristone for fibroid treatment showed an amenorrhea rate of 63–100% of fibroid patients, as well as a 74% reduction in fibroid volume over six months, with effects seen as early as three months. However the unopposed estrogen caused a 10% rate of endometrial hyperplasia, all were simple without atypia [33]. Studies with low dose mifepristone showed lower rates of hyperplasia, however it was also less therapeutic [82]. To avoid the side effect of endometrial hyperplasia, a new class of agents called SPRMs have been developed. The most well-studied SPRMs are ulipristal acetate and asoprisnil [35, 83, 84]. A study of asoprisnil 25 mg suppressed uterine bleeding in 83% of affected women by 12 weeks. In that same time period, uterine volume dropped 17%. There was noted to be some non-physiologic endometrial proliferation but no hyperplasia was noted. Even lower doses, 5 and 10 mg, showed a statistically significant improvement in fibroid symptoms, however the change was not as great as that seen with the 25 mg [35]. A recent study of oral ulipristal 5 or 10 mg, was given to women with symptomatic fibroid disease and menorrhagia [83]. When compared to leuprolide, the study showed non-inferiority for 5 mg for improvement in vaginal bleeding; 89% leuprolide vs. 90% ulipristal. The 10 mg dose was shown to be superior; 98% improvement ($p = 0.04$). The time to amenorrhea was also significantly faster with the ulipristal group, 5–7 vs. 21 days with leuprolide. Overall uterine volume reduction was similar in all three groups: ulipristal 5 mg 36%, ulipristal 10 mg 42%, and leuprolide 53%, however the changes in the ulipristal group lasted longer after discontinuation of the therapy. The side effect profile was significantly lower with ulipristal, and only about 10% of the women complained of hot flushes. About 0.5% of women using the ulipristal developed endometrial hyperplasia (simple without atypia) [83]. Notably, women with fibroids had significantly diminished fibroid regression if they were using progestin-only-pills as a birth control method post-partum [34].

Additional strategies for management

Levonorgestrel releasing intrauterine device (IUD) (Mirena®) has been shown to greatly reduce bleeding in women with fibroids. In one study all women treated with the levonorgestrel intrauterine device (LNG-IUD) for menorrhagia associated fibroids, had significant improvement in their symptoms [85]. By 6–12 months after insertion 41–57% of women were amenorrheic [85, 86]. LNG-IUD has been shown to decrease overall uterine volume by 41%, but did not decrease fibroid volume [87]. As a clinical pearl: for peri-menopausal women with menorrhagia as their major complaint related to fibroids, LNG-IUD is an excellent choice as by the time it is removed they have often completed menopause and their symptoms may not return.

Although non-steroidal anti-inflammatory drug (NSAIDS) are often used as first line treatment, they have not been found to be helpful for fibroid associated menorrhagia [88]. NSAIDS have been found helpful for control of pain related to degenerating fibroids, specifically in pregnancy [89].

Evidence-based non-surgical treatments

Uterine artery embolization (UAE), introduced in 1995 [90], is a minimally invasive procedure that, via angio-catheter and fluoroscopy, deposits particulate emboli (usually polyvinyl alcohol) into the bilateral uterine arteries, thus significantly diminishing the blood to the uterus and fibroids. The uterus which has a relatively small oxygen need is adequately perfused via the peripheral utero-ovarian arteries. Fibroids subsequently undergo necrosis. The procedure is a substitute for hysterectomy as it not indicated for women who wish to preserve their fertility. Significant improvement in menorrhagia was observed in 80–90% of women after UAE and fibroid volume was decreased by 30–46%. These improvements lasted for at least two years, but 10% of women will need another procedure in that time. UAE has a higher safety and side effect profile than hysterectomy, as major side effects are nausea, vomiting, and pain from necrosis of fibroids within the first week after the procedure while hysterectomy patients had a greater blood loss, slower resumption of daily activities and longer hospital stays [91, 92]. When compared to myomectomy there were similar rates of significant symptomatic relief, however a greater percentage of women had complete relief after myomectomy, 70% vs. 46% respectively [93]. UAE is not recommended for women who to retain fertility as there is a risk of premature ovarian failure (POF) associated with scattered particulate that travel to the utero-ovarian artery as well as higher risks of placental abnormalities leading to placenta previa, accreta, and retained placenta [94]. Bulk symptoms were significantly improved with UAE, and urinary incontinence is actually 2.6 times more likely to improve with UAE when compared to hysterectomy [95]. UAE has not been shown to improve sexual symptoms associated with fibroids [96].

Magnetic resonance-guided high-intensity focused ultrasound (MRg-FUS or MR-HIFU) has been developed and used in multi-national studies. The procedure overall appears to have a high safety profile, the most common side effects are fever, nausea, and vomiting likely secondary to necrosis of the target fibroid, and 5% of women have had minor skin burns. Original data showed that 70% of women treated had significant improvement of the menorrhagia and bulk symptoms (including urinary, defecatory, sexual, and psychosocial) at six months and 50% at one year [97]. More recent data shows relief of symptoms in almost 90% of women at 3, 6, and 12 m periods. After one year, 7% of patients sought alternative treatments [98]. The improvement of fibroid related symptoms and shrinkage of fibroids appears to be sustained and long term and has been followed as long as three years [99]. A benefit of MRg-FUS is that it may be used in the patient seeking pregnancy.

Evidence-based surgical treatments

Surgical techniques to manage fibroids have changed with the advent of the hysteroscopy. Submucosal fibroids can now be removed with relatively minimal risk avoiding the potential for abdominal scarring and adhesion formation, large blood loss and collateral damage. Submucosal fibroids are a cause of infertility and pregnancy loss and they may also cause abnormal uterine bleeding (see above). Removal of submucosal fibroids has been shown to improve bleeding for over 80% of women with type 0 and type I fibroids, that rate drops to 68% for type II [100]. Pregnancy rates and outcomes are also significantly improved with treatment of submucosal fibroids. A meta-analysis, mostly with patients undergoing ART, showed an equivalent clinical pregnancy and live birth rate between women who underwent removal of submucosal fibroids and their counterparts without fibroids [56, 57]. Submucosal fibroids greater than 4 cm are often difficult to remove hysteroscopically because of difficulties with visualization and large fluid deficits. The advent of a hysteroscopic morcellator will likely allow for the resection of larger fibroids.

Intramural fibroids, depending on their size may present with bulk symptoms, abnormal uterine bleeding or infertility. Surgical removal via laparotomy, laparoscopy, or robotic-assisted laparoscopy improved both the bulk symptoms and bleeding as assessed by the UFS-QOL. Symptoms were significantly improved to a similar rate and quality of those patients that underwent UAE (including sexual function which is not statistically improved in either). Studies have consistently shown that robotic procedures do not improve outcome measures but do decrease post-operative pain and hospital stay. While initially robotic-assisted cases had longer operative times, this difference may be more a reflection of the learning curve of a new technology rather than an intrinsic difference [101, 102]. Ultimately though, as many as 62% of women will have recurrence of symptoms and about half of those will need further treatment including hysterectomy [103]. For fertility purposes, there is strong evidence from international studies and meta-analyses that the removal of small and medium sized fibroids do not improve pregnancy rates or outcomes [57, 104]. However, evidence suggests that removal of intramural fibroids that are greater than 5 cm does significantly improve both pregnancy rates and live birth rates from 15% to 33% and 12% to 25%, respectively [105].

The definitive and final treatment for fibroid disease is hysterectomy. Approximately 600 000 hysterectomies are performed annually in the US, the percentage however that are due to fibroids has dropped from 44.2% in 2000 to 38.7% in 2004 [106]. Hysterectomy is the most common non-medical intervention performed to treat fibroids, as it makes up almost 86% of all interventions [107]. Some studies in the past had shown that there was diminished sexual pleasure potential if the cervix was removed at the time of hysterectomy. Multiple large studies have since shown that there is no difference in sexual outcomes with approach to hysterectomy including abdominal as compared to vaginally and with and without removal of the cervix [108]. Although hysterectomy is the definitive treatment for fibroids, there are cases reports of benign metastases of fibroids to distant areas of the bodies including the lungs and major blood vessels [109, 110] (see Table 7.3).

Conclusion

Recent developments have led to new options for the treatment of fibroids. While there is certainly more work that needs to be done and treatments to be developed, clinicians now have a greater understanding of the factors that affect the development, growth, and behavior of fibroids. These new insights have spurred new medical treatment options, such as aromatase inhibitors and LNG-IUD, and the development of new classes of medicines, such as the SPRMs that are on the horizon. Minimally-invasive treatment options such as UAE and MR-HIFU have been shown to be effective. Surgical tools that allow for more aggressive treatment with less invasive procedures such as the hysteroscopic morcellator are being designed and used. On the horizon are preventative treatments or treatments that will allow for regression of disease and future fertility. The physician's armamentarium now contains a multitude of evidence-based options from genetically-driven molecular targets to advanced remotely-controlled robotic surgeries. These options, developed in the laboratory are now on the forefront of effectively treating millions of women galvanizing greater fertility, better obstetric outcomes, decreasing gynecologic morbidity, and significantly improving quality of life.

Table 7.3 Effects of treatment by modality

	Bleeding	Amenorrhea	Fibroid size	Other effects
GnRH-A	↓↓	↓↓ [a]	↓30% [b]	Hot flushes. Leads to bone loss after 6 mon of use.
LNG-IUD	↓↓	↓40% [a,c]	↓40% [b,d]	
Mifepristone	↓↓	↓↓60–65%[a]	↓40–74% [b]	Endometrial hyperplasia
SPRM	↓↓	↓↓	↓15–30% [b]	Greater improvement than GnRH-a
Letrozole	Likely ↓, however no studies mention rate.	–	↓45% [b]	
Abd-Myomectomy		–	↓↓	Improves fertility if large. Peritoneal scarring
Hsc Myomectomy	↓↓	–	↓↓	Improves fertility
UAE	↓↓	–/↓	↓↓0[b]	Contraindicated if desire fertility. Can lead to premature ovarian failure (POF) and placental anomalies.
MR-HIFU	↓↓	–	↓↓	

↓ Decreased risk.
↓↓ Decreased risk, by more than 50%.
– No significant difference.
[a]Percentage of treated patients who had amenorrhea.
[b]Percentage decreased during treatment period.
[c]After 1 yr of treatment.
[d]Uterine volume decrease, there was no decrease in fibroid volume.

Acknowledgments

The authors would like to acknowledge the support and advice of Drs. Alan DeCherney, Irwin Merkatz, and Erica Banks, without whom this work would not have been possible.

References

1 Walker, C.L. and Stewart, E.A. (2005). Uterine fibroids: the elephant in the room. *Science* **308** (**5728**): 1589–1592. Epub 2005/06/11.

2 Davis, B.J., Haneke, K.E., Miner, K. et al. (2009). The fibroid growth study: determinants of therapeutic intervention. *J. Women's Health (Larchmt)* **18** (**5**): 725–732. Epub 2009/04/16.

3 Cramer, S.F. and Patel, A. (1990). The frequency of uterine leiomyomas. *Am. J. Clin. Pathol.* **94** (**4**): 435–438. Epub 1990/10/01.

4 Baird, D.D. and Dunson, D.B. (2003). Why is parity protective for uterine fibroids? *Epidemiology* **14** (**2**): 247–250. Epub 2003/02/28.

5 Huyck, K.L., Panhuysen, C.I., Cuenco, K.T. et al. (2008). The impact of race as a risk factor for symptom severity and age at diagnosis of uterine leiomyomata among affected sisters. *Am. J. Obstet. Gynecol.* **198** (**2**): 168 e1–9 e1. Epub 2008/01/30.

6 Jacoby, V.L., Fujimoto, V.Y., Giudice, L.C. et al. (2010). Racial and ethnic disparities in benign gynecologic conditions and associated surgeries. *Am. J. Obstet. Gynecol.* **202** (**6**): 514–521. Epub 2010/05/01.

7 Marshall, L.M., Spiegelman, D., Barbieri, R.L. et al. (1997). Variation in the incidence of uterine leiomyoma among premenopausal women by age and race. *Obstet. Gynecol.* **90** (**6**): 967–973. Epub 1997/12/16.

8 Laughlin, S.K., Baird, D.D., Savitz, D.A. et al. (2009). Prevalence of uterine leiomyomas in the first trimester of pregnancy: an ultrasound-screening study. *Obstet. Gynecol.* **113** (**3**): 630–635. Epub 2009/03/21.

9 Borgfeldt, C. and Andolf, E. (2000). Transvaginal ultrasonographic findings in the uterus and the endometrium: low prevalence of leiomyoma in a random sample of women age 25-40 years. *Acta Obstet Gynecol Scand.* **79** (**3**): 202–207. Epub 2000/03/15.

10 Marino, J.L., Eskenazi, B., Warner, M. et al. (2004). Uterine leiomyoma and menstrual cycle characteristics in a population-based cohort study. *Hum. Reprod.* **19** (**10**): 2350–2355. Epub 2004/07/10.

11 Chen, C.R., Buck, G.M., Courey, N.G. et al. (2001). Risk factors for uterine fibroids among women undergoing tubal sterilization. *Am. J. Epidemiol.* **153** (**1**): 20–26. Epub 2001/02/13.

12 Cook, J.D. and Walker, C.L. (2004). Treatment strategies for uterine leiomyoma: the role of hormonal modulation. *Semin. Reprod. Med.* **22** (**2**): 105–111. Epub 2004/05/28.

13 Peddada, S.D., Laughlin, S.K., Miner, K. et al. (2008). Growth of uterine leiomyomata among premenopausal black and white women. *Proc. Natl. Acad. Sci. U S A* **105** (**50**): 19887–19892. Epub 2008/12/03.

14 Flynn, M., Jamison, M., Datta, S., and Myers, E. (2006). Health care resource use for uterine fibroid tumors in the United States. *Am. J. Obstet. Gynecol.* **195** (**4**): 955–964. Epub 2006/05/26.

15 Cardozo, E.R., Clark, A.D., Banks, N.K. et al. (2011). The estimated annual cost of uterine leiomyomata in the United States. *Am. J. Obstet. Gynecol.* Epub 2012/01/17.

16 Tindall, V.R. (1987). Tumours of the corpus uteri. In: *Jeffcoate's Principles of Gynaecology*, 417–444.

17 Maguire, M.S.J. (2008). *The Endometrium: Molecular, Cellular, and Clinical Perspectives*, 2e. London, UK: Informa Healthcare.

18 Bajekal, N. and Li, T.C. (2000). Fibroids, infertility and pregnancy wastage. *Hum. Reprod. Update* **6** (**6**): 614–620. Epub 2000/12/29.

19 Wamsteker, K., Emanuel, M.H., and de Kruif, J.H. (1993). Transcervical hysteroscopic resection of submucous fibroids for abnormal uterine bleeding: results regarding the degree of intramural extension. *Obstet. Gynecol.* **82** (**5**): 736–740. Epub 1993/11/01.

20 Lasmar, R.B., Barrozo, P.R., Dias, R., and Oliveira, M.A. (2005). Submucous myomas: a new presurgical classification to evaluate the viability of hysteroscopic surgical treatment--preliminary report. *J. Minim. Invasive Gynecol.* **12** (**4**): 308–311. Epub 2005/07/23.

21 Lasmar, R.B., Xinmei, Z., Indman, P.D. et al. (2011). Feasibility of a new system of classification of submucous myomas: a multicenter study. *Fertil. Steril.* **95** (**6**): 2073–2077. Epub 2011/02/22.

22 Linehan, W.M., Walther, M.M., and Zbar, B. (2003). The genetic basis of cancer of the kidney. *J. Urol.* **170** (**6 Pt 1**): 2163–2172. Epub 2003/11/25.

23 Stewart, L., Glenn, G.M., Stratton, P. et al. (2008). Association of germline mutations in the fumarate hydratase gene and uterine fibroids in women with hereditary leiomyomatosis and renal cell cancer. *Arch. Dermatol.* **144** (**12**): 1584–1592. Epub 2008/12/17.

24 Toro, J.R., Nickerson, M.L., Wei, M.H. et al. (2003). Mutations in the fumarate hydratase gene cause hereditary leiomyomatosis and renal cell cancer in families in North America. *Am. J. Hum. Genet.* **73** (**1**): 95–106. Epub 2003/05/29.

25 Schwartz, S.M., Marshall, L.M., and Baird, D.D. (2000). Epidemiologic contributions to understanding the etiology of uterine leiomyomata. *Environ. Health Perspect.* **108** (**Suppl 5**): 821–827. Epub 2000/10/19.

26 Rackow, B.W. and Arici, A. (2006). Options for medical treatment of myomas. *Obstet. Gynecol. Clin. North Am.* **33** (**1**): 97–113. Epub 2006/03/01.

27 Gooden, K.M., Schroeder, J.C., North, K.E. et al. (2007). Val153Met polymorphism of catechol-O-methyltransferase and prevalence of uterine leiomyomata. *Reprod. Sci.* **14** (**2**): 117–120. Epub 2007/07/20.

28 Catherino, W.H. and Malik, M. (2007). Uterine leiomyomas express a molecular pattern that lowers retinoic acid exposure. *Fertil. Steril.* **87** (**6**): 1388–1398. Epub 2007/02/06.

29 Bowden, W., Skorupski, J., Kovanci, E., and Rajkovic, A. (2009). Detection of novel copy number variants in uterine leiomyomas using high-resolution SNP arrays. *Mol. Hum. Reprod.* **15** (**9**): 563–568. Epub 2009/07/02.

30 Marshall, L.M., Spiegelman, D., Manson, J.E. et al. (1998). Risk of uterine leiomyomata among premenopausal women in relation to body size and cigarette smoking. *Epidemiology* **9** (**5**): 511–517. Epub 1998/09/08.

31 Ishikawa, H., Reierstad, S., Demura, M. et al. (2009). High aromatase expression in uterine leiomyoma tissues of African-American women. *J. Clin. Endocrinol. Metab.* **94** (**5**): 1752–1756. Epub 2009/02/26.

32 Ishikawa, H., Ishi, K., Serna, V.A. et al. (2010). Progesterone is essential for maintenance and growth of uterine leiomyoma. *Endocrinology* **151** (**6**): 2433–2442. Epub 2010/04/09.

33 Steinauer, J., Pritts, E.A., Jackson, R., and Jacoby, A.F. (2004). Systematic review of mifepristone for the treatment of uterine leiomyomata. *Obstet. Gynecol.* **103** (**6**): 1331–1336. Epub 2004/06/03.

34 Laughlin, S.K., Hartmann, K.E., and Baird, D.D. (2011). Postpartum factors and natural fibroid regression. *Am. J. Obstet. Gynecol.* **204** (**6**): 496 e1–496 e6. Epub 2011/04/16.

35 Chwalisz, K., Larsen, L., Mattia-Goldberg, C. et al. (2007). A randomized, controlled trial of asoprisnil, a novel selective progesterone receptor modulator, in women with uterine leiomyomata. *Fertil. Steril.* **87** (**6**): 1399–1412. Epub 2007/02/20.

36 Cramer, S.F., Mann, L., Calianese, E. et al. (2009). Association of seedling myomas with myometrial hyperplasia. *Hum. Pathol.* **40** (**2**): 218–225. Epub 2008/09/19.

37 Leppert, P.C., Baginski, T., Prupas, C. et al. (2004). Comparative ultrastructure of collagen fibrils in uterine leiomyomas and normal myometrium. *Fertil. Steril.* **82** (**Suppl 3**): 1182–1187. Epub 2004/10/12.

38 Chegini, N. (2010). Proinflammatory and profibrotic mediators: principal effectors of leiomyoma development as a fibrotic disorder. *Semin. Reprod. Med.* **28** (**3**): 180–203. Epub 2010/04/24.

39 Chang, H.L., Senaratne, T.N., Zhang, L. et al. (2010). Uterine leiomyomas exhibit fewer stem/progenitor cell characteristics when compared with corresponding normal myometrium. *Reprod. Sci.* **17** (**2**): 158–167. Epub 2009/10/07.

40 Halder, S.K., Goodwin, J.S., and Al-Hendy, A. (2011). 1, 25-Dihydroxyvitamin D3 reduces TGF-beta 3-induced fibrosis-related gene expression in human uterine leiomyoma

cells. *J. Clin. Endocrinol. Metab.* **96** (**4**): E754–E762. Epub 2011/02/04.

41 Boynton-Jarrett, R., Rich-Edwards, J., Malspeis, S. et al. (2005). A prospective study of hypertension and risk of uterine leiomyomata. *Am. J. Epidemiol.* **161** (**7**): 628–638. Epub 2005/03/23.

42 Murta, E.F., Oliveira, G.P., Prado Fde, O. et al. (2002). Association of uterine leiomyoma and Chagas' disease. *Am. J. Trop. Med. Hyg.* **66** (**3**): 321–324. Epub 2002/07/26.

43 Parker, W.H. (2012). The utility of MRI for the surgical treatment of women with uterine fibroid tumors. *Am. J. Obstet. Gynecol.* **206** (**1**): 31–36. Epub 2011/10/11.

44 Wegienka, G., Baird, D.D., Hertz-Picciotto, I. et al. (2003). Self-reported heavy bleeding associated with uterine leiomyomata. *Obstet. Gynecol.* **101** (**3**): 431–437. Epub 2003/03/15.

45 Sehgal, N. and Haskins, A.L. (1960). The mechanism of uterine bleeding in the presence of fibromyomas. *Am. Surg.* **26**: 21–23. Epub 1960/01/01.

46 Patterson-Keels, L.M., Selvaggi, S.M., Haefner, H.K., and Randolph, J.F. Jr. (1994). Morphologic assessment of endometrium overlying submucosal leiomyomas. *J. Reprod. Med.* **39** (**8**): 579–584. Epub 1994/08/01.

47 Rackow, B.W. and Taylor, H.S. (2010). Submucosal uterine leiomyomas have a global effect on molecular determinants of endometrial receptivity. *Fertil. Steril.* **93** (**6**): 2027–2034. Epub 2008/06/17.

48 Sharma, S.P., Misra, S.D., and Mittal, V.P. (1979). Endometrial changes--a criterion for the diagnosis of submucous uterine leiomyoma. *Indian J. Pathol. Microbiol.* **22** (**1**): 33–36. Epub 1979/01/01.

49 Stewart, E.A. (2001). Uterine fibroids. *Lancet* **357** (**9252**): 293–298. Epub 2001/02/24.

50 Lippman, S.A., Warner, M., Samuels, S. et al. (2003). Uterine fibroids and gynecologic pain symptoms in a population-based study. *Fertil. Steril.* **80** (**6**): 1488–1494. Epub 2003/12/12.

51 Coyne, K.S., Margolis, M.K., Bradley, L.D. et al. (2012). Further validation of the uterine fibroid symptom and quality-of-life questionnaire. *Value Health* **15** (**1**): 135–142. Epub 2012/01/24.

52 Kjerulff, K.H., Langenberg, P., Seidman, J.D. et al. (1996). Uterine leiomyomas. Racial differences in severity, symptoms and age at diagnosis. *J. Reprod. Med.* **41** (**7**): 483–490. Epub 1996/07/01.

53 Ferrero, S., Abbamonte, L.H., Giordano, M. et al. (2006). Uterine myomas, dyspareunia, and sexual function. *Fertil. Steril.* **86** (**5**): 1504–1510. Epub 2006/10/31.

54 Ubaldi, F., Tournaye, H., Camus, M. et al. (1995). Fertility after hysteroscopic myomectomy. *Hum. Reprod. Update* **1** (**1**): 81–90. Epub 1995/01/01.

55 Ezzati, M., Norian, J.M., and Segars, J.H. (2009). Management of uterine fibroids in the patient pursuing assisted reproductive technologies. *Womens Health (Lond Engl).* **5** (**4**): 413–421. Epub 2009/07/10.

56 Pritts, E.A. (2001). Fibroids and infertility: a systematic review of the evidence. *Obstet. Gynecol. Surv.* **56** (**8**): 483–491. Epub 2001/08/10.

57 Pritts, E.A., Parker, W.H., and Olive, D.L. (2009). Fibroids and infertility: an updated systematic review of the evidence. *Fertil. Steril.* **91** (**4**): 1215–1223. Epub 2008/03/15.

58 Somigliana, E., Vercellini, P., Daguati, R. et al. (2007). Fibroids and female reproduction: a critical analysis of the evidence. *Hum. Reprod. Update* **13** (**5**): 465–476. Epub 2007/06/23.

59 Oliveira, F.G., Abdelmassih, V.G., Diamond, M.P. et al. (2004). Impact of subserosal and intramural uterine fibroids that do not distort the endometrial cavity on the outcome of in vitro fertilization-intracytoplasmic sperm injection. *Fertil. Steril.* **81** (**3**): 582–587. Epub 2004/03/24.

60 Vergani, P., Ghidini, A., Strobelt, N. et al. (1994). Do uterine leiomyomas influence pregnancy outcome? *Am. J. Perinatol.* **11** (**5**): 356–358. Epub 1994/09/01.

61 Ouyang, D.W., Economy, K.E., and Norwitz, E.R. (2006). Obstetric complications of fibroids. *Obstet. Gynecol. Clin. North Am.* **33** (**1**): 153–169. Epub 2006/03/01.

62 Shavell, V.I., Thakur, M., Sawant, A. et al. (2012). Adverse obstetric outcomes associated with sonographically identified large uterine fibroids. *Fertil. Steril.* **97** (**1**): 107–110. Epub 2011/11/22.

63 Stout, M.J., Odibo, A.O., Graseck, A.S. et al. (2010). Leiomyomas at routine second-trimester ultrasound examination and adverse obstetric outcomes. *Obstet. Gynecol.* **116** (**5**): 1056–1063. Epub 2010/10/23.

64 Qidwai, G.I., Caughey, A.B., and Jacoby, A.F. (2006). Obstetric outcomes in women with sonographically identified uterine leiomyomata. *Obstet. Gynecol.* **107** (**2 Pt 1**): 376–382. Epub 2006/02/02.

65 Rosati, P., Bellati, U., Exacoustos, C. et al. (1989). Uterine myoma in pregnancy: ultrasound study. *Int. J. Gynaecol. Obstet.* **28** (**2**): 109–117. Epub 1989/02/01.

66 Lev-Toaff, A.S., Coleman, B.G., Arger, P.H. et al. (1987). Leiomyomas in pregnancy: sonographic study. *Radiology* **164** (**2**): 375–380. Epub 1987/08/01.

67 Higham, J.M., O'Brien, P.M., and Shaw, R.W. (1990). Assessment of menstrual blood loss using a pictorial chart. *Br. J. Obstet. Gynaecol.* **97** (**8**): 734–739. Epub 1990/08/01.

68 Ware, J.E. Jr. and Sherbourne, C.D. (1992). The MOS 36-item short-form health survey (SF-36). I. Conceptual framework and item selection. *Med. Care* **30** (**6**): 473–483. Epub 1992/06/11.

69 Spies, J.B., Coyne, K., Guaou Guaou, N. et al. (2002). The UFS-QOL, a new disease-specific symptom and health-related quality of life questionnaire for leiomyomata. *Obstet. Gynecol.* **99** (**2**): 290–300. Epub 2002/01/30.

70 Parker, W.H. (2007). Uterine myomas: management. *Fertil. Steril.* **88** (**2**): 255–271. Epub 2007/07/31.

71 Schlaff, W.D., Zerhouni, E.A., Huth, J.A. et al. (1989). A placebo-controlled trial of a depot gonadotropin-releasing hormone analogue (leuprolide) in the treatment of uterine

leiomyomata. *Obstet. Gynecol.* **74** (**6**): 856–862. Epub 1989/12/01.

72 Olive, D.L., Lindheim, S.R., and Pritts, E.A. (2004). Non-surgical management of leiomyoma: impact on fertility. *Curr. Opin. Obstet. Gynecol.* **16** (**3**): 239–243. Epub 2004/05/07.

73 McCarthy-Keith, D.M., Malik, M., Britten, J. et al. (2011). Gonadotropin-releasing hormone agonist increases expression of osmotic response genes in leiomyoma cells. *Fertil. Steril.* **95** (**7**): 2383–2387. Epub 2011/04/19.

74 Xu, J., Luo, X., and Chegini, N. (2003). Differential expression, regulation, and induction of Smads, transforming growth factor-beta signal transduction pathway in leiomyoma, and myometrial smooth muscle cells and alteration by gonadotropin-releasing hormone analog. *J. Clin. Endocrinol. Metab.* **88** (**3**): 1350–1361. Epub 2003/03/12.

75 Stovall, T.G., Muneyyirci-Delale, O., Summitt, R.L. Jr., and Scialli, A.R. (1995). GnRH agonist and iron versus placebo and iron in the anemic patient before surgery for leiomyomas: a randomized controlled trial. Leuprolide acetate study group. *Obstet. Gynecol.* **86** (**1**): 65–71. Epub 1995/07/01.

76 Vercellini, P., Crosignani, P.G., Mangioni, C. et al. (1998). Treatment with a gonadotrophin releasing hormone agonist before hysterectomy for leiomyomas: results of a multicentre, randomised controlled trial. *Br. J. Obstet. Gynaecol.* **105** (**11**): 1148–1154. Epub 1998/12/16.

77 Vercellini, P., Trespidi, L., Zaina, B. et al. (2003). Gonadotropin-releasing hormone agonist treatment before abdominal myomectomy: a controlled trial. *Fertil. Steril.* **79** (**6**): 1390–1395. Epub 2003/06/12.

78 Letterie, G.S., Coddington, C.C., Winkel, C.A. et al. (1989). Efficacy of a gonadotropin-releasing hormone agonist in the treatment of uterine leiomyomata: long-term follow-up. *Fertil. Steril.* **51** (**6**): 951–956. Epub 1989/06/01.

79 Leather, A.T., Studd, J.W., Watson, N.R., and Holland, E.F. (1993). The prevention of bone loss in young women treated with GnRH analogues with "add-back" estrogen therapy. *Obstet. Gynecol.* **81** (**1**): 104–107. Epub 1993/01/01.

80 Gurates, B., Parmaksiz, C., Kilic, G. et al. (2008). Treatment of symptomatic uterine leiomyoma with letrozole. *Reprod. Biomed. Online* **17** (**4**): 569–574. Epub 2008/10/16.

81 Parsanezhad, M.E., Azmoon, M., Alborzi, S. et al. (2010). A randomized, controlled clinical trial comparing the effects of aromatase inhibitor (letrozole) and gonadotropin-releasing hormone agonist (triptorelin) on uterine leiomyoma volume and hormonal status. *Fertil. Steril.* **93** (**1**): 192–198. Epub 2009/01/13.

82 Fiscella, K., Eisinger, S.H., Meldrum, S. et al. (2006). Effect of mifepristone for symptomatic leiomyomata on quality of life and uterine size: a randomized controlled trial. *Obstet. Gynecol.* **108** (**6**): 1381–1387. Epub 2006/12/02.

83 Donnez, J., Tomaszewski, J., Vazquez, F. et al. (2012). Ulipristal acetate versus leuprolide acetate for uterine fibroids. *N. Engl. J. Med.* **366** (**5**): 421–432. Epub 2012/02/03.

84 Levens, E.D., Potlog-Nahari, C., Armstrong, A.Y. et al. (2008). CDB-2914 for uterine leiomyomata treatment: a randomized controlled trial. *Obstet. Gynecol.* **111** (**5**): 1129–1136. Epub 2008/05/02.

85 Murat Naki, M., Tekcan, C., Ozcan, N., and Cebi, M. (2010). Levonorgestrel-releasing intrauterine device insertion ameliorates leiomyoma-dependent menorrhagia among women of reproductive age without a significant regression in the uterine and leiomyoma volumes. *Fertil. Steril.* **94** (**1**): 371–374. Epub 2009/11/10.

86 Grigorieva, V., Chen-Mok, M., Tarasova, M., and Mikhailov, A. (2003). Use of a levonorgestrel-releasing intrauterine system to treat bleeding related to uterine leiomyomas. *Fertil. Steril.* **79** (**5**): 1194–1198. Epub 2003/05/10.

87 Magalhaes, J., Aldrighi, J.M., and de Lima, G.R. (2007). Uterine volume and menstrual patterns in users of the levonorgestrel-releasing intrauterine system with idiopathic menorrhagia or menorrhagia due to leiomyomas. *Contraception* **75** (**3**): 193–198. Epub 2007/02/17.

88 Ylikorkala, O. and Pekonen, F. (1986). Naproxen reduces idiopathic but not fibromyoma-induced menorrhagia. *Obstet. Gynecol.* **68** (**1**): 10–12. Epub 1986/07/01.

89 Katz, V.L., Dotters, D.J., and Droegemeuller, W. (1989). Complications of uterine leiomyomas in pregnancy. *Obstet. Gynecol.* **73** (**4**): 593–596. Epub 1989/04/01.

90 Ravina, J.H., Herbreteau, D., Ciraru-Vigneron, N. et al. (1995). Arterial embolisation to treat uterine myomata. *Lancet* **346** (**8976**): 671–672. Epub 1995/09/09.

91 Gupta, J.K., Sinha, A.S., Lumsden, M.A., and Hickey, M. (2006). Uterine artery embolization for symptomatic uterine fibroids. *Cochrane Database Syst. Rev.* (**1**): CD005073. doi: 10.1002/14651858.CD005073.pub3. Epub 2006/01/27.

92 Spies, J.B., Ascher, S.A., Roth, A.R. et al. (2001). Uterine artery embolization for leiomyomata. *Obstet. Gynecol.* **98** (**1**): 29–34. Epub 2001/06/30.

93 Mara, M., Fucikova, Z., Maskova, J. et al. (2006). Uterine fibroid embolization versus myomectomy in women wishing to preserve fertility: preliminary results of a randomized controlled trial. *Eur. J. Obstet. Gynecol. Reprod. Biol.* **126** (**2**): 226–233.

94 Pron, G., Mocarski, E., Bennett, J. et al. (2005). Pregnancy after uterine artery embolization for leiomyomata: the Ontario multicenter trial. *Obstet. Gynecol.* **105** (**1**): 67–76. Epub 2004/12/31.

95 Hehenkamp, W.J., Volkers, N.A., Birnie, E. et al. (2008). Symptomatic uterine fibroids: treatment with uterine artery embolization or hysterectomy--results from the randomized clinical embolisation versus hysterectomy (EMMY) trial. *Radiology* **246** (**3**): 823–832. Epub 2008/01/12.

96 Voogt, M.J., De Vries, J., Fonteijn, W. et al. (2009). Sexual functioning and psychological well-being after uterine artery embolization in women with symptomatic uterine fibroids. *Fertil. Steril.* **92** (**2**): 756–761.

97 Stewart, E.A., Rabinovici, J., Tempany, C.M. et al. (2006). Clinical outcomes of focused ultrasound surgery for the treatment of uterine fibroids. *Fertil. Steril.* **85** (**1**): 22–29. Epub 2006/01/18.

98 Gorny, K.R., Woodrum, D.A., Brown, D.L. et al. (2011). Magnetic resonance-guided focused ultrasound of uterine leiomyomas: review of a 12-month outcome of 130 clinical patients. *J. Vasc. Interv. Radiol.* **22** (**6**): 857–864. Epub 2011/04/13.

99 Kim, H.S., Baik, J.H., Pham, L.D., and Jacobs, M.A. (2011). MR-guided high-intensity focused ultrasound treatment for symptomatic uterine leiomyomata: long-term outcomes. *Acad. Radiol.* **18** (**8**): 970–976. Epub 2011/07/02.

100 Vercellini, P., Maddalena, S., De Giorgi, O. et al. (1999). Determinants of reproductive outcome after abdominal myomectomy for infertility. *Fertil. Steril.* **72** (**1**): 109–114. Epub 1999/07/31.

101 Liu, H., Lu, D., Wang, L. et al. (2012). Robotic surgery for benign gynaecological disease. *Cochrane Database Syst. Rev.* (**2**): CD008978. doi: 10.1002/14651858.CD008978.pub2. Epub 2012/02/18.

102 Nash, K., Feinglass, J., Zei, C. et al. (2012). Robotic-assisted laparoscopic myomectomy versus abdominal myomectomy: a comparative analysis of surgical outcomes and costs. *Arch. Gynecol. Obstet.* **285** (**2**): 435–440. Epub 2011/07/23.

103 Hanafi, M. (2005). Predictors of leiomyoma recurrence after myomectomy. *Obstet. Gynecol.* **105** (**4**): 877–881. Epub 2005/04/02.

104 Casini, M.L., Rossi, F., Agostini, R., and Unfer, V. (2006). Effects of the position of fibroids on fertility. *Gynecol. Endocrinol.* **22** (**2**): 106–109. Epub 2006/04/11.

105 Bulletti, C., Dez, D., Levi Setti, P. et al. (2004). Myomas, pregnancy outcome, and in vitro fertilization. *Ann. N. Y. Acad. Sci.* **1034**: 84–92. Epub 2005/02/26.

106 Centers for Disease Control and Prevention. CDC. http://www.cdc.gov/reproductivehealth/womensrh/00-04-FS_Hysterectomy.htm. (accessed on 23 June 2018).

107 Carls, G.S., Lee, D.W., Ozminkowski, R.J. et al. (2008). What are the total costs of surgical treatment for uterine fibroids? *J. Women's Health (Larchmt)* **17** (**7**): 1119–1132. Epub 2008/08/09.

108 Roovers, J.P., van der Bom, J.G., van der Vaart, C.H., and Heintz, A.P. (2003). Hysterectomy and sexual wellbeing: prospective observational study of vaginal hysterectomy, subtotal abdominal hysterectomy, and total abdominal hysterectomy. *BMJ* **327** (**7418**): 774–778. Epub 2003/10/04.

109 Taveira-Dasilva, A.M., Alford, C.E., Levens, E.D. et al. (2012). Favorable response to antigonadal therapy for a benign metastasizing leiomyoma. *Obstet. Gynecol.* **119** (**2 Pt 2**): 438–442. Epub 2012/01/25.

110 Peng, H.J., Zhao, B., Yao, Q.W. et al. (2011). Intravenous leiomyomatosis: CT findings. *Abdom. Imaging* Epub 2011/09/01.

8 CHAPTER 8
Endometriosis and adenomyosis

Maria Victoria Vargas[1] and Kathy Huang[2]
[1]*Department of Obstetrics and Gynecology, George Washington University Medical Center, USA*
[2]*Department of Obstetrics and Gynecology, NYU Langone Medical Center, New York, NY, USA*

CLINICAL SCENARIO

A 34-year-old woman with a history of progressive dysmenorrhea presents for evaluation. She reports progressive dysmenorrhea since menarche age 13 years. She was started on combined oral contraceptives (COCs) for management of her dysmenorrhea at age 14 years and stopped them at age 30 years. She has since been using condoms for contraception. Since stopping COCs she has developed progressively worsening dysmenorrhea, at times debilitating and causing her to miss work. In addition, she now has developed diffuse pelvic pain between her menses and pain with intercourse. She reports pain with deep penetration and has recently developed pain with entry. She desires to conceive soon and would like to avoid hormonal therapy. She wants to know her options for management.

Background

Endometriosis

Endometriosis is a common disease, estimated to affect 10% of reproductive aged women. It is defined as the presence of ectopic endometrial glands and stroma outside of the uterine cavity [1]. The most common anatomical locations affected by endometriosis are the pelvic peritoneum and the ovaries, but endometriosis can involve almost any organ including the pericardium, pleura, and the brain [2]. Symptoms of endometriosis can be debilitating, affecting work productivity and quality of life (QoF) [3, 4]. Common manifestations include painful menses, chronic pelvic pain, pain with intercourse, and infertility. In subgroups of women manifesting symptoms of endometriosis, prevalence rates are markedly increased. For example, women with chronic pelvic pain have an estimated prevalence of up to 87%, and women with infertility have an estimated prevalence of up to 50% [5]. An estimated 1/3 of women with endometriosis do not have symptoms of the disease [6].

Similar to eutopic endometrium, implants of endometriosis are hormone responsive, expressing both estrogen and progesterone receptors. In addition, implants of endometriosis produce estrogen locally through aromatase activity. Another key component of the pathology of endometriosis implants is the creation of a proinflammatory milieu secondary to the production of cytokines, prostaglandins, and metalloproteinases. Inflammation present in endometriosis lesions leads to an abnormal peritoneal environment that may impact fertility and lead to adhesions between pelvic organs. In addition, endometriotic implants release angiogenic and neurogenic growth factors leading to the expression of nerve fibers, lymphatic vessels, and blood vessels [7].

Disease severity has been historically described using the American Society of Reproductive Medicine (ASRM) endometriosis staging system [8]. Points are assigned based on factors such as lesion appearance, size, depth of invasion, and location. Endometriosis is classified as stage I (mild), stage II (minimal), stage III (moderate), and stage IV (severe). Several limitations exist with the ASRM staging system, including lack of reproducibility [9] and poor correlation of symptoms with stage of disease [10, 11]. In 2005, the Enzian system was proposed as an adjunct to the ASRM staging of endometriosis to describe deeply infiltrative disease in further detail [12]. More recently, the Endometriosis Fertility Index (EFI) was developed and validated for the prediction of spontaneous pregnancy in women with endometriosis [13, 14]. Both the ENZIAN and EFI systems have recognized clinical utility, but neither has been adopted for the staging of endometriosis in the United States.

From a clinical perspective, endometriosis is distinguished by three distinct manifestations: (i) superficial endometriosis, (ii) ovarian endometriomas, and (iii) DIE [15, 16].

Evidence-Based Obstetrics and Gynecology, First Edition. Edited by Errol R. Norwitz, Carolyn M. Zelop, David A. Miller, and David L. Keefe.

Though they can present simultaneously, these three types of endometriosis vary in severity, symptoms, and management. Endometriosis involving the superficial pelvic peritoneal surfaces is the most common form of the disease. Women who only have peritoneal endometriosis are classified as having minimal to moderate disease. However, symptom severity (pain and infertility) does not correlate with severity of disease and patients with superficial endometriosis may manifest severe symptoms. Endometriomas are pseudocysts that form from the invagination of ectopic endometrium implanted on the ovarian cortex. They are present in 17–44% of women with endometriosis. Women with endometriomas commonly experience dysmenorrhea, chronic pelvic pain, and infertility and often also have superficial disease [17]. DIE is relatively rare and is estimated to affect 1–% of all reproductive age women [18]. It is the most advanced form of endometriosis and is associated with significant distortion of pelvic anatomy. The lesions of DIE invade at least 5 mm beyond the superficial peritoneum and most commonly involve the uterosacral ligaments, the rectosigmoid colon, the vagina, and the bladder. Three to thirty-seven percent of women with DIE have intestinal involvement and many require extensive surgical intervention [19]. There is some association of depth of infiltration of lesions and symptom severity. The most predictable symptoms of DIE are menstrual dyschezia and severe dyspareunia [20].

Adenomyosis

The presence of endometrial tissue glands and stroma located within the myometrium is termed adenomyosis, or endometriosis in situ. The endometrial tissue may invade throughout the entire myometrium – *diffuse adenomyosis*, or may form a circumscribed collection – *focal adenomyosis*. The pathophysiology of adenomyosis is thought to be distinct from that of endometriosis. The most widely held theory regarding the development of adenomyosis is that the endometrial basalis layer invaginates into the myometrium when the boundary between endometrial basal layer and myometrium is disrupted. This process is thought to be facilitated by the lack of intervening submucosa between the endometrial-myometrial interface. As such, even in normal uteri, it is common that endometrium superficially invades normal myometrium [1]. Myometrial weakness caused by prior pregnancy or surgery may incite invasion by endometrial tissue [21]. In addition, impaired immunologic control of cell division at the endometrial-myometrial interface may be present [22]. Estrogen and progesterone are suspected to contribute to the development and maintenance of adenomyosis. This is suggested by the development of adenomyosis in the reproductive years and regression after menopause. In addition, adenomyosis is associated with other hormonally driven pathologies such as leiomyomas, endometriosis, and endometrial cancer [23].

The most significant risk factors of adenomyosis are parity and age. Nearly 90% of women with adenomyosis are parous, and nearly 80% of cases develop in women in their 1940s and 1950s [1]. Other risk factors include chronic endometritis, abortion, uterine trauma from childbirth, elevated BMI, early menarche, and use of the selective estrogen receptor modulator, tamoxifen. Use of combined oral contraceptives (COCs) has been associated with adenomyosis, but it is unclear whether this is because of a causal relationship or because symptoms of adenomyosis are often managed with COCs [24, 25].

About 2/3 of women with adenomyosis are symptomatic and symptom severity correlates with increasing number of ectopic foci and extent of invasion. The most common symptoms are menorrhagia (40–50%) and dysmenorrhea (15–30%) [21]. About 10% of women with adenomyosis report dyspareunia [25]. The association of infertility and adenomyosis is not completely clear, but findings suggestive of adenomyosis are being more frequently noted on imaging for women with otherwise unexplained infertility [26]. In addition, women with adenomyosis and infertility undergoing in-vitro fertilization with intracytoplasmic sperm injection have lower clinical and ongoing pregnancy rates as well as higher miscarriage rates [27].

The exact prevalence of adenomyosis is not known given that the diagnosis is usually based on histologic findings in surgical specimens. Reported incidences in hysterectomy specimens range from 20% to 60% [21, 28].

Search strategy

The following search strategy was used to identify potential studies to answer the clinical questions. A search of the MEDLINE, Embase, and the Cochrane Database of Systematic Reviews database was made from inception until January 2016. The following search terms were used: endometriosis, endometrioma, deeply infiltrating endometriosis (DIE), adenomyosis, infertility, surgery, systematic review, and meta-analysis. In addition, consensus guidelines were reviewed.

Clinical questions

1. How should patients with suspected endometriosis and adenomyosis be evaluated?
2. What non-surgical options are available for the management of pain symptoms of endometriosis and adenomyosis?
3. How effective is conservative surgery for endometriosis and adenomyosis related pain?
4. How effective is conservative surgery for the treatment of endometriosis related infertility?
5. What is the role of peri-operative medical therapy for endometriosis?
6. What is the role of ovarian preservation in women undergoing hysterectomy for endometriosis?

1. How should patients with suspected endometriosis and adenomyosis be evaluated?

Endometriosis

The formal diagnosis of endometriosis involving the abdominal cavity is through laparoscopy or laparotomy, with or without biopsy for histologic confirmation [2]. However, endometriosis can be suggested clinically with the assistance of a good history, exam, and appropriate imaging. Questions should focus on menstrual history as well as a detailed history of any pain or infertility symptoms. Severe dysmenorrhea and chronic pelvic pain are the most common symptoms of women diagnosed with endometriosis. In a study of 1000 women with endometriosis, 79% reported having dysmenorrhea and 69% reported chronic pelvic pain [29]. Women with dysmenorrhea will often report pain before the onset of their menses and sometimes lasting for days after their menses is over. Dyspareunia is reported in 45% of women with endometriosis and is associated with rectovaginal and uterosacral involvement [29, 30]. Dysuria, dyschezia, constipation, and diarrhea may also be present and can be suggestive of DIE involving the bladder and bowel respectively [31, 32]. However, these symptoms may also be present without deeply infiltrative disease [33, 34]. In cases of DIE of the rectosigmoid, cyclic hematochezia may be reported [31], and in rare cases of transmural infiltration of lesions, stenosis and even occlusion of the intestinal lumen can occur [35, 36].

Up to 50% of women with endometriosis suffer from infertility and even higher rates can be seen with worsened disease severity. In some cases, infertility is the only symptom suggesting the presence of endometriosis [5]. Thus, questions about pregnancy and prior attempts at conception should be included in the history to guide evaluation and management.

Other symptoms commonly seen with endometriosis include depression, and anxiety as well as central sensitivity syndromes such as myofascial pain syndrome, painful bladder syndrome, and irritable bowel syndrome [33, 34, 37]. Inquiry about these symptoms should also be made during the collection of the history as management for these related disorders should be simultaneously pursued in parallel to any specific therapy for endometriosis.

Depending on the severity of disease, the physical examination may vary. In the case of superficial endometriosis, lesions cannot be palpated on bimanual exam. Endometriomas may be palpable on bimanual or abdominal examination depending on the size. Adnexal tenderness may also be present. Deeply infiltrating nodules of endometriosis are often palpable on bimanual and recto-vaginal examination as uterosacral nodularity, retroflexion of the uterus, and fixation of the posterior cul-de-sac. When concomitant myofascial or painful bladder syndrome symptoms are present, levator ani pain and bladder pain may also be present.

Transvaginal ultrasonography is the initial imaging study of choice and when possible, should be performed in the late secretory phase of the menstrual cycle given that this is when the disease is most active. Superficial lesions are often not visible on transvaginal ultrasonography but endometriomas can be reliably diagnosed by ultrasound [38]. For cases of DIE, transvaginal, and transrectal ultrasonography can be useful for the identification of lesions involving the rectovaginal septum, parametrium, and utero sacral ligaments [39]. However, ultrasonography is highly operator dependent and in can lack sensitivity for smaller nodules of DIE [38]. In addition, many facilities are not able to offer transrectal sonographic imaging due to a lack of trained ultrasonographers.

T1 and T2-weighted magnetic resonance imaging (MRI) with and without fat suppression can reliably diagnose small nodules when DIE is suspected but transvaginal ultrasound is equivocal. MRI should be performed with and without gadolinium. When bladder involvement is suspected, ensuring a full bladder during MRI may enhance the ability to recognize nodules. When rectal involvement is suspected, a bowel prep followed by an antispasmodic agent to reduce artifact from peristalsis may also enhance the sensitivity of MRI [40].

In cases where bladder and/or ureteric endometriosis are suspected, cystoscopy, renal ultrasonography, and intravenous urography can assist with diagnosis. In addition, rectosigmoidoscopy should be performed, ideally during menses, if rectal infiltration is suspected [41].

Adenomyosis

Similar to endometriosis, the diagnosis of adenomyosis is formally made using histologic findings in surgical specimens. However, adenomyosis can also be suspected clinically with the assistance of history, exam, and imaging [26] .

During the collection of the history, questions should focus on menstrual history including amount of bleeding, intermenstrual bleeding, and painful menses. Severe dysmenorrhea and menorrhagia are the most common symptoms of women diagnosed with adenomyosis. Other common symptoms include intermenstrual spotting and dyspareunia. Adenomyosis does not typically cause uterine enlargement beyond 12 weeks, but in women with significant enlargement from very severe adenomyosis, large adenomyomas, and/or concomitant leiomyomas (up to 50%), pressure type symptoms may be present [21].

An estimated 12% of women with adenomyosis may report infertility and an estimated 11% of women with adenomyosis will have concomitant endometriosis. As such, associated symptoms and conditions should be addressed during the collection of the history. The physical exam may be notable for enlargement of the uterus and uterine tenderness. In addition, exam findings may suggest co-existing leiomyomas or endometriosis [25].

Transvaginal ultrasonography can be utilized to elucidate subtle myometrial findings that suggest the presence of adenomyosis. A systematic review of 14 studies found that transvaginal ultrasound had a pooled sensitivity of 79% and specificity of 85% of identifying adenomyosis using histologic diagnosis as the gold standard. Findings used to diagnose diffuse adenomyosis on ultrasound included: [1] myometrial texture heterogeneity, [2] globular asymmetric uterus, [3] small myometrial hypoechoic cysts, [4] striated projections extending from the endometrium into the myometrium, [5] ill-defined endometrial echo [6] anterior or posterior myometrial wall appearing thicker than its counterpart, [7] thickening of anterior and posterior myometrial walls with associated hypo- or hyper-echogenecity [26]. Focal adenomyosis, also known as adenomyomas, was identified by the following criteria: discrete hypoechoic nodules with poorly defined margins, elliptical shape, minimal mass effect on surrounding tissues, lack of calcifications, and presence of anechoic cysts of varying diameter [1, 26]. Similar to endometriosis, operator experience influences diagnostic accuracy and the common presence of concurrent uterine disease such as leiomyomas can limit the accuracy of transvaginal ultrasound. In these settings, MRI imaging may be complementary. The aforementioned systematic review assessing transvaginal ultrasound also assessed MRI for the diagnosis of adenomyosis. A pooled analysis of six studies showed a sensitivity of 74% and specificity of 92% for the identification of adenomyosis using histopathology for confirmatory diagnosis. Findings on MRI used to diagnose adenomyosis included (i) a myometrial mass with indistinct margins of primarily low intensity, (ii) diffuse or local widening of junctional zones on T2 weighted images, (iii) junctional zone thickness of >15 mm, (iv) subjective thickening of junctional zone, localized or diffuse, (v) ill-defined low intensity lesion, (vi) junctional zone wider than 12 mm, (vii) uterine enlargement or (viii) small hypointense myometrial spots [26].

2. What non-surgical options are available for the management of pain symptoms of endometriosis and adenomyosis?

Endometriosis

Treatment algorithms are dependent on patient symptomatology, location of lesions, desire to conserve the option for future childbearing, and plans for immediate child bearing. In patients presenting with mild to moderate pain and without the desire for immediate conception, medical therapy is appropriate. This is true even if endometriosis is suspected but not yet confirmed. First line regimens include COCs and progestins. COCs inactivate implants of endometriosis through a process of decidualization. Abundant observational data supports the use of COCs for the relief of endometriosis related pain. [42]. In addition, one large randomized control trial (RCT) showed significant improvement in endometriosis related pain with COCs when compared to placebo [43]. Regimens for oral contraceptives may be cyclic but extended cycle and continuous regimens are often used for women with severe dysmenorrhea. COCs have a good side effect profile and are generally well tolerated by patients. For women on extended cycle and continuous regimens, break through bleeding is the most common side effect [43]. For women who are not candidates for estrogen containing therapy, progestins alone are utilized. These agents inactivate endometrial implants by antagonizing the effects of estrogen. Two randomized trials showed equivalence in pain reduction of depot medroxyprogesterone (DMPA) acetate against gonadotropin releasing hormone (GnRH) agonists for pain symptoms related to endometriosis [44, 45]. In addition, women who received DMPA had less loss of bone mineral density. Other progestins have also been shown to improve symptoms related to endometriosis, such as norethindrone acetate and the levonorgestrel intrauterine device [46, 47]. One small prospective cohort study showed significant improvement in pain symptoms with the levonorgestrel intrauterine device during a three year follow-up period [48] and another RCT showed equivalence in pain reduction of the levonorgestrel intrauterine device with GnRH agonist [49] Side effects of progestins can include weight gain, edema, acne, and irregular bleeding which may limit their acceptability by patients.

For women with symptoms refractory to COCs and progestins, second line agents include GnRH agonists, such as leuprolide acetate. There is strong evidence supporting the efficacy of GnRH agonists to reduce pain related to endometriosis. However, GnRH agonists lead to a hypoestrogenic state that simulates menopause and side effects can be poorly tolerated. These include significant loss of bone mineral density and vasomotor symptoms (hot flashes) [50]. Combining GnRH agonists with low dose "add-back" hormone therapy (e.g. norethindrone acetate 5 mg daily) significantly reduces the hypoestrogenic effects and makes the regimen more tolerable for patients. In addition, with use of "add-back" therapy, bone mineral density loss is significantly reduced if not eliminated [51]. Notably, a Cochrane Review comparing GnRH agonists with other medical therapies for pain related to endometriosis found little or no difference in pain relief. GnRH agonists also have a higher cost compared to other medical therapies and as such are not typically recommended as first line medical therapy [52].

Aromatase inhibitors have been more recently introduced as a potential treatment for endometriosis-related pain. Several studies have shown that these agents reduce pain symptoms in women with endometriosis. When used alone, they share a similar side effect profile to GNRH agonists that make them difficult to tolerate. However, recent study of aromatase inhibitors with a COC showed significant pain relief with an improved acceptability [53]. This option remains promising for otherwise refractory cases but is not yet widely utilized. Androgens, such as danazol, have also been shown to significantly reduce the size endometriotic lesions and improve pain symptoms, but have significant androgenic effects making them generally not well accepted by patients [7]. There is limited data available about antiprogestins that suggest these agents could reduce pain related to endometriosis. However, a Cochrane Review found no benefit in pain reduction when compared to danazol and leuprorelin [54].

The biggest limitation of medical options for the treatment of pain related to endometriosis is the recurrence of pain after discontinuation. This is most notable is with GnRH agonists since the Food and Drug Administration (FDA) has only approved a 12-month course of GnRH therapy for the treatment of endometriosis related pain. The pain recurrence rate at five-year follow-up after discontinuing GnRH agonist therapy ranges from 53% to 73% in women with advanced disease [20].

A number of alternative therapies for pain related to endometriosis have also been studied. One randomized trial comparing acupuncture to traditional Chinese medicine met criteria for a systematic review of alternative therapies for endometriosis. This trial showed an overall reduction in pain with auricular acupuncture with the greatest benefit in cases of severe dysmenorrhea [55]. Another systematic review assessing alternative therapies for the treatment of dysmenorrhea (rather than endometriosis) identified a single trial of acupuncture vs. placebo acupuncture or no treatment and showed reduction of symptoms in the acupuncture group [56]. The same systematic review for the treatment of dysmenorrhea assessed seven trials of high frequency transcutaneous electrical nerve stimulation (TENS) therapy. High frequency TENS was found to reduce reported pain when compared to placebo TENS [56].

Adenomyosis

Though a number of imaging characteristics have been identified as being associated with a diagnosis of adenomyosis, no formal ultrasonographic or MRI criteria have been established as diagnostic. As a result, monitoring treatment effect and comparing findings among studies is challenging. In addition, there is a lack of randomized trials assessing the medical management of adenomyosis. The main objective of medical treatment is relief from pain and bleeding symptoms. Conservative therapy for symptomatic adenomyosis is similar to that for endometriosis. Combination oral contraceptives and progestin-only regimens can be used to induce endometrial atrophy and decrease endometrial prostaglandin production to improve dysmenorrhea and menorrhagia. However, no randomized controlled trials have assessed these regimens for the management of symptoms of adenomyosis [57]. Limited data suggests that the levonorgestrel-releasing intrauterine device is effective for treatment of adenomyosis-related bleeding and dysmenorrhea [58–60]. Only one randomized study has been completed. The trial compared symptoms and QoL after placement of the levonorgestrel intrauterine device vs. after hysterectomy. Both groups showed significant improvement in symptoms and QoL. However, the levonorgestrel intrauterine device group had improvement in all five QoL mean domains scores (physical health, psychological health, social relationships, environmental health, national environmental health) vs. an improvement in three of five mean domain scores (physical health, environmental health, national environmental health in the hysterectomy group [60]. The authors concluded that the symptomatic outcomes between hysterectomy and the levonorgestrel intrauterine device were comparable, but that the levonorgestrel intrauterine device may have benefits for the psychological and social aspects of QoL. The follow-up period for this trial was one year. A prospective cohort assessed symptoms and uterine volume over a three-year follow-up period in women with adenomyosis and moderate to severe dysmenorrhea and found significant improvement in symptoms and uterine volume at three years. Overall patient satisfaction was 72.5% [58]. Another prospective cohort with a 3-year follow-up period also showed an overall improvement in symptoms, pictorial blood loss, and uterine volume at 36 months. However, there was a significant increase in uterine volume, blood loss, and pain symptoms between 12 and 36 months of follow-up. The authors concluded that the benefits of the levonorgestrel intrauterine device for the treatment of symptoms of adenomyosis might decline after two years [59]. Common side effects reported with the use of the levonorgestrel intrauterine device included weight gain, ovarian cysts, and pelvic pain. In addition, there were reports of headache, acne, breast tenderness, and transient mood changes.

Several case reports and case series have reported improvement of uterine volume and symptoms, with the use of GnRH agonists for the treatment adenomyosis. In addition, there have been reports of post-treatment spontaneous conception in women with previous sub-fertility. Hypo-estrogenic side effects were common and symptoms as well as uterine volume tended to return to pretreatment levels after discontinuation of therapy [25].

A case series of 14 patients with dysmenorrhea, menorrhagia, or infertility showed significant improvement in all three symptoms after a six month trial of therapy of an intrauterine device containing danazol. Systemic levels of danazol were undetectable throughout the treatment and no side-effects typical of danazol were reported. Three of four women with infertility spontaneously conceived after completion of the trial [61].

3. How effective is conservative surgical therapy for the treatment of pain related to endometriosis?

When symptoms are refractory to medical therapy, or in circumstances that preclude the use of medical treatments, such as desire for immediate conception, surgery is typically the next recommended approach to treatment [20]. Over 20 years of reports exist of laparoscopic management of peritoneal endometriosis and endometriomas [62]. Laparoscopy rather than laparotomy is thus considered the standard of care for the surgical management of mild to moderate endometriosis. There are also increasing reports of laparoscopic management of DIE [63], even in cases where bowel resection is necessary [64]. The literature suggests a significant short-term improvement in pain with surgical treatment of endometriosis. A Cochrane Review of nine randomized trials compared laparoscopic excision, laparoscopic ablation, and diagnostic laparoscopy for the treatment of pain in women with mild to moderate disease. Operative laparoscopy was associated with decreased overall pain at 6 and 12 months of follow-up compared to diagnostic laparoscopy. Two trials collected data on peri-operative complications and none were reported in either the treatment or control groups. There was no difference in pain relief between excision vs. ablative techniques [62, 65].

In the case of endometriomas, another Cochrane Review assessed two randomized trials comparing excision vs. ablative techniques. All participants had a primary complaint of pain and an endometrioma greater than 3 cm in diameter. Laparoscopic excision of the cyst wall was associated with a reduced recurrence rate of the symptoms of dysmenorrhea, dyspareunia, and non-menstrual pelvic pain. In addition, in women with previous sub-fertility who subsequently attempted to conceive, excision of the cyst wall was associated with an increased spontaneous pregnancy rate compared with laparoscopic ablation of the endometrioma. Laparoscopic excision of the cyst wall was also associated with a reduced rate of endometrioma recurrence with a reduced requirement for further surgery [66]. There is also little data to suggest that excision therapy has benefits over expectant management for asymptomatic women with endometriomas less than 3 cm [67].

A number of studies have demonstrated relief of pain with laparoscopic excision for DIE [63, 65, 68, 69]. In 2014, Fritzer and colleagues published a systematic review of three prospective cohort studies that included a total of 128 patients. The majority of these cases were completed using a laparoscopic approach. The authors assessed surgical intervention for the management of dyspareunia in women with an 89% rate of Stage III/IV endometriosis. All three articles used standardized instruments to measure pain and quality of sex life (QoSL) before and after surgery. The follow-up periods were 12, 24, and 60 months. Significant reductions in overall pain and sexual function were seen in all three studies [70]. Complications were reported in two of the studies. One study of 22 patients reported rectovaginal fistula in 4.5% (1/22), blood transfusion in 4.5% (1/22), and temporary urinary retention in 9.1% (2/22) [71]. The other larger study of 135 patients reported blood transfusion in 3.7% (5/135), and intentional bowel entry to excise disease in 3% (4/135) [68].

Another prospective cohort study of 83 patients with rectovaginal endometriosis evaluated long-term outcomes after radical surgical excision. Though the majority of patients had improvement in symptoms, about 36% of these patients required bowel resection, and 7.2% required partial bladder resection. In addition, the study showed a 28% cumulative recurrence rate over a period of 36 months [72]. Other studies have reported similar symptom recurrence rates [73].

The available literature does suggest that laparoscopic treatment of advanced endometriosis does lead to improvement in disease and pain and thus supports the recommendation to surgically treat endometriotic lesions [74]. Whether surgical therapy has significant advantage over medical therapy for pain related to deeply infiltrative endometriosis is unclear, as very limited data is available on this topic [75]. The potentially radical nature of surgery and the associated risk of complications necessitates appropriate patient counseling prior to the decision to move forward with surgery. Women should be counseled that surgery might temporarily alleviate pain, but that recurrence is common. In addition, repeat surgery may not provide benefit beyond medical management [76]. Experts recommend a thorough pre-operative assessment, gynecological surgical expertise, and a multidisciplinary approach with urology and colorectal surgery when appropriate [7].

With regards to pre-sacral neurectomy, benefit in dysmenorrhea, dyspareunia, and chronic pelvic pain was shown in one randomized controlled trial that included women with midline pelvic pain [77]. The intervention group reported significantly higher constipation and urinary urgency over a 12-month follow-up period.

Adenomyosis

For women not desiring future fertility, endometrial ablation or resection has been shown to be effective for the management of symptoms of adenomyosis. However, in a prospective cohort of 50 women, myometrial invasion of > 2 mm predicted failure of roller ball endometrial ablation. Patients with > 2 mm of invasion were less likely to have pain reduction (23% vs. 73%; $P < 0.001$) and were less likely to report satisfaction after the procedure. A total of 46% of women with >2 mm of invasion were considered treatment failures. The authors concluded that preoperative sonography or MRI could be utilized to identify deep lesions and thereby improve patient selection [78]. In a retrospective assessment of women undergoing radiofrequency and thermal balloon ablation, dysmenorrhea, uterine length > 9 cm, age < 45 years, parity > 5, and prior tubal ligation were predictors of ablation failure [79]. A review of the literature concluded that based on these results, dysmenorrhea, and parity could be utilized, in combination with depth of invasion if known, to select appropriate women with adenomyosis for endometrial ablation as therapy [25].

Uterine artery embolization has also been used to relieve symptoms of dysmenorrhea and menorrhagia related to adenomyosis. However, success rates vary widely, ranging from 25% to 85%, and approximately 50% of patients still require eventual hysterectomy [80].

Conservative surgery with adenomyomectomy or resection of a well-defined area of adenomyosis has been described in case series and may be appropriate in women with a desire for fertility. A laparoscopic approach has been reported and peri-operative outcomes are suggested to be similar of those for laparoscopic myomectomy [26, 81]. The benefit for symptoms is unclear. A systematic review reported a pooled live birth rate of 36% after this procedure [26]. Case series and reports of combined GnRH analogue with surgical excision have shown no benefit in symptoms or reproductive outcomes with adjunctive medical therapy [25]. MRI guided focused ultrasound surgery is an experimental procedure for the treatment of symptoms of adenomyosis that allows for uterine conservation. Two case series have shown a reduction of pretreatment bleeding and pain. One showed a reduction in uterine volume. Adverse events included skin burn, nausea and vomiting, and sciatic nerve injury [25]. One live birth has been reported after this procedure [26].

Hysterectomy is considered the definitive treatment for adenomyosis. There is no role for adenexectomy unless the woman is post-menopausal or has another indication for the procedure. A vaginal or laparoscopic approach is favored due to improved outcomes, but an increased risk of bladder injury has been reported with a vaginal approach [25].

4. What is the impact of endometrioma and surgical therapy of endometrioma on fertility?

There is some evidence to suggest that the presence of an intact endometrioma per se diminishes ovarian function, but reports are conflicting [82]. One prospective study of 70 women with unilateral endometriomas who had sonographic tracking of ovulation showed a 31% lower ovulation rate from the ovaries containing the endometrioma ($p = 0.002$) [83]. However, a larger and more recent prospective study showed no difference in spontaneous ovulation in the affected ovaries of women with a unilateral endometrioma [84]. In contrast, studies assessing ovarian reserve in women with intact endometriomas using anti-Mullerian hormone (AMH) have consistently showed lower concentrations when compared to age and BMI matched controls [85, 86]. With regards to response to gonadotropic stimulation, a 2015 meta-analysis of in vitro fertilization (IVF) outcomes of women compared woman with endometriomas to women without the disease. Women with endometriomas had a lower mean of oocytes retrieved overall. However, they had comparable clinical pregnancy and live birth rates when compared to women without endometriomas [87]. Whether the presence of an endometrioma affects ovarian function is unclear, but the data does not support a negative impact of endometriomas on IVF outcomes.

For women with pain symptoms laparoscopic excision of the cyst wall is associated with a reduced recurrence rate of the symptoms of dysmenorrhea, dyspareunia, and non-menstrual pelvic pain [66]. The dilemma is that surgical excision for endometrioma has also been implicated as a cause of loss of ovarian function, though the data is conflicting. The mechanism is thought to be secondary to inadvertent removal of ovarian cortex while stripping the wall of the endometriotic pseudocyst. Multiple studies have explored the effect of surgical resection of endometriomas on ovarian reserve. A higher rate of premature ovarian failure and a younger age of menopause have been associated with prior bilateral excision of endometriomas. Two systematic reviews showed lower ovarian reserve as measured by decline in AMH concentration after surgical excision of endometriomas [88, 89]. Conversely, a more recently published systematic review of 13 studies evaluating almost 600 patients found no significant reduction in antral follicle count (AFC) in women after excisional treatment of an endometrioma [90].

With regards to spontaneous conception, a pooled analysis of two randomized controlled trials showed a pregnancy rate of 60.9% for excision vs. 23.4% with ablation or drainage of endometriomas (OR 5.11: 95% CI, 2.03–12.85) [91]. A Cochrane Review similarly showed that women with sub-fertility who attempted to conceive after excision of an endometrioma had an increased spontaneous pregnancy rate compared with laparoscopic ablation of the endometrioma [66]. However, two subsequent randomized studies assessing ovarian function after excision vs. ablative techniques showed a greater decline in AMH [92] and AFC [93] in women undergoing excisional procedures. A recent meta-analysis assessed IVF outcomes of women who underwent excisional procedures. Women with endometriomas who had excision prior to their IVF cycle had no difference in mean number of oocytes retrieved, clinical pregnancy rates, and live birth rates when compared to women who had expectant management of their endometriomas [87]. Though there is a reduction in recurrence of endometriomas with excision vs. ablative procedures, there are still reports of up to 30% recurrence rates with the excision [94]. Patients must therefore be counseled about the risk of recurrence and the potential loss of ovarian function with each procedure.

The ASRM guidelines are not firm about when to perform surgical excision of an endometrioma. In symptomatic women, most clinicians would advocate for excisional treatment, especially if the cyst is greater than 4 cm. Women should be counseled about the risk of recurrence. In women planning IVF with no pain symptoms, excision is recommended only in cases on an endometrioma >4 cm if a woman has not previously had histologic diagnosis of endometriosis. The potential benefits are improved access to follicles and avoidance of rupture and contamination of the oocytes with endometriotic fluid. Women should be counseled about the potential impact of surgery on ovarian reserve and the lack of benefit for IVF outcomes. In any circumstance, repeat procedures should be avoided if at all possible [95].

5. How effective is conservative surgery for the treatment of endometriosis related infertility?

Evidence suggests an association between endometriosis and infertility, however, a causal relationship has not yet been established. Regardless, up to 50% of women with endometriosis suffer from infertility and even higher rates can be seen with worsened disease severity. In some cases, infertility is the only symptom suggesting the presence of endometriosis [5]. There are a number of postulated mechanisms by which endometriosis may cause infertility, among the most common being distorted pelvic anatomy and the creation of a proinflammatory milieu by endometriotic implants. As a result of our limited understanding of endometriosis related infertility, no optimal therapeutic approach has been established [95].

For minimal to mild endometriosis, surgical treatment has been associated with a statistically significant, but clinically modest improvement in live birth rates compared to diagnostic laparoscopy. One RCT compared diagnostic laparoscopy with either excision or ablation of endometriotic lesions. The results showed a small but significant improvement in cumulative pregnancy rates in women who underwent excision or ablation vs. those who underwent diagnostic laparoscopy (30.7% vs. 17.7%; P = 0.006). A subsequent smaller trial showed no difference in pregnancy rates in women who had a diagnostic surgery vs. a therapeutic surgery, though the study was not powered for the primary outcome of live births [96]. A pooled analysis of the two studies estimated an OR of 1.65 (95% confidence interval (CI), 1.06–2.58) for post-surgery conception. The authors calculated a number needed to treat of 12 [91]. However, based on a conservative estimate of 30% prevalence of endometriosis in women with infertility undergoing a laparoscopy, 40 women would have to undergo surgery before one pregnancy was gained [95]. As such, both ACOG and ASRM concluded that the magnitude of benefit from laparoscopy for women with minimal to mild endometriosis is insufficient to recommend it solely for the treatment of infertility [20, 95]. The ASRM further recommends expectant management or superovulation with intrauterine insemination as first line therapy [95].

A discussion of the effect of surgical treatment of endometrioma on fertility can be found under the clinical question specifically addressing this topic.

There are no randomized trials of the impact of surgical treatment on fertility in women with advanced disease, including those with deeply infiltrative disease. However, there has been a trend to suggest surgery for infertility in the setting of Stage III of IV endometriosis, as some authors have reported high post-surgical cumulative pregnancy rates in previously sub-fertile patients [63, 69, 97]. No difference was noted in pregnancy rates when laparotomy was compared to laparoscopy [63].

One prospective cohort study compared fertility outcomes between surgical treatment and expectant management. Vercillini and colleagues assessed pregnancy rates in 105 women with rectovaginal endometriosis. Forty-one women had conservative surgery via laparotomy and 66 women had expectant management. Pregnancy rates were equivalent in the surgical and expectant management groups (24-month cumulative probabilities, 44.9% vs. 46.8%; P = 0.38) [98]. Notably, the surgical group, had a 23% rate of overall complications with one (2.2%) major complication reported. In the case of laparoscopy, complications can be reduced with experience [64]. Regardless, women requiring colorectal resection at the time of laparoscopic surgical treatment of rectovaginal endometriosis/DIE have about a 10% risk of major morbidity [64, 99, 100]. Moreover, no available data has shown a consistent benefit of either surgical approach for rectovaginal endometriosis/DIE over alternative therapies such as IVF. As such, alternatives to surgery such as assisted reproductive technology (ART), should be thoroughly examined as an option for asymptomatic or minimally symptomatic women with infertility and rectovaginal endometriosis/DIE. Surgery may be of benefit to highly symptomatic women who prefer to attempt spontaneous conception [91]. In addition, women with infertility who plan to undergo oocyte retrieval with significant anatomic distortion may require surgery for anatomic restoration to facilitate safe oocyte retrieval. Regardless, after the first surgery, the ASRM recommends referral to a specialist for ART, as further surgery does not seem to provide any fertility benefit [95].

6. What is the role of peri-operative medical therapy for endometriosis?

A Cochrane Review of 16 trials compared the efficacy of pre and post-operative medical therapy in reducing symptoms of endometriosis with surgery alone. The primary outcomes measured were pain, disease recurrence, and pregnancy rates. Two trials were assessed pre-surgical medical therapy. There was no difference in the primary outcome measures between pre-operative medical therapy vs. surgery alone. Ease of surgery could not be adequately assessed. Post-surgical treatment compared to placebo or surgery alone also showed no improvement in the primary outcomes. The authors concluded that there was insufficient data to assess the benefit of pre-surgical medical therapy and no benefit for post-surgical medical therapy (Low-quality evidence) [101].

One systematic review and a subsequent randomized controlled trial showed reduced post-operative recurrence of endometrioma and associated dysmenorrhea with 24 months of oral-contraceptive use after surgery [102, 103]. There was no persistent effect after discontinuation of use.

GnRH antagonists may have post-surgical benefit, but are not generally recommended as post-surgical treatment due to limited data, associated long-term side effects, and cost [20].

Post-surgical used of the levonorgestrel intrauterine device was assessed in a Cochrane Review which showed a reduction of post-surgical dysmenorrhea (Moderate quality evidence) [104].

Though the data is conflicting, the ASRM summary of the available literature concluded that post-operative use of medical therapy increases the time to recurrence of symptoms [74]. ACOG suggests that the use of post-operative medical therapy could be useful when residual disease is expected after surgery, when women have to pain relief after surgery, or to extend the pain-free interval after surgery [20].

7. What is the role of ovarian preservation in women undergoing hysterectomy for endometriosis?

Hysterectomy with bilateral salpingo-ophorectomy has historically been considered the definitive management of women with endometriosis who no longer desire fertility and who have failed prior medical and conservative surgical management [20]. This is based off a retrospective study with a five year follow-up period that showed relative risks of symptom recurrence of 6.1 (95% CI, 2.5–14.6) and additional surgery required of 8.1 (95% CI, 2.1–31.3) with ovarian conservation at the time of hysterectomy for endometriosis. A limitation of the study was that it did not report whether endometriosis was resected at the time of hysterectomy [105]. A subsequent retrospective study showed that in women with endometriosis who underwent hysterectomy with ovarian preservation, the two, five and seven year reoperation-free percentages were 95.7%, 86.6%, and 77.0%, respectively. In women who underwent hysterectomy without ovarian preservation, the percentages were 96.0%, 91.7%, and 91.7%, respectively. The trend toward higher rates of re-operation in the ovarian conservation group was not statistically significant. In women between 30 and 39 years of age, removal of the ovaries did not significantly improve the surgery-free time [106]. Symptom recurrence was not reported. Based on these findings, ACOG and the ASRM suggest that ovarian conservation can be considered, though the risks of recurrence should be weighed against those of surgical menopause, especially in young women [20, 74]. With regards to hormone replacement therapy (HRT) after hysterectomy with bilateral salpingo-ophorectomy, limited data suggests a slight increase in disease recurrence with the use of combined HRT [107]. In women requiring HRT, there is no advantage in terms of disease recurrence in delaying hormone replacement. Continuous combined estrogen and progestin therapy is the commonly recommended regimen, though there is no data to suggest a benefit with this regimen over estrogen alone [20, 74].

References

1 Schorge, J., Schaffer, J., Halvorson, L. et al. (2008). *Williams Gynecology*. New York, NY: McGraw Hill Medical.

2 Giudice, L.C. and Kao, L.C. (2004). Endometriosis. *Lancet* **364** (**9447**): 1789–1799.

3 Gao, X., Yeh, Y.C., Outley, J. et al. (2006). Health-related quality of life burden of women with endometriosis: a literature review. *Curr. Med. Res. Opin.* **22** (**9**): 1787–1797.

4 Nnoaham, K.E., Hummelshoj, L., Webster, P. et al. (2011). Impact of endometriosis on quality of life and work productivity: a multicenter study across ten countries. *Fertil. Steril.* **96** (**2**): 366–373.e8.

5 Ozkan, S., Murk, W., and Arici, A. (2008). Endometriosis and infertility: epidemiology and evidence-based treatments. *Ann. N. Y. Acad. Sci.* **1127**: 92–100.

6 Eskenazi, B. and Warner, M.L. (1997). Epidemiology of endometriosis. *Obstet. Gynecol. Clin. North. Am.* **24** (**2**): 235–258.

7 Ferrero, S., Alessandri, F., Racca, A., and Leone Roberti Maggiore, U. (2015). Treatment of pain associated with deep endometriosis: alternatives and evidence. *Fertil. Steril.* .

8 (1997). Revised American Society for Reproductive Medicine Classification of Endometriosis: 1996. *Fertil. Steril.* **67** (**5**): 817–821.

9 Hornstein, M.D., Gleason, R.E., Orav, J. et al. (1993). The reproducibility of the revised American fertility society classification of endometriosis. *Fertil. Steril.* **59** (**5**): 1015–1021.

10 Vercellini, P., Trespidi, L., De Giorgi, O. et al. (1996). Endometriosis and pelvic pain: relation to disease stage and localization. *Fertil. Steril.* **65** (**2**): 299–304.

11 Guzick, D.S., Silliman, N.P., Adamson, G.D. et al. (1997). Prediction of pregnancy in infertile women based on the American Society for Reproductive Medicine's revised classification of endometriosis. *Fertil. Steril.* **67** (**5**): 822–829.

12 Tuttlies, F., Keckstein, J., Ulrich, U. et al. (2005). ENZIAN-score, a classification of deep infiltrating endometriosis. *Zentralbl. Gynakol.* **127** (**5**): 275–281.

13 Tomassetti, C., Geysenbergh, B., Meuleman, C. et al. (2013). External validation of the endometriosis fertility index (EFI) staging system for predicting non-ART pregnancy after endometriosis surgery. *Hum. Reprod.* **28** (**5**): 1280–1288.

14 Adamson, G.D. and Pasta, D.J. (2010). Endometriosis fertility index: the new, validated endometriosis staging system. *Fertil. Steril.* **94** (**5**): 1609–1615.

15 Kamergorodsky, G., Ribeiro, P.A., Galvao, M.A. et al. (2009). Histologic classification of specimens from women affected by superficial endometriosis, deeply infiltrating endometriosis, and ovarian endometriomas. *Fertil. Steril.* **92** (**6**): 2074–2077.

16 Adamson, G.D. (2011). Endometriosis classification: an update. *Curr. Opin. Obstet. Gynecol.* **23** (**4**): 213–220.

17 Gelbaya, T.A. and Nardo, L.G. (2011). Evidence-based management of endometrioma. *Reprod. Biomed. Online* **23** (**1**): 15–24.

18 Koninckx, P.R. (1998). Biases in the endometriosis literature. Illustrated by 20 years of endometriosis research in Leuven. *Eur. J. Obstet. Gynecol. Reprod. Biol.* **81** (**2**): 259–271.

19 Meuleman, C., Tomassetti, C., Wolthuis, A. et al. (2014). Clinical outcome after radical excision of moderate-severe endometriosis with or without bowel resection and reanastomosis: a prospective cohort study. *Ann. Surg.* **259** (**3**): 522–531.

20 (2010). Practice Bulletin no. 114: Management of Endometriosis. *Obstet. Gynecol.* **116** (**1**): 223–236.

21 Levgur, M., Abadi, M.A., and Tucker, A. (2000). Adenomyosis: symptoms, histology, and pregnancy terminations. *Obstet. Gynecol.* **95** (**5**): 688–691.

22 Ferenczy, A. (1998). Pathophysiology of adenomyosis. *Hum. Reprod. Update* **4** (**4**): 312–322.

23 Azziz, R. (1989). Adenomyosis: current perspectives. *Obstet. Gynecol. Clin. North Am.* **16** (**1**): 221–235.

24 Templeman, C., Marshall, S.F., Ursin, G. et al. (2008). Adenomyosis and endometriosis in the California teachers study. *Fertil. Steril.* **90** (**2**): 415–424.

25 Struble, J., Reid, S., and Bedaiwy, M.A. (2015). Adenomyosis; a clinical review of a challenging Gynecologic condition. *J. Minim. Invasive Gynecol.* **23** (**2**): 164–185.

26 Maheshwari, A., Gurunath, S., Fatima, F., and Bhattacharya, S. (2012). Adenomyosis and subfertility: a systematic review of prevalence, diagnosis, treatment and fertility outcomes. *Hum. Reprod. Update* **18** (**4**): 374–392.

27 Salim, R., Riris, S., Saab, W. et al. (2012). Adenomyosis reduces pregnancy rates in infertile women undergoing IVF. *Reprod. Biomed. Online* **25** (**3**): 273–277.

28 Vavilis, D., Agorastos, T., Tzafetas, J. et al. (1997). Adenomyosis at hysterectomy: prevalence and relationship to operative findings and reproductive and menstrual factors. *Clin. Exp. Obstet. Gynecol.* **24** (**1**): 36–38.

29 Sinaii, N., Plumb, K., Cotton, L. et al. (2008). Differences in characteristics among 1,000 women with endometriosis based on extent of disease. *Fertil. Steril.* **89** (**3**): 538–545.

30 Vercellini, P., Somigliana, E., Buggio, L. et al. (2012). "I can't get no satisfaction": deep dyspareunia and sexual functioning in women with rectovaginal endometriosis. *Fertil. Steril.* **98** (**6**): 1503–11.e1.

31 Remorgida, V., Ferrero, S., Fulcheri, E. et al. (2007). Bowel endometriosis: presentation, diagnosis, and treatment. *Obstet. Gynecol. Surv.* **62** (**7**): 461–470.

32 Knabben, L., Imboden, S., Fellmann, B. et al. (2015). Urinary tract endometriosis in patients with deep infiltrating endometriosis: prevalence, symptoms, management, and proposal for a new clinical classification. *Fertil. Steril.* **103** (**1**): 147–152.

33 Stratton, P., Khachikyan, I., Sinaii, N. et al. (2015). Association of chronic pelvic pain and endometriosis with signs of sensitization and myofascial pain. *Obstet. Gynecol.* **125** (**3**): 719–728.

34 Ek, M., Roth, B., Ekstrom, P. et al. (2015). Gastrointestinal symptoms among endometriosis patients--a case-cohort study. *BMC Womens Health* **15**: 59-015-0213-2.

35 Ruffo, G., Crippa, S., Sartori, A. et al. (2014). Management of rectosigmoid obstruction due to severe bowel endometriosis. *Updates Surg.* **66** (**1**): 59–64.

36 Venable, J.H. (1972). Endometriosis of the ileum: four cases with obstruction. *Am. J. Obstet. Gynecol.* **113** (**8**): 1054–1055.

37 Chung, M.K., Chung, R.P., and Gordon, D. (2005). Interstitial cystitis and endometriosis in patients with chronic pelvic pain: the "evil twins" syndrome. *JSLS* **9** (**1**): 25–29.

38 Exacoustos, C., Manganaro, L., and Zupi, E. (2014). Imaging for the evaluation of endometriosis and adenomyosis. *Best. Pract. Res. Clin. Obstet. Gynaecol.* **28** (**5**): 655–681.

39 Abrao, M.S., Goncalves, M.O., Dias, J.A. Jr. et al. (2007). Comparison between clinical examination, transvaginal sonography and magnetic resonance imaging for the diagnosis of deep endometriosis. *Hum. Reprod.* **22** (**12**): 3092–3097.

40 Bazot, M. and Darai, E. (2005). Sonography and MR imaging for the assessment of deep pelvic endometriosis. *J. Minim. Invasive Gynecol.* **12** (**2**): 178–185. quiz 177, 186.

41 Bulun, S.E. (2009). Endometriosis. *N. Engl. J. Med.* **360** (**3**): 268–279.

42 Davis, L., Kennedy, S.S., Moore, J., and Prentice, A. (2007). Modern combined oral contraceptives for pain associated with endometriosis. *Cochrane Database Syst. Rev.* **3** (**3**): CD001019. doi: 10.1002/14651858.CD001019.

43 Harada, T., Momoeda, M., Taketani, Y. et al. (2008). Low-dose oral contraceptive pill for dysmenorrhea associated with endometriosis: a placebo-controlled, double-blind, randomized trial. *Fertil. Steril.* **90** (**5**): 1583–1588.

44 Crosignani, P.G., Luciano, A., Ray, A., and Bergqvist, A. (2006). Subcutaneous depot medroxyprogesterone acetate vs. leuprolide acetate in the treatment of endometriosis-associated pain. *Hum. Reprod.* **21** (**1**): 248–256.

45 Schlaff, W.D., Carson, S.A., Luciano, A. et al. (2006). Subcutaneous injection of depot medroxyprogesterone acetate compared with leuprolide acetate in the treatment of endometriosis-associated pain. *Fertil. Steril.* **85** (**2**): 314–325.

46 Vercellini, P., Cortesi, I., and Crosignani, P.G. (1997). Progestins for symptomatic endometriosis: a critical analysis of the evidence. *Fertil. Steril.* **68** (**3**): 393–401.

47 Vercellini, P., Frontino, G., De Giorgi, O. et al. (2003). Comparison of a levonorgestrel-releasing intrauterine device vs. expectant management after conservative surgery for symptomatic endometriosis: a pilot study. *Fertil. Steril.* **80** (**2**): 305–309.

48 Lockhat, F.B., Emembolu, J.O., and Konje, J.C. (2005). The efficacy, side-effects and continuation rates in women with symptomatic endometriosis undergoing treatment with

an intra-uterine administered progestogen (levonorgestrel): a 3 year follow-up. *Hum. Reprod.* **20** (**3**): 789–793.

49 Petta, C.A., Ferriani, R.A., Abrao, M.S. et al. (2005). Randomized clinical trial of a levonorgestrel-releasing intrauterine system and a depot GnRH analogue for the treatment of chronic pelvic pain in women with endometriosis. *Hum. Reprod.* **20** (**7**): 1993–1998.

50 Brown, J., Pan, A., and Hart, R.J. (2010). Gonadotrophin-releasing hormone analogues for pain associated with endometriosis. *Cochrane Database Syst. Rev.* (**12**): CD008475. doi: 10.1002/14651858.CD008475.pub2.

51 Surrey, E.S. and Judd, H.L. (1992). Reduction of vasomotor symptoms and bone mineral density loss with combined norethindrone and long-acting gonadotropin-releasing hormone agonist therapy of symptomatic endometriosis: a prospective randomized trial. *J. Clin. Endocrinol. Metab.* **75** (**2**): 558–563.

52 Winkel, C.A. (2000). A cost-effective approach to the management of endometriosis. *Curr. Opin. Obstet. Gynecol.* **12** (**4**): 317–320.

53 Amsterdam, L.L., Gentry, W., Jobanputra, S. et al. (2005). Anastrazole and oral contraceptives: a novel treatment for endometriosis. *Fertil. Steril.* **84** (**2**): 300–304.

54 Brown, J., Kives, S., and Akhtar, M. (2012). Progestagens and anti-progestagens for pain associated with endometriosis. *Cochrane Database Syst. Rev.* **3**: CD002122. doi: 10.1002/14651858.CD002122.pub2.

55 Zhu, X., Hamilton, K.D., and McNicol, E.D. (2011). Acupuncture for pain in endometriosis. *Cochrane Database Syst. Rev.* (**9**): CD007864. doi: 10.1002/14651858.CD007864.pub2.

56 Proctor, M.L., Smith, C.A., Farquhar, C.M., and Stones, R.W. (2002). Transcutaneous electrical nerve stimulation and acupuncture for primary dysmenorrhoea. *Cochrane Database Syst. Rev.* (**1**): CD002123. doi: 10.1002/14651858.CD002123.

57 Garcia, L. and Isaacson, K. (2011). Adenomyosis: review of the literature. *J. Minim. Invasive Gynecol.* **18** (**4**): 428–437.

58 Sheng, J., Zhang, W.Y., Zhang, J.P., and Lu, D. (2009). The LNG-IUS study on adenomyosis: a 3-year follow-up study on the efficacy and side effects of the use of levonorgestrel intrauterine system for the treatment of dysmenorrhea associated with adenomyosis. *Contraception* **79** (**3**): 189–193.

59 Cho, S., Nam, A., Kim, H. et al. (2008). Clinical effects of the levonorgestrel-releasing intrauterine device in patients with adenomyosis. *Am. J. Obstet. Gynecol.* **198** (**4**): 373.e1–373.e7.

60 Ozdegirmenci, O., Kayikcioglu, F., Akgul, M.A. et al. (2011). Comparison of levonorgestrel intrauterine system vs. hysterectomy on efficacy and quality of life in patients with adenomyosis. *Fertil. Steril.* **95** (**2**): 497–502.

61 Igarashi, M., Abe, Y., Fukuda, M. et al. (2000). Novel conservative medical therapy for uterine adenomyosis with a danazol-loaded intrauterine device. *Fertil. Steril.* **74** (**2**): 412–413.

62 Duffy, J.M., Arambage, K., Correa, F.J. et al. (2014). Laparoscopic surgery for endometriosis. *Cochrane Database Syst. Rev.* **4**: CD011031. doi: 10.1002/14651858.CD011031.pub2.

63 Crosignani, P.G., Vercellini, P., Biffignandi, F. et al. (1996). Laparoscopy vs. laparotomy in conservative surgical treatment for severe endometriosis. *Fertil. Steril.* **66** (**5**): 706–711.

64 Tarjanne, S., Heikinheimo, O., Mentula, M., and Harkki, P. (2015). Complications and long-term follow-up on colorectal resections in the treatment of deep infiltrating endometriosis extending to bowel wall. *Acta Obstet. Gynecol. Scand.* **94** (**1**): 72–79.

65 Abbott, J., Hawe, J., Hunter, D. et al. (2004). Laparoscopic excision of endometriosis: a randomized, placebo-controlled trial. *Fertil. Steril.* **82** (**4**): 878–884.

66 Hart, R.J., Hickey, M., Maouris, P., and Buckett, W. (2008). Excisional surgery vs. ablative surgery for ovarian endometriomata. *Cochrane Database Syst. Rev.* (**2**): CD004992. doi: 10.1002/14651858.CD004992.pub3.

67 Chapron, C., Vercellini, P., Barakat, H. et al. (2002). Management of ovarian endometriomas. *Hum. Reprod. Update* **8** (**6**): 591–597.

68 Abbott, J.A., Hawe, J., Clayton, R.D., and Garry, R. (2003). The effects and effectiveness of laparoscopic excision of endometriosis: a prospective study with 2-5 year follow-up. *Hum. Reprod.* **18** (**9**): 1922–1927.

69 Possover, M., Diebolder, H., Plaul, K., and Schneider, A. (2000). Laparascopically assisted vaginal resection of rectovaginal endometriosis. *Obstet. Gynecol.* **96** (**2**): 304–307.

70 Fritzer, N., Tammaa, A., Salzer, H., and Hudelist, G. (2014). Dyspareunia and quality of sex life after surgical excision of endometriosis: a systematic review. *Eur. J. Obstet. Gynecol. Reprod. Biol.* **173**: 1–6.

71 Setala, M., Harkki, P., Matomaki, J. et al. (2012). Sexual functioning, quality of life and pelvic pain 12 months after endometriosis surgery including vaginal resection. *Acta Obstet. Gynecol. Scand.* **91** (**6**): 692–698.

72 Fedele, L., Bianchi, S., Zanconato, G. et al. (2004). Long-term follow-up after conservative surgery for rectovaginal endometriosis. *Am. J. Obstet. Gynecol.* **190** (**4**): 1020–1024.

73 Guo, S.W. (2009). Recurrence of endometriosis and its control. *Hum. Reprod. Update* **15** (**4**): 441–461.

74 Practice Committee of the American Society for Reproductive Medicine (2014). Treatment of pelvic pain associated with endometriosis: a committee opinion. *Fertil. Steril.* **101** (**4**): 927–935.

75 Vercellini, P., Giudice, L.C., Evers, J.L., and Abrao, M.S. (2015). Reducing low-value care in endometriosis between limited evidence and unresolved issues: a proposal. *Hum. Reprod.* **30** (**9**): 1996–2004.

76 Vercellini, P., Frattaruolo, M.P., Somigliana, E. et al. (2013). Surgical vs. low-dose progestin treatment for endometriosis-associated severe deep dyspareunia II: effect

on sexual functioning, psychological status and health-related quality of life. *Hum. Reprod.* **28** (**5**): 1221–1230.

77 Zullo, F., Palomba, S., Zupi, E. et al. (2003). Effectiveness of presacral neurectomy in women with severe dysmenorrhea caused by endometriosis who were treated with laparoscopic conservative surgery: a 1-year prospective randomized double-blind controlled trial. *Am. J. Obstet. Gynecol.* **189** (**1**): 5–10.

78 McCausland, A.M. and McCausland, V.M. (1996). Depth of endometrial penetration in adenomyosis helps determine outcome of rollerball ablation. *Am. J. Obstet. Gynecol.* **174** (**6**): 1786–1793. 1793–4.

79 El-Nashar, S.A., Hopkins, M.R., Creedon, D.J. et al. (2009). Prediction of treatment outcomes after global endometrial ablation. *Obstet. Gynecol.* **113** (**1**): 97–106.

80 Popovic, M., Puchner, S., Berzaczy, D. et al. (2011). Uterine artery embolization for the treatment of adenomyosis: a review. *J. Vasc. Interv. Radiol.* **22** (**7**): 901–909. quiz 909.

81 Wood, C. (1998). Surgical and medical treatment of adenomyosis. *Hum. Reprod. Update* **4** (**4**): 323–336.

82 Shah, D.K., Mejia, R.B., and Lebovic, D.I. (2014). Effect of surgery for endometrioma on ovarian function. *J. Minim. Invasive Gynecol.* **21** (**2**): 203–209.

83 Benaglia, L., Somigliana, E., Vercellini, P. et al. (2009). Endometriotic ovarian cysts negatively affect the rate of spontaneous ovulation. *Hum. Reprod.* **24** (**9**): 2183–2186.

84 Leone Roberti Maggiore, U., Scala, C., Venturini, P.L. et al. (2015). Endometriotic ovarian cysts do not negatively affect the rate of spontaneous ovulation. *Hum. Reprod.* **30** (**2**): 299–307.

85 Kim, J.Y., Jee, B.C., Suh, C.S., and Kim, S.H. (2013). Preoperative serum anti-mullerian hormone level in women with ovarian endometrioma and mature cystic teratoma. *Yonsei Med. J.* **54** (**4**): 921–926.

86 Jeon, J.H., Park, S.Y., Lee, S.R. et al. (2015). Serum anti-Mullerian hormone levels before surgery in patients with ovarian Endometriomas compared to other benign ovarian cysts. *J. Menopausal Med.* **21** (**3**): 142–148.

87 Hamdan, M., Dunselman, G., Li, T.C., and Cheong, Y. (2015). The impact of endometrioma on IVF/ICSI outcomes: a systematic review and meta-analysis. *Hum. Reprod. Update* **21** (**6**): 809–825.

88 Raffi, F., Metwally, M., and Amer, S. (2012). The impact of excision of ovarian endometrioma on ovarian reserve: a systematic review and meta-analysis. *J. Clin. Endocrinol. Metab.* **97** (**9**): 3146–3154.

89 Somigliana, E., Berlanda, N., Benaglia, L. et al. (2012). Surgical excision of endometriomas and ovarian reserve: a systematic review on serum antimullerian hormone level modifications. *Fertil. Steril.* **98** (**6**): 1531–1538.

90 Muzii, L., Di Tucci, C., Di Feliciantonio, M. et al. (2014). The effect of surgery for endometrioma on ovarian reserve evaluated by antral follicle count: a systematic review and meta-analysis. *Hum. Reprod.* **29** (**10**): 2190–2198.

91 Vercellini, P., Somigliana, E., Vigano, P. et al. (2009). Surgery for endometriosis-associated infertility: a pragmatic approach. *Hum. Reprod.* **24** (**2**): 254–269.

92 Tsolakidis, D., Pados, G., Vavilis, D. et al. (2010). The impact on ovarian reserve after laparoscopic ovarian cystectomy vs. three-stage management in patients with endometriomas: a prospective randomized study. *Fertil. Steril.* **94** (**1**): 71–77.

93 Var, T., Batioglu, S., Tonguc, E., and Kahyaoglu, I. (2011). The effect of laparoscopic ovarian cystectomy vs. coagulation in bilateral endometriomas on ovarian reserve as determined by antral follicle count and ovarian volume: a prospective randomized study. *Fertil. Steril.* **95** (**7**): 2247–2250.

94 Koga, K., Takemura, Y., Osuga, Y. et al. (2006). Recurrence of ovarian endometrioma after laparoscopic excision. *Hum. Reprod.* **21** (**8**): 2171–2174.

95 Practice Committee of the American Society for Reproductive Medicine (2012). Endometriosis and infertility: a committee opinion. *Fertil. Steril.* **98** (**3**): 591–598.

96 Moini, A., Bahar, L., Ashrafinia, M. et al. (2012). Fertility outcome after operative laparoscopy vs. no treatment in infertile women with minimal or mild endometriosis. *Int. J. Fertil. Steril.* **5** (**4**): 235–240.

97 Chopin, N., Vieira, M., Borghese, B. et al. (2005). Operative management of deeply infiltrating endometriosis: results on pelvic pain symptoms according to a surgical classification. *J. Minim. Invasive Gynecol.* **12** (**2**): 106–112.

98 Vercellini, P., Pietropaolo, G., De Giorgi, O. et al. (2006). Reproductive performance in infertile women with rectovaginal endometriosis: is surgery worthwhile? *Am. J. Obstet. Gynecol.* **195** (**5**): 1303–1310.

99 De Cicco, C., Corona, R., Schonman, R. et al. (2011). Bowel resection for deep endometriosis: a systematic review. *BJOG* **118** (**3**): 285–291.

100 Darai, E., Thomassin, I., Barranger, E. et al. (2005). Feasibility and clinical outcome of laparoscopic colorectal resection for endometriosis. *Am. J. Obstet. Gynecol.* **192** (**2**): 394–400.

101 Furness, S., Yap, C., Farquhar, C., and Cheong, Y.C. (2004). Pre and post-operative medical therapy for endometriosis surgery. *Cochrane Database of Syst. Rev.* doi: 10.1002/14651858.CD003678.pub2.

102 Seracchioli, R., Mabrouk, M., Frasca, C. et al. (2010). Long-term oral contraceptive pills and postoperative pain management after laparoscopic excision of ovarian endometrioma: a randomized controlled trial. *Fertil. Steril.* **94** (**2**): 464–471.

103 Seracchioli, R., Mabrouk, M., Manuzzi, L. et al. (2009). Post-operative use of oral contraceptive pills for prevention of anatomical relapse or symptom-recurrence after conservative surgery for endometriosis. *Hum. Reprod.* **24** (**11**): 2729–2735.

104 Abou-Setta, A.M., Houston, B., Al-Inany, H.G., and Farquhar, C. (2013). Levonorgestrel-releasing intrauterine device (LNG-IUD) for symptomatic endometriosis following surgery. *Cochrane Database Syst. Rev.* (**1**): CD005072. doi: 10.1002/14651858.CD005072.pub3.

105 Namnoum, A.B., Hickman, T.N., Goodman, S.B. et al. (1995). Incidence of symptom recurrence after hysterectomy for endometriosis. *Fertil. Steril.* **64** (**5**): 898–902.

106 Shakiba, K., Bena, J.F., McGill, K.M. et al. (2008). Surgical treatment of endometriosis: a 7-year follow-up on the requirement for further surgery. *Obstet. Gynecol.* **111** (**6**): 1285–1292.

107 Matorras, R., Elorriaga, M.A., Pijoan, J.I. et al. (2002). Recurrence of endometriosis in women with bilateral adnexectomy (with or without total hysterectomy) who received hormone replacement therapy. *Fertil. Steril.* **77** (**2**): 303–308.

9

CHAPTER 9

Contraception and sterilization

Rasha S. Khoury[1] and Danielle M. Roncari[2]
[1]*Division of Family Planning and Global Women's Health, Department of Obstetrics, Gynecology & Reproductive Biology, Brigham and Women's Hospital, Harvard Medical School, Boston, MA, USA*
[2]*Division of Family Planning, Department of Obstetrics and Gynecology, Tufts University School of Medicine, Boston, MA, USA*

CLINICAL SCENARIO

A 35-year-old G5P323 presents to your clinic desiring birth control. She reports that she and her partner of five years have been sporadically using condoms. Two nights ago, she believes a condom broke during intercourse. She is wondering if there is anything she can do to prevent pregnancy at this point and is also looking for an easier, more reliable long-term method. She is fairly certain that she does not want any more children. In the past, other than condoms, she reports intermittent use of birth control pills for 10 years and more recently Depo-Provera after the birth of her last child.

Her medical history is significant for migraine headaches without aura. She denies any surgical history and is not taking any medications. She does report smoking cigarettes, approximately 1/2 pack a day. She has had five pregnancies, two spontaneous vaginal deliveries, one cesarean section, and two first trimester abortions. She denies any history of abnormal pap smears and had chlamydia that was treated seven years ago.

The patient's vital signs are within normal limits: temperature 37 C (oral), heart rate 66 beats per minute, respiratory rate 15 breaths per minute and blood pressure 115/70 mmHg (left arm). Her BMI is 28. Her last menstrual period was seven days ago. On exam, she is well appearing. She had a normal gynecological exam approximately six months ago. Her office pregnancy test is negative. You obtain a urine gonorrhea and chlamydia test per the patient's request.

Background

In 2006, approximately 49% of pregnancies in the United States (US) were unintended with 43% ending in abortion [1]. Of these unintended pregnancies, 46% were in women reporting no birth control or inconsistent use during the month they became pregnant [2]. The most popular methods of birth control among US women using contraception are the pills and female sterilization at 27.5% and 26.6% respectively [3]. The most effective methods of birth control other than female and male sterilization are long-acting reversible contraception methods (LARC) including IUC and the implant. In a prospective cohort study of nearly 1000 women, the Contraceptive Choice Project, LARC methods had an unintended pregnancy rate of 0.27 per 100 participants as compared to the pill, patch, and ring with a rate of 4.55/100 women [4]. When counseling women on birth control options, it is important to discuss method effectiveness, future pregnancy desire, a patient's medical problems, her concern over particular methods, and method related side effects and risks.

Clinical questions

In order to address the issues of most relevance to your patient and to help in searching the literature for the evidence regarding contraception methods, you structure your clinical questions as recommended in Chapter 1.

1. How should women be counseled around fertility desires, pregnancy spacing, and limiting?
2. How is contraceptive effectiveness determined and what is the effectiveness of the most common methods?
3. What are the US medical eligibility criteria for contraceptive use? What methods are women with a history of migraine and active tobacco use eligible for?
4. Who are appropriate candidates for LARC methods? Can women with a history of sexually transmitted infections (STIs) safely use these methods?
5. What are non-LARC contraceptive options?
6. What methods are available for permanent contraception (sterilization)?

Evidence-Based Obstetrics and Gynecology, First Edition. Edited by Errol R. Norwitz, Carolyn M. Zelop, David A. Miller, and David L. Keefe.

7. What are currently available methods of emergency contraception and does BMI alter effectiveness?
8. What barrier methods are currently available and what is best practice for using these methods?

General search strategy

You begin to address these questions by searching for evidence in the common electronic databases such as the Cochrane Library and MEDLINE looking specifically for systematic reviews and meta-analyses.

Searching for evidence synthesis: primary search strategy

_ Cochrane Library: ____________ AND (topic)
_ MEDLINE:

Critical Review of the Literature

1. How should women be counseled around fertility desires, pregnancy spacing and limiting?

Search Strategy

MEDLINE: (pregnancy OR birth) AND (intention OR spacing); sterilization AND counseling.

Exploring women's viewpoints toward future pregnancies is an integral component of contraceptive counseling. Schwartz et al. suggest we expand the framework around pregnancy intention from intending and not intending to become pregnant to "seeking pregnancy now, avoiding now, planning for future and avoiding forever" [5]. This allows a provider to better understand a patient's life context and meet her needs. On both ends of the spectrum, a patient who is seeking pregnancy now or avoiding forever can be offered pre-conceptual counseling and sterilization counseling respectively. For patients avoiding pregnancy now and planning pregnancy in the future a discussion of preferred timing is paramount, taking into consideration optimal pregnancy intervals for maternal and neonatal health, age, fecundity, fertility desires, health services access, family and community support, social and economic support, and individual preference. With respect to spacing after a live birth the WHO recommends a birth-to-pregnancy interval of at least 24 months but less than five years [6] (to achieve the primary outcome of risk reduction in maternal, perinatal, and infant adverse events) [7–9]. Data reviewed for the WHO consultation suggest the risk of prematurity, fetal death, small for gestational age and low birth weight are highest for birth-to-pregnancy intervals shorter than 18 months (or longer than 59 months). While the relationship between pregnancy intervals and maternal mortality is unclear, maternal morbidity does appear to be associated with very long pregnancy intervals (mainly preeclampsia) rather than very short intervals (where cesarean delivery is the only variable with a clear relationship to short pregnancy interval-related adverse events, mainly uterine rupture) [7]. The WHO birth spacing recommendation is also consistent with the WHO/UNICEF recommendation for breastfeeding for at least two years.

It is important when discussing sterilization methods to impart their permanence (and correct any misperceptions of their reversibility), the possibility of future regret, and specific information about the procedures available including risk of failure. Information should be communicated in the patient's primary language, adjusted for literacy, remain medically accurate, understandable, and unbiased. The decision to move forward with sterilization, as with any medical procedure, should involve informed consent (an understanding of the risks, benefits, and alternatives as well decision-making free of coercion). Parity and age are no longer considered criteria for sterilization though regret is associated with sterilization of women younger than 30 [10–12]. In addition to age at time of sterilization, external pressure by clinicians, partners, and others, has been correlated with post-sterilization regret [10]. However, marital status, level of education and childlessness have not been correlated with regret. [10]. The 14-years cumulative probability of regret among a cohort of US women sterilized when they were younger than 30 was found to be 20.3%, compared to 5.9% among women older than 30 [10]. Regret is also associated with unpredictable life events, such as a change in partner status, health status, or the illness/death of a child.

Risk of sterilization failure should factor into the counseling. The US Collaborative Review of Sterilization (CREST) study provided us with a cumulative 10-years probability of pregnancy after sterilization of 18/1000 (highest after clip sterilization and lowest after unipolar coagulation and postpartum partial salpingectomy – bipolar coagulation, Filshie clips, and hysteroscopic occlusion were not assessed as they were not available at that time) [12]. Failure can occur due to undetected luteal pregnancy, occlusion/transection of an incorrect structure, development of a tuboperitoneal fistula, incomplete or inadequate occlusion, device migration or slippage, and spontaneous reanastamosis/recanalization of the cut tubal ends. While one third of post sterilization pregnancies in the CREST study were ectopic pregnancies (high relative risk), sterilization has an overall protective effect on the risk of ectopic pregnancy (absolute risk of 4/1000). Complications are incredibly rare (occurring in fewer than 0.5% of cases) [13, 14]. All women requesting sterilization should be counseled on the highly effective LARC with comparably low failure rates using the (levonorgestrel intrauterine system (LNG IUS): 0.2% pregnant at one year, and implant 0.05% pregnant at one year).

2. How is contraceptive effectiveness determined and what is the effectiveness of the most common methods?

Search Strategy

_ MEDLINE: (contraception OR birth control) AND effectiveness.

Many women aren't able to determine the relative effectiveness of various birth control methods; yet most women cite effectiveness as the most important factor for choosing a contraceptive [15]. Understanding effectiveness is crucially important to making an informed choice regarding a birth control method.

Many factors contribute to overall effectiveness including the fecundity of both partners, the timing of intercourse in relation to the timing of ovulation, the method of contraception used, the intrinsic effectiveness of the contraceptive method, and the correct and continuous use of the method. The Pearl formula is one way to estimate pregnancy risk. This formula calculates a pregnancy rate per 100 women per year by dividing the number of pregnancies by the total number of months contributed by all couples, and then multiplying the quotient by 1200. Because with most methods pregnancy rates decrease with time as the more fertile or less careful couples become pregnant and drop out of the calculations, the Pearl formula does not reflect actual use. More commonly, rates of pregnancy among different methods are best calculated by reporting two different rates derived from multiple studies (i.e. the lowest rate) and the usual or typical rate.

Perfect use is the percentage of couples who have an unintended pregnancy during the first year of use despite using a method *perfectly* (both consistently and correctly). Among average couples (may not use a method consistently or correctly), typical use refers to the percentage who experience an unintended pregnancy during the first year of use. Typical use is a practical way to look at overall effectiveness when counseling patients as it more accurately reflects practice than perfect use [16]. Continuation at one year is another important component in assessing a method's overall effectiveness.

In looking at the effectiveness across methods, many providers find it useful to arrange effectiveness from least to most effective. Methods that require consistent and correct use have a wide range of effectiveness. Depicted in Table 9.1 is the percentage of women experiencing an accidental pregnancy within the first year of use of a contraceptive method along with one year continuation [16].

Table 9.1 Percentage of women experiencing an unintended pregnancy during the first year of typical use and the first year of perfect use of contraception and the percentage continuing use at the end of the first year in the United States

	Percentage of women experiencing an unintended pregnancy within the first year of use		**Percentage of women continuing use at one year**
Method	Typical use	Perfect use	
No method	85	85	
Spermicides	28	18	42
Fertility awareness-based methods	24		47
Standard days method		5	
Two day method		4	
Ovulation method		3	
Symptothermal method		0.4	
Withdrawal	22	4	46
Sponge			36
Parous women	24	20	
Nulliparous women	12	9	
Condom			
Female (fc)	21	5	41
Male	18	2	43
Diaphragm	12	6	57
Combined pill and progestin-only pill	9	0.3	67
Evra patch	9	0.3	67
NuvaRing	9	0.3	67
Depo-Provera	6	0.2	56
Intrauterine contraceptives			
ParaGard (copper T)	0.8	0.6	78
Mirena (LNG)	0.2	0.2	80
Implanon	0.05	0.05	84
Female sterilization	0.5	0.5	100
Male sterilization	0.15	0.10	100

Source: Trussell, 2011 [16].

3. What are the US medical eligibility criteria for contraceptive use? What methods are women with a history of migraine and active tobacco use eligible for?

Search Strategy

_ MEDLINE: (medical eligibility criteria) AND (contraception); contraception AND migraine; contraception AND smoking.

When counseling women on their contraceptive options it is vital to consider their medical and psychosocial context. While counseling should focus on the efficacy of each method as well as the synergy between the method's duration of action and the woman's future fertility desires, coexisting medical conditions, tobacco, alcohol, drug use, and social stressors will impact the safety profile and effectiveness of any method. Is the woman safe to choose a female user dependent method?; a male user dependent method?; an irreversible method? Does she need the method to be discrete? Can she access health care services if she experiences adverse effects?

After a thorough medical history, the CDC's US Medical Eligibility Criteria (USMEC) (2010) can be most helpful in presenting the safety profile for method initiation and continuation according to the individual woman's medical and personal characteristics. The USMEC are available in English and Spanish on the CDC website free of charge in both narrative and chart/table form. More recently they have become available as a user-friendly iPhone and iPad application available for free download [17].

For healthy young women under the age of 35 the CDC considers all contraceptive methods (hormonal and non-hormonal) safe without restriction (USMEC category 1). The risk of cardiovascular disease increases with age and might increase with combined hormonal contraceptive (CHC – pill, patch, ring) use however in the absence of other adverse clinical conditions, data suggest CHCs can be used until menopause (at age 40 the USMEC for CHCs changes to a 2 but remains safe). For women with migraines without aura the initiation of any method is category 1 or 2 (advantages outweigh risks) under 35; for women 35 and older the initiation of estrogen containing methods is category 3 (theoretical or proven risks outweigh the advantages of using the method), progestin only pills and copper IUC (category 1) and Depo-Provera (depot medroxyprogesterone acetate (DMPA)), implants and LNG IUC (category 2). It is important to take a thorough headache history to delineate headaches that are migrainous from those that are not. New headaches and changes in headache character should be evaluated. The USMEC for migraines without aura are for women without any other risk factors for stroke (risk of stroke increases with age, hypertension, and smoking). Among women with migraines those with aura (complex of neurologic symptoms that occur just before or at the onset of the migraine headache [18] have a higher risk of stroke than those without aura [19–21] and those who use CHCs are 2–4 times as likely to have an ischemic stroke as non-users with a history of migraine [20, 22–25].

Tobacco use less than 15 cigarettes per day in women 35 and older renders estrogen containing methods a category 3 and all other methods a category 1. If smoking is in fact heavier, more than or equal to 15 cigarettes per day, estrogen containing methods are category 4 (unacceptable health risk if the method is used) and all other methods category 1. CHC users who smoked were at increased risk for cardiovascular disease, especially myocardial infarction, compared to those who did not smoke. The effect appears to be dose dependent, increased risk for MI with increasing number of cigarettes smoked per day [26–29].

4. Who are appropriate candidates for LARC methods? Can women with a history of sexually transmitted infections safely use these methods?

Search Strategy

_ MEDLINE: (intrauterine contraception OR IUC) and (chlamydia OR sexually transmitted infection OR STI).

LARC methods, including IUCs and implants are the most effective methods of reversible birth control. Despite their effectiveness, uptake of these methods in the US is still relatively low. Most recent estimates are that approximately 7.7% of women rely on IUCs and 0.8% on implants [30].

There is only one commercially available implant in the US, the etonorgestrel implant. This is a one-rod subdermal system that has contraceptive efficacy for three years. There are few contraindications to the implant, and because it is a progesterone only method, it does not have any estrogen associated thrombosis risk. Insertion and removal must be done by trained providers.

Currently available IUCs in the US are the levonorgestrel IUC, a 14 and 25 mg levonorgestrel type, and the copper T 380A. In addition to high contraceptive efficacy, the levonorgestrel IUC 25 mg has the added benefit of reducing menstrual bleeding and cramping and has been shown to be an effective treatment in improving the symptoms of endometriosis [31, 32], adenomyosis [33], and uterine fibroids [34, 35].

There are many misconceptions surrounding modern use IUCs. Among these are that IUCs are not appropriate for adolescents and nulliparous women, that IUCs should only be inserted during menses and that IUCs cause infection. Modern day IUCs are safe for most women including adolescents and nulliparous women, can be inserted at any time in the menstrual cycle as long as a woman isn't pregnant and do not predispose patients to pelvic infection [36]. There is a slightly higher risk of infection the first 20 days after insertion but this risk declines to baseline after this period, suggesting the risk is related to the insertion process and a background risk of STIs. Screening for gonorrhea and chlamydia at the time of insertion is recommended for adolescents or those with risk factors, but it is not considered necessary to wait for the results before insertion since patients with positive results have no adverse effects if treated promptly [37]. Because of an overall low risk of infection associated with IUC insertion, prophylactic antibiotics have not been proven to be of benefit [38].

There also does not appear to be an association with bacterial vaginosis and presence of bacterial vaginosis is not a reason to delay IUC insertion [38]. Pelvic inflammatory disease (PID), puerperal sepsis or post-abortion sepsis within the past three months are considered contraindications and patients with purulent cervicitis should be tested and treated before insertion [36]. For patients in whom PID is suspected after insertion, appropriate cultures should be obtained, and antibiotic therapy should be administered. IUC removal is not necessary unless the patient remains symptomatic 72 hours after treatment [39].

5. What are non-LARC contraceptive options?

Search Strategy

_ MEDLINE: (hormonal contraception) AND (BMI OR weight OR bone health OR BMD).

The risk of pregnancy at one year in the absence of a contraceptive method is 85%. Non-LARC methods include barrier methods (male and female condoms) with a typical use risk of pregnancy of 18% and 21% respectively; CHCs (pills, patch, ring) or progesterone only pills (POP) with a pregnancy risk of 9% and continuation rate of 67% at one year; DMPA with typical use failure of 6% and continuation of 56% at one year [40]. CHCs are contraindicated in women that cannot take estrogen. POPs are safe for most women and unlikely to interact with other medications. To be a candidate for POPs, a patient must have reliable access to health care services, must be able to adhere to a daily medication and able to take it within a three hour window each day. DMPA has the advantage of being a mid-acting contraceptive method with injections every three months. A patient must have reliable access to health care service, as this is a provider-dependent method.

In counseling patients on DMPA, it is important to address its association with bone loss. DMPA creates a hypoestrogenic state that promotes bone resorption over bone formation. In 2004, the FDA placed a "black box" warning on DMPA labels in the US stating that "bone loss grows worse over time, may remain long after discontinuation and may be irreversible" [41]. The WHO in contrast supports the use of DMPA without restriction [42, 43]. More recent data suggest that the greatest bone loss occurs in the first 1 to two years after initiating DMPA, then stabilizes and does not appear to fall below 1 standard deviation of normal even after five years of use [44–46]. After discontinuing DMPA, bone mineral density (BMD) appears to return to baseline (within 30 months for premenopausal women) when matching for age and race, independent of the length of DMPA use or first use at a young age [44, 46–48]. The American College of Obstetricians and Gynecologists supports the use of DMPA beyond two years and states that concern over BMD should not prevent the prescription of or continuation of DMPA [49].

6. What methods are available for permanent contraception (sterilization)?

Search Strategy

_ MEDLINE: (sterilization) AND (male OR female); sterilization AND hysteroscopic.

For patients that are certain that they do not want any more children, they should be counseled on female and male permanent methods of contraception. Female sterilization (tubal ligation and occlusion) and male sterilization procedures (vasectomy) are the safest, most effective, and most cost-effective contraceptive methods. Sterilization (male and female) procedures additionally are the most widely used modern method of family planning worldwide. Among women in the US aged 15–44 using contraception, 16.5% relied on female sterilization, and 6.2% on male sterilization [50]. While male and female sterilization methods are comparable in effectiveness, male methods are simpler, safer, and less costly. When considering male sterilization it is vital to inquire about the patient's partner status to assess whether her primary partner is her only partner in order to protect her from undesired pregnancy. Sterilization's mechanism of action is preventing fertilization (the oocyte and sperm from uniting). While there are no absolute medical contraindications to sterilization, each method has different side effects and risks so medical history should be factored into procedure choice.

Female sterilization: ligation or occlusion of the fallopian tubes can be accomplished transabdominally or transcervically. The most common procedure in the US is postpartum tubal ligation (via subumbilical minilaparotomy after vaginal delivery or at time of cesarean section) followed by interval laparoscopic ligation (via fulguration, falope ring, or Filshie clip application). In November 2002, the FDA approved Essure sterilization (transcervical application of microinserts into the interstitial portion of each fallopian tube for occlusion bilaterally). This has become the safest, least invasive, irreversible contraceptive method available. Following Essure, tubal occlusion must be confirmed by hysterosalpingogram (HSG) at 12 weeks in the US (outside the US pelvic X-ray is performed to confirm microinsert placement). Backup contraception must be used until tubal occlusion is confirmed. Bilateral placement rates on the current FDA-approved device is 96.9%, with average hysteroscopic placement time of nine minutes [51, 52]. Provider experience does not seem to affect placement success rates, though does have an impact on procedure time [53]. A variety of cervical and uterine anomalies and pathology can be barriers for successful placement, however, other factors such as nulliparity, BMI, prior abdominal surgery and age do not appear to impact placement [53–56]. Essure is 99.74% effective at preventing pregnancy at five years according to the manufacturer's clinical trials. In a review of 50 000 worldwide Essure placements between 1997 and 2005, 64 pregnancies were reported to the manufacturer [57]. Upon investigation, these pregnancies were attributed to poor patient selection, poor microinsert placement, poor adherence to HSG follow-up (unconfirmed occlusion), and misinterpretation of HSG. In a recent retrospective review of hysteroscopic sterilization from 2001 to 2010, (497 305 hysteroscopic sterilization kits distributed worldwide), 748 pregnancies were reported, further supporting the Essure manufacturer age-adjusted effectiveness of 99.74% at five years [58]. Essure failures were predominantly due to patient or provider non-adherence and misinterpreted HSGs.

Male sterilization: occlusion of the bilateral vas deferens to prevent the transfer of sperm from the epididymis to the ejaculate. Performed under local anesthesia with a no-scalpel technique (NSV) (reaching the vas through a puncture site in the scrotum) [59–61]. This approach has been shown to be associated with less bleeding and pain, fewer infections, and faster return to sexual activity [62]. While NSV is safe, cheap, and effective, it is not immediate. Semen analysis performed at three months post NSV must confirm azoospermia before the couple can rely on male sterility [63] (varies by technique and age). Reliable backup contraception must be used in the interim.

7. What are currently available methods of emergency contraception and does BMI alter effectiveness?

Search Strategy

_ MEDLINE: (emergency contraception AND efficacy) AND risk factors.

Levonorgestrel 1.5 mg and ulipristal acetate are the most effective hormonal means of emergency contraception. These methods both have delay of ovulation as their primary mechanism of action [64, 65]. Levonorgestrel is a progesterone-only method that is most effective taken within 72 hours of unprotected intercourse but has some efficacy up to 120 hours [66]. Ulipristal acetate is an anti-progesterone, similar in structure to mifepristone. The usual abortifacient dose is 200 mg, but a dose of only 10 mg is effective for emergency contraception. This method may have superior efficacy as compared to levonorgestrel methods from 72 to 120 hours after intercourse [67].

Overall efficacy of these methods varies greatly depending on timing of intercourse and cycle day. Average pregnancy rates are 60–94% for the levonorgestrel method and 62–85% for ulipristal acetate [67–69]. Because the main mechanism of these methods is a delay in ovulation, it is important that women start a more effective method of birth control after taking emergency contraception.

The most effective method of emergency contraception is the copper T 380A IUC with a nearly 100% efficacy when inserted within five days of unprotected intercourse [70]. In a multicenter trial by Wu et al., of 1893 women who returned for a follow-up visit, there were no pregnancies within one month of IUC insertion. In addition, this study showed an added benefit of this method in that 94% of the subjects were continuing with the IUC at the 12 months follow-up [71]. It is unknown whether the levonorgestrel IUC would have similar efficacy.

Recent data suggests BMI may alter the efficacy of the levonorgestrel regimen and ulipristal acetate. For women with a BMI greater than 30, pregnancy rates among users of the levonorgestrel method were not significantly different than for women who used no emergency contraception. At a BMI greater than 35, ulipristal acetate appears to lose its effectiveness [72, 73]. It is not known whether increasing the standard dosage of these medications will improve effectiveness in overweight and obese women. BMI has no impact on the effectiveness of the copper T 380A IUC for emergency contraception.

8. What barrier methods are currently available and what is best practice for using these methods?

Search Strategy

_ MEDLINE: condom AND failure and sexually transmitted disease.

Barrier methods, and in particular condoms, remain a popular method of birth control in the US. Nearly nine million reproductive aged women report using condoms as a method for pregnancy and disease prevention, and condoms are the third most popular method of contraception in the US [74]. Barrier methods remain a popular option as they are non-hormonal, coital dependent, and easy to access. And for patients at risk for STIs, these methods have the added benefit of decreasing the risk of disease transmission. Their relatively low effectiveness, however, makes these methods less attractive as a primary method. It is important that these methods are used consistently and correctly to increase their effectiveness.

Both male and female condoms are available. Today's male condoms are made from latex, natural membrane, and synthetic materials. There is about a 3% risk of breakage with condoms [75] that may be reduced with the use of water-based lubricants. Petroleum-based options may increase the risk of breakage [76]. Natural membrane condoms may not provide as much STI protection as latex condoms due to small pores in the membrane [77]. Synthetic condoms are manufactured from materials such as polyurethane and have similar efficacy in pregnancy prevention as latex condoms. Their effectiveness against STI prevention has been less well studied than in latex condoms so the FDA recommends restricting their use in individuals that have a latex allergy or sensitivity [78]. Condoms containing spermicide are no longer recommended as the frequent use of nonoxynol-9 may lead to micro tears in the genitals and the risk of increased disease transmission [79].

The female condom is made from synthetic latex. The efficacy of this method is lower than that of male condoms; however, its perfect use effectiveness is comparable to perfect use with other female barrier methods including the cervical cap and diaphragm. It is thought that while breakage is less common with the female than with the male condoms, slippage is more common [75]. Other female barrier methods include diaphragms, cervical caps, and the sponge. Diaphragms and cervical caps must be fitted by a clinician while the sponge can be purchased over the counter. While the effectiveness for each of these methods is relatively low, they have the benefit of being female initiated and coital dependent.

Conclusions

The patient from this chapter was educated on her contraceptive options. She is seeking contraception that can help prevent an unintended pregnancy subsequent to unprotected intercourse (emergency contraception) as well as a highly effective long-term method (LARC or sterilization). You review her options for emergency contraception: copper IUC most effective (with the secondary advantage of being a highly effective long-term method as well), levonorgestrel 1.5 mg or ulipristal acetate. You reassure her that these methods are safe despite her medical history notable for migraines without aura and tobacco use; also the distant chlamydia infection will not impact her method eligibility.

She is interested in the copper IUC and you advise her to have it inserted today, providing her with nearly 100% efficacy in preventing pregnancy, and allowing her to have a highly effective long-term contraceptive method. You review the possible side effects mainly heavier menses and dysmenorrhea, mitigated by non-steroidal anti-inflammatory drug (NSAIDs), heat and time.

She would like to return with her partner to discuss sterilization with you at a later time. You inform her that she is a candidate for all sterilization procedures (interval laparoscopic tubal ligation and hysteroscopic occlusion with microinserts) as well as male sterilization. Should she choose hysteroscopic sterilization or male sterilization, the copper IUC can provide her back-up contraception until tubal occlusion or male azoospermia is confirmed three months post op.

References

1 Finer, L.B. and Zolna, M.R. (2011). Unintended pregnancy in the United States: incidence and disparities, 2006. *Contraception* **84**: 478–485.

2 Jones, R.K., Darroch, J.E., and Henshaw, S.K. (2002). Contraceptive use among U.S. women having abortions in 2000–2001. *Perspect. Sex. Reprod. Health* **34**: 294–303.

3 Jones, J., Mosher, W.D., and Daniels, K. (2012). Current contraceptive use in the United States, 2006–2010, and changes in patterns of use since 1995. *Natl. Health Stat. Rep.* (**60**). http://www.cdc.gov/nchs/data/nhsr/nhsr060.pdf (accessed 23 June 2018).

4 Winner, B., Peipert, J.F., Zhao, Q. et al. (2012). Effectiveness of long-acting reversible contraception. *N. Engl. J. Med.* **366**: 1998–2007.

5 Schwartz, A., Peacock, N., McRae, K. et al. (2010). Defining new categories of pregnancy intention in African-American women. *Women's Health Issues.* **20** (**6**): 371–379.

6 WHO. 2005. Department of Reproductive Health and Research (RHR). Report of a WHO Technical Consultation on Birth Spacing. Geneva, Switzerland, 13–15 June 2005.

7 Conde-Agudelo, A., Rosas-Bermúdez, A., and Kafury- Goeta, A.C. (2006). Birth spacing and risk of adverse perinatal outcomes: a meta-analysis. *JAMA* **295**: 1809–1823.

8 DaVanzo, J., Hale, L., Razzaque, A. et al. (2008). The effects of pregnancy spacing on infant and child mortality in Matlab, Bangladesh: how they vary by the type of pregnancy outcome that began the interval. *Popul. Stud. (Camb)* **62**: 131–154.

9 Rutstein, S.O. (2005). Effects of preceding birth intervals on neonatal, infant and under-five years mortality and nutritional status in developing countries: evidence from the demographic and health surveys. *Int. J. Gynaecol. Obstet.* **89**: S7–S24.

10 Hillis, S.D., Marchbanks, P.A., Tylor, L.R. et al. (1999). Post-sterilization regret: findings from the United States collaborative review of sterilization. *Obstet. Gynecol.* **93**: 889–895.

11 Curtis, K., Mohllajee, A., and Peterson, H. (2006). Regret following female sterilization at a young age: a systematic review. *Contraception* **73**: 205–210.

12 Peterson, H.B., Xia, Z., Hughes, J.M. et al. (1996). The risk of pregnancy after tubal sterilization: findings from the U.S. collaborative review of sterilization. *Am. J. Obstet. Gynecol.* **174**: 1161–1168.

13 Hulka, J.F., Phillips, J.M., Peterson, H.B. et al. (1995). Laparoscopic sterilization: American Association of Gynecologic Laparoscopists' 1993 membership survey. *J. Am. Assoc. Gynecol. Laparosc.* **2**: 137–138.

14 (1982). Minilaparotomy or laparoscopy for sterilization: a multicenter, multinational randomized study. World Health Organization, task force on female sterilization, special Programme of research, development and research training in human reproduction. *Am. J. Obstet. Gynecol.* **143**: 645–652.

15 Steiner, M.J., Trussell, J., Mehta, N. et al. (2006). Communicating contraceptive effectiveness: a randomized controlled trial to inform a World Health Organization family planning handbook. *Am. J. Obstet. Gynecol.* **195**: 85–91.

16 Trussell, J. (2011). Contraceptive efficacy. In: *Contraceptive Technology*: Twentieth Revised Edition (ed. R.A. Hatcher, J. Trussell, A.L. Nelson, et al.), 791–792. New York: Ardent Media.

17 USMEC iPhone. iPad application download: https://itunes.apple.com/WebObjects/MZStore.woa/wa/viewSoftware?id=595752188™mt=8

18 Headache Classification Subcommittee of the International Headache Society (2004). *The International Classification of Headache Disorders*, 2e, 24. Cephalagia. http://ihs-classification.org/en/02_klassifikation/02_teil1/01.02.00_migraine.html.

19 Carolei, A., Marini, C., and De Matteis, G. (1996). History of migraine and risk of cerebral ischaemia in young adults. The Italian National Research Council Study Group on Stroke in the Young. *Lancet* **347**: 1503–1506.

20 Chang, C.L., Donaghy, M., and Poulter, N. (1999). Migraine and stroke in young women: case-control study. The World Health Organisation collaborative study of cardiovascular disease and steroid hormone contraception. *Br. Med. J.* **318**: 13–18.

21 Tzourio, C., Tehindrazanarivelo, A., Iglesias, S. et al. (1995). Case-control study of migraine and risk of ischaemic stroke in young women. *Br. Med. J.* **310**: 830–833.

22 Gillum, L.A., Mamidipudi, S.K., and Johnston, S.C. (2000). Ischaemic stroke risk with oral contraceptives: a meta-analysis. *J. Am. Med. Assoc.* **284**: 72–78.

23 Schwartz, S.M., Petitti, D.B., Siscovick, D.S. et al. (1998). Stroke and use of low-dose oral contraceptives in young women: a pooled analysis of two US studies. *Stroke* **29**: 2277–2284.

24 Etminan, M., Takkouche, B., Isorna, F.C. et al. (2005). Risk of ischaemic stroke in people with migraine: systematic review and meta-analysis of observational studies. *Br. Med. J.* **330**: 63.

25 Nightingale, A.L. and Farmer, R.D. (2004). Ischaemic stroke in young women: a nested case-control study using the UK general practice research database. *Stroke* **35**: 1574–1578.

26 Khader, Y.S., Rice, J., John, L. et al. (2003). Oral contraceptive use and the risk of myocardial infarction: a meta-analysis. *Contraception* **68**: 11–17.

27 Nightingale, A.L., Lawrenson, R.A., Simpson, E.L. et al. (2000). The effects of age, body mass index, smoking and general health on the risk of venous thromboembolism in users of combined oral contraceptives. *Eur. J. Contracept. Reprod. Health Care* **5**: 265–274.

28 Tanis, B.C., van den Bosch, M.A., Kemmeren, J.M. et al. (2001). Oral contraceptives and the risk of myocardial infarction. *N. Engl. J. Med.* **345**: 1787–1793.

29 WHO (1995). Venous thromboembolic disease and combined oral contraceptives: results of international multicentre case-control study. *Lancet* **346**: 1575–1582.

30 Finer, L.B., Jerman, J., and Kavanaugh, M.L. (2012). Changes in use of long-acting contraceptive methods in the U.S., 2007–2009. *Fertil. Steril.* **98**: 893–897.

31 Vercellini, P. (1999). A levonorgestrel-releasing intrauterine system for the treatment of dysmenorrheal associated with endometriosis: a pilot study. *Fertil. Steril.* **72**: 505–508.

32 Fedele, L. (2001). Use of a levonorgestrel-releasing intrauterine device in the treatment of rectovaginal endometriosis. *Fertil. Steril.* **75**: 485–488.

33 Sheng, J., Zhang, J.P., and Lu, D. (2009). The LNG-IUS study on adenomyosis: a 3-year follow-up study on the efficacy and side effects of the use of levonorgestrel intrauterine system for the treatment of dysmenorrhea associated with adenomyosis. *Contraception* **79**: 189–193.

34 Magalhaes, J., Aldrighi, J.M., and de Lima, G.R. (2007). Uterine volume and menstrual patters in users of the levonorgestrel-releasing intrauterine system with idiopathic menorrhagia or menorrhagia due to leiomyomas. *Contraception* **75**: 193–198.

35 Rizkalla, H.F., Higgins, M., Kelehan, P. et al. (2008). Pathological findings associated with the presence of a Mirena intrauterine system at hysterectomy. *Int. J. Gynecol. Pathol.* **27**: 74–78.

36 (2011). Long-acting reversible contraception: implants and intrauterine devices. Practice bulletin no. 121. American College of Obstetricians and Gynecologists. *Obstet. Gynecol.* **118**: 184–196.

37 American College of Obstetricians and Gynecologists, ACOG Committee Opinion. Intrauterine devices and adolescents. Number 392, December 2007.

38 Martinez, F. and Arregui-Lopez, E. (2009). Infection risk and intrauterine devices. *Acta Obstet. Gynecol.* **88**: 246–250.

39 World Health Organization (2002). *Select Practice Recommendations for Contraceptive Use*. Geneva, Switzerland: WHO.

40 Trussell, J. (2007). Contraceptive efficacy. In: *Contraceptive Technology: Nineteenth Revised Edition* (ed. R.A. Hatcher, J. Trussell, A.L. Nelson, et al.). New York, NY: Ardent Media.

41 FDA Talk Paper. (November 17, 2004). Black Box Warning Added Concerning Long-Term Use of DMPA Contraceptive Injection. Available at http://web.archive.org/web/20051221195621/http://www.fda.gov/bbs/topics/ANSWERS/2004/ANS01325.html (accessed 23 June 2018).

42 WHO. (September 2005). Hormonal contraception and bone health. Family Planning. Available at http://www.who.int/reproductivehealth/publications/family_planning/pbrief1/en (accessed 23 June 2018).

43 Curtis, K.M. and Martins, S.L. (2006). Progestogen-only contraception and bone mineral density: a systematic review. *Contraception* **73**: 470–487.

44 Cromer, B.A., Bonny, A.E., Stager, M. et al. (2008). Bone mineral density in adolescent females using injectable or oral contraceptives: a 24-month prospective study. *Fertil. Steril.* **90**: 2060–2067.

45 Kaunitz, A.M., Arias, R., and Mcclung, M. (2008). Bone density recovery after depot medroxyprogesterone acetate injectable contraception use. *Contraception* **77**: 67–76.

46 Guilbert, E.R., Brown, J.P., Kaunitz, A.M. et al. (2009). The use of depot-medroxyprogesterone acetate in contraception and its potential impact on skeletal health. *Contraception* **79**: 167–177.

47 Rosenberg, L., Zhang, Y., Constant, D. et al. (2007). Bone status after cessation of use of injectable progestin contraceptives. *Contraception* **76**: 425–431.

48 Kaunitz, A.M., Miller, P.D., Rice, V.M. et al. (2006). Bone mineral density in women aged 25-35 years receiving depot medroxyprogesterone acetate: recovery following discontinuation. *Contraception* **74**: 90–99.

49 ACOG (2014). Depot Medroxyprogesterone Acetate and Bone Effects. *Committee Opinion* **602**. Available at: http://www.acog.org/Resources_And_Publications/Committee_Opinions/Committee_on_Adolescent_Health_Care/Depot_Medroxyprogesterone_Acetate_and_Bone_Effects (accessed 26 June 2018).

50 Carlson, C., Plonczynski, D.J., Yao, P. (2016). The impact of personal characteristics on contraceptive choices and use over 5 years. *SAGE Open Nursing* **2**: 1–10.

51 Palmer, S.N., Greenberg, J.A. (2009). Transcervical Sterilization: A Comparison of Essure® Permanent Birth Control System and Adiana® Permanent Contraception System. *Rev. Obstet. Gynecol.* **2** (**2**): 84–92.

52 Conceptus Inc. (2010). Conceptus(R) Receives FDA Approval on Essure's Bilateral Placement Rate to 96.9%. Published Wednesday 19 May 2010. Available at: http://www.medicalnewstoday.com/releases/189244.php (accessed 24 June 2018).

53 Cooper, J.M., Carignan, C.S., Cher, D. et al. (2003). Selective tubal occlusion procedure 2000 investigators group. Microinsert nonincisional hysteroscopic sterilization. *Obstet. Gynecol.* **102**: 59–67.

54 Nichols, M., Carter, J.F., Fylstra, D.L. et al. (2006). A comparative study of hysteroscopic sterilization performed in-office versus a hospital operating room. *J. Minim. Invasive Gynecol.* **13**: 447–450.

55 Panel, P. and Grosdemouge, I. (2010). Predictive factors of Essure implant placement failure: prospective, multicenter study of 495 patients. *Fertil. Steril.* **93**: 29–34.

56 Savage, U.K., Masters, S.J., Smid, M.C. et al. (2009). Hysteroscopic sterilization in a large group practice: experience and effectiveness. *Obstet. Gynecol.* **114**: 1227–1231.

57 Levy, B., Levie, M.D., and Childers, M.E. (2007). A summary of reported pregnancies after hysteroscopic sterilization. *J. Minim. Invasive Gynecol.* **14**: 271–274.

58 Munro, M.G., Nichols, J.E., Levy, B. et al. (2013). Hysteroscopic sterilization: ten-year retrospective analysis of worldwide pregnancy reports. *J Minim Invasive Gynecol.* **13**: S1553–S4650.

59 Xiaozhang, L. (2009). *Scalpel Versus No Scalpel Incision for Vasectomy*. Geneva: RHL Commentary. The WHO Reproductive Health Library, WHO.

60 Engender Health. No scalpel vasectomy. An illustrated guide for surgeons. http://engenderhealth.org (accessed 19 November 2013).

61 INFO Project. 2007. Family planning: a global handbook for providers. World Health Organization and Johns Hopkins Bloomberg School of Public Health/Center for Communication Programs (CCP), INFO Project: Baltimore, Geneva.

62 Cook, L.A., Pun, A., Gallo, M.F. et al. (2007). Scalpel versus no-scalpel incision for vasectomy. *Cochrane Database Syst. Rev.* 2 (Art. No.: CD004112) doi: 10.1002/14651858.CD004112.

63 Barone, M.A., Nazerali, H., Cortes, M. et al. (2003). A prospective study of time and number of ejaculations to azoospermia after vasectomy by ligation and excision. *J. Urol.* **170**: 892–896.

64 Noe, G., Croxatto, H.B., Salvatierra, A.M. et al. (2010). Contraceptive efficacy of emergency contraception with levonorgestrel given before or after ovulation. *Contraception* **81**: 414–420.

65 Brache, V., Cochon, L., Jesam, C. et al. (2010). Immediate pre-ovulatory administration of 30 mg ulipristal acetate significantly delays follicular rupture. *Hum. Reprod.* **25**: 2256–2263.

66 Rodrigues, I., Grou, F., and Joly, J. (2001). Effectiveness of emergency contraception pills between 72 and 120 hours after unprotected sexual intercourse. *Am. J. Obstet. Gynecol.* **184**: 531–537.

67 Glasier, A.F., Cameron, S.T., Fine, P.M. et al. (2010). Ulipristal acetate versus levonorgestrel for emergency contraception: a randomised non-inferiority trial and meta-analysis. *Lancet* **375**: 555–562.

68 Arowojolu, A.O., Okewole, I.A., and Adekunle, A.O. (2002). Comparative evaluation of the effectiveness and safety of two regimens of levonorgestrel for emergency contraception in Nigerians. *Contraception* **66**: 269–273.

69 Task force on postovulatory methods of fertility regulation. (1998). Randomised controlled trial of levonorgestrel versus the Yuzpe regimen of combined oral contraceptives for emergency contraception. *Lancet* **352**: 428–433.

70 Cheng, L., Gulmezoglu, A.M., Piaggio, G.G.P. et al. (2008). Interventions for emergency contraception. *Cochrane Database Syst. Rev.* 2006; 2 (Art. No.: CD001324) doi: 10.1002/14651858.CD001324.pub.3.

71 Wu, S., Godfrey, E., Wojdyla, D. et al. (2010). Copper T380A intrauterine device for emergency contraception: a prospective, multicentre, cohort clinical trial. *BJOG* **117**: 1205–1210.

72 Glasier, A., Cameron, S.T., Blithe, D. et al. (2011). Can we identify women at risk of pregnancy despite using emergency contraception? data from randomized trials of ulipristal acetate and levonorgestrel. *Contraception* **84**: 363–367.

73 Moreau, C. and Trussell, J. (2012). Results from pooled phase III studies of ulipristal acetate for emergency contraception. *Contraception* **86**: 673–680.

74 Mosher, W.D. and Jones, J. (2010). Use of contraception in the United States: 1982-2008 . National Center for Health Statistics. *Vital Health Stat. 23* 20.

75 Valappil, T., Kelaghan, J., Artz, L. et al. (2005). Female condom and male condom failure among women at high risk of sexually transmitted diseases. *Sex. Transm. Dis.* **32**: 35–43.

76 Voeller, B., Coulson, A.H., Bernstein, G.S. et al. (1989). Mineral oil lubricant causes rapid deterioration of latex condoms. *Contraception* **39**: 95–102.

77 Lytle, C.D., Routson, L.B., Seaborn, G.B. et al. (1997). An in vitro evaluation of condoms as barriers to a small virus. *Sex. Transm. Dis.* **24**: 161–164.

78 Gallo, M., Grimes, D., Lopez, L. et al. (2006). Non-latex versus latex male condoms for contraception. *Cochrane Database Syst. Rev.* 1 (Art. No.: CD003550) doi: 10.1002/14651858.CD003550.

79 Centers for Disease Control and Prevention (2000). CDC statement on study results of products containing nonoxynol-9. *MMWR Morb. Mortal. Wkly. Rep.* **49**: 717–718.

Urogynecology

10

CHAPTER 10

Pelvic floor prolapse/urinary incontinence

Scott W. Smilen[1,2], Kimberley Ferrante[1], Dianne Glass[1,2], and Dominique Malacarne[1,2]

[1]*Division of Female Pelvic Medicine and Reconstructive Pelvic Surgery, Department of Obstetrics and Gynecology, NYU Langone Medical Center, New York, NY, USA*

[2]*Division of Female Pelvic Medicine and Reconstructive Pelvic Surgery, Department of Urology, NYU Langone Medical Center, New York, NY, USA*

CLINICAL SCENARIO

A 71-year-old woman presents to her gynecologist having noted a "ball" at her vaginal opening while showering. She denies bleeding and urinary incontinence, but does urinate frequently. Her past obstetrical and gynecological history is notable for three uncomplicated term vaginal deliveries. She had normal monthly menses until menopause at age 50. Her medical history is notable for hypertension. Her surgical history is remarkable for tubal ligation following her third delivery, appendectomy at age 17 and laparoscopic cholecystectomy at age 59.

Pelvic exam is remarkable for protrusion of the anterior vaginal wall beyond the hymen while straining and descent of the cervix to near the hymen with straining. She has no palpable pelvic masses. She is referred to a urogynecologist for further evaluation and management of pelvic organ prolapse.

Background

Pelvic organ prolapse is a benign, common condition that can significantly impact a woman's life. Approximately 3% of women complain of feeling a vaginal protrusion while up to 50% of women will be found to have prolapse on examination [1]. Pelvic organ prolapse occurs in women across all age groups, with peak incidence in the 1970s [2]. Risk factors include age, parity, connective tissue disorders, menopause and conditions that increase abdominal pressure (e.g. obesity, chronic constipation) [3, 4]. Acceptable treatment options include observation (for women who are minimally symptomatic), surgery and non-surgical treatments. In the United States, approximately 300 000 surgeries per year are performed for pelvic organ prolapse [5] and a woman has about a 6% lifetime risk of having surgery for prolapse [6]. We conducted a review of pelvic organ prolapse using evidence based medicine. Clinical questions relevant to the clinical scenario were developed using the evidence based medicine format, PICO (Population, Intervention, Comparison, and Outcomes). We searched the EMBASE, CINAHL, PubMed, Medline, and Cochrane Databases as well as performed a manual search of references for each question. In this review we will discuss pelvic organ prolapse interventions, including considerations for hysterectomy vs. uterine preservation, routes of surgery and use of native tissue vs. graft materials.

Pelvic organ prolapse occurs because of weakness in the pelvic floor muscles and its supporting network of connective tissues and ligaments. Vaginal childbirth is a common inciting reason for this problem which is closely related to hernias. Some women with prolapse are asymptomatic, while others may see or feel pressure and/or protrusion, experience voiding, defecatory, or sexual dysfunction. Impairment in quality of life typically leads women to seek treatment for this problem.

When the normal pelvic supportive structures are impaired, organs including the bladder, cervix/uterus, rectum, and peritoneum/intestines, may herniate into and distend the vaginal canal. The entities associated with these areas of prolapse can be called, respectively, cystocele, uterine prolapse, rectocele, and enterocele.

Pelvic organ prolapse is considered to be a slowly progressive problem, although there are few studies evaluating its natural evolution. One study found that 78% of women had no change in their prolapse stage after 16 months of

Evidence-Based Obstetrics and Gynecology, First Edition. Edited by Errol R. Norwitz, Carolyn M. Zelop, David A. Miller, and David L. Keefe.

follow-up [7]. Therefore, many women without significant bother may be observed. Those desiring treatment can utilize a vaginal insert device (pessary) or undergo surgery. There are many different considerations for women undergoing prolapse repair surgery, and operations should be tailored toward each patient's anatomic abnormalities, considering their objectives, age, medical co-morbidities, and surgeon experience.

Clinical questions

1. Are pessaries effective in the management of pelvic organ prolapse?

Search Strategy: Pessary, pelvic organ prolapse; Meta-analysis; clinical trial; randomized controlled trial.

Databases: EMBASE, CINAHL, PubMed, Medline, Cochrane Database.

Manual Search of references.

Vaginal pessaries are effective non-surgical treatments for women with pelvic organ prolapse. Most women can be effectively fit with a pessary [8]. The risks from pessary use are very low relative to surgery, whereas the benefit may be relief of prolapse symptoms. There is also some data to suggest therapeutic effects of pessaries. Recent literature reports significant improvement in stage of disease after consistent pessary use for one year [9]. Additionally, there is data to support low likelihood of prolapse worsening during pessary use. Pessaries therefore should be considered for all women with prolapse [10]. There are many different types, sizes, and shapes of pessaries and the individual efficacies have not been extensively compared to each other. One randomized crossover trial aimed at comparing symptoms relief and change in life impact for women using the ring with support and Gelhorn pessaries revealed equivalence in clinical efficacy among the two devices [11]. Neither the optimal way to fit a pessary nor how best to manage it have been studied. It is generally recommended that women are taught to change the pessary themselves and to do so as frequently as they desire. Prolapse symptoms are usually worse during the day when patients are upright and improve at night with the supine position. Therefore, pessaries may remain out overnight with little adverse consequence. For patients unable to change their pessary, providers can do this at least every three months. When pessaries are retained over long periods of time, women will often develop manifestations of long-term foreign body use, including inflammatory discharge, ulceration, and bleeding. Various creams and gels are often recommended for regular use to decrease the occurrence of these problems. None of these strategies have been adequately studied.

2. For women with uterine prolapse desiring surgical treatment, does hysterectomy have to be performed?

Search Strategy: Uterine prolapse, hysterectomy, hysteropexy; Meta-analysis; clinical trial, randomized controlled trial.

Databases: EMBASE, CINAHL, PubMed, Medline, Cochrane Database.

Manual Search of references.

The pathology of uterine prolapse is deficiency in the supporting structures for the uterus. These include Level I apical support, the uterosacral, and cardinal ligaments, as well as widening of the genital hiatus [12]. Since uterine descent is a result of these disruptions, the uterus in theory can be re-attached to its ligamentous supports and not removed. A uterine suspension or hysteropexy procedure therefore may be utilized for these patients.

Some women may prefer hysteropexy for reasons including: preservation of fertility, body image, or patient preference [13]. Alternatively, removal of the uterus (i.e. hysterectomy) will eliminate the risk for uterine cancer (as well as cervical cancer if the cervix is removed), eliminate menstrual bleeding and provide permanent contraception.

Hysteropexy procedures may be performed vaginally, abdominally, or laparoscopically/robotically. When performed vaginally, the cervix, and upper vagina may be attached to the sacrospinous or uterosacral ligaments, typically done with sutures or graft material. Abdominal, laparoscopic or robotic routes may be utilized to shorten uterosacral ligaments and attach the cervix/upper vagina to the proximal segments of those ligaments. Alternatively, sacro-hysteropexy may be performed by attaching a piece of mesh between the anterior longitudinal ligament at the sacral promontory and the cervix [14, 15].

There are no studies that have compared the various types of hysteropexy procedures. Overall, there is a paucity of literature comparing hysteropexy to hysterectomy, however there is some data to support similar results in durability when looking at these two techniques [16]. A recent multicenter randomized non-inferiority trial looking at women with stage II prolapse or higher found that sacrospinus hysteropexy was non-inferior for anatomical recurrence of the apical compartment, bothersome bulge symptoms and repeat surgery, when compared with vaginal hysterectomy [17]. However, in other reports, hysterectomy has been demonstrated to decrease the risk for recurrent prolapse when compared to hysteropexy in women with advanced (Stage III or IV) prolapse [16].

Colpocleisis, or vaginal closure, is another alternative to hysterectomy in women with prolapse. Patients undergoing this procedure must be thoroughly counseled regarding the irreversible loss of sexual function following colpocleisis.

In such patients, this has been shown to be a very successful procedure, yielding high patient satisfaction [18].

3. Are vaginal, abdominal, and laparoscopic/robotic routes for prolapse repair effective?

Search Strategy

Vaginal prolapse, sacrocolpopexy, sacrospinous ligament fixation, uterosacral ligament suspension; Meta-analysis; Clinical trial; Randomized controlled trial.

Databases: EMBASE, CINAHL, PubMed, Medline, Cochrane Database.

Manual Search of references.

Each mode of prolapse repair has varying degrees of efficacy. There are also multiple ways to define success when looking at the efficacy of prolapse operations. Some studies look at subjective outcome measures such as patient symptoms and quality of life questionnaires. Others look at objective measures such as anatomic recurrence. In fact, a 2009 paper by Barber et al. looked at 18 different definitions of success after abdominal sacrocolpopexy and found that success varied widely based on definition. They also found that the absence of bulge symptoms correlated strongly with a patient's assessment of improvement. Prolapse past the hymen seems to be the point where women report more bulge symptoms. This study concluded that using the hymen as the "cut off point" for anatomic success seems to be reasonable [19, 20].

Although this recommendation was published in 2009, current reviews are limited to the definition of success used in the individual studies. One such review by Hill and Barber nicely summarizes success rates of apical prolapse repairs [21]. Vaginal operations include McCall culdoplasty, Iliococcygeus fixation, sacrospinous ligament fixation, uterosacral ligament suspension, and colpocleisis. Sacrocolpopexy is approached abdominally with an open, laparoscopic or robotic approach.

McCall culdoplasty involves plication of the uterosacral ligaments at the time of hysterectomy. Data on success rates of this procedure are limited to retrospective series looking at reoperation rates which range from 0% to 14% [22].

Uterosacral ligament suspension is typically performed at the time of hysterectomy as this is an intraperitoneal procedure. The uterosacral ligaments are tagged at the level of the ischial spines bilaterally and attached to the vaginal cuff to suspend the apex. This suspension varies in the types and numbers of sutures used with some surgeons using only delayed absorbable sutures, others using only permanent sutures, and some using a combination. The success rates vary widely and range from 48% to 96% [23]. When looking at success stratified by compartment, recurrent apical prolapse (POP-Q stage 2 or greater) occurred in less than 3% of patients [24]. Reoperation rates for prolapse of any compartment were 5.8% [23].

Sacrospinous ligament suspension is typically accomplished via an extraperitoneal approach. The apex can be attached to the ligament unilaterally or bilaterally and just as with a uterosacral ligament suspension, there are varying techniques in terms of number and type of suture (delayed absorbable and/or permanent). The range of anatomic success reported for this procedure is 64% to 97% [21].

The OPTIMAL trial was a randomized controlled trial comparing uterosacral ligament suspension to sacrospinous ligament suspension outcomes. The study defined success as apical prolapse no greater than 1/3 of the way down the vagina, no anterior or posterior compartment prolapse beyond the hymen, no bothersome vaginal bulge symptoms and no retreatment for prolapse. Using this objective and subjective definition, success rates were similar between groups (59.2% for uterosacral ligament suspension and 60.5% for sacrospinous) [24]. Looking at the apex alone, however, those women who underwent a uterosacral suspension were less likely to have an apical failure than those who underwent sacrospinous suspension (8.6 versus 20.8%). Overall, 18% of women had bothersome vaginal bulge symptoms and 5.1% opted for retreatment within a two-year period.

Sacrocolpopexy involves attaching the vaginal apex to the anterior longitudinal ligament overlying the sacrum. This is typically achieved with synthetic mesh. This operation can be performed by an open, laparoscopic or robotic route. Success rates of open sacrocolpopexy have been quoted to be between 78% and 100% in terms of apical support with reoperation rates for any prolapse of 4.4% with up to three-year follow-up [25]. When looking at longer term data at seven years after the initial operation, however, data suggest that almost half of the women have had a treatment failure in one or more compartments [26]. The laparoscopic approach to sacrocolpopexy was compared to the open approach in an equivalence trial by Freeman et al. and no difference was found in terms of recurrence [27]. Paraiso et al. compared the robotic approach to laparoscopic sacrocolpopexy and also did not find a difference in outcomes at one year [28]. Similar results were obtained by Anger et al., also in a randomized controlled trial comparing the two minimally invasive approaches [29].

Less commonly performed is the sacrohysteropexy. This procedure involves running mesh through the broad ligaments bilaterally and attaching it to the cervicovaginal fascia and the rectovaginal fascia. The tail of the mesh is then attached to the anterior longitudinal ligament overlying the sacrum. There is five-year outcome data on a cohort of 55 women who underwent either an open or laparoscopic uterine sparing procedure. None of the women had recurrent uterine prolapse, however 13.4% had recurrent anterior or posterior compartment prolapse [30]. This data contrasts that of Fayyad and Siozos who found reoperation rates after laparoscopic sacrohysteropexy for any prolapse at one year to be 8.5% with half of these being recurrent uterine prolapse [31]. In a recent retrospective case control study, Paek et al. compared 54 women who underwent minimally invasive hysteropexy versus 57 women who had an open procedure. They found objective success rates of 96.3% and 98.2% for minimally invasive and open sacrohysteropexies respectively at one year, and reoperation rates of 3.7 and 1.8 [32].

In summary, all modes of repair discussed have acceptable and varying degrees of effectiveness in treating pelvic organ prolapse. The approach should be a shared decision with the patient with consideration for failure rates, operating times, possible adverse events, as well as cost.

4. When repairing cystocele and rectocele vaginally, are native tissue and graft repairs effective?

Search Strategy: Cystocele, vaginal mesh, native tissue, colporrhaphy; Meta-analysis; Clinical trial; Randomized control trial.

Databases EMBASE, CINAHL, PubMed, Medline, Cochrane Database.

Manual Search of references.

When looking at effectiveness, there are both subjective and objective measures to consider. In addition, the definition of objective success has recently changed in the literature to be at or above the hymen [20]. Success also varies based on the compartment of prolapse, anterior versus posterior. There are multiple approaches which can be compared. The first is the traditional colporrhaphy which is a midline plication of the fibromuscular tissue of the vagina with absorbable suture. Posteriorly, some surgeons opt for a site-specific repair which brings together specific defects appreciated in the fibromuscular layer. Augmentations of native tissue repairs include biologic graft or mesh inlay or armed grafts/meshes. In addition meshes can be made of absorbable or permanent materials.

A recent Cochrane review by Maher et al. compared various surgeries for prolapse of the anterior wall of the vagina [33]. They looked at graft augmented repairs versus anterior colporrhaphy alone. There is conflicting evidence as to whether anatomic outcomes are equal with one trial showing a relative risk of failure of 2.09 (95% CI 1.14–3.84) for native tissue and others showing no difference in outcomes. Even in the trial with better objective outcomes, subjective results did not differ. The Cochrane review also found that absorbable mesh made from Vicryl improved objective success when compared to native tissue midline plication with a relative risk of 1.39 (95% CI 1.02–1.90) of recurrence in the native tissue group. Eight of the ten trials comparing permanent mesh to native tissue in the anterior compartment showed a 14% recurrence rate for mesh while the recurrence for colporrhaphy was 46%. Included in this analysis were mesh inlays, as well as armed meshes. However, those women who underwent repair with mesh were more likely to develop prolapse in other compartments than were those women who underwent native tissue anterior colporrhaphy (18% vs 10%, risk ratio (RR) 1.8 (95% CI 1.0–3.40). Mesh erosions occurred in 11.4% of those patients who underwent repair with permanent mesh with a reoperation rate of 6.8%. So although recurrence rates might be higher for native tissue repair, the reoperation rate for mesh exposure should be weighed against the benefit of possible better anatomic outcomes. The most powerful point seems to be in looking at quality of life outcome differences between the two groups. A variety of quality of life outcomes were reported by five studies and there were no differences found between the two types of surgery, nor were there differences on sexual function questionnaires [33].

Overall, the posterior compartment has much lower rates of recurrence than the anterior vaginal wall. Karram and Maher reviewed native tissue versus graft and mesh repairs for the posterior compartment [22]. The posterior compartment can be approached via the vagina or via the anus. Data from this review suggested that the transvaginal approach was superior. They also found that midline plication posteriorly versus a site-specific repair seemed to have superior anatomic outcomes, with failure rates of 13% and 32%, respectively, in one study. If a levatorplasty is added to the surgical procedure, this review found that those women are more likely to complain of dyspareunia. In four trials looking at biologic grafts for the repair of posterior wall defects, the addition of graft made no difference in recurrence risk. There were no studies which showed any benefit to the addition of mesh to the posterior colporrhaphy [34]. And while none of these studies showed any mesh exposure, it is unlikely that the risk of mesh extrusion is zero.

In summary, the anterior and posterior compartments vary in terms of their success rates both with native tissue repairs and with augmentations with graft and mesh. The anterior vaginal wall is more likely to fail overall than the posterior compartment and some benefit has been seen to adding graft and/or mesh to the repairs. However, these anatomic benefits must be weighed with the higher risks of mesh erosion into the vagina and higher potential for dyspareunia. For the posterior compartment, the evidence currently shows that there are no benefits to the addition of mesh and in fact the risks of the surgery are increased with the use of this augmentation.

5. For patients with prolapse and without stress urinary incontinence (SUI) undergoing prolapse repair, when is a concurrent incontinence procedure recommended?

Search Strategy: Occult stress incontinence, mid-urethral sling, suburethral sling, Burch colposuspension; Meta-analysis; Clinical trial; Randomized control trial.

Databases: EMBASE, CINAHL, PubMed, Cochrane Database.

Manual Search of references.

Women with significant prolapse (generally prolapse beyond the hymen) may have associated poor urethral support (which is typically associated with urinary incontinence), but may not manifest stress urinary incontinence (SUI) because the prolapse results in kinking of the urethra. When the prolapse with resultant kinking is relieved, SUI often results. This is referred to as occult SUI.

All women preparing for prolapse surgery should be evaluated for this possibility. This involves reducing the prolapse back to a normal anatomic position and having the patient cough with a full bladder. The occurrence of urinary incontinence in this setting should prompt a discussion of treatment options for urinary incontinence at the time of prolapse repair [35].

Data on the utility of this type of testing in predicting the presence of absence of SUI after prolapse repair is lacking. Prophylactic surgery for SUI has been shown to decrease but not eliminate the risk of SUI in women undergoing prolapse repair. Several prospective randomized studies have evaluated prophylactic surgery for SUI during abdominal or vaginal prolapse repairs. In the CARE (Colpopexy and Urinary Reduction Efforts) trial, a prospective randomized comparison of abdominal sacrocolpopexy with or without Burch urethropexy, 44% of patients who did not have a Burch versus 24% who did, met criteria for SUI at three months after surgery [36]. Similarly, in the OPUS (Outcomes following Vaginal Prolapse repair and Mid-Urethral Sling) trial, a prospective randomized comparison of vaginal prolapse repair with or without mid-urethral sling, the rate of SUI three months after surgery was 24% when slings were performed and 49% when they were not [37]. Given that the chance of SUI is not eliminated with these procedures and that these interventions come with risk of adverse events, it is important to counsel patients on risks and benefits of concomitant procedures when planning prolapse surgery.

6. Should cystoscopy be performed during pelvic organ prolapse repairs?

Search Strategy: Cystoscopy, prolapse surgery, urinary tract complication; Meta-analysis; Clinical trial Randomized control trial.

Databases: EMBASE, CINAHL, PubMed, Cochrane Database. Manual Search of references.

The incidence of urinary tract injuries during prolapse surgery ranges from approximately 3% to 5% [38]. Most prolapse procedures, but especially hysterectomy, sacrocolpopexy, uterosacral ligament suspension, and anterior colporrhaphy, present risk to the urinary tract. As such, expert consensus deems routine performance of cystoscopy during these prolapse procedures to be necessary.

Intra-operative cystoscopy should include a complete survey of the urethra, bladder, and assessment for efflux of urine from the ureteral orifices. If any injuries are identified and/or if there is no flow seen from one or both ureters, it can be addressed intra-operatively. This can significantly decrease morbidity as recognition and repair that occurs during the post-operative period is associated with poorer outcomes and delay in return to normal activities [38, 39].

References

1 Nygaard, I., Barber, M.D., Burgio, K.L. et al. (2008). Prevalence of symptomatic pelvic floor disorders in US women. *JAMA* **300** (**11**): 1311–1316.

2 Wu, J.M., Hundley, A.F., Fulton, R.G., and Myers, E.R. (2009). Forecasting the prevalence of pelvic floor disorders in U.S. women: 2010 to 2050. *Obstet. Gynecol.* **114** (**6**): 1278–1283.

3 Luber, K.M., Boero, S., and Choe, J.Y. (2001). The demographics of pelvic floor disorders: current observations and future projections. *Am. J. Obstet. Gynecol.* **184** (**7**): 1496–1501; discussion 1501-3.

4 Bump, R.C. and Norton, P.A. (1998). Epidemiology and natural history of pelvic floor dysfunction. *Obstet. Gynecol. Clin. North Am.* **25** (**4**): 723–746.

5 Weber, A.M. and Richter, H.E. (2005). Pelvic organ prolapse. *Obstet. Gynecol.* **106** (**3**): 615–634.

6 Smith, F.J., Holman, C., D'Arcy, J. et al. (2010). Lifetime risk of undergoing surgery for pelvic organ prolapse. *Obstet. Gynecol.* **116** (**5**): 1096–1100.

7 Olsen, A.L., Smith, V.J., Bergstrom, J.O. et al. (1997). Epidemiology of surgically managed pelvic organ prolapse and urinary incontinence. *Obstet. Gynecol.* **89** (**4**): 501–506.

8 Gilchrist, A.S., Campbell, W., Steele, H. et al. (2013). Outcomes of observation as therapy for pelvic organ prolapse: a study in the natural history of pelvic organ prolapse. *Neurourol. Urodyn.* **32** (**4**): 383–386.

9 Clemons, J.L., Aguilar, V.C., Tillinghast, T.A. et al. (2004). Patient satisfaction and changes in prolapse and urinary symptoms in women who were fitted successfully with a pessary for pelvic organ prolapse. *Am. J. Obstet. Gynecol.* **190** (**4**): 1025–1029.

10 Handa, V.L. and Jones, M. (2002). Do pessaries prevent the progression of pelvic organ prolapse? *Int. Urogynecol. J.* **12**: 349–352.

11 Arias, B.E., Ridgeway, B., and Barber, M.D. (2008). Complications of neglected vaginal pessaries: case presentation and literature review. *Int. Urogynecol. J. Pelvic Floor Dysfunct.* **19** (**8**): 1173–1178.

12 Cundiff, G.N., Amundsen, C.L., Bent, A.E. et al. (2007). The PESSRI study: symptom relief outcomes of a randomized crossover trial of the ring and Gelhorn pessaries. *Am. J. Obstet. Gynecol.* **196**: 405.e1–405.e8.

13 DeLancey, J.O. and Nygaard, I. (1991). Exercise-associated urinary incontinence. *JAMA* **265** (**4**): 514.

14 Korbly, N.B., Kassis, N.C., Good, M.M. et al. (2013). Patient preferences for uterine preservation and hysterectomy in women with pelvic organ prolapse. *Am. J. Obstet. Gynecol.* **209** (**5**): 470.e1–470.e6.

15 Dietz, V., van der Vaart, C.H., van der Graaf, Y. et al. (2010). One-year follow-up after sacrospinous hysteropexy and vaginal hysterectomy for uterine descent: a randomized study. *Int. Urogynecol. J.* **21** (**2**): 209–216.

16 Gutman, R.E., Nygaard, I.E., Ye, W. et al. (2013). The pelvic floor complication scale: a new instrument for reconstructive pelvic surgery. *Am. J. Obstet. Gynecol.* **208** (**1**): 81.e1–81.e9.

17 Romanzi, L.J. and Tyagi, R. (2012). Hysteropexy compared to hysterectomy for uterine prolapse surgery: does durability differ? *Int. Urogynecol. J.* **23**: 625–631.

18 Detollenaere, R.J., den Boon, J., Stekelenburg, J. et al. (2015). Sacrospinous hysteropexy versus vaginal hysterectomy with suspension of the uterosacral ligaments in women with uterine prolapse stage 2 or higher: multicentre randomized non-inferiority trial. *BMJ* **351**: h3717.

19 Fitzgerald, M.P., Richter, H.E., Sohail, S. et al. (2006). Colpocleisis: a review. *Int. Urogynecol. J. Pelvic Floor Dysfunct.* **17** (**3**): 261–271.

20 Barber, M.D., Brubaker, L., Nygaard, I. et al. (2009). Pelvic floor disorders network. Defining success after surgery for pelvic organ prolapse. *Obstet. Gynecol.* **114** (**3**): 600–609.

21 Hill, A.J. and Barber, M.D. (2015). Apical prolapse repair: weighing the risks and benefits. *Curr. Opin. Obstet. Gynecol.* **27** (**5**): 373–379.

22 Barber, M.D. and Maher, C. (2013). Apical prolapse. *Int. Urogynecol. J.* **24** (**11**): 1815–1833.

23 Margulies, R.Y., Rogers, M.A., and Morgan, D.M. (2010). Outcomes of transvaginal uterosacral ligament suspension. *Am. J. Obstet. Gynecol.* **202** (**2**): 124–134.

24 Barber, M.D., Brubaker, L., Burgio, K.L. et al. (2014). Comparison of 2 transvaginal surgical approaches and perioperative behavioral therapy for apical vaginal prolapse: the OPTIMAL randomized trial. *JAMA* **311** (**10**): 1023–1034.

25 Nygaard, I.E., McCreery, R., Brubaker, L. et al. (2004). Pelvic floor disorders network. Abdominal sacrocolpopexy: a comprehensive review. *Obstet. Gynecol.* **104** (**4**): 805–823.

26 Nygaard, I., Brubaker, L., Zyczynski, H.M. et al. (2013). Long-term outcomes following abdominal sacrocolpopexy for pelvic organ prolapse. *JAMA* **309** (**19**): 2016–2024.

27 Freeman, R.M., Pantazis, K., Thomson, A. et al. (2013). A randomized controlled trial of abdominal versus laparoscopic sacrocolpopexy for the treatment of posthysterectomy vaginal vault prolapse: LAS study. *Int. Urogynecol. J.* **24** (**3**): 377–384.

28 Paraiso, M.F., Jelovsek, J.E., Frick, A. et al. (2011). Laparoscopic compared with robotic sacrocolpopexy for vaginal prolapse: a randomized controlled trial. *Obstet. Gynecol.* **118** (**5**): 1005–1013.

29 Anger, J.T., Mueller, E.R., Tarnay, C. et al. (2014). Robotic compared with laparoscopic sacrocolpopexy: a randomized controlled trial. *Obstet. Gynecol.* **123** (**1**): 5–12.

30 Constantini, E., Lazzeri, M., Zucchi, A. et al. (2011). Five year outcome of uterus sparing surgery for pelvic organ prolapse repair: a single center experience. *Int. Urogynecol. J.* **22** (**3**): 287–292.

31 Fayyad, A.M. and Siozos, C.S. (2014). Safety and one year outcomes following vaginally assisted laparoscopic uterine sacropexy (VALUES) for advanced uterine prolapse. *Neurourol. Urodyn.* **33** (**3**): 345–349.

32 Paek, J., Lee, M., Kim, B.W., and Kwon, Y. (2015). Robotic or laparoscopic sacrohysteropexy versus open sacrohysteropexy for uterus preservation in pelvic organ prolapse. *Int. Urogynecol. J.* **27** (**4**): 593–599.

33 Maher, C., Feiner, B., Baessler, K., and Schmid, C. (2013). Surgical management of pelvic organ prolapse in women. *Cochrane Database Syst. Rev.* 30 (Art. No.: CD004014) doi: 10.1002/14651858.

34 Karram, M. and Maher, C. (2013). Surgery for posterior vaginal wall prolapse. *Int. Urogynecol. J.* **24** (**11**): 1835–1841.

35 (2015). ACOG practice bulletin no. 155: urinary incontinence in women. *Obstet. Gynecol.* **126**: e66–e81.

36 Brubaker, L., Cundiff, G.W., Fine, P. et al. (2006). Abdominal sacrocolpopexy with Burch colposuspension to reduce urinary stress incontinence. *N. Engl. J. Med.* **354** (**15**): 1557–1566.

37 Wei, J., Nygaard, I., Richter, H. et al. (2009). Pelvic floor disorders N. Outcomes following vaginal prolapse repair and mid urethral sling (OPUS) trial--design and methods. *Clin. Trials* **6** (**2**): 162–171.

38 Kwon, C.H., Goldberg, R.P., Koduri, S., and Sand, P.K. (2002). The use of intraoperative cystoscopy in major vaginal and urogynecologic surgeries. *Am. J. Obstet. Gynecol.* **187** (**6**): 1466–1471.

39 Gustilo-Ashby, A., Eric Jelovsek, J., Barber, M.D. et al. (2006). The incidence of ureteral obstruction and the value of intraoperative cystoscopy during vaginal surgery for pelvic organ prolapse. *Am. J. Obstet. Gynecol.* **194** (**5**): 1478–1485.

Reproductive endocrinology and infertility

11

CHAPTER 11
Amenorrhea

A. Reza Radjabi and David L. Keefe
Department of Obstetrics and Gynecology, NYU Langone Medical Center, New York, NY, USA

CASE SCENARIO

A 16-year-old girl was referred by her primary care physician to the gynecology service due to primary amenorrhea. She was an otherwise healthy adolescent with no significant previous medical history. On clinical examination, she had normal stature for her age, breast development appropriate to Tanner stage and scanty pubic hair. External genitalia appeared normal, but a palpable mass could be felt in the left groin. Ultrasonography (US) of the abdomen and inguinal regions demonstrated the absence of ovaries and Müllerian structures, the presence of the vagina which measured approximately 5 cm in length, and a solid mass in the left inguinal region measuring approximately 3 cm in diameter, also containing some small peripheral cystic areas and normal looking lymph nodes. The appearance of the lesion was highly suggestive of a dysgenetic gonad. The right gonad could not be visualized. A karyotype revealed the presence of 46XY complement and the diagnosis of complete androgen insensitivity syndrome (CAIS) was established (X).

Background

Definition

Amenorrhea can be a transient, intermittent, or a permanent condition resulting from dysfunction of the hypothalamus, pituitary, ovaries, uterus, or vagina. Amenorrhea can be classified as either primary or as secondary [1].

Primary amenorrhea is defined as the absence of menses at age 15 years in the presence of normal growth and secondary sexual characteristics or alternatively by age 13 years, if no menses have occurred and there is a complete absence of secondary sexual characteristics [2].

Secondary amenorrhea is defined as absence of menses for more than three months in girls or women who previously had regular menstrual cycles or six months in girls or women who had irregular menses [3, 4].

The list of possible etiologies is extensive, but most causes they fall into a limited number of categories and therefore the diagnosis of amenorrhea is subject to a logic and systematic approach. The basic principles in menstrual function provide a framework to understand the causes of amenhorrhea.

Amenorrhea can be classified based upon the level of control of the menstrual cycle; hypothalamus and pituitary, ovary, and uterus and vagina [5, 6]. In addition, steroid receptor abnormalities and deficiencies in enzymes of steroidogenesis cause primary amenorrhea at the level of the ovary and the adrenal gland [7].

The basic requirements for normal menstrual function thus include four anatomically and functionally distinct structural components – the genital outflow tract including the uterus, the ovary, the pituitary, and the hypothalamus – thus providing a natural and useful hierarchy for organizing the diagnostic evaluation of amenorrhea. Accordingly, the many causes of amenorrhea can be categorized according to the site or level of the disorder or disturbance [2, 8]. A differential diagnosis for amenorrhea can be developed based on requirements for normal menses and from the medical history and physical examination [2, 9].

Clinical questions

1. How is amenorrhea evaluated?

The first step is to obtain a comprehensive history [6]. The history surrounding the onset of amenorrhea, cyclic pelvis or lower abdominal pain or urinary complaints may provide important diagnostic clues [5, 9, 10]. The physical examination starts with the overall evaluation of the body habitus to investigate possible causes of amenorrhea arising from nutrition disorders, physical, psychological or emotional stress and obesity [5, 12]. Examination of the skin and the thyroid gland are important [7]. The presence of pubic hair is a sign of androgen production or exposure [12].

Evidence-Based Obstetrics and Gynecology, First Edition. Edited by Errol R. Norwitz, Carolyn M. Zelop, David A. Miller, and David L. Keefe.

The skin may demonstrate evidence of hypercarotenemia, acanthosis nigrans, acne, or hirsutism [13]. Signs of virilization, including deepening of the voice, increased muscle mass, clitoromegaly, fronto-temporal balding, or decreased breast size, suggest neoplasm of ovarian or adrenal origin, or ovarian hyperthecosis [9].

Examination of the breast demands special attention [14]. Breast development reflects estrogen exposure and arrested breast development suggests disruption of the hypothalamus-pituitary-ovarian (HPO) axis [9, 14]. Physical examination of the genital anatomy includes investigation of the genital outflow tract and the uterus. In women with primary amenorrhea, symptoms of obstructed menses and a blind or absent vagina may have a transverse vaginal septum or imperforate hymen. Presence of androgenization with no outflow suggests Müllerian agenesis. Scant or absent pubic hair suggests Androgen Insensitivity Syndrome (AIS) [1, 7, 8].

Menstrual physiology

The arcuate nucleus located in the medial basal hypothalamus secretes gonadotropin releasing hormones (GnRH) in a pulsatile fashion. GnRH stimulates gonadotrophs in the anterior pituitary to synthesize, store, and secrete follicle stimulating hormone (FSH) and luteinizing hormone (LH). These gonadotropins enter the peripheral circulation and act on the ovary to stimulate both follicular development and ovarian hormone production, including estrogen, progesterone, androgens, and inhibin. Inhibin blocks FSH synthesis and secretion [14, 15]. Development of mature follicle results in a rapid rise in estrogen levels, acting positively at the pituitary cogenerate a mid-cycle surge in LH release and simultaneously stimulate the development of a thickened, proliferative endometrial lining. Following ovulation, LH stimulates luteinization of the follicular granulose cell and surrounding theca cells to form the corpus luteum. The corpus luteum produces estrogen and progesterone. Progesterone changes the endometrium in a secretory pattern. If pregnancy does not occur, then progesterone and estrogen ceases, corpus lute regresses, and endometrial sloughing occurs. If pregnancy occurs then human chorionic gonadotropin (hCG) is secreted from syncytiotrophoblast and the corpus luteum is saved during early pregnancy because of similarity in the structure of hCG compared to LH [14].

2. What are the causes of amenorrhea?

Outflow tract abnormalities resulting in primary amenorrhea

Imperforate hymen and transverse vaginal septum are outflow tract malformations that typically present with acute pain in an early teenager who has breast development but fails to menstruate.

Mayer-Rokitansky-Kuester-Hauser (MRKH) syndrome, also known as Müllerian agenesis refers to congenital absence of the vagina with variable uterine development. It is usually accompanied by cervical and uterine agenesis; 7–10% of women with MRKH syndrome have a normal but obstructed or rudimentary uterus with functional endometrium, resulting in cyclic pain [2, 9]. The defect results from agenesis or hypoplasia of the Müllerian duct system [5]. Patients typically present in their late teens with normal breast development, normal pubic hair development and in most cases amenorrhea is generally the only complaint. Imaging of the urinary tract should be performed in all patients because approximately 30% of the patients have simultaneous renal anomalies. Skeletal abnormalities are also commonly associated with MRKH. Vaginal dilator therapy can usually create a functional vagina [1, 9].

Complete androgen insensitivity syndrome (CAIS) is an X-linked recessive disorder occurring in genetically affected men and resulting in phenotypic women. Testes are present and secrete normal male levels of testosterone and anti-Müllerian hormone (AMH). AMH results in regression of Müllerian structures. Masculinization fails to occur because of an androgen receptor defect. Like MRKH patients, CAIS patients present in their late teens with normal breast development and complains of amenorrhea. Patients with CAIS will have on physical exam sparse pubic and axillary hair, which differentiates CAIS from MRKH on examination, and testes are often palpable in the inguinal region or in the abdomen. Serum testosterone is usually more than 200 ng dl^{-1} which is in the normal male range and CAIS patients have 46, XY karyotype [9, 17]. CAIS patients have an incidence of gonadal malignancy of 22%, which occurs usually after age 20. For this reason gonadectomy is preformed after pubertal maturation and epiphyseal closure. Vaginal dilator therapy if offered to create functional vagina.

Outflow tract abnormalities resulting in secondary amenorrhea

Ashermann syndrome, also known as intrauterine synechiae, is most commonly associated with aggressive postpartum curettage or abortion [18]. Other risk factors than can contribute to Ashermann syndrome include uterine and cervical surgeries, including cesarean section, septoplasty, myomectomy, and cone procedures [18].

Overall the diagnosis of outflow tract abnormalities can be assisted with the instrumentation of a sonohysterogram, hysteroscopy, hysterosalpingogram, or a MRI, if there is clinical suspicion for Müllerian anomalies.

Endocrine disorders

Hypergonadotropic primary amenorrhea

Turner syndrome is caused by loss of part or all of an X chromosome [19]. Approximately 60% of Turner syndrome patients are 45, X. The other 40% include karyotype abnormalities such as 45,X/46,XX mosaics, 46,XXqi isochromosome, and 46,XXp-short arm deletion. Internal and external genitalia develop normally for females, while primordial follicles undergo accelerated atresia and oocytes are depleted before puberty [20]. This results in lack of estrogen leading to failure of breast development, osteoporosis and fractures. Appropriate estrogen replacement therapy starting in the second decade of life, and continued until the age of menopause, can help to prevent bone demineralization. Patients with Turner syndrome whose karyotype includes a Y chromosome (such as 45,X/46,XY mosaicism) are at increased risk for gonadoblastoma and therefore prophylactic gonadectomy is advised [25, 26]. Patients with Turner syndrome are at increased risk for cardiovascular malformations, including aortic valvular disease, aortic arch anomalies, pulmonary or systemic venous abnormalities, ventricular septal defects, and hypoplastic left heart syndrome. Patients are at risk for aortic dilatation and dissection, particularly during pregnancy [13, 19, 21].

Mosaicism

Mosaicism refers to heterogeneous expression of a disease at the cellular or tissue level, resulting from cell-specific differences in the expression of a mutation or the presence of a chromosome aberration. This involves partial deletions or rearrangements of one chromosome and can cause a wide range of gonadal dysfunction, from gonadal dysgenesis to premature ovarian insufficiency (POI) [9, 22, 23].

Pure gonadal dysgenesis

These disorders result in premature depletion of all ovarian oocytes and follicles early in embryonic development. All patients are phenotypic women of normal height who fail to undergo puberty. Patients with Swyer syndrome (46, XY gonadal dysgenesis) require removal of their gonadal streaks to prevent malignancy [3, 24].

CYP17 Deficiency is a rare autosomal recessive disorder that can affect 46, XY or XX individuals. The lack of 17 alpha-hydroxylase and 17.20 hydroxylase activities results in both gonadal and adrenal insufficiencies. XY individuals are phenotypic women but lack a uterus because of AMH secretion. There is an increase shift of mineralocorticoid production with hypertension, hypokalemia, and hypergonadotropic hypogonadism [24, 25].

Hypergonadotropic secondary amenorrhea

POI is defined as the development of hypergonadotropic hypogonadism before the age of 40 years [27]. The presenting symptoms are similar to those of menopause. In POI there is impaired ovarian responsiveness to exogenous or endogenous gonadotropin stimulation and it is a continuum of impaired ovarian function.

X chromosome abnormalities, including short- or long-arm deletions or mosaicism are not severe enough to cause primary gonadal dysgenesis but may manifest as POI. Obtaining a karyotype is recommended since 13% of women less than 30 years of age with spontaneous POI have abnormal karyotype, even though the majority of POI patients are idiopathic. It is important to obtain a detailed family history in POI and evaluate the risk of adrenal insufficiency, since 14% of patients with familial POI and 2% of isolated POI have permutations in the fragile X syndrome gene (FMR1) and 4% have steroidogenic cell autoimmunity [22, 27]. In addition, 20% of patients are at risk of developing autoimmune hypothyroidism and therefore women with POI should undergo adrenal and thyroid antibody testing [27].

Latrogenic premature follicular depletion can cause hypergonadotropic secondary amenorrhea [26]. This includes removal of ovarian tissue, radiation or chemotherapy, especially chemotherapy with alkylating agents.

Hypothalamic amenorrhea

Functional hypothalamic amenorrhea (FHA) is the term used to describe amenorrhea which is diagnosed after ruling out other etiologies of amenorrhea. FHA results from causes like low energy availability resulting from decreased caloric intake, nutrition disorders, excessive energy expenditure, weight loss, and/or stress [31–36]. These factors contribute to dysfunctional hypothalamic GnRH secretion, by reduced pulsatile secretion of GnRH which results further in low levels of LH, FSH, and estrogen [31, 32]. Therefore risk factors for FHA include eating disorders like anorexia nervosa [47–49]. Although amenorrhea is no longer a diagnostic criterion for anorexia nervosa as per the Diagnostic and Statistical Manual of Mental Disorders, FHA is commonly seen in this condition. The terms FHA and hypothalamic amenorrhea (HA) are often used interchangeably [53].

Absent pulsatile GnRH secretion is uncommon except in Kallmann's syndrome and in congenital GnRH deficiency. In Kallmann's syndrome genetic mutation causes a failure of olfactory and GnRH neuronal migration from the olfactory placode [28]. This syndrome is characterized by primary amenorrhea, absent breast development, presence of cervix and uterus, and anosmia. In contrast in congenital GnRH deficiency there is absence of functional hypothalamic neurons from a genetic abnormality, and it is not associated with anosmia [28]. Other central nervous system (CNS) pathologies such as hypothalamic neoplasms, trauma, hemorrhage, or cranial irradiation can interrupt the function of the HPO axis. Craniopharyngioma is the most common CNS neoplasm causing delayed puberty. An MRI should be ordered if no other cause is present [28–30].

Pituitary disorders

Most pituitary dysfunction is acquired after menarche and therefore presents with normal pubertal development followed by secondary amenorrhea. Nevertheless, in rare cases, these disorders may begin prior to puberty and result in delayed pubertal development, amenorrhea and low or normal levels of gonadotropins [5, 10, 15]. The most common cause of acquired pituitary dysfunction are pituitary adenomas and the most common adenomas secrete prolactin [11]. Excessive secretion of pituitary-derived hormones result in amenorrhea. Alternatively adenomas can be non-functioning, producing other hormones, or empty sella syndrome may also be present. In 14% of secondary amenorrhea, hyperprolactinemia is present. This rises to 90% when galactorrhea and amenorrhea are simultaneously present [11]. Through negative feedback of prolactin the GnRH secretion is suppressed, resulting in lower levels of FSH and LH. Medications that can cause hyperprolactinemia include methyldopa, verapamil, reserpine, metoclopramide, including most antiypsychotics, antidepressants, and H_2 receptor blockers. If an initial serum prolactin concentration is only slightly elevated (21–40 ng ml^{-1} [21–40 μg l^{-1} SI units]), the test should be repeated before the patient is considered to have hyperprolactinemia [39, 40]. Prolactin concentrations vary with time of day, level of stress, and breast stimulation. Prolactin levels also are affected by eating, so repeat prolactin level should be obtain after fasting. If serum prolactin remains elevated on the second sample, hyperprolactinemia is confirmed, and the next step is to determine the cause. Most patients with hyperprolactinemia have a lactotroph adenoma. Therefore, the evaluation is aimed at exclusion of pharmacologic or extrapituitary causes of hyperprolactinemia and at neuroradiologic evaluation of the hypothalamic–pituitary region. Thirty to forty percent of women with hyperprolactinemia have pituitary adenoma, although the incidence of malignancy in prolactinomas is very low [41]. Medical treatment with dopamine agonist, such as cabergoline or bromocriptine, is highly effective. Surgical resection rarely is needed. Hyperprolactinemia in postmenopausal women also can cause galactorrhea, but most postmenopausal women who have hyperprolactinemia do not have galactorrhea. Many women who have galactorrhea have normal serum prolactin concentrations. Careful physical exam of the breast must be performed, with attempted expression of the nipples. Bloody discharge suspicious for cancer requires further diagnostic testing [41]. The general differential diagnosis for galactorrhea includes drugs that inhibit hypothalamic dopamine, hypothyroidism, increased prolactin secreted from a pituitary tumor, excessive estrogen leading to a feedback with hypothalamic suppression, stress and prolactin secretion from non-pituitary sources such as lung or renal tumors. The first line treatment is the use of dopamine agonist [39, 40].

Other pituitary disorders

The pituitary gland is enlarged during pregnancy and is prone to infarction following hypovolemic shock. Damage to the pituitary can be mild or severe, and can affect the secretion of one, several, or all of its hormones. A common presentation is a combination of failure to lactate post-delivery and amenorrhea or oligomenorrhea, but any of the manifestations of hypopituitarism (e.g. hypotension, hyponatremia, hypothyroidism) can occur any time from the immediate postpartum period to years after delivery. Sheehan's syndrome results from pituitary necrosis following massive obstetric hemorrhage or lymphocytic hypophysitis. If the patient remains hypotensive after control of hemorrhage and volume replacement, she should be evaluated and treated for adrenal insufficiency immediately; evaluation of other hormonal deficiencies can be deferred until four to six weeks postpartum [8, 9].

Polycystic ovary syndrome

Polycystic ovary syndrome (PCOS) is an important cause of both menstrual irregularity and androgen excess in women [45]. When fully expressed, manifestations include irregular menstrual cycles, hirsutism, obesity, insulin resistance, and anovulatory infertility. The diagnostic criteria established by the National Institute of Health (NIH) define PCOS as hyperandrogenism and chronic anovulation in cases in which secondary causes have been excluded [46]. The Rotterdam Consensus Conference expanded the criteria by diagnosing PCOS when two of the following three criteria are present: chronic oligo-ovulation, chronic androgen access, polycystic ovaries appearing on ultrasound [44]. PCOS accounts for approximately 28% of secondary amenorrhea, but can also be a cause of primary amenorrhea [16, 42, 47]. If signs of hyperandrogenism are present, serum testosterone and dehydropepiandrosterone sulfate (DHEAS) level can guide in the search of adrenal or other androgen-producing tumors, even though androgen producing adrenal tumors are very rare and serum androgen levels are not sensitive or specific for tumors. PCOS is associated with an increased risk for Type II diabetes, hypertension, lipid abnormalities, metabolic syndrome, and endometrial cancer [37, 38, 42]. Therefore metabolic evaluation should include assessment for lipid abnormalities, impaired glucose tolerance, or diabetes [46]. In order to prevent endometrial hyperplasia and possible malignancy, withdrawal bleeding should be induced every two months, either by oral contraception or by cyclic progestins [46, 50].

Menopause

The diagnosis of the menopausal transition is made in the setting of irregular menstrual cycles and menopausal symptoms such as hot flashes, mood changes, or sleep disturbance [43]. Although serum FSH is often measured, it offers no additional information, and may be misleading. Menopause may be diagnosed clinically as 12 months of amenorrhea in a woman over age 45 years in the absence of other biological or physiological causes. The menopausal transition, or perimenopause, begins on average four years before the final menstrual period, and is marked by irregular menstrual cycles, intense hormonal fluctuations, often accompanied by vasomotor complaints, sleep disturbances, and changes in sexual function. Women between the ages of 40 and 45 years who present with irregular menstrual cycles and menopausal symptoms may be in the menopausal transition. However the recommendations for this group are the same endocrine evaluation as for any woman with oligo/amenorrhea: serum hCG, prolactin, thyroid-stimulating hormone (TSH), FSH. For women under age 40 years with irregular menses and menopausal symptoms, the recommendations extend to a complete evaluation for POI [3, 9, 43].

3. How is amenorrhea treated?

Many women are under the impression that it is dangerous not to have a menstrual period, while women with an intact endometrium should be aware the risks of unopposed estrogen action. The overall goals of management in women with amenorrhea include correcting the underlying pathology, if possible achieving fertility, and preventing complications of the disease process [43].

In hypothalamic amenorrhea and in athletic women, explaining the need for adequate caloric intake to match energy expenditure sometimes results in increased caloric intake or reduced exercise, followed by resumption of menses [51, 53]. However, many women are reluctant to modify their behaviors [52]. Non-athletic women who are underweight or who appear to have nutritional deficiencies should have nutritional counseling, and they can be referred to a multidisciplinary team specializing in the assessment and treatment of individuals with eating disorders [31, 32, 34].

Women with prolonged hypoestrogenic amenorrhea resulting from conditions such as hypothalamic amenorrhea or from POI should be offered hormone treatment in maintaining or prevention of bone loss [49, 58]. This can be either an oral contraceptive if the patient is having intermittent ovarian function and does not wish to become pregnant, or replacement doses of estrogen and progestin [55–58]. The benefits and risks of hormone treatment are different when used for these conditions when compared to menopausal women [54]. Supplemental calcium and vitamin D should be added [43].

Anatomical abnormalities will require surgical correction, if possible. A surgical correction of a vaginal outlet obstruction to allow passage of menstrual blood or the creation of a neovagina for patients with Müllerian failure is a possible surgical correction [9]. Therapy of Ashermann's syndrome or intrauterine adhesions consists of hysteroscopic lysis of adhesions followed by long-term estrogen administration to stimulate regrowth of endometrial tissue [18].

Women with PCOS have multiple abnormalities that require attention, including oligomenorrhea, hyperandrogenism, anovulatory infertility, and metabolic risk factors such as obesity, insulin resistance, dyslipidemia, and impaired glucose tolerance [37, 38, 50]. Weight loss, which can restore ovulatory cycles and improve metabolic risk, is the first-line intervention for most women. The first line management is diet and exercise for weight reduction for overweight and obese women with PCOS. Available evidence suggests that lifestyle interventions (diet, exercise, and behavioral interventions) are more effective than minimal treatment for weight loss and for improving insulin resistance and hyperandrogenism. In addition, there appear to be reproductive benefits as well. Oral contraceptives are the mainstay of pharmacologic therapy for women with PCOS for managing hyperandrogenism and menstrual dysfunction and for providing contraception [50]. Alternatives to oral estrogen-progestin contraceptives include cyclic progestin therapy, continuous progestin therapy, or a progestin-releasing intrauterine device (IUD). Cyclic progestin therapy can induce regular withdrawal uterine bleeding and reduce the risk of endometrial hyperplasia. Both continuous progestin therapy and the progestin-releasing IUD provide contraception and reduce the risk of endometrial hyperplasia. Estrogen-progestin contraceptive can also be considered as first-line pharmacologic therapy for hirsutism in most women. For women with hirsutism and contraindications to oral contraceptives (OCs), spironolactone may be used. Spironolactone acts as an antiandrogen and therefore, in women using spironolactone as monotherapy for hyperandrogenism, progestin therapy is often needed [50].

FHA can be reversed by decreasing stress, reduced exercise intensity, weight gain, or cognitive behavioral therapy for anorexia. In most cases intensive psychotherapy is required [51, 52].

Hyperprolactinemia is usually treated with dopamine agonists such as bromocriptine and cabergoline. Hypothyroidism should be treated with a suggested starting dosage of 50 µg of levothyroxine orally daily. TSH response is slow and levels should be rechecked six to eight weeks following initiation, and can be adjusted or increased in 12.5–25 µg step doses [1, 39–41].

Lastly, as in all medical conditions, patients should be adequately counseled regarding their diagnosis, the long-term implication of their diagnosis and their treatment options.

References

1 Deligeoroglou, E., Athanasopoulos, N., Tsimaris, P. et al. (2010). Evaluation and management of adolescent amenorrhea. *Ann. N.Y. Acad. Sci.* **1205**: 23.

2 Reindollar, R.H., Byrd, J.R., and McDonough, P.G. (1981). Delayed sexual development: a study of 252 patients. *Am. J. Obstet. Gynecol.* **140**: 371.

3 Practice Committee of the American Society for Reproductive Medicine (2008). Current evaluation of amenorrhea. *Fertil. Steril.* **90**: S219–S225.

4 Reindollar, R.H., Novak, M., Tho, S.P. et al. (1986). Adult-onset amenorrhea: a study of 262 patients. *Am. J. Obstet. Gynecol.* **155**: 531–543.

5 Santoro, N., Filicori, M., and Crowley, W.F. Jr. (1986). Hypogonadotropic disorders in men and women: diagnosis and therapy with pulsatile gonadotropin-releasing hormone. *Endocr. Rev.* **7**: 11.

6 Crowley, W.F. Jr. and Jameson, J.L. (1992). Clinical counterpoint: gonadotropin-releasing hormone deficiency: perspectives from clinical investigation. *Endocr. Rev.* **13**: 635.

7 Laufer, M.R., Floor, A.E., Parsons, K.E. et al. (1995). Hormone testing in women with adult-onset amenorrhea. *Gynecol. Obstet. Invest.* **40**: 200.

8 Quaynor, S.D., Stradtman, E.W. Jr., Kim, H.G. et al. (2013). Delayed puberty and estrogen resistance in a woman with estrogen receptor *α* variant. *N. Engl. J. Med.* **369**: 164.

9 Speroff, L. and Fritz, M.A. (2011). *Clinical Gynecologic Endocrinology and Infertility*, 8e. Philadelphia, PA: Lippincott Williams & Wilkins.

10 de Roux, N., Young, J., Misrahi, M. et al. (1997). A family with hypogonadotropic hypogonadism and mutations in the gonadotropin-releasing hormone receptor. *N. Engl. J. Med.* **337**: 1597.

11 Goel, P., Kahkasha, N.S. et al. (2015). Evaluation of serum prolactin level in patients of subclinical and overt hypothyroidism. *J. Clin. Diagn. Res.* **9**: BC15.

12 Rosenfield, R.L. (2013). Clinical review: Adolescent anovulation: maturational mechanisms and implications. *J. Clin. Endocrinol. Metab.* **98**: 3572.

13 Gordon, C.M., Ackerman, K.E., Berga, S.L. et al. (2017). Functional hypothalamic amenorrhea: An Endocrine Society Clinical Practice Guideline. *J. Clin. Endocrinol. Metab.* **102**: 1413.

14 Perkins, R.B., Hall, J.E., and Martin, K.A. (2001). Aetiology, previous menstrual function and patterns of neuro-endocrine disturbance as prognostic indicators in hypothalamic amenorrhoea. *Hum. Reprod.* **16**: 2198.

15 Falsetti, L., Gambera, A., Barbetti, L., and Specchia, C. (2002). Long-term follow-up of functional hypothalamic amenorrhea and prognostic factors. *J. Clin. Endocrinol. Metab.* **87**: 500.

16 Rachmiel, M., Kives, S., Atenafu, E., and Hamilton, J. (2008). Primary amenorrhea as a manifestation of polycystic ovarian syndrome in adolescents: a unique subgroup? *Arch. Pediatr. Adolesc. Med.* **162**: 521.

17 Kohmanaee, S., Dalili, S., and Rad, A.H. (2015). Pure gonadal dysgenesis (46 XX type) with a familial pattern. *Adv. Biomed. Res.* **4**: 162.

18 Broome, J.D. and Vancaillie, T.G. (1999). Fluoroscopically guided hysteroscopic division of adhesions in severe syndrome. *Obstet. Gynecol.* **93**: 1041.

19 Saenger, P. (1996). Turner's syndrome. *N. Engl. J. Med.* **335**: 1749.

20 Massarano, A.A., Adams, J.A., Preece, M.A., and Brook, C.G. (1989). Ovarian ultrasound appearances in Turner syndrome. *J. Pediatr.* **114**: 568.

21 Zhong, Q. and Layman, L.C. (2012). Genetic considerations in the patient with Turner syndrome—45 X with or without mosaicism. *Fertil. Steril.* **98**: 775.

22 de Vries, L., Behar, D.M., Smirin-Yosef, P. et al. (2014). Exome sequencing reveals SYCE1 mutation associated with Caburet S, Arboleda VA, Llano E, et al. Mutant cohesin in premature ovarian failure. *N. Engl. J. Med.* **370**: 943.

23 Bastian, C., Muller, J.B., Lortat-Jacob, S. et al. (2015). Genetic mutations and somatic anomalies in association with 46 XY gonadal dysgenesis. *Fertil. Steril.* **103**: 1297.

24 Krasna, I.H., Lee, M.L., Smilow, P. et al. (1992). Risk of malignancy in bilateral streak gonads: the role of the Y chromosome. *J. Pediatr. Surg.* **27**: 1376.

25 De Arce, M.A., Costigan, C., Gosden, J.R. et al. (1992). Further evidence consistent with Yqh as an indicator of risk of gonadal blastoma in Y-bearing mosaic Turner syndrome. *Clin. Genet.* **41**: 28.

26 Rebar, R.W. and Connolly, H.V. (1990). Clinical features of young women with hypergonadotropic amenorrhea. *Fertil. Steril.* **53**: 804.

27 Nelson, L.M., Covington, S.N., and Rebar, R.W. (2005). An update: spontaneous premature ovarian failure is not an early menopause. *Fertil. Steril.* **83**: 1327–1332.

28 Laitinen, E.M., Vaaralahti, K., Tommiska, J. et al. (2011). Incidence, phenotypic features and molecular genetics of Kallmann syndrome in Finland. *Orphanet. J. Rare Dis.* **6**: 41.

29 Perkins, R.B., Hall, J.E., and Martin, K.A. (1999). Neuroendocrine abnormalities in hypothalamic amenorrhea: spectrum, stability, and response to neurotransmitter modulation. *J. Clin. Endocrinol. Metab.* **84**: 1905.

30 Constantini, N.W. and Warren, M.P. (1995). Menstrual dysfunction in swimmers: a distinct entity. *J. Clin. Endocrinol. Metab.* **80**: 2740.

31 Couzinet, B., Young, J., Brailly, S. et al. (1999). Functional hypothalamic amenorrhoea: a partial and reversible gonadotrophin deficiency of nutritional origin. *Clin. Endocrinol. (Oxf)* **50**: 229.

32 Laughlin, G.A., Dominguez, C.E., and Yen, S.S. (1998). Nutritional and endocrine-metabolic aberrations in women with functional hypothalamic amenorrhea. *J. Clin. Endocrinol. Metab.* **83**: 25.

33 Warren, M.P., Voussoughian, F., Geer, E.B. et al. (1999). Functional hypothalamic amenorrhea: hypoleptinemia and disordered eating. *J. Clin. Endocrinol. Metab.* **84**: 873.

34 Miller, K.K., Grinspoon, S., Gleysteen, S. et al. (2004). Preservation of neuroendocrine control of reproductive function despite severe undernutrition. *J. Clin. Endocrinol. Metab.* **89**: 4434.

35 Berga, S.L., Daniels, T.L., and Giles, D.E. (1997). Women with functional hypothalamic amenorrhea but not other forms of anovulation display amplified cortisol concentrations. *Fertil. Steril.* **67**: 1024.

36 Caronia, L.M., Martin, C., Welt, C.K. et al. (2011). A genetic basis for functional hypothalamic amenorrhea. *N. Engl. J. Med.* **364**: 215.

37 Gaete, X., Vivanco, M., Eyzaguirre, F.C. et al. (2010). Menstrual cycle irregularities and their relationship with HbA1c and insulin dose in adolescents with type 1 diabetes mellitus. *Fertil. Steril.* **94**: 1822.

38 Codner, E., Merino, P.M., and Tena-Sempere, M. (2012). Female reproduction and type 1 diabetes: from mechanisms to clinical findings. *Hum. Reprod. Update* **18**: 568.

39 Kooy, A., de Greef, W.J., Vreeburg, J.T. et al. (1990). Evidence for the involvement of corticotropin-releasing factor in the inhibition of gonadotropin release induced by hyperprolactinemia. *Neuroendocrinology* **51**: 261.

40 Groff, T.R., Shulkin, B.L., Utiger, R.D., and Talbert, L.M. (1984). Amenorrhea-galactorrhea, hyperprolactinemia, and suprasellar pituitary enlargement as presenting features of primary hypothyroidism. *Obstet. Gynecol.* **63**: 86S.

41 Zacur, H.A. (1999). Indications for surgery in the treatment of hyperprolactinemia. *J. Reprod. Med.* **44**: 1127–1131.

42 Wang, J.G. and Lobo, R.A. (2008). The complex relationship between hypothalamic amenorrhea and polycystic ovary syndrome. *J. Clin. Endocrinol. Metab.* **93**: 1394.

43 American College of Obstetricians and Gynecologists (2014, 123). ACOG practice bulletin No. 141: management of menopausal symptoms. *Obstet. Gynecol.* 202–216.

44 Rotterdam ESHRE/ASRM-Sponsored PCOS consensus workshop group (2004). Revised 2003 consensus on diagnostic criteria and long-term health risks related to polycystic ovary syndrome (PCOS). *Hum. Reprod.* **19**: 41.

45 Burgers, J.A., Fong, S.L., Louwers, Y.V. et al. (2010). Oligoovulatory and anovulatory cycles in women with polycystic ovary syndrome (PCOS): what's the difference? *J. Clin. Endocrinol. Metab.* **95**: E485.

46 Legro, R.S., Arslanian, S.A., Ehrmann, D.A. et al. (2013). Diagnosis and treatment of polycystic ovary syndrome: an Endocrine Society clinical practice guideline. *J. Clin. Endocrinol. Metab.* **98**: 4565.

47 Golden, N.H., Jacobson, M.S., Schebendach, J. et al. (1997). Resumption of menses in anorexia nervosa. *Arch. Pediatr. Adolesc. Med.* **151**: 16.

48 Misra, M., Tsai, P., Anderson, E.J. et al. (2006). Nutrient intake in community-dwelling adolescent girls with anorexia nervosa and in healthy adolescents. *Am. J. Clin. Nutr.* **84**: 698.

49 Misra, M., Katzman, D., Miller, K.K. et al. (2011). Physiologic estrogen replacement increases bone density in adolescent girls with anorexia nervosa. *J. Bone Miner. Res.* **26**: 2430.

50 American College of Obstetricians and Gynecologists (2009). ACOG practice bulletin no. 108: polycystic ovary syndrome. *Obstet. Gynecol.* **114**: 936–949.

51 Berga, S.L., Marcus, M.D., Loucks, T.L. et al. (2003). Recovery of ovarian activity in women with functional hypothalamic amenorrhea who were treated with cognitive behavior therapy. *Fertil. Steril.* **80**: 976.

52 Michopoulos, V., Mancini, F., Loucks, T.L., and Berga, S.L. (2013). Neuroendocrine recovery initiated by cognitive behavioral therapy in women with functional hypothalamic amenorrhea: a randomized, controlled trial. *Fertil. Steril.* **99**: 2084.

53 Meczekalski, B., Katulski, K., Czyzyk, A. et al. (2014). Functional hypothalamic amenorrhea and its influence on women's health. *J. Endocrinol. Invest.* **37**: 1049.

54 Borges, L.E., Morgante, G., Musacchio, M.C. et al. (2007). New protocol of clomiphene citrate treatment in women with hypothalamic amenorrhea. *Gynecol. Endocrinol.* **23**: 343.

55 Djurovic, M., Pekic, S., Petakov, M. et al. (2004). Gonadotropin response to clomiphene and plasma leptin levels in weight recovered but amenorrhoeic patients with anorexia nervosa. *J. Endocrinol. Invest.* **27**: 523.

56 Warren, M.P., Brooks-Gunn, J., Fox, R.P. et al. (2003). Persistent osteopenia in ballet dancers with amenorrhea and delayed menarche despite hormone therapy: a longitudinal study. *Fertil. Steril.* **80**: 398.

57 Rickenlund, A., Carlström, K., Ekblom, B. et al. (2004). Effects of oral contraceptives on body composition and physical performance in female athletes. *J. Clin. Endocrinol. Metab.* **89**: 4364.

58 Cumming, D.C. (1996). Exercise-associated amenorrhea, low bone density, and estrogen replacement therapy. *Arch. Intern. Med.* **156**: 2193.

12

CHAPTER 12
Polycystic ovarian syndrome

Lubna Pal and Shefali Pathy
Department of Obstetrics, Gynecology and Reproductive Sciences, Yale University School of Medicine, New Haven, CT, USA

CLINICAL SCENARIO

A 22-year-old Hispanic female presents to the office for the evaluation of irregular and infrequent menses. Her menses have always been irregular and occur every two to three months. She also reports excess hair growth on her face and body, particularly the upper lip, chin and neck, and on her lower abdomen and thighs. She has been using electrolysis for the past few years for the control of facial hair. Her gynecologic history is significant for menarche at age 10, and a longstanding history of infrequent menses; her last menstrual period was two months ago and lasted 10 days. She denies any history of abnormal Pap smears or of sexually transmitted infections. She reports initiation of coitus at age 15 and acknowledges three lifetime partners. She used condoms for birth control in the past and has never been pregnant, but hopes to conceive within the next two to three years. The remainder of her medical and surgical history is unremarkable. She denies use of medications and reports no significant allergies. She acknowledges smoking ½ pack of cigarettes per day for the past four years; otherwise denies use of other recreational drugs or alcohol. She works as an assistant teacher at a local elementary school. Her family history is significant for Type II diabetes (mother and maternal grandmother) and hypertension (mother and a maternal aunt); menstrual irregularity is acknowledged for her two younger sisters. She denies history of malignancy in her family. Notably, both her sisters also have excess facial and body hair. Her physical exam is significant for a weight of 200 pounds at a height of 5 ft 2 in. (BMI 36.6 $kg\,m^{-2}$). Her waist circumference is 48 in. Her blood pressure is 130/80 mmHg and her heart rate is at 80 beats per minute. Examination demonstrates a pleasant albeit morbidly obese young Hispanic woman with gross evidence of acanthosis nigricans along the neck creases, acne under the chin and upper back, and clinical evidence of hirsutism (coarse hair along the upper lip, undersurface of chin extending onto her neck, along the anterior abdominal wall with distribution in a male pattern escutcheon, and along the upper medial aspects of her thighs). There is no evidence of scalp hair loss, nor are there any visible striae along the anterior abdominal wall. Abdominal examination confirms evidence of central obesity with no evidence of visceromegaly. On pelvic exam, her external genitalia are unremarkable with no evidence of clitoromegaly. On bimanual examination, the uterus is of normal size and adnexa are non-tender and without any palpable masses. Office urine pregnancy test was negative.

Clinical questions

1. What are the primary diagnostic criteria for PCOS?
2. What is the differential diagnosis in a woman who presents with this constellation of symptoms?
3. What is the prevalence of the disorder?
4. How do women present with PCOS?
5. How is diagnosis of PCOS established?
6. What are the recommended diagnostic tests for a patient in whom you presume PCOS?
7. In patients who are not interested in conceiving, what are the options for management?
8. What are the best treatment modalities/options for a patient whose primary concern is fertility?
9. How do you counsel this patient on the risks associated with this diagnosis? (Diabetes, cardiovascular disease, endometrial pathology including hyperplasia and even cancer). What additional tests would you recommend to her?

Evidence-Based Obstetrics and Gynecology, First Edition. Edited by Errol R. Norwitz, Carolyn M. Zelop, David A. Miller, and David L. Keefe.

Introduction

Polycystic ovarian syndrome (PCOS) is an endocrine and metabolic disorder characterized by androgen excess, ovulatory dysfunction, and/or polycystic ovaries. It was first described by Stein and Leventhal in 1935 [1]. The etiology is still unclear, and the diagnosis of PCOS is one of exclusion, i.e. other etiologies of these characteristics should be excluded before identifying this as the diagnosis. What is agreed upon is that PCOS is a *syndrome* consisting of four main features: chronic course, features of androgen excess, ovulatory dysfunction and a classic sonographic polycystic ovarian morphology (PCOM).

The prevalence of PCOS varies depending on the criteria used to make the diagnosis; however, what is known is that PCOS is a worldwide women's health issue, which is likely underappreciated given this controversy in defining it. This condition can have significant long-term health consequences, with implications for a diverse array of disorders that range from diabetes, cardiovascular disease and mental health concerns to infertility, pregnancy-related complications, to increased risk of endometrial cancer [2–5].

1. What are the diagnostic criteria for PCOS?

PubMed search: criteria for defining PCOS.

The definition of PCOS has been developed over time by various expert opinions established by leading health organizations. The three primary diagnostic criteria currently in use are: (i) the NIH criteria, developed in 1990; (ii) the Rotterdam criteria proposed at the ESHRE/ASRM conference in Rotterdam (2003); and (iii) the Androgen Excess Society (AES) criteria proposed in 2006 (Table 12.1). The primary criteria revolve around the presence or absence of features of hyperandrogenism, ovulatory dysfunction, and PCOM on ultrasound evaluation. Notably, all of the organizations require the exclusion of other endocrine disorders, which could result in a PCOS-like phenotypic presentation (see Table 12.3) [1, 6, 7].

Table 12.1 Defining PCOS.

Features	1990 NIH criteria	ESHRE/ASRM (Rotterdam) 2003	AES 2006
Hyperandrogenism (acne and/or hirsutism)	+	+	+
Hyperandrogenemia	+	+	+
Ovulatory dysfunction/menstrual abnormalities	+	+	+
Polycystic ovaries on ultrasound	–	+	+

Hirsutism and acne are commonly recognized as features of hyperandrogenism, whereas hyperandrogenemia refers to the presence of elevated circulating levels of androgens.

The NIH, in 1990 established a broad definition of PCOS, identifying the three primary characteristics as: (i) hyperandrogenism (clinical or biochemical); (ii) ovulatory dysfunction; and (iii) exclusion of other endocrine disorders that could result in the constellation of signs and symptoms [8]. In 2003, The Rotterdam conference modified the diagnostic criteria by including the ultrasonographic findings of "polycystic ovarian morphology (PCOM)" to the inclusion criteria. This addition allowed for the identification of a subset of women who would be at an increased risk of ovarian hyperstimulation when undergoing ovulation induction treatment for the management of oligo-anovulatory infertility. As per the Rotterdam criteria, PCOS diagnosis requires the presence of two of the following three criteria: (i) hyperandrogenism (clinical and/or biochemical); (ii) ovulatory dysfunction; and (iii) PCOM on sonography (evidence of any one or both of the following in *either* ovary: (i) presence of 12 or more follicles measuring 2–9 mm in diameter; *and/or* (ii) an increased ovarian volume (> 10 ml) in the absence of a dominant follicle or corpus luteum in either ovary). The most recent modification were proposed by the AES with an aim of minimizing potential for diagnostic heterogeneity that resulted from a widespread adoption of the Rotterdam criteria that allowed inclusion of milder phenotype variants of PCOS. Based on the AES criteria, diagnosis of PCOS is made in the presence of: (i) clinical and/or biochemical evidence of androgen excess; (ii) evidence of ovulatory dysfunction (either manifest as oligo-anovulation and/sonographic evidence of PCOM); and (iii) after exclusion of other causes of androgen excess or ovarian dysfunction [8]. While diagnosis of PCOS based on the Rotterdam criteria allows identification of milder phenotypes wherein PCOS diagnosis may have minimal to no health consequences. PCOS diagnosis based on AES criteria allows identification of PCOS phenotypes that are at risk for recognized long-term consequences created a broader criteria base to incorporate all women, with all phenotypes of PCOS who are at risk for the consequences. Further research is necessary to define particular risks in different ethnic groups and clearly define options for each phenotype.

2. What is the prevalence of PCOS in the population?

Keywords: PCOS, Prevalence, Epidemiology.

Epidemiology

The prevalence of PCOS varies depending on the criteria used for diagnosis. For example, using the 1990 NIH criteria, the prevalence of PCOS varies between 6.5% and 8% [8], affecting 5 million women in the US and 105 million women worldwide. While there appears to be no significant difference among various ethnic backgrounds, this may be a reflection of insufficient sample size in most studies.

In contrast, by incorporating a transvaginal ultrasound (TVUS) finding of PCOM to the Rotterdam criteria, there is an estimated 20–60% increase in prevalence in women with hirsutism and oligomenorrhea. [8, 9]. As a result, the documented prevalence of PCOS is strongly dependent on the criteria used to define the syndrome as well as on the population studied. [8]

3. How do women with PCOS present?

Keywords: Clinical presentation, PCOS.

While the etiology of PCOS is not clearly understood, and there is some debate as to the exact definition, most women will present to their providers with a combination of complaints of menstrual abnormalities, facial and /or body hair excess, and/or with fertility problems. Menstrual abnormalities usually range from amenorrhea and oligomenorrhea to menometrorrhagia. For many women, menstrual dysfunction dates back to since menarche and hence may not even be apparent to her as being "abnormal." Evaluation for other causes of menstrual abnormalities is critical, as a variety of hormonal (disorders of thyroid, pituitary, and adrenal gland) and structural (tumors secreting androgens or cortisol, as well as focal endometrial pathologies such as endometrial polyps, hyperplasia, and even cancer) disorders can result in the spectrum of menstrual dysfunction seen in PCOS.

Clinical manifestations of hyperandrogenism commonly encountered in women with PCOS include excess of facial and/or body hair, and acne. While thinning of scalp hair (female pattern hair loss or androgenetic alopecia) is more common in women with PCOS compared to the general population, its relationship to androgen excess or signaling remains unclear. Hirsutism is the presence of excessive terminally differentiated hair in a male pattern distribution (primarily midline). Sometimes this concern surfaces only on questioning, when women will report difficulty with facial hair and history of trying various methods for hair removal (including shaving, waxing, and laser). Commonly, women with PCOS acknowledge a long-standing history of some degree of acne and report having tried one or more non-prescription over the counter formulations. Often, many would also have seen a dermatologist for this issue.

Although menstrual dysfunction and symptoms of hyperandrogenism may be the reason for a woman seeking consultation, many are also concerned about their fertility potential, and this aspect merits attention. Since most women present during the reproductive years, given that ovulatory dysfunction underlies menstrual dysfunction, infertility will eventually be a concern. PCOS is the most common underlying diagnosis in women with ovulatory infertility, and may be seen in almost 80% of women with anovulatory infertility. Despite the obvious however, since infertility is often multifactorial and treatment modalities can be complex, these patients should preferentially be referred for specialty care with an infertility specialist.

4. How is PCOS diagnosed?

Keywords: PCOS, Diagnosis, Signs and Symptoms.

No single sign or symptom is pathognomonic for PCOS. Each of the prevailing diagnostic criterion emphasizes combinations of clinical and endocrine phenomenon commonly encountered in PCOS, namely: (i) hyperandrogenism (clinical and/or biochemical); (ii) oligo-ovulation characterized by menstrual disturbance; and (iii) PCOM on ultrasound. Elimination through systemic testing of additional conditions that could potentially mimic PCOS is inherent to each one of the diagnostic paradigms. Diagnosis of PCOS should therefore be considered only after other etiologies (Table 12.3) have been excluded.

A complete evaluation should begin with a complete history and physical exam. This would include a thorough menstrual history, focused history of hyperandrogenic symptoms (presence, duration and persistence, rapidity of progression, and features of virilization, such as temporal hair loss, deepening of voice, regression in breast size and clitoromegaly, that should alert one of a possible androgen secreting tumor) as well as inquiry of medication use (e.g. valproic acid as well as use of potent androgenic progestins are both associated with features of hyperandrogenism). While oligomenorrhea is the most common menstrual abnormality (menstrual length greater than 35 days and/or 8 or less menstrual periods during a year), menorrhagia (excessive and prolonged bleeding at time of menses), polymenorrhea (short menstrual cycles <21 days) and menometrorrhagia (erratic, unscheduled, and unpredictable bleeding) can all be encountered in the setting of PCOS and reflect an underlying ovulatory disturbance. Symptoms of hyperandrogenism typically encountered include acne and facial and/or body hair excess. Inquiry about pharmacologic and non-pharmacologic treatments for hirsutism and acne, such as oral contraceptives, antiandrogen treatments as well as waxing and laser therapies are important.

Physical examination should include an assessment of body habitus, features of insulin resistance (central obesity as reflected by body mass index and waist circumference, and evidence of acanthosis nigricans (AN)) are meaningful for risk quantification in addition to signs of androgen excess. Excessive terminal hair evident in a male pattern distribution (chin, upper lip, mid-abdomen, and upper/medial aspects of thighs), and acne (face, forehead, and upper back) (Figure 12.1) are common symptoms of hyperandrogenism.

Hirsutism: Unwanted hair growth is a commonly encountered complaint among women. In any setting of excessive hair growth, hypertrichosis (generalized increase in fine and non-pigmented hair with a non-sexual pattern of distribution, which commonly has a familial inheritance, but may also be associated with conditions such as malnutrition, thyroid dysfunction, and certain medications such as phenytoin,

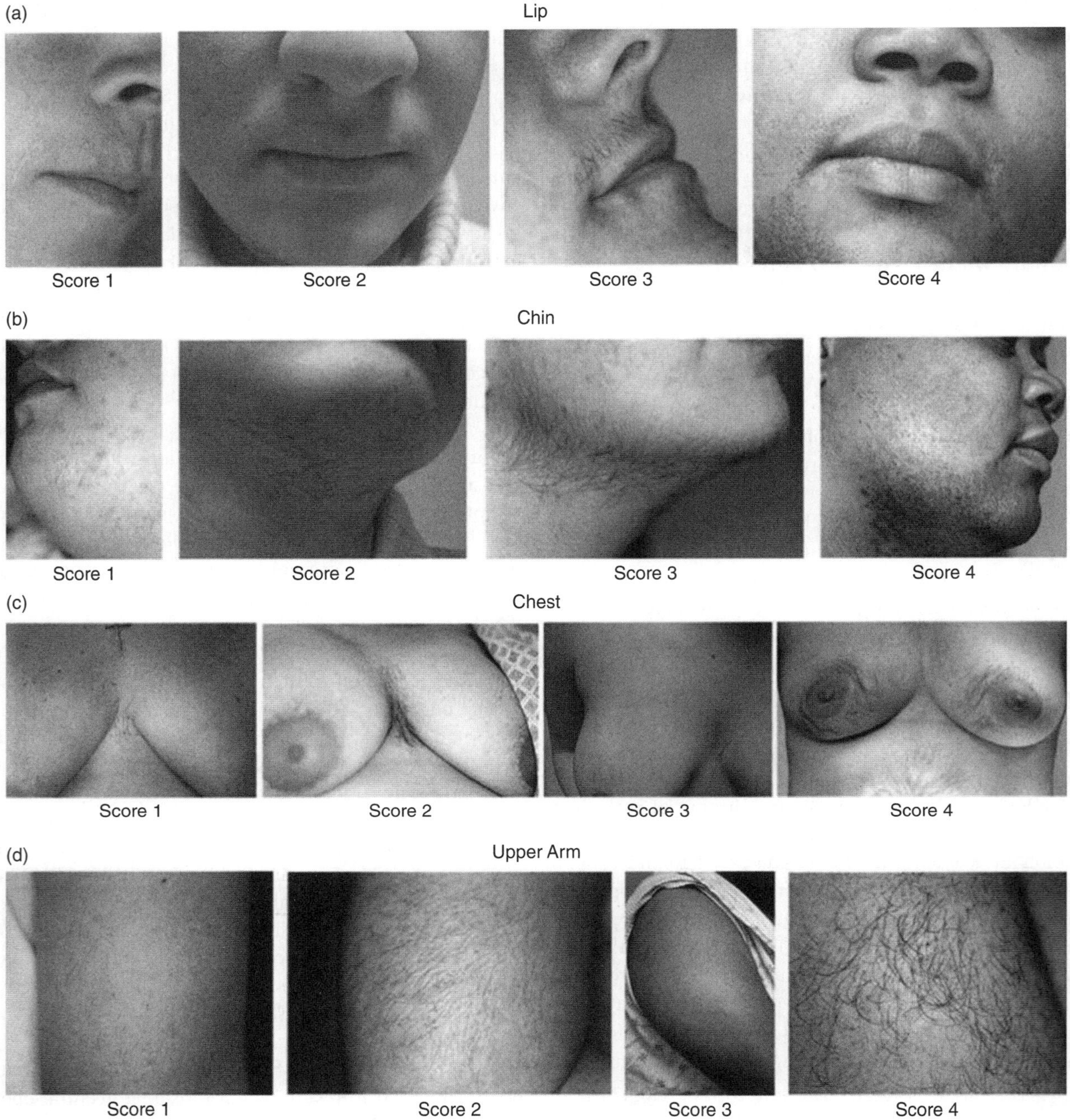

Figure 12.1 Photographs depicting facial and body terminal hair growth scored according to the modified FG method. Source: Yildliz et al., 2010 [10].

valproic acid, and minoxidil) must be distinguished from hirsutism (defined as the presence in females of terminal, or dark, coarse hairs that grow in a pattern normally seen in males). Hypertrichosis is generally not associated with androgen excess, although hyperandrogenism may exacerbate hypertrichosis. Regardless of the severity, hirsutism is a cause of much distress in the affected women and warrants further evaluation.

Excessive facial and/or body hair growth is the presenting complaint in almost 2/3rd of women with PCOS. The presence and the severity of hirsutism should be objectively quantified based on the extent and severity of excess hair growth. The Ferriman-Gallwey (FG) scoring system was developed in 1961 as a means of quantifying hirsutism for research purposes [3]. The original scoring system assessed the distribution and severity of hair growth on 11 body areas, whereas the modified scale limits assessment of hair distribution across nine facial and body areas (Table 12.2) [10]. Region-specific hair density is scored on a scale from 0 (absence of terminal hairs) to 4 (extensive terminal hair

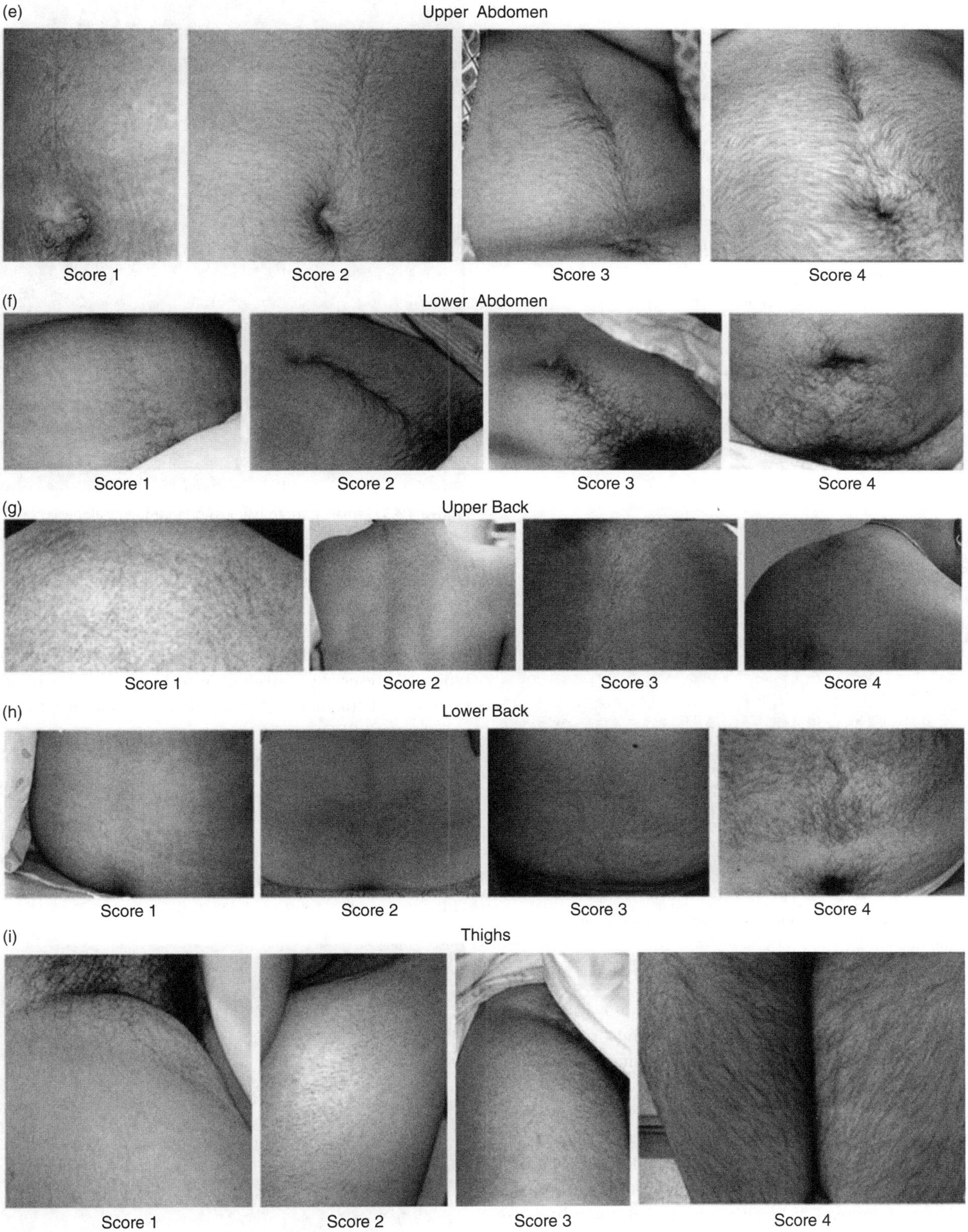

Figure 12.1 *(Continued)*

Table 12.2 Objective Assessment of Hirsutism: modified Ferriman-Gallwey (9 site) score

Region	Site	Score
Face		
	Upper lip	
	Chin	
Body		
	Mid chest	
	Upper back	
	Lower back	
	Upper abdomen	
	Lower abdomen	
	Thighs	
Total score		

Site-specific density of terminal hairs at each site is scored from 0 (absent) to 4 (dense)
Hirsutism defined as total score > 8
Source: Yildliz et al., 2010 [10].

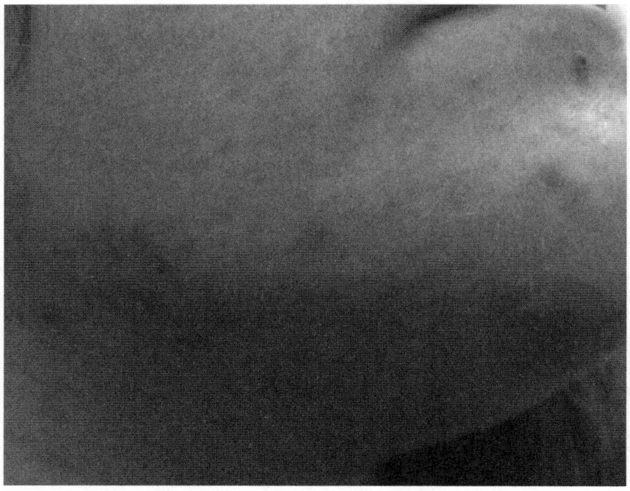

Figure 12.2 Acne – a commonly encountered symptom of hyperandrogenism.

growth). The modified FG scale is commonly utilized in clinical practice to objectively assess for the presence and severity of hirsutism and a score of >8 is commonly utilized as objective evidence of hirsutism

Acne is another prevalent symptom of hyperandrogenism noted in women with PCOS (Figure 12.2). Exaggerated effects of androgens at the level of the pilosebaceous unit are recognized to underline a predisposition to acne in this population. Forehead, face, chin, chest, and upper back are common sites and acne lesions encountered can range from papules, to pustules, cysts, and nodules.

Female pattern hair loss (Figure 12.3) or *androgenetic alopecia* is another commonly encountered, albeit less appreciated physical phenomenon evident in women with PCOS.

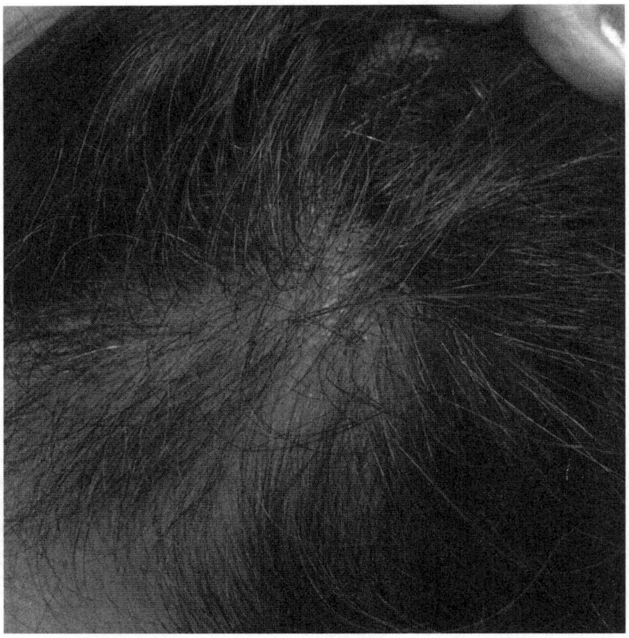

Figure 12.3 Female pattern hair loss or androgenic alopecia.

Female pattern hair loss is more common in women with PCOS compared to the general population, and classically presents as a diffuse thinning of scalp hair; the crown of the scalp is preferentially affected while the frontal hair line is typically preserved. A widening of hair parting is often an early complaint or is volunteered on questioning by many women with PCOS.

Acanthosis nigrans (AN): velvety areas of hyperpigmentation of the skin, can be found on the posterior folds of the neck, axilla, undersurface of breasts, and along the groins and suggests insulin signaling dysregulation and chronic hyperinsulinemia (Figure 12.4). While commonly encountered in women with PCOS, AN is not a diagnostic feature of PCOS,

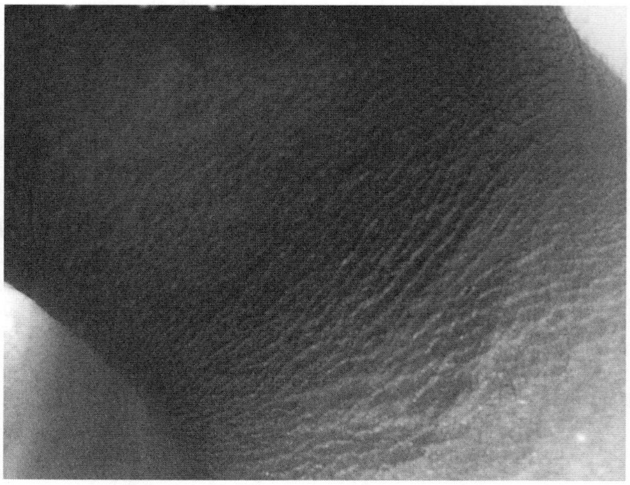

Figure 12.4 Acanthosis nigrans.

Table 12.3 Differential diagnoses for PCOS.

Adrenal dysfunction
– Non-classical congenital adrenal hyperplasia
– Cushing's syndrome
Androgen secreting tumor
– Adrenal
– Ovarian
Iatrogenic
– Androgenic progestins
– Anticonvulsants
– Androgens
Thyroid disease
– Hypothyroidism
Pituitary disorder
– Hyperprolactinemia
– ACTH secreting tumor
Miscellaneous
– Ectopic ACTH production

and is commonly seen in association with obesity and in patients with Type II diabetes.

5. What are the diagnostic tests for PCOS?

Keywords: PCOS, Diagnosis, Tests.

No single laboratory test is pathognomonic for PCOS. Diagnosis of PCOS requires not only that the individual woman meet specified diagnostic criteria (Table 12.1) but also requires an elimination of differential diagnoses that could potentially mimic PCOS. Disorders of thyroid, pituitary, adrenal gland and, androgen secreting tumors (adrenal or ovarian) can all present as PCOS (Table 12.3).

Virilization: Features such as clitoromegaly (Figure 12.5), deepening of voice, male pattern baldness, regression in breast size and an increase in muscle mass should prompt consideration of androgen secreting tumor, non-classical congenital adrenal hyperplasia and iatrogenic exposures as plausible differential diagnoses.

Laboratory evaluation for PCOS

Laboratory evaluation should focus on (i) screening for conditions that could mimic a PCOS-like picture; (ii) assessing for the presence, severity, and source of hyperandrogenism (ovarian versus adrenal); and (iii) quantifying overall health risks for the individual woman (Table 12.4).

Given the risk of future development of cardiovascular disorders, the leading fertility and endocrine organizations recommend evaluation for metabolic dysfunction including screening for dysglycemia, dyslipidemia, and for insulin resistance. By identifying those at risk for diabetes mellitus and for cardiovascular disease, preventive care strategies can be tailored to each individual.

6. In patients who are not interested in conceiving, what are the options for management?

Keywords: PCOS, treatment.

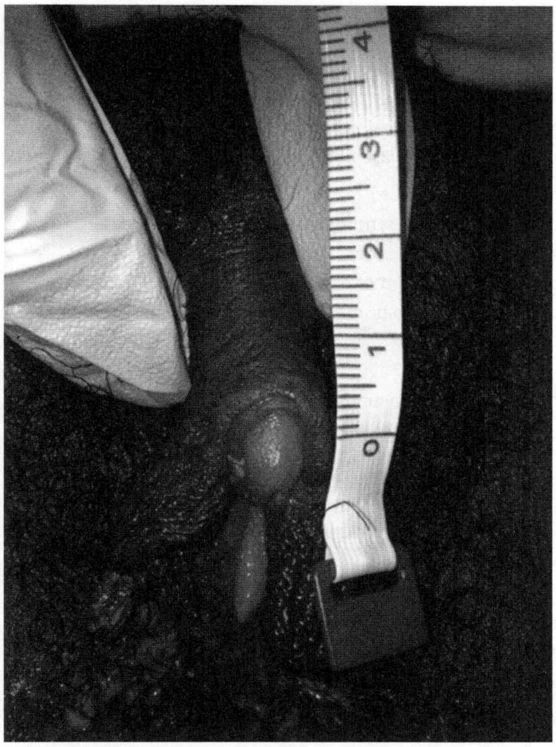

Figure 12.5 Clitoromegaly, a sign of virilization, is *not* a feature of PCOS.

Management goals should target symptoms that are bothersome to the woman, as well as pre-emptively address the covert risks that are manifest for the individual. Management strategies thus will vary depending upon the woman's presenting symptoms and her own goals. When fertility is desired, features of hyperandrogenism take the back stage. For those who are not interested in conceiving in the near future, a combination of strategies are available to address the spectrum of symptoms common to this condition.

Combined oral contraceptives (COC) are commonly utilized and also recommended as the first line strategy for managing menstrual irregularities and symptoms of hyperandrogenism [11]. For women whose dominant complaint is erratic menses, COCs offer predictable uterine bleeding and protection against endometrial hyperplasia risk; for those in whom symptoms of hyperandrogenism (particularly of acne) dominate, COC use is associated with an improvement in the severity of clinical hyperandrogenism, an effect achieved through a combination of mechanisms including (i) suppression of ovarian androgen production; (ii) decline in free circulating androgens achieved through increased hepatic production of sex hormone binding globulin (SHBG; driven by estrogen content of COC); and (iii) through mechanisms that remain unclear, attenuation of adrenal androgen production. An ever-increasing number of COC formulations are available. The choice of COC formulation for the management of hyperandrogenic symptoms should take into

Table 12.4 Laboratory evaluation in PCOS.

Tests to rule out differential diagnoses
17 Hydroxyprogesterone (17-OHP)
Screen for non-classical congenital adrenal hyperplasia (NCAH) due to 21-hydroxylase deficiency
24 hours urine free cortisol
Screen for Cushing's syndrome
Thyroid stimulating hormone
Screen for hypothyroidism
Prolactin
Screen for hyperprolactinemia
Pelvic ultrasound
– To screen for ovarian androgen secreting tumor
Tests to assess for hyperandrogenism
Total and free T
Dehydropepiandrosterone sulfate (DHEAS)
Total testosterone greater than 200–250 ng dl^{-1} is suggestive of an androgen-secreting tumor (ovarian or adrenal)
DHEAS levels greater than 6000–7000 ng ml^{-1} suggest androgen-secreting adrenal tumor
Pelvic ultrasound
– To assess for PCOM
– To screen for ovarian androgen-secreting tumor
Tests for evaluation of menstrual/ovulatory dysfunction
Pregnancy test
Luteinizing hormone (LH)
Follicle stimulating hormone (FSH)
LH-to-FSH ratio
Estradiol (E2)
E2 level allows meaningful interpretation of FSH/LH data given negative feedback of E2 at the hypothalamic–pituitary level.
Pelvic ultrasound
– To assess for ovarian morphology/antral follicle count/ovarian cysts
Anti-Müllerian hormone
> 35 pmol l^{-1} levels have been suggested to reflect PCOS diagnosis

consideration the severity of hyperandrogenism, and the pattern of hyperandrogenemia (i.e. a reduction in elevated free testosterone levels will result with any COC formulation secondary to an increase in SHBG level due to hepatic effects of the estrogen component of COC formulation; the higher the dose of estrogen, the higher the magnitude of decline in free testosterone). Overall, any and all COC formulations should offer benefit against symptoms of hyperandrogenism through mechanisms outlined; worsening of acne may, however, be experienced by some with the use of COC formulations containing androgenic progestins (such as levonorgestrel) [12]. Conversely, certain COC formulations include unique progestins with antiandrogenic effects that confer additional efficacy against symptoms of hyperandrogenism; drospirenone and cyproterone acetate are examples of antiandrogenic progestins. Despite documented benefits for symptoms of hyperandrogenism, COCs are not FDA approved to treat hirsutism; a few, however, have gained FDA approval for the management of acne.

Progestin-only approach: Endometrial protection against risk for hyperplasia and control of menstrual dysfunction can be achieved with the use of progestin-only formulations. Progesterone-only contraceptive pill, cyclic progesterone (for 10–12 days every one to three months) regimens, intramuscular or subcutaneous depot progesterone formulations and a levonogesterol intrauterine device (IUD) are available options for managing erratic menstrual bleeding and also assist in preventing endometrial hyperplasia. However, progestin formulations and regimens can themselves cause menstrual dysfunction and their efficacy against symptoms of hyperandrogenism is questionable.

Anti-androgens: While antiandrogens have been used empirically to treat hyperandrogenism and PCOS, the data on its efficacy are poor. A meta-analysis by Swiglo et al., found that antiandrogen therapy may provide some benefit in treating hirsutism [13]. They did find that combination treatment with antiandrogen and COC is superior to treatment alone with antiandrogen [1].

7. What are the best treatment modalities/options for a patient whose primary concern is fertility?

Keywords: PCOS, Treatment, Fertility-sparing.

Exploring the individual's plans for fertility is important when deciding on the treatment options. Ovulatory dysfunction is a common cause for infertility and PCOS is the most common contributor to ovulatory infertility (almost 80% of women with ovulatory infertility may meet criteria for PCOS) [7]. Despite the obvious ovulatory considerations, however, additional contributors to infertility, such as abnormal semen parameters or blocked tubes, must be ruled out for any infertile couple.

Managing ovulatory dysfunction and infertility in PCOS can be a challenge as treatment modalities themselves can pose unique risks in this population. While traditional approaches have focused on ovulation induction with agents such as clomiphene citrate (CC), and, more recently, aromatase inhibitors (AIs), there are known risks associated with medical ovulation induction in women with PCOS. Women with PCOS are more likely to develop ovarian hyperstimulation syndrome (OHSS) with fertility treatments. Additionally, women with PCOS are at an increased risk for treatment-related multiple pregnancy due to poly ovulatory responses to fertility medications Finally, women with PCOS are at increased risk of complications in pregnancy, ranging from a risk for miscarriage to risk for gestational diabetes, pre-eclampsia, fetal macrosomia, need for operative delivery including Cesarean section, as well as for neonatal complication [5, 14].

Lifestyle modification must be considered as a first-line management strategy for PCOS-related infertility. The overarching goal is to achieve a healthy pregnancy in a healthy mother. For the overweight, the obese and the insulin resistant, spontaneous ovulation can be achieved in a proportion just through judicious weight loss achieved through a combination of dietary modification and exercise. Weight reduction in overweight or obese women can result in ovulatory regulation and improvement in pregnancy outcomes [9]. In some women with PCOS, weight loss may result in spontaneous ovulation, without pharmacologic assistance [9]. Additionally, weight loss and improvement in overall health status have been shown to improve ovarian response to ovulation induction strategies, thus minimizing the likelihood of need for more aggressive treatments that are associated with risk for OHSS and multiple pregnancy risks [8].

Beyond optimizing well-being through lifestyle modifications and weight reduction (for the overweight and the obese), for those where PCOS-related ovulatory dysfunction is deemed as the primary cause for infertility, medical ovulation induction is generally regarded as the first-line management strategy. The ESHRE/ASRM PCOS Consensus Workshop Group (2008) established treatment with CC as first-line therapy for ovulation induction [13]. A selective estrogen receptor modulator (SERM), CC acts on the hypothalamus to modify the gonadotrophin releasing hormone (GnRH) pulse activity with a resulting increase in pituitary follicle stimulating hormone (FSH) secretion. In turn, the increased pituitary FSH secretion promotes follicular development and dominant follicle selection; rising estradiol levels produced by the growing follicle are responsible for a spontaneous luteinizing hormone (LH) surge with consequent ovulation. Ovulation induction is successful in approximately 70–80% of women, but the pregnancy rate is usually 50–60% [9]. CC usually is initiated between days 2–5 of the cycle and then continued for five days; recommended starting dose is 50 mg per day. In properly selected women, 50% will ovulate through the use of the 50 mg dose CC regimen; of those not responding to the starting dose of CC, another 25% will ovulate at an increased dose of CC 100 mg to a maximum daily dose of 150 mg daily for five days. Women undertaking ovulation induction with CC should undertake some degree of monitoring to determine response to therapy; strategies available range from noninvasive and cost effective approaches of basal body temperature and ovulation prediction utilizing an over-the-counter ovulation predictor kit (OPK) to more sensitive, albeit costly, strategies of serial ultrasound monitoring of follicle growth and rupture, and/or luteal-phase progesterone measurements. Measurement of the urinary LH surge using OPK can prospectively identify the periovulatory interval, which is the optimal time for intercourse to achieve conception. While a failure to detect an LH surge on serial urine monitoring using OPK is suggestive of a failed response to therapy, persistent elevated LH levels can at times contribute to false positive results on OPK testing in women with PCOS. Risk of multiple pregnancy associated with CC is generally less than 10% with the majority being twin conceptions.

If both weight loss and CC fail to induce ovulation, addition of an insulin-sensitizing agent such as metformin may be considered as an adjuvant to CC. Alternatively, switch to a different class of ovulation induction agents, such as AI, or exogenous gonadotropins can be tried. Ovarian surgery, specifically laparoscopic ovarian drilling, is an invasive yet efficacious approach to achieving spontaneous ovulation in women with PCOS who are unresponsive to CC, and *in vitro* fertilization (IVF) with embryo transfer remains a highly effective, albeit expensive, therapy for infertility management in women with PCOS. The goal would be to "develop more patient-tailored approaches based on initial screening characteristics." Treatment with CC should be limited to 6 cycles or less as a failure to achieve conception despite successful ovulation should prompt consideration of additional underpinnings to a couple's infertility and a referral to an infertility specialist is recommended at this point if not sooner. While initial recommendations were against use of metformin and other insulin-sensitizing agents except in women with documented glucose intolerance, more recent research has identified the benefits of combination treatment with metformin and CC in increasing the rate of ovulation and rate of pregnancy [7, 15]. This result can be explained by various mechanisms, including improving hyperandrogenism as well as menstrual cycle abnormalities [7]. Additionally, metformin has been shown to reduce the risk of OHSS in women with PCOS who are treated with CC [16] and those undergoing IVF [15]. Table 12.5 outlines a stepwise approach to management of ovulatory dysfunction in women with PCOS seeking fertility.

Women with PCOS are at increased risk of pregnancy complications. In a recent meta-analysis by Qin et al. (2013), the risk of gestational diabetes was found to be doubled (OR = 2.81 95% CI: 1.99–3.98), with these findings being statistically significant. [5]. Higher, albeit statistically insignificant, rates of pre-eclampsia and prematurity were additionally observed. Given that the spectrum of obstetric risks gets escalated in the setting of multiple pregnancy, the importance of avoiding risk for multiple pregnancy in women with PCOS cannot be minimized [5]. While more research is needed to confirm these findings, the importance of strict surveillance to prevent adverse outcomes is imperative.

8. How do you counsel this patient on the long term risks associated with this PCOS? What additional tests would you recommend to her?

Keywords: PCOS, Diabetes, Metabolic Syndrome, Cancer, Depression.

Table 12.5 Stepwise approach to management of PCOS related ovulatory infertility.

Step	Strategy	Considerations
1	Weight loss if baseline BMI is >30 kg m^{-2}	Safe with improved overall health; offers global risk reduction
2	Clomiphene	Overall safe with <5% risk of multiple pregnancy Resistance is well described particularly with increasing obesity and insulin resistance
3	Aromatase inhibitors	Overall safe with <5% risk of multiple pregnancy Effective in women with evidence of clomid resistance
4	Injectable gonadotropins	High risk for ovarian hyperstimulation syndrome (OHSS) Risk for multiple pregnancy is markedly increased
5	Laparoscopic ovarian drilling	Ovulatory response achieved is comparable to that seen with gonadotropins and without any risk for multiple pregnancy Surgery related risks and potential for pelvic adhesions need to be considered
6	Assisted reproduction/*in vitro* fertilization	Highly effective High risk for OHSS, but can be lowered through protocol modification Low risk of multiple pregnancy ONLY with single embryo transfer

Long-term implications of PCOS for chronic disorders is well-described (Table 12.6). In a prospective cohort study of young adults, Wang et al. found that women in their 20s with PCOS were more likely to develop diabetes and dyslipidemia [17]. Notably, this risk was increased in both normal weight as well as overweight women. Their data demonstrated a threefold increase in risk of diabetes and twofold increase in risk of dyslipidemia in women with PCOS. Altered insulin receptor signaling, chronic insulin resistance, oxidative damage to pancreatic beta cells, chronic hyperandrogenemia, and body mass excess have all been hypothesized as potential mechanisms for an increased risk for diabetes in women with PCOS [17]. Features of metabolic syndrome are commonly encountered in women with PCOS. While a *cause and effect* relationship is not entirely clear, obesity and insulin resistance, both individually and collectively, are recognized as underpinnings to the dysmetabolic milieu of PCOS. Long-term risk quantification through a thorough history and appropriate screening tests must be consistently undertaken in this population and overall risks should be individualized based upon a patient's profile and her family history. Further assessments and treatments should be guided by the patient's risk factors.

Table 12.6 Evaluation of co-existing and long term health risks in PCOS.

Screening for metabolic risk/s

Fasting insulin/Fasting glucose

Glucose-to-insulin ratio > 4.5 is suggestive of insulin resistance

Two-hour oral glucose tolerance test (OGTT) (75 g oral glucose load)

- Timed glucose (and insulin) levels at 0, 30, 60, 90, and 120 minutes

Fasting lipid profile

Screening for depressive symptoms

Screening for endometrial pathology

Endometrial biopsy

- Consider for women with longstanding oligomenorrhea, with inter menstrual intervals exceeding three months and/or for those with menometrorrhagia.

Because of the demonstrated increased risk of diabetes in women with PCOS, the ASRM and the AES have both recommended screening of all women with PCOS for diabetes with a 75 g glucose tolerance test [13]. Metformin use is an effective strategy for managing insulin resistance, in women with PCOS [18]. Beyond conferring a metabolic benefit, improvements in hyperandrogenism and ovulatory function has been shown with metformin use in women with PCOS. [18]

In addition to the cardiovascular risks posed to women, those with PCOS have a two to threefold increase in risk of developing endometrial cancer [2]. The primary risk factor for development of endometrial hyperplasia (the precursor to endometrial cancer) is the chronic anovulation that results in prolonged exposure to unopposed estrogen. Chronic hyperinsulinemia has been recently hypothesized as an additional mechanism placing women with PCOS at risk for endometrial hyperplasia and carcinoma [4]. Endometrial biopsy should be considered for women experiencing prolonged periods of oligomenorrhea (>3 months) and/or for women experiencing dysfunctional uterine bleeding. COC, continuous or cyclic progesterone therapy (oral, intramuscular, vaginal, or intrauterine) can reduce the risk of endometrial hyperplasia and malignancy by reducing endometrial exposure to unopposed estrogen. Additionally, lifestyle modification aimed at weight reduction can target obesity, one of the major risk factors for endometrial cancer. Emerging data seem to suggest that metformin use may offer endometrial protection against progression to endometrial cancer in this at-risk population, although this aspects merits better elucidation through appropriately designed clinical trials [19].

Susceptibility of women with PCOS for depressive symptoms is recognized by Dokras et al. in a meta-analysis of 10 articles assessed the prevalence of depression in women with PCOS (most of the included studies defined PCOS using the Rotterdam Criteria) [20]. Women with PCOS were 4 times more likely to exhibit abnormal depression scores (defined by Beck Depression Inventory) compared to those in the control group. Accruing data highlight the importance of assessment of psychological well-being in women with PCOS [20].

Conclusion

Case scenario

A 22-year-old Hispanic female presents to the office for the evaluation of irregular and infrequent menses. Her menses have always been irregular and occur every two to three months. She also reports excess hair growth on her face and body, particularly the upper lip, chin and neck, and on lower abdomen and her thighs. She has been using electrolysis for the past few years for the control of facial hair. Her gynecologic history is significant for menarche at age 10, and a long-standing history of infrequent menses; her last menstrual period was two months ago and lasted 10 days. She denies any history of abnormal Pap smears or of sexually transmitted infections. She reports initiation of coitus at age 15 and acknowledges three lifetime partners. She used condoms for birth control in the past and has never been pregnant, but hopes to conceive within the next two to three years. The remainder of her medical and surgical history is unremarkable. She denies use of medications and reports no significant allergies. She acknowledges smoking ½ pack of cigarettes per day for the past four years; otherwise denies use of other recreational drugs or alcohol. She works as an assistant teacher at a local elementary school. Her family history is significant for type II diabetes (mother and maternal grandmother) and hypertension (mother and a maternal aunt); menstrual irregularity is acknowledged for her two younger sisters. She denies history of malignancy in her family. Notably, both her sisters also have excess facial and body hair.

Her physical exam is significant for a weight of 200 pounds at height of 5 ft 2 in. (BMI 36.6 $kg\,m^{-2}$). Her waist circumference is 48 in. Her blood pressure is 130/80 mmHg and her heart rate is at 80 beats per minute. Examination demonstrates a pleasant albeit morbidly obese young Hispanic woman with gross evidence of acanthosis nigricans along the neck creases, of acne under the chin and upper back, and clinical evidence of hirsutism (coarse hair along the upper lip, undersurface of chin extending onto her neck, along the anterior abdominal wall with distribution in a male pattern escutcheon, and along the upper medial aspects of her thighs). There is no evidence of scalp hair loss, nor are there any visible striae along the anterior abdominal wall. Abdominal examination confirms evidence of central obesity with no evidence of visceromegaly. On pelvic exam, her external genitalia are unremarkable with no evidence of clitoromegaly. On bimanual examination, the uterus is of normal size and adnexa are non-tender and without any palpable masses. Office urine pregnancy test was negative.

Consideration #1: Does this patient have PCOS?

This patient presents with two of the recognized criteria, i.e. clinical hyperandrogenism (hirsutism) and oligo-ovulation, and hence meets all three of the diagnostic criteria for PCOS (see Table 12.1). However, given that PCOS remains a diagnosis of exclusion, differential diagnoses (see Table 12.2) need to be excluded before she is labeled as PCOS.

Consideration #2: How should evaluation proceed?

Goals of evaluation are: (i) To rule out differential diagnoses; (ii) To quantify severity of hormonal imbalance; and (iii) To individualize risk assessment based on patient profile, family history, and results of targeted testing. Investigations should aim to systematically eliminate conditions that can mimic PCOS (Table 12.2), and offer individualized risk assessment and quantification (risk for diabetes, cardiovascular disease, depression, endometrial pathology).

Consideration #3: What are her risks?

a. Clinical features of insulin resistance (central obesity and acanthosis nigricans) and a sedentary lifestyle in the setting of ethnic predisposition and a positive family history identify this patient at an enhanced risk for diabetes.

b. Central obesity, insulin resistance, sedentary lifestyle, hyperandrogenism, smoking status, in the setting of a family history of hypertension identify this young woman at an enhanced lifetime risk for cardiovascular disease. Blood pressure reading of 130/80 mmHg should be viewed with concern and monitored.

c. Chronic oligomenorrhea, obesity, and insulin resistance all are risk factors for endometrial pathology including endometrial hyperplasia and even cancer. This patient should be offered screening endometrial biopsy and choice of management must ensure endometrial protection through judicious exposure to a progestin.

d. Given the pattern of menstrual cycles, ovulatory dysfunction is apparent. Despite a negative history of sexually transmitted infections, given young age at coitus initiation and >2 lifetime partners, this patient is deemed at an increased risk for acquisition/exposure to sexually transmitted infection/s and consequently at risk for tubal disease.

Consideration #4: What management strategies could be considered for this patient?

1 Lifestyle modification must be initiated as a first-line management strategy with the goal of achieving at least a 10% decline in body mass achievable though a combination of regular physical activity and dietary modification.

2 Menstrual dysfunction is her primary presenting complaint. Normalization of abnormal menses can be achieved in a proportion of women with PCOS through weight reduction and with use of metformin. Combined hormonal contraceptive regimen offers the dual benefit of menstrual regulation and endometrial protection against hyperplasia on one hand, and benefit against features of hyperandrogenism on the other. However, benefits of combined oral contraceptives must be balanced against her personal risk for stroke and deep vein thrombosis given her smoking habit and mildly elevated blood pressure reading in the setting of obesity and a strong family history of hypertension. Smoking cessation must be underscored. Progestin only regimen may be a preferred strategy for endometrial protection until improved health parameters are achieved through smoking cessation, improved lifestyle, weight reduction, and normalization of blood pressure.

3 Low-dose combined oral contraceptives will offer benefit against hyperandrogenism. However, given concerns for vascular health (as discussed earlier), a combination of an effective progestin-only contraceptive such as Levonorgestrel IUD, and an antiandrogen (such as spironolactone) offers an effective approach to managing hirsutism with minimal iatrogenic detriment in this patient is deemed at an enhanced risk for stroke and deep vein thrombosis given her smoking habit and mildly elevated blood pressure reading in the setting of obesity and a strong family history of hypertension. Once improved health parameters are achieved through smoking cessation, improved lifestyle, weight reduction and normalization of blood pressure is achieved, consideration for a trial of a combined oral contraceptive regimen can be revisited.

4 Given the combination of features of insulin resistance and a strong family history of diabetes, assessment of glucose homeostasis by a two hour oral glucose tolerance test, and risk quantification for cardiovascular disease through screening for dyslipidemia is recommended. Metformin trial should be considered for metabolic benefit.

5 While currently not seeking fertility, counseling should address relevance of PCOS diagnosis for fertility, as well as implications of smoking, obesity and of insulin resistance for maternal and fetal well-being. Preconception optimization of overall health should be underscored. When ready to proceed with fertility management, an early assessment of tubal patency should be considered given that despite a negative history of sexually transmitted infections, young age at coitus initiation and >2 lifetime partners identify this patient at an increased risk for acquisition/exposure to sexually transmitted infections, and consequently at risk for tubal disease.

References

1 Stein, I.F. and Leventhal, N.L. (1935). Amenorrhea associated with bilateral polycystic ovaries. *Am. J. Obstet. Gynecol.* **29**: 181–191.

2 Dumesic, D.A. and Lobo, R.A. (2013). Cancer risk and PCOS. *Steroids* **78** (**8**): 782–785.

3 Ferriman, D. and Gallwey, J.D. (1961). Clinical assessment of body hair growth in women. *J. Clin. Endocrinol. Metab.* **21**: 1440–1447.

4 Li, X. and Shao, R. (2014). PCOS and obesity: insulin resistance might be a common etiology for type I endometrial carcinoma. *Am. J. Cancer Res.* **4** (**1**): 73–79.

5 Qin, J., Pang, L., Mu, L. et al. (2013). Obstetric complications in women with polycystic ovary syndrome: a systematic review and meta-analysis. *Reprod. Biol. Endocrinol.* **11**: 56.

6 ACOG Practice Bulletin Number 108. 2009 (reaffirmed 2013) PCOS Clinical Management Guidelines for Obstetricians and Gynecologists.

7 Ayaz, A., Alwan, Y., and Farooq, M. (2013). Metformin-clomiphene citrate vs clomiphene citrate alone: polycystic ovarian syndrome. *J. Hum. Reprod. Sci.* **6** (**1**): 15–18.

8 Azziz, R. (2007). *The Polycystic Ovary Syndrome, Current Concepts on Pathogenesis and Clinical Care*. Springer Science and Business Media LLC.

9 Sirmans, S. and Pate, K. (2014). Epidemiology, diagnosis, and management of polycystic ovary syndrome. *Clin. Epidemiol.* **6**: 1–13.

10 Yildliz, B.O., Bolor, S., Woods, K. et al. (2010). Visually scoring hirsuitism. *Hum. Reprod. Update* **16** (**1**): 51–64.

11 Bhattacharya, S.M. and Jha, A. (2012). Comparative study of therapeutic effects of oral contraceptive pills containing desogesterols, cyptoretone acetate and drospirenone in patients with polycystic ovary syndrome. *Fertil. Steril.* **98** (**4**): 1053–1059.

12 Schindler, A.E., Campagnoli, C., Druckmann, R. et al. (2003). Classification and pharmacology of progestins. *Maturitas* **46** (**suppl. 1**): S7–S16.

13 Swiglo, B.A., Cosma, M., Flynn, D.N. et al. (2008). Clinical review: antiandrogens for the treatment of hirsuitism: a systematic review and meta-analyses of randomized controlled trials. *J. Clin. Endocrinol. Metab.* **93**: 1153–1160.

14 McDowell, S., Kroon, B., and Yazdani, A. (2013). Clomiphene ovulation induction and higher-order multiple pregnancy. *Aust. N. Z. J. Obstet. Gynaecol.* **53** (**4**): 395–398.

15 Jungheim, E. and Odibo, A. (2010). Fertility treatment in women with polycystic ovary syndrome: a decision analysis of different oral ovulation agents. *Fertil. Steril.* **94** (**7**): 2659–2664.

16 Palomba, S., Falbo, A., and Carrillo, L. (2011). Metformin reduces risk of ovarian Hyperstimulation syndrome in patients with polycystic ovary syndrome during gonadotropin-stimulated in vitro fertilization cycles: a randomized control trial. *Fertil. Steril.* **90**: 1384–1390.

17 Wang, E., Claderone-Margalit, R., Cedars, M. et al. (2011). Polycystic ovary syndrome and risk of long term diabetes and dyslipidemia. *Obstet. Gynecol.* **117** (**1**): 6–13.

18 Thessaloniki and ESHRE/ASRM-Sponsored PCOS Consensus Workshop Group (2008). Consensus on infertility treatment related to polycystic ovary syndrome. *Fertil. Steril.* **89** (**3**): 505–522.

19 Shafiee, M.N., Khan, G., Ariffin, R. et al. (2014). Preventing endometrial cancer risk in polycystic ovarian syndrome (PCOS) women: could metformin help? *Gynecol. Oncol.* **132** (**1**): 248–253.

20 Dokras, A., Clifton, S., Futterwit, W., and Wild, R. (2011). Increased risk of abnormal depression scores in women with polycystic ovarian syndrome: a systematic review and meta-analysis. *Obstet. Gynecol.* **117** (**1**): 145–152.

13

CHAPTER 13

Recurrent pregnancy loss

H. J. A. Carp

Department Obstetrics and Gynecology, Sheba Medical Center, Tel HaShomer, Israel

CLINICAL SCENARIO

A 27-year-old Para 0 presented for investigation after four previous pregnancy losses. The first and second pregnancies terminated as intra-uterine fetal deaths at 20 and 23 weeks. Each of these pregnancies had started normally, and the fetal death was completely unexpected. In both cases nuchal translucency scanning was normal, and early ultrasound (15 week) systems scans were normal. The third pregnancy terminated as a biochemical pregnancy at five weeks with a serum human chorionic gonadotrophin (hCG) level which rose until a plateau of 600 iu, then fell. The fourth pregnancy terminated as an intrauterine death at 22 weeks.

She was diagnosed as having antiphospholipid syndrome (APS) due to a positive assay for β2 glycoprotein1 (β2GP1) dependent anticardiolipin antibodies (aCL) and lupus anticoagulant (LA) due to a prolonged activated partial thromboplastin time and Russell's Viper venom time. She was also positive for antinuclear antibodies (ANAs). In the fifth pregnancy, the patient was treated with Enoxaparin 40 mg per day from seven weeks, (after fetal heart was detected) and low dose aspirin (100 mg per day). The pregnancy terminated as a missed abortion at 10 weeks. At curettage, the abortus was karyotyped and found; to be triploid. 69XXY. The subsequent pregnancy (6th) was also treated with enoxaparin and aspirin. The course of pregnancy was normal until 32 weeks when growth retardation was detected on routine ultrasound scanning. There were no other complications of Systemic lupus erythematosus SLE or APS syndrome. At 39 weeks an attempt was made to induce labor. However, fetal monitoring revealed variable decelerations and late decelerations. The pregnancy was terminated by an urgent cesarean section. A male infant weighing 2435 g. was delivered with an Apgar score of 9/10. The postoperative period was uneventful. There were no obstetric or operative complications.

Background

Miscarriage, the commonest complication of pregnancy, is the loss of a pregnancy before fetal viability. The term therefore includes all pregnancy losses from conception up to 20 weeks in North America and 24 weeks of gestation in Europe. Although 15% of clinical pregnancies miscarry, up to 50% of conceptuses may be lost [1]. Some of these may present as biochemical pregnancies as in the third pregnancy in the above patient. Recurrent pregnancy loss (RPL), defined as the loss of three or more consecutive pregnancies, occurs in approximately 1% of couples attempting to bear children. This incidence rate is higher than would be expected if recurrences were due solely to chance, suggesting an underlying predisposition in some couples. The patient usually requires four answers, the cause of her miscarriages, the prognosis both for the next pregnancy and, whether she will ever have a live child, and what treatment can be offered to prevent a recurrence. RPL is often due to fetal abnormalities such as structural malformations [2] or chromosomal aberrations in the embryo. Maternal risk factors for RPL have included APS, maternal hereditary thrombophilias [3], structural uterine anomalies [4], maternal immune dysfunction, and endocrine abnormalities. In this patient APS was found. However, after exhaustive investigation, the cause is often unclear, the prognosis uncertain, and treatment empiric, rather than being evidence based.

Clinical questions

1. In patients with RPLs, what diagnostic tests should be performed, and which risk factors which should be assessed in order to establish a diagnosis of cause?
2. In pregnant patients with previous pregnancy losses, what is the diagnostic value of serum β-human chorionic gonadotrophin (β-hCG), or ultrasound examinations to determine the likelihood of the pregnancy developing?
3. What prognosis can be offered to the patient in the interval between pregnancies?

Evidence-Based Obstetrics and Gynecology, First Edition. Edited by Errol R. Norwitz, Carolyn M. Zelop, David A. Miller, and David L. Keefe.

4. What treatment options are available for patients with pregnancy loss and APS?
5. Which confounding factors may influence the proper assessment of results?
6. Which treatment options are effective in unexplained RPL?
7. What problems exist in using evidence based medicine (EBM) to manage RPL?

General search strategy

A literature search was performed in January 2012 for all papers available at that time in EMBASE and MEDLINE looking specifically for studies of diagnostic tests, systematic reviews, and randomized controlled trials of therapy for RPL. The following search terms were used: RPL, recurrent miscarriage, antiphospholipid antibodies, APS, RPL prognosis, Genetics of miscarriage. Reports were limited to clinical human data including guidelines. All articles considered were investigator initiated trials and published in the scientific literature. In addition, the Cochrane library was searched for systematic reviews of treatment strategies in RPL. If a systematic review was identified, recent updates were sought in the Cochrane Library, MEDLINE, and EMBASE in order to identify randomized controlled trials that became available after publication of the systematic review. However, as positive results have a better chance of being published the selection of studies used for assessment may be biased.

Critical appraisal of the literature

1. In patients with RPLs, what are diagnostic tests which should be performed, and the various risk factors which should be assessed in order to establish a diagnosis of cause?

Search Strategy

- MEDLINE and EMBASE (risk factors): RPL risk factors.
- Karyotype and RPL, APS, Thrombophilia and RPL, hormones and RPL, uterine anomalies, natural killer (NK) cells and RPL, infections, and RPL.
- AND (risk factors OR risk factors.mp) AND clinical trial AND case – control studies AND cohort studies.

There are various guidelines available with investigation protocols. These include the Royal College of Obstetricians [5], the American College of Obstetricians and Gynecologists (ACOG) [6], the European Society of Human Reproduction and Embryology (ESHRE), [7], and numerous others. However, to date there is no consensus on the optimal evaluation and management strategy. The above protocols differ as to the criteria for investigation. The ACOG protocol recommends investigation after two or more pregnancy losses, whereas the Royal College of Obstetricians and Gynaecologists (RCOG) and ESHRE protocols recommend assessment after three or more losses. The author tends to agree with the conclusions laid out by Farquharson et al. [8], that RPL needs to be much better defined before any relevant investigation or treatment protocols can be determined.

The RCOG protocol [5], was last updated in 2011. Recommendations are made for and against various factors causing miscarriage and methods of treatment are graded according to the level of evidence available. Areas lacking evidence are called "Good practice points." The guideline recommends parental karyotyping, fetal karyotyping, ultrasound or hydrosonography for uterine anomalies, APS testing, and interpretation according to the "Sapporo" criteria [9]. The guideline claims that there is insufficient evidence to assess progesterone or hCG supplementation, bacterial vaginosis, factor V Leiden (FVL) or the other hereditary thrombophilias. Assessment of Thyroid function, the glucose challenge test, antithyroid antibodies, alloimmune testing and immunotherapy, and assessment of TORCH and other infective agents are not recommended. The guideline states that a significant proportion of cases of RPL remain unexplained, despite detailed investigation, and that the prognosis for a successful future pregnancy with supportive care alone is in the region of 75%. However, the guideline takes no account of specific types of pregnancy loss, and does not distinguish between different types of patient. There are no suggestions regarding patients who subsequently miscarry despite the reassurance of a 75% prognosis for a live birth.

The ACOG guideline [6] has not been revised since 2001, and is now considered out of date. However, the guideline was less dogmatic than the RCOG guideline. Two pregnancy losses are recognized as warranting investigation. The ACOG guideline does not base its recommendations on a strictly evidence based approach, and states clearly that it should not be construed as dictating an exclusive course of treatment or procedure. The guideline states that new and controversial etiologies may be investigated or treated, if they have been discussed between physician and patient. The guideline also states that variations in practice may be justified according to the needs of the individual patient, resources, and limitations in the institution or type of practice. As the RCOG guideline, the ACOG guideline recommends parental karyotyping, and suggests that the couple should be offered prenatal diagnosis if one parent has a chromosomal aberration. The guideline abstains from giving an opinion on karyotyping of the abortus, and reserves judgment on assessment of the uterine cavity. The guideline claims that assessment of the uterine cavity is based on consensus alone, without good evidence. As in the RCOG guideline, there is said to be insufficient evidence to assess luteal phase defect, progesterone or hCG supplements. The ACOG does not recommend assessment of antithyroid antibodies, infections such as Chlamydia, mycoplasma or bacterial vaginosis. Alloimmune testing, paternal leucocyte immunization and IVIg are also not recommended.

The ESHRE guideline [7] restricts the definition of RPL to three or more consecutive miscarriages. It does take account of different types of patient as the introduction states, "The number of previous miscarriages and maternal age are the most important covariates and they have to be taken into account when planning therapeutic trials. The ideal trial should have stratification for the number of previous miscarriages and maternal age, with randomization between control and experimental treatments within each stratum". The protocol discusses investigations of cause and treatment interventions separately, and unlike the RCOG or ACOG guidelines does not quote the level of evidence for its recommendations. The protocol does recommend testing blood sugar levels and thyroid function tests, antiphospholipid antibodies (LA and aCL), parental karyotyping and assessment of the uterine cavity by pelvic ultrasound or hysterosalpingography (HSG). Hysteroscopy and laparoscopy are reserved as "advanced investigations" but the protocol does not define which patients warrant "advanced investigations." There is a category of investigations, known as investigations which should be used in the framework of a clinical trial. These include: fetal karyotyping, testing of NK cells, luteal phase endometrial biopsy, and homocysteine levels. Treatment is classified separately from investigation in this protocol. Both tender loving care and health advice such as diet, abstention, or reduction of coffee intake smoking and alcohol are described as established treatments. However, no evidence, results or references are quoted to justify calling these treatment modalities established treatment.

The author uses an approach which differentiates between patients with a good, medium, or poor prognosis. This approach has been fully described elsewhere [10].

Specific risk factors

An abnormal fetal karyotype is the only definitive cause of miscarriage. Five series have assessed the embryonic karyotype in RPL [11–15]. The mean number of miscarriages was 4.12 ± 0.48. The incidence of chromosomal aberrations varied between 25 and 57%, (mean 41.6% ± 13.9). Ogasawara et al. [12] have also shown that the incidence of chromosomal aberrations decreases as the number of miscarriages increases. Embryonic chromosomal aberrations can be found in the presence of other causes of RPL. A 30% incidence has been reported in two small series of patients with APS [12, 16]. In the present patient, the fifth pregnancy was triploid, and therefore not related to the other pregnancies. The author has reported embryonic chromosomal aberrations in four patients with hereditary thrombophilias [17].

Karyotyping of the abortus allows the patient to be given prognostic information regarding subsequent pregnancy outcomes. Two studies [12, 13] have examined the outcome of the subsequent pregnancy according to the karyotype of the miscarriage. In the series of Ogasawara et al. [12], there was a statistically significant trend for a patient with an aneuploidic abortion to have a better prognosis. The same trend was apparent in Carp et al.'s [13] series. However, repeat aneuploidy may occur and has been assessed in an observational study of the subsequent miscarriage by Sullivan et al. [15]. Of 30 patients with an aneuploid abortion, only three (10%) had a subsequent aneuploid abortion. In the author's series (unpublished), 43 abortuses were aneuploid, and a subsequent abortion was karyotyped. Only 8 of the 43 abortuses were aneuploid (19%). Hence, approximately 15% of aneuploid abortions may be followed by a subsequent aneuploid abortion. Therefore, 85% of patients with an aneuploid abortion can be assured that the prognosis is good, and that the aneuploid abortion may be a chance occurrence.

Parental karyotyping is usually investigated in the interval between pregnancies. In approximately 3–10% of couples with recurrent miscarriage, one of parents carries a balanced structural chromosomal rearrangement [18–20], most commonly a balanced reciprocal or Robertsonian translocation. Although the risk of miscarriage is often said to be greater with parental chromosomal; rearrangements, four papers which have examined the subsequent live birth rate in RPL and parental chromosomal rearrangements [18, 19, 21, 22], have reported a live birth rate of 53.6% for patients with a mean of 4.19 previous miscarriages. This is the expected rate for patients with 4.19 abortions. Patients are often advised that the presence of a parental karyotypic aberration diagnoses the cause of the miscarriage, as the aberration may be carried to the embryo in an unbalanced form. However, Carp et al. [23], have examined the karyotype of abortuses from parents with karyotypic aberrations. Thirty-nine abortuses from recurrently miscarrying couples with parental karyotypic aberrations were karyotyped. Of the 39, 17 (26%) were euploid. Another 10 (26%) had the same balanced translocation as the parent. Hence, 69% were chromosomally normal. Only five (13%) abortuses had unbalanced translocations. Seven (18%) of subsequent miscarriages were numerical aberrations unrelated to the parental chromosomal disorder (five trisomies and two embryos with monosomy X). Hence, parental karyotyping is of limited value.

APS. All the guidelines above recommend testing for anticardiphospholipid antibodies (aPL), aCL, and LA. In order to be meaningful, there should be two positive values 12 weeks apart. Most pregnancy losses in APS are in the later stages of pregnancy. Rai et al. [24] found that fetal heart activity was previously present in 86% of recurrently miscarrying women with APS, but in only 43% of recurrently miscarrying women without APS. Lockshin [25] has reported that typically pregnancies start normally, and a fetal heart is detected early in the first trimester. IUGR or second or third trimester fetal death ensues. The author [26] has found an increased prevalence of second trimester miscarriages in APS compared to women with unexplained RPLs. In the above patient aPL were assessed due to three fetal deaths in the second trimester.

Hereditary thrombophilias are genetic tendencies to thrombosis. They have been reported to predispose to thrombosis in decidual vessels, leading to fetal anoxia and possibly pregnancy loss. The hereditary thrombophilias include: antithrombin deficiency, protein C deficiency, protein S deficiency, activated protein C resistance and FVL, homozygosity for the methylenetetrahydrofolate reductase mutation (MTHFR, C677T), and the prothrombin gene (FII) mutation G20210. A meta-analysis [3] of 68 retrospective studies has reported a strong association between second trimester miscarriage and hereditary thrombophilias: FVL, FII gene mutation, and protein S deficiency. Hereditary thrombophilias have also been reported to be associated with an increased risk of early fetal loss (less than 25 weeks) in women with protein C, protein S, or antithrombin deficiencies [27] and in FVL [28]. There are five studies examining the incidence of pregnancy complications in the presence of thrombophilias. Neither Ogasawara [29], nor Carp et al. [30] found an increased subsequent miscarriage for patients. However, both Jivraj et al. [31] and Lund et al. [32] found a lower live birth rate in women with FVL and the prothrombin gene (G20210A) mutation in Lund et al.'s [32] series.

Hormone testing has not been shown to be valuable in the interval between pregnancies in RPL. There is no question that adequate hormone support is essential in early pregnancy. Progesterone enhances implantation, affects cytokine balance, inhibits NK cell activity at the feto-maternal interface, inhibits the release of arachidonic acid, prevents myometrial contractility and prevents cervical dilatation. Lutectomy prior to seven weeks causes miscarriage, and mifepristone blocks the progesterone receptor, leading to fetal death and placental separation. However, assessment of mid luteal progesterone levels have been unreliable as predictors of the progesterone status in pregnancy, as progesterone secretion is pulsatile. Blood may be drawn at a pulse peak or nadir. These may vary 10-fold. There is also a lack of correlation between plasma progesterone levels and endometrial histology.

Polycystic ovary syndrome (PCOS) has been linked to an increased risk of miscarriage, but elevated serum luteinizing hormone levels or testosterone levels do not predict an increased risk of future pregnancy loss. An elevated free androgen index may be a prognostic factor for a subsequent miscarriage in women with recurrent miscarriage [33].

A recent systematic review and meta-analysis [34] reported a strong association between (sub) clinical hypothyroidism and recurrent miscarriage (OR 2.3, 95% confidence interval (CI) 1.5–3.5). There may therefore be value in assessing thyroid function. Anti-thyroid antibodies have been linked to recurrent miscarriage. However, in the authors series [35] there was no increased prevalence of antithyroid antibodies in women with RPL. One prospective study [36] has reported that the presence of thyroid antibodies in RPL does not affect future pregnancy outcome if the patient is euthyroid.

Uterine cavity assessment can be performed by HSG, two or three dimensional ultrasound, hydrosonography or hysteroscopy. HSG, probably the most painful of the procedures, cannot differentiate between a septate uterus and a bicornuate uterus, nor determine the myometrial extension or the size of intra-uterine lesions. However, HSG has the advantage of assessing tubal patency if there is concurrent infertility. Two or three dimensional ultrasound can diagnose congenital anomalies such as a septum, fibroids, polyps, etc. and has the ability to visualize both the uterine cavity and the myometrium. A three dimensional scan facilitates the diagnosis of uterine anomalies and enables easy differentiation between subseptate and bicornuate uteri. However, ultrasound is not so accurate regarding intrauterine adhesions.

Valenzano et al. [37], have assessed transvaginal sonohysterography (SHG) in the detection of uterine anomalies. SHG was able to detect all uterine anomalies found in a study of 54 patients with primary or secondary infertility or RPL and a sonographically suspected abnormal uterus. The sensitivity and specificity of SHG were the same as for hysteroscopy.

Hysteroscopy can directly visualize intracavitary structures and directed biopsies can be obtained when indicated. A retrospective study [38] has found an association, between the hysteroscopic findings in 344 women with recurrent spontaneous abortion and major, and even minor uterine anomalies. The anomalies were shown to correlate with an increased risk of recurrent miscarriage.

Uterine anomalies have for long been known to be associated with pre-term labor, but have only recently been definitely associated with RPL. Sugiura-Ogasawara et al. [4] have performed a case controlled study on 676 patients with two or more pregnancy losses. Twenty-five (59.5%) of the 42 patients with a bicornuate or septate uterus had a successful first pregnancy after examination, compared to 1096 (71.7%) of the 1528 with normal uteri. However, the incidence of embryonic chromosome aberrations in women with and without uterine anomalies were 15.4% (2 of 13) and 57.5% (134 of 233), respectively. The author's concluded that congenital uterine anomalies have a negative impact on reproductive outcome in couples with recurrent miscarriage and are associated with further miscarriage with a normal embryonic karyotype. Chan et al. [39] carried out a systematic review to evaluate the prevalence of uterine anomalies in an unselected population, infertility, a history of miscarriage, infertility and recurrent miscarriage combined and preterm delivery. The authors identified 94 observational studies on 89 861 women. The prevalence of uterine anomalies was 5.5% in the unselected population, 13.3% (CI, 8.9–20.0) in women with a history of miscarriage and 24.5% (95% CI, 18.3–32.8) in women with miscarriage and infertility.

NK cells are large granular lymphocytes bearing the CD56+ antigen, and are part of the innate immune system. These cells have been scrutinized as to their role in the immune response to pregnancy, as they are the only lymphocytes to be found in the uterine mucosa. Uterine NK cells seem to be involved with immunosurveillance of the pregnancy, but their exact role is unclear. It has been suggested that NK cells may be responsible for remodeling of spiral arteries into utero-placental arteries, or that NK cells may be responsible for immune attack on the placenta, if lymphokine activated. Since Aoki et al.'s original report [40] showing that increased numbers of NK cells in the peripheral blood of women with RSA predict the likelihood of another miscarriage, there have been two trends, both to identify subgroups of patient with RPL and to include all patients with RPL in mega-trials. Shakhar et al. [41] have found increased numbers of peripheral NK cells in primary (patients who lose all their pregnancies), but not secondary aborters (live birth or births, followed by a string of miscarriages). Perricone et al. [42] have reported that patients with APS and RPL have higher levels of NK cells than patients with APS and no RPL. However, when all patients with RPL are assessed as a homogeneous group, it is difficult to see the association between NK cells and RPL. Tang et al. [43] carried out a literature search for relevant publications from 1950 to 2010. The study included peripheral blood and uterine NK cell numbers or activity in women with RPL, or infertility. The search identified 12 publications which fulfilled the inclusion criteria. However, there were too few women entered into the observational studies to assess whether high peripheral blood NK cell numbers or activity predicted subsequent miscarriage in women with idiopathic RPL. Similarly, the studies of uterine NK cells were not large enough to assess whether abnormal uterine NK cell density predicted subsequent miscarriage in women with idiopathic RPL. At present, more studies are needed to confirm or refute the role of NK cell assessment as a predictive test for subsequent miscarriages.

Infections such as toxoplasmosis, *Listeria monocytogenes*, mycoplasma, Chlamydia, and Parvovirus B19 have been implicated in RPL. However, the role of infection in RPL is unclear. For an infective agent to be causative, it must be asymptomatic in the interval between pregnancies, and capable of persisting in the genital tract. There is some evidence that bacterial vaginosis may predispose to second-trimester miscarriage and preterm delivery [44], but there is little evidence of an association with first trimester miscarriage. It is conceivable that infections may cause miscarriage of live embryos when the uterus contracts and expels a live embryo or fetus, or that a retroplacental hematoma may become infected. However, there are no reports of research in these subgroups of patients. At present no screening for infections has been shown to be helpful.

2. In pregnant patients with previous pregnancy losses, what is the diagnostic value of single and serial measurements of serum β-hCG or serial ultrasound examinations to determine the likelihood of the pregnancy developing?

Search strategy

- MEDLINE and EMBASE: hCG and prognosis, β-hCG and prognosis.
- AND clinical trial AND case–control studies AND cohort studies.

At the beginning of pregnancy, repeated or serial hCG measurements are the only practical test to provide information about fetal viability. hCG can be used clinically to diagnose pregnancy from nine days after the luteinizing hormone (LH) surge. In the first trimester, hCG values approximately double every two days in women with developing pregnancies [45]. If the rise of hCG is slower, pregnancy development may be abnormal, or may indicate an ectopic pregnancy. Osmanağaoğlu et al. [46] carried out a study to determine the value of β-hCG, progesterone, CA125 and their combined use in the prediction of first trimester abortions. A total of 140 singleton pregnant women between 5 and 13 weeks of gestational age whose pregnancies resulted in missed, incomplete, complete, or inevitable abortion were compared to 129 normal pregnancies. When using the free β-hCG level of 520 ng ml^{-1} as a cut-off point, the sensitivity, specificity, positive predictive value (PPV), and negative predictive value (NPV) were 91%, 82%, 46%, and 98%. When a progesterone level of 515 ng ml^{-1} was used as a cut-off point, they were 91%, 89%, 59%, and 98% respectively. The authors concluded that a single measurement of free β-hCG or progesterone levels can be useful in the prediction of first trimester spontaneous abortions. CA125 levels are not found to be an effective marker.

Others have also assessed the predictive value of progesterone levels. Al-Sebai et al. [47] assessed 358 threatened abortions before 18 weeks of pregnancy, and found a single progesterone level $\leq$ 45 nmol l^{-1} (14 ng ml^{-1}) can differentiate aborting and ongoing pregnancies with a sensitivity of 87.6% and specificity of 87.5%.

However, β-hCG and progesterone can be unreliable, as hCG comes from the trophoblast and progesterone from the corpus luteum or later from the placenta. In blighted ova, both may be high. The only test of embryonic viability is the detection of a heartbeat on ultrasound. A heartbeat can be detected from 5.5 weeks. Prior to that β-hCG and progesterone levels are the only diagnostic tests.

A large number of patients repeatedly lose blighted ova, in whom no heartbeat is ever detected. In these patients, the detection of a fetal heartbeat on ultrasound indicates that the pregnancy is developing differently to previous pregnancies. The likelihood of a pregnancy loss after the detection of a fetal heartbeat was 69/359 (14.2%) in Li et al.'s series [48] and 22.7% of 185 study patients with multiple spontaneous abortions in Laufer et al.'s series [49]. If the patient reaches the second trimester with a live fetus, she can also be assured of a good prognosis if she has had previous first trimester abortions.

3. What prognosis can be offered to the patient in the interval between pregnancies?

Search Strategy

• MEDLINE and EMBASE (risk factors): RPL prognosis.

• Recurrent Abortion, recurrent miscarriage or "recurrent pregnancy loss or recurrent spontaneous abortion or habitual abortion").mp.

• limit 5 to yr = "2009–Current".

Various predictive factors can affect the prognosis, viz. (i) Number of previous pregnancy losses. As the number of previous losses increases, the chance of a live birth decreases. The prognosis for a subsequent live birth has been quoted to be approximately 60% after three miscarriages or 80% after two miscarriages. Hence, 40% of patients with three miscarriages will suffer a fourth miscarriage. After four miscarriages, the prognosis for a live birth is 46%, and 54% will miscarry again. Therefore, 22%, ($40 \times 54\%$) of patients with three miscarriages will have two further miscarriages. In the author's series, after five pregnancy losses, the chance of a live birth is only 29%. (ii) Maternal age. Increasing age is associated with a worse prognosis, possibly due to an increased incidence of trisomy in older patients. In the author's series [12], there was a 25% incidence of embryonic chromosomal aberrations in women age 20–39, compared to a 63% incidence in women age above 40. (iii) Karyotype of previous miscarriage. The patient with an aneuploid abortion has a better chance of a live birth [12, 13]. Concurrent infertility has often been quoted as the time taken to conceive, or the need for infertility treatment. The patient with concurrent Infertility has a poorer prognosis than the patient who conceives easily. (iv) Early or late pregnancy losses, as the patient with late losses tends to have a worse prognosis.

In APS, the prognosis is also not clear, as there is no large series on the natural history of the condition. In a small series, the prognosis for a live birth has been reported to be as low as 10% without treatment [24]. There are however, three placebo controlled trials of aspirin, in APS which have been combined in a systematic review [50]. Fifty-two of 61 (86%) pregnancies developed normally in the placebo group.

4. What treatment options are available for patients with pregnancy loss and APS?

Search Strategy

• MEDLINE, EMBASE and COCHRANE DATABASE: APS therapy.

• exp recurrent abortion, recurrent miscarriage or RPL, or recurrent spontaneous abortion or habitual abortion.mp.

• exp APS/dm, dt, rt., su, th Disease Management, Drug Therapy, limit to yr="2009 – Current", limit to (EBM or meta-analysis or "systematic review") AND clinical trial AND case–control studies AND cohort studies AND meta-analysis.

Various regimens have been used to improve the prognosis in APS. These include aspirin, steroids, intravenous immunoglobulin (IVIg), heparins, and hydroxychloroquin. The combination of low molecular weight heparin and aspirin is the most widely used regimen for improving the live birth rate in women with APS. However, this regimen has never been tested in a placebo controlled trial. When Empson et al. [50] carried out a meta-analysis of all the modes of treatment, they reported that a combination of heparin and aspirin can significantly improve the live birth rate in women with recurrent miscarriage and APS. However, this conclusion was based on two trials at that time comparing aspirin to aspirin with the addition of heparins. There have since been a number of meta-analysis comparing aspirin to aspirin with the addition of heparins. The largest analysis [51] summarized five RCT's. There was a common odds ratio of 2.63 in favor of adding heparin (95% CI 1.46–4.75).

The question therefore arises as to the role of aspirin. There are three placebo controlled randomized trials assessing the subsequent live birth rate after aspirin treatment in APS [52–54]. Not one found aspirin to confer any benefit. These three papers have been combined in a meta-analysis [50]. There was no improvement in the live birth rate, (Risk Ratio (RR), 1.05; 95% CI, 0.66–1.68). Therefore, there is currently no evidence that women with the APS have improved pregnancy outcomes with low-dose aspirin.

Steroids are used infrequently to-day due to uncertainty as to efficacy, and the side effects (Cushing's syndrome, acne, osteoporosis, etc.). The efficacy of steroids has also been questioned, as two controlled studies have not confirmed a beneficial effect for glucocorticoids in APS pregnancy [55, 56]. However, there is still a place for steroids in the presence of vasculitis.

IVIg has also been used to improve the prognosis in APA. IVIg inhibits the action [57] and production of aPL [58]. Caccavo et al. (1994) have reported the inhibition of binding of anticardiolipin antibody to cardiolipin by the F(ab')2 fragment from IVIg in a dose-dependent manner. Galli et al. [59] have demonstrated the inhibition of LA activity from the F (ab')2 fragment of IVIg. Additionally, IVIg lowers the levels of aCL after each infusion [60]. However, IVIg seems to have no advantage over heparins in respect to previous live births according to grade 1 evidence from randomized trials [61–64]. However, the incidence of late complications of pregnancy such as intrauterine growth restriction, preeclampsia, and prematurity seem to be reduced with IVIg [65]. At present it seems that IVIg may have a place as a second line of treatment in patients who are refractory to heparin or who continue to suffer the late obstetric complications of APS.

Hydroxychloroquine is often used for SLE. Hydroxychloroquine may reduce the thrombosis risk associated with aPL in non-pregnant SLE patients [66]. However, there have been no trials of hydroxychloroquine in APS pregnancy.

5. Which confounding factors may influence the proper assessment of results?

Search Strategy

• MEDLINE and EMBASE: RPL confounding factors.

• AND exp. recurrent abortion recurrent miscarriage or RPL or "recurrent spontaneous abortion or habitual abortion.mp".

• limit to yr="2009–Current".

• confounding factor$.mp.

It is common practice to assess the efficacy of a treatment modality according to the outcome of the following pregnancy. However, the results may be confounded by alternative causes of miscarriage. RPL may be due to fetal or maternal factors. In the above patient APS had been diagnosed. However, the fifth pregnancy terminated as a missed abortion at 10 weeks. This seems like a failure of treatment. If the patient had been enrolled in a trial of therapy with anticoagulants, and the primary outcome measure was a live birth, she would have been classified as a failure of treatment. However, the fifth pregnancy loss was due to triploidy. The triploidy was a confounding factor. If the embryo had not been karyotyped, the diagnosis would have been missed and the patient classified as refractory APS. The diagnosis of a confounding factor, indicated that anticoagulants were still the right choice of therapy, and that should be used again.

Another confounding factor may be embryonic structural malformations which are incompatible with life. Transcervical embryoscopy has shown that aneuploid embryos have disordered growth and development (such as anencephaly and facial and limb dysplasia), and that similar abnormalities are found in up to 18% of euploid pregnancies ending in miscarriage [2]. However, fetal structural malformations have been investigated in sporadic missed abortion, but not in recurrent miscarriage.

Any severe infection can cause sporadic miscarriage. The role of infection in recurrent miscarriage is unclear. Toxoplasmosis, Mycoplasma, Chlamydia, Parvovirus B19, listeria infections and bacterial vaginosis have been implicated as causes for pregnancy loss. However, if an infection occurs, it may confound the results of any trial of treatment.

6. Which treatment options are effective in unexplained RPL?

Search Strategy

• MEDLINE, EMBASE, and COCHRANE DATABASE: RPL therapy.

• exp. recurrent abortion, recurrent miscarriage or RPL or recurrent spontaneous abortion or habitual abortion.mp. AND Disease Management, Drug Therapy, Radiotherapy, Surgery, Therapy AND EBM or meta-analysis or systematic review, OR case–control study OR cohort study OR review OR meta-analysis.

• limit to yr="2009–Current".

In the above patient, a diagnosis had been made. However, in many cases of RPL, no diagnosis can be made. Therefore some of the empirical treatment regimens are discussed.

Hormone supplementation

Progesterone supplementation has been assessed in a meta-analysis by Daya [67] (1989). Only three trials from the 1950s and 1960s met the criteria of recurrent miscarriage, randomization, and no threatened abortion at the start of treatment. No trial showed evidence of a treatment effect, but pooling the results in a meta-analysis, showed a 23% improvement in the live birth rate, (Grade I evidence). However, these papers were published in the 1950s and 1960s, there was no controlling for embryonic chromosomal aberrations, maternal age, number of miscarriages, etc. Therefore although the results are statistically significant, it is very doubtful whether they are medically or biologically significant. Fourteen years later, Oates-Whitehead et al. [68] repeated the same meta-analysis for the Cochrane database, but found the same three publications as Daya. A large multicenter study (PROMISE) is currently investigating progesterone supplementation in women with unexplained RPL.

hCG supplementation has been assessed in a meta-analysis of four trials in the Cochrane database [69]. The odds ratio for miscarriage was a statistically significant 0.26 (CI 0.14–0.52). However, the conclusions must be treated with caution as two trials assessed were not randomized, and included patients with only two prior miscarriages. Hence the evidence is at best Grade II. Since that time Carp [70] has shown that the benefit is greater in women with five or more miscarriages, in this high risk group, there was an OR of 3.45 for a live birth (CI 1.76–6.80). Figure 13.1 is an updated meta-analysis of six trials which are found in the literature. The OR for a live birth was 2.65 (CI 1.58–4.44). Although the evidence relies on some weaker trials, this is the strongest evidence for any treatment effect in unexplained RPL.

Uterine surgery for anomalies

Unfortunately, there are no published randomized trials assessing the benefits of either open or hysteroscopic surgical correction of uterine abnormalities on pregnancy outcome. The ACOG guideline recommends uterine surgery, but states that this recommendation is based on consensus alone. A review by Homer et al. [82], suggests a benefit in patients with RPL. However, Homer et al.'s review compares pregnancy outcome prior to surgery, compared to the results after surgery. It therefore suffers from selection bias. According to estimates, 65–85% of patients with bicornuate or septate uteri have a successful pregnancy outcome after metroplasty [83]. However, 59.5% of the patients with such anomalies have a successful subsequent pregnancy without surgery, with a cumulative live birthrate of 78.0%.

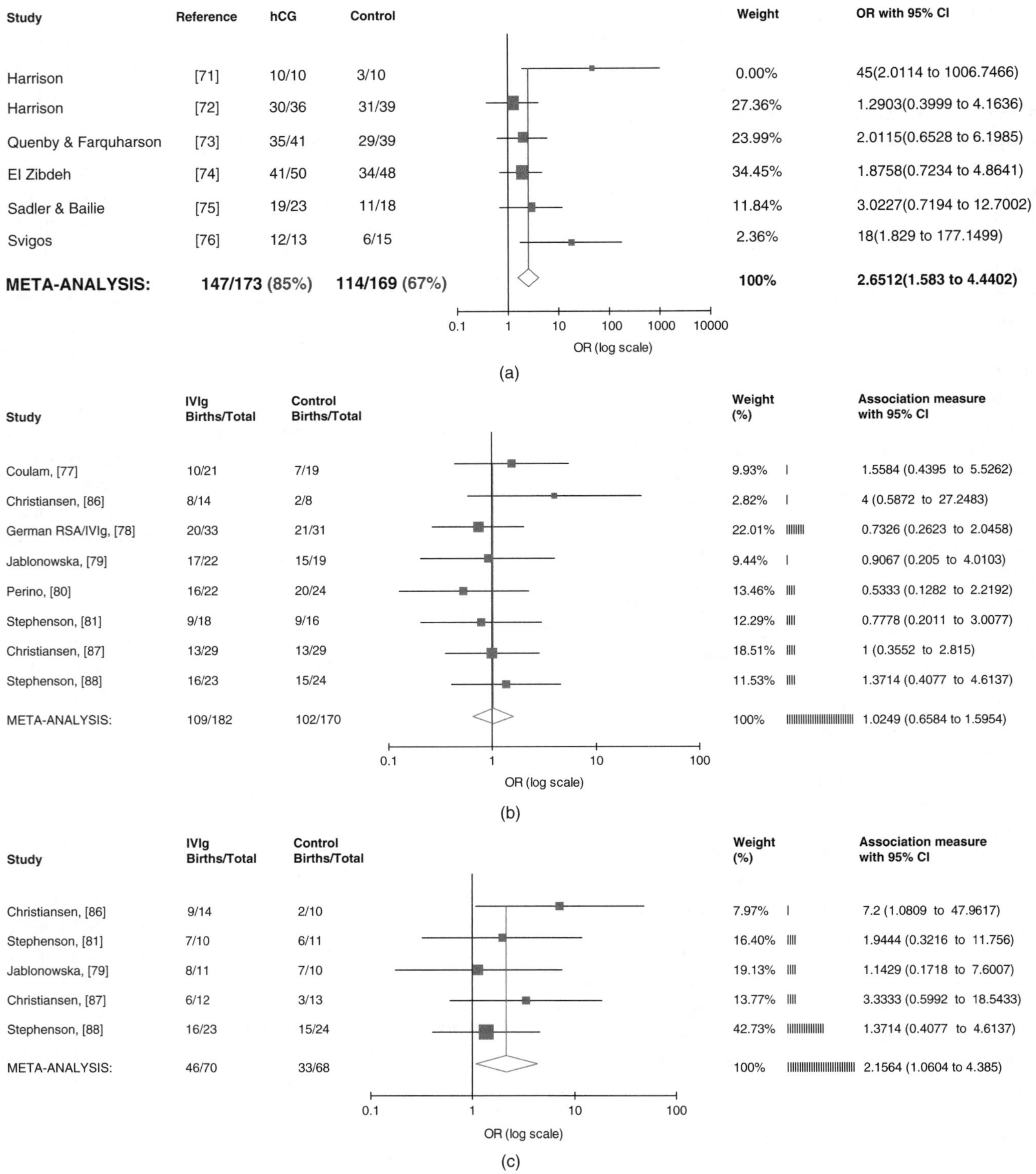

Figure 13.1 Updated meta-analysis on hCG supplementation. (a) Updated Meta-analysis on IVIG in RPL: All series analyzed as a single group. (b) Updated Meta-analysis on IVIG in RPL: Administration prior to pregnancy. (c) Updated Meta-analysis on IVIG in RPL: Secondary Aborters.

Anticoagulant therapy

The effect of anticoagulants in APS has been described above. Two topics of debate are whether anticoagulants should be used in hereditary thrombophilias or unexplained RPL. Recently three randomized trials have been published assessing Aspirin and anticoagulants in unexplained pregnancy losses [84–86]. In Kaandorp et al.'s [84] and Clark et al.'s [85] studies it was possible to do a subgroup analysis

Table 13.1 Aspirin in unexplained RPL

	Aspirin	Control	RR (CI)
Tulppala et al. [52]	22/27 (81.5%)	22/27 (81.5%)	1.0 (0.78–1.29)
Rai et al. [87]	373/556 (67.1%)	308/449 (61.7%)	1.26 (0.92–1.64)
Kaandorp et al. [84]	42/82 (51.2%)	47/81 (58.0%)	0.90 (0.66–1.22)
Visser et al. [86]	32/48 (66.7%)	35/51 (68.3%)	0.96 (0.62–1.46)
Aspirin and Enoxaparin vs. Enoxaparin and placebo			

Table 13.2 Aspirin in hereditary thrombophilias

	Aspirin	Control	RR (CI)
Kaandorp et al. [84]	11/17 (64.7%)	9/17 (52.9%)	1.3 (0.62–2.64)
Visser et al. [86]	9/15 (60%)	13/17 (76.5%)	0.68 (0.33–1.39)
Aspirin and Enoxaparin vs. Enoxaparin and placebo			

for the patients with hereditary thrombophilias. Aspirin has been assessed in unexplained pregnancy loss in Tulppala et al. [52], Rai et al. [87], Kaandorp et al. [84], and Visser et al.'s [86] series (Table 13.1). There was no effect on the live birth rate in any of the series. Tullpala et al. [52] concluded "Low dose aspirin is ineffective in the prevention of miscarriage in recurrent spontaneous abortion". The effect of aspirin in hereditary thrombophila can be determined from 31 patients in Kaandorp et al. [84] and Visser et al.'s [86] series (Table 13.2). Again there was no beneficial effect. Rai et al.'s [87] series showed a benefit in the subgroup of patients with mid trimester miscarriages. As there is not one publication showing a definite increase in the live birth rate, we felt justified in using aspirin as a control group for assessing the effect of heparins.

There is a meta-analysis of five series of heparin in unexplained pregnancy losses [88]. However, this systematic review includes series with only one pregnancy loss, and patients with and without hereditary thrombophilias as a single group. It is therefore of limited value in assessing RPL. Tables 13.3 and 13.4 shows the effect of heparins in unexplained RPL. Heparins had no beneficial effect. In hereditary thrombophilias however, the author [2003] has published a controlled trial on the effect of enoxaparin. Treatment was associated with a 25% increase in the live birth rate. Patients were matched for age and number of miscarriages. The treatment effect was also apparent in patients with five or more miscarriages (Grade II). The figures for hereditary thrombophilias can also be obtained from Kaandorp and Visser's studies. Overall there was a statistically significant odds ratio for a live birth of 1.69 (CI 1.11–2.58). A randomized trial is now necessary to confirm the results.

Immunotherapy is currently out of favor. All the guidelines above claim no evidence of effect, and that immunotherapy should not be used outside of randomized trials. Both active immunotherapy with leucocyte immunization, and passive immunization with IVIg have been summarized in a Cochrane systematic review [90] which show neither form of immunotherapy to have any beneficial effect. In the case of paternal leucocyte immunization, the figures were pulled into statistical insignificance by Ober et al.'s trial [91]. However, Ober et al.'s [91] trial has been criticized for using refrigerated rather than fresh cells, and using a suboptimal dose, If the authors had asked whether fresh cell immunization prevents pregnancy loss, there is a statistically significant benefit. Clark's meta-analysis [92] shows a statistically significant benefit when all patients

Table 13.3 Heparins in unexplained RPL

	Heparin	Control	RR (CI)
Dolitzky et al. [89] Enoxaparin vs. Aspirin	44/54 (81.5%)	42/50 (84.0%)	0.92 (0.58–1.46)
Clark et al. [85] Heparin and Aspirin vs. surveillance alone	111/143 (77.6%)	111/140 (79.3%)	0.95 (0.73–1.25)
Kaandorp et al. [84] Nandoparin and Aspirin vs. placebo	45/92 (48.9%)	47/81 (58.0%)	0.84 (0.64–1.11)
Visser et al. [86] Enoxaparin and placebo vs. Aspirin	35/51 (68.2%)	34/57 (59.6%)	1.24 (0.79–1.92)

Table 13.4 Heparins in hereditary thrombophilias.

	Heparin	Control	RR (CI)
Carp et al. [17] Non randomized Enoxaparin vs. surveillance	26/37 (70%)	22/49 (35%)	1.87 (1.07–3.28)
Kaandorp et al. [84] Nandoparin and Aspirin vs. placebo	9/13 (64.7%)	9/17 (52.9%)	1.3 (0.62–2.64)
Visser et al. [86] Enoxaparin and placebo vs. Aspirin	13/17 (76.5%)	12/19 (63.2%)	1.43 (0.36–10.46)
Total	48/67 (71.6%)	43/85 (50.6%)	1.69 (1.11–2.58)

are treated as a homogeneous group. Subgroup analyses have been performed. Daya and Gunby [93] have shown paternal leucocyte immunization (with fresh cells) to be beneficial in primary but not secondary aborters, and Carp et al. [94] have shown efficacy in women with five or more miscarriages. There is therefore grade 1 evidence for and against the use of paternal leucocyte immunization. It seems that there is a subgroup of patients with immunologically mediated miscarriages which remains to be defined.

IVIg is beset with similar problems. Porter et al.'s systematic review claims that there is no beneficial effect. Hutton et al. [95] have performed a subgroup analysis on all the trials in Porter et al.'s systematic review. Efficacy was found in secondary aborters, and when IVIg was administered prior to pregnancy. Ata et al. [96], repeated Hutton's [95] meta-analysis, and was able to reduce the results to statistical insignificance by excluding two positive trials by Christiansen et al. [97, 98]. An updated meta-analysis is shown in Figure 13.1 including Christiansen and Stephenson's [99] trials. The three meta-analysis forest plots show the importance of assessing subgroups, and not always the group as a whole.

Pregestational genetic screening (PGS) has been used in a number of series to improve the live birth rate in RPL. PGS is based on the concept, that if a large number of RPL are due to embryonic chromosomal aberrations, the replacement of a euploid embryo should increase the number of live births. However, the effectiveness of PGS remains uncertain, due to reports of low implantation and pregnancy rates following PGS [100, 101]. PGS entails a number of drawbacks. Many zygotes do not survive the biopsy. With fluorescent in situ hybridization (FISH) or polymerase chain reaction (PCR) techniques, only five chromosomes are usually assessed, and only nine in leading centers. Hence, an embryo cannot be considered euploid at PGS, only euploid for the chromosomes assessed. To ascertain that an embryo is euploid the entire genome need be assessed. This is possible with comparative genomic hybridization (CGH) microarrays. However, the arrays are presently expensive, transfer in the same cycle time-consuming, and interpretation of results difficult. This will improve in the future and PGS using an array is a promising area of research. There are a number of centers offering PGS with CGH microarrays, but there is not enough evidence available for conclusions to be drawn.

In the case of parental chromosomal aberrations, Franssen et al. [102] carried out a systematic review of the reproductive outcome after PGD in couples with RPL and a parental structural chromosome abnormality. No Randomized or cohort studies were found comparing natural conception to PGD. There were four observational studies on outcome after natural conception and 21 studies on the outcome after PGD. After natural conception, there was a 53% live birth rate in the first subsequent pregnancy (average miscarriage rate, 35%). After PGD, there were 35% live births (average miscarriage rate, 5%). Therefore although PGD reduces the number of miscarriages, there is also a reduced number of live births. The authors concluded that there is currently, insufficient evidence to recommend PGD as a method to increase live birth rates in couples with RPL and a structural chromosome abnormality.

Cytokine modulation is another new approach. Winger and Reed [103] have administered a TNF–α inhibitor either etanercept or adalimumab. There was no advantage over IVIg. Scarpellini and Sbracia [104], have published a randomized control trial (RCT) of G-CSF in 68 women with at least four consecutive primary miscarriages and negative for all clinical investigations. Thirty-five patients were randomized for G-CSF (1 μg $(\text{kg/day})^{-1}$) and 33 for placebo. In the G-CSF group, 82.8% (29/35) women delivered a healthy baby, compared to 48.5% (16/33) in the placebo group (OR = 5.1; 95%, CI 1.5–18.4).

7. What problems exist in using EBM to manage RPL?

The justification for EBM is obvious, to know whether treatment improves prognosis, and to avoid unnecessary treatments which may have side effects. With that in mind the physician can use the best available evidence (which may not always be grade 1) to make decisions about the care of individual patients. However, even grade 1 evidence may be misleading. Meta-analysis may not always be matched. The number of previous miscarriages and maternal age are two important prognostic factors for subsequent pregnancy outcome. If treatment and control groups were not matched for these factors, the results may not be meaningful. Therefore, after EBM it is always necessary to ask whether treatment may be effective in a subgroup of patients rather than all patients with RPL, e.g. IVIg is ineffective when assessed on all RPL patients [90], but effective in secondary aborters [95]. Confounding factors might not have been considered, e.g. in a trial of thrombophilia treatment, were genetic factors excluded? Evidence is used to determine treatment, but evidence may change if more trials added to a meta-analysis. Therefore patients may be denied treatment one year, and have it recommended the next year. Hence, no evidence of effect does *not* mean evidence of no effect. Guidelines are often written based on evidence with the above flaws. Guidelines, although only "Guidelines" and not definitive instructions are used by public health authorities and insurance companies restrict physicians freedom to act. Lastly, EBM gives no information about treatment failures.

There is also an ethical problem. The patient consults her physician to help her to have child. She is often told that the prognosis is excellent if RPL is unexplained. The prognosis is not excellent. As stated in question three above, 40% of patients will miscarry again after three miscarriages. As their prognosis for a live birth is 46%, 20% of patients with three miscarriages will have two further miscarriages. After five pregnancy losses, the chance of a live birth is only 29%. Additionally, the prognosis is unknown in recurrent biochemical pregnancies, after *in vitro* fertilization, APS, or in the older woman.

In the course of reviewing the literature, there are many articles and guidelines advising that treatment should not be provided if there is no evidence of effect, and that patients should be protected from unproven therapies. However, the patients want treatment to prevent pregnancy losses. How does the attitude to provide only proven treatment stand up in an era when patients have rights, such as the right to Cesarean section on demand, (which has morbidity and no evidence of effect), or the patient's right to cosmetic surgery?

References

1 Chard, T. (1991). Frequency of implantation and early pregnancy loss in natural cycles. *Baillieres Clin. Obstet. Gynaecol.* **5**: 179–189.

2 Philipp, T., Philipp, K., Reiner, A. et al. (2003). Embryoscopic and cytogenetic analysis of 233 missed abortions: factors involved in the pathogenesis of developmental defects of early failed pregnancies. *Hum. Reprod.* **18**: 1724–1732.

3 Rey, E., Kahn, S.R., David, M., and Shrier, I. (2003). Thrombophilic disorders and fetal loss: a meta-analysis. *Lancet* **361**: 901–908.

4 Sugiura-Ogasawara, M., Ozaki, Y., Kitaori, T. et al. (2010). Midline uterine defect size is correlated with miscarriage of euploid embryos in recurrent cases. *Fertil. Steril.* **93** (**6**): 1983–1988.

5 Royal College of Obstetricians and Gynaecologists (2011). *Guideline No. 17. The Management of Recurrent Miscarriage*. London: RCOG.

6 American College of Obstetricians and Gynecologists (2002). Management of recurrent early pregnancy loss, ACOG practice bulletin number 24, February 2001. *Int. J. Gynecol. Obstet.* **78**: 179–190.

7 Jauniaux, E., Farquharson, R.G., Christiansen, O.B., and Exalto, N. (2006). Evidence-based guidelines for the investigation and medical treatment of recurrent miscarriage. *Hum. Reprod.* **21** (**9**): 2216–2222.

8 Farquharson, R.G., Jauniaux, E., Exalto, N., and ESHRE Special Interest Group for Early Pregnancy (SIGEP) (2005). Updated and revised nomenclature for description of early pregnancy events. *Hum. Reprod.* **20**: 3008–3011.

9 Miyakis, S., Lockshin, M.D., Atsumi, T. et al. (2006). International consensus statement on an update of the classification criteria for definite antiphospholipid syndrome (APS). *J. Thromb. Haemost.* **4** (**2**): 295–306.

10 HJA, C. (2007). Investigation protocol for recurrent pregnancy loss. In: *Recurrent Pregnancy Loss, Causes, Controversies and Treatment* (ed. C. HJA). London, UK: Informa Healthcare Ltd.

11 Stern, J.J., Dorfman, A.D., Gutierez-Najar, A.J. et al. (1996). Frequency of abnormal karyotype among abortuses from women with and without a history of recurrent spontaneous abortion. *Fertil. Steril.* **65** (**2**): 250–253.

12 Ogasawara, M., Aoki, K., Okada, S., and Suzumori, K. (2000). Embryonic karyotype of abortuses in relation to the number of previous miscarriages. *Fertil. Steril.* **73**: 300–304.

13 Carp, H.J.A., Toder, V., Orgad, S. et al. (2001). Karyotype of the abortus in recurrent miscarriage. *Fertil. Steril.* **5**: 678–682.

14 Stephenson, M.D., Awartani, K.A., and Robinson, W.P. (2002). Cytogenetic analysis of miscarriages from couples with recurrent miscarriage: a case-control study. *Hum. Reprod.* **17**: 446–451.

15 Sullivan, A.E., Silver, R.M., LaCoursiere, D.Y. et al. (2004). Recurrent fetal aneuploidy and recurrent miscarriage. *Obstet. Gynecol.* **104**: 784–788.

16 Takakuwa, K., Asano, K., Arakawa, M. et al. (1997). Chromosome analysis of aborted conceptuses of recurrent aborters positive for anticardiolipin antibody. *Fertil. Steril.* **68**: 54–58.

17 Carp, H.J.A., Dolitzky, M., and Inbal, A. (2003). Thromboprophylaxis improves the live birth rate in women with consecutive recurrent miscarriages and hereditary thrombophilia. *J. Thromb. Hemost.* **1**: 433–438.

18 Carp, H.J.A., Feldman, B., Oelsner, G., and Schiff, E. (2004). Parental karyotype and subsequent live births in recurrent miscarriage. *Fertil. Steril.* **81**: 1296–1301.

19 Stephenson, M.D. and Sierra, S. (2006). Reproductive outcomes in recurrent pregnancy loss associated with a parental carrier of a structural chromosome rearrangement. *Hum. Reprod.* **21**: 1076–1082.

20 Barber, J.C., Cockwell, A.E., Grant, E. et al. (2010). Is karyotyping couples experiencing recurrent miscarriage worth the cost? *BJOG* **117**: 885–888.

21 Sugiura-Ogasawara, M., Ozaki, Y., Sato, T. et al. (2004). Poor prognosis of recurrent aborters with either maternal or paternal reciprocal translocations. *Fertil. Steril.* **81**: 367–373.

22 Goddijn, M., Joosten, J.H., Knegt, A.C. et al. (2004). Clinical relevance of diagnosing structural chromosome abnormalities in couples with repeated miscarriage. *Hum. Reprod.* **19**: 1013–1017.

23 Carp, H.J.A., Guetta, E., Dorf, H. et al. (2006). Embryonic karyotype in recurrent miscarriage with parental karyotypic aberrations. *Fertil. Steril.* **85**: 446–450.

24 Rai, R.S., Clifford, K., Cohen, H., and Regan, L. (1995). High prospective fetal loss rate in untreated pregnancies of women with recurrent miscarriage and antiphosspholipid antibodies. *Hum. Reprod.* **10**: 3301–3304.

25 Lockshin, M.D. (1992). Antiphospholipid antibody syndrome. *JAMA* **268**: 1451–1453.

26 Carp, H.J.A., Cohen, S., and Dulitzki, M. Antiphospholipid antibody syndrome and pregnancy. In: *Recent Advances in Obstetrics and Gynaecology* (ed. S. Dasgu), 1997. New Delhi: Jaypee Ltd.

27 Sanson, B.J., Friederich, P.W., Simioni, P. et al. (1996). The risk of abortion and stillbirth in antithrombin-, protein C-, and protein S-deficient women. *Thromb. Haemost.* **75**: 387–388.

28 Ridker, P.M., Miletich, J.P., Buring, J.E. et al. (1998). Factor V Leiden mutation as a risk factor for recurrent pregnancy loss. *Ann. Intern. Med.* **128**: 1000–1003.

29 Ogasawara, M.S., Aoki, K., Katano, K. et al. (2001). Factor XII but not protein C, protein S, antithrombin III, or factor XIII is a predictor of recurrent miscarriage. *Fertil. Steril.* **75**: 916–919.

30 Carp, H.J.A., Dolitzky, M., and Inbal, A. (2002). Hereditary thrombophilias are not associated with a decreased live birth rate in women with recurrent miscarriage. *Fertil. Steril.* **78**: 58–62.

31 Jivraj, S., Makris, M., Saravelos, S., and Li, T.C. (2009). Pregnancy outcome in women with factor V Leiden and recurrent miscarriage. *BJOG* **116** (**7**): 995–998.

32 Lund, M., Nielsen, H.S., Hviid, T.V. et al. (2010). Hereditary thrombophilia and recurrent pregnancy loss: a retrospective cohort study of pregnancy outcome and obstetric complications. *Hum. Reprod.* **25** (**12**): 2978–2984.

33 Cocksedge, K.A., Saravelos, S.H., Wang, Q. et al. (2008). Does free androgen index predict subsequent pregnancy outcome in women with recurrent miscarriage? *Hum. Reprod.* **23**: 797–802.

34 Vissenberg, R., Van Den Boogaard, E., Van Der Post, J.A. et al. (2011). Treatment of (sub) clinical thyroid dysfunction and thyroid autoimmunity before conception and in early pregnancy: a systematic review. *J. Reprod. Immunol.* **90** (**2**): 148–149.

35 Shoenfeld, Y., Carp, H.J.A., Molina, V. et al. (2006). Autoantibodies and prediction of reproductive failure. *Am. J. Reprod. Immunol.* **56** (**5–6**): 337–344.

36 Rushworth, F.H., Backos, M., Rai, R. et al. (2000). Prospective pregnancy outcome in untreated recurrent miscarriers with thyroid autoantibodies. *Hum. Reprod.* **15**: 1637–1639.

37 Valenzano, M.M., Mistrangelo, E., Lijoi, D. et al. (2006). Transvaginal sonohysterographic evaluation of uterine malformations. *Eur. J. Obstet. Gynecol. Reprod. Biol.* **124**: 246–249.

38 Valli, E., Zupi, E., Marconi, D. et al. (2001). Hysteroscopic findings in 344 women with recurrent spontaneous abortion. *J. Am. Assoc. Gynecol. Laparosc.* **8**: 398–401.

39 Chan, Y.Y., Jayaprakasan, K., Zamora, J. et al. (2011). The prevalence of congenital uterine anomalies in unselected and high-risk populations: a systematic review. *Hum. Reprod. Update* **17** (**6**): 761–771.

40 Aoki, K., Kajiura, S., Matsumoto, Y. et al. (1995). Preconceptional natural-killer-cell activity as a predictor of miscarriage. *Lancet* **345** (**8961**): 1340–1342.

41 Shakhar, K., Ben-Eliyahu, S., Loewenthal, R. et al. (2003). Differences in number and activity of peripheral natural killer cells in primary versus secondary recurrent miscarriage. *Fertil. Steril.* **80** (**2**): 368–375.

42 Perricone, C., De Carolis, C., Giacomelli, R. et al. (2007). High levels of NK cells in the peripheral blood of patients affected with anti-phospholipid syndrome and recurrent spontaneous abortion: a potential new hypothesis. *Rheumatology (Oxford)* **46** (**10**): 1574–1578.

43 Tang, A.W., Alfirevic, Z., and Quenby, S. (2011). Natural killer cells and pregnancy outcomes in women with recurrent miscarriage and infertility: a systematic review. *Hum. Reprod.* **26** (**8**): 1971–1980.

44 Leitich, H. and Kiss, H. (2007). Asymptomatic bacterial vaginosis and intermediate flora as risk factors for adverse pregnancy outcome. *Best Pract. Res. Clin. Obstet. Gynaecol.* **21**: 375–390.

45 Kadar, N., Caldwell, B.V., and Romero, R. (1981). A method of screening for ectopic pregnancy and its indications. *Obstet. Gynecol.* **58** (**2**): 162–166.

46 Osmanağaoğlu, M.A., Erdoğan, I., Eminağaoğlu, S. et al. (2010). The diagnostic value of beta-human chorionic gonadotropin, progesterone, CA125 in the prediction of abortions. *J. Obstet. Gynaecol.* **30** (**3**): 288–293.

47 Al Sebai, M.A.H., Kingsland, J.R., Diver, M. et al. (1995). The role of a single progesterone measurement in the diagnosis of early pregnancy failure and the prognosis of fetal viability. *Br. J. Obstet. Gynaecol.* **102**: 364–369.

48 Li, T.C., Makris, M., Tomsu, M. et al. (2002). Recurrent miscarriage: aetiology, management and prognosis. *Hum. Reprod. Update* **8**: 463–481.

49 Laufer, M.R., Ecker, J.L., and Hill, J.A. (1994). Pregnancy outcome following ultrasound detected fetal cardiac activity in women with a history of multiple spontaneous abortions. *J. Soc. Gynecol. Investig.* **1** (**2**): 138–142.

50 Empson, M., Lassere, M., Craig, J.C., and Scott, J.R. (2002). Recurrent pregnancy loss with antiphospholipid antibody: a systematic review of therapeutic trials. *Obstet. Gynecol.* **99**: 135–144.

51 Mak, A., Cheung, M.W.L., Cheak, A.A.C., and Chun-Man Ho, R. (2010). Combination of heparin and aspirin is superior to aspirin alone in enhancing live births in patients with recurrent pregnancy loss and positive anti-phospholipid antibodies: a meta-analysis of randomized controlled trials and meta-regression. *Rheumatology (Oxford)* **49** (**2**): 281–288.

52 Tulppala, M., Marttunen, M., Soderstrom-Anttila, V. et al. (1997). Low dose aspirin in the prevention of miscarriage in women with unexplained or autoimmune related recurrent

miscarriage: effect on prostacyclin and thromboxane A2 production. *Hum. Reprod.* **12**: 1567–1572.

53 Cowchock, S. and Reece, E.A. (1997). Do low-risk pregnant women with antiphospholipid antibodies need to be treated? Organizing Group of the Antiphospholipid Antibody Treatment Trial. *Am. J. Obstet. Gynecol.* **176**: 1099–1100.

54 Pattison, N.S., Chamley, L.W., Birdsall, M. et al. (2000). Does aspirin have a role in improving pregnancy outcome for women with the antiphospholipid syndrome? A randomized controlled trial. *Am. J. Obstet. Gynecol.* **183**: 1008–1012.

55 Lockshin, M.D., Druzin, M.L., and Qamar, T. (1989). Prednisone does not prevent recurrent fetal death in women with antiphospholipid antibody. *Am. J. Obstet. Gynecol.* **160**: 439–443.

56 Silver, R.K., MacGregor Sholl, J.S., Hobart, J.M. et al. (1993). Comparative trial of prednisone plus aspirin versus aspirin alone in the treatment of anticardiolipin antibody-positive obstetric patients. *Am. J. Obstet. Gynecol.* **169**: 1411–1417.

57 Caccavo, D., Vaccaro, F., Ferri, G.M. et al. (1994). Anti-idiotypes against antiphospholipid antibodies are present in normal polyspecific immunoglobulins for therapeutic use. *J. Autoimmun.* **7**: 537–548.

58 Sherer, Y., Levy, Y., and Shoenfeld, Y. (2000). Intravenous immunoglobulin therapy of antiphospholipid syndrome. *Rheumatology (Oxford)* **39**: 421–426.

59 Galli, M., Cortelazzo, S., and Barbui, T. (1991). In vivo efficacy of intravenous gammaglobulins in patients with lupus anticoagulant is not mediated by an anti-idiotypic mechanism. *Am. J. Hematol.* **38**: 184–188.

60 Kwak, J.Y., Quilty, E.A., Gilman-Sachs, A. et al. (1995). Intravenous immunoglobulin infusion therapy in women with recurrent spontaneous abortions of immune etiologies. *J. Reprod. Immunol.* **28**: 175–188.

61 Vaquero, E., Lazzarin, N., Valensise, H. et al. (2001). Pregnancy outcome in recurrent spontaneous abortion associated with antiphospholipid antibodies: a comparative study of intravenous immunoglobulin versus prednisone plus low-dose aspirin. *Am. J. Reprod. Immunol.* **45**: 174–179.

62 Branch, D.W., Peaceman, A.M., Druzin, M. et al. (2000). A multicenter, placebo-controlled pilot study of intravenous immune globulin treatment of antiphospholipid syndrome during pregnancy. The Pregnancy Loss Study Group. *Am. J. Obstet. Gynecol.* **182**: 122–127.

63 Triolo, G., Ferrante, A., Ciccia, F. et al. (2003). Randomized study of subcutaneous low molecular weight heparin plus aspirin versus intravenous immunoglobulin in the treatment of recurrent fetal loss associated with antiphospholipid antibodies. *Arthritis Rheum.* **48**: 728–731.

64 Dendrinos, S., Sakkas, E., and Makrakis, E. (2009). Low-molecular-weight heparin versus intravenous immunoglobulin for recurrent abortion associated with antiphospholipid antibody syndrome. *Int. J. Gynaecol. Obstet.* **104**: 223–225.

65 Carp, H.J.A., Asherson, R., and Shonfeld, Y. (2001). The role of intravenous immunoglobulin in pregnancies complicated by the antiphospholipid syndrome. *J. Clin. Rheum.* **7**: 291–294.

66 Petri, M. (1996). Thrombosis and systemic lupus erythematosus: the Hopkins lupus cohort perspective. *Scand. J. Rheumatol.* **25**: 191–193.

67 Daya, S. (1989). Efficacy of progesterone support for pregnancy in women with recurrent miscarriage. A meta-analysis of controlled trials. *Br. J. Obstet. Gynaecol.* **96**: 275–280.

68 Oates-Whitehead, R.M., Haas, D.M., and Carrier, J.A. (2003). Progestogen for preventing miscarriage. *Cochrane Database Syst. Rev.* **4**: CD003511. doi: 10.1002/14651858.CD003511.

69 Scott, J.R. and Pattison, N. (2000). Human chorionic gonadotrophin for recurrent miscarriage. *Cochrane Database Syst. Rev.* **2**: CD000101. doi: 10.1002/14651858.CD000101.

70 Carp, H.J.A. (2010). Recurrent miscarriage and hCG supplementation: a review and metaanalysis. *Gynecol. Endocrinol.* **26** (**10**): 712–716.

71 Harrison, R.F. (1985). Treatment of habitual abortion with human chorionic gonadotropin: results of open and placebo-controlled studies. *Eur. J. Obstet. Gynecol. Reprod. Biol.* **20**: 159–168.

72 Harrison, R.F. (1992). Human chorionic gonadotrophin (hCG) in the management of recurrent abortion; results of a multi-centre placebo-controlled study. *Eur. J. Obstet. Gynecol. Reprod. Biol.* **47**: 175–179.

73 Quenby, S. and Farquharson, R.G. (1994). Human chorionic gonadotropin supplementation in recurring pregnancy loss: a controlled trial. *Fertil. Steril.* **62**: 708–710.

74 El-Zibdeh, M.Y. (2005). Dydrogesterone in the reduction of recurrent spontaneous abortion. *J. Steroid Biochem. Mol. Biol.* **97** (**5**): 431–434.

75 Sandler, S.W. and Baillie, P. (1979). The use of human chorionic gonadotropin in recurrent abortion. *S. Afr. Med. J.* **19**: 832–835.

76 Svigos, J. (1982). Preliminary experience with the use of human chorionic gonadotrophin therapy in women with repeated abortion. *Clin. Reprod. Fertil.* **1**: 131–135.

77 Coulam, C.B., Krysa, L., Stern, J.J., and Bustillo, M. (1995). Intravenous immunoglobulin for treatment of recurrent pregnancy loss. *Am. J. Reprod. Immunol.* **34**: 333–337.

78 The German RSA/IVIG Group (1994). Intravenous immunoglobulin in the prevention of recurrent miscarriage. *Br. J. Obstet. Gynaecol.* **101**: 1072–1077.

79 Jablonowska, B., Selbing, A., Palfi, M. et al. (1999). Prevention of recurrent spontaneous abortion by intravenous immunoglobulin: a double-blind placebo-controlled study. *Hum. Reprod.* **14**: 838–841.

80 Perino, A., Vassiliadis, A., Vucetich, A. et al. (1997). Short-term therapy for recurrent abortion using intravenous immunoglobulins: results of a double-blind placebo-controlled Italian study. *Hum. Reprod.* **12**: 2388–2392.

81 Stephenson, M.D., Dreher, K., Houlihan, E., and Wu, V. (1998). Prevention of unexplained recurrent spontaneous abortion using intravenous immunoglobulin: a prospective, randomized, double-blinded, placebo-controlled trial. *Am. J. Reprod. Immunol.* **39**: 82–88.

82 Homer, H.A., Li, T.C., and Cooke, I.D. (2000). The septate uterus: a review of management and reproductive outcome. *Fertil. Steril.* **73** (**1**): 1–14.

83 Sugiura-Ogasawara, M., Ozaki, Y., Katano, K. et al. (2011). Uterine anomaly and recurrent pregnancy loss. *Semin. Reprod. Med.* **29** (**6**): 514–521.

84 Kaandorp, S.P., Goddijn, M., van der Post, J.A. et al. (2010). Aspirin plus heparin or aspirin alone in women with recurrent miscarriage. *N. Engl. J. Med.* **362** (**17**): 1586–1596.

85 Clark, P., Walker, I.D., Langhorne, P. et al. (2010). SPIN (Scottish Pregnancy Intervention) study: a multicenter, randomized controlled trial of low-molecular-weight heparin and low-dose aspirin in women with recurrent miscarriage. *Blood* **115** (**21**): 4162–4167.

86 Visser, J., Ulander, V.M., Helmerhorst, F.M. et al. (2011). Thromboprophylaxis for recurrent miscarriage in women with or without thrombophilia. HABENOX: a randomised multicentre trial. *Thromb. Haemost.* **105** (**2**): 295–301.

87 Rai, R., Backos, M., Baxter, N. et al. (2000). Recurrent miscarriage – an aspirin a day? *Hum. Reprod.* **15** (**10**): 2220–2223.

88 Mantha, S., Bauer, K.A., and Zwicker, J.I. (2010). Low molecular weight heparin to achieve live birth following unexplained pregnancy loss: a systematic review. *Thromb. Haemost.* **8**: 263–268.

89 Dolitzky, M., Inbal, A., Segal, Y. et al. (2006). A randomized study of thromboprophylaxis in women with unexplained consecutive recurrent miscarriages. *Fertil. Steril.* **86** (**2**): 362–366.

90 Porter, T.F., LaCoursiere, Y., and Scott, J.R. (2006). Immunotherapy for recurrent miscarriage. *Cochrane Database Syst. Rev.* **2**: CD000112. doi: 10.1002/14651858.CD000112.pub2.

91 Ober, C., Karrison, T., Odem, R.R. et al. (1999). Mononuclear-cell immunisation in prevention of recurrent miscarriages: a randomised trial. *Lancet* **354**: 365–369.

92 Clark, D.A., Coulam, C.B., Daya, S., and Chaouat, G. (2001). Unexplained sporadic and recurrent miscarriage in the new millennium: a critical analysis of immune mechanisms and treatment. *Human Reprod Update* **7**: 501–511.

93 Daya, S. and Gunby, J. (1994). The effectiveness of allogeneic leucocyte .Immunization in unexplained primary recurrent spontaneous abortion. *Am. J. Reprod. Immunol.* **32**: 294–302.

94 Carp, H.J.A., Toder, V., Torchinsky, A. et al. (1997). Allogenic leukocyte immunization after five or more miscarriages. Recurrent Miscarriage Immunotherapy Trialists Group. *Hum. Reprod.* **12** (**2**): 250–255.

95 Hutton, B., Sharma, R., Fergusson, D. et al. (2006). Use of intravenous immunoglobulin for treatment of recurrent miscarriage: a systematic review. *Br. J. Obstet. Gynaecol.* **114**: 134–142.

96 Ata, B., Tan, S.L., Shehata, F. et al. (2011). A systematic review of intravenous immunoglobulin for treatment of unexplained recurrent miscarriage. *Fertil. Steril.* **95** (**3**): 1080–1085.

97 Christiansen, O.B., Mathiesen, O., Husth, M. et al. (1995). Placebo-controlled trial of treatment of unexplained secondary recurrent spontaneous abortions and recurrent late spontaneous abortions with i.v. immunoglobulin. *Hum. Reprod.* **10**: 2690–2695.

98 Christiansen, O.B., Pedersen, B., Rosgaard, A., and Husth, M. (2002). A randomized, double-blind, placebo-controlled trial of intravenous immunoglobulin in the prevention of recurrent miscarriage: evidence for a therapeutic effect in women with secondary recurrent miscarriage. *Hum. Reprod.* **17** (**3**): 809–816.

99 Stephenson, M.D., Kutteh, W.H., Purkiss, S. et al. (2010). Intravenous immunoglobulin and idiopathic secondary recurrent miscarriage: a multicentered randomized placebo-controlled trial. *Hum. Reprod.* **25** (**9**): 2203–2209.

100 Hardarson, T., Hanson, C., Lundin, K. et al. (2008). Preimplantation genetic screening in women of advanced maternal age caused a decrease in clinical pregnancy rate: a randomized controlled trial. *Hum. Reprod.* (**12**): 2806–2812.

101 Staessen, C., Verpoest, W., Donoso, P. et al. (2008). Preimplantation genetic screening does not improve delivery rate in women under the age of 36 following single-embryo transfer. *Hum. Reprod.* (**12**): 2818–2825.

102 Franssen, M.T., Musters, A.M., van der Veen, F. et al. (2011). Reproductive outcome after PGD in couples with recurrent miscarriage carrying a structural chromosome abnormality: a systematic review. *Hum. Reprod. Update* **17** (**4**): 467–475.

103 Winger, E.E. and Reed, J.L. (2008). Treatment with tumor necrosis factor inhibitors and intravenous immunoglobulin improves live birth rates in women with recurrentspontaneous abortion. *Am. J. Reprod. Immunol.* **60** (**1**): 8–16.

104 Scarpellini, F. and Sbracia, M. (2009). Use of granulocyte colony-stimulating factor for the treatment of unexplained recurrent miscarriage: a randomised controlled trial. *Hum. Reprod.* **24** (**11**): 2703–2708.

CHAPTER 14
Unexplained infertility

Anne-Sophie Boes[1], Diane De Neubourg[1], Karen Peeraer[1], Carla Tomassetti[1], Christel Meuleman[1], and Thomas D'Hooghe[2]
[1]*Leuven University Fertility Centre (LUFC), UZ Leuven, Leuven, Belgium*
[2]*Division of Reproductive Medicine and Biology, Department of Obstetrics and Gynecology, University of Leuven, Leuven, Belgium*

CASE SCENARIO

A 28-year-old female is referred to the fertility clinic because of primary subfertility since 15 months. She is married since five years. She stopped the oral contraceptive pill 15 months ago. Her menarche was at the age of 13. She has a regular cycle of 28–30 days. In her medical history she had an appendectomy at the age of 12. She has no history of any clinical disease. She never smoked. She drinks alcohol only on occasions (+/−2 units per week). Her family history reveals no relevant medical issues. The coitus frequency is twice a week, with special timing around ovulation. No problems are noticed during sexual intercourse. Her body mass index is 20.8. Her secondary sexual signs are normal. There is no symptom of hirsutism, acne or any other systemic disease. Laboratory findings including serum follicle-stimulating hormone (FSH), luteinizing hormone (LH), prolactin, thyroid-stimulating hormone (TSH), androgens, progesterone, estradiol, anti-Müllerian hormone (AMH) are within normal ranges. Mid-luteal phase serum progesterone shows an adequate ovulation. Transvaginal ultrasound is normal. Hysterosalpingography (HSG) reveals a normal uterine cavity with a unilateral blocked tube. To confirm this finding a diagnostic laparoscopy with chromopertubation is planned. During the operation minimal adhesions in the right iliac fossa secondary to the appendectomy are found. There are no signs of tubal adhesions or endometriosis. A chromopertubation shows bilateral patent tubes. Evaluation of her 30-year-old partner reveals normal semen analysis. In conclusion, no obvious cause of the subfertility is found. The couple questions their prognosis and management options giving them the best chance to conceive.

Background

Subfertility is defined as the failure to achieve a successful pregnancy after 12 months or more of regular unprotected intercourse in women less than 35 years of age, and after six months of regular intercourse without use of contraception in women 35 years and older [1]. It affects 13–15% of couples worldwide [2]. Many disorders can lead to subfertility. The most common causes of subfertility are ovulatory disorders, tubal disease and semen abnormalities, each accounting for the source of subfertility in approximately 25% of the couples. Other causes such as endometriosis, cervical factor and uterine abnormalities can explain subfertility in approximately 10% of the couples. About 15% of the couples are classified as having unexplained subfertility. The diagnosis of unexplained subfertility is made when the couple has tried to conceive for at least one year (or six months in women 35 years and older) without success despite evidence of ovulation, tubal patency and normal semen parameters [3–6]. The management of unexplained subfertility is empiric as correctable abnormalities lack. Proposed treatment regiments include expectant management, ovarian stimulation with oral or injectable medications, intrauterine insemination (IUI), and assisted reproductive technologies (ART).

Clinical questions

When starting a treatment for unexplained infertility, the effectiveness of each treatment option should be evaluated. The following clinical questions are relevant to search the literature for the evidence regarding management strategy.

1. In patients with unexplained subfertility (population), what proportion of patients (prognosis) will conceive spontaneously (outcome)?

Evidence-Based Obstetrics and Gynecology, First Edition. Edited by Errol R. Norwitz, Carolyn M. Zelop, David A. Miller, and David L. Keefe.

2. What is the effectiveness (outcome) of ovarian stimulation (OS) agents (intervention) against other treatment options (control) in couples with unexplained subfertility (population)?

a. Clomiphene citrate (CC)

b. Gonadotropins

c. Aromatase inhibitors

3. What is the effectiveness (outcome) of intra-uterine insemination (intervention) against other treatment options (control) in couples with unexplained subfertility (population)?

4. What is the effectiveness (outcome) of *in vitro* fertilization (IVF) (intervention) against other treatment options (control) in couples with unexplained subfertility (population)?

5. What is the benefit (outcome) of laparoscopy (intervention) in women with unexplained subfertility (population)?

Furthermore, it is important to use internationally accepted terms and definitions, recently developed by the World Health Organization (WHO) [7].

General search strategy

Literature searches were performed in the common electronic databases such as Pubmed, MEDLINE, Embase and the Cochrane Library. We looked for systematic reviews, meta-analyses and randomized controlled trials (RCTs). Evidence-based clinical practice guidelines for treatment of subfertility were retrieved from the European Society of Human Reproduction and Embryology (ESHRE), Royal College of Obstetricians and Gynaecologists (RCOG), the American College of Obstetricians and Gynaecologists (ACOG), and the WHO.

Searching for evidence synthesis

Primary search strategy

A combination of medical subject headings and text words were used to find articles related to unexplained subfertility. The terms used were "subfertility," "unexplained subfertility," "definition of subfertility," "treatment options," "conservative management," "expectant management," "Clomiphene Citrate," "gonadotropins," "aromatase inhibitors," "intrauterine insemination," "ovarian stimulation," "assisted reproductive technology," "in vitro fertilization," "laparoscopy." These terms were combined using "AND".

Critical review of the literature

1. In patients with unexplained subfertility (population), what proportion of patients (prognosis) will conceive spontaneously (outcome)?

In a review of studies of unexplained subfertility, the average cycle fecundity over three years of follow-up in the untreated control groups was 1.8% in 11 non-randomized studies and 3.8% in 6 randomized studies [8]. Therefore, effective fertility treatment for unexplained subfertility must demonstrate an increase in the pregnancy rate above this baseline fecundability. With expectant management, 14–28% of couples will achieve a successful pregnancy within 12 months [9–11]. Pregnancy rates are lower when the duration of infertility exceeds three years and the female partner is more than 35 years of age. If the duration of infertility is less than two years, the prognosis is relatively good even without therapy, unless the female partner is more than 35 years. Treatment has generally been indicated if duration is more than two years or the female is more than 35 years of age [11]. In conclusion, couples should have tried expectant treatment before medically assisted reproduction is considered. The chance of such a pregnancy depends mainly on patient's age, duration of infertility and history of any other pregnancy in the same relationship [12].

2. What is the effectiveness (outcome) of ovarian stimulation (intervention) against other treatment options (control) in couples with unexplained subfertility (population)?

a. Clomiphene citrate

Ovulation induction with CC is effective for the treatment of subfertility associated with oligo-ovulation. It increases the likelihood of ovulation approximately 10-fold and pregnancy approximately sixfold [13]. In ovulatory women with unexplained infertility the role of CC is controversial. It has been suggested that the empiric use of CC in ovulatory women can cause alterations in the normal endocrinology of ovulation [14]. The effectiveness of the treatment can only be judged by the evidence of RCTs where placebo or no treatment has been used in the control group.

CC combined with intercourse has been evaluated in different trials. Three level-I RCTs and one case–control study showed a significant but small effect of CC: approximately one additional pregnancy in 40 CC cycles (95% CI, 20–202) compared with untreated control cycles [15–18]. The latest RCT reported on live-birth rates and showed that CC offered inferior live-birth rates than expectant management: 26/192 (14%) women in the clomiphene group and 32/193 (17%) women in the control group. Compared with expectant management, the odds ratio for a live birth was 0.79 (95% CI 0.45–1.38) after CC [19]. The most reliable evidence comes from a systematic review, which showed data relating to 1159 participants from seven trials [20]. There was no evidence that CC was more effective than no treatment or placebo for live birth (odds ratio 0.79, 95% CI 0.45–1.38; P = 0.41) or for clinical pregnancy per woman randomized both with IUI (OR 2.40, 95% CI 0.70–8.19; P = 0.16), without IUI (OR 1.03, 95% CI 0.64–1.66; P = 0.91) and without IUI but using human chorionic gonadotropin (hCG) (OR 1.66, 95% CI 0.56–4.80; P = 0.35). The number of cycles in the studies ranged from four to six. The clinical heterogeneity and variable methodological quality of the studies should be noticed. In one study surgically treated endometriosis was present in 40% of the patients [21]. There was also some discrepancy in the use of hCG as an ovulation-trigger. Despite the lack of homogeneity among the studies, it is important to counsel patients regarding the effectiveness of CC. Realistic expectations should be clearly defined prior treatment. Possible side-effects such as transient hot flushes and visual disturbances of CC should also be discussed. Multiple pregnancies occur in 8–10% of cases and ovarian cysts in 5–10% [22]. A case-cohort study has suggested a link with ovarian cancer when used for more than 12 months [23].

In conclusion, these data suggest no evidence that CC has an effect on pregnancy rate in women with unexplained subfertility and would therefore not recommend CC as a treatment for unexplained subfertility.

b. Gonadotropins

Gonadotropins have an established role in women with anovulation with resistance to CC [24]. The role of gonadotropins in women with normal ovulatory function is not clear.

There are no RCTs which compare gonadotropins with expectant management. Therefore the question should be rephrased: does gonadotropin therapy offer benefit over anti-estrogen therapy such as CC in couples with unexplained subfertility? The use of gonadotropin therapy must be justifiable on the grounds of robust evidence of its effectiveness as it is linked to higher risks than CC, such as ovarian hyperstimulation syndrome (OHSS), multiple pregnancy and miscarriage. Also there are increased costs associated with gonadotropin therapy. A recent review of a Cochrane database reviewed the evidence of oral anti-estrogens versus gonadotropins (either human menopausal gonadotropins or recombinant FSH) with intercourse or IUI in the treatment of unexplained subfertility [25]. Five RCTs, including a total of 231 identified couples with unexplained subfertility, were included [26–30]. CC was compared with human menopausal gonadotropins (hMG) in two studies. The results of the two studies as a whole were not significantly different in live-birth rate per couple (OR 0.51, 95% CI 0.18–1.47). Clinical pregnancy rate per woman was examined in three studies, two comparing CC versus hMG and one comparing CC versus high purity urinary gonadotropins. There was a statistically significant higher pregnancy rate with the hMG group when the data from the three studies were combined (OR 0.44, 95% CI 0.19–0.99). The meta-analysis was repeated excluding the trials with co-intervention of an hCG trigger injection (given only in the gonadotropin group). The results were not statistically significant (OR 0.33, 95% CI 0.09–1.20). Pregnancy rate per cycle was reported in five trials. Main pregnancy rate per cycle was 8% (CC) and 25% (gonadotropins), indicating a benefit associated with gonadotropins, although the confidence intervals of all five trials crossed the line of no effect.

Miscarriage rate per pregnancy (defined as a woman being clinically pregnant who does not deliver a live baby) was reported in three studies, one comparing CC versus hMG, one comparing CC versus high purity urinary gonadotropins and one comparing CC with recombinant FSH (rFSH). The results as a whole were not statistically significant (OR 0.46 95% CI 0.06–3.33).

Three trials reported on multiple birth rate per pregnancy (defined as a woman who delivers two or more babies in one pregnancy), one comparing CC versus hMG, one comparing CC versus high purity urinary gonadotropins and one comparing CC with rFSH. The rate of multiple pregnancies after OS with CC was 1/11 (9%) compared to 5/22 (22.7%) after OS with gonadotropins. The results as a whole were not statistically significant (OR 0.37, 95% CI 0.06–2.43).

OHSS was reported in none of the trials, neither was cancellation due to overstimulation. Important considerations should be made about the trials. They all used a different regiment with regard to the treatment that was being prescribed. Almost all trials used an hCG trigger in the gonadotropin groups, but most of the CC groups did not receive hCG. When the trials with this important co-intervention were excluded from the meta-analysis, no significant differences were apparent between gonadotropins and anti-estrogens for the primary outcome.

Cost of treatment is also an important factor when choosing the method of treatment. A retrospective analysis suggested that though gonadotropins were more likely to produce pregnancy, the cost per pregnancy was less in the CC group as opposed to the gonadotropin group. In their study CC was more cost-effective [8].

Although there might be a benefit associated with gonadotropins this review showed that there was insufficient evidence to prefer either of the methods comparing pregnancy or live-birth rates. In conclusion, further RCTs are needed to answer this question.

c. Aromatase inhibitors

Aromatase inhibitors have been successfully used to induce ovulation. In contrast to CC they do not deplete estrogen receptors and therefore have no adverse effect on endometrium or endocervix and they result in lower serum estrogen concentrations. They are also associated with good pregnancy rates and with a lower incidence of multiple pregnancies than CC [31].

There are no trials comparing the use of aromatase inhibitors versus placebo in unexplained subfertility.

A systematic review and meta-analysis of five RCTs compared the efficacy of aromatase inhibitors (letrozole or anastrozole) versus CC for unexplained subfertility. A total of 273 patients were included. Two of the trials compared anastrozole versus CC and three compared letrozole and CC. There was no significant difference observed for live pregnancies between the compared arms (pooled OR 0.87, 95% CI, 0.46–1.65). The methodological qualities of the trials were not highly scored and OS with FSH was also included where aromatase inhibitor and CC were used [32].

The use of aromatase inhibitors as a standard treatment for unexplained subfertility should not be recommended.

3. What is the effectiveness (outcome) of intra-uterine insemination (intervention) against other treatment options (control) in couples with unexplained subfertility (population)?

In couples with unexplained subfertility IUI is a commonly used treatment. Does IUI improve the live birth rate compared with timed intercourse (TI) or expectant management, both with or without OS?

A Cochrane review examined truly RCTs with at least one of the following comparisons: IUI versus TI, both in a natural cycle; IUI versus TI, both in a stimulated cycle; IUI in a natural cycle versus IUI in a stimulated cycle; IUI with OS versus TI in a natural cycle; IUI in a natural cycle versus TI with OS. Only couples with unexplained subfertility were included [33].

One trial compared IUI versus TI or expectant management in a natural cycle [19]. In the IUI group live birth rate was 23% versus 16% in the expectant management group. This was not significantly different (OR 1.60, 95% CI 0.92–2.78). Pregnancy rates did not significantly differ between IUI in natural cycle and expectant management (OR 1.53, 95% CI 0.88–2.64).

Six trials compared IUI with TI in stimulated cycles [28, 34–38]. Only two of the six trials reported on live birth rate and found no significant difference between live birth rate after IUI compared with TI (OR 1.59, 95% CI 0.88–2.88). The two studies were statistical heterogeneous and had insufficient power [34, 38]. One study included a population with poor prognosis because all patients had previously received fertility treatment [38]. Pregnancy rate per couple was reported in all six trials. There was a statistically increased pregnancy rate after IUI if all cycles were analyzed (OR 1.68, 95% CI 1.13–2.50). The number of treatment cycles was also analyzed. There was no significant difference in pregnancy rate when analyzing the first treatment cycle. Cumulative pregnancy rates increased with a rising number of treatment cycles per couple but the optimal number of treatment cycles needed was unable to be determined. The number needed to treat was calculated. Approximately 13 couples need to undergo a treatment with one to three cycles of IUI and OS to have one additional pregnancy.

Four RCTs compared IUI with OS versus IUI in natural cycle and showed a significant increase in live birth rate (OR 2.07, 95% CI 1.22–3.50) [39–42]. Also, clinical pregnancy per woman was significantly higher in IUI combined with OS (OR 2.14, 95% CI 1.26–3.61). Approximately nine couples need to be treated with IUI and OS for approximately four cycles to result in one additional live birth compared to the control group.

Two RCTs compared IUI with OS versus TI or expectant management in a natural cycle. There was no evidence of a difference in live birth rate per couple (OR 0.82, 95% CI 0.45–1.49) or pregnancy rate [21, 43]. One RCT compared IUI in natural cycle versus TI with OS and showed a marginal but significant increase in live births for IUI in natural cycle (OR 1.95, 95% CI 1.10–3.44) and a small significant effect in the ongoing pregnancy rate (OR 1.77, 95% CI 1.01–3.08) [19].

In conclusion, there is evidence that IUI with OS increases the live birth rate compared to IUI alone. The likelihood of pregnancy was also increased for treatment with IUI and OS compared to TI combined with OS. One adequately powered multicenter trial showed no evidence of effect of IUI in natural cycle compared with expectant management. Some studies also seriously questioned the role of IUI in stimulated cycle over six months of expectant management. There was insufficient information on several important outcomes including multiple pregnancies, miscarriage, ectopic pregnancies and risk of ovarian hyperstimulation for treatment with OS. Therefore couples should be fully informed about the risks of IUI and OS as well as alternative treatment options.

As mentioned previously, there is no evidence that CC is more effective than no treatment or placebo for live birth (odds ratio 0.79, 95% CI 0.45–1.38; $P = 0.41$) or for clinical pregnancy per woman randomized both with IUI (OR 2.40, 95% CI 0.70–8.19; $P = 0.16$), without IUI (OR 1.03, 95% CI 0.64–1.66; $P = 0.91$) and without IUI but using hCG (OR 1.66, 95% CI 0.56–4.80; $P = 0.35$) [19].

A prospective randomized trial compared CC and letrozole for OS before IUI in unexplained infertility. A total of 412 infertile women with unexplained infertility were included. Patients were randomized to treatment with 100 mg of CC daily (207 patients, 404 cycles) or 5 mg of letrozole daily (205 patients, 400 cycles) for five days starting on day 3 of menses. The IUI was done approximately 36 hours after hCG injection. The total number of follicles during stimulation was statistically significantly greater in the CC group. There was no statistically significant difference in pretreatment endometrial thickness between the two groups or endometrial thickness at the time of hCG administration. Serum estradiol and progesterone concentrations were statistically significantly higher in the CC group. The days to hCG injection were similar in both groups. Pregnancy occurred in 73 out of 205 patients (400 cycles) in the letrozole group (35.6% and 18.2%, respectively) and 78 out of 207 patients (404 cycles) (37.6% and 19.3%, respectively) in the CC group; the differences were not statistically significant. This study found no superiority between letrozole and CC for inducing ovulation in women with unexplained infertility before IUI [44].

One review evaluated the use of gonadotropins versus CC with IUI to define the best stimulation protocol [45]. Meta-analyses showed higher pregnancy rates in couples treated with gonadotropins versus CC (OR 1.8, 95% CI 1.2–2.7). There was no significant increase in multiple pregnancies (4% for gonadotropin treatment versus 2% for CC). There was no significant difference between anti-oestrogens and aromatase inhibitors (OR 1.2, 95% CI 0.64–2.1). The same could be concluded comparing different types of gonadotropins. Adding a gonadotropin-releasing hormone (GnRH) agonist did not improve pregnancy rates (OR 0.98, 95% CI 0.6–1.6), although it resulted in significantly higher multiple pregnancy rates improved pregnancy rates (OR 2.9 95% CI 1.0–8). There was no convincing evidence of adding a GnRH antagonist to gonadotropins (OR 1.5 95% CI 0.83–2.8). Doubling the dose of gonadotropins did not show better results (OR 1.2 95% 0.67–1.9) but increased the rates for multiple pregnancy and OHSS.

Gonadotropins seem to be the most effective drugs when IUI is combined with OS. Low dose protocols are advised since pregnancy rates do not differ from pregnancy rates with high dose regimen. Low dose gonadotropins are important to limit multiple pregnancy and OHSS.

4. What is the effectiveness (outcome) of *in vitro* fertilization (intervention) against other treatment options (control) in couples with unexplained subfertility (population)?

IVF is widely accepted as a method of treatment for unexplained subfertility. It is considered as the most effective method but is expensive and has important adverse effects. The 12th annual ESHRE publication on European Data on ART reports clinical pregnancy rates per transfer of 32.5%. The mean delivery rate per transfer was 20.4%. The pregnancy and delivery rates decreased with advancing age (≥35 years). Adverse effects are multiple pregnancy and OHSS. The total multiple delivery rates was 21.7% and in 1% of all stimulated cycles OHSS was recorded [46].

Among women with unexplained subfertility the American Society for Reproductive Medicine/Society for Assisted Reproductive Technology Registry (ASRM/SART) reported a live-birth rate of 30.4% [47]. It is important to evaluate the effectiveness of IVF versus other less-invasive treatment options in women with unexplained subfertility, as the high cost and adverse effects are not negligible.

A review of RCTs examined the effectiveness of IVF [48]. In trials where IVF was compared to expectant management life birth rate (LBR) per woman or couple was significantly higher with a single cycle of IVF (45.8%) than with expectant management (3.7%) (OR 22.00, 95% CI 2.56–189.37). So was the pregnancy rate per woman or couple (OR 3.24, 95% CI 1.07–9.80) [49]. There were no comparative data about IVF versus CC.

Studies compared IVF with IUI in natural cycle and showed no evidence of a significant difference in LBR between IVF (6 cycles) and IUI alone (6 cycles) (OR 1.96, 95% CI 0.88–4.36): 40.7% LFB with IVF versus 25.9% with IUI [40]. In studies comparing IVF versus IUI with OS in women who did not previously underwent IUI with OS (treatment-naïve women), LBR per woman did not differ significantly (OR 1.09, 95% CI 0.74–1.59; 2 RCTs, 234 women) [40, 50]. LBR was significantly higher in those who underwent IVF compared to IUI and OS in a large RCT of women pretreated with IUI and CC (OR 2.66, 95% CI 1.94–3.63, 1 RCT, 341 women) [51]. There was no evidence of a significant difference in multiple pregnancy rate between the two treatments (OR 0.64, 95% CI 0.31–1.29; 3 RCTs, 351 women [40, 50, 51]. There was no evidence of a significant difference of OHSS (OR 1.53, 95% CI 0.25–9.49, 1 RCT, 118 women, respectively) [49].

Due to paucity of data from RCTs the effectiveness of IVF for unexplained infertility relative to expectant management, CC and IUI alone remains unproven. IVF may be more effective than IUI with OS but results have to be interpreted with caution. Adverse events and the costs associated with these interventions have not been adequately assessed [52]. Clinicians and couples should balance the invasive nature of IVF and related costs against chances of success with other treatment modalities.

5. What is the benefit (outcome) of laparoscopy (intervention) in women with unexplained subfertility (population)?

The use of laparoscopy in couples with unexplained subfertility is still a subject of debate, although it is generally accepted as the gold standard in diagnosing tubal pathology and other intra-abdominal causes of infertility. It is often the final test in the infertility work up. Laparoscopy reveals abnormal findings in 21–68% of the cases after normal HSG [53–59]. These findings include adhesions and minimal/mild endometriosis. An appropriate surgical treatment can be given during diagnostic laparoscopy, enhancing the chance of spontaneous conception. The clinical value of these laparoscopic treatments depends on the effect to pregnancy rates. The laparoscopic findings can also change the decision of which treatment should be applied. Whether this change of treatment is effective needs to be assessed.

There are no studies comparing fecundity rate after laparoscopic adhesiolysis with no treatment. Only one non-randomized study compared open adhesiolysis versus no treatment. Sixty-nine infertile women having periadnexal adhesions were treated by laparotomy and salpingo-ovariolysis and 78 were not treated. There was a highly significant cumulative pregnancy rate at 12 and 24 months follow-up in the treated group compared to the non-treatment group (32% and 45% versus 11% and 16%) [60]. These findings suggest that adhesiolysis might be associated with higher spontaneous pregnancy rates. Whether laparoscopic adhesiolysis enhances pregnancy rates after IUI has never been studied.

Two RCTs compared laparoscopic ablation of minimal and mild endometriosis with no treatment. In one study 341 infertile patients with minimal and mild endometriosis were randomized to laparoscopic ablation or expectant management. Laparoscopic ablation of minimal and mild endometriosis doubled the cumulative fecundity rate after a follow-up period of 36 weeks: 30.7% in the treatment group versus 17.7% in the no treatment group [61]. In a smaller study 100 infertile patients with minimal and mild endometriosis were randomized to laparoscopic surgery or expectant management. There was no difference in fecundity rate between the treatment and no treatment group after a follow-up period of one year: 24% versus 29% respectively. We notice the lack of power as a result of the study's small sample size [62]. The results of these two RCTs were combined into a meta-analysis. This analysis showed that surgical treatment is favorable instead of expectant management (OR 1.7; 95% CI 1.1–2.5) [63]. Whether laparoscopic treatment prior to IUI with OS will increase pregnancy rates should be determined by further studies.

There is a growing tendency for bypassing diagnostic laparoscopy in couples suspected of having unexplained infertility including a normal HSG. Some authors recommend treatment by three to six cycles of combined gonadotropins and IUI and if unsuccessful immediately switch to IVF instead of finalizing the infertility work up by diagnostic laparoscopy. They claim this approach would be the most cost-effective and efficient treatment protocol [64, 65]. In our experience, laparoscopy can still be beneficial before the start of treatment of IUI since we reported a 50% prevalence of endometriosis in women with a regular ovulatory cycle whose husbands have normal sperm [66], and indirect evidence suggests that the pregnancy rate after IUI is better after endometriosis surgery than in women not operated for endometriosis [67]. Randomized controlled trials are needed to confirm this statement.

Conclusions

Given the younger age of the patient and the duration of the subfertility, the prognosis of this couple is relatively good. An expectant management for up to two years of subfertility can be recommended. Inducing ovulation with CC or aromatase inhibitors in women with regular menstruation does not appreciably increase pregnancy rate. Ovarian stimulation using gonadotropins has been shown to increase clinical pregnancy rates. Low dose protocols are advised to limit multiple pregnancy and OHSS. Although the efficacy of IUI is not robust, six cycles of gonadotropin-stimulated IUI can be recommended following expectant management. Several reports found improved pregnancy rates, but some recent studies found no benefit of IUI. IVF is associated with a significant increase in pregnancy rates but should be the final resort due to its invasive nature and related costs. IVF is probably the best option for women who are more than 40 years of age, but some cycles of gonadotropin stimulation and IUI can be offered before progressing to IVF. Diagnostic laparoscopy should be strongly considered in couples with unexplained subfertility because laparoscopic surgery of the most frequently found abnormalities leads to higher spontaneous fecundity rates and possibly higher pregnancy rates after IUI. Further studies should be performed to assess whether delaying or bypassing entirely diagnostic laparoscopy is more cost-effective.

References

1 Practice Committee of the American Society for Reproductive Medicine (2008). Definitions of infertility and recurrent pregnancy loss. *Fertil. Steril.* **90**: S60.

2 World Health Organization: Report of the Meeting on the Prevention of Infertility at the Primary Health Care Level. WHO, Geneva, 1984. 12–16 December 1983. WHO/MCH/1984.4.

3 Collins, J.A. and Crosignani, P.G. (1992). Unexplained infertility: a review of diagnosis, prognosis, treatment efficacy and management. *Int. J. Gynaecol. Obstet.* **39**: 267–275.

4 Templeton, A.A. and Penney, G.C. (1982). The incidence, characteristics, and prognosis of patients whose infertility is unexplained. *Fertil. Steril.* **37**: 175–182.

5 Guzick, D.S., Grefenstette, I., Baffone, K. et al. (1994). Infertility evaluation in fertile women: a model for assessing the efficacy of infertility testing. *Hum. Reprod.* **9**: 2306–2310.

6 Moghissi, K.S. and Wallach, E.E. (1983). Unexplained infertility. *Fertil. Steril.* **39**: 5–21.

7 Zegers-Hochschild, F., Adamson, G.D., de Mouzon, J. et al. (2009). International Committee for Monitoring Assisted Reproductive Technology (ICMART) and the World Health Organization (WHO) revised glossary of ART terminology, 2009. *Fertil. Steril.* **92**: 1520–1524.

8 Guzick, D.S., Sullivan, M.W., Adamson, G.D. et al. (1998). Efficacy of treatment for unexplained subfertility. *Fertil. Steril.* **70**: 207–213.

9 Snick, H.K.A., Snick, T.S., Evers, J.L.H., and Collins, J.A. (1997). The spontaneous pregnancy prognosis in untreated subfertile couples: the Walcheren primary care study. *Hum. Reprod.* **12**: 1582–1588.

10 Gleicher, N., Vanderlaan, B., Pratt, D., and Karande, V. (1996). Background pregnancy rates in infertile population. *Hum. Reprod.* **11**: 1011–1012.

11 Collins, J.A., Burrows, E.A., and Wilan, A.R. (1995). The prognosis for live birth among untreated infertile couples. *Fertil. Steril.* **64**: 22.

12 Royal College of Obstetricians and Gynaecologists Infertility Guideline Group (1998). *The Management of Infertility in Secondary Care*. London: RCOG.

13 Hughes, E., Collins, J., and Vandekerckhove, P. (2000). Clomiphene citrate for ovulation induction in women with oligo-amenorrhoea. *Cochrane Database Syst. Rev.*2 (Art. No.: CD000056) doi: 10.1002/14651858.CD000056.

14 Randall, J.M. and Templeton, A. (1991). The effects of clomiphene citrate upon ovulation and endocrinology when administered to patients with unexplained infertility. *Hum. Reprod.* **6**: 659–664.

15 Fisch, P., Casper, R.F., Brown, S.E. et al. (1989). Unexplained infertility: evaluation of treatment with clomiphene citrate and human chorionic gonadotropin. *Fertil. Steril.* **51**: 828–833.

16 Glazener, C.M., Coulson, C., Lambert, P.A. et al. (1990). Clomiphene treatment for women with unexplained infertility: placebo-controlled study of hormonal responses and conception rates. *Gynecol. Endocrinol.* **4**: 75–83.

17 Harrison, R.F. and O'Moore, R.R. (1983). The use of clomiphene citrate with and without human chorionic gonadotropin. *Irish Med. J.* **76**: 273–274.

18 Fujii, S., Fukui, A., Fukushi, Y. et al. (1997). The effects of clomiphene citrate on normally ovulatory women. *Fertil. Steril.* **68**: 997–999.

19 Bhattacharya, S., Harrild, K., Mollison, J. et al. (2008). Clomiphene citrate or unstimulated intrauterine insemination compared with expectant management for unexplained subfertility: pragmatic randomized controlled trial. *Br. Med. J.* **a716**: 337.

20 Hughes, E., Brown, J., Collins, J., and Vandekerckhove, P. (2010). Clomiphene citrate for unexplained subfertility in women. *Cochrane Database Syst. Rev.*1 (Art. No.: CD000057) doi: 10.1002/14651858.CD000057.pub2.

21 Deaton, J., Gibson, M., Blackmer, K. et al. (1990). A randomized, controlled trial of clomiphene citrate and intrauterine insemination in couples with unexplained infertility or surgically corrected endometriosis. *Fertil. Steril.* **54**: 1083–1088.

22 Tarlatzis, B. and Grimbizis, G. (1998). Future use of clomiphene in ovarian stimulation. Will clomiphene persist in the 21st century? *Hum. Reprod.* **13**: 2356–2358.

23 Rossing, M.A., Tang, M.R., Flagg, E.W. et al. (2004). A case-control study of ovarian cancer in relation to infertility and the use of ovulation-inducing drugs. *Am. J. Epidemiol.* **160**: 1070–1078.

24 Hughes, E., Collins, J., and Vandekerckhove, P. (2000). GnRH hormone analogue as an adjunct to gonadotrophin therapy for clomiphene-resistant polycystic ovarian syndrome. *Cochrane Database Syst. Rev.*2 (Art. No.: CD000097) doi: 10.1002/14651858.CD000097.

25 Athaullah, N., Proctor, M., and Johnson, N.P. (2009). Oral versus injectable ovulation induction agents for unexplained subfertility. *Cochrane Database Syst. Rev.*3 (Art. No.: CD003052) doi: 10.1002/14651858.CD003052.

26 Balash, J., Ballesca, J.L., Pimentel, C. et al. (1994). Late low dose pure FSH for ovarian stimulation in IUI insemination cycles. *Hum. Reprod.* **9**: 1863–1866.

27 Echocard, R., Mathieu, C., Royere, D. et al. (2000). A randomized prospective study comparing pregnancy rates after CC and hMG before IUI. *Fertil. Steril.* **73**: 90–93.

28 Karlstrom, P.O., Bergh, T., and Lundkvist, O. (1993). A prospective randomized controlled trial of artificial insemination versus intercourse in cycles stimulated with human menopausal gonadotrophin or clomiphene citrate. *Fertil. Steril.* **59**: 554–559.

29 Karlstrom, P.O., Berkurezion, M., Bergh, T., and Lundkvist, O. (1998). An extended prospective randomized trial of artificial insemination versus intercourse in cycles stimulated with human menopausal gonadotropins (hMG) or clomiphene citrate (CC). *Fertil. Steril.* **70 (suppl 1)**: S420.

30 Nakajima, A.K., Smith, L.L., Wong, B. et al. (1999). A randomized trial of CC plus IUI versus rFSH plus IUI for the treatment of subfertility. *Fertil. Steril.* **72**: 208.

31 Casper, R.F. and Mitwally, M.F. (2006). Review: aromatase inhibitors for ovulation induction. *J. Clin. Endocrinol. Metab.* **91**: 760–771.

32 Polyzos, N.P., Tzioras, S., Mauri, D. et al. (2008). Treatment of unexplained infertility with aromatase inhibitors or clomiphene citrate: a systematic review and meta-analysis. *Obstet. Gynecol. Surv.* **63**: 472–479.

33 Badawy, A., Elnashar, A., and Totongy, M. (2009). Clomiphene citrate or aromatase inhibitors for superovulation in women with unexplained infertility undergoing intrauterine insemination: a prospective randomized trial. *Fertil. Steril.* **92**: 1355–1359.

34 Veltman-Verhulst, S.M., Cohlen, B.J., Hughes, E., and Heineman, M.J. (2012). Intra-uterine insemination for unexplained subfertility. *Cochrane Database of Syst. Rev.*9 (Art. No. : CD001838) doi: 10.1002/14651858.CD001838.pub4.

35 Arcaini, L., Bianchi, S., Baglioni, A. et al. (1996). Superovulation and intrauterine insemination vs. superovulation alone in the treatment of unexplained infertility. A randomized study. *J. Reprod. Med.* **41**: 614–618.

36 Chung, C.C., Fleming, R., Jamieson, M.E. et al. (1995). Randomized comparison of ovulation induction with and without intrauterine insemination in the treatment of unexplained infertility. *Hum. Reprod.* **10**: 3139–3141.

37 Crosignani, P.G., Walters, D.E., and Soliani, A. (1991). The ESHRE multicentre trial on the treatment of unexplained infertility: a preliminary report. *Hum. Reprod.* **6**: 953–958.

38 Janko, P., Hruzik, P., Pruzinec, J. et al. (1998). Induction of ovulation with or without intrauterine insemination in cases of unexplained sterility. *Fertil. Steril.* **70**: S442.

39 Melis, G.B., Paoletti, A.M., Ajossa, S. et al. (1995). Ovulation induction with gonadotropins as sole treatment in infertile couples with open tubes: a randomized prospective comparison

between intrauterine insemination and timed vaginal intercourse. *Fertil. Steril.* **64**: 1088–1093.

40 Arici, A., Byrd, W., Bradshaw, K. et al. (1994). Evaluation of clomiphene citrate and human chorionic gonadotropin treatment: a prospective, randomized, crossover study during intrauterine insemination cycles. *Fertil. Steril.* **61**: 314–318.

41 Goverde, A.J., McDonnell, J., Vermeiden, J.P. et al. (2000). Intrauterine insemination or in-vitro fertilisation in idiopathic subfertility and male subfertility: a randomised trial and cost-effectiveness analysis. *Lancet* **355**: 13–18.

42 Guzick, D., Carson, S., Coutifaris, C. et al. (1999). Efficacy of superovulation and intrauterine insemination in the treatment of infertility. *N. Engl. J. Med.* **340**: 177–183.

43 Murdoch, A.P., Harris, M., Mahroo, M. et al. (1991). Gamete intrafallopian transfer (GIFT) compared with intrauterine insemination in the treatment of unexplained infertility. *BJOG* **98**: 1107–1111.

44 Steures, P., van der Steeg, J.W., Hompes, P.G. et al. (2006). Intrauterine insemination with controlled ovarian hyperstimulation versus expectant management for couples with unexplained subfertility and an intermediate prognosis: a randomised clinical trial. *Lancet* **368**: 216–221.

45 Cantineau, A.E. and Cohlen, B.J. (2009). Ovarian stimulation protocols (anti-oestrogens, gonadotrophins with and without GnRH agonists/antagonists) for intrauterine insemination (IUI) in women with subfertility. *Cochrane Database of Syst. Rev.*2 (Art. No.: CD005356) doi: 10.1002/14651858.CD005356.pub2.

46 Ferraretti, A.P., Goossens, V., de Mouzon, J. et al. (2012). Assisted reproductive technology in Europe, 2008: results generated from European registers by ESHRE. European IVF-monitoring (EIM); Consortium for European Society of Human Reproduction and Embryology (ESHRE). *Hum. Reprod.* **27**: 2571–2584.

47 The Practice Committee of the American Society for Reproductive Medicine (ASRM) (2006). Effectiveness and treatment for unexplained infertility. *Fertil. Steril.* **86**: S111.

48 Pandian, Z., Gibreel, A., and Bhattacharya, S. (2012). In vitro fertilisation for unexplained subfertility. *Cochrane Database of Syst. Rev.*4 (Art. No. : CD003357) doi: 10.1002/14651858.CD003357.pub3.

49 Hughes, E.G., Beecroft, M.L., Wilkie, V. et al. (2004). A multicentre randomized controlled trial of expectant management versus IVF in women with fallopian tube patency. *Hum. Reprod.* **19**: 1105–1109.

50 Custers, I.M., König, T.E., Broekmans, F.J. et al. (2011). Couples with unexplained subfertility and unfavorable prognosis: a randomized pilot trial comparing the effectiveness of in vitro fertilization with elective single embryo transfer versus intrauterine insemination with controlled ovarian stimulation. *Fertil. Steril.* **96**: 1107–1111.

51 Reindollar, R.H., Regan, M.M., Neumann, P.J. et al. (2009). A randomized clinical trial to evaluate optimal treatment for unexplained infertility: the fast track and standard treatment (FASTT) trial. *Fertil. Steril.* **94**: 888–899.

52 van Rumste MME, Custers IM, Koks CA, van Weering HGI, Beckers NGM, Scheffer GJ, et al. IVF with single embryo transfer versus IUI with ovarian hyperstimulation in couples with unexplained subfertility, an economic analysis. Abstracts of the 25th Annual Meeting of ESHRE, Amsterdam, the Netherlands 28 June–1 July 2009; 25:0–110 Oral.

53 Tanahatoe, S.J., Hompes, P.G.A., and Lambalk, C.B. (2003). Investigation of the infertile couple: should diagnostic laparoscopy be performed in the infertility work up programme in patients undergoing intrauterine insemination? *Hum. Reprod.* **18**: 8–11.

54 Al Badawi, I.A., Fluker, M.R., and Bebbington, M.W. (1999). Diagnostic laparoscopy in infertile women with normal hysterosalpingograms. *J. Reprod. Med.* **44**: 953–957.

55 Corson, S.L., Cheng, A., and Gutmann, J.N. (2000). Laparoscopy in the "normal" infertile patient: a question revisited. *J. Am. Assoc. Gynecol. Laparosc.* **7**: 317–324.

56 Cundiff, G., Carr, B.R., and Marshburn, P.B. (1995). Infertile couples with a normal hysterosalpingogram. Reproductive outcome and its relationship to clinical and laparoscopic findings. *J. Reprod. Med.* **40**: 19–24.

57 Henig, I., Prough, S.G., Cheatwood, M., and DeLong, E. (1991). Hysterosalpingography, laparoscopy and hysteroscopy in infertility. A comparative study. *J. Reprod. Med.* **36**: 573–575.

58 Opsahl, M.S., Miller, B., and Klein, T.A. (1993). The predictive value of hysterosalpingography for tubal and peritoneal infertility factors. *Fertil. Steril.* **60**: 444–448.

59 Wood, G.P. (1983). Laparoscopic examination of the normal infertile woman. *Obstet. Gynecol.* **62**: 642–643.

60 Tulandi, T., Collins, J.A., Burrows, E. et al. (1990). Treatment-dependent and treatment-independent pregnancy among women with periadnexal adhesions. *Am. J. Obstet. Gynecol.* **162**: 354–357.

61 Marcoux, S., Maheux, R., and Berube, S. (1997). Laparoscopic surgery in infertile women with minimal or mild endometriosis. Canadian Collaborative Group on Endometriosis. *N. Engl. J. Med.* **337**: 217–222.

62 Parazzini, F. (1999). Ablation of lesions or no treatment in minimal-mild endometriosis in infertile women: a randomized trial. Gruppo Italiano per lo Studio dell'Endometriosi. *Hum. Reprod.* **14**: 1332–1334.

63 Olive, D.L. and Pritts, E.A. (2002). The treatment of endometriosis: a review of the evidence. *Ann. N. Y. Acad. Sci.* **955**: 360–406.

64 Balasch, J. (2000). Investigation of the infertile couple: investigation of the infertile couple in the era of assisted reproductive technology: a time for reappraisal. *Hum. Reprod.* **15**: 2251–2257.

65 Fatum, M., Laufer, N., and Simon, A. (2002). Investigation of the infertile couple: should diagnostic laparoscopy be performed after normal hysterosalpingography in treating infertility suspected to be of unknown origin? *Hum. Reprod.* **17**: 1–3.

66 Meuleman, C., Vandenabeele, B., Fieuws, S. et al. (2009). High prevalence of endometriosis in infertile women with normal ovulation and normospermic partners. *Fertil. Steril.* **92**: 68–74.

67 Werbrouck, E., Spiessens, C., Meuleman, C., and D'Hooghe, T.M. (2006). No difference in cycle pregnancy rate and in cumulative live birth rate between women with surgically treated minimal – mild endometriosis and women with unexplained infertility after controlled ovarian hyperstimulation (COH) and intrauterine insemination (IUI). *Fertil. Steril.* **86**: 566–571.

15

CHAPTER 15
Menopause and HRT

Jenna Friedenthal[1], Frederick Naftolin[1], Lila Nachtigall[2], and Steven Goldstein[2]
[1] *Department of Obstetrics and Gynecology, New York University, New York, NY, USA*
[2] *Department of Obstetrics and Gynecology, NYU Langone Medical Center, New York, NY, USA*

CASE SCENARIO

A 54-year-old Caucasian G2P2002 accountant with last menstrual period (LMP) eight months prior presents with six to eight moderate to severe hot flushes a day, increasing in intensity over the last few months and disturbing her sleep and seriously interfering with her work. She has tried several over-the-counter preparations, which often work for a few weeks, and then lose effect.

She has otherwise been well. She was hospitalized only for her normal spontaneous deliveries 22 and 24 years ago. She has had regular physical exams, with negative pap smears to date and has had six negative mammographic studies. Her review of systems is negative except for poor sleep and subsequent headache. She is sexually active with her husband of 26 years, and has had no problems with sexual function.

She recently saw her primary care physician and had normal routine blood work, including liver function tests (LFTs) thyroid and lipids. Her follicle stimulating hormone (FSH) is reported at 76 mIU ml^{-1} and her serum estradiol at <20 pg ml^{-1}. Both parents are alive and well at ages 78 and 79.

Physical Exam is as follows:

Blood pressure (BP) 110/70 Height: 5.2 in. Weight: 116 lbs
Breast: neg findings. No L < S > K palpable
Pelvic: normal size uterus, no fibroids, ovaries not felt, normal vulva
Vagina: pale with absent rugae
Pap smear is normal, with poor maturation index

The diagnosis was impending menopause, symptomatic.

Patient was offered choices of transdermal estrogen with cyclic progesterone or conjugated equine estrogen (CEE)/bazedoxifene (BZA), and when told there would be no menses with the latter, chose CEE/BZA.

She returns as requested in five months, very happy to report she has had no flushes since being on the medication for three weeks. She has had no bleeding and her exam is normal, including a return of vaginal rugae. Patient is kept on the same medication and told to return in one year, and to phone if any bleeding occurs or any other abnormal finding is evidenced. A mammogram is ordered for one year, before her return.

Overview

Menopause is defined as the permanent cessation of menstrual periods. It is determined retrospectively after one year of complete amenorrhea and is caused by a loss of ovarian follicle recruitment [1]. In the United States, the average age of menopause, i.e. the age at which the final menses occurs, is 51, with smokers experiencing menopause on average two years earlier than non-smokers.

Prior to menopause, women experience the menstrual transition, also known as perimenopause. During this time there is irregular follicle recruitment with increased numbers of multiple dominant follicles and wide swings of estradiol, menstrual cycles become more irregular and unpredictable, with eventual cessation of menses. Women begin experiencing symptoms during perimenopause included but not limited to hot flushes and vaginal dryness. There exist both short and long term consequences of the estrogen loss associated with menopause, as described below.

Search strategy

A review of the most updated literature was performed using Medline and the Cochrane library. Search phrases included "menopause," "perimenopause," "menopause physiology," "hormone treatment," "management of menopause,"

Evidence-Based Obstetrics and Gynecology, First Edition. Edited by Errol R. Norwitz, Carolyn M. Zelop, David A. Miller, and David L. Keefe.

"symptoms of menopause," and "long term consequences and menopause."

Clinical questions

1. What are the endocrinological changes associated with perimenopause and menopause?
2. What are the clinical symptoms associated with menopause?
3. What are the short and long term sequelae of menopause on the female body?
4. What is the role for ultrasonography in the menopausal patient?
5. What are the current treatment options and indications for treatment?

Discussion of the evidence

1. What are the endocrinological changes associated with perimenopause and menopause?

Normal reproductive physiology

Before one can understand the hormonal and endocrine changes associated with menopause, it is important to briefly review normal, pre-menopausal reproductive physiology. During the follicular phase, FSH is secreted by the pituitary in order to stimulate follicle growth and granulosa cell development. The granulosa cells convert androgens to estradiol, stopping the anti-follicular effect of androgen and inhibiting FSH secretion; it is this balance that leads to the development of a single follicle ready for ovulation. The ovary also produces both Inhibin A and Inhibin B, which fine-tune negative feedback inhibition of FSH by acting on the pituitary gonadotrophes [2]. As the follicle(s) near maturation the rising estrogen levels trigger the luteinizing hormone (LH) surge and ovulation; the luteal phase then ensues, including progesterone and estradiol; progesterone assists in preparation of the uterine endometrium for pregnancy, while also inhibiting gonadotrophin releasing hormone analogue (GnRH) pulse frequency [3]. If a woman becomes pregnant, beta human chorionic gonadotrophin (bHCG) maintains the corpus luteum past its usual two-week lifespan, until the implanted embryo's placenta takes over. In the absence of conception, the corpus luteum involutes, and progesterone and estradiol levels fall and menstruation ensues. The pulses of GnRH secretion become more frequent and smaller, raising the levels of circulating FSH and stimulating the already activated follicles that will contribute to the coming follicular phase of the cycle. Had pregnancy ensued, the progesterone and estrogen from the embryo-placenta would have blocked menstruation and the rise of hypothalamic-pituitary secretion [4].

Ovarian aging with menopause

One of the first hormonal indications of perimenopause is a rising FSH; this is secondary to decreasing production of Inhibin B by granulosa cells in antral follicles. As ovarian function and antral follicle count declines, Inhibin B levels fall, allowing for rising levels of gonadotropins [5]. Rising FSH drives increased recruitment of follicles, with consequential increase in the rate of follicle loss during perimenopause [6, 7].

In addition, estradiol levels also fall with decline in functional ovarian reserve; this results in further disinhibition of GnRH pulsatility, increased sensitivity of gonadotropins to GnRH, and increased levels of FSH as mentioned [8]. Rance et al. suggest that the increase in GnRH may be mediated by increases in neurokinin B and kisspeptin, both stimulatory peptides, and decreasing levels of dynorphin, an inhibitory neuropeptide [2, 9].

In addition to Inhibin A and B, anti-Müllerian hormone (AMH) is a glycoprotein also produced by granulosa cells in preantral and small antral follicles [10]. AMH inhibits the stimulatory actions of FSH follicle recruitment [11]; as the number of antral follicles decreases with age, so too do AMH levels also decrease, reaching undetectable levels at menopause [12]. As such, AMH has become increasingly popular as a measure for ovarian reserve and as an index for menopause [13].

Hypothalamic changes with menopause

Beyond ovarian aging and its hormonal consequences, several studies have also suggested that the hypothalamic-pituitary unit itself is affected by aging and also contributes to menopause independent of gonadal feedback. Studies by Hall et al. suggest that in menopause, GnRH pulse frequency decreases, while overall levels of GnRH increase in a compensatory manner [14]. Additionally, LH and FSH levels fall significantly in the post-menopausal patient, independent of ovarian steroid response [15]. The pituitary itself also becomes less sensitive to GnRH, with significant decreases in both LH and FSH responses in older versus younger postmenopausal women [8]. Interestingly, estrogen-negative feedback appears to remain intact in postmenopausal women, while estrogen-positive feedback may be lost during perimenopause [16, 17].

In sum, the hormonal and neuro-endocrine changes associated with menopause are complex and are still being studied currently. What we believe we understand to date is that with aging, follicle count, and ovarian reserve decreases. This leads to falling levels of Inhibin B and estradiol, which in turn leads to rising levels of FSH in an attempt to preserve normal ovarian function. Eventually, these mechanisms fail as ovarian reserve diminishes, and menopause ensues.

2. What are the clinical symptoms associated with menopause?

Much of our information regarding the clinical manifestations of menopause comes from longitudinal studies of perimenopausal patients, one of the largest being the Study of Women's Health Across the Nation (SWAN), a multi-site longitudinal study of mid-life aging in over 3000 women of diverse racial and ethnic groups [18]. In addition, a "state-of-the-science" meeting in 2005 gathered the world's experts to determine which midlife symptoms were most likely to be caused by menopause as compared to aging alone; symptoms were evaluated on their proximity to the menopause as well as their relationship to estrogen [19, 20].

The symptoms associated with menopause actually begin in the perimenopausal period, which begins approximately two to eight years preceding menopause and continues to approximately one year after the final menses [21]. Symptomatology varies widely in onset, duration, and quality, and an individualized approach should be taken when managing patients.

Uterine bleeding

Mirroring the hormonal fluctuations occurring during perimenopause, menstrual cycles are also in flux at this time and become increasingly irregular. A change in menstrual pattern is the most common symptom of perimenopause [22]. More specifically, cycles tend to become shorter, leading to increasing frequency of menses. However longer cycles are also possible [23], and as perimenopause proceeds, the tendency toward oligomenorrhea increases [24].

Bleeding tends to be heavier in early perimenopause, becoming increasingly lighter as the transition progresses toward the final menstrual period. It is important to note that despite this irregularity, heavy, prolonged bleeding as well as heavy inter-menstrual bleeds are not normal and warrant further clinical evaluation.

Vasomotor symptoms

Vasomotor symptoms are the second-most common symptom of perimenopause/menopause, with as many as 85% of perimenopausal women experiencing night sweats, hot flushes, and sleep disturbances secondary to vasomotor symptoms [19]. Also known as hot flushes or hot flashes, vasomotor symptoms (VMSs) are generally defined as episodes of intense heat and sweating, accompanied by flushing of the head, neck, chest, and/or upper back [25]. The intensity, quality, and duration of hot flushes vary widely among patients from several minutes of extreme heat in the upper body and face to perspiration, chills, clamminess, anxiety, and palpitations [26].

Vasomotor symptoms are generally milder in early perimenopause and tend to worsen significantly throughout the late perimenopausal period [27]. A recent study by Avis et al. found that the earlier that VMS began in the pre/perimenopausal transition, the longer the total duration of symptoms, while women who were post-menopausal when vasomotor symptoms began had the shortest duration of vasomotor symptoms (median 3.4 years); on average, VMS lasted more than seven years for more than half of subjects and persisted for 4.5 years after their final menses [28]. In addition, several studies have shown a correlation between vasomotor symptoms and cardiovascular disease as well as greater degree of bone loss and increased bone turnover [29, 30]. Hot flashes generally stop within four to five years of onset; however, some women report continuation of vasomotor symptoms for many years, and their impact on quality of life should not be underestimated.

Genitourinary syndrome

Estrogen receptors are present along the vulva, vagina, bladder, and pelvic floor; in these organs, estrogen plays an important role in collagen synthesis and turnover [31]. As such, as estrogen levels decrease during the menopausal state, changes in the vulva, vagina, and pelvic floor are common. In 2014, a consensus conference was held, bringing together the International Society for the Study of Women's Sexual Health and the North American Menopause Society with the goal of reviewing terminology to more accurately encompass the genitourinary symptoms of menopause [32]. Members created the term "genitourinary syndrome of menopause" to describe the collection of symptoms associated with the genitourinary changes of menopause. These include loss of vaginal rugae and elasticity, thinning of vaginal epithelium, vulvar or vaginal irritation, burning, or itching, increased tissue friability and bleeding, and shortening/narrowing of the vagina and entroitus. Other symptoms include genital dryness, decreased lubrication, discomfort with sexual activity, post-coital bleeding, and decreased arousal, as well as urinary symptoms such as urinary frequency/urgency and dysuria. Vaginal pH becomes more alkaline, increasing risk for infection. Altogether, these symptoms may significantly affect quality of life, from pain, and bleeding to sexual dissatisfaction. These atrophic changes can be treated effectively and safely with very low dose estrogens delivered to the vagina.

Sleep disturbances, depressed mood, cognitive changes

Women report difficulty sleeping more frequently than men; this appears to worsen with aging, with women reporting increasing sleep symptoms associated with aging as compared to men [33]. Hot flashes occur more commonly during the night, causing sleep disturbance. However, studies suggest that approximately 40% of perimenopausal women experience sleep disturbance even in the absence of hot flashes [34].

In addition to sleep disturbance, recent studies have shown that menopause is associated with increased risk for depression; one study suggests as high as a 14-fold increase in the rate of onset of major depressive disorder during the 24 months surrounding the final menses, suggesting an increased risk for depression in both the perimenopausal as well as early postmenopausal period [35]. Although there are several environmental stressors and life events occurring at the time of menopause that may serve to contribute to or exacerbate depressive symptoms, studies have shown that variability in estrogen levels during the menopause transition leads to changes in the serotenergic and noradrenergic systems within the central nervous system, more specifically within the amygdala, hippocampus, and hypothalamus, all of which are involved in regulating affect [36]. Women in menopause also complain of changes in cognition, most predominantly difficulty with memory. Results from the SWAN study report that perimenopausal women were more likely to report difficulty remembering than premenopausal women [37]. In addition, increases in anxiety and depression associated with menopause have been shown to have detrimental effects on cognition [38].

3. What are the short and long term sequelae of menopause on the female body?

There are several important long-term consequences of estrogen depletion after menopause. These include bone loss, cardiovascular disease, and cognitive decline. Other common long-term effects of estrogen loss include skin changes, alteration in body composition, and impaired balance.

Bone loss

Estrogens decrease bone resorption and lower the rate of bone remodeling. Thus, when estrogen or androgen levels decrease, as in menopause, there is an associated increase in bone turnover with increased osteoclast and osteoblast activity. However, this activity is unbalanced. More specifically, estrogens and androgens act defensively against oxidative stress on bone; decreasing levels of these hormones, concomitant with a rise in reactive oxygen species associated with aging, lead to increased oxidative stress on bone, resulting in increased bone resorption and risk for osteoporosis [39].

Cardiovascular disease

Estrogen plays an important role in cardioprotection. Several studies have shown that rates of cardiovascular disease rise during the menopausal period; in addition, falling estrogen levels in patients having undergone oophorectomy have been associated with the onset of atherosclerosis [40]. A study by Shi et al. [41] evaluated the effect of oophorectomy with subsequent estrogen replacement on cortical ischema-reperfusion injury in rats. Shi found that those rats having undergone oophorectomy that were then treated with estrogen replacement had a decrease in lesion size during reperfusion as compared with controls, suggesting that estrogen plays a protective role in cortical ischemic damage. Similar studies have been performed in cardiac tissue and have shown that pre-treating mice with estrogen decreased levels of cardiac necrosis and macrophage recruitment while increasing rates of coronary flow [42, 43].

Estrogen may exert its cardioprotective effects in a number of ways. Research has suggested that estradiol may help to stabilize endothelial cells via dampening of locally acting tumor necrosis factor (TNF)-alpha induced apoptosis [44]. In addition, estrogen may inhibit the production of inflammatory cytokines, such as IL-6, which are associated with atherosclerotic disease [45]; a recent study by Pratap et al. suggests that the decline in estrogen associated with menopause promotes a concomitant decline in certain immune and intra-cellular signaling pathways and antioxidant activity. These effects were mitigated with estrogen treatment [46]. Estrogen also enhances endothelial nitric oxide synthesis raising nitric oxide and resulting in heightened vasodilation.

Cognitive decline

Estrogen receptors have been discovered throughout the brain but are known to have specific importance in the prefrontal cortex and hippocampus. Estrogen induces spinogenesis and synaptogenesis and is involved in a number of signal transduction pathways in the brain. Specifically, estrogen increases N-methyl-D-aspartate (NMDA) receptor binding and expression; it also activates hippocampal AKT (a kinase regulating numerous cellular processes in the brain), via the PI13K pathway, leading to spinogenesis and protein translation [47].

During the menopausal transition, declining estrogen levels are associated with increased risk for cognitive decline and dementia. Studies have shown this association exists even in the pre-menopausal state in patients who underwent oophorectomy, further implicating estrogen as a critical factor in neuroprotection and prevention of cognitive decline [48].

4. What is the role for ultrasonography in the menopausal patient?

The vaginal probe has revolutionized gynecology. Previously, early equipment was a tool of the obstetrician. It had barely enough resolution to do very limited things such as measure biparietal diameter, establish fetal presentation and localize the placenta. The vaginal probe gives a degree of image magnification that is as if we are doing ultrasound through a low-power microscope. This has been termed "sonomicroscopy." We are able to see things with transvaginal ultrasound that one could not image with their naked eye if you could hold the structure at arms length and squint at it. This has allowed great utilization in fields like menopause. For purposes of this chapter, we will concentrate on the role of ultrasound in patients with postmenopausal bleeding and incidental ultrasound findings in postmenopausal women and their significance.

Postmenopausal bleeding is "endometrial cancer until proven otherwise." The incidence of malignancy ranges from 1–14%. Obviously, this will depend on such factors such as years since menopause, and the classic risk factors such as obesity, hypertension, diabetes and low parity. All women's healthcare providers, however, realize that any such bleeding in postmenopausal patients will require prompt evaluation. Early observational studies of postmenopausal women with bleeding found that, for an endometrial thickness on transvaginal ultrasound of ≤ 5 mm, the incidence of endometrial cancer approached 0. Subsequently, several large prospective trials were performed to validate this concept, that is that in postmenopausal women with bleeding, a thin distinct endometrial echo could reliably exclude cancer and thus allow such patients to avoid any further endometrial evaluation with its risk, discomfort and expense. These trials combined found that, for an endometrial echo ≤ 4 mm, there were three cases of cancer in 2,752 patients for an incidence of 1 in 917. Based on this, in 2009, The American College of Obstetricians and Gynecologists in their Committee opinion entitled "The role of transvaginal ultrasound in the evaluation of postmenopausal bleeding," stated that, when present, a thin, distinct endometrial echo on transvaginal ultrasound that is 4 mm or less has a risk of malignancy that does not require endometrial biopsy. Furthermore, if one does a biopsy on such patients with a thin, distinct endometrial echo on transvaginal ultrasound, it is common to not successfully obtain tissue or when tissue is present, it is often so scant that it cannot be evaluated histologically. It is essential, however, to realize that not all uteri lend themselves to a meaningful enough ultrasound examination to produce a reliable endometrial echo. Patients who have coexisting fibroids, previous surgery, adenomyosis, marked obesity and even an axial orientation of the uterus can result in the inability to find a reliable endometrial echo. It is in such cases that fluid enhancement by infusing saline (a procedure known as sonohysterography) can easily highlight the endometrial cavity in what has become a simple painless office procedure. Sonohysterography, therefore, should be thought of as a subset of transvaginal ultrasonography to be used when the endometrial echo is either not well visualized or not thin and distinct. This allows differentiation into no anatomic pathology which may not have been appreciated without saline infusion, a globally thick endometrial echo in which a blind endometrial biopsy is appropriate, or focal abnormalities such as polyps or focal thickening, which are best approached with the direct visualization of hysteroscopy.

It is unfortunate that in clinical practice many healthcare providers have assumed without validation that if an endometrial echo ≤ 4 mm is indicative of no cancer that endometrial echoes > 4 mm are problematic. All of the above work was done on patients with postmenopausal bleeding. Often a thick endometrial echo is encountered incidentally when imaging is performed for another reason. The incidence of thick endometrial echo in non-bleeding patients was best characterized by a Danish study where asymptomatic non-bleeding polyps discovered on sonohysterography in post menopausal women was actually 13%! Furthermore, in a multicenter Italian study of 1,152 polyps in asymptomatic postmenopausal women diagnosed by sonohysterography, only one cancer was found in a polyp and three cancers thought to be polyps on sonohysterography but actually represented focal pathology. The incidence of serious complications of operative hysteroscopy in such non-bleeding postmenopausal patients is reported to be as high as 3.6%. Furthermore, a German study showed that even if endometrial cancers are detected in asymptomatic postmenopausal women there is no prognostic advantage over those patients with cancer who had uterine bleeding for less than eight weeks at the time of diagnosis.

Thus, for the negligible risk that an asymptomatic polyp might harbor cancer (less than 1 in 1,000) or that polypoid tissue mistaken for a polyp might be malignant (less than 3 in 1,000) there is no advantage prognostically not to wait until such patients bleed. Finally, such an approach, spares the other 996 out of 1,000 any intervention and its risk, discomfort and expense.

Thus, the take home message is that for postmenopausal bleeding, a thin distinct endometrial echo ≤ 4 mm excludes cancer but there is no validation that a thick echo in a non-bleeding patient requires automatic intervention. Of course, in patients at high risk (hypertension, obesity or diabetes), it may be appropriate for them to be individualized.

Postmenopausal cysts that are asymptomatic and incidental have also gone through a learning curve. Dating back to the early days of ultrasound, such cysts were often felt to be cancer until proven otherwise. Once again, small early observational ultrasound studies found the incidence of cancer in unilocular simple cysts in postmenopausal women to approach 0. Subsequent large prospective studies mainly from ovarian cancer screening trials confirmed the incidence of malignancy in simple postmenopausal cysts to approach 0 as well as placing the overall incidence of such simple cysts in postmenopausal women to be as high as 18%! As a result, a consensus conference held by the Society of Radiologists in Ultrasound in 2009 recommended that such simple cysts up to 7 cm be followed, not removed surgically. The recommendation was that those above 7 cm not necessarily be removed but have "alternative imaging" such as MRI because of concern about ultrasound potentially missing small solid areas or mural nodules. In 2013, ACOG reaffirmed its position that such masses are invariably benign and can be managed expectantly up to a size of 10 cm.

Finally, the incidental finding of endometrial fluid collections discovered in postmenopausal women deserves discussion. In the 1980's, on transabdominal ultrasound, the presence of endometrial fluid was said to be associated with a risk of gynecologic malignancy as high as 75%! With the vaginal probe, fluid is easily seen regardless of its location. Subsequent study has revealed that endometrial fluid is actually a naturally occurring sonohysterogram and allows excellent visualization of the surrounding endometrial tissue. If this is thin and symmetric, the fluid is felt to be a transudate associated with some degree of cervical stenosis. If there is a focal abnormality then there is the possibility that the fluid represents blood that is not clinically apparent, secondary to cervical stenosis. This will require further evaluation.

In summary, transvaginal ultrasound when used appropriately in postmenopausal patients can reduce surgical intervention in many and allow appropriate triage in others who will require further evaluation.

5. What are the current treatment options and indications for treatment?

The two primary indications for treatment endorsed by the American College of Obstetricians and Gynecologists are vasomotor and vaginal symptoms [1]. However, almost all women can safely and effectively take estrogen if started within five to seven years of the LMP for short term (e.g. seven years duration). Treatment options may first be sub-categorized by hormonal vs non-hormonal. Within the hormonal treatment category, most include estrogen alone as well as estrogen combined with progestin; for each of these, several options exist in terms of dosing and mode of transmission (oral, transdermal, etc). In addition, selective estrogen receptor modulators (SERMs) have been investigated in the treatment of menopausal symptoms for their agonist/antagonist qualities. Specifically, the SERM BZA has been shown to have protective, agonist effects on bone while providing antagonistic effects on the breast and uterus [49, 50]. As such, estrogen combined with BZA has been developed and Food and Drug Administration (FDA) approved for the treatment of menopausal symptoms. An additional SERM, ospemifene, has also been studied for its beneficial effects for the treatment of dyspareunia in menopausal patients. Non-hormonal options include selective serotonin reuptake inhibitors (SSRIs), serotonin and norepinephrine reuptake inhibitors (SNRIs), Gabapentin; more recently phytoestrogens have also been studied for the SERM-like activity. However, phytoestrogens are currently not FDA approved for the treatment of menopause. Below is a review of the most recent studies evaluating the effectiveness of different treatment modalities on the symptoms/disease processes associated with menopause.

A double-blind, placebo-controlled, randomized trial by Caan et al. showed that while both low-dose estrogen and venlafaxine improve quality of life in patients with VMS, estrogen performed better [51]. In addition, a study by Lobo et al. [52] evaluated NZA/conjugated estrogens for the treatment of menopausal symptoms and overall safety. Their large multi-center, randomized, double-blind, placebo-controlled trial showed that the combination of bazedoxifine at 20 mg combined with conjugated estrogens at either 0.625 or 0.45 mg significantly reduced the frequency and severity of hot flushes while also improving measures of vaginal atrophy. BZA/conjugated estrogen (CE) also improved lipid parameters, with no effect on incidence of breast pain or adverse events. These results highlight BZA/CE as a promising new treatment alternative for managing menopausal symptoms.

Several studies have also evaluated the effects of hormone therapy on neuronal activity as well as on mood and cognition. Smith et al. measured cholinergic activity in the hippocampus of 50 postmenopausal women who were on early long-term hormone treatment and found that hormone therapy was associated with preservation of cholinergic neuronal activity [53]. Moses et al. showed that administration of estrogen plus progestin significantly increased cortical serotonin receptor ($5\text{-HT}_{2A}R$) binding potential; alterations in this system (e.g. decreased receptor activity) have been associated with depression and Alzheimer's [54]. Additionally, results from the KEEPS-Cognitive and Affective Study [55] suggest that for women having undergone menopause recently (within three years of the LMP), treatment with conjugated equine estrogens was associated with beneficial mood effects and no effect on cognition. This is important, as previous literature suggested that treatment with conjugated equine estrogens was associated with adverse cognitive effects in a small subset of their post-menopausal population [56]. However, the subjects in these studies were distant in age from their LMP; other studies therefore explain this discrepancy by suggesting the importance of initiating hormone therapy shortly after menopause, i.e. during the "critical window [57]."

This critical window also appears to apply to the effects of hormone therapy on cardiovascular disease. A study published in JAMA by Rossouw et al. found that women who began hormone treatment closer to their LMP tended to have decreased risk for cardiovascular disease when compared to women who began hormone therapy further away in timing from the menopause [58]. In addition, Manson et al. [59] evaluated the effect of estrogen treatment on coronary artery calcified plaque; such plaque is a known marker for overall plaque burden and is predictive of future risk for cardiovascular events. Manson found that women on estrogen treatment had significantly lower coronary artery calcified plaque burden than controls. Of note, women enrolled in the study were aged 50–59 years, reinforcing the notion that earlier initiation of hormone therapy leads to more advantageous results.

References

1 The American College of Obstetricians and Gynecologists (2014). ACOG Practice Bulletin No. 141: management of menopausal symptoms. *Obstet. Gynecol.* **123** (**1**): 202–216.

2 Hall, J. (2015). Endocrinology of the menopause. *Endocrinol. Metab. Clin. North Am.* **44** (**3**): 485–496.

3 Filicori, M., Butler, J.P., and Crowley, W.F. (1984). Neuroendocrine regulation of the corpus luteum in the human. Evidence for pulsatile progesterone secretion. *J. Clin. Invest.* **73**: 1638–1647.

4 Welt, C.K., Martin, K.A., Taylor, A.E. et al. (1997). Frequency modulation of follicle-stimulating hormone (FSH) during the luteal-follicular transition: evidence for FSH control of inhibin B in normal women. *J. Clin. Endocrinol. Metab.* **82**: 2645–2652.

5 Gill, S., Lavoie, H.B., Bo-Abbas, Y., and Hall, J. (2002). Negative feedback effects of gonadal steroids are preserved with aging in postmenopausal women. *J. Clin. Endocrinol. Metab.* **87** (**5**): 2297–2302.

6 Gosden, R.G. and Faddy, M.J. (1994). Ovarian aging, follicular depletion, and steroidogenesis. *Exp. Gerontol.* **29** (**3–4**): 265–274.

7 Gougeon, A. (1998). Ovarian follicular growth in humans: ovarian ageing and population of growing follicles. *Maturitas* **30** (**2**): 137–142.

8 Shaw, N.D., Histed, S.N., Srouji, S.S. et al. (2010). Estrogen negative feedback on gonadotropin secretion: evidence for a direct pituitary effect in women. *J. Clin. Endocrinol. Metab.* **95** (**4**): 1955–1961.

9 Rance, N., Krajewsi, S., Smith, M. et al. (2010). Neurokinin B and the hypothalamic regulation of reproduction. *Brain Res.* **1364**: 116–128.

10 Vigier, B., Tran, D., Legeai, L. et al. (1984). Origin of anti-Mullerian hormone in bovine freemartin fetuses. *J. Reprod. Fertil.* **70** (**2**): 473–479.

11 Durlinger, A.L., Gruijters, M.J., Kramer, P. et al. (2001). Anti-Mullerian hormone attenuates the effects of FSH on follicle development in the mouse ovary. *Endocrinology* **142** (**11**): 4891–4899.

12 de Vet, A., Laven, J.S., de Jong, F.H. et al. (2002). Antimullerian hormone serum levels: a putative marker for ovarian aging. *Fertil. Steril.* **77** (**2**): 357–362.

13 Van Disseldorp, J., Broekmans, F.J., Peeters, P.H. et al. (2008). The association between vascular function-related genes and age at natural menopause. *Menopause* **15** (**3**): 511–516.

14 Hall, J.E., Lavoie, H.B., Marsh, E.E., and Martin, K.A. (2000). Decrease in gonadotropin-releasing hormone (GnRH) pulse frequency with aging in postmenopauseal women. *J. Clin. Endocrinol. Metab.* **85** (**5**): 1794–8000.

15 Santoro, N., Banwell, T., Tortoriello, D. et al. (1998). Effects of aging and gonadal failure on the hypothalamic-pituitary axis in women. *Am. J. Obstet. Gynecol.* **178** (**4**): 732–741.

16 Gill, S., Lavoie, H.B., Bo-Abbas, Y., and Hall, J.E. (2002). Negative feedback effets of gonadal steroids are preserved with aging in postmenopausal women. *J. Clin. Endocrinol Metab.* **87** (**5**): 2297–2302.

17 Fujimoto, V.Y., Klein, N.A., Battaglia, D.E. et al. (1996). The anterior pituitary response to a gonadotrophin-releasing hormone challenge test in normal older reproductive-age women. *Fertil. Steril.* **65** (**3**): 539–544.

18 Study of Women's Health Across the Nation (SWAN). SWAN Study. Epidemiology Data Center, n.d. Web. 23 Sept. 2015. University of Pittsburgh: Pittsburgh, PA.

19 (2005). Proceedings from the NIH State-of-the-Science Conference on Management of Menopause-Related Symptoms, March 21–23, 2005, Bethesda, Maryland, USA. *Am. J. Med.* **118** (**Suppl 12B**): 1–171.

20 Santoro, N., Epperson, C.N., and Mathews, S.B. (2015 Sep). Menopausal symptoms and their management. *Endocrinol. Metab. Clin. North Am.* **44** (**3**): 497–515.

21 MicKinlay, S.M., Brambilla, D.J., and Posner, J.G. (1992). The normal menopause transition. *Maturitas* **14** (**2**): 103–115.

22 Nachtigall, L. (1998). The symptoms of perimenopause. *Clin. Obstet. Gynecol.* **41** (**4**): 921–927.

23 Paramsothy, P., Harlow, S.D., Greendale, G.A. et al. (2014 Nov). Bleeding patterns during the menopausal transition in the multi-ethnic study of Women's health across the nation (SWAN): a prospective cohort study. *BJOG* **121** (**12**): 1564–1573.

24 Santoro, N., Brown, J.R., Adel, T., and Skurnick, J.H. (1996). Characterization of reproductive hormonal dynamics in the perimenopause. *J. Clin. Endocrinol. Metab.* **81** (**4**): 1495–1501.

25 Thurston, R.C. and Joffe, H. (2011). Vasomotor symptoms and menopause: findings from the study of Women's Health across the Nation. *Obstet. Gynecol. Clin. North Am.* **38** (**3**): 489–501.

26 Freedman, R.R. (2001). Physiology of hot flashes. *Am. J. Hum. Biol.* **13**: 453–464.

27 Gold, E., Colvin, A., Avis, N. et al. (2006). Longitudinal analysis of the association between vasomotor symptoms and race/ethnicity across the menopausal transition: study of Women's Health across the Nation. *Am. J. Public Health* **97** (**7**): 1226–1235.

28 Avis, N., Crawford, S., Bromberger, J. et al. (2015). Duration of vasomotor symtpoms over the menopause transition. *JAMA Intern. Med.* **175** (**4**): 531–539.

29 Thurston, R.C., Sutton-Tyrrell, K., Everson-Rose, S.A. et al. (2011). Hot flashes and carotid intima media thickness among midlife women. *Menopause* **18** (**4**): 352–358.

30 Crandall, C.J., Tseng, C.H., Crawford, S.L. et al. (2011). Association of menopausal vasomotor symptoms with increased bone turnover during the menopausal transition. *J. Bone Miner. Res.* **26** (**4**): 840–849.

31 Weber, M.A., Kleijn, M.H., Langendam, M. et al. (2015). Local oestrogen for pelvic floor disorders: a systematic review. *PLoS One* **10** (**9**): e0136265.

32 Portman, D.J., Gass, M.L., and Vulvovaginal Atrophy Terminology Consensus Conference Panel (2014). Genitourinary syndrome of menopause: new terminology for vulvovaginal atrophy from the International Society for the Study of Women's Sexual Health and the North American Menopause Society. *Menopause* **21** (**10**): 1063–1068.

33 Ohayon, M.M., Carskadon, M.A., Guilleminault, C., and Vitiello, M.V. (2004). Meta-analysis of quantitative sleep parameters from childhood to old age in healthy individuals: developing normative sleep values across the human lifespan. *Sleep* **27** (**7**): 1255–1273.

34 Kravitz, H.M., Ganza, P.A., Bromberger, J. et al. (2003). Sleep difficulty in women at midlife: a community survey of sleep and the menopausal transition. *Menopause* **10** (**1**): 19–28.

35 Schmidt, P.J., Haq, N., and Rubinow, D.R. (2004). A longitudinal evaluation of the relationship between reproductive status and mood in perimenopausal women. *Am. J. Psychiatry* **161** (**12**): 2238–2244.

36 Amin, Z., Canil, T., and Epperson, C.N. (2005). Effect of estrogen-serotonin interactions on mood and cognition. *Behav. Cogn. Neurosci. Rev.* **4** (**1**): 43–58.

37 Gold, E.B., Sternfeld, B., Kelsey, J.L. et al. (2000). Relation of demographic and lifestyle factors to symptoms in a multi-racial/ethnic population of women 40-55 years of age. *Am. J. Epidemiol.* **152** (**5**): 463–473.

38 Greendale, G.A., Derby, C.A., and Maki, P.M. (2011). Perimenopause and cognition. *Obstet. Gynecol. Clin. North Am.* **38** (**3**): 519–535.

39 Manolagas, S. (2010). From estrogen-centric to aging and oxidative stress: a revised perspective of the pathogenesis of osteoporosis. *Endocr. Rev.* **31** (**3**): 266–300.

40 Colditz, G.A., Willett, W.C., Stampfer, M.J. et al. (1987). Menopause and the risk of coronary heart disease in women. *N. Engl. J. Med.* **316** (**18**): 1105–1110.

41 Shi, J., Bui, J.D., Yang, J.D. et al. (2001). Estrogens decrease reperfusion-associated cortical ischemic damage: an MRI analysis in a transient focal ischemia model. *Stroke* **32** (**4**): 987–992.

42 Squadrito, F., Altavilla, D., Squadrito, G. et al. (1997). 17Beta-oestradiol reduces cardiac leukocyte accumulation in myocardial ischaemia reperfusion injury in rat. *Eur. J. Pharmacol.* **335** (**2–3**): 185–192.

43 Zhai, P., Eurell, T.E., Cotthaus, R. et al. (2000). Effect of estrogen on global myocardial ischemia-reperfusion injury in female rats. *Am. J. Physiol. Heart Circ. Physiol.* **279** (**6**): H2766–H2775.

44 Spyridopoulos, I., Sullivan, A.B., Kearney, M. et al. (1997). Estrogen-receptor-mediated inhibition of human endothelial cell apoptosis. Estadiol as a survival factor. *Circulation* **95** (**6**): 1505–1514.

45 Sukovich, D.A., Kauser, K., Shirley, F.D. et al. (1998). Expression of interleukin-6 in atherosclerotic lesions of male ApoE-knockout mice: inhibition by 17beta-estradiol. *Arterioscler. Thromb. Vasc. Biol.* **18** (**9**): 1498–1505.

46 Pratap, U.P., Sharma, H.R., Mohanty, A. et al. (2015). Estrogen upregulates inflammatory signals through NF-kB, IFN-y, and nitric oxide via Akt/mTOR pathway in the lymph node lymphocytes of middle-aged female rats. *Int. Immunopharmacol.* **29** (**2**): 591–598. pii: S1567-5769(15)30127-2.

47 Hara, Y., Waters, E.M., BS, M.E., and Morrison, J.H. (2015). Estrogen effects on cognitive and synaptic health over the lifecourse. *Physiol. Rev.* **95** (**3**): 785–807.

48 Rocca, W.A., Bower, J.H., Maraganore, D.M. et al. (2007). Increased risk of cognitive impairment or dementia in women who underwent oophorectomy before menopause. *Neurology* **69** (**11**): 1074–1083.

49 Komm, B.S., Kharode, Y.P., Bodine, P.V. et al. (2005). Bazedoxifene acetate: a selective estogen receptor modulator with improved selectivity. *Endocrinology* **146** (**9**): 3999 –4008.

50 Ronkin, S., Northington, R., Baracat, E. et al. (2005). Endometrial effects of bazedoxifene acetate, a novel selective estrogen receptor modulator, I postmenopausal women. *Obstet. Gynecol.* **105** (**6**): 1397–1404.

51 Caan, B., LaCroix, A.Z., Joffe, H. et al. (2015). Effects of estrogen and venlafaxine on menopause-related quality of life in healthy postmenopausal women with hot flashes: a placebo-controlled randomized trial. *Menopause* **22** (**6**): 607–615.

52 Lobo, R.A., Pinkerton, J.V., Gass, M.L. et al. (2009). Evaluation of bazedoxifene/conjugated estrogens for the treatment of menopausal symptoms and effects on metabolic parameters and overall safety profile. *Fertil. Steril.* **92** (**3**): 1025–1038.

53 Smith, Y.R., Bowen, L., Love, T.M. et al. (2011). Early initiation of hormone therapy in menopausal women is associated with increased hippocampal and posterior cingulate cholinergic activity. *J. Clin. Endocrinol. Metab.* **96** (**11**): E1761–E1770.

54 Moses, E.L., Drevets, W.C., Smith, G. et al. (2000). Effects of estradiol and progesterone administration on human serotonin 2A receptor binding: a PET study. *Biol. Psychiatry* **48** (**8**): 854–860.

55 Gleason, C.E., Dowling, N.M., Wharton, W. et al. (2015). Effects of hormone therapy on cognition and mood in recently postmenopausal women: findings from the randomized, controlled KEEPS-cognitive and affective study. *PLoS Med.* **12** (**6**): e1001833; discussion e1001833.

56 Rapp, S.R., Espeland, M.A., Shumaker, S.A. et al. (2003). Effect of estrogen plus progestin on global cognitive function in postmenopausal women: the Women's Health Initiative Memory Study: a randomized controlled trial. *JAMA* **289** (**20**): 2663–2672.

57 Resnick, S.M. and Henderson, V.W. (2002). Hormone therapy and risk of Alzheimer disease: a critical time. *JAMA* **288** (**17**): 2170–2172.

58 Rossouw, J.E., Prentice, R.L., Manson, J.E. et al. (2007). Postmenopausal hormone therapy and risk of cardiovascular disease by age and years since menopause. *JAMA* **297** (**13**): 1465–1477.

59 Manson, J.E., Allison, M.A., Rossow, J.E. et al. (2007). Estrogen therapy and coronary-artery calcification. *N. Engl. J. Med.* **356** (**25**): 2591–2602.

Gynecologic oncology

16 CHAPTER 16

Cervical cancer

Jovana Y. Martin[1], Britt K. Erickson[2], and Warner K. Huh[2]
[1]*Department of Obstetrics and Gynecology, University of Alabama at Birmingham, Birmingham, AL, USA*
[2]*Division of Gynecologic Oncology, University of Alabama at Birmingham, Birmingham, AL, USA*

CLINICAL SCENARIO

A 60-year-old woman presents to her primary care physician with post-menopausal vaginal bleeding. The bleeding is painless, and is heaviest after intercourse. Her past obstetrical and gynecological history is notable for three uncomplicated term vaginal deliveries followed by tubal sterilization. She had normal monthly menses until menopause at age 55. Her most recent cervical cytology screening test was during her last pregnancy 25 years ago and she cannot recall if it was normal or abnormal. Her medical history is otherwise unremarkable and her social history is notable for a 20 pack-year history of smoking.

Pelvic exam is remarkable for a 3 cm friable mass on the anterior lip of her cervix. She has no other palpable pelvic masses. A biopsy is performed and pathology shows invasive squamous cell carcinoma. She is referred to a gynecologic oncologist for 1B1 cervical cancer and ultimately undergoes a radical hysterectomy, bilateral salpingo-oophorectomy, pelvic, and para-aortic lymph node dissection.

Background

Cervical cancer is the second most common cancer among females worldwide, with an incidence of almost 500 000 new cases per year [1]. Cervical cancer typically presents in the fourth to fifth decade of life [1] with a variable clinical presentation ranging from no symptoms to abnormal vaginal bleeding, vaginal discharge, or pelvic pain. On physical exam an exophytic mass, ulcerative mass, or grossly normal appearing cervix can be seen. Cervical cancer is clinically staged and treatment options and outcomes are dependent on the stage at diagnosis.

Infection with the Human Papillomavirus (HPV) is necessary for the development of both pre-invasive disease of the cervix, known as cervical intraepithelial neoplasia (CIN), and cervical cancer [2, 3]. HPV infection can be divided into high-risk and low-risk types. It is the high-risk types that cause high grade CIN and invasive disease.

Squamous cell carcinoma is the most common histological type of cervical cancer, accounting for 80% of cervical cancers [4, 5] followed by adenocarcinoma and adenosquamous carcinoma, which account for 15% of cervical cancers [4]. The remaining 5% of cervical cancers consist of rare histological types [4]. Recent trends have shown a significant decline in both the incidence and mortality of cervical cancer in many developed and some developing countries [6, 7]. These trends are related to large population based screening programs that have been implemented to detect pre-invasive disease of the cervix.

Clinical questions

1. In women (population), are there environmental, genetic, or behavioral risk factors (exposure) that increase their risk of developing cervical cancer (outcome)?

Search Strategy: Cervical Neoplasm; Risk factors; Sexually Transmitted Disease STD; Tobacco use; Immune suppression; Oral contraception; Meta-analysis; Clinical trial; Randomized controlled trial.

Databases: EMBASE, CINAHL, PubMed, Medline, Cochrane Database.

Manual Search of references

While high-risk HPV infection is necessary for the development of cervical cancer [2], there are other environmental and behavioral factors that alter the course of CIN and affect progression to invasive cancer (Table 16.1). These risk factors can largely be grouped into those that increase the rate of HPV acquisition and those that affect HPV persistence. Age of sexual debut, number of sexual partners, and history of infection with other STDs have been shown in the literature to increase HPV acquisition, whereas tobacco use and immunosuppression affect HPV persistence.

Evidence-Based Obstetrics and Gynecology, First Edition. Edited by Errol R. Norwitz, Carolyn M. Zelop, David A. Miller, and David L. Keefe.

A number of epidemiological studies have shown a strong correlation between early age of first sexual intercourse and HPV prevalence [8, 9]. In addition to increasing the risk of HPV infection, early age of sexual intercourse also increases the risk for cervical cancer [5, 10]. This age related susceptibility is secondary to cellular changes within the transformation zone which begin during menarche [11]. Specifically, cells transform from columnar to squamous epithelium, a process known as metaplasia. Metaplastic cells in the transformation zone are especially susceptible to HPV infection, and thus HPV exposure at an early age corresponds to increasing rates of HPV infection [12].

Another component of sexual history that increases the risk of HPV infection is number of sexual partners. There has been a clear association with an increasing number of sexual partners and HPV infection [5, 9, 10, 13–15]. Herrero et al., in a large case-control study, reported a 1.7 times greater risk for cervical cancer with six or more lifetime partners compared to women with one lifetime partner [10]. More recently, a prospective cohort study examined risk factors for newly acquired HPV infections and found that risk of HPV infection increased 10-fold for each new sexual partner per month [14].

Previously it was thought that co-infection with other STDs increased the rate of HPV infection and cervical cancer risk, [10] however most studies were confounded by other elements of the sexual history making a causative relationship difficult to establish [10]. Despite this, there have been data showing an association between Herpes Simplex Virus type 2 (HSV 2) and Chlamydia *trachomatis* (C. *trachomatis*) and HPV infection. Smith et al. performed a pooled analysis and adjusted for sexual behavior confounders and found an association between HSV 2 seropositivity and cervical cancer suggesting a carcinogenic mechanism exists between these two viruses [14, 16].

Epidemiologic and case-control studies have shown that co-infection with chlamydia is associated with an increased risk for cervical cancer [17–20]. Co-infection with chlamydia may affect HPV persistence secondary to a chronic inflammatory state [21] or by micro-abrasions, which allow HPV access to the basal epithelium [22]. A nested case-control study of 182 women with invasive cervical cancer found that serum antibodies to C. *trachomatis* was associated with a twofold increase risk of invasive squamous cell carcinoma [17].

Historically, oral contraceptive use was thought to contribute to cervical cancer risk through various hormonal pathways [23, 24]. A recent meta-analysis supported this view and also suggested that increased duration of use was proportional to increasing cervical cancer risk [25]. In addition, this study noted that cessation of hormonal contraceptive use was associated with a return to baseline risk for cervical cancer [25]. Follow-up studies have failed to show hormonal contraceptive use as an independent risk factor for cervical cancer and have suggested that differences in sexual behavioral patterns likely account for the previously observed differences in cervical cancer risk [26, 27].

Most infected females will clear their HPV infection within two years [14]. However, factors that affect persistence, such as tobacco use and immunodeficiency, alter this clearance rate and thus put women at risk for CIN and cervical cancer. Carcinogens from tobacco use have been found in cervical tissue and are thought to impair immunity and disrupt normal cell division [28, 29]. Several studies have shown that tobacco use increases cervical cancer risk and that this risk is correlated to the number of pack-years smoked [29–32]. Increased risk exists even in former smokers [30]. The data correlating tobacco use and cervical cancer risk has been so convincing that The International Agency for Research on Cancer (IARC), an agency that performs global investigations using evidence based medicine regarding potential human carcinogens, declared tobacco use as a human carcinogen and risk factor for cervical cancer [33].

Because cervical cancer is caused by a viral infection, a competent immune system plays an important role in preventing the progression of HPV infection to CIN and cervical cancer. Conversely, population based trials have

Table 16.1 Cervical cancer risk factors

	Risk factor	Mechanism
Infection with high-risk HPV types	Established high-risk HPV types: 16, 18, 31, 33, 35, 39, 45, 51, 52, 56, 58, 59, 66 Probably high-risk HPV types: 26, 53, 67, 68, 70, 73, 82	Overexpression of oncoproteins E6 and E7 affect tumor suppressors p53 and pRB leading to loss of control of the cell cycle
HPV acquisition	Age at first intercourse	Age related susceptibility of the transformation zone to HPV
	Increasing number of sexual partners	Increased exposure to HPV
	Co-infection with chlamydia, genital herpes simplex virus	Pro-inflammatory state; allows HPV access to basal epithelium
HPV persistence	Tobacco use	Impaired immunity; disruption of normal cell division
	Immunosuppression	Impaired immunity

shown that patients who are immunocompromised, such as women with Human Immunodeficiency Virus (HIV), have high rates of HPV persistence [34, 35]. Higher HIV viral loads and lower CD4 counts are correlated with persistence [36]. Moreover, rates of CIN are higher in HIV positive women, independent of other risk factors [37]. Although data is conflicting regarding the risk of cervical cancer in women with well-controlled HIV, retrospective case-control studies have shown that the degree of immunosuppression correlates with an increased risk of invasive disease [38].

2. In women with HPV infections (population) are there certain HPV types (exposure) which are more likely to cause cervical cancer (outcome) than other HPV types (comparison)?

Search Strategy: *HPV; Cervical cancer; CIN; Meta-analysis; Clinical trial, Randomized controlled trial.*

Databases: EMBASE, CINAHL, PubMed, Medline, Cochrane Database.

Manual Search of references.

Forty types of HPV can affect the anogenital tract [39]. Thirteen HPV types have been established as oncogenic [40] while an additional seven types are probably oncogenic [41] (Table 16.1). With the advent of more sensitive HPV DNA detection methods, it is now recognized that high-risk HPV DNA is detected in almost 100% of cervical cancers [2, 42]. HPV types 16, 18, 45, 31 have consistently been shown to be the most common high-risk oncogenic types in cervical cancer [3]. Specifically, HPV 16 and HPV 18 are detected in 60–70% of cervical cancers [43]. This may be due, in part, to their slower clearance rates compared to other HPV types [44]. Oncoproteins E6 and E7 are overexpressed in cells infected with HPV 16 and 18. These proteins in turn affect tumor suppressor proteins pRB and p53, leading to loss of control of the cell cycle and consequently increase the risk of developing malignancy [11, 39, 45].

The implications of identifying the HPV types with the most oncogenic potential have been widespread. In order to decrease the burden of HPV disease globally, prophylactic vaccines against HPV 16 and 18 have been developed. A meta-analysis of 13 randomized controlled trials found that prophylactic HPV vaccines have been effective in reducing both vaccine-targeted HPV infections and pre-invasive cervical disease [46]. Data regarding the effects of vaccination on morbidity and mortality due to cervical cancer is limited due to the recent introduction of large scale vaccination programs.

3. For women in the general population, what is the sensitivity and specificity of cervical cytology compared to primary HPV testing (diagnostic test) for the detection of CIN and cervical cancer (outcomes)?

Search Strategy: Cervical neoplasm; Screening; HPV; Pap smear; Cytology; Sensitivity; Specificity; Meta-analysis; Clinical trial; Randomized controlled trial.

Databases: EMBASE, CINAHL, PubMed, Medline, Cochrane Database.

Manual Search of references.

In the 1940s, George Papanicolaou and his colleague Herbert Traut reported that malignant cervical cells could be detected with vaginal cytological evaluation [47]. This method of cytological testing became known as the Papanicolaou, or "Pap" smear. In the decades that followed, population based studies described the utility of the Pap smear in screening programs to prevent morbidity and mortality from cervical cancer [48–50]. Public health efforts throughout the world have led to the widespread implementation of cervical cancer screening with the Pap smear.

A Pap smear is performed by gently sampling the transformation zone with a brush and/or a spatula to collect cervical epithelial cells. These cells may either be immediately transfixed to a slide (conventional cytology) or suspended in a preservation solution for delayed fixation (liquid based cytology). The slide is then evaluated by a clinician or cytopathologist. The spectrum of epithelial cell changes in a Pap smear range from a normal appearance to koilocytosis (clearing of cytoplasm around the nucleus typical of HPV infection), cellular dysplasia, and features suggestive of carcinoma. Dysplastic changes are then characterized as low-grade or high-grade, guiding the evaluation for underlying CIN.

While Pap smears have historically been the basis of cervical cancer screening, they are not without limitations. The specificity of a Pap smear is high (i.e. low number of false-positive test results). However, the sensitivity of Pap smears is only moderate (i.e. high number of false-negative test results) leading to missed CIN and cervical cancer diagnoses. More specifically, a systematic review reported the mean sensitivity and specificity of Pap smears to be 47% (range 30–87%) and 95% (range 86–100%), respectively [51]. This moderate sensitivity is further supported by a recent meta-analysis which reported that 30% of women with invasive cervical cancer had at least one normal Pap smear in the six years prior to being diagnosed with cervical cancer [52].

In addition to its moderate sensitivity, the Pap smears have other limitations. Pap smears have considerable interobserver and intraobserver variability [53–55]. A randomized control trial, reported the agreement between clinicians (interobserver variability) for a series of Pap smears to be 60% [54], while another study reported that clinicians agree with their own Pap smear diagnosis (intraobserver variability) only 78% of the time [55].

Given the limitations of Pap smear testing, as well as the improved understanding of the role of HPV in CIN and cervical cancer, screening methods directly testing HPV have been developed. Several HPV DNA tests are now commercially available to detect 13–14 of the most common high-risk (i.e. cancer causing) HPV types, using a variety of molecular techniques [56].

Primary HPV testing for cervical cancer screening appears promising. Several randomized controlled trials and population based studies have shown that HPV testing has a higher sensitivity, but lower specificity when compared to Pap smear testing [57–62]. A systematic review reported the sensitivity of HPV testing to range from 86% to 97.3% and the specificity to range from 83% to 95.2% [63]. Because primary HPV testing has lower specificity, more women undergoing this method of screening will be referred for colposcopy [59, 64]. One systematic review reported that immediate referral to colposcopy with primary HPV screening was 5.8% compared to 2.5% with cytological screening [63].

In addition to improved sensitivity, there are other advantages to primary HPV testing. Unlike in cytological testing, primary HPV testing is highly reproducible since it does not require clinician interpretation. Two randomized controlled trials found that HPV testing allows for earlier detection of pre-invasive cervical disease and cervical cancer compared to cytology [57, 61]. A negative high-risk HPV test result is protective against future cervical cancer risk [58, 61]; with a cumulative rate of CIN2+ development over six years of less than 1% in those with an HPV negative screening test compared to a 1.4% cumulative rate of CIN2+ development in those with negative cervical cytology only [61]. The protective effect of negative primary HPV testing allows for more time between screening intervals.

Globally, clinical trials continue to explore the ideal method for cervical cancer screening and subsequent follow-up management of abnormal test results in an attempt to improve detection rates while minimizing morbidity due to overtreatment.

4. In women with early stage cervical cancer (population) does surgery compared with radiation therapy (intervention) affect recurrence and survival (outcome)?

Search Strategy: Cervical neoplasm; Hysterectomy; Radical hysterectomy; Radiation therapy; Chemoradiation; Chemotherapy; Meta-analysis; Clinical trial; Randomized control trial.

Databases: EMBASE, CINAHL, PubMed, Medline, Database. Manual Search of references.

Cervical cancer starts in the cervix and grows locally, extending to surrounding tissues. It is clinically staged using physical exam findings and imaging. Although it may affect prognosis, surgical pathology does not play a role in cervical cancer staging. Like other malignancies, cervical cancer is either early stage, locally advanced, or widely metastatic (Table 16.2). Early stage disease (stage 1) includes cancer that is confined to the cervix only. Locally advanced disease refers to spread of the tumor to the tissue lateral to the cervix, known as the parametrium (stage 2). In some cases the tumor can spread further to the pelvic side wall or to the vagina (stage 3). Obstruction of the ureters, as determined by various imaging modalities, is specifically considered stage 3B. Metastatic cervical cancer (stage 4) implies spread to distant organs.

Cervical cancer treatment is dependent on the stage at diagnosis. Treatment modalities for cervical cancer consist of surgery or radiotherapy. Since cervical cancer grows locally, surgery is acceptable if surgical margins free of disease are obtainable. Surgical management can include fertility sparing procedures, such as a cold knife conization

Table 16.2 2008 International Federation of Gynecology and Obstetrics (FIGO) staging: carcinoma of the cervix uteri [65]

Stage I	The carcinoma is strictly confined to the cervix
IA	Invasive carcinoma which can be diagnosed only by microscopy, with deepest invasion ≤5 mm and largest extension ≤7 mm
IA1	Measured stromal invasion of ≤3.0 mm in depth and extension of ≤7.0 mm
IA2	Measured stromal invasions of >3.0 mm and not >5.0 mm with an extension of not >7.0 mm
IB	Clinically visible lesions limited to the cervix uteri or pre-clinical cancers greater than Stage IA
IB1	Clinically visible lesion ≤4.0 cm in greatest dimension
IB2	Clinically visible lesion >4.0 cm in greatest dimension
Stage II	Cervical carcinoma invades beyond the uterus, but not to the pelvic wall or to the lower third of the vagina
IIA	Without parametrial involvement
IIA1	Clinically visible lesion ≤4.0 cm in greatest dimension
IIA2	Clinically visible lesion >4.0 cm in greatest dimension
IIB	With obvious parametrial involvement
Stage III	The tumor extends to the pelvic wall and/or involves the lower third of the vagina and/or causes hydronephrosis or non-functioning kidney
IIIA	Tumor involves the lower third of the vagina, with no extension to pelvic wall
IIIB	Extension to pelvic wall and/or hydronephrosis or non-functioning kidney
Stage IV	The carcinoma has extended beyond the true pelvis or has involved (biopsy proven) the mucosa of the bladder or rectum.
IVA	Spread of the growth to adjacent organs
IVB	Spread to distant organs

(CKC) of the cervix for microinvasive disease or radical trachelectomy (where the uterine cervix and upper portion of the vagina are removed) with pelvic lymphadenectomy for early disease [66]. If fertility preservation is not desired than an extrafascial (simple) hysterectomy is performed for microinvasive disease [67]. If the cancer stage is greater than microinvasive (1A1), more extensive surgery is required. Compared to a simple hysterectomy, a radical hysterectomy requires excision of the uterosacral ligaments and ligation of the uterine artery at its origin so that the cardinal ligaments can be removed. These maneuvers allow for complete dissection of the parametrium [68]. A radical hysterectomy with pelvic lymphadenectomy is a treatment option if the tumor is confined to the cervix [66, 69, 70]. Although lymph node status does not affect staging, pelvic lymphadenectomy is performed at the time of radical hysterectomy to determine the need for further therapy [66].

Cervical cancer is a radiosensitive disease [71]. Randomized controlled trials have shown that the concurrent use of chemotherapy and radiation, known as chemoradiation, increases the sensitivity of cervical cancer to radiation effects [72, 73]. Consequently, chemoradiation reduces cervical cancer recurrence rates and improves overall survival compared to radiation alone [72–74]. Radiation therapy for cervical cancer consists of external beam radiation to the whole pelvis followed by brachytherapy. Brachytherapy is a method of radiation therapy where the source of radiation is placed in the upper vagina, which allows for the delivery of high doses of radiation to the cervix [75].

Chemoradiation can be used in all stages of cervical cancer. For early disease, equal cure rates are seen with radical hysterectomy and pelvic lymphadenectomy and primary chemoradiation therapy [76–79]. A randomized controlled trial randomized 343 patients with early stage cervical cancer to receive either surgery or chemoradiation and found that the overall five-year survival was not statistically different, 84% in the surgery group compared to 88% in the chemoradiation group and recurrence rates were the same for both groups [76]. Overall morbidity was 28% in the surgery group compared to 12% in the chemoradiation group [76]. However, chemoradiation therapy can be associated with a lifetime of post-radiation complications secondary to chronic radiation damage to irradiated bowel, bladder, and vagina [76]. For early stage cervical cancer, treatment methods can be selected on a per patient basis with chemoradiation therapy typically being reserved for patients unfit for surgery [66].

While early stage disease can be treated with chemoradiation or surgery, the standard treatment for advanced cervical cancer that involves the parametrium, lower third of the vagina, the pelvic sidewall, or is locally metastatic is chemoradiation. On the other hand, widely metastatic cervical cancer is considered incurable. Palliative measures may be taken in widely metastatic disease to alleviate symptoms either with systemic chemotherapy or chemoradiation therapy [80].

Summary

Persistent infection with high-risk HPV can lead to the development of cervical cancer. The most common oncogenic HPV types are HPV 16, 18, 45, and 31. There are risk factors that affect HPV acquisition such as early age at first sexual intercourse, increasing number of partners, and co-infection with chlamydia. Other risk factors affect HPV persistence such as tobacco use and immunodeficiency. Since the implementation of cervical cancer screening programs there has been a decrease in cervical cancer incidence. Traditional screening was performed exclusively with Pap smears; however, with improved understanding of the role of HPV in CIN and cervical cancer, HPV DNA testing methods have become available and are currently being integrated into cervical screening methods. Cervical cancer treatment options are determined by clinical stage at diagnosis. Early stage cervical cancer can be treated with hysterectomy or chemoradiation with no difference in survival while advanced stage cervical cancer is primarily treated with chemoradiation.

Acknowledgements

The following research grant is acknowledged: National Institutes of Health NRSA grant #T32CA091078.

References

1 Kamangar, F., Dores, G.M., and Anderson, W.F. (2006). Patterns of cancer incidence, mortality, and prevalence across five continents: defining priorities to reduce cancer disparities in different geographic regions of the world. *Journal of Clinical Oncology* **24** (**14**): 2137–2150.

2 Walboomers, J.M.M., Jacobs, M.V., Manos, M.M. et al. (1999). Human papillomavirus is a necessary cause of invasive cervical cancer worldwide. *The Journal of Pathology* **189** (**1**): 12–19.

3 Bosch, F.X., Manos, M.M., Muñoz, N. et al. (1995). Prevalence of human papillomavirus in cervical cancer: a worldwide perspective. *Journal of the National Cancer Institute* **87** (**11**): 796–802.

4 ACOG (2002). ACOG practice bulletin no. 35: diagnosis and treatment of cervical carcinomas. *Obstetrics and Gynecology* **99** (**5, Part 1**): 855–867.

5 International Collaboration of Epidemiological Studies of Cervical Cancer (2007). Comparison of risk factors for invasive squamous cell carcinoma and adenocarcinoma of the cervix: collaborative reanalysis of individual data on 8,097 women with squamous cell carcinoma and 1,374 women with adenocarcinoma from 12 epidemiological studies. *International Journal of Cancer* **120** (**4**): 885–891.

6 Nieminen, P., Kallio, M., and Hakama, M. (1995). The effect of mass screening on incidence and mortality of squamous and

adenocarcinoma of cervix uteri. *Obstetrics and Gynecology* **85** (**6**): 1017–1021.

7 Cantor, S.B., Atkinson, E.N., Cardenas-Turanzas, M. et al. (2005). Natural history of cervical intraepithelial neoplasia: a meta-analysis. *Acta Cytologica* **49** (**4**): 405–415.

8 Franco, E.L., Villa, L.L., Ruiz, A., and Costa, M.C. (1995). Transmission of cervical human papillomavirus infection by sexual activity: differences between low and high oncogenic risk types. *Journal of Infectious Diseases* **172** (**3**): 756–763.

9 Hariri, S., Unger, E.R., Sternberg, M. et al. (2011). Prevalence of genital human papillomavirus among females in the United States, the National Health and Nutrition Examination Survey, 2003–2006. *Journal of Infectious Diseases* **204** (**4**): 566–573.

10 Herrero, R., Brinton, L.A., Reeves, W.C. et al. (1990). Sexual behavior, venereal diseases, hygiene practices, and invasive cervical cancer in a high-risk population. *Cancer* **65** (**2**): 380–386.

11 Schiffman, M., Castle, P.E., Jeronimo, J. et al. (2007). Human papillomavirus and cervical cancer. *The Lancet* **370** (**9590**): 890–907.

12 Moscicki, A.-B., Schiffman, M., Kjaer, S., and Villa, L.L. (2006). Chapter 5: updating the natural history of HPV and anogenital cancer. *Vaccine* **24** (**Supplement 3**): S42–S51.

13 Berrington de Gonzalez, A., Sweetland, S., and Green, J. (2004). Comparison of risk factors for squamous cell and adenocarcinomas of the cervix: a meta-analysis. *British Journal of Cancer* **90** (**9**): 1787–1791.

14 Moscicki, A., Hills, N., Shiboski, S. et al. (2001). Risks for incident human papillomavirus infection and low-grade squamous intraepithelial lesion development in young females. *JAMA* **285** (**23**): 2995–3002.

15 Winer, R.L., Lee, S.-K., Hughes, J.P. et al. (2003). Genital human papillomavirus infection: incidence and risk factors in a cohort of female university students. *American Journal of Epidemiology* **157** (**3**): 218–226.

16 Smith, J.S., Herrero, R., Bosetti, C. et al. (2002). Herpes simplex virus-2 as a human papillomavirus cofactor in the etiology of invasive cervical cancer. *Journal of the National Cancer Institute* **94** (**21**): 1604–1613.

17 Koskela, P., Anttila, T., Bjørge, T. et al. (2000). Chlamydia trachomatis infection as a risk factor for invasive cervical cancer. *International Journal of Cancer* **85** (**1**): 35–39.

18 Lehtinen, M., Ault, K.A., Lyytikainen, E. et al. (2011). Chlamydia trachomatis infection and risk of cervical intraepithelial neoplasia. *Sexually Transmitted Infections* **87** (**5**): 372–376.

19 Smith, J.S., Bosetti, C., Muñoz, N. et al. (2004). Chlamydia trachomatis and invasive cervical cancer: a pooled analysis of the IARC multicentric case-control study. *International Journal of Cancer* **111** (**3**): 431–439.

20 Wallin, K.-L., Wiklund, F., Luostarinen, T. et al. (2002). A population-based prospective study of *Chlamydia trachomatis* infection and cervical carcinoma. *International Journal of Cancer* **101** (**4**): 371–374.

21 Samoff, E., Koumans, E.H., Markowitz, L.E. et al. (2005). Association of Chlamydia trachomatis with persistence of high-risk types of human papillomavirus in a cohort of female adolescents. *American Journal of Epidemiology* **162** (**7**): 668–675.

22 Silins, I., Ryd, W., Strand, A. et al. (2005). Chlamydia trachomatis infection and persistence of human papillomavirus. *International Journal of Cancer* **116** (**1**): 110–115.

23 Castle, P.E., Walker, J.L., Schiffman, M., and Wheeler, C.M. (2005). Hormonal contraceptive use, pregnancy and parity, and the risk of cervical intraepithelial neoplasia 3 among oncogenic HPV DNA-positive women with equivocal or mildly abnormal cytology. *International Journal of Cancer* **117** (**6**): 1007–1012.

24 Muñoz, N., Franceschi, S., Bosetti, C. et al. (2002). Role of parity and human papillomavirus in cervical cancer: the IARC multicentric case-control study. *The Lancet* **359** (**9312**): 1093–1101.

25 International Collaboration of Epidemiological Studies of Cervical Cancer (2007). Cervical cancer and hormonal contraceptives: collaborative reanalysis of individual data for 16,573 women with cervical cancer and 35,509 women without cervical cancer from 24 epidemiological studies. *The Lancet* **370** (**9599**): 1609–1621.

26 Longatto-Filho, A., Hammes, L.S., Sarian, L.O. et al. (2011). Hormonal contraceptives and the length of their use are not independent risk factors for high-risk HPV infections or high-grade CIN. *Gynecologic and Obstetric Investigation* **71** (**2**): 93–103.

27 Syrjänen, K., Shabalova, I., Petrovichev, N. et al. (2006). Oral contraceptives are not an independent risk factor for cervical intraepithelial neoplasia or high-risk human papillomavirus infections. *Anticancer Research* **26** (**6C**): 4729–4740.

28 Waggoner, S.E., Darcy, K.M., Fuhrman, B. et al. (2006). Association between cigarette smoking and prognosis in locally advanced cervical carcinoma treated with chemoradiation: A Gynecologic Oncology Group study. *Gynecologic Oncology* **103** (**3**): 853–858.

29 Haverkos Harry, W., Soon, G., Steckley Stacey, L., and Pickworth, W. (2003). Cigarette smoking and cervical cancer: Part I: a meta-analysis. *Biomedicine & Pharmacotherapy* **57** (**2**): 67–77.

30 International Collaboration of Epidemiological Studies of Cervical Cancer (2006). Carcinoma of the cervix and tobacco smoking: collaborative reanalysis of individual data on 13,541 women with carcinoma of the cervix and 23,017 women without carcinoma of the cervix from 23 epidemiological studies. *International Journal of Cancer* **118** (**6**): 1481–1495.

31 Louie, K.S., Castellsague, X., de Sanjose, S. et al. (2011). Smoking and passive smoking in cervical cancer risk: pooled analysis of couples from the IARC multicentric case–control studies. *Cancer Epidemiology Biomarkers & Prevention* **20** (**7**): 1379–1390.

32 McIntyre-Seltman, K., Castle, P.E., Guido, R. et al. (2005). Smoking is a risk factor for cervical intraepithelial neoplasia grade 3 among oncogenic human papillomavirus DNA–positive women with equivocal or mildly abnormal cytology. *Cancer Epidemiology Biomarkers & Prevention* **14** (**5**): 1165–1170.

33 World Health Organization, International Agency for Research on Cancer (IARC) (2004). Tobacco smoke and involuntary smoking. *IARC Monographs on the Evaluation of Carcinogenic Risks to Humans* **83**: 1–1438.

34 Denny, L., Boa, R., Williamson, A.L. et al. (2008). Human papillomavirus infection and cervical disease in human immunodeficiency virus-1 infected women. *Obstetrics and Gynecology* **111** (**6**): 1380–1387.

35 Moodley, J., Hoffman, M., Carrara, H. et al. (2006). HIV and pre-neoplastic and neoplastic lesions of the cervix in South Africa: a case-control study. *BMC Cancer* **6** (**1**): 135.

36 Strickler, H.D., Burk, R.D., Fazzari, M. et al. (2005). Natural history and possible reactivation of human papillomavirus in human immunodeficiency virus-positive women. *Journal of the National Cancer Institute* **97** (**8**): 577–586.

37 Wright, T.C. Jr., Ellerbrock, T.V., Chiasson, M.A. et al. (1994). Cervical intraepithelial neoplasia in women infected with human immunodeficiency virus: prevalence, risk factors, and validity of Papanicolaou smears. New York Cervical Disease Study. *Obstetrics and Gynecology* **84** (**4**): 591–597.

38 Leitao, M.M., White, P., and Cracchiolo, B. (2008). Cervical cancer in patients infected with the human immunodeficiency virus. *Cancer* **112** (**12**): 2683–2689.

39 Muñoz, N., Castellsagué, X., de González, A.B., and Gissmann, L. (2006). Chapter 1: HPV in the etiology of human cancer. *Vaccine* **24** (**Supplement 3**): S1–S10.

40 IARC (2007). Human papillomaviruses. IARC monographs on the evaluation of carcinogenic risks to humans/World Health Organization. *International Agency for Research on Cancer* **90**: 1–636. Epub 2008/03/22.

41 Bouvard, V., Baan, R., Straif, K. et al. (2009). A review of human carcinogens Part B: biological agents. *Lancet Oncology* **10** (**4**): 321–322.

42 Bosch, F.X. and de Sanjosé, S. (2007). The epidemiology of human papillomavirus infection and cervical cancer. *Disease Markers* **23** (**4**): 213–227.

43 Wheeler, C.M., Hunt, W.C., Joste, N.E. et al. (2009). Human papillomavirus genotype distributions: implications for vaccination and cancer screening in the United States. *Journal of the National Cancer Institute* **101** (**7**): 475–487.

44 Ramanakumar, A.V., Goncalves, O., Richardson, H. et al. (2010). Human papillomavirus (HPV) types 16, 18, 31, 45 DNA loads and HPV-16 integration in persistent and transient infections in young women. *BMC Infectious Diseases* **10**: 326.

45 Guan, P., Howell-Jones, R., Li, N. et al. (2012). Human papillomavirus types in 115,789 HPV-positive women: a meta-analysis from cervical infection to cancer. *International Journal of Cancer* **131** (**10**): 2349–2359.

46 Lu, B., Kumar, A., Castellsague, X., and Giuliano, A. (2011). Efficacy and safety of prophylactic vaccines against cervical HPV infection and diseases among women: a systematic review & Meta-analysis. *BMC Infectious Diseases* **11** (**1**): 13.

47 Papanicolaou, G.N. and Traut, H.F. (1997). The diagnostic value of vaginal smears in carcinoma of the uterus. 1941. *Archives of Pathology & Laboratory Medicine* **121** (**3**): 211–224.

48 Erickson, C.C., Everett, B.E., Graves, L.M. et al. (1956). Population screening for uterine cancer by vaginal cytology: preliminary summary of results of first examination of 108,000 women and second testing of 33,000 women. *JAMA* **162** (**3**): 167–173.

49 Lundin, F.E., Christopherson, W.M., Mendez, W.M., and Parker, J.E. (1965). Morbidity from cervical cancer: effects of cervical cytology and socioeconomic status. *Journal of the National Cancer Institute* **35** (**6**): 1015–1025.

50 Christopherson, W.M., Lundin, F.E., Mendez, W.M., and Parker, J.E. (1976). Cervical cancer control. A study of morbidity and mortality trends over a twenty-one-year period. *Cancer* **38** (**3**): 1357–1366.

51 Nanda, K., McCrory, D.C., Myers, E.R. et al. (2000). Accuracy of the papanicolaou test in screening for and follow-up of cervical cytologic abnormalities: a systematic review. *Annals of Internal Medicine* **132** (**10**): 810–819.

52 Spence, A.R., Goggin, P., and Franco, E.L. (2007). Process of care failures in invasive cervical cancer: systematic review and meta-analysis. *Preventive Medicine* **45** (**2–3**): 93–106.

53 Renshaw, A.A. (2002). Measuring sensitivity in gynecologic cytology: a review. *Cancer Cytopathology* **96** (**4**): 210–217.

54 Schiffman, M. and Solomon, D. (2003). Findings to date from the ASCUS-LSIL triage study (ALTS). *Archives of Pathology & Laboratory Medicine* **127** (**8**): 946–949.

55 Klinkhamer, P.J., Vooijs, G.P., and de Haan, A.F. (1988). Intraobserver and interobserver variability in the diagnosis of epithelial abnormalities in cervical smears. *Acta Cytologica* **32** (**6**): 794–800.

56 Arney, A. and Bennett, K.M. (2010). Molecular diagnostics of human papillomavirus. *Lab Medicine* **41** (**9**): 523–530.

57 Bulkmans, N.W.J., Berkhof, J., Rozendaal, L. et al. (2007). Human papillomavirus DNA testing for the detection of cervical intraepithelial neoplasia grade 3 and cancer: 5-year follow-up of a randomised controlled implementation trial. *The Lancet* **370** (**9601**): 1764–1772.

58 Kitchener, H.C., Gilham, C., Sargent, A. et al. (2011). A comparison of HPV DNA testing and liquid based cytology over three rounds of primary cervical screening: extended follow up in the ARTISTIC trial. *European Journal of Cancer* **47** (**6**): 864–871.

59 Mayrand, M.H., Duarte-Franco, E., Coutlée, F. et al. (2006). Randomized controlled trial of human papillomavirus testing versus pap cytology in the primary screening for cervical cancer precursors: design, methods and preliminary accrual results of the Canadian cervical cancer screening trial (CCCaST). *International Journal of Cancer* **119** (**3**): 615–623.

60 Rijkaart, D.C., Berkhof, J., Rozendaal, L. et al. (2012). Human papillomavirus testing for the detection of high-grade cervical intraepithelial neoplasia and cancer: final results of the POBASCAM randomised controlled trial. *The Lancet Oncology* **13** (**1**): 78–88.

61 Ronco, G., Giorgi-Rossi, P., Carozzi, F. et al. (2010). Efficacy of human papillomavirus testing for the detection of invasive cervical cancers and cervical intraepithelial neoplasia: a randomised controlled trial. *The Lancet Oncology* **11** (**3**): 249–257.

62 Castle, P.E., Stoler, M.H., Wright, T.C. Jr. et al. (2011). Performance of carcinogenic human papillomavirus (HPV) testing and HPV16 or HPV18 genotyping for cervical cancer screening of women aged 25 years and older: a subanalysis of the ATHENA study. *The Lancet Oncology* **12** (**9**): 880–890.

63 Whitlock, E.P., Vesco, K.K., Eder, M. et al. (2011). Liquid-based cytology and human papillomavirus testing to screen for cervical cancer: a systematic review for the U.S. preventive services task force. *Annals of Internal Medicine* **155** (**10**): 687–697.

64 Dillner, J., Rebolj, M., Birembaut, P. et al. (2008). Long term predictive values of cytology and human papillomavirus testing in cervical cancer screening: joint European cohort study. *BMJ* **337**: a1754.

65 Pecorelli, S. (2009). Revised FIGO staging for carcinoma of the vulva, cervix, and endometrium. *International Journal of Gynecology & Obstetrics* **105** (**2**): 103–104.

66 Greer, B.E., Koh, W.-J., Abu-Rustum, N.R. et al. (2010). Cervical cancer. *Journal of the National Comprehensive Cancer Network* **8** (**12**): 1388–1416.

67 Takeshima, N., Yanoh, K., Tabata, T. et al. (1999). Assessment of the revised International Federation of Gynecology and Obstetrics Staging for early invasive squamous cervical cancer. *Gynecologic Oncology* **74** (**2**): 165–169.

68 Querleu, D. and Morrow, C.P. (2008). Classification of radical hysterectomy. *The Lancet Oncology* **9** (**3**): 297–303.

69 Buckley, S.L., Tritz, D.M., Van Le, L. et al. (1996). Lymph node metastases and prognosis in patients with stage IA2Cervical cancer. *Gynecologic Oncology* **63** (**1**): 4–9.

70 Kodama, J., Mizutani, Y., Hongo, A. et al. (2002). Optimal surgery and diagnostic approach of stage IA2 squamous cell carcinoma of the cervix. *European Journal of Obstetrics & Gynecology and Reproductive Biology* **101** (**2**): 192–195.

71 Eifel, P.J. (1993). Radiotherapy versus radical surgery for gynecologic neoplasms: carcinomas of the cervix and vulva. *Frontiers of Radiation Therapy and Oncology* **27**: 130–142.

72 Eifel, P.J., Winter, K., Morris, M. et al. (2004). Pelvic irradiation with concurrent chemotherapy versus pelvic and para-aortic irradiation for high-risk cervical cancer: an update of radiation therapy oncology group trial (RTOG) 90-01. *Journal of Clinical Oncology* **22** (**5**): 872–880.

73 Morris, M., Eifel, P.J., Lu, J. et al. (1999). Pelvic radiation with concurrent chemotherapy compared with pelvic and para-aortic radiation for high-risk cervical cancer. *New England Journal of Medicine* **340** (**15**): 1137–1143.

74 Rose, P.G., Bundy, B.N., Watkins, E.B. et al. (1999). Concurrent cisplatin-based radiotherapy and chemotherapy for locally advanced cervical cancer. *New England Journal of Medicine* **340** (**15**): 1144–1153.

75 Eifel, P.J., Moughan, J., Owen, J. et al. (1999). Patterns of radiotherapy practice for patients with squamous carcinoma of the uterine cervix: patterns of care study. *International Journal of Radiation Oncology, Biology, Physics* **43** (**2**): 351–358.

76 Landoni, F., Maneo, A., Colombo, A. et al. (1997). Randomised study of radical surgery versus radiotherapy for stage Ib-IIa cervical cancer. *The Lancet* **350** (**9077**): 535–540.

77 Newton, M. (1975). Radical hysterectomy or radiotherapy for stage I cervical cancer. A prospective comparison with 5 and 10 years follow-up. *American Journal of Obstetrics and Gynecology* **123** (**5**): 535–542.

78 Piver, M.S., Marchetti, D.L., Patton, T. et al. (1988). Radical hysterectomy and pelvic lymphadenectomy versus radiation therapy for small (less than or equal to 3 cm) stage IB cervical carcinoma. *American Journal of Clinical Oncology* **11** (**1**): 21–24.

79 Morley, G.W. and Seski, J.C. (1976). Radical pelvic surgery versus radiation therapy for stage I carcinoma of the cervix (exclusive of microinvasion). *American Journal of Obstetrics and Gynecology* **126** (**7**): 785–798.

80 Long, H.J. (2007). Management of metastatic cervical cancer: review of the literature. *Journal of Clinical Oncology* **25** (**20**): 2966–2974.

17

CHAPTER 17
Vulval/vaginal cancer

Jessica Lee and John P. Curtin
Division of Gynecologic Oncology, Department of Obstetrics and Gynecology, NYU Langone Medical Center, New York, NY, USA

CLINICAL SCENARIO

A 61-year-old female presented to the clinic for an initial visit after not having seen a gynecologist for five years. She stated that at her prior visit, she complained of vulvar pruritis and was prescribed a cream that she used for six months. The pruritis transiently improved but then worsened. She also had intermittent vaginal spotting. She had never been tested for human immunodeficiency virus (HIV). She believed that her prior pap smear was normal, but has a history of abnormal pap smears. She has hypertension and is a current smoker with a 30 pack-year history. She has 20 prior sexual partners but is not currently sexually active.

On examination, she appeared in no distress. Her abdomen was soft and nontender. Examination of her lymphatic system was significant for firm, fixed left inguinal lymph nodes with nonpalpable right inguinal lymph nodes. Pelvic examination revealed a 4 cm ulcerated, raised lesion on the left labium minus extending into the lower third of the left vaginal wall and a separate 5 cm raised lesion on the posterior fourchette extending to the external anal sphincter.

A punch biopsy was taken of the left vulvar lesion and a fine needle aspiration of the inguinal lymph node was performed. Both specimens returned as moderately differentiated squamous cell carcinoma.

Background

Vulvar cancer is the fourth most common gynecologic cancer accounting for 5% of female genital tract malignancies. According to the American Cancer Society, 5950 new cases of vulvar cancer with 1110 deaths from vulvar cancer are estimated for 2016 [1]. Although there are various histologic subtypes of vulvar cancer, the majority of cases are squamous cell carcinomas. The signs and symptoms of vulvar cancer are similar despite different histologic subtypes. Patients may present with pruritis but often are asymptomatic. On visual inspection of the vulva, a lesion, ulcer, or mass will be present most commonly on the labia majora and may also involve the labia minora, perineum, clitoris, and mons. A punch biopsy of a suspicious vulvar lesion in the outpatient setting can efficiently diagnose a vulvar malignancy.

Primary vaginal cancer comprises approximately 3% of gynecologic malignancies. The American Cancer Society estimates 4620 new cases with 950 deaths from vaginal cancer for 2016 [1]. While primary vaginal cancers are rare, metastatic disease to the vagina via lymphatic or hematogeneous spread or local extension from adjacent gynecologic structures is not uncommon. Most patients present with vaginal bleeding or discharge but many are asymptomatic. Tumors occur in the upper third of the vagina in 50% of cases with the posterior wall of the upper third of the vagina being the most common site of primary vaginal cancer [2]. A thorough speculum exam is typically required to fully visualize the lesion. As with vulvar cancer, a biopsy of any suspicious vaginal lesion either in the outpatient setting or in the operating room can diagnose the malignancy.

General search strategy

You begin to address the topics of vulvar and vaginal carcinoma by searching for evidence in the common electronic databases such as MEDLINE and EMBASE, looking specifically for large population studies for prognostic factors and prospective studies for treatments. In addition, you search the Cochrane Library looking for systematic reviews of treatment strategies in vulvar and vaginal carcinoma. When a systematic review is identified, you also search for recent updates on the Cochrane Library and on MEDLINE and EMBASE to identify more trials that have become available after the publication date of the systematic review.

Evidence-Based Obstetrics and Gynecology, First Edition. Edited by Errol R. Norwitz, Carolyn M. Zelop, David A. Miller, and David L. Keefe.

Critical appraisal of the literature

Clinical questions

1. How does immunosuppression (prognostic factor) contribute to the development of preinvasive or invasive cancer (outcome) in women (population)?

Search Strategy

- MEDLINE and EMBASE: (immunosupp*): *explode* vulvar cancer OR vaginal cancer AND (immunosupp* OR immunosupp*.mp) AND population studies AND cohort studies AND meta-analysis.
- Hand-searching (immunosuppression): references listed in the articles obtained.

Vulvar and vaginal cancers and their preinvasive precursors are considered to be highly associated with the human papillomavirus (HPV). An estimated 40–50% of vulvar cancers and 64–91% of vaginal cancers have been linked to HPV [3]. Although at least 70% of women are infected with HPV in their lifetime, most infections are asymptomatic and spontaneously clear within 12–18 months. Less than 10% of women have a persistent infection, which in turn may develop into invasive cancer [4].

Since the majority of vulvar and vaginal cancers are HPV-related, an immunocompromised state can render one's immune system unable to clear the infection, thereby increasing the risk of developing these cancers. The majority of the data on immunosuppression and vulvovaginal cancers are on patients with HIV infections and acquired immune deficiency syndrome (AIDS), with an increasing number of studies on patients after organ transplantations and patients on renal dialysis. Due to the rarity of vulvar and vaginal cancers, epidemiologic studies require a large cohort of patients to adequately assess for potential risk factors. Thanks to large HIV/AIDS and transplant registries and databases, these types of population studies can be conducted [5–12].

Table 17.1 lists the results of several multicenter cohort studies and the reported standardized incidence ratios (SIRs) of preinvasive and invasive vulvovaginal cancers, comparing their incidence rates in immunosuppressed patients and the general population. The SIRs vary considerably among the studies, and this variance is likely due to the overall low incidence of vulvar and vaginal cancers. However, the SIRs are consistently high throughout the studies: the lowest SIR is still over two for vaginal cancer in Engels et al. [10], and the highest SIR is over 26 for vulvar cancer in Adami et al. [6]. These studies strongly suggest a potential role of an impaired immune system in increasing the rate of development of invasive vulvar and vaginal cancers.

In addition, multiple studies have demonstrated associations between low CD4 counts and increased risks of both invasive and preinvasive vulvar and vaginal cancers [9, 13–15]. Chaturvedi et al. in their study of cancer registry data found an elevated relative risk of 4.91 (95% confidence interval 1.02–23.60) with each 100 cells mm^{-3} decline in CD4 count, suggesting that there may be a relationship between the severity of immunosuppression and cancer risk. The authors also compared patients who were 4–27 months after AIDS onset and 28–60 months after onset and discovered that vulvar and vaginal cancer incidences were significantly elevated in the 28–60 month group but not in the 4–27 month group [9]. This may be due to both the role of long-term immunosuppression in increasing cancer risk as well as the natural slow progression of HPV infection to invasive disease.

Smoking, which has been considered to enhance immunosuppression, is also a known risk factor for vulvovaginal cancers. Daling et al. in a tumor-based registry study found

Table 17.1 Results of multicenter cohort studies and standardized incidence ratios (SIRs) of preinvasive and invasive vulvovaginal cancers

Reference	Year	*n* (Patients)	Risk factor	Invasive vulvar cancer SIR	Preinvasive vulvar cancer SIR	Invasive vaginal cancer SIR	Preinvasive vaginal cancer SIR
Frisch et al. [5]	2000	309 365	HIV/AIDS	5.8[a]	3.9[b]	5.8[a]	3.9[b]
Adami et al. [6]	2006	5931	Solid organ transplant	26.2	NR	16.4	NR
Vajdic et al. [7]	2006	28 855	Solid organ transplant	22.2	NR	NR	NR
Grulich et al. [8]	2007	444 172	HIV/AIDS	6.45[a]	NR	6.45[a]	NR
Grulich et al. [8]	2007	31 977	Solid organ transplant	22.76[a]	NR	22.76[a]	NR
Chaturvedi et al. [9]	2009	499 230	AIDS	5.8[a]	27.2[b]	5.8[a]	27.2[b]
Engels et al. [10]	2011	175 732	Solid organ transplant	7.6	NR	2.35	NR
Skov Dalgaard et al. [11]	2013	241 817	ESRD	5.81[a]	NR	5.81[a]	NR
Madeleine et al. [12]	2013	187 649	Solid organ transplant	7.3	20.3	NR	10.6

SIR, Standardized incidence ratios; HIV, human immunodeficiency virus; AIDS, acquired immune deficiency syndrome; ESRD, end stage renal disease; NR, not reported.

[a]Reported as invasive vulvar cancer or vaginal cancer.

[b]reported as preinvasive vulvar cancer or vaginal cancer.

that 59.5% of vulvar cancer patients and 42.0% of vaginal cancer patients were current smokers compared with 26.8% of control patients [16]. Mabuchi et al. saw an increasing risk associated with an increasing number of cigarettes smoked a day [17]. Madsen et al. categorized vulvar cancer cases by high-risk HPV involvement and discovered that tobacco smoking had only a significant risk on the incidence of high-risk HPV-associated vulvar cancer and not on HPV-negative vulvar cancer cases. The authors suggested that the role of tobacco smoking is limited to vulvar cancer associated with HPV, possibly due to a biologic interaction between tobacco smoking and viral proteins [18]. The exact mechanisms of how smoking increases the risk of vulvovaginal cancer has yet to be elucidated, but early studies have implicated that smoking decreases the numbers of T-cell lymphocytes which produce cytokines that ultimately combat HPV infections [19].

Additionally, the therapeutic role of imiquimod, an immune response modulator, demonstrates the role of the immune system in clearing HPV-infected cells when used as medical management of vulvovaginal dysplasia. Imiquimod *in vivo* raises levels of various cytokines to increase the potency of natural killer cells and also activates T cells and Langerhans cells to target HPV-infected cells [20]. Two randomized controlled trials have shown objective responses with imiquimod compared to placebo control: Van Seters et al. found a 35% response rate with imiquimod compared with a 0% response rate with placebo [21] and Mathiesen et al. achieved an 81% response rate with imiquimod compared with 0% response with placebo [22].

The causative role of HPV infections with high-risk subtypes allows for specific targeting of these viruses to prevent HPV-related cancers including cervical and anal malignancies. There are now three available HPV vaccines in the United States: the bivalent Cervarix® which protects against HPV-16 and -18, the quadrivalent Gardasil that includes HPV-6, -11, -16, and -18, and the recently approved nonavalent Gardasil-9 that adds HPV-31, -33, -45, -52, and -58 to the quadrivalent Gardasil. The phase III randomized controlled FUTURE I trial showed that the quadrivalent vaccine was 100% effective in preventing vaginal, vulvar, perineal, and perianal intraepithelial lesions with an average follow up of three years [23]. Saraiya et al. found in the Center for Disease Control (CDC) Cancer Registry Data that universal administration of the bivalent HPV vaccine can prevent 55.1% of vaginal cancers and 48.6% of vulvar cancers in the United States and report that many more cancer cases could be avoided with the nonavalent vaccine [24]. Given the promising data on HPV vaccines, many organizations including the CDC, the American College of Obstetrics and Gynecology, and the Society of Gynecologic Oncology have endorsed the universal administration of HPV vaccines to females 9–26 years of age. The HPV vaccine consists of recombinant HPV L1-specific DNA fragments, and therefore can be safely given to immunocompromised patients without risk of infection.

In summary, immunosuppression significantly increases the risk of preinvasive and invasive vulvar and vaginal cancers as demonstrated in multiple large cohort studies. This relationship is likely due to a decreased ability to clear HPV infections, thereby allowing HPV infections to progress to preinvasive then invasive cancers. The severity of immunosuppression indicated by low CD4 counts may correspond to higher rates of vulvar and vaginal cancers. HPV vaccines can be safely administered to immunocompromised patients and can potentially prevent the development of these neoplasms.

2. In patients with early stage vulvar cancer (population), what is the role of sentinel lymph node dissection (intervention) compared to inguinofemoral lymph node dissection (comparison) in detecting lymph node metastasis (outcome)?

Search Strategy

- MEDLINE and EMBASE: (sentinel node): *explode* vulvar cancer OR vaginal cancer AND (sentinel node OR sentinel node.mp) AND clinical trial AND cohort studies AND meta-analysis
- Hand-searching (sentinel node): references listed in the articles obtained.

Classical standard treatment for early-stage vulvar carcinoma with a depth of invasion of greater than 1 mm consists of wide local excision or partial/complete vulvectomy with complete inguinofemoral lymphadenectomy (CIL). The procedure is efficacious but CIL is associated with significant morbidity including lymphedema, cellulitis, and wound breakdown. Previous studies have reported lymphedema rates of 19–37.2%, cellulitis rates of 4.5–39%, and wound breakdown rates of 7.4–29.0% [25–28]. Although the complication rates are high, only 25–35% of patients with early stage disease will have lymph node metastases [29–31], therefore 65–75% of patients will be at risk for significant morbidity without benefitting from CIL. In response to the significant surgical morbidities associated with CIL coupled with the low rate of lymph node metastases, techniques in sentinel lymph node dissections (SLNDs) were developed, and now SLND is a component of the standard surgical management for early stage vulvar carcinoma.

Candidates for SLND are patients with squamous cell carcinoma of the vulva characterized as unifocal tumors with a depth of invasion greater than 1 mm and size less than 4 cm and with clinically uninvolved inguinal lymph nodes. Preoperatively, patients undergo peritumoral injections with technetium-99m sulfur colloid followed by lymphoscintigraphy to detect the presence of a sentinel node. Prior to skin incision, patients receive peritumoral injections with isosulfan blue dye and intraoperatively, the sentinel node is identified with the aid of a handheld gamma counter detecting increased activity as well as the visualization of blue afferent lymphatic channels and/or blue-stained lymph nodes. Studies have been performed with technetium-99m alone, isosulfan blue dye alone, and the two together have been shown to improve sentinel node detection rates. A meta-analysis of 24 pooled studies showed that detection rates for technetium-99m alone were 94.0%, for blue dye alone 95%, and for technetium-99m and blue dye together 97.7% [32].

Multiple prospective and retrospective studies have been performed to evaluate the detection rates and false negative rates of SLND. Table 17.2 summarizes the findings of all studies with at least 50 subjects [28, 31–43]. In most of these studies, patients underwent SLND followed by CIL to calculate the false negative rate, defined as a negative lymph node on SLND but a positive lymph node on CIL. Minimizing the false negative rate is paramount as failure to resect a positive lymph node can lead to a groin recurrence, which is almost always fatal. Therefore, it is important that a negative sentinel node represent a negative inguinofemoral lymph node basin. Two large prospective landmark trials with 855 combined patients showed that SLND had a high sensitivity and low false negative rate [28, 42]. One of these studies, Levenback et al. found that the false negative rate was significantly lower with tumors <4.0 cm compared with tumors ≥4.0 cm (2.0% vs 7.4%) [42].

Long-term follow up results of one of the landmark trials with a median follow-up time of 105 months found the rate of groin recurrences in patients with negative sentinel lymph nodes to be 2.5% [44]. Robison et al. in their prospective study found a groin recurrence rate of 5.2% in patients with negative sentinel lymph nodes after a median follow-up period of 58.3 months [43]. These are comparable to the historically reported 5–5.8% groin recurrence rates in patients after negative CIL [45, 46].

Van der Zee et al. examined the complication rates with SLND compared with CIL and found dramatic differences in rates of lymphedema, wound breakdown, cellulitis, and recurrent erysipelas with SLND. Performing SLND was able to decrease rates of lymphedema from 25.2% to 1.9%, wound breakdown from 34.0% to 11.7%, cellulitis from 21.3% to 4.5%, and recurrent erysipelas from 16.2% to 0.4% [28].

The Cochrane review on SLND in vulvar cancer evaluated 34 studies and concluded that SLND with technetium-based tests reduced the need for CIL by 70% in women with early vulvar cancer. Technetium-99m and blue dye together was superior to either modality alone in detecting a sentinel node. However, the review was unable conclude if there was a survival difference between patients with negative SLND and patients with negative CIL [47].

Several cost analyses have shown that performing SLND to be cheaper than CIL and when taking the decreased rates of complications into account, sentinel lymph node dissections are even more economically advantageous [48–50]. Interestingly, Farrell et al. surveyed women with vulvar carcinoma who had undergone CIL if they had a choice of upfront surgical management, whether they would opt for SLND or CIL [51]. The potential for missing a positive lymph node due to a false negative sentinel lymph node and the high possibility of developing lymphedema after CIL were discussed with the subjects. The study found that 68% of subjects did not want to take any risk of missing a positive groin lymph node and opted for CIL.

In conclusion, SLND with wide local excision and partial/complete vulvectomy is the standard treatment for early stage vulvar carcinoma with clinically negative lymph nodes due to low false negative rates, low rates of groin recurrences and reduced complication rates. Limited research

Table 17.2 Summary of studies performed to evaluate the detection rates and false negative rates of Sentinel lymph node dissections (SLND)

Reference	Year	*n* (Patients)	Type of study	Detection agent	Detection rate, %	False negative rate, %
Ansink et al. [33]	1999	51	Prospective	BD	82	3.9
De Hullu et al. [31]	2000	59	Prospective	Tc + BD	100	0.0
Levenback et al. [34]	2001	52	Prospective	BD	88	0.0
Vidal-Sicart et al. [35]	2007	50	Prospective	Tc	98	0.0
Van der Zee et al. [28]	2008	403	Prospective	Tc + BD	100	6.0
Johann et al. [36]	2008	63	Retrospective	Tc + BD	95	2.2
Hampl et al. [37]	2008	119	Prospective	Tc ± BD	98.3	2.5
Lindell et al. [38]	2010	77	Retrospective	Tc ± BD	98	2.7
Radziszewski et al. [39]	2010	56	Prospective	Tc ± BD	99	17.0
Devaja et al. [40]	2011	60	Prospective	Tc + BD	98.3	0.0
Garcia-Iglesias et al. [41]	2012	76	Prospective	Tc + BD	100	0.0
Levenback et al. [42]	2012	452	Prospective	Tc ± BD	92	6 (2% if tumor size <2 cm)
Robison et al. [43]	2014	69	Prospective	Tc + BD	93	NR

Tc, Technetium-99m; BD, blue dye; NR, not reported.

suggests that some patients may prefer CIL to ensure that all lymph nodes are pathologically examined, highlighting the importance of preoperative counseling so that patients can make an informed decision.

For vaginal cancer, the role of SLND is still under investigation. Due to the rarity of vaginal cancer, large prospective trials are difficult to design. A small number of prospective studies have been published with one to seven patients that have shown promising results high detection rates and low false negative rates [52–54]. Further research is necessary prior to recommending SLND as standard of care for early stage vaginal cancer.

3. In patients with unresectable locally advanced vulvar cancer (population), does concurrent chemotherapy with radiation therapy (intervention) compared to primary surgery (comparison) improve clinical response (outcome)?

Search Strategy

- MEDLINE and EMBASE: (chemotherapy OR chemoradiation): *explode* advanced vulvar cancer OR advanced vaginal cancer AND (chemotherapy OR chemotherapy.mp OR chemoradiation OR chemoradiation.mp) AND clinical trial AND cohort studies AND meta-analysis.
- Hand-searching (chemotherapy OR chemoradiation): references listed in the articles obtained.

For early stage vulvar cancer, surgical resection with curative intent is the preferred treatment. For locally advanced vulvar cancer characterized by either fixed or ulcerated groin lymph nodes or close proximity to the urethra, vagina or anus, more extensive surgical procedures are needed to excise the tumor burden with adequate margins. The standard procedure consist of an en-bloc radical vulvectomy and bilateral inguinofemoral lymphadenectomy and possibly pelvic exenteration with a formation of a colostomy or urinary diversion, which carries an operative mortality of up to 10% [55] as well as significant physical and psychological morbidity detrimentally affecting quality of life.

As an alternative primary treatment method for locally advanced vulvar cancer, Boronow and Hacker independently introduced regimens of radiation therapy followed by surgical resection to avoid pelvic exenteration by decreasing the preoperative tumor burden [56, 57]. After the benefits of concurrent chemoradiotherapy were seen in other types of cancer including cervical cancer, two prospective phase II trials by the Gynecologic Oncology Group (GOG) evaluated the efficacy of preoperative chemoradiation followed by surgical resection [58, 59]. Montana et al. found that in patients with unresectable groin lymph nodes, a course of chemotherapy consisting of cisplatin and 5-fluorouracil and external beam radiation therapy was well tolerated and resulted in a 95% resectability rate after chemoradiation [58]. A subsequent GOG study by Moore et al. included patients with locally advanced vulvar cancer not amenable to surgical resection by radical vulvectomy and treated them with cisplatin alone with a 20% higher dose of external beam radiation than in Montana et al. This regimen was also well tolerated and following chemoradiation, 64% of patients had a complete clinical response and 50% had a complete pathological response at the time of surgery [59]. A subsequent retrospective study utilizing chemotherapy and intensity-modulated radiation therapy (IMRT) have shown promising results with a complete pathologic response rate of 64% and a lower rate of severe toxicity, suggesting that IMRT by delivering higher but targeted radiation doses can yield similar response rates while sparing patients from radiation-related toxicities [60]. A small Cochrane review of three studies reported no significant difference in overall survival or treatment-related toxicity when primary chemoradiation was compared with primary surgery [61].

The use of preoperative chemotherapy alone without radiation has also been studied. An early European prospective study with neoadjuvant chemotherapy treated patients with bleomycin, lomustine, and methotrexate and found a tumor response rate of 64% but with over 20% of the patients experiencing severe toxicity [62]. A follow-up study treated patients again with bleomycin, lomustine, and methotrexate but at lower doses. Results of this study demonstrated a comparable response rate of 56% but a higher rate of severe toxicity of 40% [63]. Smaller subsequent studies with different chemotherapy regimens have shown more promising results including Domingues et al., which showed a 60% response rate with bleomycin alone and lower toxicity rates [64].

In summary, primary treatment for patients with locally advanced vulvar cancer either presenting with fixed or ulcerated groin nodes or involving important structures such as the urethra and anus has moved away from radical surgery likely requiring an exenterative procedure to preoperative chemotherapy or chemoradiation followed by less extensive surgical resections. Studies evaluating preoperative chemotherapy and chemoradiation have demonstrated favorable tumor response rates that have prevented exenterations; however optimal chemotherapy or chemoradiation regimens have not yet been established. There are no prospective randomized studies comparing neoadjuvant chemotherapy alone to chemoradiation, therefore it is difficult to establish whether one is superior over the other.

For vaginal cancer, primary surgery is rarely performed due to the close proximity of vaginal tumors to critical organs and the high risk of significant complications. The mainstay of treatment is typically definitive radiation therapy with concurrent cisplatin-based chemotherapy. Due to the rarity of vaginal cancers, the majority of studies are retrospective; however one prospective study of 11 patients with stage II vaginal cancer evaluated the use of neoadjuvant chemotherapy with cisplatin and paclitaxel followed by surgery and demonstrated that this treatment method was feasible and safe with a low rate of complications and a high survival rate

[65]. The remainder of the literature on vaginal carcinoma is largely retrospective. The largest population-based study of 8222 patients from the National Cancer Data Base found that the additions of concurrent chemotherapy and brachytherapy were independently associated with improved survival for vaginal cancer of all stages [66]. Another study of 2517 patients from the Surveillance, Epidemiology, and End Result (SEER) database found brachytherapy with external beam radiation therapy to be superior to external beam radiation therapy alone, and the number of women who needed to be treated with brachytherapy to prevent a death from vaginal cancer to be eight [67]. Although prospective data is very limited regarding the optimal treatment for vaginal carcinoma, chemoradiation with brachytherapy is typically utilized although neoadjuvant chemotherapy followed by surgical resection has shown promise.

Conclusions

You refer the patient to a gynecologic oncologist who initiated chemoradiation given her inguinal node involvement. After she completed the course of upfront chemoradiation, her inguinal nodes were no longer palpable and her vulvar lesions were significantly smaller. She then underwent a successful radical vulvectomy and bilateral inguinofemoral lymphadenectomy with final pathology only showing disease in the vulvectomy specimen with negative margins. She has been without evidence of disease for 12 months. She has also quit smoking after receiving smoking cessation counseling.

Vulvar and vaginal cancers are rare conditions that are infrequently encountered by general gynecologists. However, survival rates significantly improve with early detection. During routine pelvic examination, the vulva and vagina should be thoroughly examined especially in immunocompromised patients. Any abnormal appearing lesion on the vulva or vagina should be biopsied prior to the initiation of topical treatments. Early stage vulvar cancer with clinically negative groin nodes can safely undergo sentinel lymph node dissections to reduce the operative morbidity and long-term sequelae associated complete node dissections. Locally advanced vulvar cancers can be treated with upfront chemoradiation or chemotherapy in order to decrease the tumor burden prior to surgical resection. Vaginal cancers are most often treated with primary chemoradiation with data demonstrating improved survival with the addition of brachytherapy.

References

1 Siegel, R.L., Miller, K.D., and Jemal, A. (2016). Cancer statistics, 2016. *CA Cancer J. Clin.* **66** (**1**): 7–30.

2 Hiniker, S.M., Roux, A., Murphy, J.D. et al. (2013). Primary squamous cell carcinoma of the vagina: prognostic factors, treatment patterns, and outcomes. *Gynecol. Oncol.* **131** (**2**): 380–385.

3 Bosch, F.X., Broker, T.R., Forman, D. et al. (2013). Comprehensive control of human papillomavirus infections and related diseases. *Vaccine* **31** (**Suppl 8**): I1–I31.

4 Hampl, M., Sarajuuri, H., Wentzensen, N. et al. (2006). Effect of human papillomavirus vaccines on vulvar, vaginal, and anal intraepithelial lesions and vulvar cancer. *Obstet. Gynecol.* **108** (**6**): 1361–1368.

5 Frisch, M., Biggar, R.J., and Goedert, J.J. (2000). Human papillomavirus-associated cancers in patients with human immunodeficiency virus infection and acquired immunodeficiency syndrome. *J. Natl. Cancer Inst.* **92** (**18**): 1500–1510.

6 Adami, J., Gabel, H., Lindelof, B. et al. (2003). Cancer risk following organ transplantation: a nationwide cohort study in Sweden. *Br. J. Cancer* **89** (**7**): 1221–1227.

7 Vajdic, C.M., McDonald, S.P., McCredie, M.R. et al. (2006). Cancer incidence before and after kidney transplantation. *JAMA* **296** (**23**): 2823–2831.

8 Grulich, A.E., van Leeuwen, M.T., Falster, M.O., and Vajdic, C.M. Incidence of cancers in people with HIV/AIDS compared with immunosuppressed transplant recipients: a meta-analysis. *Lancet* **370** (**9581**): 59–67.

9 Chaturvedi, A.K., Madeleine, M.M., Biggar, R.J., and Engels, E.A. (2009). Risk of human papillomavirus-associated cancers among persons with AIDS. *J. Natl. Cancer Inst.* **101** (**16**): 1120–1130.

10 Engels, E.A., Pfeiffer, R.M., Fraumeni, J.F. Jr. et al. (2011). Spectrum of cancer risk among US solid organ transplant recipients. *JAMA* **306** (**17**): 1891–1901.

11 Skov Dalgaard, L., Fassel, U., Ostergaard, L.J. et al. (2013). Risk of human papillomavirus-related cancers among kidney transplant recipients and patients receiving chronic dialysis--an observational cohort study. *BMC Nephrol.* **14**: 137.

12 Madeleine, M.M., Finch, J.L., Lynch, C.F. et al. (2013). HPV-related cancers after solid organ transplantation in the United States. *Am. J. Transplant.* **13** (**12**): 3202–3209.

13 Jamieson, D.J., Paramsothy, P., Cu-Uvin, S., and Duerr, A. (2006). Vulvar, vaginal, and perianal intraepithelial neoplasia in women with or at risk for human immunodeficiency virus. *Obstet. Gynecol.* **107** (**5**): 1023–1028.

14 Massad, L.S., Silverberg, M.J., Springer, G. et al. (2004). Effect of antiretroviral therapy on the incidence of genital warts and vulvar neoplasia among women with the human immunodeficiency virus. *Am. J. Obstet. Gynecol.* **190** (**5**): 1241–1248.

15 Massad, L.S., Xie, X., Darragh, T. et al. (2011). Genital warts and vulvar intraepithelial neoplasia: natural history and effects of treatment and human immunodeficiency virus infection. *Obstet. Gynecol.* **118** (**4**): 831–839.

16 Daling, J.R., Sherman, K.J., Hislop, T.G. et al. (1992). Cigarette smoking and the risk of anogenital cancer. *Am. J. Epidemiol.* **135** (**2**): 180–189.

17 Mabuchi, K., Bross, D.S., and Kessler, I.I. (1985). Epidemiology of cancer of the vulva. A case-control study. *Cancer* **55** (**8**): 1843–1848.

18 Madsen, B.S., Jensen, H.L., van den Brule, A.J. et al. (2008). Risk factors for invasive squamous cell carcinoma of the vulva

and vagina–population-based case-control study in Denmark. *Int. J. Cancer* **122** (**12**): 2827–2834.

19 Hussain, S.K., Madeleine, M.M., Johnson, L.G. et al. (2008). Cervical and vulvar cancer risk in relation to the joint effects of cigarette smoking and genetic variation in interleukin 2. *Cancer Epidemiol. Biomarkers Prev.* **17** (**7**): 1790–1799.

20 de Witte, C.J., van de Sande, A.J., van Beekhuizen, H.J. et al. (2015). Imiquimod in cervical, vaginal and vulvar intraepithelial neoplasia: a review. *Gynecol. Oncol.* **139** (**2**): 377–384.

21 van Seters, M., van Beurden, M., ten Kate, F.J. et al. (2008). Treatment of vulvar intraepithelial neoplasia with topical imiquimod. *N. Engl. J. Med.* **358** (**14**): 1465–1473.

22 Mathiesen, O., Buus, S.K., and Cramers, M. (2007). Topical imiquimod can reverse vulvar intraepithelial neoplasia: a randomised, double-blinded study. *Gynecol. Oncol.* **107** (**2**): 219–222.

23 Garland, S.M., Hernandez-Avila, M., Wheeler, C.M. et al. (2007). Quadrivalent vaccine against human papillomavirus to prevent anogenital diseases. *N. Engl. J. Med.* **356** (**19**): 1928–1943.

24 Saraiya, M., Unger, E.R., Thompson, T.D. et al. (2015). US assessment of HPV types in cancers: implications for current and 9-valent HPV vaccines. *J. Natl. Cancer Inst.* **107** (**6**): djv086.

25 Rouzier, R., Haddad, B., Dubernard, G. et al. (2003). Inguinofemoral dissection for carcinoma of the vulva: effect of modifications of extent and technique on morbidity and survival. *J. Am. Coll. Surg.* **196** (**3**): 442–450.

26 Stehman, F.B., Bundy, B.N., Dvoretsky, P.M., and Creasman, W.T. (1992). Early stage I carcinoma of the vulva treated with ipsilateral superficial inguinal lymphadenectomy and modified radical hemivulvectomy: a prospective study of the Gynecologic Oncology Group. *Obstet. Gynecol.* **79** (**4**): 490–497.

27 Gaarenstroom, K.N., Kenter, G.G., Trimbos, J.B. et al. (2003). Postoperative complications after vulvectomy and inguinofemoral lymphadenectomy using separate groin incisions. *Int. J. Gynecol. Cancer* **13** (**4**): 522–527.

28 Van der Zee, A.G., Oonk, M.H., De Hullu, J.A. et al. (2008). Sentinel node dissection is safe in the treatment of early-stage vulvar cancer. *J. Clin. Oncol.* **26** (**6**): 884–889.

29 Hacker, N.F., Leuchter, R.S., Berek, J.S. et al. (1981). Radical vulvectomy and bilateral inguinal lymphadenectomy through separate groin incisions. *Obstet. Gynecol.* **58** (**5**): 574–579.

30 Bell, J.G., Lea, J.S., and Reid, G.C. (2000). Complete groin lymphadenectomy with preservation of the fascia lata in the treatment of vulvar carcinoma. *Gynecol. Oncol.* **77** (**2**): 314–318.

31 de Hullu, J.A., Hollema, H., Piers, D.A. et al. (2000). Sentinel lymph node procedure is highly accurate in squamous cell carcinoma of the vulva. *J. Clin. Oncol.* **18** (**15**): 2811–2816.

32 Meads, C., Sutton, A.J., Rosenthal, A.N. et al. (2014). Sentinel lymph node biopsy in vulval cancer: systematic review and meta-analysis. *Br. J. Cancer* **110** (**12**): 2837–2846.

33 Ansink, A.C., Sie-Go, D.M., van der Velden, J. et al. (1999). Identification of sentinel lymph nodes in vulvar carcinoma patients with the aid of a patent blue V injection: a multicenter study. *Cancer* **86** (**4**): 652–656.

34 Levenback, C., Coleman, R.L., Burke, T.W. et al. (2001). Intraoperative lymphatic mapping and sentinel node identification with blue dye in patients with vulvar cancer. *Gynecol. Oncol.* **83** (**2**): 276–281.

35 Vidal-Sicart, S., Puig-Tintore, L.M., Lejarcegui, J.A. et al. (2007). Validation and application of the sentinel lymph node concept in malignant vulvar tumours. *Eur. J. Nucl. Med. Mol. Imaging* **34** (**3**): 384–391.

36 Johann, S., Klaeser, B., Krause, T., and Mueller, M.D. (2008). Comparison of outcome and recurrence-free survival after sentinel lymph node biopsy and lymphadenectomy in vulvar cancer. *Gynecol. Oncol.* **110** (**3**): 324–328.

37 Hampl, M., Hantschmann, P., Michels, W., and Hillemanns, P. (2008). Validation of the accuracy of the sentinel lymph node procedure in patients with vulvar cancer: results of a multicenter study in Germany. *Gynecol. Oncol.* **111** (**2**): 282–288.

38 Lindell, G., Jonsson, C., Ehrsson, R.J. et al. (2010). Evaluation of preoperative lymphoscintigraphy and sentinel node procedure in vulvar cancer. *Eur. J. Obstet. Gynecol. Reprod. Biol.* **152** (**1**): 91–95.

39 Radziszewski, J., Kowalewska, M., Jedrzejczak, T. et al. (2010). The accuracy of the sentinel lymph node concept in early stage squamous cell vulvar carcinoma. *Gynecol. Oncol.* **116** (**3**): 473–477.

40 Devaja, O., Mehra, G., Coutts, M. et al. (2011). A prospective study of sentinel lymph node detection in vulval carcinoma: is it time for a change in clinical practice? *Int. J. Gynecol. Cancer* **21** (**3**): 559–564.

41 Garcia-Iglesias, A., Rodriguez-Martin, M.O., Ruano, R. et al. (2012). Sentinel node disection in the treatment of early stages of vulvar cancer. *Eur. J. Gynaecol. Oncol.* **33** (**2**): 151–154.

42 Levenback, C.F., Ali, S., Coleman, R.L. et al. (2012). Lymphatic mapping and sentinel lymph node biopsy in women with squamous cell carcinoma of the vulva: a gynecologic oncology group study. *J. Clin. Oncol.* **30** (**31**): 3786–3791.

43 Robison, K., Roque, D., McCourt, C. et al. (2014). Long-term follow-up of vulvar cancer patients evaluated with sentinel lymph node biopsy alone. *Gynecol. Oncol.* **133** (**3**): 416–420.

44 Te Grootenhuis, N.C., van der Zee, A.G., van Doorn, H.C. et al. (2016). Sentinel nodes in vulvar cancer: long-term follow-up of the GROningen INternational Study on Sentinel nodes in Vulvar cancer (GROINSS-V) I. *Gynecol. Oncol.* **140** (**1**): 8–14.

45 Stehman, F.B., Bundy, B.N., Ball, H., and Clarke-Pearson, D.L. (1996). Sites of failure and times to failure in carcinoma of the vulva treated conservatively: a Gynecologic Oncology Group study. *Am. J. Obstet. Gynecol.* **174** (**4**): 1128–1132. discussion 1132–3.

46 Burke, T.W., Levenback, C., Coleman, R.L. et al. (1995). Surgical therapy of T1 and T2 vulvar carcinoma: further experience with radical wide excision and selective inguinal lymphadenectomy. *Gynecol. Oncol.* **57** (**2**): 215–220.

47 Lawrie, T.A., Patel, A., Martin-Hirsch, P.P. et al. (2014). Sentinel node assessment for diagnosis of groin lymph node involvement in vulval cancer. *Cochrane Database Syst. Rev.* (**6**): Cd010409. doi: 10.1002/14651858.

48 Sutton, A.J., Barton, P., Sundar, S. et al. (2013). Cost-effectiveness of sentinel lymph node biopsy vs inguinofemoral lymphadenectomy in women with vulval cancer. *Br. J. Cancer* **109** (**10**): 2533–2547.

49 Erickson, B.K., Divine, L.M., Leath, C.A. 3rd, and Straughn, J.M. Jr. (2014). Cost-effectiveness analysis of sentinel lymph node biopsy in the treatment of early-stage vulvar cancer. *Int. J. Gynecol. Cancer* **24** (**8**): 1480–1485.

50 McCann, G.A., Cohn, D.E., Jewell, E.L., and Havrilesky, L.J. (2015). Lymphatic mapping and sentinel lymph node dissection compared to complete lymphadenectomy in the management of early-stage vulvar cancer: a cost-utility analysis. *Gynecol. Oncol.* **136** (**2**): 300–304.

51 Farrell, R., Gebski, V., and Hacker, N.F. (2014). Quality of life after complete lymphadenectomy for vulvar cancer: do women prefer sentinel lymph node biopsy? *Int. J. Gynecol. Cancer* **24** (**4**): 813–819.

52 van Dam, P., Sonnemans, H., van Dam, P.J. et al. (2004). Sentinel node detection in patients with vaginal carcinoma. *Gynecol. Oncol.* **92** (**1**): 89–92.

53 Frumovitz, M., Gayed, I.W., Jhingran, A. et al. (2008). Lymphatic mapping and sentinel lymph node detection in women with vaginal cancer. *Gynecol. Oncol.* **108** (**3**): 478–481.

54 Hertel, H., Soergel, P., Muecke, J. et al. (2013). Is there a place for sentinel technique in treatment of vaginal cancer?: feasibility, clinical experience and results. *Int. J. Gynecol. Cancer* **23** (**9**): 1692–1698.

55 Geisler, J.P., Manahan, K.J., and Buller, R.E. (2006). Neoadjuvant chemotherapy in vulvar cancer: avoiding primary exenteration. *Gynecol. Oncol.* **100** (**1**): 53–57.

56 Boronow, R.C., Hickman, B.T., Reagan, M.T. et al. (1987). Combined therapy as an alternative to exenteration for locally advanced vulvovaginal cancer. II. Results, complications, and dosimetric and surgical considerations. *Am. J. Clin. Oncol.* **10** (**2**): 171–181.

57 Hacker, N.F., Berek, J.S., Juillard, G.J., and Lagasse, L.D. (1984). Preoperative radiation therapy for locally advanced vulvar cancer. *Cancer* **54** (**10**): 2056–2061.

58 Montana, G.S., Thomas, G.M., Moore, D.H. et al. (2000). Preoperative chemo-radiation for carcinoma of the vulva with N2/N3 nodes: a gynecologic oncology group study. *Int. J. Radiat. Oncol. Biol. Phys.* **48** (**4**): 1007–1013.

59 Moore, D.H., Ali, S., Koh, W.J. et al. (2012). A phase II trial of radiation therapy and weekly cisplatin chemotherapy for the treatment of locally-advanced squamous cell carcinoma of the vulva: a gynecologic oncology group study. *Gynecol. Oncol.* **124** (**3**): 529–533.

60 Beriwal, S., Shukla, G., Shinde, A. et al. (2013). Preoperative intensity modulated radiation therapy and chemotherapy for locally advanced vulvar carcinoma: analysis of pattern of relapse. *Int. J. Radiat. Oncol. Biol. Phys.* **85** (**5**): 1269–1274.

61 Shylasree, T.S., Bryant, A., and Howells, R.E. (2011). Chemoradiation for advanced primary vulval cancer. *Cochrane Database Syst. Rev.* (**4**): Cd003752. doi: 10.1002/14651858.

62 Durrant, K.R., Mangioni, C., Lacave, A.J. et al. (1990). Bleomycin, methotrexate, and CCNU in advanced inoperable squamous cell carcinoma of the vulva: a phase II study of the EORTC Gynaecological Cancer Cooperative Group (GCCG). *Gynecol. Oncol.* **37** (**3**): 359–362.

63 Wagenaar, H.C., Colombo, N., Vergote, I. et al. (2001). Bleomycin, methotrexate, and CCNU in locally advanced or recurrent, inoperable, squamous-cell carcinoma of the vulva: an EORTC Gynaecological Cancer Cooperative Group Study. European Organization for Research and Treatment of Cancer. *Gynecol. Oncol.* **81** (**3**): 348–354.

64 Domingues, A.P., Mota, F., Durao, M. et al. (2010). Neoadjuvant chemotherapy in advanced vulvar cancer. *Int. J. Gynecol. Cancer* **20** (**2**): 294–298.

65 Benedetti Panici, P., Bellati, F., Plotti, F. et al. (2008). Neoadjuvant chemotherapy followed by radical surgery in patients affected by vaginal carcinoma. *Gynecol. Oncol.* **111** (**2**): 307–311.

66 Rajagopalan, M.S., Xu, K.M., Lin, J.F. et al. (2014). Adoption and impact of concurrent chemoradiation therapy for vaginal cancer: a National Cancer Data Base (NCDB) study. *Gynecol. Oncol.* **135** (**3**): 495–502.

67 Orton, A., Boothe, D., Williams, N. et al. Brachytherapy improves survival in primary vaginal cancer. *Gynecol. Oncol.*

18

CHAPTER 18

Endometrial cancer

Stephanie V. Blank and Zachary P. Schwartz

Division of Gynecologic Oncology, Department of Obstetrics and Gynecology, NYU Langone Medical Center, New York, NY, USA

CLINICAL SCENARIO

A 44-year-old nulliparous woman presents with intermenstrual bleeding and irregular cycles. Work up includes an endometrial biopsy which reveals Federation of Gynecology and Obstetrics (FIGO) grade 1 endometrioid endometrial carcinoma. She is otherwise healthy, with no past medical or surgical history and no medications. The patient has no knowledge of paternal family history; her mother, who was adopted, had colon cancer at 45. Physical exam is notable for a heart rate of 80, blood pressure (BP) of 120/70 and body mass index (BMI) of 26. Abdomen is soft, non-tender and pelvic exam reveals a mobile, well supported uterus of normal size, shape, and contour. She presents for definitive surgical management.

Clinical questions

1. In women with low grade endometrial cancer (population), what is the evidence for and against (comparison) lymph node dissection (intervention) in relation to prognosis (outcome)?

Approximately 2.8% of women will develop endometrial cancer over their lifetimes; this represents a rate of about 25 per 100 000 women per year. Of these newly diagnosed endometrial cancers, an estimated 67% will be localized to the uterus [1]. Additionally, an estimated 75% of all endometrial cancers are low grade [2]. In the case of patients diagnosed with endometrial cancer, the standard method of staging and treatment is total hysterectomy, bilateral salpingo-oophorectomy, peritoneal cytology and pelvic and para-aortic lymph node dissection [3]. While few would argue about the role of removal of uterus, tubes, and ovaries, there remains great debate as to the role for and necessity of lymph node dissection in patients with low risk endometrial cancer.

The argument supporting lymph node dissection rests on the following principles:

1. *The belief that the risk of nodal metastases in these patients warrants the dissection*:

Creasman's landmark study found an estimated rate of lymph node metastases in patients who are clinically low grade of upwards of 9% [4], but notably, there were no lymph node metastases in patients with tumors invading less than one third of the myometrium. Mariani et al. which established the "Mayo Criteria" for identifying low-risk endometrial cancer cases noted that in even low-risk endometrial cancer cases, the risk of nodal metastasis was seen in up to 5% of cases [5]. These percentile risks are felt to be high enough by some to warrant this process.

2. *The possibility that the cancer will be upgraded or upstaged when the uterus is removed:*

In a prospective randomized study by Benedetti et al., patients with low-grade endometrial cancer were assigned to either receive complete pelvic lymphadenectomy or no lymphadenectomy at all. This study found that, indeed, those with complete pelvic lymphadenectomies had improved surgical staging, with significantly more patients found to have nodal metastasis, thereby upstaging their clinical low-grade status [6]. Finding this higher stage status is important because it has large implications for potential need for and exposure to adjuvant therapies.

3. *The belief that there is inherent therapeutic benefit to nodal dissection among these patients:*

This benefit is twofold: (i) nodal dissection allows select patients to potentially avoid treatment and the adverse effects of such treatment when nodes are negative and (ii) an upgraded staging based on positive nodes identifies patients who would benefit from adjuvant therapy.

The treatment distinction between patients with positive nodes versus those with negative nodes is based on the idea that patients with positive lymph nodes are immediately placed within an advanced stage requiring chemotherapy. They therefore get appropriate treatment based on that

Evidence-Based Obstetrics and Gynecology, First Edition. Edited by Errol R. Norwitz, Carolyn M. Zelop, David A. Miller, and David L. Keefe.

knowledge. On the other hand, a patient with no positive nodes has the potential to be followed with surveillance alone. This is based on Gynecologic Oncology Group 99 study by Keys et al. which evaluated patients who had complete surgical staging, including pelvic and para-aortic lymph node dissections and were without evidence of lymph node metastases. These patients were placed in low, intermediate, and high-risk groups based on age, histology, depth of invasion, and lymphovascular space invasion. Those in the intermediate and high-risk groups were randomized to either no treatment or whole pelvic radiation therapy. While no statistically significant difference was noted in expected four year survival between the two groups, there was a significant difference in evidence of pelvic and vaginal recurrences after treatment (12% in no treatment versus 3% in treatment arm, Relative hazard: 0.42, $p = 0.007$) [7]. This conclusion was again supported by the Post-Operative Radiation Therapy in Endometrial Carcinoma (PORTEC) trial in 2000 which found patients with low grade endometrial cancer randomized to either radiation or placebo had similar five year overall survival (81% vs. 85%, $p = 0.31$) but had a decrease in locoregional recurrence (4% vs. 14%, $p = <0.001$) [8]. Thus, with surgical staging, the patient is able to be definitively placed within a low, intermediate, and high risk group and be given the opportunity for treatment that decreases overall locoregional recurrence of disease.

The counter argument to lymphadenectomy is based upon the idea that despite the possibility of upstaging patients with this procedure, patients have no difference in progression for free or overall survival despite lymphadenectomies [6, 9]. In Benedetti et al. study mentioned above, 514 patients with Stage I endometrial carcinoma were randomized to receive pelvic lymphadenectomy vs. no lymphadenectomy. Despite finding increased evidence of nodal metastasis in patients having undergone pelvic lymphadenectomy versus those that didn't (13.3% vs. 3.2%, $p = 0.001$), there was no notable difference in five-year disease free survival and overall survival (81% vs. 85.9% and 81.7 vs. 90.0%, respectively). Of note, the treatments were not standardized in these trials, thereby limiting the interpretation of the role of lymphadenectomy.

The landmark, international, randomized ASTEC trial further helped support this conclusion [9]. This study randomized 1408 women with suspected low-grade endometrial cancer confined to the uterus to either total abdominal hysterectomy, bilateral salpingo-oophorectomy, washings, and palpation of para-aortic lymph nodes compared to the same procedure, but with added pelvic lymph node dissection and possible para-aortic lymph node dissection based on the discretion of the surgeon. The study then took a step further than the Benedetti et al. study and controlled for post-surgery treatment by randomizing those patients with intermediate or high-risk cancer into the whole pelvic radiation versus no radiation, with both groups being able to possibly receive vaginal vault radiation therapy. In the end, after controlling for baseline characteristics and pathology details, the study found that Hazard Ratio for overall survival was 1.04 (0.74–1.45; $p = 0.83$) and for recurrence free survival was 1.25 (0.93–1.66; $p = 0.14$). Thus, the conclusions of this study demonstrated no difference in survival or recurrence of disease whether or not lymph node dissection was performed.

Now, while this ASTEC trial was strongly powered and had the strength of being randomize-controlled, many aspects have been called into question. Often cited concerns regarding this study include selection bias based on the European locale of the study and the ability of the surgeon to decide on whether or not para-aortics were performed as well as inappropriate randomization within the radiation treatment arms [3, 10]. European guidelines rarely require para-aortic lymph node dissections [11] and given that this study was performed entirely within Europe, it is suggested that surgical inexperience with full staging would bias the practitioner against said staging. Additionally, and perhaps one of the most controversial aspects of this study, is that survival was evaluated after patients received radiation treatment randomization. In this study, those who were randomized to receive radiation were only those who were deemed intermediate or high-risk cancer patients based on uterine pathology only. There was no consideration of lymph node status. In addition, by the nature of this randomization, approximately 50% of patients with intermediate or high-risk cancers did not receive whole pelvic radiation. Thus, the outcomes of the patients receiving lymphadenectomies could very much be confounded by whether or not they received appropriate adjuvant therapy. Additionally, there is no way to tell whether lymphadenectomies would change outcomes with adjuvant therapy because lymphadenopathy was not considered in triaging patients to treatment.

Lymph node dissection in patients with low-grade endometrial cancer remains controversial. Lymph node dissection introduces surgical risks including lymphedema and damage to major nerves and blood vessels [12]. But, regarding oncologic outcomes, studies either suggest that this process has no benefit or some. There is little to suggest that it has a negative impact on oncologic outcomes, but cost and impact on quality of life (for which there is a paucity of data) must be considered. At present, there is not an evidence-based answer to this clinical question.

Some have recommended sentinel lymph node dissection for low grade endometrial cancer as a means to obtain the prognostic and treatment-driving information that comes from pathologic evaluation of the lymph nodes all while minimizing the morbidity associated with full lymph node dissections [13]. Studies have suggested that using this methodology, despite its diminished invasiveness does not negatively impact the disease free survival, progression free survival and overall survival when comparing low-grade disease [14, 15]. These studies are small however and there is very little long-term follow-up as yet. As such, lymph node evaluation via complete staging remains the standard of care.

2. In women with endometrial cancer (population) what is the evidence regarding minimally invasive surgery (intervention) in relation to adequacy of surgery, quality of life and oncologic outcomes (outcome)?

The surgical management of early stage endometrial cancer has, historically, been limited to laparotomy, total abdominal hysterectomy, bilateral salpingo-oophorectomy and lymph node dissection [3]. In the early 1990s, however, small case studies started to establish laparoscopy as a safe, effective mode of surgical staging of endometrial cancer [16, 17]. Since then, multiple studies continued to support the efficacy, safety and beneficial outcomes of minimally invasive surgical techniques in early clinical stage endometrial cancers. These minimally invasive techniques include laparoscopic staging with total laparoscopic hysterectomy or laparoscopic assisted vaginal hysterectomy and, more recently, robotic assisted laparoscopic approaches.

Since the establishment of laparoscopy as a viable surgical staging tool, multiple prospective studies – many randomized – have evaluated just how effective this tool is in staging endometrial cancer [18–23]. Holub et al. [18] in 2002 is an example of one such study that evaluated 92 women who completed laparoscopically assisted vaginal hysterectomy as well as bilateral salpingo-oophorectomy, and lymph node dissection compared to an abdominal approach control group of 24 patients. They found an increase in time for laparoscopy (an average of 38 more minutes, $p = <0.0001$) but importantly they also found a significantly shorter hospital course (an average of 3.6 days shorter, $p = <0.0001$) for laparoscopy compared to laparotomy. They also found no statistically significant difference in complications, estimated blood loss, and number of lymph nodes removed.

Malur et al. [24] similarly evaluated patients undergoing laparoscopically assisted vaginal hysterectomy, bilateral salpingo-oophorectomy and lymph node dissection (assuming tumor was more than 1/3 invaded through the myometrium). They compared 37 patients via laparoscopy versus 33 patients via laparotomy. They similarly found a statistically significant decline in length of stay, blood loss, and length of time until first bowel movement. They also noted no statistically significant difference in disease recurrence or long-term survival over a three year period.

Further studies looked at laparoscopy alone as a methodology for hysterectomy, bilateral salpingo-oophorectomy and lymph node dissections. Important studies such as Kuoppala et al. [19] and Malzoni et al. [25] compared patients with laparoscopy ($n = 40$ and $n = 81$, respectively) alone versus laparotomy ($n = 40$ and $n = 78$, respectively). Like previous studies mentioned above, both studies found a statistically significant increase in the duration of surgery but they also noted a significant decline in blood loss and length of post-operative hospitalization. In the Kuoppala et al. study they interestingly found a statistically higher number of lymph nodes removed in the laparoscopic group. Survival and recurrence, however, wasn't compared in this trial between the two groups so the significance of the increased number of nodes is hard to interpret. The Malzoni et al. group did compare rates of recurrence, overall survival rates and disease free survival. They had a median duration of follow-up of 38.5 months. They found no statistically significant difference in rates of recurrence in laparoscopy versus laparotomy (8.6% vs. 11.5%), rates of overall survival (93.2% vs. 91.1%, $p = 0.31$), or disease free survival (91.4% vs. 88.5%, $p = 0.28$). Thus, both studies demonstrated surgical benefits of laparoscopy over laparotomy and Malzoni et al. found that despite this surgical benefit, there was no decline in survival or recurrence outcomes.

Now, while the above-mentioned studies have all importantly demonstrated the merits of laparoscopic surgery in clinically early stage endometrial cancer, all of these studies have had small cohorts of participants. As such, the laparoscopy (LAP2) trial by Walker et al. [21] was designed to further evaluate these methodologies on a larger scale. This landmark trial randomized 2616 patients into laparoscopic ($n = 1682$) and open laparotomy ($n = 920$) groups. Both groups underwent total hysterectomy, bilateral salpingo-oophorectomy, pelvic cytology, and pelvic and para-aortic lymph node dissections. This study found a longer median operative time in laparoscopy compared to laparotomy (204 vs. 140 min, $p < 0.001$) but, as with previous smaller studies, they found fewer post-operative adverse events in laparoscopic cases (14% vs. 21%) and hospitalizations greater than two days were significantly less in laparoscopic cases (52% vs. 94%, $p < 0.0001$). Interestingly, they found that surgeons were unable to remove both pelvic and para-aortic lymph nodes in 8% of laparoscopic cases, as opposed to only 4% in open cases ($p < 0.0001$). This did not seem to affect outcomes, however, with no notable difference in the detection of advanced stage disease between groups, which occurred in 17% of patients in both groups ($p = 0.841$).

This same study cohort was further evaluated for recurrence and survival by Walker and colleagues in 2012 [26]. In this analysis, 1696 from the laparoscopy group and 920 from the laparotomy group were followed for a median follow-up of 59.3 months. While the study did not meet its initial objective of establishing the non-inferiority of laparoscopy compared to laparotomy, it did find no statistical difference in three-year estimated cumulative incidence of recurrence for patients in the laparotomy arm versus the laparoscopy arm (10.24% vs. 11.39%, lower 90%, −1.278; 95% upper bound, 3.996). The five-year overall survival in both arms was exactly the same at 84.8%. Although not confirming the noninferiority of laparoscopy vs laparotomy, LAP 2 did establish a minimally invasive approach as standard of care for endometrial cancer, demonstrating reduced surgical morbidity with laparoscopy and similar oncologic outcomes between the two groups.

Zullo et al. [27] performed a meta-analysis of eight randomized controlled trials comparing laparotomy to laparoscopy for endometrial cancer, finding no difference in intraoperative complication rates between the two groups (Risk Ratio (RR), 1.25; 95% CI, 0.99–1.56; p = 0.062). They did find a significant advantage to laparoscopy over laparotomy with decreased rates of post-operative complications (RR, 0.71; 95% CI, 0.63–0.79; p = 0.016). There was an increased operative time in laparoscopy (weighted mean difference (WMD) = 51.46; 95% CI, 46.56–58.36; $P < 0.0001$) but a decreased blood loss (WMD = 17.82; 95% CI, −20.86 to −14.79; $p < 0.0001$). They also found no difference in number of pelvic lymph nodes (WMD = 0.79; 95% CI 0.57–2.16; p = 0.141) or number of para-aortic lymph nodes (WMD = 0.22; 95% CI −0.68 to 1.13; p = 0.625) removed. Thus, when evaluating the previously demonstrated randomized controlled trials as a total group, similar findings were demonstrated among most all of them – increased operating time but decreased blood loss, decreased post-operative complications and similar staging amongst both surgical approaches.

While decreased post-operative complications presumes a benefit to the quality of life of each individual participant undergoing laparoscopy, a study by Kornblith et al. in 2009 specifically addressed this question. Kornblith et al. [28] utilizing the same population of patients from the LAP 2 trial evaluated 802 patients who were randomly assigned to laparoscopy (n = 535) and laparotomy (n = 267) for surgical staging. These patients were given Quality of Life assessments at baseline and at one week post-operation, three week, six week, and six month intervals. They found that at each post-operative interval up to six weeks, patients undergoing laparoscopy had better physical functioning (p = 0.006), less pain ($p < 0.001$), less interference with overall quality of life ($p < 0.001$), earlier resumption of normal activities (p = 0.003), and earlier return to work (p = 0.04). Most of these differences in quality of life, however, were no longer seen at six months from the date of surgery. At this point, patients having undergone laparotomy had similar levels of quality of life in most all metrics as their laparoscopic counterparts. The one measurement of quality of life that remained statistically significant at six months was the improved body image in the laparoscopic patients over the laparotomy patients ($p < 0.001$).

Despite the prior gold standard of clinically early stage endometrial cancer being laparotomy with hysterectomy, bilateral salpingo-oophorectomy and lymph node dissection, studies now have demonstrated time and again that the same oncologic outcomes can be achieved through laparoscopic approaches. Similar levels of lymph nodes collected, recurrence rates, and overall survival are all achieved with reproducible decreases in operative blood loss, length of hospital stays, and decreases in postoperative complications. This is also achieved with short-term benefits in quality of life and long-term benefits of improved body image. As such, minimally invasive surgery is a well-supported methodology of surgery for clinically early stage endometrial cancer with many advantages over laparotomy.

3. In premenopausal woman with endometrial cancer (population), what is the evidence for and against ovarian removal (intervention) in relation to prognosis (outcome)?

Endometrial cancer is usually perceived as a disease of post-menopausal women. Indeed, the most recent Surveillance, Epidemiology, and End Results Database (SEER) puts the average age of diagnosis at 64 years old [1]. However, almost one quarter of these women who were diagnosed prior to the age of menopause [1]. The current gold standard for staging includes bilateral oophorectomy [29]. Oophorectomy is performed to remove potential occult concurrent ovarian cancer or metastases to the ovaries as well as remove the primary source of estrogen that might contribute to recurrence given endometrial cancer's estrogen responsiveness. This procedure, however, forces a number of young women to undergo surgical menopause with resulting sterility and decline in bone, cardiovascular health and potentially, longevity. As such, debate surrounds whether oophorectomy is required for premenopausal women in clinically early stage endometrial cancer.

The primary argument for the removal of both ovaries in women with endometrial cancer comes from the definitive work on the natural pathologic spread of metastasis in early Stage I endometrial cancer by Creasman et al. in 1987 [4]. This study found that of the 621 patients that they evaluated, 5% of all early stage endometrial cancer patients had metastatic spread to the adnexa. Further studies have evaluated the risk for concurrent ovarian or metastatic endometrial cancer to the adnexa specifically within younger pre-menopausal women. They found an incidence of concurrent malignancy within the adnexa ranging between 11% and 29% [30–32]. These studies were, however, small and retrospective and were not limited to patients with clinically stage 1 endometrial cancer. Despite the limitations of these studies, this information has historically supported the argument for bilateral oophorectomy in premenopausal women with endometrial cancer.

Bilateral oophorectomy in general has been shown to negatively impact metabolic and cardiovascular risk in premenopausal women. A large Norwegian study by Dorum et al. [33] evaluated 463 women before the age of 50 years old who had undergone bilateral oophorectomies compared to 789 age matched controls that had not. They found that the women undergoing bilateral oophorectomies were significantly more likely to develop metabolic syndrome as defined by the International Diabetes Federation's definition (47% vs. 36%, p = 0.001) and by the National Cholesterol Education Program/Adult Treatment Panel (NCEP/ATP III) definition (35% vs. 25%, p = 0.002). Furthermore, when evaluating these patients' cardiovascular risk using the Framingham Risk Score, they found that there was a significantly higher proportion of individuals with clinically significant scores in those who underwent a bilateral oophorectomy compared to controls (22% vs. 15%, p =0.005). Another study by the same group [34] looked patients undergoing bilateral oophorectomy as a risk reducing measure due to familial risks of breast and ovarian cancer with similar findings.

Rocca et al. [35] evaluated 1097 In a large population-based cohort analysis, premenopausal women who underwent bilateral oophorectomy for non-malignant etiologies and compared them to 2390 referent women who did not receive an oophorectomy. Those who underwent a bilateral oophorectomy prior to 45 years old were found to have a significantly higher mortality than those who did not (hazard ratio [HR] 1.67 [95% CI 1.16–2.40], p = 0.006). This difference was attributable primarily to non-cancer related deaths (64% vs. 59%, p = 0.009) and not from cancers overall (33% vs. 37%, p = 0.25). Thus, the prospect of removing both ovaries in a premenopausal woman is not an entirely benign process.

These consequences of premenopausal bilateral oophorectomy coupled with the overall excellent prognosis associated with early stage endometrial cancer led clinicians to consider ovarian preservation for premenopausal endometrial cancer patients. Lee et al. [36] found that 7.3% of 260 patients diagnosed with endometrial cancer over a 12-year period had coexisting ovarian malignancy (19 out of 260 patients). 12 of these patients had metastatic carcinoma while the remaining seven had synchronous primaries. They noted, however, that among the subgroup of patients with no visible evidence of extrauterine disease, the coexisting rate was only 0.97% (2 patients out of 206). These data caused authors to conclude that intraoperative evidence of extrauterine disease was a statistically significant predictor of coexisting ovarian malignancy (odds ratio (OR) = 542.1; 95% CI, 57.18 –5129.23). And, importantly, this study found that while 30% of their study population was made up of patients less than 45 years old, not a single patient in this premenopausal age group had any evidence of co-existing ovarian disease when the ovaries appeared grossly normal intraoperatively.

Similarly, Akbayir et al. [37] evaluated 499 patients who underwent surgical treatment for clinical stage I endometrial cancer over a 10 year period and found. Coexisting ovarian malignancy in premenopausal patients was low at 9% and only 5% in patients younger than age 45. This group further noted that intraoperative evaluation was predictive of ovarian pathology with sensitivity of 99.6%, specificity of 78.8, positive predictive value of 98.5% and a negative predictive value of 92.9%.

The actual practice of ovarian preservation in premenopausal endometrial cancer patients was reviewed by Lee et al. [38] in 2009. This group studied 175 endometrial cancer patients over 14 tertiary care hospitals who underwent ovarian sparing surgery with a median follow-up time was 55.0 months finding recurrence free survival of 94.3% and overall survival of 93.3%. Additionally, there were no disease recurrences in patients with Stage I endometrioid adenocarcinoma.

The same group [39], in 2013, further expounded upon these findings in 2013 when they evaluated a cohort of patients across 20 Korean tertiary care hospitals who underwent surgical staging for Stage IA, IB, and II endometrioid endometrial cancer. They identified 176 of 495 patients who underwent ovarian preserving surgery. They compared those undergoing ovarian preservation versus those who had bilateral oophorectomies. Median follow-up duration was 49.0 months and found that the Kaplan-Meier and the log rank test showed no statistically significant difference in recurrence-free survival (p = 0.742) and overall survival (p = 0.462).

Wright et al. [40] evaluated 3269 women from the SEER who underwent surgical treatment for stage 1 endometrioid carcinoma and uterine adenocarcinoma not otherwise specified. They found that of these 3269 women, 402 had ovarian preserving treatment. They compared both groups via Cox proportional hazards models and Kaplan-Meier curves. They found that ovarian preservation had no effect on cancer specific survival (HR = 0.58; 95% CI, 0.14–2.44) or overall survival (HR = 0.68; 95% CI, 0.34–1.35). They interestingly also demonstrated that these findings were unchanged when patients who had undergone pelvic radiation were excluded.

While there is good evidence to suggest that even young patients with clinically early stage endometrial cancer still have a decently high risk of coexisting malignancies in their ovaries, the studies mentioned above point to the fact that the prospect of ovarian removal comes with real metabolic and cardiovascular risks. And, while the risk of coexisting adnexal cancer is real, these studies show that this coexisting ovarian cancer is usually clinically evident in the operating room. And, it has now also been further demonstrated that those patients with younger age and non-surgically evident ovarian disease who maintain their ovaries have similar rates of recurrence and overall survival as those who have them removed. Thus, there is real evidence to suggest that ovarian preservation might be a viable option – particularly in those with age less than 45, no evidence of extrauterine disease, and with endometrioid histology.

4. In premenopausal woman with endometrial cancer (population), what is the sensitivity and specificity (test) of immunohistochemical evaluation for mismatch repair proteins in diagnosing Lynch syndrome?

Lynch syndrome, also known as Hereditary Non-Polyposis Colorectal Cancer, is a well-described autosomal dominant familial cancer susceptibility disorder caused by a germline mutation in of the mismatch repair genes, MSH2, MLH1, MSH6, and PMS2 [41]. While this disorder was originally described as a cause of familial lower colorectal cancers, making up to 1–2% of all colorectal cancers [42], this disorder also places women at significant risk for endometrial cancer and ovarian cancer, among other malignancies. The cumulative lifetime risk for endometrial cancer in women with Lynch syndrome is between 30% and 45% with a mean age of presentation at 50 years old and between 6% and 14% cumulative lifetime risk for ovarian cancer [43]. Importantly, this endometrial cancer often presents about 10 years earlier than sporadic endometrial cancer with age of presentation often between 48 and 62 years old [44].

The typical manner by which patients have been identified as being at-risk for Lynch syndrome was through two primary sets of criteria significantly beholden to family pedigrees – The Amsterdam Criteria II and the Revised Bethesda Criteria. The Amsterdam Criteria relies heavily upon having had at least three relatives with Lynch syndrome related cancers in order to stratify patients into at-risk populations needing to undergo intensive screening or prophylactic treatments. While this screening test has an excellent specificity at 98%, it's sensitivity is only 22% [45]. A response to the Amsterdam Criteria is the Revised Bethesda Criteria. It is designed to screen and select those with newly diagnosed Lynch syndrome related cancers who have family members with similar Lynch-related tumors. This has a higher sensitivity 82% but has a lower specificity at 77% [46]. This test, however, functions to stratify patients as to whether or not they should undergo further genetic testing of their tumor – specifically via microsatellite instability genetic testing. This criteria therefore coupled with microsatellite instability testing increases the specificity of the overall screening.

Now, while microsatellite instability is one method by which a patient and her tumor can be identified as carrying a Lynch syndrome mismatch repair, immunohistochemistry is the alternative. Immunohistochemistry for Lynch syndrome is the process by which color or fluorescent-tagged antibodies are directed toward any of the MSH2, MLH1, MSH6, and PMS2 gene expressed proteins. Tissue is then exposed to this these antibodies and if a particular area under microscopy fails to stain, it reveals that there is a deficiency in that gene's expressed protein – as would happen in Lynch. This therefore often strongly suggests Lynch diagnosis of the tumor. Based on the gene deficiency, the Lynch diagnosis is further confirmed via either polymerase chain reaction-based methylation testing or via whole gene sequencing. This process is often preferred over microsatellite instability testing based on its relative cost accessibility and ease of interpretation [47].

Despite the utility and accessibility of the test, it is also very important to evaluate the sensitivity and specificity of immunohistochemistry in identifying true Lynch syndrome in endometrial cancer patients. Perhaps the most involved study to date evaluating immunohistochemistry in patients with endometrial cancer is that of Hampel et al. in 2006 [48]. They evaluated 543 patients who had a new diagnosis of endometrial cancer. All of the tumors underwent microsatellite instability testing and those that were positive for Lynch defects were evaluated by immunohistochemistry. Those that tested negative for microsatellite instabilities were tested by immunohistochemistry if the patients' clinical picture was concerning for Lynch. This study found that the estimated sensitivity of this immunohistochemistry was between 90% and 96% in identifying high risk microsatellite instabilities. This study did not fully address the specificity of this test given that it did not fully evaluate the patients who had both negative microsatellite instability and a negative immunohistochemistry.

Indeed, the only routinely studied sensitivity and specificity of immunohistochemistry in Lynch syndrome is based on the evaluation of colorectal tumor tissue. In the most recent position statement by Evaluation of Genomic Applications in Practice and Prevention (EGAPP) Working Group [49], there were only nine studies with a total of 149 patients. These however demonstrated a sensitivity of this test at 83%. Two studies were identified that showed the specificity of the test to be 89%.

Thus, while there is no clearly evident information available regarding the specificity of immunohistochemistry in endometrial cancer specifically, a large, well-developed, recent study places the sensitivity for this test at greater than 90%. The specificity is not clear, but the information can be extrapolated from our colorectal cancer date, which places the specificity of this test at 89%. Thus, this test not only has significant practical and financial benefits to its use, it also has a high sensitivity and specificity. Thus, it is appears to be a very useful tool in the process of diagnosing potential Lynch syndrome in women with endometrial cancer – especially those who are premenopausal.

References

1 Surveillance, Epidemiology and End Resukts Program (2018). *SEER Cancer Statistics Factsheets: UterineCancer*. Bethesda, MD: National Cancer Institute http://seer.cancer.gov/statfacts/html/corp.html.

2 American College of Obstetrics and Gynecology (2015). *Endometrial Cancer*. ACOG Practice Bulletin. Number 149.

3 Burke, W.M., Orr, J., Leitao, M. et al. (2014). Endometrial cancer: a review and current management strategies: part I. *Gynecologic Oncology* **134**: 385–392.

4 Creasman, W.T., Morrow, C.P., Bundy, B.N. et al. (1987). Surgical pathological spread patterns of endometrial cancer: a gynecologic oncology group study. *Cancer* **60**: 2035–2041.

5 Mariani, A., Web, M.J., Keeney, G.L. et al. (2000). Low-risk corpus cancer: is lymphadenectomy or radiation necessary? *American Journal of Obstetrics and Gynecology* **182**: 1502–1519.

6 Benedetti Panici, P., Basile, S., Maneschi, F. et al. (2008). Systematic pelvic lymphadenectomy vs no lymphadenectomy in early-stage endometrial carcinoma: randomized clinical trial. *Journal of the National Cancer Institute* **100**: 1707–1716.

7 Keys, H.M., Roberts, J.A., Brunetto, V.L. et al. (2004). A phase III trial of surgery with or without adjunctive external pelvic radiation therapy in intermediate risk endometrial adenocarcinoma: a Gynecologic oncology group study. *Gynecologic Oncology* **92**: 744–751.

8 Creutzberg, C.L., van Putten, W.L.J., Koper, P.C.M. et al. (2000). Surgery and postoperative radiotherapy versus surgery alone for patients with stage-1 endometrial carcinoma: multicenter randomised trial. *The Lancet* **355**: 1404–1411.

9 Kitchener, H., Swart, A.M.C., Qian, W. et al. (2009). Efficacy of systemic pelvic lymphadenectomy in endometrial cancer (MRC ASTEC trial): a randomised study. *The Lancet* **373**: 125–136.

10 Todo, Y. and Sakuragi, N. (2012). Methodological considerations in the analysis of the therapeutic significance of lymphadenectomy in endometrial cancer. *Taiwanese Journal of Obstetrics & Gynecology* **52**: 8–12.

11 Colombo, N., Preti, E., Landoni, F. et al. (2011). ESMO guidelines working group. Endometrial cancer: ESMO clinical practice guidelines for diagnosis, treatment and follow-up. *Annals of Oncology* **22**: vi35–vi39.

12 Abu-Rustum, N.R. et al. (2006). The incidence of symptomatic lower-extremity lymphedema following treatment of uterine corpus malignancies: a 12-year experience at Memorial Sloan-Kettering Cancer Center. *Gynecologic Oncology* **103** (**2**): 714–718.

13 Abu-Rustum, N.R. (2014). Sentinel lymph node mapping for endometrial cancer: a modern approach to surgical staging. *JNCCN* **12** (**2**): 288–297.

14 Tschernichovsky, R., Diver, E.J., Schorge, J.O., and Goodman, A. (2016). The role of lymphadenectomy versus sentinel lymph node biopsy in early-stage endometrial cancer: a review of the literature. *American Journal of Clinical Oncology* **39**: 516–521.

15 Schiavone, M.B., Scelzo, C., Straight, C. et al. (2017). Survival of patients with serous uterine carcinoma undergoing sentinel lymph node mapping. *Annals of Surgical Oncology* doi: 10.1245/s10434-017-5816-4 [Epub ahead of print].

16 Childers, J.M., Brzechffa, P.R., Hatch, K.D., and Surwit, E.A. (1993). Laparoscopically assisted surgical staging (LASS) of endometrial cancer. *Gynecologic Oncology* **53**: 33–38.

17 Spirtos, N.M., Schlaerth, J.B., Spirtos, T.W. et al. (1995). Laparoscopic bilateral pelvic and paraaortic lymph node sampling: an evolving technique. *American Journal of Obstetrics and Gynecology* **173**: 105–111.

18 Holub, Z., Jabor, A., Bartos, P. et al. (2002). Laparoscopic pelvic lymphadenectomy in the surgical treatment of endometrial cancer: results of a multicenter study. *JSLS* **6**: 125–131.

19 Kuoppala, T., Tomas, E., and Heinonen, P.K. (2004). Clinical outcome and complications of laparoscopic surgery compared with traditional surgery in women with endometrial cancer. *Archives of Gynecology and Obstetrics* **270**: 25–30.

20 Bijen, C.B., Briet, J.M., de Bock, G.H. et al. (2009). Total laparoscopic hysterectomy versus abdominal hysterectomy in the treatment of patients with early stage endometrial cancer: a randomized multi center study. *BMC Cancer* **9**: 23.

21 Walker, J.L., Piedmonte, M.R., Spirtos, N.M. et al. (2009). Laparoscopy compared with laparotomy for comprehensive surgical staging of uterine cancer: Gynecologic oncology group study LAP2. *Journal of Clinical Oncology* **27**: 5331–5336.

22 Kondalsamy-Chennakesavan, S., Janda, M., Gebski, V. et al. (2012). Risk factors to predict the incidence of surgical adverse events following open or laparoscopic surgery for apparent early stage endometrial cancer: results from a randomised controlled trial. *European Journal of Cancer* **48**: 2155–2162.

23 Lu, Q., Liu, H., Liu, C. et al. (2013). Comparison of laparoscopy and laparotomy for management of endometrial carcinoma: a prospective randomized study with 11-year experience. *Journal of Cancer Research and Clinical Oncology* **139**: 1853–1859.

24 Malur, S., Possover, M., Michels, W., and Schneider, A. (2001). Laparoscopic-assisted vaginal versus abdominal surgery in patients with endometrial cancer—a prospective randomized trial. *Gynecologic Oncology* **80**: 239–244.

25 Malzoni, M., Tinelli, R., Cosentino, F. et al. (2009). Total laparoscopic hysterectomy versus abdominal hysterectomy with lymphadenectomy for early-stage endometrial cancer: a prospective randomized study. *Gynecologic Oncology* **12**: 126–133.

26 Walker, J.L., Piedmonte, M.R., Spirtos, N.M. et al. (2012). Recurrence and survival after random assignment to laparoscopy versus laparotomy for comprehensive surgical staging of uterine cancer: Gynecologic oncology group LAP2 study. *Journal of Clinical Oncology* **30** (**7**): 695–700.

27 Zullo, F., Falbo, A., and Palomba, S. (2012). Safety of laparoscopy vs laparotomy in the surgical staging of endometrial cancer: a systemic review and metaanalysis of randomized controlled trials. *AJOG* **207** (**2**): 94–100.

28 Kornblith, A.B., Huang, H.Q., Walker, J.L. et al. (2009). Quality of life in patients with endometrial cancer undergoing laparoscopic International Federation of Gynecology and Obstetrics staging compared with laparotomy: a Gynecologic oncology group study. *Journal of Clinical Oncology* **27** (**32**): 5337–5342.

29 National Comprehensive Cancer Center (NCCN). NCCN Clinical Practice Guidelines in Oncology: Uterine Neoplasms. http://www.nccn.org/professionals/physician_gls/f_guidelines.asp#uterine; 2016.

30 Crissman, J.D., Azoury, R.S., Barnes, A.E., and Schellhas, H.F. (1981). Endometrial carcinoma in women 40 years of age or younger. *Obstetrics and Gynecology* **57** (**6**): 699–704.

31 Evans-Metcalf, E.R., Brooks, S.E., Reale, F.R., and Baker, S.P. (1998). Profile of women 45 years of age and younger with endometrial cancer. *Obstetrics and Gynecology* **91** (**3**): 349–354.

32 Gitsch, G., Hanzal, E., Jensen, D., and Hacker, N.E. (1995). Endometrial cancer in premenopausal women 45 years and younger. *Obstetrics and Gynecology* **85** (**4**): 504–508.

33 Dorum, A., Tonstad, S., Liavaag, A.H. et al. (2008). Bilateral oophorectomy before 50 years of age is significanty associated with the metabolic syndrome and Framingham risk score: a controlled population-based study (HUNT-2). *Gynecologic Oncology* **109**: 377–383.

34 Michelsen, T.M., Pripp, A.H., Tonstad, S. et al. (2008). Metabolic syndrome after risk-reducing salpingo-oophorectomy in women at high risk for hereditary breast ovarian cancer: a controlled observational study. *European Journal of Cancer* **45**: 82–89.

35 Rocca, W.A., Grossardt, B.R., de Andrade, M. et al. (2006). Survival patterns after oophorectomy in premenopausal women: a population-based cohort study. *Lancet Oncology* **7**: 821 –828.

36 Lee, T.S., Jung, J.Y., Kim, J.W. et al. (2006). Feasibility of ovarian preservation in patients with early stage endometrial carcinoma. *Gynecologic Oncology* **104**: 52–57.

37 Akbayir, O., Kuru, O., Goksedef, P. et al. (2012). Coexisting ovarian malignancy in patients with clinical stage I endometrial carcinoma. *Archives of Gynecology and Obstetrics* **286**: 1241–1245.

38 Lee, T.S., Kim, J.W., Kim, T.J. et al. (2009). Ovarian preservation during the surgical treatment of early stage endometrial cancer: a nation-wide study conducted by the Korean Gynecologic oncology group. *Gynecologic Oncology* **115**: 26–31.

39 Lee, T.S., Lee, J., Kim, J. et al. (2013). Outcomes of ovarian preservation in a cohort of premenopausal women with early stage endometrial cancer: a Korean Gynecologic oncology group study. *Gynecologic Oncology* **131**: 289–293.

40 Wright, J.D., Buck, A.M., Shah, M. et al. (2009). Saftey of ovarian preservation in premenopausal women with endometrial cancer. *Journal of Clinical Oncology* **27**: 1214–1219.

41 Lynch, H.T. and de la Chapelle, A. (2003). Hereditary colorectal cancer. *New England Journal of Medicine* **348**: 919–932.

42 Barnetson, R.A., Tenesa, A., Farrington, S.M. et al. (2006). Identification and survival of carriers of mutations in DNA mismatch repair genes in colon cancer. *New England Journal of Medicine* **354** (**26**): 2751–2763.

43 Barrow, E., Hill, J., and Evans, D.G. (2013). Cancer risk in lynch syndrome. *Familial Cancer* **12**: 229–240.

44 Giardiello, F.M., Allen, J.I., Axibund, J.E. et al. (2014). Guidelines on genetic evaluation and management of lynch syndrome: a consensus statement by the US multi-society task force on colorectal cancer. *American Journal of Gastroenterology* **109**: 1159–1179.

45 Vasen, H.F.A., Watson, P., Mecklin, J. et al. (1999). New clinical criteria for hereditary Nonpolyposis colorectal cancer (HNPCC, lynch syndrome) proposed by the international collaborative group on HNPCC. *Gastroenterology* **116**: 1453–1456.

46 Umar, A., Boland, R., Terdiman, J.P. et al. (2004). Revised Bethesda guidelines for hereditary nonpolyposis colorectal cancer (lynch syndrome) and microsatellite instability. *Journal of the National Cancer Institute* **96**: 261–268.

47 Mills, A.M. and Longacre, T.A. (2016). Lynch syndrome screening in the gynecologic tract: current state of the art. *American Journal of Surgical Pathology* **40**: e35–e44.

48 Hampel, H., Frankel, W., Panescu, J. et al. (2006). Screening for lynch syndrome (hereditary nonpolyposis colorectal cancer) among endometrial cancer patients. *Cancer Research* **66** (**15**): 7810–7817.

49 EGAPP Working Group (2009). Recommendations from the EGAPP working group: genetic testing strategies in newly diagnosed individuals with colorectal cancer aimed at reducing morbidity and mortality from lynch syndrome in relatives. *Genetics in Medicine* **11** (**1**): 35–41.

19 CHAPTER 19

Cervical dysplasia and HPV

Mila de Moura Behar Pontremoli Salcedo[1] and Kathleen M. Schmeler[2]

[1]*Department of Gynecology and Obstetrics, Federal University of Health Sciences (UFCSPA)/Santa Casa de Porto Alegre, Porto Alegre, RS, Brazil*

[2]*Department of Gynecologic Oncology and Reproductive Medicine, The University of Texas, MD Anderson Cancer Center, Houston, TX, USA*

CASE SCENARIO

A 28-year-old gravida 0 female presents to the gynecologist for routine screening. She undergoes a Pap test that shows high-grade squamous intraepithelial lesion (HSIL). Colposcopy is performed with a large acetowhite lesion noted. Biopsy returns cervical intraepithelial neoplasia (CIN 3) with a focus of adenocarcinoma-in-situ (AIS). She asks what caused this and how she could have prevented it. She would also like to know the probability of this lesion progressing to cancer. You recommend a cold knife cone (conization, CKC) biopsy of the cervix. She would like to have children in the future and asks how the recommended treatment will affect her ability to become pregnant and deliver at term. After all her questions are answered, she agrees to the procedure. On the morning of surgery, the patient is noted to have a positive pregnancy test.

Background

Cervical dysplasia or CIN is a premalignant condition of the cervix. It is caused by the human papillomavirus (HPV) and is usually detected by screening with cytology (Pap test) [1]. Women with low-grade CIN have minimal potential of progression to malignancy. However, women with high-grade CIN can develop invasive cervical cancer if left untreated. The goal of management of CIN is to prevent progression to invasive cancer while avoiding overtreatment of lesions that are likely to regress [2].

Clinical questions

In order to address the issues of most relevance to your patient and to help in searching the literature for the evidence regarding cervical dysplasia and HPV issues, you structure your clinical questions as recommended in Chapter 1.

1. What is the chance of developing cervical dysplasia if infected with the HPV?
2. What are the risk factors for cervical dysplasia?
3. How effective are the HPV vaccines in preventing cervical dysplasia and cancer?
4. What is the risk of recurrence and progression to cancer with and without treatment for CIN 2 and 3?
5. In women diagnosed with AIS (population), what is the risk of recurrence and progression to cancer (outcomes)?
6. In patients who have undergone treatment for cervical dysplasia (population), what are the subsequent risks of preterm delivery and other adverse obstetrical outcomes (outcomes)?
7. How is cervical dysplasia managed (intervention) in pregnant patients (population)?

General search strategy

You begin to address these questions by searching for evidence in the common electronic databases such as the Cochrane Library and MEDLINE looking specifically for systematic reviews and meta-analyses. The Cochrane Library is particularly rich in high-quality systematic review evidence on numerous aspects of cervical dysplasia. In fact, this group's review productivity was the model for the development of the Cochrane Library. When a systematic review is identified, you also search for recent updates on the Cochrane Library and also search MEDLINE and EMBASE to identify randomized controlled trials that became available after the publication date of the systematic review. In addition, access to relevant, updated and evidence-based clinical practice guidelines (CPGs) on cervical dysplasia are

Evidence-Based Obstetrics and Gynecology, First Edition. Edited by Errol R. Norwitz, Carolyn M. Zelop, David A. Miller, and David L. Keefe.

accessed to determine the consensus rating of areas lacking evidence.

Searching for evidence synthesis

Primary search strategy

• Cochrane Library: (cervical dysplasia odds ratio (OR) CIN) AND (topic)

• MEDLINE: (cervical dysplasia OR CIN) AND MEDLINE AND (systematic review OR meta-analysis OR meta-analysis) AND adult AND (topic).

• Consensus guidelines for the management and follow-up of patients with cervical dysplasia are provided by:
  - American Society for Colposcopy and Cervical Pathology (ASCCP) Consensus Guidelines (www.asccp.org) [3]
  - National Comprehensive Cancer Network (NCCN) Clinical Practice Guidelines in Oncology: Cervical Cancer Screening (www.nccn.org) [4]

Critical review of the literature

1. In patients infected with HPV (population), what proportion of patients will develop cervical dysplasia (outcome)?

Search Strategy:

MEDLINE: (cervical dysplasia OR CIN) AND HPV.

There are three categories of CIN based on histological changes:

• CIN 1 includes mild dysplasia and condyloma (anogenital warts).

• CIN 2 includes moderate dysplasia.

• CIN 3 includes severe dysplasia and carcinoma-in-situ (CIS).

CIN is graded based on the extent of abnormal cell proliferation of the basal layer of the cervical epithelium. CIN 1 is considered a low-grade lesion, and CIN 2 and 3 are considered high-grade lesions. In CIN 1, proliferation occurs up to the lower third of the epithelium. In CIN 2, proliferation occurs up to the upper two thirds; and in CIN 3, proliferation occurs in more than the upper two-thirds of the epithelium. In CIS, the entire epithelium is abnormal [5–7].

CIN and cervical cancer are caused by HPV [8]. HPV is a small DNA virus that is sexually transmitted. The initial infection usually occurs during adolescence, and up to 80% of sexually active people become infected at least once during their lifetime. The large majority of HPV infections clear without treatment, however, in some patients the infection persists and can develop into CIN and possibly cancer [9].

HPV is central to the pathogenesis of cervical cancer, with the virus detected in the vast majority of the cases [10]. Furthermore, HPV has also been associated with other malignancies including cancer of the vulva, vagina, anus, oropharynx, and penis [9, 11, 12]. To date, more than 100 HPV subtypes have been identified [13]. Approximately 40 of these are associated with anogenital infections, and include both low-risk and high-risk types. The most common low-risk types are HPV 6 and 11, which account for more than 90% of cases of anogenital condyloma or genital warts. HPV 16 and 18 are the most common high-risk types and account for 70% of cervical cancer cases. Prophylactic vaccines are currently available to protect against HPV [14, 15].

In the United States, 3.5 million (7%) of the 50 million Pap tests performed each year are abnormal and require additional testing. Approximately 300 000 of these women (8.6% of women with abnormal Pap tests) are subsequently diagnosed with CIN 2 or 3 [16, 17]. The cost associated with the diagnosis and treatment of cervical dysplasia and genital warts in the United States is estimated to be $3 billion per year.

CIN 1 with Low-Grade Cervical Cytology:

Given the high rates of spontaneous regression, CIN 1 is usually managed expectantly. This is particularly true if the diagnosis of CIN 1 is preceded by low-grade cervical cytology, i.e. atypical squamous cells of undetermined significance (ASCUS) or low-grade squamous intraepithelial lesion (LSIL). These patients can undergo co-testing with cytology and HPV testing at 12 months or repeat cytology alone at 12 month if patient is 21–24 years old [1, 3].

CIN 1 with High-Grade Cervical Cytology:

If the diagnosis of CIN 1 is preceded by cytology showing HSIL or atypical glandular cells (AGC), there is a higher chance of underlying CIN 2/3 or worse, and more aggressive management should be considered. In patients who have completed childbearing, an excisional procedure is recommended. In women who desire future fertility, close follow-up with cytology and colposcopy at six months is performed [1, 3].

How are CIN 2 & 3 Managed?

Given the lower rates of spontaneous regression and higher rates of progression, it is recommended that most women with CIN 2 or CIN 3 undergo treatment. Both ablative and excisional procedures are used, with similar efficacy rates (>90% cure) in properly selected patients [1–3, 18].

Ablative Procedures:

Ablative procedures are solely for the treatment of CIN and do not provide further diagnostic information. To qualify for ablative therapy, there should be no suspicion of glandular or invasive squamous disease. Specific criteria for ablative therapies include [1, 3]:

• Satisfactory colposcopy (visualization of entire cervical squamocolumnar junction)

• Biopsy confirming presence of CIN; abnormal cytology alone is not sufficient

• Negative endocervical curettage.

The most common ablative procedures used in the United States are cryotherapy and laser ablation:

Cryotherapy:

Cryotherapy cools the ectocervix with a metal cryoprobe using a refrigerant gas, either carbon dioxide or nitrous oxide. The ectocervix is cooled to −20°C causing crystallization of intracellular water that destroys the lesion. A freeze-thaw-freeze-thaw cycle is used where the cervix is frozen for three minutes, allowed to thaw and then frozen again for three minutes [19, 20]. Cryotherapy can be performed in the office setting.

Laser Ablation:

Laser ablation of CIN can be performed by physicians with specialized training. A carbon dioxide laser is directed at the cervical lesion under colposcopic guidance. Water in the tissue absorbs the laser energy, and the tissue is destroyed by vaporization. The lesion is typically ablated to a depth of 5 mm. Several safety procedures must be followed including the use of protective eyewear by all personnel in the procedure room, the use of a blackened or brushed speculum to avoid damage to surrounding tissues by misdirected laser beams, and using wet towels and cloth drapes to prevent fires.

Excisional Procedures:

Excisional procedures have the advantage over ablative procedures of providing a pathologic specimen for further diagnostic information. The specific indications for an excisional procedure over an ablative procedure include:

- Suspected microinvasion
- Unsatisfactory colposcopy (the transformation zone is not fully visualized)
- Lack of correlation between the cytology and colposcopy/biopsies
- Suspected AIS
- Unable to rule out invasive disease
- Lesion extending into the endocervical canal
- Endocervical curettage showing CIN or a glandular abnormality
- Recurrence after an ablative or previous excisional procedure.

The standard procedures used in the United States include cold knife conization (CKC), laser conization, and loop electrosurgical excision procedure (LEEP), also called large loop excision of the transformation zone (LLETZ). In both procedures, the cervix is infiltrated with an anesthetic/vasoconstrictor solution and a cone shaped piece of the cervix inclusive of the transformation zone is removed [21]. This is often followed by an endocervical curettage (ECC) above the cone bed. There is no evidence that one technique is significantly more effective than the other with regards to treatment failures or procedure-related morbidity [20].

Cold Knife Conization:

Cold knife conization (CKC) is performed with a scalpel under general or regional anesthesia in the operating room. CKC is recommended in patients with suspected microinvasion or AIS as the margins can be evaluated without cautery artifact.

Laser Conization:

Laser conization uses a carbon dioxide laser to excise a cone-shaped piece of the cervix. It is usually performed in the operating room under general or regional anesthesia. The laser allows greater flexibility in managing the ectocervical component of the disease because if its ability to combine the vaporization and conization techniques.

LEEP/LLETZ:

The LEEP or LLETZ procedure utilizes a thin wire in the shape of a loop with an electrosurgical generator. The loops are available in a variety of shapes and sizes, allowing individualization of the cone specimen removed in order to avoid excessive excision. This procedure has the advantage of being performed in the office setting.

2. What are the risk factors for cervical dysplasia?

HPV infection is necessary but not sufficient to develop CIN. Most HPV infections are spontaneously cleared by the immune system within one to two years without treatment. Approximately 60% of CIN 1 lesions regress without treatment and less than 1% progress to cancer. However, it is estimated that 5% of CIN 2 and 12% of CIN 3 cases will progress to invasive cancer if untreated [2]. In general, it takes 10 years for CIN to progress to cancer, allowing a significant time period for the detection and treatment of CIN [22]. Progression from CIN to cancer requires persistent HPV infection [9]. Co-factors associated with persistent HPV infection and disease progression include smoking [23], HIV infection and other types of immunosuppression [24].

The risk factors for CIN are the same as the risk factors for HPV infection and cervical cancer. They include [4, 25, 26]:

- Early onset of sexual activity
- Multiple sexual partners
- High-risk sexual partner (i.e. a partner with multiple sexual partners or known HPV infection)
- History of other sexually transmitted infections
- History of vulvar, vaginal, or anal dysplasia
- Immunosuppression
- Cigarette smoking.

3. How effective are the HPV vaccines in preventing cervical dysplasia and cancer?

Approximately 70% of cervical cancers are caused by HPV types 16 and 18. In addition, 90% of genital warts are caused by HPV types 6 and 11. Currently available prophylactic vaccines include Gardasil, which is a quadrivalent vaccine targeting HPV types 6, 11, 16 and 18, and Cervarix, a bivalent vaccine that targets HPV types 16 and 18. Gardasil and Cervarix are administered in three doses at time 0, and at one to two and six months of follow-up, In the United States, it is currently recommended that HPV immunization be offered to girls and boys 11–12 years of age, but can be administered as early as nine years. Catch up-vaccination should be offered to females and males aged 13–26 years who have not been previously vaccinated (http://www.cdc.gov/vaccines/hcp/acip-recs/vacc-specific/hpv.html.) The vaccine is most effective if given prior to sexual debut and exposure to HPV. There are several clinical trials showing the efficacy of these prophylactic vaccines [14, 15].

4. In women diagnosed with CIN 2 and CIN 3 (population), what is the risk of recurrence and progression to cancer (outcomes)?

What is the risk of recurrence following treatment of CIN 2/3?

The rate of recurrent or persistent disease is 5–17% following excisional or ablative treatment for CIN 2 or 3. There are no significant differences in efficacy between the different treatment modalities described [18]. Factors associated with recurrent/persistent disease include:

- Large lesion size
- Endocervical gland involvement
- Positive margins.

Patients who have positive margins on the excised specimens or in the concomitant ECC specimen can undergo a repeat excisional procedure or be followed closely with cytology and endocervical sampling in four to six months [1, 27, 28]. The recommended surveillance following ablation or excision for CIN 2 or 3 with negative margins and ECC consists of HPV testing and cervical cytology (co-testing) at 12 and 24 months [1]. Women diagnosed with CIN 2 or 3 require annual surveillance for 20 years [1, 29].

5. In women diagnosed with AIS (population), what is the risk of recurrence and progression to cancer (outcomes)?

AIS of the cervix is a preinvasive glandular condition, and the precursor to invasive cervical adenocarcinoma. It is less common than squamous cervical dysplasia, representing approximately 25% of preinvasive cervical disease [30]. Most lesions are contiguous, but 10–15% of patients with AIS have multifocal disease with "skip" lesions making management more challenging [31]. In women with known or suspected AIS, cervical conization with ECC is recommended to make or confirm the diagnosis, assess the extent of disease, and exclude invasive disease. CKC is preferred over LEEP in order to adequately assess the margins, but LEEP is also acceptable. If positive margins are noted on the cone specimen, a repeat CKC is recommended. Given the possibility of skip lesions, hysterectomy is recommended following conization for women with AIS who have completed childbearing. If the patient desires future fertility, conservative management with conization alone is acceptable, provided negative cone margins are obtained [1].

The best evidence for AIS outcomes is a meta-analysis by Salani et al. [32] evaluating 1278 women from 33 studies. They noted that a positive conization margin was associated with a significant increase in the risk of residual disease at hysterectomy (OR = 4.01). In addition, of the 671 patients followed up with surveillance only, 2.6% with negative margins and 19.4% with positive margins developed a recurrence (OR = 2.48). They also found invasive adenocarcinoma to be more commonly associated with positive margins (5.2%) compared with negative margins (0.1%). They concluded that patients with positive margins following conization for AIS are significantly more likely to have residual or recurrent disease, whereas those with negative margins can be managed conservatively.

6. In patients who have undergone treatment for cervical dysplasia (population), what are the subsequent risks of preterm delivery and other adverse obstetrical outcomes (outcomes)?

Search Strategy:

- Cochrane and MEDLINE: cervical dysplasia OR CIN OR LEEP OR cold knife cone AND pregnancy loss OR spontaneous abortion.

Excisional and ablative procedures for cervical dysplasia are often performed in reproductive age women and may impact future fertility and pregnancy outcomes [33–35]. Potential adverse effects include cervical stenosis, infertility, second trimester pregnancy loss, preterm premature rupture of membranes (PPROM), and preterm delivery. Several studies have shown that previous conization increases preterm labor and second trimester pregnancy loss [33, 34, 36].

Kyrgiou et al. performed a meta-analysis evaluating the obstetrical outcomes following treatment of intraepithelial and early invasive cervical lesions. In this systematic review of 27 studies, the authors found that CKC was significantly associated with preterm delivery before 37 weeks gestation (relative risk (RR) = 2.59), low birthweight below 2500 g (RR = 2.53), and cesarean section (RR = 3.17). LEEP was found to be significantly associated with preterm delivery (RR = 1.70), low birthweight (RR = 1.82), and PPROM (RR = 2.69). Of note, there were no increased obstetric risks in patients undergoing laser ablation. The authors concluded that all excisional procedures to treat cervical dysplasia are associated with similar pregnancy related morbidity, without apparent neonatal morbidity [33].

A subsequent Norwegian population-based cohort study by Albrechtsen and colleagues compared 15 108 births in women who had previously undergone cervical conization (cold knife, laser, or LEEP) with 2 164 006 births in women who had no CIN treatment, and 57 136 births in women who underwent cervical conization after their index pregnancy. The proportion of preterm delivery was 17.2% in women who gave birth after conization compared with 6.7% who gave birth before conization and 6.2% in women who had not undergone conization. Furthermore, they noted a significantly higher rate of preterm delivery prior to 24 weeks gestation in the group that underwent previous conization (1.5%) compared with the groups that had no cervical dysplasia (0.4%) or underwent treatment after their index pregnancy (0.4%). The relative risk of delivery was 4.4 at 24–27 weeks, 3.4 at 28–32 weeks, 2.5 at 33–36 weeks. The authors concluded that cervical conization increases the risk of preterm delivery, especially at early gestational ages when the clinical significance is highest. However, the study was limited by the lack of stratification by type of conization [34].

An additional meta-analysis by Arbyn et al. [35] reviewed 20 studies encompassing over 12 000 births. They found CKC to be associated with a significant increase in perinatal mortality (RR = 2.78), extreme preterm delivery (<28 weeks) (RR = 5.33), severe preterm delivery (<32 weeks) (RR = 2.78), and low birthweight (<2000 g) (RR = 2.86). In this study, LEEP and cryotherapy were not associated with increased preterm delivery or perinatal mortality. However, a subsequent study by Noehr et al. [37] noted an overall twofold increase in the risk of spontaneous preterm delivery subsequent to LEEP treatment.

Other factors associated with preterm delivery include a greater depth of excision at conization (>10 mm cervical canal) and repeat conizations, with two or more conizations increasing the rate of preterm delivery two- to fivefold when compared with one conization [38–40]. Preterm delivery may also been associated with a short interval between conization and conception. A nested case control study by Himes et al. [41] found increased rates of preterm delivery in women with a 2.5-month interval between conization (LEEP or CKC) and conception, versus a 10.5-month interval. In contrast, other studies have shown no difference in preterm delivery rates in women with a short interval between conization and conception [38].

In summary, women who are planning future pregnancy should be treated with the method that best diagnoses and/or treats their CIN2/3, yet incurs the lowest risk of adverse effects on obstetrical outcomes. The treatment of CIN does not appear to impair fertility in most women but excisional procedures may increase second trimester pregnancy loss and preterm labor. Women undergoing cervical conization should be counseled on these potential associated adverse effects.

7. How is cervical dysplasia managed (intervention) in pregnant patients (population)?

Search Strategy:

- MEDLINE: cervical dysplasia OR cervical cancer OR CIN OR LEEP OR cold knife cone AND pregnancy.

There are high rates of spontaneous postpartum regression of cervical dysplasia and very low rates (<0.5%) of progression of CIN 2/3 to invasive cancer [42–44]. A large study by Yost and colleagues [42] evaluated 153 patients with CIN 2 (n = 82) or 3 (n = 71) diagnosed during pregnancy. The regression rates were 68% for CIN 2 and 70% for CIN 3. None of the CIN lesions progressed to invasive carcinoma. There were no differences in regression rates between women who had a vaginal delivery (n = 130) compared with cesarean section (n = 23). The authors concluded that given the high rates of regression, conservative management during pregnancy is recommended unless invasive cancer is suspected [42, 45].

Current recommendations [3, 4] state that pregnant patients diagnosed with ASCUS on cytology do not need colposcopy or monitoring during pregnancy, and can wait until the postpartum period for further evaluation and follow-up. For pregnant women LSIL or HSIL on cytology, colposcopy with referral to a colposcopist with experience and familiarity with the colposcopic changes noted during pregnancy is recommended. Any lesions concerning for high-grade dysplasia or malignancy should be biopsied. Endocervical curettage should never be performed during pregnancy due to the risk of bleeding and disrupting the pregnancy. If the patient is diagnosed with CIN 2 or 3 on biopsy, repeat colposcopy is performed each trimester to ensure the lesion is not worsening with biopsies only obtained if progression to invasive disease is suspected. Excisional procedures should only be performed if invasive disease is suspected. In general, the treatment of CIN 2/3 is avoided during pregnancy due to the increased risk of adverse pregnancy outcomes including heavy vaginal bleeding and spontaneous abortion. If conization is required during pregnancy, it should be performed in the operating room, with removal of a shallow cone to rule out invasive disease. Cervical dysplasia is not an indication for cesarean section, and the mode of delivery should be based on obstetrical factors. Patients with cervical dysplasia should undergo repeat cytology and colposcopy six weeks postpartum.

Conclusions

Cervical cancer is one of the leading causes of cancer and cancer-related deaths among women worldwide. More than 85% of cases and deaths occur in the developing world where the availability of effective screening is limited. Cervical cancer screening and HPV prophylactic vaccines are required to reduce these cases and deaths.

CIN is a premalignant condition of the uterine cervix. Low-grade lesions (CIN 1) have a great chance to regress, while high-grade lesions (CIN 2/3 and AIS) are at high risk of progression to malignancy. Cervical dysplasia affects women of childbearing age. For women who desire future fertility, conservative management with cervical conization is considered a feasible option. High-grade dysplasia has a high rate of cure when the entire lesion has been excised. However, the treatment can be challenging, particularly in women with AIS, repeat conizations are often required until negative margins are obtained. The large and repeat cervical conizations are known to be associated with adverse obstetrical outcomes, including preterm delivery and very low birth weight infants. Women diagnosed with CIN 2/3 or AIS require surveillance for 20 years, to prevent lesions and their possible progression to invasive cancer.

Conflicts of Interest

None were reported.

References

1 Massad, L.S., Einstein, M.H., Huh, W.K. et al. (2013). 2012 updated consensus guidelines for the management of abnormal cervical cancer screening tests and cancer precursors. *Journal of Lower Genital Tract Disease* **17** (**5 Suppl 1**): S1–S27.

2 Ostör, A.G. (1993). Natural history of cervical intraepithelial neoplasia: a critical review. *International Journal of Gynecological Pathology* **12**: 186–192.

3 American Society for Colposcopy and Cervical Pathology (ASCCP) 2006 Consensus Guidelines. Available at: www.asccp.org. Accessed 3 July 2018.

4 National Comprehensive Cancer Network (NCCN) Clinical Practice Guidelines in Oncology: Cervical Cancer Screening. Version 1.2012. Available at: www.nccn.org. Accessed March 30, 2014.

5 Richart, R.M. (1973). Cervical intraepithelial neoplasia. *Pathology Annual* **8**: 301–328.

6 Luff, R.D. (1992). The Bethesda system for reporting cervical/vaginal cytologic diagnoses. Report of the 1991 Bethesda workshop. *American Journal of Clinical Pathology* **98** (**2**): 152–154.

7 Solomon, D., Davey, D., Kurman, R. et al. (2002). The 2001 Bethesda system. Terminology for reporting results of cervical cytology. *JAMA* **287**: 2114–2119.

8 Walboomers, J.M., Jacobs, M.C., Manos, M.M. et al. (1999). Human papillomavirus is a necessary cause of invasive cervical cancer worldwide. *The Journal of Pathology* **189** (**1**): 12–19.

9 Schiffman, M., Castle, P.E., Jeronimo, J. et al. (2007). Human papillomavirus and cervical cancer. *Lancet* **370**: 890.

10 zur Hausen, H. (2009). Papillomavirus in the causation of human cancers – a brief historical account. *Virology* **384**: 260–265.

11 Kreimer, A.R., Clifford, G.M., Boyle, P., and Franceschi, S. (2005). Human papillpmavirus types in head and neck squamous cell carcinomas worldwide: a systematic review. *Cancer Epidemiology, Biomarkers & Prevention* **14**: 467.

12 Jemal, A., Bray, F., Center, M.M. et al. (2011). Global cancer statistics. *CA: a Cancer Journal for Clinicians* **61** (**2**): 69–90. doi: 10.3322/caac.20107.

13 de Villiers, E.M., Fauquet, C., Broker, T.R. et al. (2004). Classification of papillomaviruses. *Virology* **324** (**1**): 17.

14 (2007). Quadrivalent vaccine against human papillomavirus to prevent high-grade cervical lesions. *The New England Journal of Medicine* **356** (**19**): 1915–1927. FUTURE II Study Group.

15 Paavonen, J., Naud, P., Salmeron, J. et al. (2009). Efficacy of human papillomavirus (HPV)-16/18 AS04-adjuvanted vaccine against cervical infection and precancer caused by oncogenic HPV types (PATRICIA): final analysis of a double-blind, randomised study in young women. *Lancet* **374** (**9686**): 301–314.

16 Kurman, R.J., Henson, D.E., Herbst, A.L. et al. (1994). Interim guidelines for management of abnormal cervical cytology. The 1992 National Cancer Institute workshop. *JAMA* **271** (**23**): 1866.

17 Mahdavi, A. and Monk, B.J. (2005). Vaccines against human papillomavirus and cervical cancer: promises and challenges. *The Oncologist* **10** (**7**): 528.

18 Soutter, W.P., de Barros Lopes, A., Fletcher, A. et al. (1997). Invasive cervical cancer after conservative therapy for cervical intraepithelial neoplasia. *Lancet* **349** (**9057**): 978.

19 Hatch, K.D. (1995). Cryotherapy. *Baillière's Clinical Obstetrics and Gynaecology* **9** (**1**): 133.

20 Martin-Hirsch, P.P., Paraskevaidis, E., Bryant, A., and Dickinson, H.O. (2013). Surgery for cervical intraepithelial neoplasia. *Cochrane Database of Systematic Reviews* doi: 10.1002/14651858.CD001318.pub2.

21 Martin-Hirsch, P.P. and Bryant, A. (2013). Interventions for preventing blood loss during the treatment of cervical intraepithelial neoplasia. *Cochrane Database of Systematic Reviews* **12**: CD001421. doi: 10.1002/14651858.CD001421.pub3.

22 Chang, A.R. (1990). Carcinoma in situ of the cervix and its malignant potential. A lesson from New Zealand. *Cytopathology* **1** (**6**): 321–328.

23 Castle, P.E., Wacholder, S., Lorincz, A.T. et al. (2002). A prospective study of high-grade cervical neoplasia risk among human papillomavirus-infected women. *Journal of the National Cancer Institute* **94** (**18**): 1406.

24 National Cancer Institute (NCI). National Institutes of Health 2014 Cervical Cancer Treatment. Available at: http://www.cancer.gov. Accessed May 06, 2014.

25 Boyle, D.C.M. and Smith, J.R. (1999). Infection and cervical intraepithelial neoplasia. *International Journal of Gynecological Cancer* **9**: 177–186.

26 Schoell, W.M.J., Janicek, M.F., and Mirhashemi, R. (1999). Epidemiology and biology of cervical cancer. *Seminars in Surgical Oncology* **16**: 203–211.

27 MF, M., Tortolero-Luna, G., Cook, E. et al. (1998). A randomized clinical trial of cryotherapy, laser vaporization, and loop electrosurgical excision for treatment of squamous intraepithelial lesions of the cervix. *Obstetrics and Gynecology* **92** (**5**): 737–744.

28 Ghaem-Maghami, S., Sagi, S., Majeed, G., and Soutter, W.P. (2007). Incomplete excision of cervical intraepithelial neoplasia and risk of treatment failure: a meta-analysis. *The Lancet Oncology* **8** (**11**): 985.

29 Soutter, W.P., Sasieni, P., and Panoskaltsis, T. (2006). Long-term risk of invasive cervical cancer after treatment of squamous cervical intraepithelial neoplasia. *International Journal of Cancer* **118** (**8**): 2048.

30 Wang, S.S., Sherman, M.E., Hildesheim, A. et al. (2004). Cervical adenocarcinoma and squamous cell carcinoma incidence trends among white women and black women in the United States for 1976-2000. *Cancer* **100** (**5**): 1035–1044. PubMed PMID: 14983s500.

31 Wolf, J.K., Levenback, C., Malpica, A. et al. (1996). Adenocarcinoma in situ of the cervix: significance of cone biopsy margins. *Obstetrics and Gynecology* **88** (**1**): 82–86. PubMed PMID: 8684768.

32 Salani, R., Puri, I., and Bristow, R.E. (2009). Adenocarcinoma in situ of the uterine cervix: a metaanalysis of 1278 patients

evaluating the predictive value of conization margin status. *American Journal of Obstetrics and Gynecology* **200** (**2**): 182 e1–182 e5. PubMed PMID: 19019325.

33 Kyrgiou, M., Koliopoulos, G., Martin-Hirsch, P. et al. (2006). Obstetric outcomes after conservative treatment for intraepithelial or early invasive cervical lesions: systematic review and meta-analysis. *Lancet* **367** (**9509**): 489–498. PubMed PMID: 16473126. Epub 2006/02/14. eng.

34 Albrechtsen, S., Rasmussen, S., Thoresen, S. et al. (2008). Pregnancy outcome in women before and after cervical conisation: population based cohort study. *BMJ* **337**: a1343. doi: 10.1136/bmj.a1343.

35 Arbyn, M., Kyrgiou, M., Simoens, C. et al. (2008). Perinatal mortality and other severe adverse pregnancy outcomes associated with treatment of cervical intraepithelial neoplasia: meta-analysis. *BMJ* **337**: a1284. doi: 10.1136/bmj.a1284.

36 Sjoborg, K.D., Vistad, I., Myhr, S.S. et al. (2007). Pregnancy outcome after cervical cone excision: a case-control study. *Acta Obstetricia et Gynecologica Scandinavica* **86** (**4**): 423–428. PubMed PMID: 17486463.

37 Noehr, B., Jensen, A., Frederiksen, K. et al. (2009). Loop electrosurgical excision of the cervix and subsequent risk for spontaneous preterm delivery: a population-based study of singleton deliveries during a 9-year period. *American Journal of Obstetrics and Gynecology* **201** (**1**): 33 e1–33 e6. PubMed PMID: 19345930.

38 Noehr, B., Jensen, A., Frederiksen, K. et al. (2009). Depth of cervical cone removed by loop electrosurgical excision procedure and subsequent risk of spontaneous preterm delivery. *Obstetrics and Gynecology* **114** (**6**): 1232–1238. PubMed PMID: 19935024.

39 Jakobsson, M., Gissler, M., Paavonen, J., and Tapper, A.M. (2009). Loop electrosurgical excision procedure and the risk for preterm birth. *Obstetrics and Gynecology* **114** (**3**): 504–510. PubMed PMID: 19701027.

40 Ortoft, G., Henriksen, T., Hansen, E., and Petersen, L. (2010). After conisation of the cervix, the perinatal mortality as a result of preterm delivery increases in subsequent pregnancy. *BJOG : An International Journal of Obstetrics and Gynaecology* **117** (**3**): 258–267. PubMed PMID: 19943823.

41 Himes, K.P. and Simhan, H.N. (2007). Time from cervical conization to pregnancy and preterm birth. *Obstetrics and Gynecology* **109** (**2 Pt 1**): 314–319. PubMed PMID: 17267830.

42 Yost, N.P., Santoso, J.T., McIntire, D.D., and Iliya, F.A. (1999). Postpartum regression rates of antepartum cervical intraepithelial neoplasia II and III lesions. *Obstetrics and Gynecology* **93** (**3**): 359–362. PubMed PMID: 10074979.

43 Kiguchi, K., Bibbo, M., Hasegawa, T. et al. (1981). Dysplasia during pregnancy: a cytologic follow-up study. *Journal of Reproductive Medicine* **26** (**2**): 66–72.

44 Paraskevaidis, E., Koliopoulos, G., Kalantaridou, S. et al. (2002). Management and evolution of cervical intraepithelial neoplasia during pregnancy and postpartum. *European Journal of Obstetrics, Gynecology, and Reproductive Biology* **104** (**1**): 67.

45 Economos, K., Perez Veridiano, N., Delke, I. et al. (1993). Abnormal cervical cytology in pregnancy: a 17-year experience. *Obstetrics and Gynecology* **81** (**6**): 915–918. PubMed PMID: 8497355.

SECTION 2
Obstetrics

Carolyn M. Zelop

General obstetrics

20 CHAPTER 20
Preconception care

Haywood Brown
Morsani College of Medicine, University of South Florida Health Center, Tampa, FL, USA

Introduction

The primary aim of preconception and interconception care is to improve maternal health and birth outcome for mother, infant and family through prevention and interventions. Preconception care is defined by interventions that aim to identify and modify biomedical, behavioral, and social risks to a woman's health through prevention and management. These interventions focus on risk factors that can be modified and/or eliminated prior to conception or in early pregnancy in order to impact overall pregnancy health and birth outcome. The preconception period identifies the time period that these interventions are most helpful. The interconception period is the time between pregnancies that is generally around 18–24 months postpartum when a woman can improve her health status especially if the prior pregnancy was associated with an adverse maternal, obstetrical or birth outcome [1]. In November 2004, the Centers for Disease Control (CDC) launched the Preconception Health and Health Care Initiative which included experts and representatives from over 35 national, state and local organizations and representatives from 22 CDC programs concerned with the health of women and infants. In June 2005, the CDC created a select panel on Preconception Care with the goal to develop recommendations to improve preconception health and care. Recommendations and goals from that summit were released in a report in April 2006. A second submit was held in October 2007 and in December 2008 was highlighted in published supplements focused on preconception health [2].

The essential elements of preconception health promotion and intervention are as follows:

1. Screening for medical and social risk factors
2. Counseling based on age, race, medical, and/or genetic history
3. Providing appropriate immunizations such as rubella and varicella
4. Prescribing intervention aimed at improving overall pregnancy outcome and adult health such as achieving a healthy weight, diabetes control, eliminating inappropriate prescription and non-prescription medications and habits (smoking)
5. General health education

CLINICAL VIGNETTE

A 37-year-old P0 has Type II diabetes for five years that is under fair control with Metformin. She has a body mass index (BMI) of 35 $cm\,m^{-3}$ and is considering infertility treatment because of ovulatory dysfunction. Key components to be considered in her preconception care include the following:

a. Maternal age
b. Pregestational diabetes
c. Obesity
d. Medications

CLINICAL VIGNETTE

A 24-year-old G2 P1102 recently delivered a term female infant with an open neural tube defect (NTD) that was diagnosed late in pregnancy. A prior delivery three years ago was delivered at 33 weeks after preterm premature rupture of membranes. Key components of interconception counseling should include the following:

a. Recurrence risk for NTDs
b. Folic acid recommendations
c. Recurrence risk for preterm delivery
d. Progesterone recommendations

Evidence-Based Obstetrics and Gynecology, First Edition. Edited by Errol R. Norwitz, Carolyn M. Zelop, David A. Miller, and David L. Keefe.

Background and rationale for preconception/interconception care

The concept of preconception counseling can be traced to ancient and biblical writings. In writing by Plutarch, "....all the care that was possible; he ordered the maidens to exercise themselves with wrestling, running, throwing the quoit, and casting the dart, to the end that the fruit they conceived might, in strong and healthy bodies, take firmer root and find better growth, and withal that they, with this greater vigor, might be the more able to undergo the pains of child-bearing" [3]. In a report by Jones and Smith published six months after their initial report on fetal alcohol syndrome (FAS), they presented an "historical review" containing several anecdotes implying that the ancient Greeks and Romans had a rudimentary awareness of the association between maternal alcoholism and abnormal development [4]. One of these anecdotes was an alleged Carthaginian law forbidding bridal couples to drink wine on their wedding night so as to avoid the conception of defective children.

It is estimated that approximately 50% of all pregnancies in the United States are unintended or unplanned [5]. Most births occur during the active reproductive years. In fact, by age 25, 50% of women have had at least one birth and by age 44, >85% of women have given birth at least once. Yet while most women in the reproductive years have seen a health care provider within the prior year preconception counseling may not necessarily be included as a component of that visit [6]. In a Kaiser Family Foundation report in 2005 which surveyed 2766 women >18 years of age, only 55% indicated that they talked to a provider about diet, exercise or nutrition in the past three years, 43% had talked about calcium intake and only 33% and 20% has talked about smoking and alcohol use, respectively [7]. In the US adult population an estimated 7.8% have been diagnosed with diabetes [8], 25% with hypertension [9] and 33% with obesity as defined by a BMI > 30 [10]. For reproductive age women these are conditions that lend themselves to evidenced based interventions and strategies which lead to improved pregnancy outcome and infant health.

The CDC Preconception Health and Health Care Recommendations derived from the first national summit were as follows [2]:

1. Each woman, man, and couple should be encouraged to have a reproductive life plan.

2. Increase public awareness of the importance of preconception health behaviors and services by using information that is relevant across various age groups, literacy levels, and cultural/ethnic groups.

3. As a part of primary care visits, provide risk assessment and educational and health promotion counseling to all women of childbearing age to reduce reproductive risks and improve pregnancy outcome.

4. Increase the proportion of women who receive interventions as follow-up to preconception risk screening, focusing on high priority interventions (i.e. those with evidence of effectiveness and greatest potential impact).

5. Use the interconception period to provide additional intensive interventions to women who have had a previous pregnancy that ended in an adverse outcome (i.e. infant death, fetal losses, birth defects, low birth weight, or preterm birth).

6. Offer, as a component of maternity care, one prepregnancy visit for couples and persons planning a pregnancy.

7. Increase public and private health insurance coverage for women with low incomes to improve access to preventive women's health and preconception and interconception care.

8. Integrate components of preconception health into existing local public health and related programs, including an emphasis on interconception interventions for women with previous adverse outcomes.

9. Increase the evidence base and promote the use of the evidence to improve preconception health.

10. Maximize public health surveillance.

The evidence for folic acid

There is strong evidence for daily consumption of adequate amounts of folic acid prior to conception and the first trimester of pregnancy in reducing the risk for NTDs. Folate is a water soluble vitamin essential for synthesis of thymidylate to thymidine which is needed for DNA synthesis. Folic acid is the synthetic form of folate which must be reduced to the biologically active form L-5-methyl – THF [11].

Supplementation with folate to prevent NTD was first shown in 1980 by Smithells and colleagues, who gave a multivitamin containing 360 mcg per daily to women who had given birth to a prior child with a NTD [12]. While the expected recurrence risk for offspring in this group of women was expected to be approximately 5%, the actual recurrence for NTD was only 0.6% for those women who received the supplemental folate [12].

In 1992 the US Public Health Service issued a recommendation that all females of childbearing age consume 400 mcg of folic acid daily [13]. In 1998 the Institute of Medicine confirmed that reproductive age women capable of pregnancy consume 400 mcg of folic acid daily from supplements or fortified foods or both in addition to natural folate received from diet [14]. In the US mandatory fortification of grain products began in January 1998 and this was followed by a drop in the prevalence of spina bifida by 22.9% [15]. Fortification of grain products increase folate levels by 100 mcg per day however this is well short of the 400 mcg recommended for reproductive age women. In addition, although the recommendation for folate supplementation for reproductive age women was confirmed by the IOM subsequent assessment showed that only 37% of non-pregnant women age 18–45 years were in compliance with this recommendation by taking a daily vitamin containing folic acid [16]. These recommendations were reinforced by the US Preventive Service Task Force in 2009 which issued a Grade A recommendation that counseling be provided to reproductive age women encouraging folic acid consumption prior to pregnancy [17].

Normal maternal serum folate levels of >7 ng ml^{-1} ensure robust cell division for the embryo and the fetus. Adequate levels of folate correlate with the lowest prevalence of NTDs which include anencephaly, spina bifida and encephalocele [18]. The daily preconception consumption of 400 mcg of folic acid reduces the risk for NTD by 50–80% [19]. Closure of the anterior and posterior neuropore forming the neural tube is complete by 28 days' of embryogenesis or 42 days conception based on last normal menses [20].

Several notable trials point to the effectiveness of folic acid supplementation in the reduction of NTDs. A randomized trial conducted by the Medical Research Group Council Vitamin Study Research Group demonstrated reduction in the recurrence risk for NTDs of 72% for women receiving a preconception supplement of 4000 mcg per day of folic acid [21]. Another important randomized trial in women with no prior history of a previous offspring with NTD was conducted by Czeizel and Dudas in Hungary. For those women who received preconception folic acid, NTD occurred in 0 of 2471 women supplemented with 800 mcg per day of folic acid compared to 6 of 2391 women who did not take folic acid [22]. In a population based study in China, women in various geographical regions were given 400 mcg per day of folic acid while others were not given a supplement. For those receiving supplemental folic acid the reduction in the occurrence of NTDs by 79% for a rate of 0.65% in high incidence regions compared to 41% in low incidence regions with a rate of 0.08% [23]. Other studies further suggest that perhaps not all NTDs are folate sensitive or folate resistant and that may be up 25% of NTDs [24].

Folate is potential beneficial for other congenital defects however the evidence is less strong. There is reasonable evidence that supplementation with folate reduces the risk for congenital heart defects [25]. In a study by Czeizel in women supplemented with 800 mcg of folic acid per day there was reduced occurrence of conotruncal cardiac anomalies and urinary tract anomalies such as renal agenesis, cystic kidney, and ureteropelvic junction defects [26]. The cardiac defect risk reduction was 52% or a relative risk of 0.58 compared to controls [26]. A California population based case control study showed a 30% reduction in conotruncal cardiac defects for women using a vitamin with folic acid in early pregnancy [27].

The Evidence for chronic diseases

The incidence of chronic medical disorders such as diabetes, hypertension, and obesity has steadily increased over the past several decades in reproductive age women. These conditions not only complicate pregnancy health and outcome but also long-term adult health.

It has been shown that preconception control of pregestational diabetes lowers the risk for congenital anomalies especially congenital heart and neural tube. In 2010, there were approximately 1.9 million new cases of diabetes diagnosed in adults age 20 years or older. Diabetes affects 25.8 million adults in the United States [8]. Of those 20 and older with diabetes, 12.6 million are women. National survey data from 2007 to 2009 indicated that diabetes affected 7.1% of non-Hispanic whites, 8.4% of Asian Americans, 11.8% of Hispanics, and 12.6% of non-Hispanic blacks [8].

Preconception counseling for women with diabetes continues to be suboptimal despite the evidence that suggest the importance of adequate control of diabetes in preparation for pregnancy to the benefit of the fetus and the mother. A population based study from North of England investigated the association of preconception counseling with markers of care in women with pregestational diabetes. Preconception counseling was associated with better glycemic control three months preconception (Odd Ratio (OR) 1.91, 95% CI 1.10–3.04) and in the first trimester (OR 2.05, 95% CI 1.39–3.03) and a higher preconception folic acid intake (4.88, 95% CI 3.26–7.30). Adverse pregnancy outcome was less likely in the group of women receiving preconception counseling, 6% compared to 10% [28]. In other trials, proactive counseling in teen girls [29] and women [30] with Type 1 diabetes showed sustained improvement and knowledge about planned pregnancy. These studies are relevant in view of the fact than approximately one half of pregnancies including pregnancies in teens with Type 1 diabetes are unplanned.

The risk for structural congenital abnormalities in women with pregestational diabetes is increased four to eightfold over the background risk for anomalies of 1–2% for the general population [31]. The type of abnormalities associated with diabetes are considered multifactorial in origin and include abnormalities of the central nervous system (CNS) such as NTDs, cardiovascular system as well as genitourinary and limb defects. In 1981, Miller et al. compared the frequency of congenital abnormalities based on hemoglobin A1c (HgbA1c) and determined that for those diabetes with a HgbA1c less than 8.5% the rate of abnormalities was 3.4% compared to 22.4% for those with a HgbA1c above 8.5% [32]. Similarly, Lucas et al. found that the risk for congenital abnormalities was nil with a HgbA1c less than 7%, 14% for those with a HgbA1c between 7.2% and 9.1%, 23% with a HbA1c between 9.2% and 11.1%, and 25% with a HbA1c greater than 11.2% [33]. Hemoglobin A1c reflects the level of hyperglycemia over the past several weeks in the red cells. During embryogenesis, hyperglycemia produces a teratogenic effect through disturbance in the metabolism of inositol, prostaglandins, and reactive oxygen species [34]. This leads to excessive oxygen radicals acting upon susceptible fetal tissues which inhibit prostacyclin [35]. Depression of prostacyclin leads to overproduction of thromboxanes and other prostaglandins which lead to disruption of vascularization of developing embryonic tissues and structural defects.

Euglycemia and normal HbA1c levels for several weeks prior to conception and during early embryogenesis could potentially prevent >100 000 pregnancy losses and birth defects annually in the United States [36]. Preconception care aimed at normalizing the HgBA1c has proven to be beneficial in this regard [37].

Preconception evaluation in pregestational diabetes should focus on tight glycemic control with fasting glucose levels below 100 mg/dl and postprandial glucose levels no greater than 120–140 mg mg/dl. This level of euglycemia should result in normalizing to HbA1c to <6.5%. Emphasis should be placed on following an appropriately diet, focused glucose monitoring with defined goals, exercise, and weight loss prior to conception. Hypoglycemic medications, insulin or oral, should be adjusted to a regimen consistent with the goals of achieving euglycemia along with the life-style modifications. Insulin management has been the mainstay of management for poorly controlled diabetes but recent years have seen a rise in the use of the oral agents, glucophage, and glyburide. Glyburide has a favorable safety profile, a Pregnancy Category B classification and crosses the placenta in minimal amounts. Glucophage is also a Pregnancy Category B drug and women on this medication for preconception control of diabetes or insulin resistance can be safely continued throughout pregnancy. Glucophage increases insulin sensitivity and is commonly used for women with polycystic ovary syndrome (PCOS) and insulin resistance to improve ovulation for those women undergoing ovulation induction. For women with Type I diabetes subject to unstable blood sugars consideration should be given to preconception management with insulin pump in the motivated patient. In a study comparing those on insulin pump versus conventional insulin injections HbA1c levels were not significantly different, 7.5 vs. 7.6, respectively [38]. However, HbA1c during organogenesis was better (6.9% vs. 8.5%) and neither group experienced pregnancy loss or a major congenital malformation [38, 39].

Women with diabetes contemplating pregnancy should also be screened for vascular, renal, and ophthalmologic complications prior to pregnancy. For example, women with proliferative retinopathy should be treated with laser prior to pregnancy to prevent further ophthalmologic deterioration during pregnancy. Abnormal renal function increases the risk for hypertensive complications during pregnancy. Women with Type I diabetes should be screened with thyroid stimulating hormone (TSH) for hypothyroidism which occurs in 40% of young women with Type I diabetes.

Chronic hypertension should be controlled prior to pregnancy with the appropriate medications. The goal for blood pressure (BP) control is for the systolic BP to be less than 140 mmHg and the diastolic BP less than 90 mmHg. Chronic hypertension is classified as mild (systolic BP 140–159 mmHg or diastolic BP 90–109 mmHg) or as severe (systolic BP of 160 mmHg or diastolic BP 110 mmHg or greater). The maternal complications associated with chronic hypertension include worsening hypertension and superimposed preeclampsia which predisposes the women to cerebral vascular accident (CVA). The fetal risk includes fetal growth restriction, placental abruption, preterm delivery as a result of worsening maternal condition, cesarean delivery, and perinatal death.

Renal and cardiovascular function should be evaluated prior to pregnancy for end organ damage and a plan of management outlined with the patient. In a population study of 30 000 pregnant women with chronic hypertension maternal mortality was significantly higher compared to normotensive women (OR, 4.8; 95% CI, 3.1–7.6), and a higher risk demonstrated for CVAs (OR, 5.3; 95% CI, 3.7–7.5), pulmonary edema (OR, 5.2; 95% CI 3.9–6.7), and renal failure (OR, 6.0; 95% CI, 4.4–8.1) [40]. The risk for cesarean delivery even for women with uncomplicated chronic hypertension is increased threefold over normotensive women (OR, 2.7; 95% CI, 2.4–3.0) and the risk for postpartum hemorrhage increased twofold (OR, 2.2; 95% CI, 1.4–3.7) [41]. With regard to the fetus the risk for small for gestational age (SGA) infants is increased in women with chronic hypertension [42]. Perinatal mortality is greater than the general population [43]. In another study the risk for stillbirth for women with chronic hypertension was twofold increased (OR 2.04, 95% CI, 1.48–2.82), as was the risk for neonatal death (OR, 2.5, 95% CI, 1.69–3.74) [44].

The preconception evaluation of women with chronic hypertension should include a serum creatinine and urinary proteinuria along with a protein/creatinine ratio or 24-hour urine for protein and creatinine clearance to provide a baseline assessment of renal function. For those with severe hypertension a baseline electrocardiogram (ECG) and ophthalmological exam further defines cardiovascular risk. The risk for cardiomegaly, ischemic heart disease, retinopathy, and renal disease is greater for women with long standing hypertension and especially for those women of advanced reproductive age [45]. For example women with advanced reproductive age, severe hypertension, and a family history of coronary artery disease are at greater risk for myocardial infarction with pregnancy [46]. Women over 40 have a 30-fold higher risk for myocardial infarction compared with pregnancy women less than age 20 years [46]. For these women an exercise echocardiogram may be indicated in addition to an ECG to evaluate cardiovascular reserve. Acute myocardial events have been reported in older women who achieved pregnancy after *in vitro* fertilization [47].

Antihypertensive therapy should be adjusted by maximizing with a single medication to achieve the desired goals for BP control. Women on angiotensin-converting enzyme

(ACE) inhibitors should discontinue this medication prior to pregnancy because of the known teratogenicity associated with the drug. ACE inhibitors have been associated with fetal renal abnormalities, dysmorphia, and stillbirth [48, 49]. Although fetal renal function is not significant until the end of the first trimester, ACE inhibitors used in the first trimester have been associated with major fetal anomalies of the cardiovascular (Risk Ratio (RR), 3.72, 95% CI, 1.89–7.30) and CNS (RR, 4.39, 95% CI, 1.37–14.0) [50]. Currently recommended antihypertensive medications appropriate for use during pregnancy include labetalol, a combined alpha-blocker and beta-blocker which have been extensively studied. Studies indicate that oral beta blockers compared with placebo in women with mild to moderate hypertension decreased the progression to severe hypertension and need for additional medications. However, beta blockers were associated with a higher risk for SGA infants (RR, 1.36; 95% CI, 1.02–1.82) [51]. Calcium-channel blockers have also been used extensively in chronic hypertension and has comparable efficacy to methyldopa for control of hypertension [52]. Diuretics have also been shown to not adversely impact perinatal outcome [53]. In contrast to early thoughts that diuretic use leads to blunting the physiologic increase in plasma volume, no adverse effects have been shown in women who used hydrochlorothiazide prior to pregnancy and continued the medication through conception and throughout pregnancy either alone or in combination [54].

Cardiac disease has become a leading cause of maternal morbidity and indirect mortality [46, 55]. Reasons for the rise in cardiac disease as a complication of pregnancy include the increased incidence of obesity, hypertension, and diabetes in reproductive age women and the fact that women with corrected congenital heart disease have reached the age of reproduction and become pregnant.

Preconception evaluation is essential in order to prevent maternal morbidity and mortality and adverse perinatal outcome. For women with functional class I (asymptomatic) and II (symptoms with greater than normal activity) New York Heart Association classification pregnancy is usually well tolerated and pregnancy outcome favorable. However, for women with Class III (symptoms with normal activity) or Class IV (symptoms at bed rest) the prognosis for successful pregnancy outcome is poor and in some instances contraindicated because of the significant risk for maternal mortality. Conditions considered at high risk for mortality include: pulmonary hypertension, severe systemic ventricular dysfunction, aortic root dilation (more than 4 cm) and severe left-sided obstructive lesions. These conditions carry a mortality of up to 25% to 50% [56].

For women with Class I and II the base line evaluation at a minimum should include and ECG and echocardiogram to evaluate cardiac status and ejection fraction depending on the underlying condition so that counseling can be directed toward potential risk. For women with Class III or IV disease or through imaging studies in the prepregnancy evaluation of women with Class I and II determined to have evidence of more advanced disease than expected and/or pulmonary hypertension, or severe systemic ventricular dysfunction (ejection fraction <40%) counseling should directed toward risk for morbidity and mortality or against pregnancy depending on the level of concern. For these women a more extensive evaluation might be indicated to include stress testing, magnetic resonance imaging and possibly cardiac catheterization to further define risk of cardiac decompensation.

For women with corrected congenital heart disease genetic counseling should emphasize the recurrence risk for the offspring and potential for cardiac decompensation. Women with congenital heart conditions constitute more than 50% of all cardiac disease in pregnancy [57]. The risk for recurrence should be emphasized when the father has congenital heart disease as well. Even with corrected lesions and seemingly normal cardiac status the hemodynamic changes of pregnancy can unmask a compensated defect leading to arrhythmia, heart failure, or death [58].

Preconception counseling is important for the woman who is overweight or obese. Obesity is defined by a BMI > 30 kgm^{-2}. Over 67% of adult Americans are overweight, 26% are obese or morbidly obese [59].

In 2010, adult obesity rates increased and reached 30% in 12 states [60]. The rate of obesity in adult women age 20–39 years in the US has been reported to be as high as 35.5% [59, 61, 62].

A review by Ehrenberg et al. indicated a 70% increase in prepregnancy obesity from 1994 to 2003. [63] Prepregnancy obesity has adverse effects on the fetus and infant, with associations observed between maternal obesity and spontaneous abortion, fetal death, macrosomia, shoulder dystocia, and childhood obesity [64, 65].

In a review by Cedergren et al. comparing women with a BMI > 40 $kg\,m^{-2}$ to normal weight mothers, preeclampsia was increased fivefold, stillbirth after 28 weeks increased approximately threefold and early neonatal death increased approximately three and one half fold over normal weight mothers [66].

Studies indicate that obese women are more likely to have infants with structural congenital anomalies. A large population based study by Watson et al. suggested that obese women were more likely than average-weight women to have an infant with spina bifida (unadjusted odds ratio [OR]: 3.5; 95% confidence interval [CI]; 1.2–10.3), omphalocele (OR: 3.3; 95% CI: 1.0–10.3), heart defects (OR: 2.0; 95% CI: 1.2–3.4), and multiple anomalies (OR: 2.0; 95% CI: 1.0–3.8). Overweight women were more likely than average-weight women to have infants with heart defects (OR: 2.0; 95% CI: 1.2–3.1) and multiple anomalies (OR: 1.9; 95% CI: 1.1–3.4) [67]. Other data also has shown an association between obesity and NTDs and congenital heart defects [68–70].

However, Biggio et al. noted that while the prevalence of maternal obesity and anomaly has increased, maternal weight was not independently associated with an increase in congenital anomalies [71]. A total of 41, 902 pregnancies were examined over three five year periods and maternal weight, BMI, diabetes status and incidence of congenital anomalies were compared. The association between obesity and anomalies was related to the concomitant relationship with diabetes and obesity. In the multivariable logistic model, the major factor contributing to the increased rate of congenital anomalies was the prevalence of pregestational diabetes (OR 3.8, 95% CI 2.1–6.6). The risk for anomalies for obesity increased from 0% in the period 1991–1994 to 6.1% for the period 2002–2004, while the rate of congenital anomalies related to diabetes increased from 3.3% in 1991–1994 to 9.2% for 2002–2004 [71].

A randomized trial of postpartum or interconception care counseling on diet and exercise lead to a significant proportion of women returning to the prepregnancy weight from 30% to 50% [72].

Medications/teratogens

A list of known teratogenic medication is shown in Table 20.1. Some specific medications used in the management of women with chronic diseases require special mention such as anticonvulsants for seizure disorder and warfarin compounds for anticoagulation.

Evidence suggest that most mediations used in the management of seizure disorders have the potential for teratogenicity. These medications include carbamazepine, primidone, phenytoin, and valproate. Therefore these medications should be avoided in the preconception period and throughout the first trimester if possible. For control of women with active seizures monotherapy is preferable. Women should be evaluated in the preconception period in collaboration with a neurologist as to whether there is a need for medications based on type of seizure and last known seizure. If a woman has been seizure free for more than two years and has a normal electroencephalogram (EEG) seizure strong consideration should be given to discontinuing the medications prior to pregnancy and in the first trimester. Recent studies suggest that lamotrigine is the most appropriate first line therapy for partial seizures [73] and to be associated with the lowest risk for major anomalies [72–75].

Table 20.1 Drugs and medications with known teratogenic potential

Medications
Angiotensin-converting enzyme (ACE) inhibitors (e.g. lisinopril, captopril)
Antibiotics
Tetracycline
Streptomycin
Kanamycin
Anti-seizure
Valproic acid
Phenytoin
Carbamazepine
Primidone
Trimethadione
Coumadin derivatives
Isotretinoin
Lithium
Methotrexate and aminopterin (folic acid antagonists)
Others
Thalidomide and leflunomide
Diethylstilbestrol (DES)

Women on Coumadin should discontinue this medication in the preconception period and be converted to heparin for anticoagulation. Coumadin use in the first trimester may result in the fetal warfarin syndrome which include growth restriction, nasal hypoplasia, stippled epiphyses, CNS defects and developmental deficiencies in up to 25% more for exposure during the critical period of development [76]. The critical period of exposure is between the sixth to ninth weeks of gestation [76]. The only condition where there is potentially an acceptable risk benefit for continuation of warfarin during pregnancy are those with mechanical heart valves where the risk for thromboembolism is significantly increased if warfarin anticoagulation is discontinued.

Antipsychotic and antianxiety medications are commonly used by reproductive women with various anxiety, depressive, and psychotic conditions. The only medication with high suspicion for teratogenicity is lithium. The toxicity of lithium in relation to cardiac abnormalities and Ebstein's anomaly was first described in two 1988 reports [77]. However subsequent reports by Cohen et al. in 1994 [78] and Leonard in 1995 [79] suggested that the risk teratogenicity after first trimester exposure to lithium is lower than previously reported especially for women with carefully controlled therapy. However, it is still recommended that treatment with lithium be avoided during the period of cardiac organogenesis [79].

Benzodiazepines freely cross the placenta and accumulates in the fetus during organogenesis [80]. A meta-analysis of cohort and case-control studies of first trimester exposure to benzodiazepines and major malformations showed no relationship to major malformations (OR 0.90, 95% CI 0.61–1.35) or oral clefts (OR 1.19, 95% CI 0.34–4.15) [81]. Data from nine case control studies did show a relationship with major defects (OR 3.01, 95% CI 1.32–6.84) and oral clefts (OR 1.79, 95% CI 1.13–2.82) [81]. While the teratogenicity of benzodiazepines is controversial use of these medications throughout pregnancy has been associated with neonatal withdrawal. Women using these medications should be counseled to use the lowest possible dose to control symptoms.

In contrast, the class of antidepressant labeled as selective serotonin reuptake inhibitor (SSRI) have extensive reproductive studies in rats and rabbits without evidence of teratogenicity [82]. A prospective study comparing pregnancy outcome of 228 exposures to fluoxetine compared to 254 controls showed a similar rate of spontaneous abortion (10% vs. 8.5%, respectively) and structural anomalies (5.5% vs. 4.0%) [83]. The primary conclusion of meta-analysis by Addis et al. based on available data was that SSRIs are not associated with structural defects with first trimester exposure [84].

The exception to these conclusions may be with the SSRI, paroxetine in which animal and human pregnancy experience suggested no major teratogenic risk. However, more recent reports suggest a relationship with first trimester exposure and cardiac defects which prompted a Food and Drug Administration (FDA) warning in 2005 advising health care professionals to discuss the potential risk of birth defects with patients taking Paxil who plan to become pregnant or are in their first three months of pregnancy. The risk of heart defects in babies whose mothers had taken Paxil early in pregnancy was about 2%, compared to a 1% risk in the whole population. In one study, the risk of heart defects in babies whose mothers had taken Paxil in the first three months of pregnancy was 1.5%, compared to 1% in babies whose mothers had taken other antidepressants in the first three months of pregnancy [85].

Women taking prednisone and prednisolone during the first trimester might have an increased risk for oral clefts according to a meta-analysis report which showed an OR 3.03, CI 1.08–8.54 and case control studies (OR 3.35, 95% CI 1.97–5.69) [86]. Women who require these medications to control disease such as collagen/rheumatoid conditions and asthma should be so advised risk.

Isotretinoin is a vitamin A isomer for treatment of severe acne. This medication has proven teratogenicity in animals [87] and human studies [88]. Approximately 38% of women using isotretinoin are age 13–19 years [89]. It is important that women using isotretinoin medications avoid pregnancy and if planning pregnancy this medication should be discontinued at least one month prior to conception.

Substance abuse and environmental toxins

Alcohol is one of the oldest teratogens known to mankind. In 1981 a comprehensive report on FAS was published describing the patterns of anomalies [90]. Mild forms of FAS typically might be manifest by low birth weight and can occur with daily consumption as little as two drinks or 1 oz of absolute alcohol per day in early pregnancy. The complete syndrome with the constellation of anomalies can been seen when maternal consumption is four to five drinks per day or 60–75 ml of absolute alcohol. The incidence of FAS is estimated to be between 1/300 and 1/2000 births with 30–40% of the offspring of alcoholic mothers expected to show the classic features of the syndrome depending on the population [91]. The mechanism by which alcohol produces a teratogen effect has been theorized to be related to acetaldehyde, a metabolic byproduct of ethanol [91]. The anomalies associated with FAS include: craniofacial dysmorphology, prenatal, and antenatal growth restriction, CNS dysfunction and various other anomalies [92]. Researchers have not been able to find an absolute association between paternal alcohol consumption and birth weight, [93] or structural anomalies [94]. A safe level of maternal alcohol consumption during embryogenesis and throughout pregnancy is unclear A prospective study between 1974 and 1977 at the Kaiser Permanente Health Maintenance Organization in Northern California who conducted to determine whether light to moderate consumption of alcohol during pregnancy was associated with congenital defects. The total rate of anomalies was similar between non-drinkers and light (less than one drink per day) or moderate drinkers (one to two drinks per day) at 78.1/1000, 77.3/1000 and 83.2/1000, respectively [95]. **Nonetheless, current recommendations advise against any alcohol use during pregnancy.**

Cigarette smoking during pregnancy has numerous adverse effects for mother and fetus and smoking cessation is associated with reduced risk for prematurity, low birth weight, growth restriction, and perinatal death [96]. Relationship between cigarette smoking and birth defects is contradictory. A report in 2003 from the Teratology Society concluded that smoking is not associated with major congenital malformations [97]. Counseling and education on smoking cessation before and during pregnancy increase smoking cessation rates in numerous trials. Medications used for smoking cessation include bupropion, Chantix and various forms of nicotine replacement. Both bupropion [98] and Chantix [99] have shown benefit for smoking cessation during pregnancy and have not been associated with teratogenicity. While nicotine replacement has the potential for imposing a nicotine induced reduction in uterine blood flow such risk when balanced against the continued use of cigarettes with numerous known by-products including carbon monoxide would suggest benefit for the woman who is unable to achieve smoking cessation without such medications [100].

Various recreational drugs including cocaine, cannabinoids and methamphetamine have in various case reports been linked to birth defects. However, most series of cocaine exposed women have found no association with major and minor structural anomalies after controlling for various maternal characteristics [101]. There is some evidence that marijuana might potentiate the fetal effects of alcohol, however, no pattern of malformations has been observed primarily from in utero exposure to marijuana [102]. Shortening gestation and fetal growth restriction are associated with recreation drug use however, socio-environmental factors in addition to these exposures contribute to these outcomes. There is evidence that illicit substance exposure during pregnancy predisposes children to developmental and hyperactivity disorders [102, 103].

Conclusions

According to a CDC report in 2006, preconception counseling should be included as a component of standard primary care [36]. Unfortunately, evidence suggests that most primary care practitioners including obstetricians and gynecologist do not take advantage of such opportunities. In fact, only one of six obstetricians/gynecologist or family medicine physicians provide preconception care to the majority of women for whom they provide prenatal care [104]. Preconception counseling allows a women and her partner the opportunity to develop not only a preconception plan for improved pregnancy health but also a reproductive life plan to improve long-term adult health. This is the responsibility of all clinicians providing care to women of reproductive age especially those with chronic diseases (Table 20.2). In a randomized trial of women screened with a preconception survey at the time of a negative pregnancy test an average of nine risks factors that could potentially impact pregnancy health were identified [105]. Through preconception education reproductive age women can be provided with evidence-based recommendations that lead to a healthier pregnancy outcome with a planned or unplanned pregnancy. As such, preventative measures such as weight loss with the goal of achieving an healthy weigh prior to pregnancy, taking a vitamin that contains at least the minimal daily requirement of folic acid at least eight weeks prior to conception, elimination of smoking and alcohol and stabilization of medical conditions such as diabetes and hypertension with the use of safe and effective medications should be incorporated into the health and reproductive planning for all reproductive age adults.

Table 20.2 Major components of a routine preconception visit for reproductive women

History
Medical/surgical (chronic diseases)
Family (cardiovascular, diabetes, cancer, etc.)
Genetic (hereditary disorders, congenital anomalies)
Psychosocial (habits, exposures, fitness and nutrition, partner)
Reproductive (obstetric, gynecologic, contraceptive)
Medications (prescription, non-prescription, vitamins)
Immunization/vaccination
Examination
Weight, height (BMI), blood pressure, pulse
Physical (limited or complete)
Laboratory testing
Specific to condition or age appropriate screenings (i.e. HgA1c for diabetes)

References

1 Centers for Disease Control and Prevention (2006). Recommendations to improve preconception health and health care-United States: a report of the CDC/ATDSR preconception care work group and select panel on preconception care. *MMWR* **55** (**RR-6**): 1–21.

2 Jack, B. and Atrash, H.K. (2008). Guest editors. Preconception health and health care: the clinical content of preconception care. *Am. J. Obstet. Gynecol.* **199**: S257–S395.

3 Plutarch (1932). *Lycurgus 14* (ed. J. Dryden), 59–60. New York, NY: Random House.

4 Jones, K.L. and Smith, D.W. (1973). Recognition of the fetal alcohol syndrome in early infancy. *Lancet* **2**: 999–1001.

5 Henshaw, S.K. (1998). Unintended pregnancy in the United States. *Fam. Plann. Perspect.* **30** (**1**): 24–29.

6 Atrash, H., Jack, B.W., Johnson, K. et al. (2008). Where is the "W"oman in MCH? *Am. J. Obstet. Gynecol.* **1999** (**Suppl 2**): S259–S265.

7 Women and Health Care (2005). *Key Findings from the Kaiser Women's Health Survey Kaiser Family Foundation*, VI. Washington DC.

8 Centers for Disease Control and Prevention (2011). *National diabetes fact sheet: national estimates and general information on diabetes and prediabetes in the United States*. Atlanta, GA: US Department of Health and Human Services.

9 Chobanian, A.V., Bakris, G.L., Black, H.R. et al. (2003). Seventh report of the Joint National Committee on prevention, detection, evaluation and treatment of high blood pressure. *Hypertension* **42** (**6**): 1206–1252.

10 Ogden, C.L., Carroll, M.D., Curtin, L.R. et al. (2006). Prevalence of overweight and obesity in the United States, 1999-2004. *JAMA* **295** (**13**): 1549–1555.

11 Simpson, J.L., Bailey, L.B., Pietrzik, K. et al. (2010). Micronutrients and women of reproductive potential: required dietary intake and consequences of dietary deficiency or excess. Part I-Folate, vitamin b12, vitamin B6. *J. Matern. Fetal Neonatal Med.* doi: 10.3109/14767051003678234.

12 Smithells, R.W., Sheppard, S., Schorah, C.J. et al. (1980). Possible prevention of neural-tube defects by periconceptional vitamin supplementation. *Lancet* **1** (**8164**): 339–340.

13 Centers for Disease Control and Prevention (1992). Recommendations for the use of folic acid to reduce the number of cases of spina bifida and other neural tube defects. *MMWR Recomm. Rep.* **41** (**RR-14**): 1–7.

14 Institute of Medicine. Food and Nutrition Board (1998). *Dietary Reference Intakes for Tiamin, Riboflavin, Niacin, Vitamin B6, Folate, Vitamin B12, Pantothenic Acid, Biotin, and Choline*. Washington DC: National Academy Press.

15 Honein, M.A., Paulozzi, L.J., Mathews, T.J. et al. (2001). Impact of folic acid fortification of the US food supply on the occurrence of neural tube defects. *JAMA* **285** (**23**): 2981–2986.

16 March of dimes foundation. *Improving Preconception Health: Womens' Knowledge and Use of Folic Acid.* March of Dimes. website: http://www.marchofdimes.com/peristats/pdfdocs/2007_FA_report.pdf.Published 2007, Accessed February 15, 2012.

17 US Preventive Services Task Force (2009). Folic acid for the prevention of neural tube defects: US Preventive Services Task Force recommendation statement. *Ann. Intern. Med.* **150** (**9**): 626–631.

18 Daly, L.E., Kirke, P.N., Molly, A. et al. (1995). Folate levels and neural tube defects. Implications for prevention. *JAMA* **274** (**21**): 1698–1702.

19 Centers for Disease Control and Prevention (2008). Use of supplements containing folic acid among women of childbearing age-United States, 2007. *MMWR Morb. Mortal. Wkly. Rep.* **57** (**1**): 5–8.

20 Kauwell, G.P.A., Diaz, M., Yang, Q., and Bailey, L.B. (2010). Folate: recommended intakes, consumption, and status. In: *Folate in Health and Diseases*, 2e (ed. L.B. Bailey), 467–490. Boca Raton, FL: CRC Press, Taylor and Francis Group.

21 MRC Vitamin Study Research Group (1991). Prevention of neural tube defects: results of the Medical Research Council vitamin study. *Lancet* **338** (**8760**): 131–137.

22 Czeizel, A.E. and Dudas, I. (1992). Prevention of the first occurrence of neural tube defects by preiconceptional vitamin supplementation. *N. Engl. J. Med.* **327** (**26**): 1832–1835.

23 Berry, R.J., Li, Z., Erickson, J.D. et al. (1999). Prevention of neural tube defects with folic acid in China. Cina-US collaborative project for neural tube defect prevention. *N. Engl. J. Med.* **341** (**20**): 1485–1490. Erratum in: N Engl J Med. 1999; 341 (24):1864.

24 Mills, J.L., Rhoads, G.G., Simpson, J.L. et al. (1989). The absence of a relation between the periconceptional use of vitamins and neural-tube defects. National Institute of Child Health and Human Developmental and Neural Tube Defects Study Group. *N. Engl. J. Med.* **321** (**7**): 430–435.

25 Botto, L.D., Mulinare, J., and Erickson, J.D. (2003). Do multivitamin or folic acid supplements reduce the risk for congenital heart defects? Evidence and gaps. *Am. J. Med. Genet.* **121A** (**2**): 95–101.

26 Czeizel, A.E. (1996). Reduction of urinary tract and cardiovascular defects by periconceptional multivitamin supplementation. *Am. J. Med. Genet.* **62** (**2**): 179–183.

27 Shaw, G.M., O'Malley, C.D., Wasserman, C.R. et al. (1995). Maternal periconceptional use of multivitamins and reduced risk for conotruncal heart defects and limb deficiencies among offspring. *Am. J. Med. Genet.* **59** (**4**): 536–545.

28 Tripathi, A., Rankin, J., Aarvold, J. et al. (2010). Preconception counseling in women with diabetes: a population-based study in the North of England. *Diabetes Care* **33**: 586–588.

29 Charron_Erochownik, D., Ferons-Hannan, M., Sereika, S., and Becker, D. (2008). Randomized efficacy trial of early preconception counseling for diabetic teens (READY-girls). *Diabetes Care* **31**: 1327–1330.

30 Willhoite, M.B., Bennert, H.W. Jr., Palmomaki, G.E. et al. (1993). The impact of preconception counseling on pregnancy outcome: the experience of the Maine Diabetes in Pregnancy Program. *Diabetes Care* **16**: 450–455.

31 Reece, A.E., Sivan, E., Francis, G. et al. (1998). Pregnancy outcomes among women with and without diabetes microvascular disease (White's classes B to FR) versus non-diabetic controls. *Am. J. Perinatol.* **15**: 549.

32 Miller, E., Hafre, J.W., Cloherty, P. et al. (1981). Elevated maternal hemoglobin A1c in early pregnancy and major congenital anomalies in infants of diabetic mothers. *N. Engl. J. Med.* **304**: 1331.

33 Lucas, M.J., Leveno, K.J., Williams, M.L. et al. (1989). Early pregnancy glycosylated hemoglobin, severity of diabetes, and fetal malformations. *Am. J. Obstet. Gynecol.* **161**: 426–431.

34 Eriksson, U.J., Borg, L.A., Cederberg, J. et al. (2000). Pathogenesis of diabetes-induced congenital malformations. *Ups. J. Med. Sci.* **105**: 53.

35 Warso, M.A. and Lands, W.E.M. (1983). Lipid peroxidation in relation to prostacyclin and thromboxane physiology and pathophysiology. *Br. Med. Bull.* **39**: 277.

36 Johnson, K., Posner, S.F., Biermann, J. et al. (2006). Recommendations to improve preconception health and health care-United States. A report of the CDC/ATSDR Preconception Care Work Group and the Select Panel on Preconception Care. *MMWR Recomm. Rep.* **55** (**R-6**).

37 Pearson, D.W., Dernahhan, D., Lee, R. et al. (2007). The relationship between pre-pregnancy care and early pregnancy loss, major congenital anomalies or perinatal death in type I diabetes mellitus. *Br. J. Obstet. Gynecol.* **114**: 104–107.

38 Hieronimus, S., Cupelli, C., Bongain, A. et al. (2005). Pregnancy in type 1 diabetes: insulin pump versus intensified conventional therapy. *Gynecol. Obstet. Fertil.* **33**: 389–394.

39 Farrar, D., Tuffnell, D.J., and West, J. (2007). Continuous subcutaneous insulin infusion versus multiple daily injections of insulin for pregnant women with diabetes. *Cochrane Database Syst. Rev.* **18** (**3**): CD005542. doi: 10.1002/14651858. Epub 2007 Jul 18.

40 Gilbert, W.M., Young, A.L., and Danielsen, B. (2007). Pregnancy outcomes in women with chronic hypertension; a population based study. *J. Reprod. Med.* **52**: 1046–1051.

41 Vanek, M., Sheiner, E., Levy, A., and Mazor, M. (2004). Chronic hypertension and the risk for adverse pregnancy outcome after superimposed preeclampsia. *Int. J. Gynaecol. Obstet.* **86**: 7–11.

42 Vanek, Gilbert, Zetterstrom, K. et al. (2006). Chronic hypertension as a risk factor for offspring to be small for gestational age. *Acta Obstet. Gynecol. Scand.* **85**: 1046–1050.

43 Vanek, Allen, V.M., Joseph, K. et al. (2004). The effect of hypertensive disorders in pregnancy on small for gestational age and stillbirth; a population based study. *BMC Pregnancy Childbirth* **4**: 17.

44 Zetterson, K., Lindeberg, S.N., Haglund, B., and Hanson, U. (2008). The association of maternal chronic hypertension with perinatal death in male and female offspring; a record linkage study of 866, 188 women. *BJOG* **115**: 1436–1442.

45 (2000). Report of the National High Blood Pressure Education Program Working Group on High Blood Pressure in Pregnancy. *Am. J. Obset. Gynecol.* **183**: S1–S22.

46 James, A.H., Jamison, M.G., Biswas, M.S. et al. (2006). Acute myocardial infarction in pregnancy: a United States population-based study. *Circulation* **113**: 1564–1571.

47 Karadag, B. and Roffi, M. (2009). Postpartal dissection of all coronary arteries in an in vitro-fertilized postmenopausal woman. *Tex. Hear. Inst. J.* **36**: 168–170.

48 Hanssens, M., Keirse, M.J., Vankelecom, F., and Van Assche, F.A. (1991). Fetal and neonatal effects of treatment with angiotensin-converting enzyme inhibitors in pregnancy. *Obstet. Gynecol.* **78**: 128–135.

49 Pryde, P.G., Sedman, A.B., Nugent, C.E., and Barr, M. Jr. (1993). Angiotensin converting enzyme inhibitor fetopathy. *J. Am. Soc. Nephrol.* **3**: 1575–1582.

50 Cooper, W.O., Hernandez-Diaz, S., Arbogast, P.G. et al. (2006). Major congenital malformations after first trimester exposure to ACE inhibitors. *N. Engl. J. Med.* **354**: 2443–2451.

51 Magee, L. and Duley, L. (2003). Oral beta blockers for mild to moderated hypertension during pregnancy. *Cochrane Database Syst. Rev.* (**3**): C002863. doi: 10.1002/14651858.CD002863.

52 Abalos, E., Duley, L., Steyn, D.W., and Henderson-Smart, D.J. (2007). Antihypertensive drug therapy for mild to moderate hypertension during pregnancy. *Cochrane Database Syst. Rev.* (**1**): CD002252. doi: 10.1002/14641858.CD002252.pub2 (metaanalysis).

53 Collins, R., Yusuf, S., and Peto, R. (1985). Overview of randomized trials of diuretics in pregnancy. *Br. Med. J.* **290**: 17–23.

54 Sibai, B.M., Grosman, R.A., and Grossman, H.G. (1984). Effects of diuretics on plasma volume in pregnancies with long-term hypertension. *Am. J. Obstet. Gynecol.* **150**: 831–835.

55 Lewis, G. (2011). Saving Mothers' Lives: reviewing maternal deaths to make motherhood safer: 2006-2008. The Eighth report of the Confidential Enquiries into Maternal Deaths in the United Kingdom. *BJOG* **111** (**Suppl 1**): 1–203.

56 Berg, C.J., Callaghan, W.M., Syveson, C., and Henderson, Z. (2010). Pregnancy related mortality in the United States, 1998 to 2005. *Obstet. Gynecol.* **116**: 1302–1309.

57 Merz, W.M., Keyver-Pail, M.D., Baumgarten, G.L. et al. (2011). Spectrum of cardiovascular findings during pregnancy and parturition at a tertiary referral center. *J. Perinat. Med.* **39**: 251–256.

58 Drenthen, W., Pierper, P.G., Roos-Hesselink, J.W. et al. (2007). Outcome of pregnancy in women with congenital heart disease: a literature review. *J. Am. Coll. Cardiol.* **49**: 2303–2311.

59 Flegal, K.M., Carroll, M.D., Ogden, C.L., and Johnson, C.L. (2002). Prevalence and trends in obesity among US adults, 1999-2000. *JAMA* **288**: 1723–1727.

60 Centers for Disease Control. US Obesity Trends by State 1985–2010. Data from the National Health and Examination Survey (NHANES). July 2011.

61 Flegal, K.M., Carroll, M.D., Ogden, C.L., and Curtin, L.R. (2010). Prevalence and trend in obesity among US adults, 1999-2008. *JAMA* **303**: 235–241.

62 Ogden, C.L., Carroll, M.D., Mcdowell, M.A., and Flegal, K.M. (2007). Obesity among adults in the United States: no change since 2003-2004. *NCHS Data Brief* No. 1. Hyattsville (MD): National Center for Health Statistics.

63 Ehrenberg, H.M., Dierker, L., Milluzzi, C., and Mercer, B.M. (2002). Prevalence of maternal obesity in an urban center. *Am. J. Obstet. Gynecol.* **187**: 1189–1193.

64 American College of Obstetricians and Gynecologists (2005). Committee on obstetric practice. Obesity in pregnancy. *Obstet. Gynecol.* **106**: 671–675.

65 Davies, G.A., Maxwell, C., McLeod, L. et al. (2010). Obesity in pregnancy. *J. Obstet. Gynaecol. Can.* **32**: 165–173.

66 Cedergren, M.I. (2004). Maternal morbid obesity and the risk of adverse pregnancy outcomes. *Obstet. Gynecol.* **103**: 219–224.

67 Watson, M.L., Rasmussen, S.A., Honein, M.A. et al. (2003). Maternal obesity and the risk for birth defects. *Pediatrics* **111**: 1152–1158.

68 Rasmussen, S.A., Chu, S.Y., Kim, S.Y. et al. (2008). Maternal obesity and risk of neural tube defects: a metaanalysis. *Am. J. Obstet. Gynecol.* **198**: 611–619.

69 Stothard, K.J., Tennant, P.W., Bell, R., and Rankin, J. (2009). Maternal overweight and obesity and the risk of congenital anomalies: a systematic review and meta-analysis. *JAMA* **301**: 636–650.

70 Mills, J.L., Troendle, J., Conley, M.R. et al. (2010). Maternal obesity and congenital heart defects: a population-based study. *Am. J. Clin. Nutr.* 1543–1549.

71 Biggio, J.R., Chapman, V., Neely, C. et al. (2010). Fetal anomalies in obese women: the contribution of diabetes. *Obstet. Gynecol.* **115**: 290–296.

72 Kinnunen, T.I., Pasanen, M., Aittasalo, M. et al. (2007). Reducing postpartum weight retention-a pilot in primary health care. *Nutr. J.* **6**: 21–30.

73 French, J.A. (2007). First-choice drug for newly diagnosed epilepsy. *Lancet* **369**: 970–971.

74 Morrell, M.J. (1996). The new antiepileptic drugs and women, efficacy, reproductive health, pregnancy and fetal outcome. *Epilepsia* **37** (**Suppl 6**): S34–S44.

75 Marson, A.G., Al-Kharusi, A.M., Appleton, R. et al. (2007). The SANAD study of effectiveness of carvamazepine, gabapentin, lamotrigine, oxcarbazepine, or tropiramate for treatment of partial epilepsy: an unblended randomized controlled trial. *Lancet* **369**: 1000–1015.

76 Hall, J.G., Pauli, R.M., and Wilson, K.M. (1980). Maternal and fetal sequelae of anticoagulation during pregnancy. *Am. J. Med.* **68**: 122–140.

77 Warkany, J. (1988). Teratogen update: lithium. *Teratology* **38**: 593–596. Kallen B. comments on teratogen update Lithium 1988; 38:597.

78 Cohen, L.S., Friedman, J.M., Jefferson, J.W. et al. (1994). A reevaluation of risk of in utero exposure to lithium. *JAMA* **271**: 146–150.

79 Leonard, A., Hantson, P.H., and Gerber, G. (1995). Mutagenicity, carcinogenicity and teratogenicity of lithium compounds. *Mutat. Res.* **339**: 131–137.

80 Jauniaux, E., Jurkovic, D., Lees, C. et al. (1996). In-vivo study of diazepam transfer across the first trimester human placenta. *Hum. Reprod.* **11**: 889–892.

81 Dolovich, L.R., Addis, A., Vaillancourt, J.M.R. et al. (1998). Benzodiazepine use in pregnancy and major malformations or oral cleft: meta-analysis of cohort and case controlled studies. *BMJ* **317**: 839–843.

82 Prozac (2000). *Product Information*. Indiana, USA: Dista Products, Eli Lilly & Co.

83 Chambers, C.D., Johnson, D.A., Dick, L.M. et al. (1996). Birth outcomes in pregnant women taking fluoxetine. *N. Engl. J. Med.* **335**: 1010–1015.

84 Addis, A. and Koren, G. (2000). Safety of fluoxetine during the first trimester of pregnancy: a meta-analytical review of epidemiological studies. *Psychol. Med.* **30**: 89–94.

85 Wurst, K.E., Poole, C., Ephross, S.A. et al. (2010). First trimester paroxetine use and the prevalence of congenital, specifically cardiac, defects: a meta-analysis of epidemiological studies. *Birth Defects Res. A Clin. Mol. Teratol.* **88**: 159–170. (Study WEUSRTP 2280).*GlaxoSmithKline Local Label.

86 Park-Wyllie, L., Mazzotta, P., Pastuszak, A. et al. (2000). Birth defects after maternal exposure to corticosteroids: prospective cohort study and meta-analysis of epidemiological studies. *Teratology* **62**: 385–382.

87 Kamm, J.J. (1982). Toxicology, carcinogenicity, and teratogenicity of some orally administered retinoids. *J. Am. Acad. Dermatol.* **6**: 652–659.

88 Lammer, E.J., Chen, D.T., Hoar, R.M. et al. (1985). Retinoic acid embryopathy. *N. Engl. J. Med.* **313**: 837–841.

89 Anonymous (1983). Adverse effects with isotretinoin. *FDA Bull.* **13**: 21–23.

90 Abel, E.L. (1981. As cited in Anonymous. Alcohol and the fetus – is zero the only option? Lancet, 1983). *Fetal Alcohol Syndrome, Volume 1: An Annotated and Comprehensive Bibliography*, vol. **1**, 682–683. Boca Raton, FL: CRC Press.

91 Council on Scientific Affairs (1983). American Medical Association. Fetal effects of maternal alcohol use. *JAMA* **249**: 2517–2521.

92 American Council on Science and Health (1982). Alcohol Use During Pregnancy. *Nutr. Today* **17**: 29–32.

93 Rubin, D.H., Leventhal, J.M., Krasilnikoff, P.A. et al. (1986). Fathers' drinking (and smoking) and infants birth weight. *N. Engl. J. Med.* **315**: 1551.

94 Little, R.E. and Sling, C.F. (1986). Association of father's drinking and infant's birth weight. *N. Engl. J. Med.* **314**: 1644–1645.

95 Mills, J.L. and Graubard, B.I. (1987). Is moderate drinking during pregnancy associated with an increased risk for malformations? *Pediatrics* **80**: 309–314.

96 Lumley, J., Oliver, S.S., Chamberlain, C. et al. (2009). Interventions for promoting smoking cessation during pregnancy. *Cochrane Database Syst. Rev.* (**3**): DC001055. doi: 10.1002/14651858.

97 Adams, J. (2003). Statement of the Public Affairs Committee of the Teratology Society on the importance of smoking cessation during pregnancy. *Birth Defects Res. Part A Clin. Mol. Teratol.* **67**: 985–989.

98 Chan, B., Einarson, A., and Koren, G. (2005). Effectiveness of bupropion for smoking cessation during pregnancy. *J. Addict. Dis.* **24**: 19–23.

99 Cahill, K., Stead, L.F., and Lancaster, T. (2007). Nicotine receptor partial agonists for smoking cessation. *Cochrane Database Syst. Rev.* (**1**): CD006103.

100 Dempsey, D.A. and Benowitz, N.L. (2001). Risks and benefits of nicotine to aid smoking cessation in pregnancy. *Drug Saf.* **24**: 277–322.

101 Zuckerman, B., Frank, D.A., Hingson, R. et al. (1989). Effects of maternal marijuana and cocaine use on fetal growth. *N. Engl. J. Med.* **320**: 762–768.

102 Goldschmidt, L., Day, N.L., and Richardson, G.A. (2000). Effects of prenatal marijuana exposure on child behavior problems at age 10. *Neurotoxicol. Teratol.* **22**: 325–336.

103 Day, N.L., Richardson, G.A., Goldschmidt, L. et al. (1994). Effect of prenatal marijuana exposure on the cognitive development of offspring at age three. *Neurotoxicol. Teratol.* **16**: 169–175.

104 Henderson, J.T., Weisman, C.S., and Grason, H. (2002). Are two doctors better than one? Women's physician use and appropriate care. *Womens Health Issues* **12**: 136–149.

105 Jack, B.W., Culpepper, L., Babcock, J. et al. (1998). Addressing preconception risks identified at the time of a negative pregnancy test: a randomized trial. *J. Fam. Pract.* **47**: 33–38.

21 CHAPTER 21

Prenatal diagnosis

Lisa C. Zuckerwise[1], Karen Archabald[2], and Joshua Copel[1]

[1]*Department of Obstetrics, Gynecology & Reproductive Sciences, Division of Maternal-Fetal Medicine, Yale School of Medicine, New Haven, CT, USA*

[2]*Legacy Health, Portland, OR, USA*

> **CLINICAL SCENARIO**
>
> A 36-year-old G1P0 presents for her first prenatal visit to her obstetrician's office at 12 weeks' gestation based on her last menstrual period. She reports an uncomplicated pregnancy to date. Her primary objective for today's visit is to discuss her screening options for aneuploidy. In the office, she has an ultrasound to assess nuchal translucency (NT), which appears abnormally thickened with a value of 4 mm. She would like more information and asks whether she should continue with further screening tests or move toward a diagnostic procedure.

Background

Screening for aneuploidy has become an important part of routine obstetrical care. In 2007, the American College of Obstetricians and Gynecologists (ACOG) recommended that all women, regardless of maternal age, be offered aneuploidy screening before 20 weeks of gestation and be given the option of invasive testing [1, 2]. Options for screening and diagnosis depend on the gestational age at time of presentation for care as well as patient preference and availability of resources. This chapter will discuss the advantages and limitations of the various methodologies available.

Clinical questions

1. In pregnant women at high-risk for aneuploidy based on personal history or screening, what is the sensitivity and specificity of cell-free fetal DNA (cfDNA) analysis for detection of Trisomy 21 and Trisomy 18? What about in low-risk women?

Cell-free fetal DNA can be detected in maternal blood during pregnancy [3]. These small fragments of DNA actually derive from placental cells, so they more accurately reflect the DNA makeup of the placenta. The first report of cfDNA to diagnose Trisomy 21 occurred in 2008 and was by the massively parallel shotgun sequencing technique. Other techniques for analyzing cfDNA have been validated by various laboratories, including selective sequencing of target chromosomes and single nucleotide polymorphism (SNP)-based methods. These all rely on next-generation sequencing technology and advanced bioinformatics analysis and possess similarly high sensitivities and specificities for detection of Trisomy 21 and Trisomy 18 [4–6]. An early nested case control study of a cohort of 4664 high-risk pregnancies for Trisomy 21 in 27 centers validated the use of cfDNA as a diagnostic tool. Women were classified as high-risk based on maternal age, family history or a positive serum and/or sonographic screening test. cfDNA was compared to conventional karyotype analysis. Trisomy 21 was detected in 98.6% (209/212) of positive cases, the false-positive rate was 0.20% (3/1471), and the testing failed in 13 pregnancies (0.8%). Subsequent larger studies and meta-analyses have confirmed that cfDNA analysis is a very powerful screening tool for both Trisomy 21 and Trisomy 18 in the high-risk population, with an overall sensitivity and specificity of >99% [7, 8].

In low-risk women, the prevalence of aneuploidy is considerably lower. As a result, while the sensitivity and specificity of any given screening test are unchanged, the clinical significance of a positive test is altered. This is important when considering the use of circulating free DNA (cfDNA) in the low-risk obstetric population. Based on this principle, both the Society for Maternal-Fetal Medicine and the ACOGs currently recommend conventional screening methods as the most appropriate choice for first-line screening in the routine obstetric population. [9]. Despite this recommendation, there is a growing body of evidence that cfDNA analysis remains a powerful tool for detecting Trisomy 21 and Trisomy 18 even in the general obstetric population. A primary series of almost 2000 women at multiple centers presenting

Evidence-Based Obstetrics and Gynecology, First Edition. Edited by Errol R. Norwitz, Carolyn M. Zelop, David A. Miller, and David L. Keefe.

for routine prenatal care compared performance of standard aneuploidy screening (serum biochemical assays with or without NT measurement) with cfDNA in order to primarily assess the rates of false positive results. In this low-risk population with a mean age of 29.6 years, the false positive rates were significantly lower for cfDNA than with standard screening for Trisomy 21 (0.3% versus 3.6%) and for Trisomy 18 (0.2% versus 0.6%). Positive predictive values were also favorable for cfDNA compared to standard screening, with positive predictive value (PPV) of 45.5% versus 4.2% for Trisomy 21 and PPV of 40.0% versus 8.3% for trisomy 18, [4]. For counseling purposes as well as clinical applicability, it is important to recognize that based on these findings in the low-risk (i.e. younger age) population, there is still less than 50% chance of a fetus actually having Trisomy 21 or trisomy 18 with a positive cfDNA result. A subsequent larger prospective, multicenter, blinded study compared standard screening (NT and biochemical analytes) with cfDNA testing in a routine obstetric population. The average age of the more than 15 000 women included was 30.7 years. In this study, the sensitivity of standard screening for detecting Trisomy 21 was 78.9%, compared to 100% (38 of 38) for cfDNA. False positive rates were 5.4% in the standard screening and 0.06% in the cfDNA groups, and positive predictive values were 3.4% for standard screening, compared to 80.9% for cfDNA. All of these results were statistically significant [10]. While the positive predictive value in this study was higher than previously reported, it is still a function of the overall prevalence in the given population. Individual patient positive predictive values can be calculated with a tool found at http://www.perinatalquality.org/Vendors/NSGC/NIPT.

In order to obtain a meaningful result from cfDNA analysis, there must be an adequate fraction of fetal DNA (fetal fraction) in the maternal blood. In most patients, samples drawn after 10 weeks gestation will provide adequate fetal fractions, meaning >8% of fetal DNA; however, in some cases, there will be fetal fraction too low to report (0–4%) or an intermediate amount (4–8%), where a result can be given but with compromised sensitivity. Low fetal fraction is associated with maternal obesity, and multiple studies have demonstrated an inverse relationship between fetal fraction and maternal weight [11–13]. One large study of 22 384 pregnant patients who underwent cfDNA testing found that about 20% of women weighing over 130 kg and 30% weighing over 140 kg have a fetal fraction less than 4% [11]. While this is clinically important in itself, given the increasing prevalence of obesity in the general population, there is also evidence that a failed result for cfDNA is associated with aneuploidy. In a large prospective study on performance of cfDNA to detect trisomy, which included over 18 000 patients, those with failed results due to low fetal fraction (<4%) had an aneuploidy risk of 4.7%, which was significantly higher than the overall cohort rate of 0.4% [10]. This increased risk of aneuploidy in fetuses with failed cfDNA results has been reported in smaller studies as well [14], highlighting the importance of genetic counseling following failed results, including a recommendation for either repeat cfDNA analysis or invasive testing for aneuploidy.

2. In pregnant women at low or average risk of aneuploidy, what is the sensitivity and specificity of non-invasive first trimester, second trimester, and combined screening for Trisomy 21 and Trisomy 18?

Serum screening for fetal aneuploidy was introduced in the 1980s when low serum AFP in the second trimester was noted to be associated with an elevated risk of Trisomy 21 [15]. The type of noninvasive risk assessment for aneuploidy recommended depends on the time a woman presents for prenatal care and the availability of laboratory and ultrasonographic services, as well as her aneuploidy risk. Testing options include a combination of first and/or second trimester maternal serum analytes with or without the addition of ultrasonographic assessment, ultimately leading to an assignment of risk of both Trisomy 21 and Trisomy 18. Based on the risk calculation and discussion with the patient, further screening or diagnostic testing can subsequently be offered.

First trimester combined screening

First trimester combined screening includes: (i) sonographic measurement of the fetal crown–rump length and NT; and (ii) serum levels of pregnancy-associated plasma protein A (PAPP-A) and either total or free-β human chorionic gonadotropin (hCG). Prospective studies from the United States and Europe have revealed detection rates for Trisomy 21 with NT alone ranging from 54% to 79% (see Table 21.1). A meta-analysis assessing the role of NT as a screening tool

Table 21.1 Detection rate of Trisomy 21 with first trimester screening given 5% screen positive rate.

	NT	1st trimester serum	1st trimester combined
Snijders 1998 (n = 96 127) (83)	77%		
Wald 2003 SURUSS (n = 47 053) (20)	63%		86%
Wapner 2005(BUN Trial) (n = 8216) (84)	67%	69%	79%
Malone 2005 (FASTER) (n = 33 557) (7)	70%	70%	87%
Bindra 2002 (OSCAR) (n = 14 383) (85)	79%	60%	90%
Crossley 2002 (n = 17 229)(86)	54%	55%	82%
Ghaffari 2011 (n = 13 706) (87)			94% (4.8% SPR)
Guanciali-Franchi 2011 (n = 7292) (28)			81% (4% SPR)

for aneuploidy including 30 studies and 16 311 patients found an overall detection rate of 77% with a 5.9% screen positive rate [15]. Compared to euploid pregnancies [16], Trisomy 21 pregnancies have decreased levels of PAPP-A and increased levels of hCG [16, 17]; however, first trimester serum screening with these two serum analytes without ultrasound detects only 55–70% of cases (Table 21.1). When both serum markers and NT are combined, sensitivity and specificity of the screening for Trisomy 21 improves significantly (Table 21.1). In the United States, the First and Second Trimester Evaluation of Risk (FASTER) trial found that combined first trimester screening at 11 weeks increased the detection rate of Trisomy 21–87% with a screen positive rate of 5%. [18] Maintaining a 5% screen positive rate, the detection rate decreases marginally to 85% when testing is performed at 12 weeks gestation and to 82% at 13 weeks gestation [18]. Two additional large multicenter trials; the Biochemistry, Ultrasound, Nuchal Translucency (BUN) study from the United States and the Serum, Urine, and Ultrasound Screening Study (SURUSS) trial completed in the United Kingdom and Austria, found detection rates of Trisomy 21 of 86% and 79%, respectively with a set screen positive rate of 5%. For women who present early to prenatal care in centers where NT is available, first trimester combined screening is a powerful tool in early detection of Trisomy 21.

First trimester combined screening can also be used for the detection of Trisomy 18. In the first trimester, Trisomy 18 pregnancies have lower levels of maternal serum hCG and PAPP-A and a higher NT than euploid counterparts [19]. The FASTER trial found that with combination of first trimester NT and a serum screen positive for either Trisomy 21 (risk of 1 : 300), Trisomy 18 (risk of 1 : 100), or a cystic hygroma there was an 82% detection rate of Trisomy 18 with a screen positive rate of 6% [20]. In the BUN trial, the combination of NT, serum screening, and maternal age detected 90.9% of Trisomy18 with a screen positive rate of 2% [21].

In addition to combined screening with NT and maternal serum markers in the first trimester, additional sonographic markers including absent nasal bone, abnormal flow in the ductus venosus and tricuspid regurgitation have been proposed as adjunct screening tools. In an initial observational study of 701 women who were high-risk secondary to increased NT and maternal age, the nasal bone was noted to be absent in 73% of Trisomy 21fetuses and only in 0.5% of unaffected fetuses [22]. Presence or absence of the nasal bone has subsequently been well studied, with a wide range of sensitivities reported ranging from as low as 7.7% to up to 65% of aneuploidy [23, 24]. Overall, the available data suggests that in low-risk women, nasal bone screening adds little to first trimester combined screening [25–30].

Combined first and second trimester screening

There are several different approaches to combined first and second trimester screening, which are detailed below. Table 21.2 provides a comparison of screening detection rates between these different options.

Fully integrated screening

The full integrated screen includes first trimester combined screening with ultrasound measurement of NT and maternal serum PAPP-A between 10 and 13 weeks as well as second trimester assessment of α-fetoprotein (AFP), unconjugated estriol (uE3), hCG and inhibin-A [31, 32]. Between 15 and 19 weeks, pregnancies with Trisomy 21 are associated with lower maternal serum alpha-fetoprotein (MSAFP) [15], higher hCG [33], reduced levels of uE3 [34] and higher inhibin A than their euploid counterparts [35]. In contrast, pregnancies with Trisomy 18 are associated with decreased levels of AFP and uE3 [36, 37].

For true "Fully Integrated Screening," results are only given after both first and second trimester testing is completed. The FASTER trial found that the fully integrated test has a detection rate of Trisomy 21 of 95% with a 5% screen positive rate [18]. The SURUSS trial found similar detection rate of 94% with a 5% screen positive rate [38]. (Table 21.2) A more recent prospective study comparing methods of combined first and second trimester screening

Table 21.2 Detection rate of trisomy 21 with combined first and second trimester screening.

	1st trimester combined	Full integrated	Serum integrated	Stepwise sequential	Contingent	Quad screen
Malone 2005 (FASTER) (n = 33 546) (7)	87%	96%	88%	95%		81%
Cuckle 2008 (FASTER) (n = 32 355) (31)		93%		93%	92%	
Wald 2003 (SURUSS) (n = 47 053) (20)	86%	94%	87%			83%
Wald 2006 (SURUSS) Model (32)				90% (2.25% SPR)	90% (2.42% SPR)	
Platt 2004 (BUN) (n = 4325) (88)	79%			98% (17% SPR)		
Guanciali-Franchi 2011 (n = 7292) (28)	81% (4% SPR)	90% (3.4% SPR)		90% (5.2%SPR)	90% (2.6% SPR)	

found a detection rate of 90% with a screen positive rate of 3.4% [39]. The major drawback to this method of screening is that results are not given until the second trimester when diagnosis by CVS is no longer available and when pregnancies are more visible to others. Women have different reasons for undergoing aneuploidy screening; some women prefer early detection in order to facilitate safer elective termination while others desire reassurance regarding the health of the fetus. Depending on the wishes of the woman, waiting until the second trimester for results may not be the most logical option [40].

Serum integrated screening

The serum integrated test involves first trimester PAPP-A combined with a second trimester quadruple screen (AFP, uE3, hCG, inhibin-A). This test is most appropriate in places where NT is not readily available, and can also be used for women who have had blood drawn for first trimester screening at the appropriate time, but whose fetuses cannot have NT measured for technical reasons (usually either due to fetal position or because the crown rump length (CRL) of the fetus is above accepted cutoffs). The FASTER trial found an 86% detection rate of Trisomy 21 at a 5% screen positive rate [18] for serum integrated screening, while the SURUSS trial found an 87% detection rate at a 5% screen positive rate [38]. A meta-analysis of serum integrated screening for Trisomy18 found that by combining first trimester PAPP-A with second trimester AFP, uE3, and hCG at a risk cutoff of 1:100 the detection rate was 90% with a screen positive rate of 0.1% [41].

Stepwise sequential screening

Stepwise sequential screening involves the initial calculation of risk from the ultrasound measurement of NT, maternal PAPP-A and hCG between 11 and 13 weeks. Women with pregnancies at high-risk are offered immediate invasive prenatal diagnosis with CVS, while the remainder go on to have second trimester testing. After completion of second trimester testing, the risk is recalculated to include second trimester markers and a new risk is assigned. This form of testing has the advantage of providing an early diagnosis for a substantial proportion of affected pregnancies. Analysis of the FASTER data reports a detection rate of Trisomy 21 of 92% with a 5% screen positive rate. A computer model based on the SURUSS data found a detection rate of 90% with a 2.25% screen positive rate. However, the majority of women have testing in both trimesters.

Contingent screening

Contingent screening involves the initial calculation of risk from the ultrasound measurement of NT, PAPP-A and hCG between 11 and 13 weeks. Based on these results, pregnancies are classified as high, medium, or low-risk. Women at high-risk can immediately be offered CVS. Women with a low-risk (negative) screen have no further testing. Women with borderline initial risk, which should be a predetermined range, go on to have quadruple screening with AFP, hCG, uE3 and inhibin at 15–18 weeks. A final risk is calculated that combines the first and second trimester screening results. The final result is considered positive if the risk is greater than 1 in 270.

Predetermination of risk cutoffs is essential to the success of this approach. The initial first trimester cutoff should identify the majority of cases of Trisomy 21 while maintaining a low false positive rate. Studies to date have defined a first trimester false positive rate of 0.5% or a risk of >1 : 30 as high-risk [39, 42, 43]. The FASTER trial found a 60% detection rate for Trisomy 21 in the first trimester with a screen positive rate of 1.2%. Modeling from the SURUSS trial predicted a 66% detection rate with a false positive rate of 2.42%. Finally, Guanciali found a detection rate of 82% with a screen positive rate of 4% [39]. By deferring subsequent testing in the low-risk group only, this should minimize the number of affected pregnancies missed, while also limiting the number of patients who go on to have second trimester testing. Cutoffs used in the above studies range from <1 : 1200 [39] to >1 : 1500 [42]. The intermediate cutoff is the range between these two cutoffs (e.g. between 1 : 30 and 1 : 1500) and should identify many of the remaining cases of aneuploidy while minimizing the number of invasive procedures.

Contingent screening decreases the number of women who require second trimester testing. Cost effectiveness models from both the SURUSS and FASTER trials have found that contingent screening may be the most cost effective method, because it decreases the number of women who need second trimester blood work, while maintaining a high aneuploidy detection rate [44, 45].

Second trimester screening

At present, the most sensitive conventional risk assessment tool for low-risk women who present for prenatal care after 14 weeks of gestation is the Quadruple Screen. The Quadruple Screen measures serum levels of MSAFP, hCG, uE3, and inhibin-A.

Using a risk cutoff of 1 : 300 as positive, the detection rate of Trisomy 21 using the quadruple screen in the FASTER trial was 85% at an 8.5% screen positive rate [18]. Data from the same trial evaluated detection of Trisomy 18. Using a risk cutoff of 1 : 100 as positive detection the Quadruple Screen detection rate was 100% with a screen positive rate of 0.3% [20]. Although these detection rates are not as high as the first trimester or integrated screens, in a patient who presents for prenatal care in the second trimester they provide valuable information that can assist when counseling a patient regarding the advisability of diagnostic procedures.

3. How does the second trimester genetic ultrasound affect the sensitivity and specificity of first and second trimester screening?

The second trimester anatomic sonogram is optimally completed between 16 and 20 weeks gestation, as fetal anatomy can usually be visualized and amniocentesis and termination remain options. The identification of major structural malformations associated with aneuploidy identifies women with pregnancies at high-risk for aneuploidy and should prompt discussion of genetic amniocentesis. The most common structural anomalies associated with Trisomy 21 include cardiac defects (specifically ventricular septal defect and atrioventricular septal defect), duodenal atresia, cystic hygroma, cerebral ventriculomegaly, and hydrops fetalis [46, 47]. In a case control study of 142 fetuses with Trisomy 21 and 930 euploid controls, the presence of any of the above structural anomalies was associated with a likelihood ratio (LR) of 25 for Trisomy 21 [47]. Major structural anomalies associated with Trisomy 18 include cardiac malformations (specifically double outlet right ventricle, ventricular septal defects, atrioventricular septal defect), meningomyelocele, omphalocele, clenched hands, rocker bottom feet, cleft lip or palate, cystic hygroma or nuchal thickening and hydrops fetalis [46, 48].

In addition to major structural anomalies, second trimester sonography can also identify markers for aneuploidy. These markers are anatomic findings that are not structural abnormalities, but are more common in fetuses with aneuploidy than in the normal population, and are associated with a statistically significant risk for fetal aneuploidy. Common markers associated with Trisomy 21 and their associated LRs are listed in Table 21.3. LR can be used to modify the risk based on serum screening and maternal age. A large meta-analysis completed by Aagaard-Tillery suggested that nuchal thickening and hyperechoic bowel have the strongest association with Trisomy 21 (see Table 21.3). Based on pooled analysis of sonographic studies, absent nasal bone in the second trimester is also a valuable marker, as absent nasal bone is found in approximately 0.9% of euploid pregnancies and 37% of Trisomy 21 pregnancies resulting in a likelihood ratio of 41.1 for Trisomy 21 [53]. Based on results from the FASTER trial, when sonographic markers are combined, the LR of Trisomy 21 increases from 3.1 with one marker to 21 with 2 markers, and 170 with 3 markers [52].

Trisomy 18 is associated with multiple second trimester sonographic findings that result in a detection rate of approximately 80% by ultrasound alone [48, 54]. In addition to the structural anomalies listed above, sonographic markers commonly associated with Trisomy 18 include nuchal thickening, brachycephaly, early onset fetal growth restriction, shortened long bones predominantly in the lower extremities, single umbilical artery, and choroid plexus cysts (CPC) [49, 55]. A review of the literature including 27 451 pregnancies found that CPCs are found in approximately 50% of fetuses with Trisomy 18 and 0.87% of the general population [56]. In the same study, the LR of a fetus with an isolated finding of CPC having Trisomy 18 was found to be 0.03. When seen in the presence of one additional abnormality, the LR increases to 0.4, and with two additional abnormalities the LR increases to 20.5 [56]. Other studies have shown an increase in the LR of Trisomy 18 in the presence of an isolated CPC to be 7.1 [57] to 13.8 [58]. A meta-analysis including data from 427 032 low-risk pregnancies of whom 2830 had an isolated CPC and 15 had Trisomy 18, an isolated CPC was associated with a 1 in 189 chance of Trisomy 18, with a relative risk of 8.6 [59]. Given these data, the presence of CPC should prompt a thorough search for further markers and consideration of diagnostic testing depending on maternal age and a priori risk as well as patient preference. The findings of an isolated CPC may place a previously "low-risk" pregnancy into a "high-risk"

Table 21.3 Likelihood ratios (LR) of trisomy 21 with detection of isolated sonographic markers.

Marker	Nyberg 1998 (n = 1042) [47]	Nyberg 2001 (n = 8830) [49]	Smith-Bindman 2001 (n= > 131 000) [50]	Bromley 2002 (n = 820) [51]	Aagaard-Tillery 2009 [52]
Nuchal thickening	18.6	11	17	Infinite	49 (n = 6676)
Hyperechoic bowel	5.5	6.7	6.1	Not recorded	38 (n = 7833)
Short humerus	2.5	5.1	7.5	5.8	5.0 (n = 3866)
Short femur	2.2	1.5	2.7	1.2	4.6 (n = 7817)
Echogenic intracardiac focus	2	1.8	2.8	1.4	6.3 (n = 7778)
Pyelectasis	1.5	1.5	1.9	1.5	5.5 (n = 7832)
Normal	0.4	0.4	Not recorded	0.2	0.41 (n = 7842)

category. Women should be informed of these results so they may make an informed decision regarding diagnostic testing [60].

4. In pregnant women at high-risk for aneuploidy, what is the sensitivity and specificity of diagnostic testing including chorionic villous sampling (CVS) and amniocentesis for detection of Trisomy 21 and Trisomy 18? What other genetic abnormalities can be diagnosed? What are the associated risks to the pregnancy?

Women generally choose to undergo invasive testing based on abnormal aneuploidy screening or a personal history that puts them a risk for having an aneuploid fetus that they deem high enough to warrant the potential harms of invasive testing. Depending on the timing of the decision to proceed with diagnostic testing, the two invasive methods are chorionic villous sampling and amniocentesis. While a karyotype can also be obtained from fetal blood, cordocentesis is rarely used for this purpose.

Chorionic villous sampling

CVS is commonly performed between 10 and 13 weeks gestation. Two components of the chorionic villi can be analyzed: the cytotrophoblast, which has a high mitotic index and can be analyzed immediately (direct method), and the mesenchymal core, which contains the fetal blood capillaries and requires culture prior to analysis (culture method). Using a combination of both methods, the US collaborative study on CVS found a 99.7% rate of successful cytogenetic diagnosis with only 1.1% of patients requiring either repeat CVS or amniocentesis [61]. The indications for further testing included lab failure, maternal cell contamination, or mosaicism. Subsequent studies have confirmed this high accuracy [62, 63].

When CVS first became a common procedure, a prospective randomized trial of 2650 women completed in Canada found similar loss rates between CVS and amniocentesis at 7.6% and 7.0% respectively with a Risk Ratio (RR) of 1.10 (95% CI 0.92–1.30) [64]. At the same time, a multicenter nonrandomized trial in the United States including 2235 women comparing transcervical CVS to second trimester amniocentesis found no statistical difference in pregnancy loss following CVS compared with amniocentesis [65]. A large Danish randomized trial including 1068 women assigned to transcervical CVS, 1078 women to transabdominal CVS, and 1158 to second trimester amniocentesis found a similar rates of loss between transabdominal CVS (6.3%) and amniocentesis (6.4%), but a significantly higher rate of loss in the transcervical approach (10.9%), resulting in a RR of fetal loss for transcervical CVS of 1.3 (95% CI 1.1–1.7) [66]. A separate, larger randomized trial comparing transabdominal (n = 1929) to transvaginal (n = 1944) CVS failed to detect a significant difference in fetal loss between the two approaches (2.3% versus 2.5%, difference 0.26%, 95% confidence interval −0.5 to 1.0%) [67]. Importantly this study followed pregnancies to 28 weeks gestation, therefore accounting for both early and late losses following the procedures.

Since completion of these early trials, CVS has become more common and operator experience has increased. A single institution retrospective study of amniocentesis and CVS between 1983 and 2003 found that the overall loss rate was significantly higher for CVS (3.12%) compared to amniocentesis (0.83%) (adjusted odds ratio [aOR] 4.23, 95% CI 2.29–7.81) [66, 68]; however, in the final five years of the study there was no difference between the two procedures (aOR 1.03, 95% CI 0.23–4.52) [63]. Other studies have also shown that complication rate decreases with operator experience [69, 70]. In the hands of experienced operators, the loss rate of CVS seems to be comparable to that of amniocentesis. The most recent data looking at risk of invasive testing further supports the safety of both CVS and amniocentesis. In fact, a large Danish registry-based study looking prospectively at the effects of both CVS and amniocentesis on the risk of pregnancy loss suggests that invasive testing by either method does not significantly increase the risk of pregnancy loss after accounting for the baseline risk of a given patient [71]. This cohort included 147 987 women with singleton pregnancies who all underwent first trimester screening. A total of 5072 women underwent CVS and 1082 underwent amniocentesis. The authors performed propensity score stratification to assess the risk of fetal loss based on maternal characteristics as well as the screening test results and found no difference between any groups in risk of miscarriage or stillbirth following either diagnostic procedure.

Amniocentesis

Amniocentesis for genetic evaluation is commonly performed between 15 and 18 weeks gestation, as earlier amniocentesis has been associated with increased risk of miscarriage and talipes equinovarus [72, 73]. The cells obtained from the amniotic fluid are derived from the fetal respiratory tract, urinary tract, gastrointestinal tract, and placenta. These cells are cultured and subsequently undergo karyotypic analysis. This type of analysis is considered the gold standard for diagnosis of trisomy, as the accuracy of karyotypic analysis from amniocentesis is 99.4–99.8% [74]; however, results typically take 10–14 days to return. Fluorescence in situ hybridization (FISH) can be used to detect common aneuploidies associated with chromosomes 13, 18, 21, X and Y with sensitivity of 98.7– 100% within 24–48 hours [75, 76]. FISH cannot reliably detect mosaics, translocations, and rare aneuploidies and is therefore most appropriate if used when quick results are desired and a common aneuploidy is suspected based on prior screening or sonographic findings. Patients should be counseled that normal FISH results are not the final results, and final results are based on full culture, with microarray (vide infra).

The major complication of amniocentesis is miscarriage. A randomized trial of 4606 low-risk women in Denmark in 1986 found a 1% procedure related loss rate [77]. Subsequent studies have shown a significantly lower loss rate. An analysis of the FASTER trial estimated the procedure-related loss rate after amniocentesis to be 0.06% [78]. A single institution retrospective cohort study of 58 436 women found the loss rate attributable to amniocentesis to be 0.13% [79]. A systematic review including the data from the FASTER trial and four other studies with controls found the associated loss rate attributable to amniocentesis to be 0.6% [80]. These results were similar to a meta-analysis of 68 119 amniocentesis from controlled and uncontrolled studies that also found a procedure related risk of excess pregnancy loss of 0.6% [81]. As noted above, even more recent data from a large population study failed to demonstrate an increase in risk of pregnancy loss following CVS or amniocentesis for diagnosis of aneuploidy [71].

Chromosome microarray analysis

Chromosome microarray analysis is a method of searching for small genomic deletions or duplications, referred to as copy-number variants, which are too small to be detected by conventional karyotyping. This technology has been used in the pediatric population with congenital structural or neurodevelopmental anomalies with success in identifying pathogenic copy-number variants [82, 83]. For prenatal diagnosis, microarray analysis provides information in addition to karyotyping. In the largest prospective study to date, Wapner and colleagues enrolled over 4400 women undergoing diagnostic amniocentesis and compared conventional karyotyping with microarray analysis. They found clinically significant deletions or duplications in 6.0% of samples from fetuses with structural abnormalities and normal karyotype results, and also in 1.7% (1 in 60) of normal-appearing fetuses [84]. These results suggest that it is appropriate to offer diagnostic testing with chromosome microarray analysis to all patients undergoing invasive testing, as available data suggests that there is important incremental information that is often provided by microarray testing. At least, chromosome microarray analysis should be offered to all patient undergoing invasive testing.

5. In pregnant women, what is the sensitivity and specificity of elevated MSAFP and second trimester ultrasound in the detection of neural tube defect (NTD)s?

In addition to screening for aneuploidy, sonographic, and serum screening for NTDs should be offered to all women in the second trimester [85]. NTDs are cranial or spinal structural anomalies caused by abnormal closure of the embryologic neural tube thought to be secondary to a combination of genetic and environmental factors. NTDs can be isolated or can occur in conjunction with a genetic syndrome. The overall prevalence of NTD defects worldwide has decreased over the past century [86]. After folic acid fortification of cereal grain products was mandated in the United States in 1998, the prevalence of anencephaly decreased from 2.2 to 1.8 per 10 000 births and the prevalence of spina bifida decreased from 4.9 to 3.2 per 10 000 births [87]. Despite this decrease, NTDs remain one of the most common birth defects.

Maternal serum alpha-fetoprotein screening (MSAFP)

An observational study of 18 985 women in the United Kingdom found that by using 2.5 multiple of the median (MoM) as a positive screen, elevated MSAFP between 16 and 18 weeks of pregnancy identified 88% of cases of anencephaly, 79% of cases of open spina bifida with a 3% false screen positive rate [88]. Using a cutoff of 2.5 MoM, a meta-analysis of 22 English and Chinese language studies that included 684 140 pregnant women screened for NTD with MSAFP during the second trimester found the sensitivity and specificity of MSAFP screening to be 75.1 and 97.7%, respectively [89]. Because other conditions can cause elevated AFP, including fetal abdominal wall defects, diseases leading to skin breakdown, and fetal nephrotic syndrome, elevated MSAFP alone is not diagnostic of an open NTD and further testing is warranted.

Ultrasound

Routine second trimester ultrasound has been proposed as an alternative to serum MSAFP as a screening tool for open neural tube defect (ONTD). A routine second trimester ultrasound includes examination of the fetal spine and intracranial anatomy [90]. Anencephaly is easily diagnosed in the second and third trimester and is characterized by absence of the cranial vault. Open NTD is diagnosed sonographically by either direct visualization of the spinal defect or by the associated changes in the brain including scalloping of the parietal bones ("lemon sign") and anterior curving of the cerebellar hemispheres resulting in obliteration of the cisterna magna ("banana sign") [91].

A prospective multi-center trial in Scandinavia of 27 844 low-risk women reported a 79.4% detection rate of NTDs with routine second trimester ultrasound [92]. A more recent review of the efficacy of screening ultrasound in prenatal diagnosis of low-risk women in 18 European countries including 1.3 million births found an 88% overall detection rate of NTD with second trimester ultrasound [93].

Studies comparing the effectiveness of serum screening with MSAFP and routine second trimester ultrasound suggest ultrasound may be more sensitive and specific. A retrospective single institution study of 66 cases of NTD reported the sensitivity of MSAFP to be 66%, which increased to 86% if dating was confirmed by ultrasound. In the same cohort, routine second trimester ultrasound detected 100% of cases [94]. A retrospective review of 219 000 pregnancies in California with 189 cases of NTD found a false negative rate of

25% in the 102 cases of NTD who had MSAFP performed, which would have led to failure to diagnose 38% of spina bifida, 8% of anencephaly, and 67% of encephalocele cases prenatally, with a 0.9% screen positive rate in the normal population. This study used 2.5 MoM as its definition of an elevated MSAFP. Using a lower cut-off of 2.0 MoM would have improved the detection rate overall to 83%, with a screen positive rate of 2.7%. In the subset of 130 women who had routine second trimester ultrasonography without knowledge of MSAFP 96% of NTD were diagnosed [95]. Although in experienced hands ultrasound may be more sensitive in detecting NTD, MSAFP continues to play an important role when access to ultrasound is limited by access to trained sonologists/sonographers, late presentation for prenatal care, or other situations.

Amniocentesis

In cases where NTD is suspected based on either serum screening or routine second trimester ultrasound, diagnostic testing is indicated. Historically, the standard diagnostic test for NTD was amniocentesis with evaluation of amniotic fluid α-fetoprotein (AFAFP) and acetylcholinesterase (AChE) levels. A retrospective cohort study in Denmark including 9964 women with singleton pregnancies who underwent amniocentesis for increased risk of NTD, advanced maternal age, increased risk or chromosomal abnormalities, or parental anxiety found that amniotic fluid AChE level identified 100% of cases of anencephaly [17] and 100% of cases of open spina bifida [30] with a false positive rate of 0.22% [96]. In women at high-risk for ONTD secondary to family history or elevated MSAFP, ultrasound has been found to be equally as effective at identifying ONTD without the risk of pregnancy loss associated with amniocentesis. A single institution study of 2257 consecutive high-risk women found that targeted ultrasound alone was 97% sensitive (66 of 68) (95% CI 0.898–0.996) and 100% (95% CI 0.998–1.0) specific in diagnosing open NTD [97]. Given the accuracy of ultrasound in ONTD diagnosis, amniocentesis should be reserved for cases where diagnosis is difficult via ultrasound or when the parents choose amniocentesis to evaluate for chromosomal abnormalities.

Conclusion

You tell your patient that given her advanced maternal age and abnormal NT measurement, she is an appropriate candidate for screening with fetal cfDNA analysis or diagnostic testing with CVS. You discuss that cfDNA analysis is the most sensitive and specific screening test for Trisomy 21 and Trisomy 18, but that invasive testing by CVS is the only way to diagnose aneuploidy definitively in the first trimester. Additionally, you recommend that should she opt for CVS, she should consider chromosome microarray analysis to evaluate for clinically significant chromosome duplications or deletions. You explain that conventional first trimester screening is an alternative option, and the specificity of NT for detecting aneuploidy increases with the addition of serum screening. Should she opt for this, a subsequent plan for contingency screening will further increase her detection rate. The patient decides to proceed with cfDNA analysis. She receives a result of <1/10 000 risk of Trisomy 21 and Trisomy 18 and she declines CVS. She has a second trimester ultrasound without structural anomalies or markers of aneuploidy and declines amniocentesis.

References

1 American College of Obstetricians and Gynecologists ACOG practice bulletin No. 88 December 2007. Invasive prenatal testing for aneuploidy. *Obstetrics and Gynecology* **2007**, **110** (**6**): 1459.

2 American College of Obstetricians and Gynecologists (2007). ACOG practice bulletin No. 77: screening for fetal chromosomal abnormalities. *Obstetrics and Gynecology* **109**: 217–227.

3 Lo, Y.D. et al. (1997). Presence of fetal DNA in maternal plasma and serum. *The Lancet* **350** (**9076**): 485–487.

4 Bianchi, D.W. et al. (2014). DNA sequencing versus standard prenatal aneuploidy screening. *The New England Journal of Medicine* **370** (**9**): 799–808.

5 Sparks, A.B. et al. (2012). Selective analysis of cell-free DNA in maternal blood for evaluation of fetal trisomy. *Prenatal Diagnosis* **32** (**1**): 3–9.

6 Chiu, R.W. et al. (2008). Noninvasive prenatal diagnosis of fetal chromosomal aneuploidy by massively parallel genomic sequencing of DNA in maternal plasma. *Proceedings of the National Academy of Sciences* **105** (**51**): 20458–20463.

7 Gil, M.M. et al. (2015). Analysis of cell-free DNA in maternal blood in screening for fetal aneuploidies: updated meta-analysis. *Ultrasound in Obstetrics & Gynecology* **45** (**3**): 249–266.

8 Porreco, R.P. et al. (2014). Noninvasive prenatal screening for fetal trisomies 21, 18, 13 and the common sex chromosome aneuploidies from maternal blood using massively parallel genomic sequencing of DNA. *American Journal of Obstetrics and Gynecology* **211** (**4**): 365 e1–365 e12.

9 Practice Bulletin No. 145 (2014). Antepartum Fetal Surveillance. *Obstetrics & Gynecology* **124** (**1**): 182–192.

10 Norton, M.E. et al. (2015). Cell-free DNA analysis for noninvasive examination of trisomy. *The New England Journal of Medicine* **372** (**17**): 1589–1597.

11 Wang, E. et al. (2013). Gestational age and maternal weight effects on fetal cell-free DNA in maternal plasma. *Prenatal Diagnosis* **33** (**7**): 662–666.

12 Ashoor, G. et al. (2012). Fetal fraction in maternal plasma cell-free DNA at 11–13 weeks' gestation: effect of maternal and fetal factors. *Fetal Diagnosis and Therapy* **31** (**4**): 237–243.

13 Wataganara, T. et al. (2004). Inverse correlation between maternal weight and second trimester circulating cell-free fetal DNA levels. *Obstetrics & Gynecology* **104** (**3**): 545–550.

14 Pergament, E. et al. (2014). Single-nucleotide polymorphism–based noninvasive prenatal screening in a high-risk and low-risk cohort. *Obstetrics & Gynecology* **124** (**2, PART 1**): 210–218.

15 Merkatz, I.R. et al. (1984). An association between low maternal serum α-fetoprotein and fetal chromosomal abnormalities. *American Journal of Obstetrics and Gynecology* **148** (**7**): 886–894.

16 Canick, J.A. and Kellner, L.H. (1999). First trimester screening for aneuploidy: serum biochemical markers. In: *Seminars in Perinatology*. Elsevier.

17 Malone, F.D. et al. (2005). First-trimester septated cystic hygroma: prevalence, natural history, and pediatric outcome. *Obstetrics & Gynecology* **106** (**2**): 288–294.

18 Malone, F.D. et al. (2005). First-trimester or second-trimester screening, or both, for Down's syndrome. *New England Journal of Medicine* **353** (**19**): 2001–2011.

19 Tul, N. et al. (1999). Screening for trisomy 18 by fetal nuchal translucency and maternal serum free β-hCG and PAPP-A at 10–14 weeks of gestation. *Prenatal Diagnosis* **19** (**11**): 1035–1042.

20 Breathnach, F.M. et al. (2007). First-and second-trimester screening: detection of aneuploidies other than down syndrome. *Obstetrics & Gynecology* **110** (**3**): 651–657.

21 Wapner, R. et al. (2003). First-trimester screening for trisomies 21 and 18. *New England Journal of Medicine* **349** (**15**): 1405–1413.

22 Cicero, S. et al. (2001). Absence of nasal bone in fetuses with trisomy 21 at 11–14 weeks of gestation: an observational study. *The Lancet* **358** (**9294**): 1665–1667.

23 Rosen, T. et al. (2007). First-trimester ultrasound assessment of the nasal bone to screen for aneuploidy. *Obstetrics & Gynecology* **110** (**2, Part 1**): 399–404.

24 Malone, F.D. et al. (2004). First-trimester nasal bone evaluation for aneuploidy in the general population. *Obstetrics & Gynecology* **104** (**6**): 1222–1228.

25 Prefumo, F. et al. (2006). First-trimester nuchal translucency, nasal bones, and trisomy 21 in selected and unselected populations. *American Journal of Obstetrics and Gynecology* **194** (**3**): 828–833.

26 Ramos-Corpas, D., Santiago, J.C., and Montoya, F. (2006). Ultrasonographic evaluation of fetal nasal bone in a low-risk population at 11–13+ 6 gestational weeks. *Prenatal Diagnosis* **26** (**2**): 112–117.

27 Matias, A. et al. (1998). Screening for chromosomal abnormalities at 10–14 weeks: the role of ductus venosus blood flow. *Ultrasound in Obstetrics and Gynecology* **12** (**6**): 380–384.

28 Malone, F.D. and D'Alton, M.E. (2003). First-trimester sonographic screening for down syndrome. *Obstetrics & Gynecology* **102** (**5, Part 1**): 1066–1079.

29 Hecher, K. (2001). Assessment of ductus venosus flow during the first and early second trimesters: what can we expect? *Ultrasound in Obstetrics & Gynecology* **17** (**4**): 285–287.

30 Falcon, O. et al. (2006). Fetal tricuspid regurgitation at the 11+ 0 to 13+ 6-week scan: association with chromosomal defects and reproducibility of the method. *Ultrasound in Obstetrics & Gynecology* **27** (**6**): 609–612.

31 Wald, N. et al. (2003). First and second trimester antenatal screening for Down's syndrome: the results of the Serum, Urine and Ultrasound Screening Study (SURUSS). *Journal of Medical Screening* **10** (**2**): 56–87.

32 Wald, N., Watt, H., and Hackshaw, A. (1999). Integrated screening for Down's syndrome based on tests performed during the first and second trimesters. *New England Journal of Medicine* **341** (**7**): 461–467.

33 Bogart, M.H., Pandian, M., and Jones, O. (1987). Abnormal maternal serum chorionic gonadotropin levels in pregnancies with fetal chromosome abnormalities. *Prenatal Diagnosis* **7** (**9**): 623–630.

34 Canick, J.A. et al. (1988). Low second trimester maternal serum unconjugated oestriol in pregnancies with Down's syndrome. *BJOG: An International Journal of Obstetrics & Gynaecology* **95** (**4**): 330–333.

35 Renier, M.A. et al. (1998). Second trimester maternal dimeric inhibin-a in the multiple-marker screening test for Down's syndrome. *Human Reproduction* **13** (**3**): 744–748.

36 Palomaki, G.E. et al. (1995). Risk-based prenatal screening for trisomy 18 using alpha-fetoprotein, unconjugated oestriol and human chorionic gonadotropin. *Prenatal Diagnosis* **15** (**8**): 713–723.

37 Barkai, G. et al. (1993). Expanding multiple marker screening for Down's syndrome to include Edward's syndrome. *Prenatal Diagnosis* **13** (**9**): 843–850.

38 Wald, N. et al. (2004). SURUSS in perspective. *BJOG: An International Journal of Obstetrics & Gynaecology* **111** (**6**): 521–531.

39 Guanciali-Franchi, P. et al. (2011). Comparison of combined, stepwise sequential, contingent, and integrated screening in 7292 high-risk pregnant women. *Prenatal Diagnosis* **31** (**11**): 1077–1081.

40 Copel, J.A. and Bahado-Singh, R.O. (1999). Prenatal screening for Down's syndrome – a search for the family's values. *New England Journal of Medicine* **341** (**7**): 521–522.

41 Palomaki, G.E. et al. (2003). Maternal serum–integrated screening for trisomy 18 using both first-and second-trimester markers. *Prenatal Diagnosis* **23** (**3**): 243–247.

42 Cuckle, H.S. et al. (2008). Contingent screening for Down syndrome-results from the FaSTER trial. *Prenatal Diagnosis* **28** (**2**): 89–94.

43 Wald, N.J., Rudnicka, A.R., and Bestwick, J.P. (2006). Sequential and contingent prenatal screening for Down syndrome. *Prenatal Diagnosis* **26** (**9**): 769–777.

44 Gekas, J. et al. (2009). Comparison of different strategies in prenatal screening for Down's syndrome: cost effectiveness analysis of computer simulation. *BMJ* doi: 10.1136/bmj.b138.

45 Ball, R.H. et al. (2007). First-and second-trimester evaluation of risk for Down syndrome. *Obstetrics & Gynecology* **110** (**1**): 10–17.

46 Papp, C. et al. (2008). Ultrasonographic findings of fetal aneuploidies in the second trimester–our experiences. *Fetal Diagnosis and Therapy* **23** (**2**): 105–113.

47 Nyberg, D. et al. (1998). Age-adjusted ultrasound risk assessment for fetal Down's syndrome during the second

trimester: description of the method and analysis of 142 cases. *Ultrasound in Obstetrics & Gynecology* **12** (**1**): 8–14.

48 Nyberg, D.A. et al. (1993). Prenatal sonographic findings of trisomy 18: review of 47 cases. *Journal of Ultrasound in Medicine* **12** (**2**): 103–113.

49 Nyberg, D.A. and Souter, V.L. (2001). Sonographic markers of fetal trisomies: second trimester. *Journal of Ultrasound in Medicine* **20** (**6**): 655–674.

50 Smith-Bindman, R., Hosmer, W., Feldstein, V.A. et al. (2001). Second trimester ultrasound to detect fetuses with down syndrome. *JAMA* **285** (**8**): 1044–1055.

51 Bromley, B., Leiberman, E., Shipp, T.D. et al. (2002). The genetic sonogram. *Journal of Ultrasound in Medicine* **21**: 1087–1096.

52 Aagaard-Tillery, K.M. et al. (2009). Role of second-trimester genetic sonography after Down syndrome screening. *Obstetrics & Gynecology* **114** (**6**): 1189–1196.

53 Sonek, J. et al. (2006). Nasal bone assessment in prenatal screening for trisomy 21. *American Journal of Obstetrics and Gynecology* **195** (**5**): 1219–1230.

54 Shields, L.E. et al. (1998). Ultrasonographic diagnosis of trisomy 18: is it practical in the early second trimester? *Journal of Ultrasound in Medicine* **17** (**5**): 327–331.

55 Hill, L.M. (1996). The sonographic detection of trisomies 13, 18, and 21. *Clinical Obstetrics and Gynecology* **39** (**4**): 831–850.

56 Snijders, R.J., Shawa, L., and Nicolaides, K.H. (1994). Fetal choroid plexus cysts and trisomy 18: assessment of risk based on ultrasound findings and maternal age. *Prenatal Diagnosis* **14** (**12**): 1119–1127.

57 Ghidini, A. et al. (2000). Isolated fetal choroid plexus cysts: role of ultrasonography in establishment of the risk of trisomy 18. *American Journal of Obstetrics and Gynecology* **182** (**4**): 972–977.

58 Yoder, P.R. et al. (1999). The second-trimester fetus with isolated choroid plexus cysts: a meta-analysis of risk of trisomies 18 and 21. *Obstetrics & Gynecology* **93** (**5**): 869–872.

59 Walkinshaw, S.A. (2000). Fetal choroid plexus cysts: are we there yet? *Prenatal Diagnosis* **20** (**8**): 657–662.

60 Doubilet, P.M. et al. (2004). Choroid plexus cyst and echogenic Intracardiac focus in women at low risk for chromosomal anomalies the obligation to inform the mother. *Journal of Ultrasound in Medicine* **23** (**7**): 883–885.

61 Ledbetter, D. et al. (1992). Cytogenetic results from the US Collaborative Study on CVS. *Prenatal Diagnosis* **12** (**5**): 317–345.

62 Pittalis, M. et al. (1994). The predictive value of cytogenetic diagnosis after CVS based on 4860 cases with both direct and culture methods. *Prenatal Diagnosis* **14** (**4**): 267–278.

63 Hahnemann, J.M. and Vejerslev, L.O. (1997). Accuracy of cytogenetic findings on chorionic villus sampling (CVS)—diagnostic consequences of CVS Mosaicism and non-Mosaic Discrepancy in Centres contributing to EUCROMIC 1986–1992. *Prenatal Diagnosis* **17** (**9**): 801–820.

64 Group, CCC-ACT (1989). Multicentre randomised clinical trial of chorion villus sampling and amniocentesis: first report. *The Lancet* **333** (**8628**): 1–6.

65 Rhoads, G.G. et al. (1989). The safety and efficacy of chorionic villus sampling for early prenatal diagnosis of cytogenetic abnormalities. *New England Journal of Medicine* **320** (**10**): 609–617.

66 Smidt-Jensen, S. et al. (1992). Randomised comparison of amniocentesis and transabdominal and transcervical chorionic villus sampling. *The Lancet* **340** (**8830**): 1237–1244.

67 Jackson, L.G. et al. (1992). A randomized comparison of transcervical and transabdominal chorionic-villus sampling. *New England Journal of Medicine* **327** (**9**): 594–598.

68 Caughey, A.B., Hopkins, L.M., and Norton, M.E. (2006). Chorionic villus sampling compared with amniocentesis and the difference in the rate of pregnancy loss. *Obstetrics & Gynecology* **108** (**3, Part 1**): 612–616.

69 Saura, R. et al. (1994). Operator experience and fetal loss rate in transabdominal CVS. *Prenatal Diagnosis* **14** (**1**): 70–71.

70 Wijnberger, L.D., van der Schouw, Y.T., and Christiaens, G.C. (2000). Learning in medicine: chorionic villus sampling. *Prenatal Diagnosis* **20** (**3**): 241–246.

71 Wulff, C.B. et al. (2016). Risk of fetal loss associated with invasive testing following combined first-trimester screening for Down syndrome: a national cohort of 147 987 singleton pregnancies. *Ultrasound in Obstetrics & Gynecology* **47** (**1**): 38–44.

72 Early, T.C. and M-TATC Group (1998). Randomised trial to assess safety and fetal outcome of early and midtrimester amniocentesis. *The Lancet* **351** (**9098**): 242–247.

73 Philip, J. et al. (2004). Late first-trimester invasive prenatal diagnosis: results of an international randomized trial. *Obstetrics & Gynecology* **103** (**6**): 1164–1173.

74 Group, NNRfAS (1976). Midtrimester amniocentesis for prenatal diagnosis. *JAMA: The Journal of the American Medical Association* **236** (**13**): 1471–1476.

75 Sawa, R. et al. (2001). Rapid detection of chromosome aneuploidies by prenatal interphase FISH (fluorescence in situ hybridization) and its clinical utility in Japan. *Journal of Obstetrics and Gynaecology Research* **27** (**1**): 41–47.

76 Schoonmaker, M. (2001). Prenatal diagnosis using interphase fluorescence in situ hybridization (FISH): 2-year multi-center retrospective study and review of the literature. *Prenatal Diagnosis* **21**: 293–301.

77 Tabor, A. et al. (1986). Randomised controlled trial of genetic amniocentesis in 4606 low-risk women. *The Lancet* **327** (**8493**): 1287–1293.

78 Eddleman, K.A. et al. (2006). Pregnancy loss rates after midtrimester amniocentesis. *Obstetrics & Gynecology* **108** (**5**): 1067–1072.

79 Odibo, A.O. et al. (2008). Revisiting the fetal loss rate after second-trimester genetic amniocentesis: a single center's 16-year experience. *Obstetrics & Gynecology* **111** (**3**): 589–595.

80 Mujezinovic, F. and Alfirevic, Z. (2007). Procedure-related complications of amniocentesis and chorionic villous sampling: a systematic review. *Obstetrics & Gynecology* **110** (**3**): 687–694.

81 Seeds, J.W. (2004). Diagnostic mid trimester amniocentesis: how safe? *American Journal of Obstetrics and Gynecology* **191** (**2**): 607–615.

82 Sagoo, G.S. et al. (2009). Array CGH in patients with learning disability (mental retardation) and congenital anomalies: updated systematic review and meta-analysis of 19 studies and 13, 926 subjects. *Genetics in Medicine* **11** (**3**): 139–146.

83 Shaffer, L.G. et al. (2006). Targeted genomic microarray analysis for identification of chromosome abnormalities in 1500 consecutive clinical cases. *The Journal of Pediatrics* **149** (**1**): 98–102. e5.

84 Wapner, R.J. et al. (2012). Chromosomal microarray versus karyotyping for prenatal diagnosis. *The New England Journal of Medicine* **367** (**23**): 2175–2184.

85 Cheschier, N. (2003). ACOG practice bulletin. Neural tube defects. Number 44 July 2003.(Replaces committee opinion number 252, March 2001). *International Journal of Gynaecology and Obstetrics: the Official Organ of the International Federation of Gynaecology and Obstetrics* **83** (**1**): 123–133.

86 Frey, L. and Hauser, W.A. (2003). Epidemiology of neural tube defects. *Epilepsia* **44** (**s3**): 4–13.

87 Mosley, B.S. et al. (2009). Neural tube defects and maternal folate intake among pregnancies conceived after folic acid fortification in the United States. *American Journal of Epidemiology* **169** (**1**): 9–17.

88 Wald, N.J. et al. (1977). Maternal serum-alpha-fetoprotein measurement in antenatal screening for anencephaly and spina bifida in early pregnancy. Report of UK collaborative study on alpha-fetoprotein in relation to neural-tube defects. *Lancet* **1** (**8026**): 1323–1332.

89 Wang, Z.P. et al. (2009). The effectiveness of prenatal serum biomarker screening for neural tube defects in second trimester pregnant women: a meta-analysis. *Prenatal Diagnosis* **29** (**10**): 960–965.

90 American College of Obstetricians and Gynecologists (2009). ACOG practice bulletin No. 101: ultrasonography in pregnancy. *Obstetrics and Gynecology* **113** (**2 Pt 1**): 451.

91 Nicolaides, K. et al. (1986). Ultrasound screening for spina bifida: cranial and cerebellar signs. *The Lancet* **328** (**8498**): 72–74.

92 Jørgensen, F.S. et al. (1999). MULTISCAN-A Scandinavian multicenter second trimester obstetric ultrasound and serum screening study. *Acta Obstetricia et Gynecologica Scandinavica* **78** (**6**): 501–510.

93 Boyd, P.A. et al. (2008). Survey of prenatal screening policies in Europe for structural malformations and chromosome anomalies, and their impact on detection and termination rates for neural tube defects and Down's syndrome. *BJOG: An International Journal of Obstetrics & Gynaecology* **115** (**6**): 689–696.

94 Dashe, J.S. et al. (2006). Alpha-fetoprotein detection of neural tube defects and the impact of standard ultrasound. *American Journal of Obstetrics and Gynecology* **195** (**6**): 1623–1628.

95 Norem, C.T. et al. (2005). Routine ultrasonography compared with maternal serum alpha-fetoprotein for neural tube defect screening. *Obstetrics & Gynecology* **106** (**4**): 747–752.

96 Loft, A.G.R. et al. (1993). A comparison of amniotic fluid alpha-fetoprotein and acetylcholinesterase in the prenatal diagnosis of open neural tube defects and anterior abdominal wall defects. *Prenatal Diagnosis* **13** (**2**): 93–109.

97 Lennon, C.A. and Gray, D.L. (1999). Sensitivity and specificity of ultrasound for the detection of neural tube and Ventral Wall defects in a high-risk population. *Obstetrics & Gynecology* **94** (**4**): 562–566.

22

CHAPTER 22
Hyperemesis gravidarum

Veronica Gillispie and Sherri Longo
Ochsner Health System, New Orleans, LA, USA

> **CLINICAL SCENARIO**
>
> A 25-year old primigravida at 10 weeks gestation presents to your office complaining of intractable emesis throughout the day. She complains of dizziness and decreased urination. She reports being able to drink some broth and some crackers. Patient has previously been treated for severe nausea and emesis earlier in the pregnancy. Today, in the office, her vitals include a blood pressure (BP) of 90/80 mmHg and a pulse of 110. Her urine shows ketones. How would you manage her?

Incidence

Nausea and vomiting begins in the first trimester, usually starting at six to eight weeks gestation. Most frequently the symptoms peak at nine weeks gestation and dissipate by 12 weeks [1]. Hyperemesis gravidarum (HG) is a more severe form of nausea and vomiting associated with pregnancy.

The definition for HG is variable but most commonly accepted as intractable vomiting of at least three episodes in a day, a weight loss of greater than 5% of prepregnancy weight, acute starvation manifested as ketonuria, and electrolyte imbalance most commonly hypokalemia [2–4]. HG is a multifactorial condition involving gastrointestinal, hormonal, and genetic factors.

Severe nausea and emesis in pregnancy is common with an incidence of 50–80%. The incidence of HG, however, is rare and occurs in about 0.3–2% of pregnancies [2]. Most patients with HG have resolution of symptoms by 20th week of gestation. HG is the most common reason for hospitalization in the first trimester of pregnancy and is the second most common reason to be hospitalized throughout the entire pregnancy [5, 6]. The hospital readmission rate for HG is 25% [7]. In the past, the mortality rate of HG was about 10%. Now, however, maternal death is rare due to intervention with intravenous (IV) fluid [8].

Etiology

The etiology of HG is unknown. The underlying pathogenesis is not well understood but theories include hormonal, genetic, psychological, and environmental components. Hormonally, HG is thought to be caused by high levels of estrogen, low levels of prolactin, and high levels of human chorionic gonadotropin (hCG). hCG is thought to contribute to HG by stimulating the ovary to produce estrogen, and estrogen increases nausea and emesis [2]. hCG's contribution to HG is further supported by the fact that hCG levels are higher in multiple gestations and molar pregnancies which have a higher incidence of HG [9]. It has also been hypothesized by several investigators that various hCG isoforms secreted by different ethnic groups may affect HG pathogenesis [10, 11].

A large prospective study by Torgersen et al. suggested that women with the purging type of bulimia nervosa had a higher risk for nausea and vomiting during pregnancy than women without eating disorders [12]. Family history and a history of HG in a prior pregnancy are also considered risk factors for HG. Smoking seems to decrease the risk for HG [13].

Helicobacter pylori is a Gram-negative flagellated spiral bacterium that increases the risk for gastric pathology by colonizing the stomach. *H. pylori* is known to be a factor in gastrointestinal diseases. Pregnant women are thought to have a predisposition for *H. pylori* because elevated hCG causes a shift in pH, decreased gastrointestinal motility, and the altered cell mediated immune system [13].

There have been many studies that suggest a significant positive association between *H. pylori* and HG. In 2009, Sandven et al. published a systematic review and meta-analysis of case-control studies and demonstrated that the presence of *H. pylori* is associated with an increased risk of HG [14]. Lin Li et al. published a meta-analysis that included 32 articles with an overall conclusion that there is an association between *H. pylori* and HG. The mechanism by which *H. pylori*

Evidence-Based Obstetrics and Gynecology, First Edition. Edited by Errol R. Norwitz, Carolyn M. Zelop, David A. Miller, and David L. Keefe.

causes HG remains unclear, however some possible reasons include hormonal changes in early pregnancy resulting in a shift in gastrointestinal pH, mood changes affecting immune system with an increased risk for infection, and prolonged gastric emptying [15].

However, it remains unclear as to whether treating *H. pylori* will improve the symptoms of nausea and vomiting of pregnancy [16].

Biochemical thyroid axis abnormalities are frequently seen in HG patients and most commonly referred to as gestational transient thyrotoxicosis but, clinical hyperthyroidism is rare in this population. hCG is a structural homology to thyroid stimulating hormone (TSH) and suppresses TSH release. The hCG effect at the TSH receptor sites may contribute to the hyperthyroidism [8].

Over the years, investigators have proposed that there are underlying psychological or social factors that lead to HG. There has been reported a possible psychosomatic etiology to HG with patients having higher levels of anxiety with HG [17]. Some authors suggest that HG is more common in patients that are immature, dependent, depressed or hysterical but this hypothesis has not been studied [18]. There is no quality data to support the resurfacing hypothesis of a primary psychological basis for HG.

While some people have proposed a psychiatric component to HG, some studies suggest otherwise. D'Orazio et al. published in 2011 a pilot study that suggested pregnant women with HG were not more likely to have psychiatric symptoms or disturbances worse than pregnant women with normal nausea and vomiting [19]. More research is needed to determine if there is an association between psychiatric illness and HG.

Effects of hyperemesis gravidarum

Though the short-term and long-term effects of HG on the fetus have not been well established, a large meta-analysis conducted by Veenendaal et al. did identify several trends [20].

Effects on the fetus

Fetal growth restriction can result as a consequence of HG. In the meta-analysis, when low birth weight (LBW) was defined as a weight of less than 2500 g, 6.4% of HG pregnancies experienced LBW infants, compared to 5% of pregnancies not affected by HG. Not surprisingly, findings are similar when comparing the rate of small for gestational age (SGA) infants. 17.9% of pregnancies affected by HG gave birth to an infant that was SGA, compared to 12.7% of pregnancies not affected. The etiology of LBW and SGA is unclear but is most likely a result of poor maternal weight gain during the pregnancy. It is also unclear if the trend for LBW and SGA is associated with adverse outcomes as the rate of perinatal death does not seem to differ in pregnancies affected by HG versus pregnancies not affected [20].

Effects on the pregnancy

In the large meta-analysis, having HG during pregnancy was found to be associated with an increased risk of preterm delivery. 7.4% of HG pregnancies resulted in preterm delivery. This was compared to 5.8% of pregnancies not affected by HG. Again, the clinical significance, however, is unclear but the increase in preterm deliveries may also contribute to the increased rate of LBW and SGA infants in pregnancies affected by HG [20].

Effects on the mother

The effect of HG on the mother is related to the severity of symptoms. The most detrimental side effect of HG is Wernicke's encephalopathy [21]. Though rare, there have been case reports of Wernicke's encephalopathy in pregnancy related to HG. Wernicke's encephalopathy is a condition in which patients experience altered mental status due to severe thiamine deficiency. The treatment is to give high doses of thiamine but if left untreated, can lead to irreversible neurologic damage.

Because of the persistent vomiting experienced by pregnant women with HG, additional potential side effects requiring medical attention are splenic avulsion, esophageal rupture, Mallory-Weiss tears, pneumothorax or peripheral neuropathy secondary to decreased Vitamins B6 and B12 [22].

Though there are several studies that show the effect of nutrition and weight gain in pregnancy on long-term maternal health, to date, there are no studies evaluating the long-term health risks to women that experienced HG during pregnancy.

Differential diagnoses

The diagnosis of HG is made by clinical evaluation and supported by laboratory evaluation. The clinical symptoms associated with HG are intractable nausea and vomiting with an inability to tolerate solids or liquids resulting in weight loss. Laboratory evaluation often shows electrolyte disturbances including a metabolic acidosis. In addition to clinical symptoms, the diagnosis can be made by a validated questionnaire such as the Pregnancy Unique Quantification of Emesis (PUQE) questionnaire [23]. This is a three question self-administered questionnaire that quantifies the frequency of symptoms for pregnant women experiencing nausea and vomiting. The scoring system then stratifies the symptoms into mild, moderate, or severe. The results can be used to assist in distinguishing nausea and vomiting in pregnancy from HG.

Because the symptoms associated with HG can be non-specific, it is important to consider other diagnoses that can cause nausea and vomiting in pregnancy. A logical way to consider these etiologies is to divide them into systems (See Tables 22.1–22.3, and 22.4).

The differential diagnoses include gastrointestinal conditions (ex. appendicitis, small bowel obstruction, cholecystitis, and pancreatitis), endocrine disorders (ex. diabetic ketoacidosis, thyrotoxicosis, and hyperparathyroidism), neurologic conditions (pseudotumor cerebri, migraines, and vestibular lesions), biliary tract disease, hepatitis, pyelonephritis, and other pregnancy-related conditions such as acute fatty liver disease of pregnancy or pre-eclampsia [1, 25].

Laboratory Evaluation

As discussed above, the diagnosis of HG is made by clinical suspicion. Laboratory results demonstrating a metabolic acidosis help to support the diagnosis. Laboratory evaluation including a complete blood count, liver function tests, electrolytes, thyroid function tests, and urinalysis are important for ruling out other causes of nausea and vomiting in pregnancy. Other tests such as amylase and lipase may need to be added if concerned for other possible causes of the nausea and emesis. An ultrasound should be performed to rule out other pregnancy related causes of HG such as multiple gestation and molar pregnancy.

Treatment options: outpatient versus inpatient treatment

The location of treatment of HG is dependent on the severity but usually results in hospitalization. There have been some reports of patients being managed outpatient using home health services but from a patient safety standpoint in-patient care is the best [26].

Treatment of nausea and vomiting in pregnancy can be addressed in a variety of modalities. The first priority in treating HG is to treat the most detrimental manifestations. Dehydration is a hallmark of HG and must be treated first. This also includes addressing associated electrolyte disturbances. Because of the inability to tolerate oral intake, most patients will require intravenous hydration. Although there are no randomized controlled trials (RCTs) that delineate one type of fluid over another as superior, there are some key concepts regarding hydration that should be remembered. Sodium chloride 0.9% intravenous fluid is preferable to dextrose containing fluids as to not precipitate Wernicke's encephalopathy [27]. Because thiamine requirements increase in pregnancy and approximately 60% of patients with HG will have thiamine deficiency, they are at increased risk for Wernicke's encephalopathy [28]. Intravenous hydration treated with glucose containing fluid can worsen thiamine deficiency and increase the risk for development of Wernicke's encephalopathy. The rate of hydration with normal saline, as well as avoidance of

Table 22.1 Differential diagnosis of persistent vomiting in pregnancy

Gastrointestinal
- Gastroenteritis
- Biliary tract disease
- Hepatitis
- Intestinal obstruction
- Peptic ulcer disease
- Pancreatitis
- Appendicitis

Genitourinary tract
- Pyelonephritis
- Uremia
- Torsion
- Kidney stones
- Degenerating uterine leiomyoma

Metabolic
- Diabetic ketoacidosis
- Porphyria
- Addison's disease
- Hyperthyroidism

Neurologic disorders
- Pseudotumor cerebri
- Vestibular lesions
- Migraine headaches
- Tumors of the central nervous system

Miscellaneous
- Drug toxicity or intolerance

Pregnancy-related conditions
- Acute fatty liver of pregnancy

Preeclampsia

Source: Goodwin (1998) [24].

Table 22.2 Laboratory abnormalities in hyperemesis

Laboratory abnormality	%	Usual range from given limit of normal
Free T4 Index elevated	60	13–40
Free T3 Index elevated	10	225–350
TSH suppressed	60	<0.4 mU ml^{-1}
Sodium low	30	125–134
Potassium low	15	2.3–3.1
Chloride low	25	80–98
Bicarbonate high	15	27–34
Bicarbonate low	8	14–22
ALT or AST high	40	41–324
T. Bili > 1.0	20	1.1–5.3
Amylase high	10	151–391
Lipase high	10	70–200

TSH, thyrotropin; ALT, alanine amino transferase; AST, aspartate amino transferase; T. Bili, total bilirubin.
Source: Goodwin (1998) [24].

Table 22.3 Randomized trials of antiemetics in pregnancy

Agent	Number of trials	Benefit
Nausea or vomiting		
Bendectin	3	+
Pyridoxine	6	+
Meclizine	4	+
Promethazine	2	+
Hydroxyzine	1	+
Timethobenzamide	1	+
Thielpyrazine	1	+
Mepyramine	1	+
Dimenhydrinate	1	+
Hyperemesis gravidarum		
Intramuscular		
ACTH	1	–
Powdered ginger	1	+
Ondansetron	1	–

ACTH, adrenocorticotropic hormone.
Source: Goodwin (1998) [24].

Table 22.4 Medrol dosing schedule

Day	Morning (mg)	Midday (mg)	Bedtime (mg)
1	16	16	16
2	16	16	16
3	16	16	16
4	16	8	16
5	16	8	8
6	8	8	8
7	8	4	8
8	8	4	4
9	8	4	
10	8	4	
11	8		
12	8		
13	4		
14	4		

Source: Goodwin (1998) [24].

higher concentrations of sodium, should also be taken into consideration as rapid correction of hyponatremia can lead to central pontine myelinolysis.

In addition to intravenous hydration, electrolyte abnormalities including thiamine deficiency, should be addressed. Listed below are formulas for correcting sodium and potassium deficiencies: [29]

$$\text{Sodium deficit} = \text{Total body water}^{*} \times (\text{desired sodium level} - \text{present concentration})$$

*total body water is about half of body weight in women

$$\text{Potassium deficit} = 50^{*} \times (4 - \text{present concentration})$$

*100 should be used in obese women

Usually, the sodium infuses at a rate of 0.5 mEQ/l per hour and the potassium infuses at a rate of 10 mEQ per hour not to exceed a maximum of 140 mEQ per day [29].

Thiamine should be replaced intravenously 100 mg in Normal Saline over 30–60 minutes. Once tolerating oral intake it can be replaced at 25–50 mg three times per day [1]. After the immediate treatment of dehydration and the electrolyte disturbances seen in HG, the next step is to address the nausea and vomiting.

Non-pharmacologic treatment

Dietary

There are no RCTs to show the effectiveness of dietary changes in improving nausea and vomiting associated with pregnancy. It is recommended that pregnant women recognize and avoid foods that trigger their nausea. Additionally, women may benefit from eating small, frequent meals. Some women may also find benefit in increasing their intake of protein and carbohydrates.

Herbal options

Ginger is commonly recommended as an herbal option to battle nausea and vomiting of pregnancy. Though the exact mechanism of action is unknown, ginger is thought to work as an antagonist on serotonergic receptors [30]. There are no RCTs to show the benefit of ginger in treating HG. However, in a large meta-analysis conducted by Maggie Thomson et al., when 1 g per day of ginger was taken for four days, nausea and vomiting in pregnancy was improved compared to placebo, with the most commonly observed side effect being acid reflux [31]. There are no teratogenic effects of ginger in animal studies [32].

Hypnosis and acupuncture

Hypnosis and acupuncture have both been proposed as alternatives to medication for treatment of HG. There are no RCTs to demonstrate the effectiveness of hypnosis for treatment of nausea and vomiting associated with pregnancy, though a large literature review was conducted by McCormack, and most of the studies reported positive findings [33]. However, the lack of appropriate trials leaves this therapeutic option as theoretical benefit.

Acupuncture has also been used to treat nausea and vomiting associated with pregnancy. Again, there is a lack of RCTs to demonstrate the effectiveness of this approach. However, in a Cochrane Review conducted by Matthews et al, they found there was no statistically significant difference when comparing P6 acupressure to placebo, auricular acupressure to placebo, or when acupuncture, P6 acupuncture, sham acupuncture, or no treatment was compared. There was no statistically significant improvement when comparing the groups [34].

Pharmacologic treatment

Studies have suggested that taking a multivitamin starting at time of conception may decrease the risk for nausea and vomiting of pregnancy, which will decrease the rare risk for progression to HG [35]. Pharmacologic therapy includes antiemetics such as antihistamines, phenothiazines, metoclopramide, Ondansetron, and Vitamin B6.

First line pharmacotherapy for nausea and vomiting of pregnancy is the combination of pyridoxine 10 mg and one half of 25 mg of doxylamine (antihistamine) administered orally every eight hours [3, 16]. Pyridoxine has a half-life of 15–20 days and the usual upper intake level is 100 mg per day [8]. As of 2013, the Food and Drug Administration (FDA) approved the use of Diclegis® (doxylamine succinate and pyridoxine hydrochloride) for the treatment of nausea and vomiting in pregnancy. Of note, Diclegis® has not been studied in women with HG [36]. Multiple case-control and cohort studies involving over 170 000 exposures, have demonstrated the safety of pyridoxine and doxylamine [37]. A recent systematic review of randomized clinical trials had the conclusion that nausea is improved but not emesis with Vitamin B6 [34].

The American College of Obstetricians and Gynecologists (ACOG) recommends the following intravenous medications as first line antiemetic therapy: promethazine, metoclopramide, and dimenhydrinate [38]. Promethazine is a phenothiazine. Phenothiazines are dopamine antagonists that inhibit emesis by blocking the chemoreceptor trigger area and the gastrointestinal tract D_2 receptors. Promethazine (Phenergan) is usually administered as 25 mg orally, rectally, or intravenously, every four to six hours. An alternative phenothiazine is prochlorperazine (Compazine), which is administered 5–10 mg orally every six hours, 12.5 mg intramuscularly or intravenously, three times a day, or 25 mg rectally followed six hours later with an oral dose [1].

Metoclopramide (Reglan) is a dopamine antagonist. Metoclopramide acts directly on the gastrointestinal tract and also in the central chemoreceptor trigger area.

Metoclopramide is usually administered orally but can be administered intramuscularly, or intravenously 5 – 10 mg every eight hours [16]. Some other examples of dopamine antagonists are trimethobenzamide (Tigan), Droperidol, and (Inapsine) [2].

Tan et al. performed a RCT that compared intravenous promethazine to intravenous metoclopramide in the treatment of HG and each had similar reduction in nausea and emesis. But the group that received intravenous metoclopramide had fewer side effects which included drowsiness, dystonia, dizziness, and treatment curtailment [39].

Dimenhydrinate is an anti-histamine. The mechanism of antihistamines for the decrease in emesis is by inhibition of histamine at the histamine$_1$-receptor and by the vestibular system [2]. Antihistamines are considered safe in pregnancy. This has been supported by a meta-analysis of greater than 200 000 pregnant women who demonstrated no teratogenicity after being treated for nausea and emesis with antihistamines during pregnancy [41]. There are no RCTs comparing the use of oral vs. parenteral antihistamines for hospitalized HG patients. Antihistamines can be combined with other antiemetic medications to reduce the risk for extrapyramidal side effects. The most common side effect for the antihistamines is drowsiness.

Safety of these medications is of importance for the protection of the fetus. There has been documentation of isolated reports of cleft palate, limb, cardiac, and skeletal abnormalities in case reports [40]. Mazzotta et al. performed a meta-analysis of observational studies published in 2000 that demonstrated no increased risk for teratogenicity with the phenothiazines including perphenazine, prochlorperazine, promethazine, and chlorpromazine [41]. Additionally, the analysis by Gill demonstrated that there was no evidence of teratogenicity among the following medications: antihistamines, dopamine antagonists, seratonin antagonists, and phenothiazines [40]. A large database in 2009 including 3458 women treated in the first trimester with metoclopramide provides quality safety evidence [42]. Of note, in 2009 The USA FDA placed a black warning on metoclopramide secondary to reports of tardive dyskinesia especially if long-term use and high doses [43].

Ondansetron is a selective 5-HT3 serotonin receptor antagonist, which acts peripherally on the vagus nerve and small bowel, as well as on the central chemoreceptor inhibitory action to prevent emesis [3]. Most of the studies investigating the safety of ondansetron in pregnancy have not reported an increased risk for fetal abnormalities. Einarson et al. published a case series in 2004 that reported a 3.6% risk for major malformations in the ondansetron group which was not significantly different from the two control groups [44]. Pasternak published in 2013 a study from a historical cohort of 608 385 pregnancies in Denmark and concluded ondansetron taken during pregnancy was not associated with a significant increased risk for poor fetal outcome including major malformations [45]. But, two recent studies published in 2014 determined a statistically significant but small clinical risk for cardiac malformations in ondansetron exposed infants [46, 47]. The FDA and the World Health Organization in 2012, released reports suggesting ondansetron may contribute to the development of serotonin syndrome in at risk patients [48, 49]. The FDA subsequently published requirements for follow-up of patients receiving ondansetron even though many felt the concern was an overestimation and that more studies were indicated [48]. There is a report that suggested a possible association with first trimester exposure to ondansetron and cleft palate [50]. However, to date, there is not enough data to make a firm conclusion on fetal safety with ondansetron administration.

A study performed by Sullivan et al. 1996 demonstrated no difference in treatment of HG between Ondansetron and promethazine [51]. Abas et al. published in 2014 a double-blind RCT that compared intravenous ondansetron to metoclopramide in women treated for HG and found similar efficacy but lower side effects including drowsiness and xerostomia in the ondansetron group [52]. In 2012, US FDA removed the 32 mg single intravenous ondansetron dose secondary to the risk of QT interval prolongation that can result in torsades de pointes [53]. Ondansetron dosages include 4–8 mg every six to eight hours orally, 8 mg intravenous over 15 minutes every 12 hours, or 1 mg per hour continuous up to 24 hours [16].

Droperidol is a butyrophenone that has been used in HG treatment. Turcotte et al. in 2001, demonstrated there was no difference between a control group (n = 54) and the treatment group (droperidol and diphenhydramine, n = 28) for treatment of HG [54]. Ferreira et al. in 2003 reported there was no significant difference in major malformations between the treatment groups (two different doses of droperidol each combined with diphenhydramine, n = 101) and control group (n = 54) [55]. Droperidol has been used less frequently secondary to the side effects including risk for a prolonged QT interval on electrocardiographic (ECG) testing and torsades de pointes which is a potentially fatal arrhythmia. FDA has now issued a black box warning and recommends all patients have a 12 lead ECG before, during, and three hours after treatment [56, 57].

Corticosteroid administration for HG is controversial. Safari et al found oral promethazine and steroids had similar efficacy but there were less readmission rates in the steroid group [58]. Ziaei et al. concluded that oral prednisolone was less effective than promethazine at 48 hours but there was similar efficacy between the two medications by seven days of treatment [59]. Some studies have suggested an increased risk for cleft lip and palate with steroid use in first trimester. But a review by Fraser et al. came to the conclusion that the teratogenic risk of corticosteroids is extremely low [60]. Corticosteroids are not first line management for HG but rather should be considered after intravenous hydration and antiemetic therapy has not been successful. There are several available regimens that include methylprednisolone 48 mg intravenous or PO daily for three days [38], or hydrocortisone 100 mg intravenous twice a day followed by prednisolone 40–50 mg PO daily once improvement is seen [1]. If no resolution of symptoms after three days, corticosteroid therapy is discontinued.

If a patient has not improved with rehydration, antiemetics, and recommended dietary guidelines, consideration should be given for enteral nutrition. If the patient does not respond to enteral nutrition, parenteral nutrition is recommended.

In some cases of HG, enteral feedings via nasogastric or jejunostomy feeding tubes is required for patients to receive adequate nutrition. If a patient does not respond to feeding tube nutrition, consideration for invasive treatment involving peripherally inserted central catheters (PICC lines) may be indicated. The presence of PICC lines increase complications including infections, endocarditis, and thrombosis. Nuthalapaty et al. published a retrospective study of 85 pregnant patients with central catheters and reported that 25% developed major complications including infection [61]. Holmgren et al. published a case series of 33 women with HG treated with PICC for feeding and 66% had thromboembolic or infective complications [62].

This condition is multifactorial and therefore treatment should be diverse ranging from dietary to psychoanalytical therapy. The treatment options should be individualized based on the clinical status and response of the patient.

Key recommendations

The following recommendations are based on good and consistent scientific evidence (Level A):

- The short-term and long-term effects of HG have not been well established. However, there is a concern for low-birth weight infants when a pregnancy is affected by HG. Additionally, pregnant women suffering from HG are at risk for Wernicke's encephalopathy by HG (Level A).
- Because HG is a clinical diagnosis, a thorough evaluation to rule out other differential diagnoses should be performed (Level A).
- First line pharmacotherapy is the combination of pyridoxine and doxylamine.

The following recommendations are based on limited or inconsistent scientific evidence (Level B):

- *H. pylori* may cause HG but unclear if treatment improves the symptoms of nausea and emesis *Promethazine and metoclopramine intravenous have similar efficacy.
- Corticosteroid administration may be of benefit after refractory HG.
- Non-pharmacologic options such as dietary changes, use of ginger, hypnosis, and acupuncture have shown promise as alternative treatment options for nausea and vomiting associated with pregnancies. However, there are no RCTs to show their efficacy in the treatment of HG.

The following recommendations are based primarily on consensus and expert opinion (Level C):

- Treatment of HG should begin with intravenous hydration and correction of electrolyte disturbances, including thiamine deficiency. Intravenous hydration should initially be corrected with Normal Saline instead of a glucose containing solution so as not to precipitate Wernicke's encephalopathy.
- Dietary recommendations include small, frequent meals, increased protein and carbohydrate intake, and avoid foods that may trigger nausea.

References

1 Sheba, J. (2011). Management of nausea and vomiting of pregnancy. *BMJ* **342**: d3606. doi: 10.1136/BMJ.d3606. 1–8. (Level III).

2 Niebyl, J. (2010). Nausea and vomiting in pregnancy. *N. Engl. J. Med.* **363** (**16**): 1544–1550. (Level III).

3 Sonkusare, S. (2011). The clinical management of hyperemesis gravidarum. *Arch. Gynecol. Obstet.* **283**: 1183–1192. (Level III).

4 Niemeijer, M.N. and Grooten, I.J. (2014). Diagnostic markers for hyperemesis gravidarum: a systematic review and metaanalysis. *Am. J. Obstet. Gynecol.* **211** (**2**): 150.e1–150.e15. (Systematic Review and Meta-Analysis).

5 Adams, M.M., Harlass, F.E., Sarno, A.P. et al. (1994). Antenatal hospitalization among enlisted service-women, 1987–1990. *Obstet. Gynecol.* **84**: 35–39. (Level II-3).

6 Gazmararian, J.A., Petersen, R., Jamieson, D.J. et al. (2002). Hospitalizations during pregnancy among managed care enrollees. *Obstet. Gynecol.* **100**: 94–100. (Level II-2).

7 Fell, D.B., Dodds, L., Joseph, K.S. et al. (2006). Risk factors for hyperemesis gravidarum requiring hospital admission during pregnancy. *Obstet. Gynecol.* **107**: 277–284. (Level II-2).

8 Tan, P. and Omar, S. (2011). Contemporary approaches to hyperemesis during pregnancy. *Curr. Opin. Obstet. Gynecol.* **23**: 87093. (Level III).

9 Binu, P. (2003). Hyperemesis gravidarum: literature review. *Wis. Med. J.* **102** (**3**): 46–51. (Literature Review).

10 Tsuruta, E., Tada, H., Tamaki, H. et al. (1995). Pathogenic role of asaio human chorionic gonadotropin in gestational thyrotoxicosis. *J Clin. Endocrinol. Metab.* **80**: 350–355.

11 Vilming, B. and Nesheim, B.I. (2000). Hyperemesis gravidarum in contemporary population in Oslo. *Acta Obset. Gynecol. Scand.* **79**: 640–643. (Level II–2).

12 Torgersen, L., Von Hollie, A., Reichborn-Kjennerud, T. et al. (2008). Nausea and vomiting of pregnancy in women with bulimia nervosa and eating disorders not otherwise specified. *Int. J. Eat. Disord.* **41**: 722–727. (Level II-2).

13 Sonkusare, S. (2008). Hyperemesis gravidarum: a review. *Med. J. Malaysia* **62** (**3**): 272–277. (Medical Review).

14 Sandven, I., Abdelnoor, M., Nesheim, B., and Melby, K.K. (2009). Helicobacter pylori infection and hyperemesis gravidarum: a systematic review and meta-analysis of case-control studies. *Acta Obstet. Gynecol.* **88** (**11**): 1190–1200. (Systematic Review and Meta-Analysis).

15 Li, L., Li, L., Zhou, X. et al. (2015). Helicobacter pylori infection is associated with an increased risk of hyperemesis gravidarum: a meta-analysis. *Gastroenterol. Res. Pract.* 1, 278905–13. (Meta-Analysis).

16 Association of Professors of Gynecology and Obstetrics (2011). *APGO Educational Series on women's Health Issues. Nausea and Vomiting of Pregnancy*, 1–26. Boston, MA: Jespersen & Associates, LLC.

17 Zechnich, R. and Hammer, T. (1982). Brief psychotherapy for hyperemesis gravidarum. *Am. Fam. Physician* **26** (**5**): 179–181. (Level III).

18 Eliakim, R., Abulafia, O., and Sherer, D. (2000). Hyperemesis gravidarum: a current review. *Am. J. Perinatol.* **17** (**4**): 207–218. (Literature Review).

19 D'Orazio, L.M., Meyerowitz, B.E., Korst, L.M. et al. (2011 Jan). Evidence against a link between hyperemesis gravidarum and personality characteristics from an ethnically diverse sample of pregnant women: a pilot study. *J. Womens Health* **20** (**1**): 137–144. (Level II-2).

20 Veenendaal, M.V.E., van Abeelen, A.F.M., Painter, R.C. et al. (2011). Consequences of hyperemesis gravidarum for offspring: a systematic review and meta-analysis. *BJOG.* **118**: 1302–1313. (Meta-analysis).

21 Lavin, P.J., Smith, D., Kori, S.H., and Ellenberger, C. Jr. (1983). Wernicke's encephalopathy: a predictable complication of hyperemesis gravidarum. *Obstet. Gynecol.* **62** (**3 Suppl**): 13s–15s. (Level III).

22 Goodwin, T.M. (2008). Hyperemesis gravidarum. *Obstet. Gynecol. Clin. North Am.* **35** (**3**): 401–417.

23 Koren, G., Boskovic, R., Hard, M. et al. (2002). Motherisk – PUQE (pregnancy unique quantification of emesis and nausea) scoring system for nausea and vomiting of pregnancy. *Am. J. Obstet. Gynecol.* **186** (**5 Suppl Understanding**): S228–S231. (Level II-2).

24 Goodwin, T.M. Hyperemesis gravidarum. *Clin. Obstet. Gynecol.* **1998**, **41** (**3**): 597–605.

25 Management of hyperemesis gravidarum. Drug Therapy Bull. 2013; **51** (**11**): 126–129. (Review)

26 Jennings-Sanders, A. (2009). A case study approach to hyperemesis gravidarum: home care implications. *Home Healthc. Nurse.* **27** (**6**): 347–351; quiz 352-3. doi: 10.1097/01.NHH.0000356824.48175.3f. (Level III).

27 Bottomley, C. and Bourne, T. (2009). Management strategies for hyperemesis. *Best Pract. Res. Clin. Obstet. Gynaecol.* **23** (**4**): 549–564. (Review).

28 van Stuijvenberg, M.E., Schabort, I., Labadariois, D., and Nel, J.T. (1995). The nutritional status and treatment of patients with hyperemesis gravidarum. *Am. J. Obstet. Gynecol.* **172** (**5**): 1585–1591. (Level II-1).

29 Tamay, A.G. and Kuscu, N.K. (2011). Hyperemesis gravidarum: current aspect. *J. Obstet. Gynecol.* **31**: 708–712. (Review).

30 White, B. (2007). Ginger: an overview. *Am. Fam. Physician* **75** (**11**): 1689–1691. (Review).

31 Thomson, M., Corbin, R., and Leung, L. (2014). Effects of ginger for nausea and vomiting in early pregnancy: a meta-analysis. *J. Am. Board Fam. Med.* **27** (**1**): 115–122. doi: 10.3122/jabfm.2014.01.130167. (Meta-analysis).

32 Weidner, M.S. and Sigwart, K. (2001. Jan-Feb). Investigation in the teratogenic potential of a zingiber officinale extract in the rat. *Reprod. Toxicol.* **15** (**1**): 75–80.

33 McCormack, D. (2010). Hypnosis for hyperemesis gravidarum. *J. Obstet. Gynaecol.* **30** (**7**): 647–653. doi: 10.3109/01443615.2010.509825. (Review).

34 Matthews, A., Haas, D.M., O'Mathuna, D.P. et al. (2014). Interventions for nausea and vomiting in early pregnancy.

Cochrane Database Syst. Rev. (**Issue 3**. Art. No.:): CD007575. doi: 10.1002/14651858.CD007575.pub3. (repeat as 37).

35 Czeizel, A.E., Dudas, I., Fritz, G. et al. (1992). The effect of periconceptual multivitamin-mineral supplementation on vertigo, nausea and vomiting in the first trimester of pregnancy. *Arch. Gynecol. Obstet.* **251**: 181–185.

36 Duchesnay USA, Inc. Diclegis®. Prescribing Information. Rev 4/2013. https://www.diclegis.com/pdf/Diclegis_Full_Prescribing_Information.pdf. Last accessed: January 1, 2016.

37 Quinla, J.D. and Hill, D.A. (2003). Nausea and vomiting of pregnancy. *Am. Fam. Physician* **68** (**1**): 121–128. (Review).

38 ACOG (American College of Obstetrics and Gynecology) (2015). Practice Bulletin: Nausea and vomiting of pregnancy. *Obstet. Gynecol.* **153**: 1–13.

39 Tan, P.C., Khine, P.P., Vallikkannu, N., and Omar, S.Z. (2010). Promethazine compared with metoclopramide for hyeremesis gravidarum: a randomized controlled trial. *Obstet. Gynecol.* **115** (**5**): 978–981. doi: 10.1097/AOG.obo13e3181d99290. (Level I).

40 Gill, S.K. and Einarson, A. (2007). The safety of drugs for the treatment of nausea and vomiting of pregnancy. *Expert Opin. Drug Saf.* **6** (**6**): 685–694.

41 Mazzotta, P. and Magee, L.A. (2000). A risk-benefit assessment of pharmacological and non-pharmacological treatments for nausea and vomiting of pregnancy. *Drugs* **59** (**4**): 781–800. (Review).

42 Matok, I., Gorodischer, R., Koren, G. et al. (2009). The safety of metoclopramide use in the first trimester of pregnancy. *N. Engl. J. Med.* **360** (**24**): 2528–2535. doi: 10.1056/NEJMoa0807154. (LevelII-2).

43 US Food and Drug Administration. Boxed warning and risk mitigation strategy for metoclopramide; 2009. http://www.fda.gov/NewsEvents/Newsroom/PressAnnouncements/2009/ucm149533.httm.

44 Einarson, A., Maltepe, C., Navioz, Y. et al. The safety of ondansetron for nausea and vomiting of pregnancy: a prospective comparative study. *BJOG* **2004**, **111** (**9**): 940–943. (Level II-2).

45 Pasternak, B., Svanstrom, H., and Hivid, A. (2013). Ondansetron in pregnancy and risk of adverse fetal outcomes. *N. Eng. J. Med.* **368** (**9**): 814–823.

46 Danielsson, B., Wikner, B.N., and Källén, B. (2014). Use of ondansetron during pregnancy and congenital malformations in the infant. *Reprod. Toxicol.* **50**: 134–137.

47 Koren, G. (2014 Feb). Scary science: ondansetron safety in pregnancy-two opposing results from the same Danish registry. *Ther. Drug Monit.* **36** (**1**): 1–2.

48 US Food and Drug Administration. FDA Drug Safety Communication: Abnormal Heart Rhythms May be Associated With Use of Zofran (ondansetron). http://www.fda.gov/Drugs/DrugSafety/ucm271913.htm. Accessed January 29,2015.

49 World Health Organization (2012). Ondansetron and serotonin syndrome. *WHO Pharmaceuticals Newsletter* **3**: 16.

50 Anderka, M., Mitchell, A.A., Louik, C. et al. (2012). Medications used to treat nausea and vomiting of pregnancy and the risk of selected birth defects. National Birth Defects Prevention Study. *Birth Defects Res. A Clin. Mol. Teraol.* **94**: 22–30. (Level II-2) Pubmed.

51 Sullivan, C.A., Johnson, C.A., Roach, H. et al. (1996). A Pilot study of intravenous ondansetron for hyperemesis gravidarum. *Am. J. Obstet Gynecol.* **174** (**5**): 1565–1568. (Level I).

52 Abas, M.N., Tan, P.C., Azmi, N., and Omar, S.Z. (2014 Jun). Ondansetron compared with metoclopramide for hyperemesis gravidarum: a randomized controlled trial. *Obstet. Gynecol.* **123** (**6**): 1272–1279. (Level I).

53 US Food and Drug Administration (2012). *FDA Drug Safety Communication: Updated Information on 32 mg Intravenous Ondansetron (Zofran) Dose and Pre-mixed Ondansetron Products.* Silver Spring (MD): FDA.

54 Turcotte, V., Ferreira, E., and Duperron, L. (2001). Utilite de droperidol et de la diphenhydramine dans l'hyperemesis gravidarum. *J. SOGC* **23**: 133–139.

55 Ferreira, E., Bussiere, J.F., Turcotte, V., and Duperron, L. (2003). Ouellet. Case-control study comparing droperidol plus diphenhydramine in hyperemesis gravidarum. *J. Pharm. Techno.* **19**: 349–354. (Level II-2).

56 Kao, L.W., Kirk, M.A., Evers, S.J., and Rosenfeld, S.H. (2003). Droperidol, QT prolongation and sudden death: what is the evidence? *Ann. Emerg. Med.* **41**: 546–557. (Level III).

57 U.S. Food and Drug Administration (2001). *Inapsine (Droperidol) Dear Healthcare Professional Letter Dec 2001.* Silver Spring (MD): FDA (Level III).

58 Safari, H.R., Fassett, M.J., Souter, I.C. et al. (1998). The efficacy of methylprednisolone in the treatment of hyperemesis gravidarum: a randomized, double-blind, controlled study. *Am. J. Obstet. Gynecol.* **179** (**4**): 921–924. (Level I).

59 Ziaei, S., Hosseiney, F.S., and Faqhihzadeh, S. (2004). The efficacy low dose of prednisolone in the treatment of hyperemesis gravidarum. *Acta Obstet. Gynecol. Scand.* **83** (**3**): 272–275. (Level I).

60 Fraser, F.C. and Sajoo, A. (1995 Jan). Teratogenic potential of corticosteroids in humans. *Teratology* **51** (**1**): 45–46. (Level III).

61 Nuthalapty, F.S., Beck, M.M., and Mabie, W.C. (2009). Complications of central venous catheters during pregnancy and postpartum: a case series. *Am. J. Obstet. Gynecol.* **201** (**3**): 311.e1–311.e5. doi: 10.1016/j.ajog.2009.06.020. (Level III).

62 Holmgren, C., Aagaard-Tillery, K.M., Silver, R.M. et al. (2008 Jan). Hyperemesis in pregnancy: an evaluation of treatment strategies with maternal and neonatal outcomes. *Am. J. Obstet. Gynecol.* **198** (**1**): 56.e1–56.e4. doi: 10.1016/j.ajog.2007.06.004.

23

CHAPTER 23
Drugs and medication in pregnancy

Maisa N. Feghali and Steve N. Caritis
Division of Maternal-Fetal Medicine, Department of Obstetrics, Gynecology and Reproductive Sciences, Magee Women's Hospital of UPMC, Pittsburgh, PA, USA

CLINICAL SCENARIO

A 28-year-old female currently 12 weeks pregnant presents to the office for consultation about her seizure disorder. She was diagnosed with grand mal seizures five years ago and reports taking lamotrigine for seizure control. On average, she has one or two seizures per year and her last seizure occurred four months ago. This is her first pregnancy. She is otherwise a healthy woman with no other medical problems. She reports limited compliance with her medication because of a recent change in her work schedule.

On examination, she appears in no distress and reports mild nausea and vomiting since finding out she was pregnant. These symptoms occur daily but have not caused any weight loss or change in activity.

She has been reading material on the Internet and is concerned about how pregnancy will affect her seizure control. She is also aware that several treatments for seizures have fetal effects wishes to discuss her medications with you.

Background

Various medications are used during pregnancy despite a lack of testing in this specific setting. Drug labeling usually involves information on fetal safety, but lacks recommendation on dosing, efficacy and maternal safety for use during pregnancy. In most circumstances, providers treat pregnant women with the standard adult dose despite the fact that dosing, safety and efficacy were determined in healthy, and mostly male, individuals. In some instances, treatment may be withheld from pregnant women due to concerns about maternal or fetal safety. Recent advances in clinical therapeutics in pregnancy suggest a myriad of physiologic and metabolic changes affecting disease processes in pregnancy. Consequently, dose adjustments may be required for medications used during pregnancy.

Clinical questions

1. What are the major physiologic changes occurring during pregnancy?
2. How do the physiologic changes of pregnancy affect drug disposition?
3. How does the placenta affect drug therapy during pregnancy?
4. What are the fetal risks with maternal pharmacotherapy?

Critical appraisal of the literature

1. What are the major physiologic changes occurring during pregnancy?

The physiologic changes associated with pregnancy are multifold and often vary with advancing gestation. Maternal physiology evolves during the course of pregnancy to adjust for the development and growth of the placenta and fetus [1, 2].

Cardiovascular physiology is significantly altered during pregnancy. Cardiac output starts increasing early in pregnancy then plateaus at 28 weeks around $7\,l\,min^{-1}$, remaining at this level until delivery where it increases further [3]. A parallel increase is also noted for stroke volume [3]. A gradual increase is also seen with maternal heart rate reaching 90 beats per min at rest in the third trimester [3]. Furthermore, plasma volume increases approximately 40% throughout pregnancy reaching 3.5 l at 38 weeks of gestation [3]. An increase in red blood mass is also noted, yet at a slower pace, resulting in the common finding of "physiologic" anemia in a large proportion of pregnant women. Progesterone and relaxin are thought to contribute to the observed systemic vasodilation in early pregnancy [1, 4]. Dilation of the renal vasculature, increase in glomerular

Evidence-Based Obstetrics and Gynecology, First Edition. Edited by Errol R. Norwitz, Carolyn M. Zelop, David A. Miller, and David L. Keefe.

filtration rate (GFR) and renal plasma flow (RPF) are also observed [5]. GFR is 1.6-fold higher in pregnancy compared to preconceptional and postpartum values [1]. Differences have been noted in the clearance of renally eliminated drugs that could be explained by the previously described changes in blood flow and filtration. The effects of renal changes on drug disposition during pregnancy are discussed later in the chapter.

Pulmonary function in pregnancy is affected by physiologic and anatomic changes. Functional residual capacity is decreased whereas minute ventilation and tidal volume are increased by approximately a third compared to non-pregnant individuals [6]. These changes underline the finding of mild hyperventilation in two thirds of normal pregnancies.

Total hepatic perfusion is also notably increased during pregnancy. Nakai et al. used Doppler ultrasonography to assess hepatic blood flow during the third trimester of pregnancy and nonpregnant subjects [7]. In their study, hepatic artery blood flow was not significantly increased. The authors concluded that increased hepatic perfusion is likely due to higher portal venous return [7]. In theory, an increase in hepatic perfusion could lead to higher extraction of drugs by the liver and in consequence decreased systemic bioavailability. Nonetheless, studies of drugs with high rates of hepatic extraction show variable effects on their systemic availability. This suggests the presence of additional mechanisms affecting the pharmacokinetic properties of these drugs.

Pregnancy is also associated with delayed gastric emptying [8], decreased intestinal motility [9] and decreased gastric acid secretion [10]. In early pregnancy, a well-known early gastrointestinal change is pregnancy is nausea and vomiting. Almost two thirds of pregnant women report nausea and vomiting during the first trimester [11–13]. For some women, the symptoms may persist beyond that time mark. Treatment of nausea and vomiting of pregnancy (NVP) has been limited by fears of teratogenicity, despite a lack of suggestive data, and the minimal efficacy of most anti-emetics. A potential consequence of NVP is decreased intake of medications in cases with pre-pregnancy conditions requiring chronic treatment. This may be the underlying mechanism of worsening disease status during the first trimester in cases such as seizure disorders.

2. How do the physiologic changes of pregnancy affect drug disposition? (Table 23.1)

a. Drug Absorption

Theoretically, the slower intestinal motility and decreased gastric acid secretion in pregnancy could alter drug absorption and oral bioavailability. However, no confirmatory evidence validates these assumptions. In fact, in studies on ß-lactam antibiotics used for asymptomatic bacteriuria, no difference was noted in bioavailability of the drugs (given orally and intravenously) between late pregnancy and postpartum [30, 31]. Little information is available on changes in drug absorption for inhaled agents. A small observational study found that the minimum alveolar concentration of inhaled isoflurane was reduced by 28% in pregnant women at 8–12 weeks of gestation compared to nonpregnant controls [32]. The mechanisms underlying this change are not well defined but could be related to pulmonary function changes occurring during early pregnancy.

b. Drug Distribution

Decreased plasma protein levels during pregnancy lead to an increase in the free fraction of most medications. The decreased concentrations of albumin and alpha 1-acid glycoprotein (AAG) may result from the dilutional effect of increased plasma volume or the increased urinary protein excretion noted during pregnancy [33–35]. The increased free drug fraction may lead to higher drug clearance secondary to higher hepatic extraction or renal elimination. Another reason behind changes in free drug fraction is related to the different concentrations of both albumin and AAG between the maternal and fetal circulations. AAG is two-thirds lower and albumin higher in fetal plasma [36]. This difference presents a gradient between maternal and fetal circulations and may alter drug distribution. Indinavir and saquinavir are examples of differential distribution, due to lower fetal AAG concentration, with higher drug concentrations in umbilical cord samples compared to maternal samples [37].

c. Drug Metabolism

Drug metabolism can be divided into phase I and phase II, which differ by the specialized enzymes involved in drug disposition. Phase I reactions usually involve oxidation whereas phase II reactions are mainly conjugative. Changes in drug metabolism can have implications for drug dosage in pregnancy. In drugs with a narrow therapeutic window, an increased clearance during pregnancy can lead to subtherapeutic concentrations and worsening disease control. Conversely, to avoid increased toxicity, drug doses may need to be adjusted in the postpartum period, when pregnancy-related metabolic enzyme activity changes resolve.

A. Phase I metabolism

Oxidative phase I reactions are predominantly carried out by the cytochrome P450 (CYP) system. It includes a number of enzymes that differ in their substrates. CYP3A is the major P450 enzyme; it is located in the gut and liver and carries out 30% of the P450 complex's activity. In fact, it is involved in the metabolism of more than 50% of the currently known drugs [38, 39]. CYP3A activity is increased during pregnancy. The clearance of Midazolam, one of CYP3A's selective substrates is doubled during pregnancy compared to postpartum [28]. Similarly, metabolism of other CYP3A substrates increases during pregnancy. For example, the clearance of dextromethorphan, a cough suppressant, increases by almost

Table 23.1 Pregnancy induced pharmacokinetic changes for selected drugs

	Half-life	Clearance	Protein binding (%)	Bioavailability	Time during pregnancy change noted	Reference
Antimicrobials						
Cefatrizine	Decreased (1.5 h)	Increases	60	43%	19–24 weeks	[14]
Amoxicillin	Decreased (1.2 h)	Increases		95	Delivery	[15]
Cefuroxime	Decreased (44 min)	Increases		30–50	Delivery	[16]
Zidovudine	Unchanged (1.1 h)	Increases	<25	63	Delivery	[17]
Saquinavir	Unchanged (9–15 h)		98		Delivery	[18]
Lopinavir	Unchanged (5–6 h)	Decreases	99	37	30–36 weeks	[19]
Nelfinavir	Unchanged (3–5 h)		98		2nd and 3rd trimester	[20]
Ritonavir	Unchanged (3–5 h)		99		Delivery	[21]
Glucose lowering agents						
Glyburide	Unchanged (4 h)	Increases	98	Decreases	28–38 weeks	[19]
Metformin	Increased (7 h)	Increases	Negligible	40–60	2nd and 3rd trimester	[22]
Cardiovascular agents						
Digoxin	Decreased (38 h)	Increases	33	60	3rd trimester	[23]
Labetalol	Decreased (1.7 h)	Increases	60	30	3rd trimester	[24]
Atenolol	Decreased (4.8 h)	Increases		60	2nd and 3rd trimester	[25]
Nifedipine (rapid release)	Decreased (rapid release 1.3 h, extended release 2–5 h)	Increases	98	50	3rd trimester	[26, 27]
Nifedipine (extended release)	Decreased (2–5 h)					
Anti-seizure agents						
Lamotrigine	15–24 h	Increases	98	55	Throughout pregnancy	[28]
Levetiracetam		Increases	<10	99	2nd and 3rd trimester	[29]

40% [39], and that of nelfinavir, an anti-retroviral, by almost a third [40, 41]. CPY3A activity is altered by pregnancy but the enzyme's activity is also impacted by the maternal genotype. A recent study on the pharmacokinetics of nifedipine used for tocolysis revealed a genetic variability in the CYP3A5 enzyme [42]. The authors were able to determine a specific allele that influenced oral clearance of the drug and concluded that high expressors of the specific allele had an oral clearance rate almost four times as high as expressors of other allele variants [42].

The second most common enzyme in the CYP complex is CYP2D6. Two phenotypes of the enzyme's activity have been described. A poor metabolizer (PM) phenotype, which is associated with low enzyme activity, and an ultrarapid metabolism phenotype, associated with high enzyme activity [39]. The PM phenotype is an autosomal recessive trait with variable representation in different ethnic groups [43]. With standard doses of medications, individuals with the PM phenotype are expected to have higher concentrations of a specific drug whereas ultrametabolizers would have lower drug levels. In parallel with individual variation in phenotype, CYPD26 activity appears to undergo a gradual increase during pregnancy and resolves following delivery [43]. Changes in enzyme activity leading to lower drug levels have been associated with worsened control of disease such as recurring symptoms of depression in patients receiving fluoxetine during pregnancy [39].

In contrast to previously mentioned enzymes, some of the components of the CYP complex demonstrate decreased activity during pregnancy. Using caffeine as a substrate, CYP1A2 undergoes a gradual decrease in enzymatic activity during pregnancy [38]. Other substrates of the drug include ondansetron and theophylline. The latter has a narrow therapeutic index and a decrease in its clearance during the third trimester could lead to higher rates of toxicity [44–46]. Given the available evidence, it may necessary to use lower doses of medications metabolized by CYP1A2 during pregnancy. However, further studies are needed to fully describe the changes affecting CYP1A2 substrates before recommending specific dosing adjustments.

B. Phase II metabolism

An example of phase II metabolism is Uridine 5′-Diphosphate Glucuronosyltransferase (UGT). Numerous isoforms of the enzyme have been described. One of the substrates of UGT1A4 is the anti-seizure medication lamotrigine. The drug is almost exclusively metabolized by N-glucuronidation by UGT1A4 in the liver [47]. In one study, lamotrigine clearance was 360% higher in the third trimester compared to pre-pregnancy [48]. Along those findings, another study compared serum drug concentration to dose during pregnancy and postpartum in women receiving lamotrigine as monotherapy for seizure control [48]. The ratio was one fourth and two-thirds, respectively, in the first and third trimester, compared to postpartum [48]. In this study, five women required increased doses of the drug to achieve seizure control during pregnancy. Dose adjustments were reversed in the postpartum period to avoid drug toxicity [48].

d. Drug Elimination

Renal drug excretion depends on GFR, tubular secretion, and reabsorption. GFR is 50% higher by the first trimester and continues to increase until the last week of pregnancy, whereby it decreases to postpartum levels [48]. If a drug were solely excreted by glomerular filtration, its renal clearance is expected to parallel changes in GFR during pregnancy. For example, pregnancy effects on the gastrointestinal track reduce oral availability of ampicillin, while increased renal elimination due to the increase in GFR further reduces its serum concentration, [49–51]. Similar changes have been described for cefazolin and clindamycin, commonly used in pregnancy [30, 52]. However, even in cases where drugs exhibit low protein binding and are not metabolized before excretion, such as antibiotics, changes in renal clearance during pregnancy varies widely [53, 54]. More specifically, the clearance of lithium is doubled during the third trimester compared to preconception [55]. By comparison, the clearance of digoxin, which is 80% cleared, is merely 20–30% higher during the third trimester compared to postpartum [56, 57]. Furthermore, the clearance of atenolol is only 12% higher across pregnancy [28, 58]. With evidence of large variation in renal clearance between different drugs, it is not possible to make assumptions about the effect of pregnancy on the clearance of renally eliminated drugs. Further studies are needed to elaborate the various metabolic and physiologic processes underlying these findings and assess the role of tubular secretion and reabsorption.

3. How does the placenta affect drug therapy during pregnancy?

Fetal development is dependent upon the transport of nutrients by the placenta toward the fetal side and that of products of fetal metabolism for elimination by the mother [25]. In addition, the placenta produces and secretes hormones, which affect the maternal physiology and endocrine state [56, 59]. The transport role is mediated by the syncytiotrophoblasts, the functional cell of the placenta. These cells have a polarized plasma membrane consisting of a brush border at the maternal side and a border membrane on the fetal side. Compounds transported between mother and fetus are carried by the maternal circulation within the uterine vasculature directly through the intervillous spaces and then the syncytiotrophoblasts. Thereafter, blood flows from the fetal side of the placental villi through the fetal capillary endothelium to reach the fetal circulation (Figure 23.1). Most xenobiotics cross the placental barrier by simple diffusion. Protein binding, degree of ionization, lipid solubility, and molecular weight all affect transport. In fact, small, lipid soluble, unionized, and poorly protein bound molecules cross the placenta easily. For other substrates, the placenta facilitates maternal to fetal transport through the polarized expression of various transporters [60]. Transporters enable transport of specific endogenous substrates (such as cytokines, nucleoside analogs, and steroid hormones); however, exogenous compounds with similar structures may also interact with these transporters.

A number of placental drug transporters have been identified including the family of multi-drug resistance proteins (MRPs). However, phosphoglycoprotein (P-gp) and breast cancer resistance protein (BCRP) are the most studied so far and will be discussed in greater detail. P-gp is expressed on the apical microvillous surface whereas BCRP is mostly identified on the basolateral membrane and fetal blood vessels [61–64]. Their polarized distribution may reflect a difference in their role. Transporters on the apical membrane are thought to allow selective substrates to be transmitted to the fetus and hence may protect the fetus by extruding harmful xenobiotics. Both transporters have a wide number of substrates. Those of P-gp include endogenous compounds such as cortisol, aldosterone, and bilirubin as well as various drugs such as antibiotics, antiretrovirals, and steroids [65, 66]. Substrates of BCRP include antibiotics, antiretrovirals, calcium channel blockers, estrogen, and prophyrins [65, 67, 68]. These transporters have a number of overlapping substrates for which they have differing affinities [69, 70].

A small number of studies have examined the gestational changes of placental drug transporters. P-gp protein and its associated gene expression are elevated early in pregnancy and decrease near term [71, 72]. Investigations of BCRP changes have yielded inconsistent results with reported increase, decrease, or unchanged expression with advancing gestation [73, 74]. These differences may be related to the different tissues used in each study. Furthermore, evidence on the regulation of placental drug transporters expression is scarce. Both estrogen and progesterone appear to increase expression of P-gp and BCRP in trophoblast cell lines [66, 75, 76]. *In vivo* studies describe an increase in maternal and fetal glucocorticoids with advancing gestation in parallel with a decrease in P-gp. Surprisingly, studies investigating a possible direct link demonstrate that prolonged exposure to dexamethasone increased P-gp and decreased BCRP expression in mice [77, 78]. By comparison, treatment of trophoblast cells with inflammatory cytokines or simulated infection in pregnant rats resulted in decreased P-gp and BCRP expression [79, 80]. Also, P-gp and BCRP expression is lower in preterm placentas and placentas from women with preeclampsia compared to term placentas from

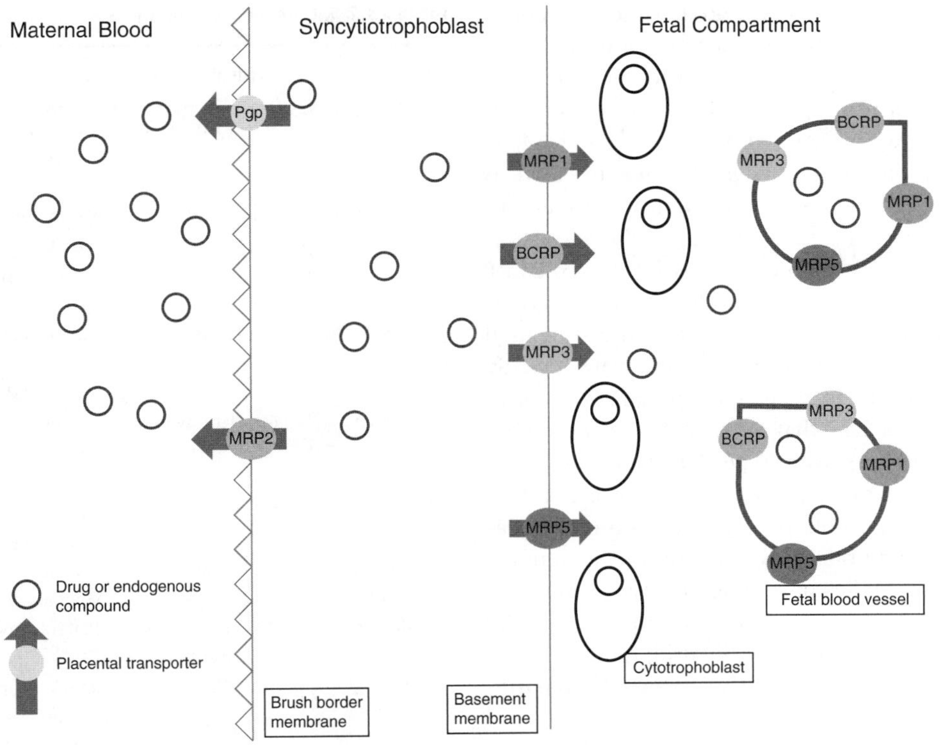

Figure 23.1 Mechanism of placental drug transport. Pgp, phosphoglycoprotein; MRP, multi-resistance protein; BCRP, breast cancer resistance protein.

uncomplicated pregnancies, suggesting a role for hypoxia in mediating these transporters [77].

Selective serotonin reuptake inhibitors (SSRIs) including fluoxetine, sertraline, and paroxetine inhibit P-gp in vitro [81]. Along with a decrease in P-gp expression late in gestation, an inhibition of its function may result in fetal and maternal consequences. The most recent guidelines for treatment of depression during pregnancy recommend using the lowest effective dose of SSRIs [82]. Maternal SSRI use in the first and third trimester has been linked to congenital anomalies and neonatal complications, respectively [83]. A clear link between inhibition of P-gp, neonatal pulmonary hypertension or tachypnea and prenatal exposure to SSRIs remains to be determined. Anti-seizure drugs appear to exhibit an inhibitory effect on carnitine placental transport [84, 85]. Carnitine deficiency has been linked to apnea, cardiac arrest, and cardiac hypertrophy [86]. Carnitine is mainly actively transported through two transporters [86–88]. One of these transporters, carinitine/organic cation transporter (OCTN2) is located on the apical membrane of the syncytiotrophoblasts and is inhibited by some anti-seizure drugs such as valproic acid and phenytoin [89, 90].

On the other hand, treating the fetus in-utero with maternally administered medications presents the opposite challenge i.e. maximizing fetal drug exposure while limiting maternal drug exposure. Fetal tachycardia is an example of transplacental pharmacotherapy whose objective is to avoid possible fetal cardiac decompensation. The main agent used for treatment is digoxin. The maternal clearance of the drug is increased during pregnancy due partly to an increase in renal filtration and an increase in transport by P-gp across the apical membrane of proximal renal tubular epithelium. These changes lead to lower maternal serum concentrations [86]. At the level of the placenta, P-gp extrudes digoxin, decreasing fetal concentration. In the setting of fetal tachycardia, increased maternal digoxin dosage is needed to overcome the physiologic changes in drug clearance both by the mother and placenta [28, 91]. Increasing the maternal dosage however is complicated by a narrow therapeutic index for digoxin and a well-defined toxicity profile.

Furthermore, an example of P-gp function manipulation is illustrated by anti-retroviral medications. The current recommended regimen for human immunodeficiency virus (HIV) treatment is pregnancy is highly-active anti-retroviral therapy (HAART). Anti-retrovirals are expected to cross the placenta into the fetal circulation to prevent fetal infection [91]. Protease inhibitors, a component of HAART, are necessary for viral control in HIV infection. However, a number of protease inhibitors have high affinity for P-gp and are excluded from fetal circulation, therefore decreasing their efficacy [92]. To overcome this effect, protease inhibitors such as saquinavir, lopinavir, and nelfinavir, may be co-administered with ritonavir. The latter has limited functional antiretroviral efficacy, but is chemically related to other protease inhibitors. It can occupy the transporter and limit its capacity to extrude other protease inhibitors. In addition, oral co-administration of ritonavir increases bioavailability saquinavir [93]. This is likely due to inhibition of liver metabolism by CYP3A4 [94, 95].

Despite these promising findings, further research is needed to develop techniques for drug transporter manipulation.

On the other hand, a more recent study has linked BCRP to transplacental transport of Glyburide. The pharmacokinetic and pharmacodynamic characteristics of the drug, used for the treatment of diabetes in pregnancy, were recently studied by Hebert et al. In pregnancy, plasma concentration of glyburide was half that seen with the same dose in non-pregnant subjects with Type 2 diabetes [23]. The authors suggested the findings were due to an increase in hepatic or intestinal metabolism [23]. In addition, transplacental passage of glyburide was thought to be minimal [23]. More recently, studies have described the presence of glyburide and its metabolites in fetal circulation and BCRP was identified as the transporter for the drug [96].

4. What are the fetal risks with maternal pharmacotherapy?

The overall risk of congenital malformations is 2–4%. However, only 10% of malformations are linked to drug exposure. Still, fetal risk remains a major concern with drug use during pregnancy. This apprehension was validated by milestone studies linking thalidomide and isotretinoin to severe malformations and branding them as teratogens. A detailed review of teratology is beyond the scope of this text. The discussion will be limited to the main principles of teratogenicity and fetal toxicity with a review of pertinent examples. For a drug to be labeled as a teratogen, it needs to affect the normal development of fetal organs [23, 97]. This can manifest either structurally or functionally [98] and malformations can vary in severity from being life threatening, to having serious cosmetic or functional consequences [99]. Despite a well-known link between certain drugs and fetal malformations, the number of teratogens with effects limited to first trimester exposure is numbered as listed in Table 23.2. A more pertinent concern with maternal pharmacotherapy is fetal and neonatal toxicity, which occur with later exposure (Table 23.3). The maternal-to-fetal transfer of drugs and the intrinsic toxicity of the drug determine fetal toxicity.

Warfarin is a known teratogen. Early exposure between 6 and 10 weeks of gestation can lead to fetal warfarin syndrome. This consists of variable findings including nasal hypoplasia, microcephaly, hydrocephalus, corpus callosum agenesis, microphthalmia, limb hypoplasia, and stippled epiphyses. Exposure later in pregnancy is associated with fetal hemorrhage particularly in the brain, which can present as ventral or dorsal midline dysplasia, and hemarthroses [100]. Fetal effects of warfarin are likely dose-dependent and the use of the drug in pregnancy is generally limited to second and early third trimester use in women with mechanical heart valves [101].

Table 23.2 Most common teratogens

Agent	Critical period	Effect
Androgens	8th–13th week	Labial fusion, clitoral hypertrophy, masculinization of female fetus
Anticonvulsants	1st trimester	Neural tube defects, cardiac defects, cleft lip and palate, microcephaly, craniofacial defects
Diethylstilbestrol	10–13 week	Vaginal adenocarcinoma, abnormalities of lower mullerian tract
Isotretinoin	6th–13th weeks	Abortion, CNS malformations, cardiac facial dysmorphism, etc.
Lithium	1st trimester	Cardiac defect (Ebstein anomaly)
Methotrexate	1st trimester	CNS and limb malformations
Misoprostol	1st trimester	Moebius sequence
Thalidomide	20–36 days post conception	Bilateral amelia or phocomelia
Warfarin	6th–9th week	Fetal Warfarin Syndrome (facial anomalies and epiphyseal stippling)

Angiotensin-converting enzyme (ACE) [102] inhibitors are also fetal teratogens whose impact on the fetus appears to [103] differ according to timing of exposure during pregnancy. Infants exposed to ACE inhibitors during the first trimester may have increased rates of cardiovascular and central nervous system (CNS) malformations [103]. Exposure in the second or third trimesters impacts the fetal kidneys and may cause oligohydramnios, anuria, renal failure, and death [104]. These concerns have led to the avoidance of ACE inhibitors use during pregnancy.

In women with epilepsy taking one anti-seizure medication the risk of birth defects (4–6%), is almost double the general population, [105, 106]. However, more than 90% of infants born to women with epilepsy are healthy. Early exposure, during the third to eighth week, carries the highest risk for malformations [107]. The risk for malformations also increases with polytherapy and higher total daily doses [108]. Older studies did not find a significant difference in the risk of malformations between different anti-seizure drugs [109]. Another report focused on neonates with fetal anticonvulsant syndrome and found that a majority were exposed to valproic acid alone [109]. In addition, neonates exposed to anti-seizure drugs in utero had a higher risk of lower birthweight, body length, and head circumference when compared to neonates born to mother without epilepsy [110]. Despite these risks, uncontrolled seizures in

Table 23.3 Common fetal drug toxicities

Agent	Toxicity
Angiotensin-converting enzyme inhibitors and angiotensin II receptor antagonists	Renal impairment, renal tubular dysplasia, anuria, oligohydramnios
Anticonvulsants	Hemorrhagic disease of the newborn
Antithyroid drugs (propylthiouracil and methimazole)	Fetal and neonatal goiter and hypothyroidism, aplasia cutis (with methimazole)
Beta adrenergic blockers	Growth delay, bradycardia
Iodine	Fetal hypothyroidism
Ketamine	CNS depression
Lithium	Newborn toxicity
Narcotics	Addiction, withdrawal
Non-steroidal anti-inflammatory drugs (NSAIDs)	Oligohydramnios, ductal closure
Sedative/hypnotics	Hypotonia, sedation, withdrawal
Selective serotonin reuptake inhibitors (SSRIs)	Persistent pulmonary hypertension
Sulfonamides	Hyperbilirubinemia
Sulfonylurea	Hypoglycemia
Warfarin	CNS defects

pregnancy pose a risk to the mother and her fetus. Contemporary strategies in pregnant women with seizures include selection of a single agent that best controls seizures and demonstrates a reasonable safety profile for the fetus.

Maternal pharmacotherapy may not only be associated with fetal malformations but also may affect newborn development and function. For example, a common consequence of maternal treatment with psychoactive drugs is neonatal withdrawal. This effect is commonly seen with opiate and sedative use as well as with SSRIs. Almost a third of neonates exposed to SSRIs exhibit symptoms consistent with withdrawal [111]. These findings have been mostly reported with infants exposed to paroxetine, but symptoms have been linked to all SSRIs [112]. In response to this risk, some women prefer to taper their SSRIs during the third trimester to avoid neonatal effects, despite an increase in recurrence of depressive symptoms and severe depression during the third trimester of pregnancy and the postpartum period.

The intrauterine environment is known to play a role in the origin of adult disease including hypertension, coronary disease, and diabetes [104, 113]. While undernutrition is the most commonly studied trigger [114], in utero drug exposure has evolved as a novel influence on remote adult-onset disease. Animal studies have described the influence of maternal glucocorticoid treatment during pregnancy on the function of the hypothalamic pituitary axis function of guinea pigs (ref). The offspring demonstrated blunted cortisol response to physical stress and the findings persisted in future generations without repeated treatment. Also, glucocorticoid treatment of sheep during gestation has been linked to delayed CNS myelination in the offspring and increased insulin response to glucose challenge in adulthood [115]. Furthermore, antiepileptic drug use during pregnancy has been linked to delays in early infant development [106, 116, 117]. Valproic acid is more likely associated with lower cognitive testing scores and a higher requirement for educational support in school-aged children compared to other anti-seizure medications [105].

Despite realistic concerns for fetal risks, avoiding drug use and drug studies during pregnancy is not possible. Instead, studies should focus on women already receiving treatment. Animal studies to assess for teratogenicity should be carried out, since all known human teratogens also exhibit their effects in animals. Attempts should be made to perform epidemiologic studies to assess for less severe malformations and fetal toxicities, since the more severe fetal effects are more likely to be described in small case reports or cohort studies. Also, long-term follow-up studies should be conducted to determine the role of drug exposure in the fetal origin of adult disease.

Conclusion

- Pregnancy involves various changes in normal physiology and disease. It logically follows, that drug disposition and effects are altered. (Level B, Class I).
- Historically, concerns about fetal safety have limited pharmacotherapy during pregnancy and have hampered drug studies during pregnancy. (Level C).
- Although these concerns have validity, pregnant women require medications for medical disorders and pregnancy does not eliminate the need for therapy. (Level B, Class I).
- Recent studies on pharmacology in pregnancy highlight the complexity of drug distribution and response in light of the dynamic process of gestation. (Level B, Class I).
- To extrapolate drug dosage and expected responses from non-pregnant populations is inappropriate and may cause harm for pregnant women. (Level B, Class IIb).
- Rather, a structured approach to study the pharmacokinetic and pharmacodynamic properties of drugs used in pregnancy should be followed. (Level B, Class I).

References

1 Hill, C.C. and Pickinpaugh, J. (2008). Physiologic changes in pregnancy. *Surg. Clin. North Am.* **88** (**2**): 391–401. vii.

2 Granger, J.P. (2002). Maternal and fetal adaptations during pregnancy: lessons in regulatory and integrative physiology. *Am. J. Physiol. Regul. Integr. Comp. Physiol.* **283** (**6**): R1289–R1292.

3 Pirani, B.B., Campbell, D.M., and MacGillivray, I. (1973). Plasma volume in normal first pregnancy. *J. Obstet. Gynaecol. Br. Commonw.* **80** (**10**): 884–887.

4 Davison, J.M. (1985). The effect of pregnancy on kidney function in renal allograft recipients. *Kidney Int.* **27** (**1**): 74–79.

5 Lindheimer, M.D., Davison, J.M., and Katz, A.I. (2001). The kidney and hypertension in pregnancy: twenty exciting years. *Semin. Nephrol.* **21** (**2**): 173–189.

6 Bonica, J.J. and McDonald, J.S. (eds.) (1995). *Principles and Practice of Obstetric Analgesia and Anesthesia,* 2nde. Baltimore, MD: Williams and Wilkins.

7 Nakai, A., Sekiya, I., Oua, A. et al. (2002). Assessment of the hepatic arterial and portal venous blood flows during pregnancy with Doppler ultrasonography. *Arch. Gynecol. Obstet.* **266** (**1**): 25–29.

8 Hunt, J.N. and Murray, F.A. (1958). Gastric function in pregnancy. *J. Obstet. Gynaecol. Br. Emp.* **65** (**1**): 78–83.

9 Parry, E., Shields, R., and Turnbull, A.C. (1970). Transit time in the small intestine in pregnancy. *J. Obstet. Gynaecol. Br. Commonw.* **77** (**10**): 900–901.

10 Gryboski, W.A. and Spiro, H.M. (1956). The effect of pregnancy on gastric secretion. *N. Engl. J. Med.* **255** (**24**): 1131–1134.

11 Gadsby, R., Barnie-Adshead, A.M., and Jagger, C. (1993). A prospective study of nausea and vomiting during pregnancy. *Br. J. Gen. Pract.* **43** (**371**): 245–248.

12 Vellacott, I.D., Cooke, E.J., and James, C.E. (1988). Nausea and vomiting in early pregnancy. *Int. J. Gynaecol. Obstet.* **27** (**1**): 57–62.

13 Weigel, R.M. and Weigel, M.M. (1989). Nausea and vomiting of early pregnancy and pregnancy outcome. A meta-analytical review. *Br. J. Obstet. Gynaecol.* **96** (**11**): 1312–1318.

14 Feghali, M.N. and Mattison, D.R. (2011). Clinical therapeutics in pregnancy. *J. Biomed. Biotechnol.* **2011**: 783528.

15 Papantoniou, N. et al. (2007). Pharmacokinetics of oral cefatrizine in pregnant and non-pregnant women with reference to fetal distribution. *Fetal Diagn. Ther.* **22** (**2**): 100–106.

16 Philipson, A. (1979). Pharmacokinetics of antibiotics in pregnancy and labour. *Clin. Pharmacokinet.* **4** (**4**): 297–309.

17 Philipson, A. and Stiernstedt, G. (1982). Pharmacokinetics of cefuroxime in pregnancy. *Am. J. Obstet. Gynecol.* **142** (**7**): 823–828.

18 Moodley, J. et al. (1998). Pharmacokinetics and antiretroviral activity of lamivudine alone or when coadministered with zidovudine in human immunodeficiency virus type 1-infected pregnant women and their offspring. *J. Infect. Dis.* **178** (**5**): 1327–1333.

19 Mirochnick, M. et al. (2007). Pharmacokinetics of oral zidovudine administered during labour: a preliminary study. *HIV Med.* **8** (**7**): 451–456.

20 Stek, A.M. et al. (2006). Reduced lopinavir exposure during pregnancy. *AIDS* **20** (**15**): 1931–1939.

21 Kosel, B.W. et al. (2003). Pharmacokinetics of nelfinavir and indinavir in HIV-1-infected pregnant women. *AIDS* **17** (**8**): 1195–1199.

22 Eyal, S. et al. (2010). Pharmacokinetics of metformin during pregnancy. *Drug Metab. Dispos.* **38** (**5**): 833–840.

23 Hebert, M.F. et al. (2009). Are we optimizing gestational diabetes treatment with glyburide? The pharmacologic basis for better clinical practice. *Clin. Pharmacol. Ther.* **85** (**6**): 607–614.

24 Fischer, J.H. et al. (2014). Influence of gestational age and body weight on the pharmacokinetics of labetalol in pregnancy. *Clin. Pharmacokinet.* **53** (**4**): 373–383.

25 Hebert, M.F. et al. (2005). Pharmacokinetics and pharmacodynamics of atenolol during pregnancy and postpartum. *J. Clin. Pharmacol.* **45** (**1**): 25–33.

26 Haas, D.M. et al. (2013). Nifedipine pharmacokinetics are influenced by CYP3A5 genotype when used as a preterm labor tocolytic. *Am. J. Perinatol.* **30** (**4**): 275–281.

27 Prevost, R.R. et al. (1992). Oral nifedipine pharmacokinetics in pregnancy-induced hypertension. *Pharmacotherapy* **12** (**3**): 174–177.

28 Hebert, M.F. et al. (2008). Effects of pregnancy on CYP3A and P-glycoprotein activities as measured by disposition of midazolam and digoxin: a University of Washington specialized center of research study. *Clin. Pharmacol. Ther.* **84** (**2**): 248–253.

29 Tomson, T. et al. (2007). Pharmacokinetics of levetiracetam during pregnancy, delivery, in the neonatal period, and lactation. *Epilepsia* **48** (**6**): 1111–1116.

30 Philipson, A. (1977). Pharmacokinetics of ampicillin during pregnancy. *J. Infect. Dis.* **136** (**3**): 370–376.

31 Philipson, A., Stiernstedt, G., and Ehrnebo, M. (1987). Comparison of the pharmacokinetics of cephradine and cefazolin in pregnant and non-pregnant women. *Clin. Pharmacokinet.* **12** (**2**): 136–144.

32 Chan, M.T., Mainland, P., and Gin, T. (1996). Minimum alveolar concentration of halothane and enflurane are decreased in early pregnancy. *Anesthesiology* **85** (**4**): 782–786.

33 Cheung, C.K. et al. (1989). Urinary excretion of transferrin by non-insulin-dependent diabetics: a marker for early complications? *Clin. Chem.* **35** (**8**): 1672–1674.

34 Erman, A. et al. (1992). Enhanced urinary albumin excretion after 35 weeks of gestation and during labour in normal pregnancy. *Scand. J. Clin. Lab. Invest.* **52** (**5**): 409–413.

35 Hayashi, M. et al. (2002). Changes in urinary excretion of six biochemical parameters in normotensive pregnancy and preeclampsia. *Am. J. Kidney Dis.* **39** (**2**): 392–400.

36 Hill, M.D. and Abramson, F.P. (1988). The significance of plasma protein binding on the fetal/maternal distribution of drugs at steady-state. *Clin. Pharmacokinet.* **14** (**3**): 156–170.

37 Sudhakaran, S. et al. (2007). Differential protein binding of indinavir and saquinavir in matched maternal and umbilical cord plasma. *Br. J. Clin. Pharmacol.* **63** (**3**): 315–321.

38 Hodge, L.S. and Tracy, T.S. (2007). Alterations in drug disposition during pregnancy: implications for drug therapy. *Expert. Opin. Drug. Metab. Toxicol.* **3** (**4**): 557–571.

39 Tracy, T.S. et al. (2005). Temporal changes in drug metabolism (CYP1A2, CYP2D6 and CYP3A activity) during pregnancy. *Am. J. Obstet. Gynecol.* **192** (**2**): 633–639.

40 Hirt, D. et al. (2006). Pregnancy-related effects on nelfinavir-M8 pharmacokinetics: a population study with 133 women. *Antimicrob. Agents Chemother.* **50** (**6**): 2079–2086.

41 Villani, P. et al. (2006). Pharmacokinetics of nelfinavir in HIV-1-infected pregnant and nonpregnant women. *Br. J. Clin. Pharmacol.* **62** (**3**): 309–315.

42 Haas, D.M. et al. (2012). Nifedipine pharmacokinetics are influenced by CYP3A5 genotype when used as a preterm labor tocolytic. *Am. J. Perinatol.*

43 Tamminga, W.J. et al. (1999). CYP2D6 and CYP2C19 activity in a large population of Dutch healthy volunteers: indications for oral contraceptive-related gender differences. *Eur. J. Clin. Pharmacol.* **55** (**3**): 177–184.

44 Tsutsumi, K. et al. (2001). The effect of pregnancy on cytochrome P4501A2, xanthine oxidase, and N-acetyltransferase activities in humans. *Clin. Pharmacol. Ther.* **70** (**2**): 121–125.

45 Brazier, J.L. et al. (1983). Pharmacokinetics of caffeine during and after pregnancy. *Dev. Pharmacol. Ther.* **6** (**5**): 315–322.

46 Grosso, L.M. and Bracken, M.B. (2005). Caffeine metabolism, genetics, and perinatal outcomes: a review of exposure assessment considerations during pregnancy. *Ann. Epidemiol.* **15** (**6**): 460–466.

47 Carter, B.L., Driscoll, C.E., and Smith, G.D. (1986). Theophylline clearance during pregnancy. *Obstet. Gynecol.* **68** (**4**): 555–559.

48 Pennell, P.B. et al. (2004). The impact of pregnancy and childbirth on the metabolism of lamotrigine. *Neurology* **62** (**2**): 292–295.

49 Davison, J.M. and Dunlop, W. (1980). Renal hemodynamics and tubular function normal human pregnancy. *Kidney Int.* **18** (**2**): 152–161.

50 Dunlop, W. (1981). Serial changes in renal haemodynamics during normal human pregnancy. *Br. J. Obstet. Gynaecol.* **88** (**1**): 1–9.

51 Davison, J.M., Dunlop, W., and Ezimokhai, M. (1980). 24-hour creatinine clearance during the third trimester of normal pregnancy. *Br. J. Obstet. Gynaecol.* **87** (**2**): 106–109.

52 Chamberlain, A. et al. (1993). Pharmacokinetics of ampicillin and sulbactam in pregnancy. *Am. J. Obstet. Gynecol.* **168** (**2**): 667–673.

53 Allegaert, K. et al. (2009). Cefazolin pharmacokinetics in maternal plasma and amniotic fluid during pregnancy. *Am. J. Obstet. Gynecol.* **200** (**2**): 170.e1–170.e7.

54 Muller, A.E. et al. (2010). Pharmacokinetics of clindamycin in pregnant women in the peripartum period. *Antimicrob. Agents Chemother.* **54** (**5**): 2175–2181.

55 Anderson, G.D. (2005). Pregnancy-induced changes in pharmacokinetics: a mechanistic-based approach. *Clin. Pharmacokinet.* **44** (**10**): 989–1008.

56 Syme, M.R., Paxton, J.W., and Keelan, J.A. (2004). Drug transfer and metabolism by the human placenta. *Clin. Pharmacokinet.* **43** (**8**): 487–514.

57 Schou, M., Amdisen, A., and Steenstrup, O.R. (1973). Lithium and pregnancy. II. Hazards to women given lithium during pregnancy and delivery. *Br. Med. J.* **2** (**5859**): 137–138.

58 Luxford, A.M. and Kellaway, G.S. (1983). Pharmacokinetics of digoxin in pregnancy. *Eur. J. Clin. Pharmacol.* **25** (**1**): 117–121.

59 St-Pierre, M.V. et al. (2000). Expression of members of the multidrug resistance protein family in human term placenta. *Am. J. Physiol. Regul. Integr. Comp. Physiol.* **279** (**4**): R1495–R1503.

60 Ushijima, K. et al. (2001). Placental transport of bile acids: analysis of bile acids in maternal serum and urine, umbilical cord blood, and amniotic fluid. *Kurume Med. J.* **48** (**2**): 87–91.

61 Enders, A.C. and Blankenship, T.N. (1999). Comparative placental structure. *Adv. Drug Deliv. Rev.* **38** (**1**): 3–15.

62 Nagashige, M. et al. (2003). Basal membrane localization of MRP1 in human placental trophoblast. *Placenta* **24** (**10**): 951–958.

63 Mylona, P., Hoyland, J.A., and Sibley, C.P. (1999). Sites of mRNA expression of the cystic fibrosis (CF) and multidrug resistance (MDR1) genes in the human placenta of early pregnancy: no evidence for complementary expression. *Placenta* **20** (**5–6**): 493–496.

64 Meyer Zu Schwabedissen, H.E. et al. (2005). Expression, localization, and function of MRP5 (ABCC5), a transporter for cyclic nucleotides, in human placenta and cultured human trophoblasts: effects of gestational age and cellular differentiation. *Am. J. Pathol.* **166** (**1**): 39–48.

65 Raggers, R.J. et al. (1999). The human multidrug resistance protein MRP1 translocates sphingolipid analogs across the plasma membrane. *J. Cell Sci.* **112** (**Pt 3**): 415–422.

66 Yeboah, D. et al. (2006). Expression of breast cancer resistance protein (BCRP/ABCG2) in human placenta throughout gestation and at term before and after labor. *Can. J. Physiol. Pharmacol.* **84** (**12**): 1251–1258.

67 Lee, Y.J. et al. (2005). Investigation of efflux transport of dehydroepiandrosterone sulfate and mitoxantrone at the mouse blood-brain barrier: a minor role of breast cancer resistance protein. *J. Pharmacol. Exp. Ther.* **312** (**1**): 44–52.

68 Zhou, S.F. (2008). Structure, function and regulation of P-glycoprotein and its clinical relevance in drug disposition. *Xenobiotica* **38** (**7–8**): 802–832.

69 Robey, R.W. et al. (2009). ABCG2: a perspective. *Adv. Drug Deliv. Rev.* **61** (**1**): 3–13.

70 Polgar, O., Robey, R.W., and Bates, S.E. (2008). ABCG2: structure, function and role in drug response. *Expert Opin. Drug Metab. Toxicol.* **4** (**1**): 1–15.

71 Schinkel, A.H. and Jonker, J.W. (2003). Mammalian drug efflux transporters of the ATP binding cassette (ABC) family: an overview. *Adv. Drug Deliv. Rev.* **55** (**1**): 3–29.

72 Doyle, L.A. et al. (1998). A multidrug resistance transporter from human MCF-7 breast cancer cells. *Proc. Natl. Acad. Sci. U.S.A* **95** (**26**): 15665–15670.

73 Sun, M. et al. (2006). Expression of the multidrug resistance P-glycoprotein, (ABCB1 glycoprotein) in the human placenta decreases with advancing gestation. *Placenta* **27** (**6–7**): 602–609.

74 Gil, S. et al. (2005). P-glycoprotein expression of the human placenta during pregnancy. *Placenta* **26** (**2–3**): 268–270.

75 Mathias, A.A., Hitti, J., and Unadkat, J.D. (2005). P-glycoprotein and breast cancer resistance protein expression in human placentae of various gestational ages. *Am. J. Physiol. Regul. Integr. Comp. Physiol.* **289** (**4**): R963–R969.

76 Meyer zu Schwabedissen, H.E. et al. (2006). Direct mass spectrometric identification of ABCB1 (P-glycoprotein/MDR1) from the apical membrane fraction of human placenta using fourier transform ion cyclotron mass spectrometry. *Pharmacogenet. Genomics* **16** (**6**): 385–389.

77 Evseenko, D.A., Paxton, J.W., and Keelan, J.A. (2007). Independent regulation of apical and basolateral drug transporter expression and function in placental trophoblasts by cytokines, steroids, and growth factors. *Drug Metab. Dispos.* **35** (**4**): 595–601.

78 Coles, L.D. et al. (2009). Estradiol and progesterone-mediated regulation of P-gp in P-gp overexpressing cells (NCI-ADR-RES) and placental cells (JAR). *Mol. Pharm.* **6** (**6**): 1816–1825.

79 Petropoulos, S., Gibb, W., and Matthews, S.G. (2010). Effect of glucocorticoids on regulation of placental multidrug resistance phosphoglycoprotein (P-gp) in the mouse. *Placenta* **31** (**9**): 803–810.

80 Petropoulos, S., Gibb, W., and Matthews, S.G. (2011). Glucocorticoid regulation of placental breast cancer resistance protein (Bcrp1) in the mouse. *Reprod. Sci.* **18** (**7**): 631–639.

81 Mason, C.W. et al. (2011). ATP-binding cassette transporter expression in human placenta as a function of pregnancy condition. *Drug Metab. Dispos.* **39** (**6**): 1000–1007.

82 Weiss, J. et al. (2003). Inhibition of P-glycoprotein by newer antidepressants. *J. Pharmacol. Exp. Ther.* **305** (**1**): 197–204.

83 Evans, J. et al. (2001). Cohort study of depressed mood during pregnancy and after childbirth. *BMJ* **323** (**7307**): 257–260.

84 Chambers, C.D. et al. (1996). Birth outcomes in pregnant women taking fluoxetine. *N. Engl. J. Med.* **335** (**14**): 1010–1015.

85 Tuccori, M. et al. (2009). Safety concerns associated with the use of serotonin reuptake inhibitors and other serotonergic/noradrenergic antidepressants during pregnancy: a review. *Clin. Ther.* **31** (**Pt 1**): 1426–1453.

86 Wu, S.P. et al. (2004). Interaction between anticonvulsants and human placental carnitine transporter. *Epilepsia* **45** (**3**): 204–210.

87 Siu, K.L. and Lee, W.H. (2004). Maternal diclofenac sodium ingestion and severe neonatal pulmonary hypertension. *J. Paediatr. Child Health* **40** (**3**): 152–153.

88 Pons, R. and De Vivo, D.C. (1995). Primary and secondary carnitine deficiency syndromes. *J. Child Neurol.* **10** (**Suppl 2**): S8–S24.

89 Tamai, I. et al. (1998). Molecular and functional identification of sodium ion-dependent, high affinity human carnitine transporter OCTN2. *J. Biol. Chem.* **273** (**32**): 20378–20382.

90 Nakanishi, T. et al. (2001). Na+- and Cl–coupled active transport of carnitine by the amino acid transporter ATB(0,+) from mouse colon expressed in HRPE cells and Xenopus oocytes. *J. Physiol.* **532** (**Pt 2**): 297–304.

91 Azancot-Benisty, A. et al. (1992). Clinical and pharmacologic study of fetal supraventricular tachyarrhythmias. *J. Pediatr.* **121** (**4**): 608–613.

92 Mirochnick, M. (2000). Antiretroviral pharmacology in pregnant women and their newborns. *Ann. N. Y. Acad. Sci.* **918**: 287–297.

93 Huisman, M.T., Smit, J.W., and Schinkel, A.H. (2000). Significance of P-glycoprotein for the pharmacology and clinical use of HIV protease inhibitors. *AIDS* **14** (**3**): 237–242.

94 Kaufmann, G.R. et al. (1998). Treatment response and durability of a double protease inhibitor therapy with saquinavir and ritonavir in an observational cohort of HIV-1-infected individuals. *AIDS* **12** (**13**): 1625–1630.

95 Koudriakova, T. et al. (1998). Metabolism of the human immunodeficiency virus protease inhibitors indinavir and ritonavir by human intestinal microsomes and expressed cytochrome P4503A4/3A5: mechanism-based inactivation of cytochrome P4503A by ritonavir. *Drug Metab. Dispos.* **26** (**6**): 552–561.

96 Langer, O. et al. (2000). A comparison of glyburide and insulin in women with gestational diabetes mellitus. *N. Engl. J. Med.* **343** (**16**): 1134–1138.

97 Gedeon, C. et al. (2006). Transport of glyburide by placental ABC transporters: implications in fetal drug exposure. *Placenta* **27** (**11–12**): 1096–1102.

98 Moore, K. (1988). *The Developing Human: Clinically Oriented Embryology*, 4e. Philadelphia: W.B. Saunders.

99 Schardein, J. (1993). *Chemically Induced Birth Defects*, 2e. New York, NY: Marcel Dekker.

100 Koren, G., Pastuszak, A., and Ito, S. (1998). Drugs in pregnancy. *N. Engl. J. Med.* **338** (**16**): 1128–1137.

101 Cotrufo, M. et al. (2002). Risk of warfarin during pregnancy with mechanical valve prostheses. *Obstet. Gynecol.* **99** (**1**): 35–40.

102 Barker, D.J. (1995). The fetal and infant origins of disease. *Eur. J. Clin. Invest.* **25** (**7**): 457–463.

103 Will, B.R. and Brace, R.A. (1985). Physiological effects of pH changes on colloid osmotic pressures. *Am. J. Physiol.* **248** (**6 Pt 2**): H890–H893.

104 Barker, D.J. (1995). Fetal origins of coronary heart disease. *BMJ* **311** (**6998**): 171–174.

105 Bromley, R. (2009). *Foetal Exposure to Antiepileptic Drugs: Cognitive Outcomes in the Child*. University of Liverpool.

106 Cummings, C. et al. (2011). Neurodevelopment of children exposed in utero to lamotrigine, sodium valproate and carbamazepine. *Arch. Dis. Child* **96** (**7**): 643–647.

107 Yerby, M.S. (2000). Quality of life, epilepsy advances, and the evolving role of anticonvulsants in women with epilepsy. *Neurology* **55** (**5 Suppl 1**): S21–S31; discussion S54-8.

108 Dansky, L. (1995). The teratogenetic effects of epilepsy and anticonvulsant drugs. In: *Epilepsy* (ed. A. Hopkins and G. Cascino), 535–555. New York, NY: Demos.

109 Kaneko, S. et al. (1999). Congenital malformations due to antiepileptic drugs. *Epilepsy Res.* **33** (**2–3**): 145–158.

110 Moore, S.J. et al. (2000). A clinical study of 57 children with fetal anticonvulsant syndromes. *J. Med. Genet.* **37** (**7**): 489–497.

111 Hvas, C.L. et al. (2000). Epilepsy and pregnancy: effect of antiepileptic drugs and lifestyle on birthweight. *BJOG* **107** (**7**): 896–902.

112 Levinson-Castiel, R. et al. (2006). Neonatal abstinence syndrome after in utero exposure to selective serotonin reuptake inhibitors in term infants. *Arch. Pediatr. Adolesc. Med.* **160** (**2**): 173–176.

113 Law, C.M. and Shiell, A.W. (1996). Is blood pressure inversely related to birth weight? The strength of evidence from a systematic review of the literature. *J. Hypertens.* **14** (**8**): 935–941.

114 Gallaher, B.W. et al. (1998). Fetal programming of insulin-like growth factor (IGF)-I and IGF-binding protein-3: evidence for an altered response to undernutrition in late gestation following exposure to periconceptual undernutrition in the sheep. *J. Endocrinol.* **159** (**3**): 501–508.

115 Newnham, J.P. (2001). Is prenatal glucocorticoid administration another origin of adult disease? *Clin. Exp. Pharmacol. Physiol.* **28** (**11**): 957–961.

116 Meador, K.J. et al. (2009). Cognitive function at 3 years of age after fetal exposure to antiepileptic drugs. *N. Engl. J. Med.* **360** (**16**): 1597–1605.

117 Thomas, S.V. et al. (2008). Motor and mental development of infants exposed to antiepileptic drugs in utero. *Epilepsy Behav.* **13** (**1**): 229–236.

Maternal complications

CHAPTER 24
Asthma

Jennifer A. Namazy[1] and Michael Schatz[2]
[1] *Scripps Clinic, San Diego, CA, USA*
[2] *Kaiser Permanente, San Diego, CA, USA*

CLINICAL SCENARIO

A 25-year-old woman, Gravida 1 Parity 0, with a history of asthma presents to clinic profoundly short of breath. She is an estimated 27 weeks gestation. She was recently prescribed an inhaled corticosteroid but has been afraid to use the medication for fear of its possible effects on her unborn baby. As a result, she is currently using an inhaled short-acting beta-agonist three to four times a day. In the last two years she has received multiple courses of oral corticosteroids for acute attacks of asthma. One of these episodes occurred after she had visited a friend's house with two cats. She is a nonsmoker, has no pets at home, and has never been evaluated for allergies before. She has a history of eczema.

The positive findings on physical exam are: scattered end-expiratory wheezes and erythematous maculopapular plaques in the popliteal fossa bilaterally. Spirometry revealed an FEV_1 of 75% of predicted which increased to FEV_1 of 88% of predicted after administration of an inhaled bronchodilator.

Background

Asthma is the most common chronic medical condition to affect pregnancy, with a prevalence of self-reported asthma in the United States between 8.4% and 8.8% [1]. It has been suggested that asthma may have an effect on pregnancy outcomes, and also that pregnancy may affect the course of asthma. Both poor asthma control and asthma medications may be potential mechanisms for adverse perinatal outcomes.

Clinical questions

The issues most relevant to the patient include: pregnancy outcomes in pregnant asthmatics, severity/control and its effect on perinatal outcomes, and the safety of inhaled corticosteroids. You structure your clinical questions as follows.

1. In pregnant women with asthma (population), is there a higher risk of adverse perinatal outcomes such as low birth weight, preterm birth, congenital malformations, perinatal mortality, and pre-eclampsia (outcomes)?
2. In pregnant women with asthma (population), does asthma control (risk factor) influence the occurrence of low birth weight, preterm birth, congenital malformations, perinatal mortality, and pre-eclampsia (outcomes)?
3. In pregnant women with asthma (population), does inhaled corticosteroid or beta-agonist use lead to adverse outcomes such as low birth weight, preterm birth, congenital malformations, perinatal mortality, and pre-eclampsia (outcomes)?

General search strategy

You begin to address the topic of asthma during pregnancy by searching for evidence in electronic databases looking for cohort studies prospective or retrospective in design addressing perinatal outcomes. Randomized controlled trials with pregnant asthmatic subjects are rarely performed but can be searched for as well.

1. In pregnant women with asthma (population), is there a higher risk of adverse perinatal outcomes such as low birth weight, preterm birth, congenital malformations, perinatal mortality, and pre-eclampsia (outcomes)?

A recent meta-analysis from Murphy et al., derived from a substantial body of literature spanning several decades and including very large numbers of pregnant women, (over 1 000 000 for low birth weight and over 250 000 for preterm labor), indicates that pregnant women with asthma are at a significantly increased risk of a range of adverse perinatal outcomes including low birth weight and preterm birth [2] (Table 24.1).

Evidence-Based Obstetrics and Gynecology, First Edition. Edited by Errol R. Norwitz, Carolyn M. Zelop, David A. Miller, and David L. Keefe.

Table 24.1 Adverse fetal outcomes reported to be increased in infants of asthmatic women

Low birth weight
Preterm birth
Small for gestational age
Congenital anomalies
Stillbirth
Low APGAR scores at birth

Low birth weight, independent of prematurity, is a significant contributor to neonatal morbidity and mortality and therefore represents a significant public health issue. Recent interest in the developmental origins of adult disease has revealed that small size at birth is also a predictor for the development of and/or death from diseases in adult life, including diabetes, cardiovascular disease, atherosclerosis, hypertension, stroke, and coronary heart disease [3–5]. In their meta-analysis, data were reported in 13 publications with over one million subjects, and this meta-analysis indicated that maternal asthma reduces fetal growth, with statistically increased risks of low birth weight and small for gestational age. The risk of having a low birth weight baby was increased by 46% in women with asthma compared to women without asthma (relative risk [RR] 1.46, 95% confidence interval [CI] 1.22, 1.75). The mean birth weight of infants of mothers with asthma was 93 g lower (95% CI 160, 25 g) than that of infants of control mothers [2].

Preterm birth is the leading cause of neonatal mortality in developed countries and is associated with significant neonatal morbidity from diseases such as cerebral palsy. The meta-analysis of 18 publications reported that maternal asthma significantly increases the risk of preterm delivery prior to 37 weeks (RR 1.41, 95% CI 1.23, 1.62) [2]. In contrast, recent data from a retrospective examination of a database which included over 17 000 births, demonstrated no significant increase in preterm delivery in pregnancies complicated by asthma (n = 1944) when compared with the normal population [6].

The meta-analysis by Murphy et al. found that the risk of congenital anomalies in women with asthma was not significantly increased compared to control women without asthma (R 1.08, 95% CI 1.00, 1.16) [2]. However, a recent retrospective study, which included a cohort of 41 637 pregnancies of women with and without asthma, found that maternal asthma was associated with an increased risk of any congenital malformation. (OR = 1.30; 95% CI: 1.20–1.40) [7].

Murphy et al. found the risk of perinatal mortality (a combination of still births and neonatal deaths) in infants of asthmatic mothers to be significantly increased compared to control mothers (RR 1.25, 95% CI 1.05, 1.50), with the overall effect size being intermediate between that observed for still birth and neonatal death [2]. This result was largely driven by a recent large Canadian database study with over 13 000 women with asthma and 28 000 controls, which reported a significantly increased risk of perinatal mortality in women with asthma [8].

Pre-eclampsia, a multi-organ disease that is characterized by the presence of both hypertension and proteinuria in later pregnancy, is the leading cause of maternal mortality during pregnancy, and in severe cases is associated with significant morbidity for both the mother and the neonate. Recent work suggests that the development of any type of hypertension in pregnancy is predictive for future cardiovascular and cerebrovascular disease later in life in the mother [9]. Murphy et al. found that maternal asthma significantly increases the risk of pre-eclampsia, by at least 50% [2].

2. In pregnant women with asthma (population), does asthma control (risk factor) influence the occurrence of outcomes such as low birth weight, preterm birth, congenital malformations, perinatal mortality, and pre-eclampsia (outcomes)?

Uncontrolled asthma can lead to hypoxia and other physiologic abnormalities that could lead to decreased fetal blood oxygen and resulting abnormal growth and development of the fetus. Another recent meta-analysis sought to investigate if asthma exacerbations, oral corticosteroid use, or asthma severity, all components of poor asthma control, are associated with prematurity and intrauterine growth restriction (IUGR).

Data from this meta-analysis found a significantly increased risk of low birth weight infants of those subjects experiencing asthma exacerbation during pregnancy (RR 3.02 [1.87, 4.89]) and using oral corticosteroids during pregnancy (RR 1.41, 95% CI [1.04, 1.93]). Overall, the risk of early low birth weight or preterm delivery was not increased in women with moderate/severe asthma compared to women with mild asthma (in publication). Murphy et al., reported in a recent meta-analysis an increased risk of low birth weight in women who had an asthma exacerbation during pregnancy (RR 2.54, 95% CI 1.52–4.25) compared with women without asthma. This meta-analysis also reported a non-significant trend of increased preterm delivery in asthmatics with exacerbations during pregnancy (RR 1.54 [0.89, 2.69]) and an increased relative risk of preterm delivery (RR 1.51, 95% CI [1.15, 1.98]) in those asthmatic women using oral corticosteroids during pregnancy [10]. Firoozi et al., investigated the effect of the severity of asthma during pregnancy on the risk of a small for gestational infants, low birth weight and preterm birth. Their retrospective cohort study included over 13 000 subjects and demonstrated an increased risk of small for gestational age infants in the moderate and severe asthmatic groups. There was no increased risk of low birth weight or preterm delivery in these groups [11].

Dombrowski et al. found no significant effect of mild asthma or moderate-severe asthma on preterm delivery (at either <32 weeks or <37 weeks gestation), compared to controls without asthma. However, when the sub-group of women with severe asthma (FEV_1 < 60% predicted and/or used oral steroids in the four weeks prior to study enrolment) was compared with controls, there was a significantly increased risk of preterm delivery (adjusted OR 2.2, 95% CI 1.2, 4.2) [12].

Stenius-Aarniala et al. compared data from 47 patients with an attack of asthma during pregnancy to data from 457 asthmatics with no recorded acute exacerbation and 237 healthy subjects. The authors found no increased incidence of congenital malformations in the infants of asthma women with exacerbations during pregnancy. [13]. However, a more recent cohort of over 4000 pregnancies found an increased risk of total congenital malformations in the infants of pregnant asthmatic women who had an asthma exacerbation during pregnancy (1.48, 95% CI, 1.04–2.09) compared to infants of women who did not experience an exacerbation [14].

Stenius Aarniala et al. did not find any increased risk of perinatal death in those women with an attack of asthma during pregnancy [13]. Similarly, a more recent study of 146 pregnant women with asthma exacerbations during pregnancy found that there was no increased risk of stillbirth in those women with severe exacerbations during pregnancy [15]. Two smaller retrospective studies also found that severe asthma was not associated with an increased risk of perinatal death compared with mild asthmatics and controls [16, 17]. This was supported by a more recent prospective study conducted at 16 centers of the Maternal-Fetal Medicine Units Network of the National Institute of Child Health and Human Development in over 2000 pregnant asthmatics. The authors found no increased risk of perinatal mortality when comparing moderate to severe asthmatics to those with milder disease [12]. One of the largest retrospective database studies found in a cohort of 13 100 and 28 042 single pregnancies in women with and without asthma and increased risk of perinatal mortality (OR 1.35, 95% CI 1.08–1.67) [18]. In follow-up, the authors used a 2-stage sampling cohort design and found that the increased risk of perinatal mortality did not remain significant after adjusting for cigarette smoking (OR 1.12, 95% CI 0.87–1.45) [19].

A large prospective cohort study specifically examined the effect of asthma severity on pre-eclampsia and found that women with moderate to severe symptoms during pregnancy were at increased risk of pre-eclampsia, suggesting a role of active maternal inflammation [20]. A recent study from Schatz et al. found a significant association between hypertension during pregnancy and lower FEV_1 after adjustment for covariates. The mean percent predicted FEV_1 was lower, and the proportion of women with FEV_1 < 80% was higher, in women with hypertension during pregnancy compared to those without hypertension [21].

Data from a case control study which investigated the relationship between maternal asthma, pre-eclampsia and preterm delivery, did not indicate a greater risk of pre-eclampsia among women with physician-diagnosed asthma [22]. However, there was a significant association between pre-eclampsia and asthma among a sub-group group of women who experienced symptoms during pregnancy and had received their diagnosis more than 10 years earlier [22]. Findings from other studies have shown that women with asthma exacerbations during pregnancy, a marker of poor control, had similar risk of pre-eclampsia to women with asthma who did not have exacerbations in pregnancy [10, 23]. These data suggest that inherent asthma severity, rather than control or exacerbations, may be related to the increased risk of pre-eclampsia in asthmatic women. This would support a common pathogenesis theory for this increased risk, which is supported by two types of observations. First, pre-eclampsia has been associated with airway hyperresponsiveness. When measurements were made in postpartum women, those who had pre-eclampsia during pregnancy had significantly increased airway hyperresponsiveness compared to women with previously normotensive pregnancies. This was observed even in non-asthmatic women, and the authors suggested that a possible explanation for the association between pre-eclampsia and asthma was mast cell infiltration of the smooth muscle in both the lungs and myometrium [24]. Another mechanism which has been proposed to contribute to pre-eclampsia in women with asthma is vascular hyperreactivity leading to changes in utero-placental blood flow which have been observed *in vitro* in placentae from women with moderate and severe asthma [25] and women with pre-eclampsia [26].

3. In pregnant women with asthma (population), does inhaled corticosteroid or short-acting beta-agonist use lead to adverse outcomes such as low birth weight, preterm birth, pre-eclampsia, perinatal mortality or congenital malformations?

An integral part of management of asthma during pregnancy is the use of common asthma medications such as inhaled corticosteroids and inhaled beta-agonists (Table 24.2). Asthma medications must also be considered as a cause of increased adverse perinatal outcomes in the infants of asthmatic mothers (Table 24.3).

Inhaled corticosteroids

Inhaled corticosteroids are the mainstay of controller therapy during pregnancy. Many studies have shown no increased perinatal risks (including pre-eclampsia, preterm birth, low birth weight, and congenital malformations) associated with inhaled corticosteroids. Bracken et al., reported in a cohort of 872 pregnant asthmatics that oral corticosteroid use

Table 24.2 Steps of asthma therapy during pregnancy

Step	Preferred controller medication	Alternative controller medication
1	None	–
2	Low dose ICS	LTRA, theophylline
3	Medium dose ICS	Low dose ICS + either LABA, LTRA or theophylline
4	Medium dose ICS + LABA	Medium dose ICS + LTRA or theophylline
5	High dose ICS + LABA	–
6	High dose ICS + LABA + oral prednisone	–

ICS, inhaled corticosteroids; LTRA, leukotriene-receptor antagonists; LABA, long-acting beta agonists.
Source: Data from Schatz and Dombrowski (2009) [27, 28].

Table 24.3 Safety of commonly used medications for the treatment of asthma during pregnancy

Drug category	Specific drug (FDA category)	Perinatal outcome
Inhaled bronchodilators Short-acting Bronchodilators	Albuterol (C)	Reassuring human data; some associations with specific malformations but may be chance or confounding by severity
Long-acting bronchodilators	Formoterol (C) Salmeterol (C)	Small amount of human data has been reassuring
Theophylline		No increase in congenital malformations; toxicity may be an issue
Systemic corticosteroids		Associated with oral clefts, low birth weight, preterm birth, pre-eclampsia, and intrauterine growth retardation. Some of these effects may be confounding by severity.
Inhaled corticosteroids	Budesonide (B) Beclomethasone (C) Fluticasone (C) Mometasone (C) Triamcinolon (C)	Substantial reassuring data. Risk of increased malformations with high dose, but may be confounding by severity. Most data for budesonide.
Leukotriene receptor Antagonist	Montelukast (B) Zafirlukast (B)	Moderate amount of reassuring data
5-LO Inhibitor	Zileuton (C)	Animal studies not reassuring; no human data
Anti-IgE	Omalizumab (C)	Increased risk of low birth weight and preterm birth, but may be confounding by severity

FDA, Food and Drug Administration.
Adapted from Schatz et al. (2014) [29].

(in 52 women) but not inhaled corticosteroid use (in 176 women) was associated with an increased risk of preterm delivery. These authors found no increased risk of IUGR, in subjects using inhaled corticosteroids [30]. These findings were supported by a larger, more recent prospective study of 2123 asthmatic patients, that found no significant relationships between the use of inhaled corticosteroids and adverse perinatal outcomes including pre-eclampsia, perinatal mortality, low birth weight, and preterm birth [31]. Clark et al. found an increased risk of small for gestational age only in male infants of asthmatic mothers treated with bronchodilators and inhaled corticosteroids [32].

In a prospective cohort of 1708 pregnant women, 656 with an asthma diagnosis and 1052 with symptoms but no diagnosis, inhaled corticosteroid use was not associated with pre-eclampsia [20]. A nested case-control study of 302 cases of pregnancy induced hypertension and 165 cases of pre-eclampsia were identified. Use of inhaled corticosteroids from conception until date of outcome was not associated with an increased risk of pregnancy induced hypertension or pre-eclampsia, and no significant dose-response relation was observed between inhaled corticosteroids and pregnancy induced hypertension or pre-eclampsia [33].

A recent, large retrospective cohort study of 13 280 pregnancies of women with asthma found that those women who used >1000 mcg d^{-1} of inhaled corticosteroid were significantly more likely to have a baby with a malformation compared with controls (adjusted RR, 1.63, 95% CI, 1.02, 2.60) [34]. This was supported by an earlier study of 24 750 infants whose mothers reported the use of anti-asthmatic drugs in early pregnancy. The use of inhaled corticosteroids was associated with an increased risk of orofacial clefts (1.39, 95% CI 1.04, 1.87) [35]. However, confounding by severity is a possible explanation for the results found in these studies. A randomized, double-blind, placebo-controlled trial included 7241 patients with mild-moderate persistent asthma for less than two years who received 400 mcg of budesonide or placebo once daily. Of the 196 pregnancies reported, there was no increased risk of congenital malformations compared with controls [36].

In terms of prenatal mortality, Breton et al. investigated whether asthmatic women exposed to inhaled corticosteroids during pregnancy were at greater risk of perinatal mortality than asthmatic women not exposed. Women exposed to inhaled corticosteroids at any dose had a no significant increased risk of perinatal mortality (OR 1.07, 95% CI 0.70–1.61). The use of greater than 250 mcg d^{-1} inhaled corticosteroid was associated with a non-significant 52% increased risk of perinatal mortality (OR 1.52, 95% CI 0.62–3.76) [8].

Because it has the most published human gestational safety data, budesonide is considered the preferred inhaled corticosteroid for asthma during pregnancy. However, no data suggest that the other inhaled corticosteroid preparations are unsafe. Therefore, inhaled corticosteroids other than budesonide may be continued in patients who were well controlled by these agents prior to pregnancy, especially if it is thought that changing formulations may jeopardize asthma control.

Inhaled beta-agonists

Inhaled short-acting beta-agonists are the rescue therapy of choice for asthma during pregnancy. Inhaled albuterol is the first-choice short-acting beta-agonist for pregnant women because it has been studied the most extensively, [31] although other agents may be used if uniquely helpful or well tolerated. In one recent case-control study, the use of bronchodilators during pregnancy was associated with an increased risk of gastroschisis among infants (OR, 2.1; 95% CI, 1.2–3.6) [37]. Also, in another cohort study involving 4558 women, there was in increased risk of cardiac defects in infants of mothers exposed to bronchodilators during pregnancy (OR, 1.4; 95% CI, 1.1–1.7) [35]. A more recent case-control study also supported this association (OR 2.20; 95% CI, 1.05, 4.61) [38]. However, these observations may be a result of confounding. Asthma exacerbations may be associated with both increased use of bronchodilators and congenital malformations. In addition, factors such as obesity or lower household socioeconomic status may be associated with both more severe asthma requiring more bronchodilators and congenital malformations.

Long-acting beta-agonists are the preferred add-on controller therapy for asthma during pregnancy. This therapy should be added on when patients' symptoms are not controlled with the use of medium-dose inhaled corticosteroids. Because long-acting and short-acting inhaled beta-agonists have similar pharmacology and toxicology, long-acting beta-agonists are expected to have a safety profile similar to that of albuterol. Two long-acting beta-agonists are available: salmeterol and formoterol. Limited observational data exist on their use during pregnancy. A recent retrospective cohort of 13 117 pregnancies found that women using long-acting beta-agonists during pregnancy were at an increased risk of major congenital malformations (OR 1.31, 95% CI 0.74–2.31). This observation was not seen with short-acting beta-agonists. However, asthma severity as a potential confounder could not be ruled out [39]. A possible association between long-acting beta-agonists and an increased risk of severe and even fatal asthma exacerbations has been observed in non-pregnant patients. As a result, long-acting beta-agonists are no longer recommended as monotherapy for the treatment of asthma and are available in fixed combination preparations with inhaled corticosteroids. Expert panels suggest that the benefits of the use of long-acting beta-agonists appear to outweigh the risks as long as they are used concurrently with inhaled corticosteroids [27].

Conclusion

Asthma is a common medical problem that may worsen during pregnancy. In addition to affecting maternal quality of life, uncontrolled asthma may lead to adverse perinatal outcomes. Awareness of proper treatment options for asthma during pregnancy is important for clinicians who care for pregnant patients.

Key conclusions

Asthma course may worsen, improve or remain unchanged during pregnancy Grade B.

Maternal asthma, especially if severe or uncontrolled, has been associated with adverse perinatal outcomes Grade B.
Safety data for commonly used asthma medications have been largely reassuring Grade B.

References

1 Kwon, H.L., Triche, E., Belanger, K., and Bracken, M. (2006). The epidemiology of asthma during pregnancy: prevalence, diagnosis, and symptoms. *Immunol. Allergy Clin. North Am.* **26** (**1**).

2 Murphy, V., Namazy, J., Powell, H. et al. (2011). A meta-analysis of adverse perinatal outcomes in women with asthma. *Br. J. Obstet. Gynaecol.* **118** (**11**): 1314–1323.

3 Barker, D.J., Hales, C.N., Fall, C.H. et al. (1993). Type 2 (non-insulin-dependent) diabetes mellitus, hypertension and hyperlipidaemia (syndrome X): relation to reduced fetal growth. *Diabetologia* **36** (**1**): 62–67.

4 Barker, D.J. and Lackland, D.T. (2003). Prenatal influences on stroke mortality in England and Wales. *Stroke* **34** (**7**): 1598–1602.

5 Barker, D., Osmond, C., Golding, J. et al. (1989). Growth in utero, blood pressure in childhood and adult life, and mortality from cardiovascular disease. *BMJ* **298** (**6673**): 564–567.

6 Clifton, V.L., Hodyl, N.A., Murphy, V.E. et al. (2010). Effect of maternal asthma, inhaled glucocorticoids and cigarette use during pregnancy on the newborn insulin-like growth factor axis. *Growth Horm. IGF Res.* **20** (**1**): 39–48.

7 Blais, L.K.F., Elfthouh, N., and Forget, A. (2010). Effect of maternal asthma on the risk of specific congenital malformations: a population-based cohort study. *Birth Defects Res. A Clin. Mol. Teratol.* **88** (**4**): 216–222.

8 Breton, M.C., Beauchesne, M.F., Lemiere, C. et al. (2010). Risk of perinatal mortality associated with inhaled corticosteroid use for the treatment of asthma during pregnancy. *J. Allergy. Clin. Immunol.* **126** (**4**): 772–7.e2.

9 Garovic, V. and Hayman, S. (2007). Hypertension in pregnancy: an emerging risk factor for cardiovascular disease. *Nat. Clin. Pract. Nephrol.* **3** (**11**): 613–622.

10 Murphy, V.E., Clifton, V.L., and Gibson, P.G. (2006). Asthma exacerbations during pregnancy: incidence and association with adverse pregnancy outcomes. *Thorax* **61** (**2**): 169–176.

11 Firoozi, F., Lemiere, C., Ducharme, F.M. et al. (2010). Effect of maternal moderate to severe asthma on perinatal outcomes. *Respir. Med.* **104** (**9**): 1278–1287.

12 Dombrowski, M.P., Schatz, M., Wise, R. et al. (2004). Asthma during pregnancy. *Obstet. Gynecol.* **103** (**1**): 5–12.

13 Stenius-Aarniala, B.S., Hedman, J., and Teramo, K.A. (1996). Acute asthma during pregnancy. *Thorax* **51** (**4**): 411–414.

14 Blais, L. and Forget, A. (2008). Asthma exacerbations during the first trimester of pregnancy and the risk of congenital malformations among asthmatic women. *J. Allergy Clin. Immunol.* **121** (**6**): 1379–1384, 84.e1.

15 Murphy, V.E., Gibson, P., Talbot, P.I., and Clifton, V.L. (2005). Severe asthma exacerbations during pregnancy. *Obstet. Gynecol.* **106** (**5 Pt 1**): 1046–1054.

16 Jana, N., Vasishta, K., Saha, S.C., and Khunnu, B. (1995). Effect of bronchial asthma on the course of pregnancy, labour and perinatal outcome. *J. Obstet. Gynaecol. (Tokyo 1995)* **21** (**3**): 227–232.

17 Greenberger, P.A. and Patterson, R. (1988). The outcome of pregnancy complicated by severe asthma. *Allergy Proc.* **9** (**5**): 539–543.

18 Breton, M.-C., Beauchesne, M.-F., Lemiere, C. et al. (2009). Risk of perinatal mortality associated with asthma during pregnancy. *Thorax* **64** (**2**): 101–106.

19 Breton, M., Beauchesne, M.F., Lemiere, C. et al. (2010). Risk of perinatal mortality associated with asthma durng pregnancy: 2-stage sampling cohort study. *Ann. Allergy Asthma. Immunol.* **105** (**3**): 211–217.

20 Triche, E.W., Saftlas, A.F., Belanger, K. et al. (2004). Association of asthma diagnosis, severity, symptoms, and treatment with risk of pre-eclampsia. *Obstet. Gynecol.* **104** (**3**): 585–593.

21 Schatz, M., Dombrowski, M.P., Wise, R. et al. (2006). Spirometry is related to perinatal outcomes in pregnant women with asthma. *Am. J. Obstet. Gynecol.* **194** (**1**): 120–126.

22 Rudra, C.B., Williams, M.A., Frederick, I.O., and Luthy, D.A. (2006). Maternal asthma and risk of pre-eclampsia: a case-control study. *J. Reprod. Med.* **51** (**2**): 94–100.

23 Tata, L.J., Lewis, S.A., McKeever, T.M. et al. (2007). A comprehensive analysis of adverse obstetric and pediatric complications in women with asthma. *Am. J. Respir. Crit. Care Med.* **175** (**10**): 991–997.

24 Siddiqui, S., Goodman, N., McKenna, S. et al. (2008). Pre-eclampsia is associated with airway hyperresponsiveness. *BJOG* **115**: 520–522.

25 Clifton, V.L., Giles, W.B., Smith, R. et al. (2001). Alterations of placental vascular function in asthmatic pregnancies. *Am. J. Respir. Crit. Care Med.* **164** (**4**): 546–553.

26 Read, M., Leitch, I., Giles, W. et al. (1999). U46619-mediated vasoconstriction of the fetal placental vasculature in vitro in normal and hypertensive pregnancies. *J. Hypertens.* **17** (**3**): 389–396.

27 Busse, W.W. (2005). NAEPP expert panel report. Managing asthma during pregnancy: recommendations for pharmacologic treatment-2004 update. *J. Allergy Clin. Immunol.* **115** (**1**): 34–46.

28 Schatz, M. and Dombrowski, M. (2009). Clinical practice. Asthma in pregnancy. *N. Engl. J. Med.* **360**: 1862–1869.

29 Schatz, M., Zeiger, R.S., Falkoff, R. et al. (2014). Asthma and allergic diseases during pregnancy. In: *Middleton's Allergy: Principles and Practice*, 8e (ed. N.F. Adkinson, B.S. Bochner, A.W. Burks, et al.), 951–969. St. Louis, MO: Mosby.

30 Bracken, M.B., Triche, E.W., Belanger, K. et al. (2003). Asthma symptoms, severity, and drug therapy: a prospective study of effects on 2205 pregnancies. *Obstet. Gynecol.* **102** (**4**): 739–752.

31 Schatz, M., Dombrowski, M.P., Wise, R. et al. (2004). The relationship of asthma medication use to perinatal outcomes. *J. Allergy Clin. Immunol.* **113** (**6**): 1040–1045.

32 Clark, P., Crawford, H., Sims, J.L. et al. (1976). Memorial resolution on the death of William Shainline Middleton, MD. *Wis. Med. J.* **75** (**1**): 28–29.

33 Martel, M.J., Rey, E., Beauchesne, M.F. et al. (2005). Use of inhaled corticosteroids during pregnancy and risk of pregnancy induced hypertension: nested case-control study. *BMJ* **330** (**7485**): 230.

34 Blais, L., Beauchesne, M.F., Lemiere, C., and Elftouh, N. (2009). High doses of inhaled corticosteroids during the first trimester of pregnancy and congenital malformations. *J. Allergy Clin. Immunol.* **124** (**6**): 1229–1234.

35 Kallen, B. and Otterblad Olausson, P. (2007). Use of anti-asthmatic drugs during pregnancy. 3. Congenital malformations in the infants. *Eur. J. Clin. Pharmacol.* **63** (**4**): 383–388.

36 Silverman, M., Sheffer, A., Diaz, P.V. et al. (2005). Outcome of pregnancy in a randomized controlled study of patients with asthma exposed to budesonide. *Ann. Allergy Asthma Immunol.* **95** (**6**): 566–570.

37 Lin, S., Munsie, J., Herdt-Losavio, M. et al. (2008). Maternal asthma medication use and the risk of gastroschisis. *Am. J. Epidemiol.* **168**: 73–79.

38 Lin, S., Herdt-Losavio, M., Gensburg, L. et al. (2009). Maternal, asthma medication use, and the risk of congenital heart defects. *Birth Defects Res. A Clin. Mol. Teratol.* **85** (**2**): 161–168.

39 Eltonsy, S., Forget, A., and Blais, L. (2011). Beta-agonists use during pregnancy and the risk of congenital malformations. *Birth Defects Res.* **91**: 937–947.

25

CHAPTER 25
Hypertensive disorders of pregnancy

Andrei Rebarber
Mount Sinai St. Luke's and Mount Sinai West, Mount Sinai Beth Israel, The Mount Sinai Hospital, Obstetrics, Gynecology and Reproductive Sciences, New York, NY, USA

CLINICAL SCENARIO

A 41-year-old P0000 presents for routine prenatal visit at 27 3/7 weeks and is noted to have an elevated blood pressure (BP) of 160/105 mmHg. Her prenatal care is notable for the pregnancy being conceived with *in vitro* fertilization (IVF) using donor sperm due to male factor issues as well as oligoovulation. She has no medical problems except that her starting body mass index (BMI) in the pregnancy was noted to be 39 with an initial office BP at eight weeks gestation was noted to be 135/85. At the time of presentation to the office she denies headache, visual changes, or right upper quadrant pain. Urine dipstick protein is noted to be +1 protein. She reports having an argument with her spouse this morning and states the she has been under a lot of pressure at work due to her profession as a trial lawyer. The fetus is assessed to have a normal heart rate of 154 bpm by Doptone. Fundal height is noted to measure 29 cm. She states she frustrated at this office visit that it took so long to be seen and states that she has a very important meeting she needs to attend following her prenatal care visit. Blood pressure is repeated and now noted to be 155/103 mmHg after sitting in the examining room 15–20 minutes after initially obtained result.

Background

Hypertensive disorders of pregnancy have plague humanity throughout its history based upon multiple historical accounts, however, it was only in the later part of the nineteenth century with the introduction of the ability to measure blood pressure that the constellation of symptoms was link to elevation of blood pressure. Current clinical management schemes have determined that hypertensive disorders of pregnancy can be broken down into four main categories of disease states: pre-eclampsia/eclampsia, gestational hypertension, chronic hypertension, and superimposed pre-eclampsia on preexisting hypertension.

Pre-eclampsia is a multi-system disorder characterized by the new onset of hypertension and proteinuria and/or end-organ dysfunction after 20 weeks in a patient who was previously noted to be normotensive. Patients diagnosed with this condition are at increased risk for maternal and/or fetal mortality or serious morbidity. Patients often present with symptoms of persistent headaches, visual changes, peripheral edema of upper and lower extremities, and possible right upper quadrant pain. Current criteria for the diagnosis of pre-eclampsia involves the association of sustained hypertensive blood pressure associated with thrombocytopenia, altered liver function, the new development of renal insufficiency, pulmonary edema, or new onset cerebral or visual changes. Pre-eclampsia can be diagnosis with and without severe features and terminology such as "mild pre-eclampsia" should no longer be used in clinical practice (Table 25.1). It is important to note that recent American College of Obstetricians and Gynecologists (ACOG) criteria [1] for the diagnosis of severe disease has removed proteinuria as an essential feature. Additionally, other notable changes include that fact that they have removed proteinuria $>5\,g\,day^{-1}$ and fetal growth restriction as criteria for the diagnosis of severe disease. Finally, oliguria is no longer used as a factor indicative of severe pre-eclampsia.

The prevalence of pre-eclampsia in the United States is about 3.4%, but 1.5-fold to 2-fold higher in first pregnancies. The age-period-cohort analysis showed a strong age effect, with women at the extremes of maternal age having the greatest risk of pre-eclampsia [2]. Late onset disease (≥34 weeks) is more prevalent than early onset disease (<34 weeks) in one population-based study: 2.7% versus 0.3%, respectively). Also, as expected in this dataset it was noted that women with early-onset and late-onset pre-eclampsia have significantly higher rates of specific maternal morbidity compared with women without early-onset and late-onset disease. Maternal death rates were higher among women with early-onset (42.1/100 000 deliveries) and late-onset pre-eclampsia (11.2/100 000) compared with women without pre-eclampsia (4.2/100 000) [3].

Evidence-Based Obstetrics and Gynecology, First Edition. Edited by Errol R. Norwitz, Carolyn M. Zelop, David A. Miller, and David L. Keefe.

Table 25.1 Criteria for the diagnosis of pre-eclampsia

Systolic blood pressure ≥ 140 mmHg or diastolic blood pressure ≥ 90 mmHg on two occasions at least four hours apart after 20 weeks of gestation in a previously normotensive patient
If systolic blood pressure is ≥160 mmHg or diastolic blood pressure is ≥110 mmHg, confirmation within minutes is sufficient
And
Proteinuria ≥ 0.3 g in a 24-h urine specimen or protein (mg dl^{-1})/creatinine (mg dl^{-1}) ratio ≥ 0.3
Dipstick ≥1+ if a quantitative measurement is unavailable
In patients with new-onset hypertension without proteinuria, the new onset of any of the following is diagnostic of pre-eclampsia:
Platelet count <100 000/μl
Serum creatinine > 1.1 mg dl^{-1} or doubling of serum creatinine in the absence of other renal disease
Liver transaminases at least twice the normal concentrations
Pulmonary edema
Cerebral or visual symptoms

Severe features of pre-eclampsia includes any of these findings:

- *Systolic blood pressure of 160 mmHg or higher, or diastolic blood pressure of 110 mmHg or higher on two occasions at least four hours apart while the patient is on bed rest (unless antihypertensive therapy is initiated before this time)*
- *Thrombocytopenia (platelets < 100 000/μl*
- *Impaired liver function as indicated by abnormally elevated blood concentrations of liver enzymes (to twice normal concentration), severe persistent right upper quadrant or epigastric pain unresponsive to medication and not accounted for by alternative diagnosis, or both*
- *Progressive renal insufficiency (Serum creatinine concentration > 1.1 mg dl^{-1} or a doubling of the serum creatinine concentration in the absence of other renal disease)*
- *Pulmonary edema*
- *New onset cerebral or visual disturbances*

From Uptodate – American College of Obstetricians and Gynecologists and Task Force on Hypertension in Pregnancy (2013) [1].

Along with hemorrhage, cardiovascular conditions, and thromboembolism, pre-eclampsia in one of the four leading causes of maternal death in the United States [4]. Women with pre-eclampsia are at increased risk for developing multiple life threatening complications including but not limited to: eclampsia, coagulopathy, placental abruption, hemorrhage, acute kidney damage, liver failure, hepatic capsular rupture, pulmonary edema and cardiovascular collapse, and cerebral hemorrhage. Atypical presentation of pre-eclampsia includes: onset of symptoms prior to 20 weeks gestation, hemolysis, elevated liver enzymes and low platelet (HELLP) syndrome patients (i.e. HELLP is an acronym that refers to a syndrome characterized by Hemolysis with a microangiopathic blood smear, Elevated Liver enzymes, and a Low Platelet count), or delayed postpartum onset after 48 hours postpartum. Pre-eclampsia prior to 20 weeks gestation is often due to a molar gestation (i.e. complete or partial) or associated with a preexisting medical condition (e.g. lupus nephritis, thrombotic thrombocytopenic purpura, hemolytic-uremic syndrome, antiphospholipid syndrome, acute fatty liver of pregnancy). The precise criteria for HELLP are necessary for predicting maternal complication and current ACOG guidelines have adopted the Tennessee classification [5]. It requires the presence of *all* of the following criteria to diagnose HELLP: (i) microangiopathic hemolytic anemia with characteristic schistocytes (also called helmet cells) on blood smear. Other signs suggestive of hemolysis include an elevated indirect bilirubin level and a low serum haptoglobin concentration (≤25 mg dl^{-1}); (ii) platelet count ≤100 000 cells/microl, (iii) total bilirubin ≥1.2 mg dl^{-1} (20.52 μmol l^{-1}); and (iv) serum aspartate aminotransferase (AST) >2 times upper limit of normal for local laboratory (usually >70 international units l^{-1}). Alanine aminotransferase (ALT) levels may be used instead of, or in addition to, AST levels. An advantage of the AST is that it is a single test that reflects both hepatocellular necrosis and red cell hemolysis. Hypertension (blood pressure ≥140/90 mmHg) and/or proteinuria are present in approximately 85% of cases, but they may be absent in women with otherwise severe HELLP syndrome [6]. The most common definition for delayed postpartum pre-eclampsia can be defined as signs and symptoms of the disease often leading to readmission greater than two days but prior to six weeks after delivery. In a recent retrospective cohort study of patients who were discharged and later readmitted with the diagnosis of delayed postpartum pre-eclampsia (more than two days to six weeks or less after delivery) the authors noted that 96 (63.2%) patients had no antecedent diagnosis of hypertensive disease in the current pregnancy. Twenty-two patients (14.5%) developed postpartum eclampsia, and more than 90% of these patients presented within seven days after discharge from the hospital. The most common presenting symptom was headache in 105 (69.1%) patients. This study highlights the fact that education about the possibility of delayed postpartum pre-eclampsia and eclampsia should occur after delivery, whether or not patients develop hypertensive disease before discharge from the hospital [7].

In a recent meta-analysis of patients with prior history of pre-eclampsia it was noted that data showed that 20.7% of patients developed hypertensive disorder in a subsequent pregnancy. Recurrence manifested as pre-eclampsia in 13.8% of the studies (95% confidence interval (CI),13.6–14.1%), gestational hypertension in 8.6% of the studies (95% CI, 8.4–8.8%) and HELLPs syndrome in 0.2% of the studies (95% CI, 0.16–0.25%). Recurrence increased with decreasing gestational age at delivery in the index pregnancy. If the hypertensive disorder of pregnancy recurred, in general it was milder, regarding maximum diastolic blood pressure, proteinuria, the use of oral antihypertensive and anticonvulsive medication, the delivery of a small-for-gestational-age child, premature delivery, and perinatal death [8]. Women with pregnancies complicated by either pre-eclampsia, growth restriction, preterm delivery, abruptio placentae, and/or stillbirth can all be sequelae of impaired placental function are at increased risk of developing one of the other disorders in future pregnancies. It is interesting to note that early onset pre-eclampsia is more likely to be associated with one of these adverse events in a subsequent pregnancy, even if normotensive, than late onset pre-eclampsia [9]. Most available evidence does not support an association between inherited thrombophilia and pre-eclampsia and screening for these conditions is not advised at this time [10, 11]. However, based upon the Sydney criteria for the diagnosis of Antiphospholipid Antibody Syndrome, screening for antiphospholipid antibodies is reasonable in the setting of ≥1 preterm deliveries of a morphologically normal infant before 34 weeks of gestation due to severe pre-eclampsia, eclampsia, or features consistent with placental insufficiency. The three main types of antiphospholipid antibodies (aPL) of concern to obstetricians are lupus anticoagulants (LAs), anticardiolipin antibodies (aCL), and anti-beta-2-glycoprotein-1 antibodies. Other antibody specificities have been proposed, but have not proven to be predictive in clinical studies [12]. No test performed in early pregnancy performs clinically well enough for selecting women who are likely to develop pre-eclampsia in current practice. Low-dose aspirin (60–81 mg) daily is the only drug for which there is some evidence of benefit in reducing the risk of pre-eclampsia when administered throughout the second and third trimesters to women at high risk for developing the disease. For women at low risk for development of pre-eclampsia, available evidence does not support use of low-dose aspirin for prevention of pre-eclampsia, but a modest (approximately 10%) reduction in the risk of pre-eclampsia and its sequelae (growth restriction, preterm birth) is possible for women at moderate to high risk of developing the disease. US Preventive Services Task Force (USPSTF) criteria for high risk include: Previous pregnancy with pre-eclampsia, especially early onset and with an adverse outcome, multifetal gestation, chronic hypertension, Type 1 or 2 diabetes mellitus, renal disease, autoimmune disease (antiphospholipid syndrome, systemic lupus erythematosus) USPSTF criteria for moderate risk include: nulliparity, obesity (BMI >30 kg m^{-2}), family history of pre-eclampsia in mother or sister, age ≥35 years, sociodemographic characteristics (African-American, low socioeconomic level), personal risk factors (e.g. history of low birthweight or small for gestational age (SGA), previous adverse pregnancy outcome, >10 year pregnancy interval) [13]. Treatment is begun at 12 weeks of gestation, however, adverse effects from earlier initiation (e.g. preconception) have not been reported.

Gestational hypertension (aka pregnancy induced hypertension) has been defined as hypertension without proteinuria or other signs/symptoms of pre-eclampsia that develops after 20 weeks of gestation. This state does not persist after 12 weeks postpartum and is regarded as a transient state. While this diagnosis may often be benign with usually a high successful pregnancy outcome, this entity can worsen to severe blood pressure elevations or even progress to fulfill criteria for pre-eclampsia. Therefore, even when blood pressure elevations are noted to be mild enhanced surveillance is indicated. Ten to 50% of women initially diagnosed with gestational hypertension go on to develop pre-eclampsia in one to five weeks [14]. Clinical risk factors associated with increased risk for progression include: diagnosis prior to 34 weeks gestation, mean systolic blood pressure of >135 mmHg on 24 hour blood pressure monitoring, abnormal uterine artery Doppler velocimetry, and/or elevated uric acid levels >5.2 mg dl^{-1} [15, 16]. Management of women with preterm gestational hypertension is controversial as it balances maternal and fetal morbidities. The HYPITAT-II trial from the Netherlands attempted to address this question by randomly assigning 703 women with non-severe hypertensive disorders of pregnancy at 34–36$^{6/7}$ weeks to delivery within 24 hours of diagnosis(n = 352) or to expectant management (n = 351) with delivery at 37 weeks or upon development of features of severe pre-eclampsia. The composite adverse maternal outcome (thromboembolic complications, HELLP syndrome, eclampsia, placental abruption) occurred in four (1.1%) of 352 women allocated to immediate delivery versus 11 (3.1%) of 351 women allocated to expectant monitoring (relative risk [RR] 0.36, 95% CI 0.12–1.11; p = 0.069). However, immediate delivery resulted in more cases of neonatal respiratory distress syndrome (5.7% versus 1.7%) [17]. Based upon this data and others we advise close monitoring of pregnancies with non-severe gestational hypertension and manage these patients expectantly as outpatient and deliver them when their clinical situation deteriorates or at term as consistent with ACOG guidelines [18]. Recently, the Antenatal Late Preterm Steroids (ALPSs) Trial randomly assigned women at 34–36$^{5/7}$ weeks of gestation at high risk for late preterm birth to receive a first course of antenatal betamethasone or placebo and found that the frequency of a composite outcome of neonatal respiratory problems was reduced in the betamethasone group [19]. Based on these data, we believe offering a first course of antenatal corticosteroids to patients diagnosed with gestational hypertension between 34 and 37 weeks may be considered and should be individualized based on severity of blood pressure and other comorbidities. We generally perform twice weekly antepartum visits with antenatal testing, our preferred test of choice is the sonographic portion of the biophysical profile with reflex nonstress test (NST) testing as indicated [20]. We instruct patients to promptly report any symptoms suggestive of pre-eclampsia (headache, visual changes, epigastric, or right upper quadrant pain). We also review signs suggestive of possible fetal impairment, such as decreased fetal movement and vaginal bleeding, and signs of preterm labor. Women may maintain most of their normal physical activities but advise against exercise. We do not prescribe antihypertensive drugs for treatment of gestational hypertension unless hypertension is severe (systolic >160 mmHg or diastolic >110 mmHg) at which point these patients are generally hospitalized and delivered if >34 weeks. For those pregnancies <34 weeks administration of antenatal steroids, and in the hospital monitoring is a reasonable approach. Patients who develop pre-eclampsia or have abnormal results on antepartum fetal testing are managed according to usual standards for these pregnancy complications. Additionally, this condition may also be a harbinger for future development of chronic hypertension in the nonpregnant state later on in life, and therefore is a useful marker for follow-up and preventative medicine decisions.

Chronic/pre-existing hypertension may be secondary to an identifiable etiology (i.e. Secondary) or due to an unknown component (i.e. Essential). It is defined as systolic pressure ≥140 mmHg and/or diastolic pressure ≥90 mmHg that antedates pregnancy or exists prior to the twentieth week of pregnancy (on at least two occasions) or persists longer than 12 weeks postpartum. Women with uncomplicated preexisting hypertension who are normotensive or mildly hypertensive on medication usually continue their therapy or have their antihypertensive agents tapered and/or stopped during pregnancy, with close monitoring of the maternal blood pressure response. Acceptable blood pressures include systolic <140–159 or diastolic <90–99 mmHg. It is not uncommon in the second trimester due to the normal decrease in blood pressure to decrease or even taper medication during the pregnancy. Neither the patient nor the fetus appears to be at risk from mild hypertension during pregnancy. Furthermore, controlled studies have not demonstrated that lowering the blood pressure with antihypertensive medications reduces the risk of pre-eclampsia or abruption, or improves fetal or maternal outcome. However, recent data has suggested that treatment during pregnancy may be associated with maternal benefit of decreasing the incidence of severe hypertension in pregnancy [21]. Eight to 13 women would need to be treated with an antihypertensive drug to prevent one episode of severe hypertension [22]. Overall, concerns of the potential fetal harm from anti-hypertensive therapy has not been proven, and therefore, a reasonable approach is to consider the patients comorbidities and symptoms when determining whether to treat mild to moderate blood pressure elevations. All antihypertensive drugs cross the placenta. There are no data from large well-designed randomized trials on which to base a recommendation for use of one drug over another. Our preference is to start treatment with labetalol. A long-acting calcium channel blocker such as nifedipine can be added as a second line treatment. These drugs have been used extensively during pregnancy and appear to be reasonably safe and effective [23]. There is some observational evidence that aggressive lowering of blood pressure, or even the medication itself, can affect fetal growth and therefore we advise serial growth assessment in pregnancy every four weeks. In the absence of superimposed pre-eclampsia or fetal growth restriction, the need for, and frequency of, antepartum fetal assessment is controversial [24, 25]. There are insufficient data to recommend one testing modality over another, or to make conclusions about when testing should begin and how frequently it should be repeated. We recommend initiating daily fetal movement counts starting at 28 weeks gestation and weekly use of the sonographic portion of the biophysical profile with reflex NST testing as indicated [20] starting at 32 weeks until delivery or increased surveillance as warranted by other clinical factors.

Superimposed pre-eclampsia on pre-existing hypertension has been defined as onset of either proteinuria or end-organ dysfunction after 20 weeks of gestation in a woman with chronic/pre-existing hypertension. This entity presents unique challenges as the clinical picture may at times be confusing. Once pre-eclampsia superimposed on chronic hypertension is determined to be present clinicians must next determine whether the superimposed pre-eclampsia is with or without severe features in order to determine the level of intervention necessary. For patients with chronic hypertension and superimposed pre-eclampsia but without severe features, expectant management until 37 weeks is generally advised. Patients with chronic hypertension diagnosed with superimposed pre-eclampsia with severe features should follow management algorithms noted in below including use of antenatal steroids, delivery prior to 34 weeks or earlier based on the clinical scenario, administration of magnesium sulfate prior to delivery for seizure prophylaxis and prior to 32 weeks for neuroprotection as indicated. For patients who present with severe and morbid features such as: uncontrollable severe hypertension, eclampsia, pulmonary edema, abruptio placenta, coagulopathy, and/or non-reassuring fetal status we advise delivery once maternal status is stabilized regardless of gestational age or administration of corticosteroid administration [1].

Clinical questions

1. What clinical risk factors does this patient possess to develop hypertensive disorder of pregnancy?

Multiple risk factors have been described to be associated with the development of pre-eclampsia in pregnancy. The extent of risk varies depending on the individual risk factor. In our above patient the described risk factors include her nulliparity, advanced maternal age, use of assisted reproductive technology (particularly donor egg IVF), obesity, and finally the borderline elevated blood pressures noted at the initial prenatal visit. It is unclear why nulliparity is a risk factor but research suggests that this may be related to paternal antigen exposure and possibly an immune mediated phenomenon affecting normal placental invasion. Maternal age ≥40 has been associated with a relative risk of 1.68, 95% CI 1.23–2.29 for primiparas) based upon a recent meta-analysis [26]. This may be secondary to the fact that older women tend to have additional medical risk factors, such as diabetes mellitus and chronic hypertension, but also seems to be independently associated with risk as well. Interestingly, blood pressure at initial prenatal visit ≥130/80 mmHg at the first prenatal visit is independently associated with an increased risk of superimposed pre-eclampsia, estimated relative risk range of 1.38–2.37 [26]. The mechanism whereby obesity imparts an increased risk for pre-eclampsia is not known. Insulin resistance, hyperlipidemia, and subclinical inflammation, have all been implicated as resulting in an increased incidence of pre-eclampsia in obese gravidas. A systematic review of 13 cohort studies comprising nearly 1.4 million women found that the risk of pre-eclampsia doubled with each 5–7 $kg\,m^{-2}$ increase in prepregnancy BMI [27]. This relationship persisted in studies that excluded women with chronic hypertension, diabetes mellitus, or multiple gestations, or after adjustment for other confounders. Cohort studies of women who underwent bariatric surgery suggest that weight loss significantly reduces the risk of pre-eclampsia [28]. Even among singleton gestations, IVF has been associated with an increased risk of multiple pregnancy complications such as pre-eclampsia, however, the absolute increase in risk has generally been small and most such pregnancies have normal outcomes. A cohort study of over 500 000 women attempted to determine the risk of pre-eclampsia in women undergoing Assisted Reproductive Technologies (ART), including IVF, compared with women who had a natural conception. After adjusting for several other risk factors the study noted that women undergoing ART had a small increase in odds of pre-eclampsia in their second and third pregnancies compared with women who did not require ART (OR 1.3 (1.1–1.6) for second pregnancy and 1.8 (1.2–2.6) for third pregnancy) [29]. A more comprehensive table of risk factors is noted in Table 25.2, however historical risk factors only predict about 30% of women who will develop pre-eclampsia [30]. The ACOG recommends taking a detailed medical history to assess a patient's risks for developing pre-eclampsia but recommends against the use of laboratory and imaging screening tests [31].

2. Is she a candidate for inpatient or outpatient evaluation?

Initial hospitalization with close maternal/fetal monitoring upon diagnosis of pre-eclampsia is important to establish the severity of the disease. After the initial clinical and laboratory evaluation, outpatient care may be an option for women with stable nonsevere pre-eclampsia after careful counseling [32]. However, there are few papers addressing the outcome of outpatient management of pre-eclamptic women and often these studies are not powered to provide clear insight into the outcome measures of most concern. In the first descriptive nonrandomized study by Barton et al. [33] 592 women with singleton pregnancies complicated by mild gestational hypertension (with and without proteinuria) at the gestational age of 24–36 weeks were reviewed. All patients had persistent elevations in blood pressure (systolic ≥140 mmHg or diastolic ≥90 mmHg) on evaluation by the enrolling physician. Patients with

Table 25.2 Factors associated with an increased risk of developing pre-eclampsia

Nulliparity
Pre-eclampsia in a previous pregnancy
Age >40 years or <18 years
Family history of pre-eclampsia
Chronic hypertension
Chronic renal disease
Antiphospholipid antibody syndrome or inherited thrombophilia
Vascular or connective tissue disease
Diabetes mellitus (pregestational and gestational)
Multifetal gestation
High body mass index
Black race
Male partner whose mother or previous partner had pre-eclampsia
Hydrops fetalis
Unexplained fetal growth restriction
Woman herself was small for gestational age
Fetal growth restriction, abruptio placentae, or fetal demise in a previous pregnancy
Prolonged interpregnancy interval
Partner related factors (new partner, limited sperm exposure [e.g. previous use of barrier contraception])
Hydatidiform mole
Susceptibility genes

By comparison, smoking decreases the risk of pre-eclampsia.

associated medical and obstetric complications (other than gestational hypertension) were excluded. After enrollment in this outpatient service patients received education on the hypertensive disease process and related subjective symptoms of pre-eclampsia and were instructed on the use of an automated data recorder. Outpatient evaluations included four times daily automated blood pressure and pulse measurement and daily weight, fetal kick counts, duration of rest/sleep periods, and assessment of proteinuria. Objective and subjective data were then transmitted by phone to a perinatal center daily. In general, patients received twice weekly antenatal evaluation with nonstress testing and frequent amniotic fluid assessment. Indications for hospitalization included worsening of blood pressure, abnormal hematologic parameters, or fetal compromise. Indications for delivery included worsening maternal or fetal condition, spontaneous labor or a favorable cervix at term. However, all clinical decisions regarding management and timing of delivery were at the discretion of the referring physicians. Gestational hypertension with proteinuria(n = 104) was associated with a lower gestational age at delivery, shorter pregnancy prolongation, lower birth weight, and an increased requirement for antepartum hospitalization compared with pregnancies with gestational hypertension but absent proteinuria. There were four stillbirths; two were associated with severe congenital malformations, one at 29 weeks' gestation in a pregnancy complicated by abruptio placentae and another at 34 weeks' gestation with unknown cause. The pregnancy prolongation in their study from enrollment to delivery was comparable to previously published inpatient trials. As this was a descriptive analysis no control group was available to assess safety, limited conclusion can be drawn from this study. Additionally, the setting was highly controlled in an established outpatient program with highly compliant patients. In another Australian paper by Turnbell et al. [34] the authors recruited 395 women to their randomized control trial (RCT) trial though they initially powered the study to recruit 576 patients. The study was designed to test the hypothesis that an alternative to hospital admissions, antenatal day care, will decrease the number of specified interventions and investigations, result in no differences in clinical outcome, lead to greater satisfaction and psychological wellbeing, and be more cost-effective. The trial participants were randomly assigned in a ratio of two to one between day care and antenatal ward, stratified for non-proteinuric hypertension, proteinuric hypertension, and preterm premature rupture of membranes (PPROM). Ultimately they recruited 263 patients [66·6%] assigned day care and 132 patients [33.4%] assigned to inpatient care, representing 65·8% of the target sample size. It is difficult from the data present to select out the hypertension patients only from the PPROM patients in the trial and clearly again it is underpowered to assess maternal and fetal outcomes to determine whether this approach is safe when compared to hospitalization. Finally, a systematic Cochrane review of three trials published in 2009 [35] with a total of 504 women with various complications of pregnancy observed no major differences in clinical outcomes for mothers or babies between antenatal day units or hospital admission. Outpatient care in these trial was provided in the patient's home or, where available, at an antenatal day care unit. Two studies were carried out in the United Kingdom in the 1980s and the third trial was already cited above as the Australian trial. The authors conclude that randomized trials to date have been too small to assess the effect of day care units on important clinical outcomes [36, 37], however, some evidence that women preferred day care to hospital admission exist based on the data reviewed. Based upon the cited data above patients can be offered outpatient monitoring but should be able to comply with frequent maternal and fetal evaluations (every one to three days) after extensive counseling on limited data regarding safety present. Outpatients should be aware of the signs and symptoms of pre-eclampsia and they should monitor fetal movements daily. They should be told to call immediately if they develop symptoms of pre-eclampsia. As with any pregnancy, decreased fetal movement, vaginal bleeding, abdominal pain, rupture of membranes, or uterine contractions should be reported immediately, as well. Home blood pressure monitoring on several occasions throughout the day should be advised with blood pressure logs and communication with provider on a frequent based with at least twice weekly office visit accompanies by antenatal testing. Restricted activity is often recommended; however, there is no evidence that bedrest improves pregnancy outcome or delays progression of disease. In fact data suggests that bedrest in the hospital setting has been shown to increases the risk of venous thromboembolism and therefore this intervention should be used judiciously. At this time given the paucity of safety data we do not manage patients with pre-eclampsia without severe features as outpatients except under select circumstances but do feel comfortable with patients diagnosed with gestational hypertension to be managed as outpatients as delineated above.

3. How should pre-eclampsia with severe features be managed?

Pre-eclampsia with severe features is generally regarded as an indication for delivery in the following settings: before fetal viability, at $\geq 34^{0/7}$ weeks of gestation, or when the maternal or fetal condition is unstable, regardless of gestational age. Between 24 and 34 weeks we offer expectant management in the appropriately selected candidates. Expectant management of pre-eclampsia with severe features is associated with better maternal and fetal outcomes after 28 weeks than those of pregnancies between 24 and 28 weeks gestation. Expectant management of pre-eclampsia with severe features should be undertaken primarily in tertiary care settings with level 3 neonatal intensive care units

(NICUs) with maternal fetal medicine specialists involved in the counseling and care of patients given the potential untoward complications that can occur. Patient are counseled regarding the lack of maternal benefit and the significant maternal risks involved in this approach (i.e. seizures, pulmonary edema, hypertensive encephalopathy, stroke, renal failure, hepatic failure or rupture, retinal detachment or cortical blindness, disseminated intravascular coagulation, placental abruption, and death) [38]. The outcome of conservative management of pre-eclampsia with severe features was initially evaluated in two small randomized trials published in the 1990s. The pregnancies were at 28–34 weeks in the initial trial performed in South Africa [39] and 28–32 weeks in a subsequent US trial [40], and the diagnosis of pre-eclampsia with severe features was based on blood pressure criteria alone. Both trials reported significant prolongation of pregnancy and improvement in neonatal outcome with expectant management, with no increase in the rate of maternal complications. Prolongation of pregnancy averaged 15.4 days (range 4–36 days) in the larger of these trials ($n = 95$) [40] and 7.1 days in the smaller trial ($n = 38$) [39]. In the larger US trial, there was no eclampsia or perinatal death in either group. The two groups had similar incidences of abruptio placentae (4.1% vs. 4.3%) and similar days of postpartum hospital stay. The expectant management group had a significantly higher gestational age at delivery (32.9 ± 1.5 vs. 30.8 ± 1.7 weeks, $p < 0.0001$), higher birth weight, lower incidence of admission to the NICU (76% vs. 100%, $p = 0.002$), lower mean days of hospitalization in the intensive care unit (20.2 ± 14 vs. 36.6 ± 17.4, $p < 0.0001$), and lower incidence of neonatal complications [40].

A more recent larger randomized trial [41] evaluated 267 patients randomized to prompt delivery (PD) $n = 133$ and expectant management (EXM) $n = 134$ at 28–33 weeks of gestation with severe pre-eclampsia based on blood pressure criteria plus proteinuria >5 g or end-organ symptoms (headache, visual disturbances, epigastric pain, tinnitus), but excluded those with HELLP, renal failure, pulmonary edema, and other comorbidities. Pregnancy prolongation was 2.2 days for the PD group vs. 10.3 days for the EXM group ($P = 0.0001$). In general, in the PD group, pregnancies were treated with a course of antenatal corticosteroids followed by delivery in 24–72 hours. The rate of perinatal mortality (9.4% vs. 8.7%; $P = 0.81$; RR, 0.91; 95% CI, 0.34–1.93) was not improved with expectant management, and neither was the composite of neonatal morbidities (56.4% vs. 55.6%; $P = 0.89$; RR, 01.01; 95% CI, 0.81–1.26). There was no significant difference in maternal morbidity in the EXM group compared with the PD group (25.2% vs. 20.3%; $P = 0.34$; RR, 1.24; 95% CI, 0.79–1.94). However, small gestational age (21.7% vs. 9.4%; $P = 0.005$; RR, 2.27; 95% CI, 1.21–4.14) and abruption were more common with expectant management (RR, 5.07; 95% CI, 1.13–22.7; $P = 0.01$). There were no maternal deaths. The lack of benefit from expectant management compared with the previous two trials may have been due to selection of patients at the most severe end of disease spectrum. In addition, 40% of patients in the expectant management group were delivered for uncontrollable hypertension (compared to 6% in an earlier trial [40]). This later point suggests that more aggressive attempts at blood pressure control might have resulted in greater prolongation of pregnancy, however, this is purely based upon conjecture.

Based upon this data we still believe that expectant management of pre-eclampsia with severe features is a reasonable approach between 24 and 34 weeks in the following two circumstances in order to improve gestational age and hopefully improve neonatal outcome. In the setting of pre-eclampsia with severe features based upon blood pressure criteria alone or in the setting of transient laboratory abnormalities we find it reasonable to delay delivery. Use of hypertensive agents should only be used to prevent stroke range blood pressures [42]. Reasonable efforts should be made to delay delivery for 48 hours to complete a full course of steroids. However, intervention will be necessary if maternal or fetal status deteriorates [43].

4. Should postpartum counseling include the long term maternal risk of cardiovascular disease (CVD)?

CVD is the leading cause of death in women in the United States [44]. CVD involves four main categories: (i) Coronary heart disease (CHD) clinically manifested by myocardial infarction (MI), angina pectoris, heart failure (HF), and coronary death; (ii) Cerebrovascular disease clinically manifested by stroke and transient ischemic attack; (iii) Peripheral artery disease clinically manifested by intermittent claudication; and (iv) Aortic atherosclerosis and thoracic or abdominal aortic aneurysm. The presence of vascular disease in one of these categories increases the likelihood of disease presence in one of the other categories. One of the risk factors for CVD that is unique to women, and has only recently been recognized, is that of pregnancy and related complications during gestation. Multiple case control and cohort studies over the past decade have highlighted the association of hypertensive disease of pregnancy and its predictive risk for the future development of CVD. Two large systematic reviews recently published evaluated the relationship between a prior obstetrical history of pre-eclampsia and the risk of later CVD in women. Bellamy et al. [45] noted in their meta-analysis of cohort papers published over a 46 year period (providing a dataset of over 3.4 million women with 198 252 affected by pre-eclampsia and 29 495 episodes of CVD and cancer) that after having pre-eclampsia, women have an increased risk of vascular disease. The relative risks (95% CIs) for hypertension were 3.70 (2.70–5.05) after 14.1 years weighted mean follow-up, for ischemic heart disease 2.16 (1.86–2.52) after 11.7 years, for stroke 1.81 (1.45–2.27) after 10.4 years, and for venous thromboembolism 1.79 (1.37–2.33) after 4.7 years. No increase in risk of any cancer was found. Overall mortality after pre-eclampsia was increased: 1.49 (1.05–2.14) after 14.5 years. In a recent paper by McDonald SD et al. [46], their meta-analysis of both cohort and case control trials (with a total of 116 175 women with and 2 259 576 women without pre-eclampsia/eclampsia) concluded that a history of pre-eclampsia/eclampsia approximately double the risk of early cardiac, cerebrovascular, and peripheral arterial disease, and cardiovascular mortality. Interestingly, in this analysis using a meta-regression evaluation the authors also noted a graded relationship between the severity of pre-eclampsia/eclampsia and the risk of cardiac disease (mild: RR 2.00, 1.83–2.19, moderate: RR 2.99, 2.51–3.58, severe: RR 5.36, 3.96–7.27, $P < 0.0001$). The authors defined pre-eclampsia as "mild" if the pregnancy had an uncomplicated course, "moderate" if pre-eclampsia was complicated by fetal growth restriction or maternal seizures and "severe" if pre-eclampsia was complicated by preterm delivery or fetal demise. This association they suggested might reflect a common cause for pre-eclampsia and CVD, or an effect of pre-eclampsia on disease development, or both. Additionally, several studies have noted that the future risk of CVD is affected by the severity of the condition, its timing in gestation (term vs. preterm), and the number of episodes or pre-eclampsia [47, 48]. Various authors have hypothesized that increased insulin resistance, sympathetic hyperactivity, proinflammatory environment, endothelial cell dysfunction, and the abnormal lipid profile in pre-eclamptic women results an early manifestation of the metabolic syndrome thus putting affected woman at increased risk of CVD [49]. The greatest risk for future development of CVD has been noted in women which suffered from both pre-eclampsia and a growth restricted newborn [50]. In this study the authors found that the metabolic syndrome was present in 7.5% of women who delivered SGA infants, 15.6% of former pulmonary embolism (PE) women, and 19.8% of women after pregnancy complicated by both SGA and PE.

The American Heart Association considers a history of hypertensive disease associated with pregnancy a significant risk factor for development of CVD [44]. Multiple medical specialty organizations have advised that modifiable risk factors should be discussed with patients at their annual examinations, particularly in patients with known risks for CVD, such as patients who had developed a history of hypertensive disease of pregnancy. For example, in the Nurses' Health Study of over 120 000 female nurses followed for over 20 years, women who maintained a desirable body weight, ate a healthy diet, exercise regularly, and did not smoke cigarettes experienced an 84% reduction in their risk of clinical CVD events [51].

References

1 American College of Obstetricians and Gynecologists, Task Force on Hypertension in Pregnancy (2013). Hypertension in pregnancy. Report of the American College of Obstetricians and Gynecologists' Task Force on Hypertension in Pregnancy. *Obstet. Gynecol.* **122**: 1122.

2 Ananth, C.V., Keyes, K.M., and Wapner, R.J. (2013). Pre-eclampsia rates in the United States, 1980-2010: age-period-cohort analysis. *BMJ* **347**: f6564.

3 Lisonkova, S., Sabr, Y., Mayer, C. et al. (2014). Maternal morbidity associated with early-onset and late-onset pre-eclampsia. *Obstet. Gynecol.* **124** (**4**): 771–781.

4 AP, M.K.A., Berg, C.J., Liu, X. et al. (2011). Changes in pregnancy mortality ascertainment: United States, 1999-2005. *Obstet. Gynecol.* **118** (**1**): 104.

5 Sibai, B.M., Ramadan, M.K., Usta, I. et al. (1993). Maternal morbidity and mortality in 442 pregnancies with hemolysis, elevated liver enzymes, and low platelets (HELLP syndrome). *Am. J. Obstet. Gynecol.* **169** (**4**): 1000.

6 Sibai, B.M. (2004). Diagnosis, controversies, and management of the syndrome of hemolysis, elevated liver enzymes, and low platelet count. *Obstet. Gynecol.* **103** (**5 Pt 1**): 981.

7 Al-Safi, Z., Imudia, A.N., Filetti, L.C. et al. (2011). Delayed postpartum pre-eclampsia and eclampsia: demographics, clinical course, and complications. *Obstet. Gynecol.* **118** (**5**): 1102.

8 van Oostwaard, M.F., Langenveld, J., Schuit, E. et al. (2015). Recurrence of hypertensive disorders of pregnancy: an individual patient data metaanalysis. *Am. J. Obstet. Gynecol.* **212** (**5**): 624.e1.

9 Chang, J.J., Muglia, L.J., and Macones, G.A. (2010). Association of early-onset pre-eclampsia in first pregnancy with normotensive second pregnancy outcomes: a population-based study. *BJOG* **117** (**8**): 946.

10 Said, J.M., Higgins, J.R., Moses, E.K. et al. (2010). Inherited thrombophilia polymorphisms and pregnancy outcomes in nulliparous women. *Obstet. Gynecol.* **115** (**1**): 5.

11 Dizon-Townson, D., Miller, C., Sibai, B. et al. (2005). The relationship of the factor V Leiden mutation and pregnancy outcomes for mother and fetus. *Obstet. Gynecol.* **106** (**3**): 517.

12 Miyakis, S., Lockshin, M.D., Atsumi, T. et al. (2006). International consensus statement on an update of the classification criteria for definite antiphospholipid syndrome (APS). *J. Thromb. Haemost.* **4** (**2**): 295.

13 ML, L.F. and U.S. Preventive Services Task Force (2014). Low-dose aspirin use for the prevention of morbidity and mortality from pre-eclampsia: U.S. Preventive Services Task Force recommendation statement. *Ann. Intern. Med.* **161** (**11**): 819.

14 Barton, J.R., O'Brien, J.M., Bergauer, N.K. et al. (2001). Mild gestational hypertension remote from term: progression and outcome. *Am. J. Obstet. Gynecol.* **184** (**5**): 979.

15 Melamed, N., Ray, J.G., Hladunewich, M. et al. (2014 Jul). Gestational hypertension and pre-eclampsia: are they the same disease? *J. Obstet. Gynaecol. Can.* (**7**): 36, 642–37.

16 Wu, Y., Xiong, X., Fraser, W.D., and Luo, Z.C. (2015 Jun). Association of uric acid with progression to pre-eclampsia and development of adverse conditions in gestational hypertensive pregnancies. *Am. J. Hypertens* **25** (**6**): 711–717. Epub 2012 Mar 01.

17 Broekhuijsen, K., van Baaren, G.J., van Pampus, M.G. et al., HYPITAT-II Study Group (2015). Immediate delivery versus expectant monitoring for hypertensive disorders of pregnancy between 34 and 37 weeks of gestation (HYPITAT-II): an open-label, randomised controlled trial. *Lancet.* **385** (**9986**): 2492.

18 American College of Obstetricians and Gynecologists Committee on Obstetric Practice. ACOG Committee Opinion #560, 2013. *Medically Indicated Late Preterm and Early Term Deliveries.*

19 Gyamfi-Bannerman, C., Thom, E.A., Blackwell, S.C. et al., NICHD Maternal–Fetal Medicine Units Network(2016). Antenatal betamethasone for women at risk for late preterm delivery. *N. Engl. J. Med.* **374** (**14**): 1311.

20 Manning, F.A., Morrison, I., Lange, I.R., Harman, C.R., Chamberlain, P.F. (1987). Fetal biophysical profile scoring: selective use of the nonstress test. *Am. J. Obstet. Gynecol.* **156** (**3**): 709.

21 Magee, L.A., von Dadelszen, P., Rey, E. et al. (2015). Less-tight versus tight control of hypertension in pregnancy. *N. Engl. J. Med.* **372** (**5**): 407–417.

22 Firoz, T., Magee, L.A., MacDonell, K. et al. (2014). Oral antihypertensive therapy for severe hypertension in pregnancy and postpartum: a systematic review. *BJOG* **121** (**10**): 1210–1218. discussion 1220. Epub 2014 May 16.

23 Signore, C., Freeman, R.K., and Spong, C.Y. (2009). Antenatal testing-a reevaluation: executive summary of a Eunice Kennedy Shriver National Institute of Child Health and Human Development workshop. *Obstet. Gynecol.* **113** (**3**): 687–701.

24 Duckitt, K. and Harrington, D. (2005). Risk factors for pre-eclampsia at antenatal booking: systematic review of controlled studies. *BMJ* **330** (**7491**): 565.

25 O'Brien, T.E., Ray, J.G., and Chan, W.S. (2003). Maternal body mass index and the risk of pre-eclampsia: a systematic overview. *Epidemiology* **14** (**3**): 368–374.

26 Maggard, M.A., Yermilov, I., Li, Z. et al. (2008). Pregnancy and fertility following bariatric surgery: a systematic review. *JAMA* **300** (**19**): 2286.

27 Tandberg, A., Klungsøyr, K., Romundstad, L.B., and Skjærven, R. (2015). Pre-eclampsia and assisted reproductive technologies: consequences of advanced maternal age, interbirth intervals, new partner and smoking habits. *BJOG* **122** (**7**): 915.

28 Leslie, K., Thilaganathan, B., and Papageorghiou, A. (2011). Early prediction and prevention of pre-eclampsia. *Best Pract. Res. Clin. Obstet. Gynaecol.* **25** (**3**): 343–354. Epub 2011 Mar 4.

29 American College of Obstetricians and Gynecologists Committee on Obstetric Practice (2015 Sep). Committee Opinion No. 638: First-trimester risk assessment for early-onset preeclampsia. *Obstet. Gynecol.* **126** (**3**): e25–e27.

30 Barton, J.R., Istwan, N.B., Rhea, D. et al. (2006). Cost-savings analysis of an outpatient management program for women with pregnancy-related hypertensive conditions. *Dis. Manag.* **9** (**4**): 236.

31 Barton, J.R., Stanziano, G.J., and Sibai, B.M. (1994). Monitored outpatient management of mild gestational hypertension remote from term. *Am. J. Obstet. Gynecol.* **170** (**3**): 765.

32 Turnbull, D.A., Wilkinson, C., Gerard, K. et al. (2004). Clinical, psychosocial, and economic effects of antenatal day care for three medical complications of pregnancy: a randomised controlled trial of 395 women. *Lancet* **363** (**9415**): 1104.

33 Waugh, J., Bosio, P., Shennan, A., and Halligan, A. (2001). Inpatient monitoring on an outpatient basis: managing hypertensive pregnancies in the community using automated technologies. *J. Soc. Gynecol. Investig.* **8** (**1**): 14–17.

34 Helewa, M., Heaman, M., Robinson, M.A., and Thompson, L. (1993). Community-based home-care program for the management of pre-eclampsia: an alternative. *CMAJ* **149** (**6**): 829–834.

35 Dowswell, T., Middleton, P., and Weeks, A. (2009). Antenatal day care units versus hospital admission for women with complicated pregnancy. *Cochrane Database Syst Rev.* doi: 10.1002/14651858.CD001803.pub2.

36 Magee, L.A., Yong, P.J., Espinosa, V. et al. (2009). Expectant management of severe pre-eclampsia remote from term: a structured systematic review. *Hypertens Pregnancy* **28** (**3**): 312.

37 Odendaal, H.J., Pattinson, R.C., Bam, R. et al. (1990). Aggressive or expectant management for patients with severe pre-eclampsia between 28-34 weeks' gestation: a randomized controlled trial. *Obstet. Gynecol.* **76**: 1070.

38 Sibai, B.M., Mercer, B.M., Schiff, E., and Friedman, S.A. (1994). Aggressive versus expectant management of severe pre-eclampsia at 28 to 32 weeks' gestation: a randomized controlled trial. *Am. J. Obstet. Gynecol.* **171**: 818.

39 Vigil-De Gracia, P., Reyes Tejada, O., Calle Miñaca, A. et al. (2013). Expectant management of severe pre-eclampsia remote from term: the MEXPRE Latin Study, a randomized, multicenter clinical trial. *Am. J. Obstet. Gynecol.* **209** (**5**): 425.e1.

40 Sibai, B.M., Barton, J.R., Akl, S. et al. (1992). A randomized prospective comparison of nifedipine and bed rest versus bed rest alone in the management of pre-eclampsia remote from term. *Am. J. Obstet. Gynecol.* **167** (**4 Pt 1**): 879.

41 Roberts, D. and Dalziel, S. (2006). Antenatal corticosteroids for accelerating fetal lung maturation for women at risk of preterm birth. *Cochrane Database Syst. Rev.* doi: 10.1002/14651858.CD004454.pub2.

42 Mosca, L., Benjamin, E.J., Berra, K. et al. (2011). Effectiveness-based guidelines for the prevention of cardiovascular disease in women – 2011 update: a guideline from the american heart association. *Circulation* **123** (**11**): 1243.

43 Bellamy, L., Casas, J.P., Hingorani, A.D., and Williams, D.J. (2007). Pre-eclampsia and risk of cardiovascular disease and cancer in later life: systematic review and meta-analysis. *BMJ* **335** (**7627**): 974.

44 SD, M.D., Malinowski, A., Zhou, Q. et al. (2008). Cardiovascular sequelae of pre-eclampsia/eclampsia: a systematic review and meta-analyses. *Am. Heart J.* **156** (**5**): 918.

45 Kessous, R., Shoham-Vardi, I., Pariente, G. et al. (2015). Long-term maternal atherosclerotic morbidity in women with pre-eclampsia. *Heart* **101** (**6**): 442–446. Epub 2015 Jan 6.

46 Mongraw-Chaffin, M.L., Cirillo, P.M., and Cohn, B.A. (2010 Jul). Pre-eclampsia and cardiovascular disease death: prospective evidence from the child health and development studies cohort. *Hypertension* **56** (**1**): 166–171. Epub 2010 Jun 1.

47 Norwitz ER and Repke JT. Pre-eclampsia: management and prognosis. Uptodate Literature Review current through: June 2018. This topic last updated: June 26, 2018. Available at: https://www.uptodate.com/contents/preeclampsia-management-and-prognosis

48 Hooijschuur, M.C., Ghossein-Doha, C., Al-Nasiry, S., and Spaanderman, M.E. (2015 Sep). Maternal metabolic syndrome, pre-eclampsia, and small for gestational age infancy. *Am. J. Obstet. Gynecol.* **213** (**3**): 370.e1–370.e7. Epub 2015 May 22.

49 Stampfer, M.J., Hu, F.B., Manson, J.E. et al. (2000). Primary prevention of coronary heart disease in women through diet and lifestyle. *N. Engl. J. Med.* **343** (**1**): 16.

50 Saudan, P., Brown, M.A., Buddle, M.L., and Jones, M. (1998). Does gestational hypertension become pre-eclampsia? *Br. J. Obstet. Gynaecol.* **105** (**11**): 1177.

51 Abalos, E., Duley, L., and Steyn, D.W. (2014). Antihypertensive drug therapy for mild to moderate hypertension during pregnancy. *Cochrane Database Syst. Rev.* doi: 10.1002/14651858.CD002252.pub2.

26

CHAPTER 26

Cardiovascular disease

Megan L. Jones[1] and Michael R. Foley[2]
[1] *The University of Ohio Wexner Medical Center, Columbus, OH, USA*
[2] *Banner University Medical Center Phoenix, Obstetrics and Gynecology, University of Arizona College of Medicine Phoenix, Phoenix, AZ, USA*

Introduction

Physiologic changes of pregnancy

The physiologic changes of pregnancy create a state of high flow and low resistance. Beginning in the first trimester, cardiac output rises due to an increased stroke volume, and the addition of an increased heart rate by the second trimester intensifies this value [1]. By mid-second trimester cardiac output has increased by 25–50%, and this remains stable throughout the duration of pregnancy [2]. Additionally, preload is increased due to a 40–50% increase in blood volume [1]. Systemic vascular resistance (SVR) falls by six weeks gestation, which accounts for the fall in systolic and diastolic blood pressure by 5 and 10 mmHg, respectively, throughout the first half of pregnancy. This subsequently rises to pre-pregnant values in the third trimester [1, 2].

Normal physical exam findings in pregnant women reflect the state of high flow and low resistance. Distended neck veins, prominent left and right ventricular impulses, systolic ejection murmur, peripheral edema, and trace pulmonary edema can be normal. However, given the similarity of normal findings with heart failure, evaluation of a patient with cardiac disease in pregnancy can be complicated [3].

The hemodynamic changes in pregnancy will also be reflected in imaging and electrical studies. Frontal axis leads in an electrocardiogram (ECG) will show mild left axis deviation (15–20%), and nonspecific ST segment and T wave abnormalities are seen in 4–14% of pregnancies [4, 5]. During echocardiography, pregnant women should be positioned in the left lateral decubitus to avoid inferior vena cava (IVC) compression by the gravid uterus, which can alter measurements. In general, eccentric hypertrophy is seen with a stable increase in the ratio of wall thickness to ventricular radius. Left ventricular systolic and diastolic function is relatively stable, but a slight increase in ejection fraction (EF) can be observed. Physiologic regurgitation is common due to the increase in blood volume and chamber dimensions. Asymptomatic pericardial effusions have been observed in up to 40% of pregnant women, especially primigravidas and those with more than 12 kg weight gain [6].

During labor, the effects of pain, sympathetic tone, and uterine contractions further increase cardiac output, SVR, and blood pressure. Relief of IVC compression and auto-transfusion following delivery promotes a further increase in cardiac output. The hemodynamic changes of pregnancy will typically resolve by two weeks postpartum but can take up to six weeks in some patients [1].

Epidemiology of cardiac disease

The prevalence of cardiac disease among reproductive age women in the United States is 1%, and pregnancy can create significant morbidity and mortality for these women. With regards to pregnancy, cardiac disease is identified in 0.1% of those in developed countries and 0.6% in developing countries [7]. Cardiac disease can be divided into acquired and congenital lesions, and the prevalence of each of these categories varies among developing versus developed countries. Acquired valvular lesions from the sequelae of rheumatic heart disease account for 60–80% of cardiac disease in pregnancy in developing countries. Whereas this held true for developed countries also until the last decade, there has been a shift toward a higher prevalence of congenital cardiac disease in pregnancy in developed regions. This is attributed to advancements in technology and success of reparative surgery, which has allowed more women to live to reproductive ages [8]. Despite this shift, acquired cardiac disease is still rising in developed regions due to prolongation of pregnancy and the increased prevalence of hypertension, diabetes, and hypercholesterolemia in women of advanced maternal age, which places further risk for the onset of cardiac disease during pregnancy [9]. Regardless of etiology, cardiac disease is collectively the most common indirect

Evidence-Based Obstetrics and Gynecology, First Edition. Edited by Errol R. Norwitz, Carolyn M. Zelop, David A. Miller, and David L. Keefe.

cause of maternal death, contributing to 9% mortality in developing countries, 36% mortality in developed countries, and 18% of ICU admissions across the United States [7, 10]. Therefore, thoughtful assessment, counseling, and management must be employed for optimal care of these pregnant women.

Risk assessment models for pregnant women with cardiac disease

The New York Heart Association (NYHA) created a classification system in 1994 to categorize functional status related to cardiac disease in a general population. Class I describes those with cardiac disease who have no limitations of physical activity and minimal symptoms with ordinary activity. Class II describes those with slight limitation in activity and significant symptoms with ordinary activity. Class III describes those with marked limitation in activity and significant symptoms with less than ordinary activity. Class IV describes those with discomfort performing any activity and significant symptoms at rest [11].

Risk assessment of cardiac disease in pregnancy is a priority for the obstetrician. The NYHA functional classification remains useful to assess and describe women who become pregnant; however, risk assessment models specific to pregnant women with cardiac disease have been proposed to aid in predicting the risk of maternal cardiac events given the condition, maternal history, and current functional status.

The risk for complications associated with pregnancy in women with heart disease (CARPREG risk score) was created from a retrospective evaluation of risks and predictors of cardiac complications in pregnant women with cardiac disease [12].

Four predictors were identified, and each was given 1 point:

- Poor functional class (NYHA class III or IV) or cyanosis.
- Previous cardiovascular event including heart failure, transient ischemic attack, stroke, or arrhythmia.
- Left heart obstruction (mitral valve area <2 cm^2, aortic valve area <1.5 cm^2, or peak left ventricular (LV) outflow gradient >30 mmHg).
- Left ventricular systolic dysfunction (EF <40%).

Subsequently, these findings were applied prospectively to a group of 562 women with 617 pregnancies who had congenital *or* acquired cardiac disease. The overall rate of cardiac events (pulmonary edema, arrhythmia requiring treatment, stroke, cardiac arrest, or death) was 13%, and about half of these occurred in the antepartum period. The rate of events predicted by the risk score of 0, 1, or >2 points was very congruent with the rates observed in the retrospective analysis: 0 points (4% versus 5%); 1 point (26% versus 27%); >2 points (62% versus 75%) [13]. Furthermore, specific analysis of the CARPREG risk score in 53 women with congenital cardiac disease in 90 pregnancies elicited an overall rate of cardiac events to be 25%. Congruency with no statistical difference was observed among the actual incidence of events and rates predicted by the CARPREG risk score [14] (Table 26.1).

The risk score for cardiac complications during completed pregnancies in women with congenital heart disease (Zwangerschap bij vrouwen met een Aangeboren HARtAfwijking-II; ZAHARA risk score) was created from a retrospective cohort study of 714 women with congenital cardiac disease in 1302 pregnancies [15]. This risk score has not been validated in further studies, however (Table 26.2).

The following factors are scored from a weighted system:

- Mechanical heart valve (4.25 points).
- Severe left heart obstruction (mean pressure gradient >50 mmHg or aortic valve area <1.0 cm^2) (2.5 points).
- History of arrhythmia (1.5 points).

Table 26.1 CARPREG risk prediction score for a cardiac event during pregnancy

Risk predictors	Points
Poor functional class (NYHA class III or IV) or cyanosis	1
Previous cardiovascular event: heart failure, transient ischemic attack, stroke, or arrhythmia	1
Left heart obstruction:	1
Mitral valve area <2 cm^2, aortic valve area <1.5 cm^2, or peak left ventricular outflow gradient >30 mmHg	
Left ventricular systolic dysfunction (ejection fraction <40%)	1

Score: 0 points = 5% risk; 1 = 27% risk; ≥2 = 75% risk.

Table 26.2 ZAHARA risk prediction score for a cardiac event during pregnancy

Risk predictors	Points
Mechanical heart valve	4.25
Severe left heart obstruction (mean pressure gradient >50 mmHg or aortic valve area <1.0 cm^2)	2.5
History or arrhythmia	1.5
History of cardiac medication use before pregnancy	1.5
History of cyanotic heart disease – corrected and uncorrected	1
Moderate-to-severe pulmonary or systemic atrioventricular valve regurgitation	0.75
Symptomatic heart failure before pregnancy (NYHA class ≥2)	0.75

Score: 0–0.5 points = 3% risk; 0.51–1.5 = 8% risk; 1.51–2.5 = 18% risk; 2.51–3.5 = 43% risk; ≥3.51 = 70% risk.

- History of cardiac medication use before pregnancy (1.5 points).
- History of cyanotic heart disease – corrected and uncorrected (1.0 points).
- Moderate-to-severe pulmonary or systemic atrioventricular valve regurgitation (0.75 points).
- Symptomatic heart failure before pregnancy (NYHA class >2) (0.75 points).

The summation of an individual score is used to predict the risk of a cardiac event that is divided into five categories: 0–0.5 points (3%); 0.51–1.5 points (8%); 1.51–2.5 points (18%); 2.51–3.5% (43%); >3.51 (70%) [15].

The World Health Organization (WHO) created a classification system that separates cardiac disease into four categories, and specific risks are assigned for each category. A large prospective study from the European Registry on Pregnancy and Heart Disease applied the WHO classification system to 1321 pregnancies, and this model showed statistical significance in comparing maternal morbidity among classes. Although statistical significance was not observed among classes for maternal mortality, risk prediction was still considered excellent [16]. The European Society of Cardiology (ESC) adopted this classification system into their guidelines for management of cardiac disease in pregnancy, which were published in 2011 [17].

Class I includes conditions associated with no detectable increased risk of maternal mortality and no/mild increase in morbidity. Cardiology follow-up should occur one or two times during pregnancy.

- Uncomplicated, small patent ductus arteriosus (PDA), mild pulmonic stenosis, or mitral valve prolapse.
- Successfully repaired simple lesions (atrial septal defect or ventricular septal defect (ASD/VSD), PDA, or anomalous pulmonary venous drainage).
- Isolated atrial or ventricular ectopic beats.

Class II includes conditions associated with a small increased risk of maternal mortality or a moderate increase in morbidity. Cardiology follow-up should occur every trimester.

- Unrepaired ASD/VSD.
- Repaired tetralogy of Fallot (TOF) or coarctation.
- Arrhythmias.
- Mild LV dysfunction.
- Hypertrophic cardiomyopathy (HCM).
- Native or bioprosthetic valvular heart disease not considered WHO I or IV.
- Marfan syndrome with aortic diameter <40 mm without aortic dissection.
- Bicuspid aortic valve with ascending aortic diameter <45 mm.

Class III includes conditions associated with significant increased risk of maternal mortality or severe morbidity. Cardiology follow-up should occur every four to eight weeks.

- Mechanical valve.
- Systemic right ventricle.
- Fontan circulation.
- Unrepaired cyanotic heart disease.
- Complex congenital cardiac disease.
- Bicuspid aortic valve with ascending aortic diameter 45–50 mm.
- Marfan syndrome with aortic root diameter 40–45 mm.

Class IV includes conditions associated with extremely high risk of maternal mortality or severe morbidity, for which pregnancy is contra-indicated. If pregnancy occurs and termination is declined, then cardiology follow-up every four to eight weeks should occur.

- Severe mitral stenosis or symptomatic severe aortic stenosis.
- Bicuspid aortic valve with ascending aortic diameter >50 mm.
- Marfan syndrome with aortic root diameter >45 mm.
- Severe systemic ventricular systolic dysfunction (LV EF <30% or NYHA class III–IV).
- Native severe coarctation.
- Significant pulmonary arterial hypertension (pulmonary artery systolic pressure >25 mmHg at rest or >30 mmHg with exercise).

During comparison of these risk assessment models, the WHO classification system has proven superiority in risk prediction. In a prospective study of 203 women with congenital cardiac disease in 213 pregnancies, CARPREG and ZAHARA risk scores were calculated for each pregnancy along with identification of WHO classification. Each risk assessment model performed sufficiently for risk estimation, but the WHO classification had the best performance [18]. Similarly, a retrospective study applied each of the three assessment models to 190 women with congenital cardiac disease in 268 pregnancies from 1985 to 2011 and found excellent performance of each model with superiority of the WHO classification system in discrimination and calibration [19].

Acquired cardiac disease

CASE SCENARIO

A 24-year-old gravida two, para one at 21 weeks gestation presents to the obstetrical triage area with dyspnea and palpitations. She is afebrile with normal blood pressure, but her heart rate is 110, respirations 24, and oxygen saturation is 91% on room air. Fetal heart tones are present. She has yet to establish care with an obstetric provider this pregnancy, but her last pregnancy two years prior was uncomplicated and elicited a term vaginal delivery of a healthy neonate. She reports a history of mitral stenosis, for which she last saw the cardiologist in her previous pregnancy. Other than her current symptoms, she has remained asymptomatic for many years. Echocardiography reveals a mitral valve area of 1.3 cm^2, normal LV function (EF 45%), a gradient across the mitral valve of 55 mmHg, and moderate left atrial hypertrophy (42 $ml\,m^{-2}$). Chest X-ray suggests patchy shadowing with air bronchograms, indicative of moderate pulmonary edema.

Clinical questions and critical review of the literature

1. What are the common etiologies for acquired valvular lesions in pregnant women?

Search Strategy: MEDLINE: pregnancy AND heart valve AND maternal.

Mitral and aortic diseases are common acquired lesions, which can be stenotic or regurgitant, in contrast to pulmonic disease, which is largely congenital. Mitral stenosis is the most common valvular lesion in pregnancy, with a majority of cases attributed to rheumatic disease, especially in developing countries [8]. These lesions can go unnoticed throughout a lifetime, but the increased blood volume and hemodynamic changes of pregnancy can initiate new symptoms and exacerbate the condition [6]. Rheumatic disease can also cause mitral regurgitation, but the most common etiology of this lesion in reproductive age women is mitral valve prolapse. Others include infective endocarditis (IE) and functional regurgitation from left ventricle dilation during pregnancy [20]. Aortic stenosis and regurgitation are most frequently caused by congenital bicuspid aortic valve, but they have also been associated with IE and rheumatic disease. Among all cases of mitral lesions caused by rheumatic disease, 5% will also have aortic lesions. Aortic regurgitation can be acquired from connective tissue disorders such as Marfan syndrome as well [21].

2. What should pre-conception counseling entail for women with cardiac disease?

Search Strategy: MEDLINE: pregnancy AND heart disease AND maternal AND counseling.

Young girls with cardiac disease should be counseled regarding effective contraception to avoid the morbidity and mortality associated with pregnancy. Once a woman is contemplating pregnancy, further discussion should include the risks of maternal mortality and cardiac complications during pregnancy along with obstetric complications, risks of fetal and neonatal morbidity and mortality, risks of inheritance of cardiac disease to the offspring, and the anticipated course of antepartum surveillance [22]. Each patient will have a unique risk profile based upon the type of lesion, severity, and current functional status. This lends to the importance of a detailed history and physical exam, with attention focused on functional status, signs and symptoms of cardiac dysfunction (dyspnea, orthopnea, and peripheral edema), prior cardiac events, and prior surgery. The risk assessment models discussed previously can aid in providing accurate predictions of expected complications in pregnancy.

Additionally, structural and functional assessment of the heart should be performed with an echocardiogram prior to pregnancy before hemodynamic changes alter the study. Specifically, valve structure and function, lesion severity, ventricular function, and pulmonary artery systolic pressure should be evaluated. Cardiac surgery during pregnancy should be avoided; therefore, women should perform any necessary procedure or surgery prior to pregnancy if indications are present. These interventions can also help improve fertility, tolerance of the physiologic changes of pregnancy, and maternal and fetal morbidity and mortality [20].

3. What is the appropriate antepartum management for a woman with an acquired cardiac lesion?

Search Strategy: MEDLINE: pregnancy AND heart valve AND maternal.

Women achieving pregnancy with acquired cardiac disease or valvular lesions should have ongoing evaluation and care by an obstetrician trained and skilled for managing these conditions, a cardiologist, and anesthesiology consultation to confirm plans and recommendations for labor and delivery management. Typically, prenatal evaluation occurs every four weeks until 28 weeks gestation, then every two weeks until 36 weeks gestation and weekly thereafter. Cardiology evaluation every four to eight weeks is recommended with echocardiogram to assess cardiac structure and function. If a woman has severe disease or is symptomatic, more frequent assessment is necessary [2].

Evaluation of a symptomatic patient with cardiac disease can be challenging in pregnancy given the similarity of normal physiologic symptoms of pregnancy, such as fatigue, dyspnea, and peripheral edema. Onset of symptoms due to cardiac pathology tends to be highest in the second half of pregnancy and peripartum period when cardiac output and blood volume are highest. Echocardiography is imperative in the evaluation to assess valvular and ventricular function for comparison with prior studies [7]. Most lesions are known ahead of time, but echocardiography can distinguish a new cardiac diagnosis if pregnancy physiology has revealed an unrecognized lesion [20]. Chest X-ray and ECG are reasonable alternatives when echocardiogram is unavailable, but these are also optimal studies to use in conjunction with echocardiogram for assessment of lung fields and chamber morphology. If cardiac assessment is reassuring, then other etiologies of infection, pulmonary embolus, or asthma exacerbation should be evaluated [7].

If pre-conception genetic counseling was not performed, then arranging this early in pregnancy is ideal. Fetal echocardiography from 19 to 22 weeks gestation should be offered to a pregnant woman when either parent is affected. Nuchal fold thickness measurement in the first trimester has a 99% negative predictive value for ruling out cardiac disease with a reassuring value [23]. Both studies can help distinguish those fetuses at risk for inherited cardiac disease.

4. What are the maternal and obstetric risks associated with valvular lesions in pregnancy?

Search Strategy: MEDLINE: pregnancy AND valve disease AND maternal AND risks.

Acquired valvular lesions can create a myriad of maternal and obstetric complications in pregnancy, which can be related to the type and severity of lesion in addition to the alteration in hemodynamics from the physiologic changes of pregnancy. Risk assessment models can help predict the onset of these complications, but prompt assessment and treatment must be employed.

Mitral stenosis is graded on the measurement of the valve diameter, which is obtained from echocardiography. A normal mitral valve diameter is 4–6 cm^2, and abnormalities are diagnosed with the following values: >1.5 cm^2 (mild disease), 1–1.49 cm^2 (moderate disease), and <1.0 cm^2 (severe disease) [24]. Mild disease is typically associated with NYHA class I–II (symptoms with strenuous activity). Moderate disease is most frequently associated with NYHA class III (symptoms with ordinary or less than ordinary activity), and severe disease is associated with NYHA class IV (symptoms at rest) [7].

Generally, stenotic lesions are poorly tolerated in pregnancy due to the increased volume and intensification of gradients across valves. Multiple small studies have shown that a decreased mitral valve area and more advanced functional class before pregnancy are strongly associated with decompensation and maternal complications [25–27]. Mild disease rarely precipitates symptoms, but those with moderate or severe disease (mitral valve area <1.5 cm^2) are at a significantly increased risk for arrhythmias, pulmonary edema, and heart failure, which can be progressive and typically onset in the second half of pregnancy. If an arrhythmia onsets, then the additional risk of a thromboembolic event arises [26, 27]. Overall mortality for mitral stenosis is 1–3% in developed nations, but developing countries can observe maternal mortality up to 30% [20]. Therefore, avoidance of pregnancy or treatment prior to pregnancy should occur in women with moderate to severe disease.

Similarly, maternal complications linked to aortic stenosis depend on the severity of the lesion and presence of symptoms. Those with mild to moderate disease without symptoms can generally tolerate pregnancy well, and the rate of complications is extremely low [28, 30]. Severe disease is characterized by an aortic diameter <1 cm^2 or gradient >50 mmHg, and this carries significant risk for heart failure (10%) and arrhythmias (3–25%) [20, 29]. Mortality is actually rare given the escalation of appropriate management [26, 28, 29]. Careful attention to symptoms in women with severe aortic stenosis guides management. Even in women with critical measurements that remain asymptomatic, have a normal blood pressure response to exercise testing, no evidence of severe LV hypertrophy or a progressive lesion, pregnancy can be tolerated well, and pre-pregnant treatment might not be necessary. However, if any of these factors are identified, then pregnancy should be avoided until proper treatment is employed [29–31].

Regurgitant lesions are often better tolerated in pregnancy than stenotic lesions. The physiologic changes of pregnancy create a decrease in SVR and increased cardiac output, which aid in propagating blood flow in a forward direction [6, 20]. Maternal cardiac risk associated with aortic and mitral regurgitation is dependent upon symptoms, regurgitation severity, and LV function. Increased symptoms and suboptimal LV function can precipitate heart failure in pregnancy [7, 32]. Arrhythmias are of more concern in an asymptomatic woman with preserved LV function, and progressive worsening of regurgitation is always a risk in any woman with baseline disease [15, 33]. If severe symptoms or LV dysfunction are present, then valve repair or replacement prior to pregnancy is warranted. Otherwise, pregnancy can be advised with close observation and risk counseling [20].

5. When is intervention necessary for valvular lesions in pregnancy? What treatment options are available?

Search Strategy: *MEDLINE*: pregnancy AND valve disease AND treatment.

Proper assessment of valvular function prior to pregnancy is vital to properly plan for treatment interventions necessary before conception occurs. If indicated, procedures performed prior to pregnancy can optimize functional status, decrease symptoms, and help avoid obstetrical complications. When lesions are mild and symptoms are minimal, medical management and intensive follow-up throughout pregnancy can be maintained. There are no randomized controlled trials to evaluate the efficacy of interventions for cardiac disease in pregnancy. Most recommendations are made from observational studies, which have limitations and selection bias to account for [8].

When symptoms of volume overload present in women with stenotic lesions, primary goals are to reduce activity, volume, and cardiac workload. Pulmonary and peripheral edema, pulmonary hypertension, dyspnea and fatigue from an inadequate cardiac output due to cardiac dysfunction, and arrhythmias from dilated chambers with blood flow stasis are signs and symptoms of significant decompensation. These women should be counseled to minimize activity, which exacerbates symptoms, and to rest. Oral diuretics, such as thiazides and furosemide, may be initiated along with β1-specific receptor antagonists. If a woman develops atrial fibrillation, anticoagulation, along with a β-receptor antagonist or non-dihydropyridine calcium channel antagonist for rate control, should commence [21, 34]. Digoxin can be used in refractory cases [7, 35]. If echocardiography shows significantly dilated chambers (left atrium >40 ml m^{-2}), low cardiac output or a woman has symptoms of congestive heart failure, then anticoagulation should also be considered [21, 34].

If women with moderate to severe mitral stenosis (mitral valve area <1.2 cm^2) are considered NYHA class III–IV, perform pathologic exercise tests or have pulmonary arterial pressures >50 mmHg, then intervention prior to pregnancy is recommended. These women have a 60% risk for deterioration in pregnancy, and treatment helps optimize functional status and obstetric outcomes [27]. If not performed prior to pregnancy, then treatment during pregnancy is reserved for women meeting the same criteria or having progressive disease despite medical therapy optimization [7, 21, 34].

Percutaneous balloon mitral commissurotomy is the preferred treatment option if echocardiography confirms a mobile, non-calcified valve and no left atrial thrombus, which are contra-indications to the procedure [6]. Fluoroscopy is necessary for the technique, so optimal timing for treatment is beyond 14 weeks, abdominal shielding is recommended, and using the Inoue balloon catheter can facilitate a shorter procedure time. All these factors help minimize radiation effects to the fetus. Total fetal radiation exposure <5 rad is optimal for an entire pregnancy, and approximately 0.2 rad is administered with abdominal shielding and an average fluoroscopy time of 16 minutes [7, 21, 34, 36]. There has been tremendous success with balloon commissurotomy performed in pregnancy. Mitral valve area has been shown to increase from 1 to 2 cm^2, which is similar to the efficacy seen in non-pregnant patients [37–40]. Additionally, functional status, pulmonary artery pressure, and pressure gradient across the valve have shown improvement [7, 38, 41–43].

The fewest complications are observed with balloon commissurotomy. Maternal mortality is rare, with rates as low as <1%. However, minor risks of tamponade, hemorrhage, transient atrial fibrillation, worsening mitral regurgitation, and pulmonary edema have been reported [37, 41–43]. Fetal effects have been favorable [44, 45], but most studies report increased risks of stillbirth, growth restriction, and preterm birth, despite treatment [27, 46, 47]. This might be related to the underlying disease or late timing of intervention that prevents the fetus from gaining all the physiologic benefit in such a short time. Nevertheless, offspring have shown normal growth and development following the procedure for up to seven years [44, 45, 48–52]. In developing countries or when percutaneous procedures are unavailable, closed mitral commissurotomy is preferred, with a slightly higher maternal mortality (2.5%) [7]. Fetal mortality for percutaneous and closed procedures remains <10%, but this rises to 10–30% when open-heart surgery is performed for commissurotomy or valve replacement. These procedures should be reserved for refractory cases when a mother's life is threatened [7, 21, 34, 53, 54].

In severe aortic stenosis (aortic valve area <1 cm^2), an additional factor of symptoms, significant LV dysfunction or hypertrophy, or progressive stenosis will merit the need for intervention prior to conception to avoid the high probability of deterioration and to optimize maternal, fetal, and obstetric outcomes. Additionally, valve gradient >50 mmHg should prompt pre-conception treatment [21, 34]. Otherwise, pregnancy is usually tolerated well in women with severe aortic stenosis without any additional complications [28, 34]. If pregnancy commences prior to intervention, rest and medical management should be maximized. If no improvement is observed, nonetheless, balloon valvuloplasty can be performed in non-calcified valves with minimal regurgitation [57]. The same principles apply to timing of the procedure and precautions taken for fetal radiation exposure as for mitral valve balloon commissurotomy, but there is little data that reports efficacy and maternal and fetal outcomes following this procedure [7, 21, 55, 56]. If valvuloplasty is unable to be performed, then early delivery of the fetus followed by valve replacement should be executed due to the 30% fetal mortality risk associated with valve replacement surgery [2, 57].

Regurgitant lesions are better tolerated than stenotic lesions in pregnant women; therefore, thresholds for intervention are much higher. Volume overload can be managed with oral diuretics, and symptoms can be minimized with rest and limitations of activity. If severe regurgitation stimulates compromised LV function or significant symptoms of heart failure (NYHA class III–IV) refractory to medical management, then surgery is an option. Valve repair is preferred over replacement to avoid the risks of thrombosis and anticoagulation [20, 34]. Fetal mortality can reach 30% with open surgery and cardiopulmonary bypass, so the risks and benefits of early delivery prior to surgery should be discussed [21, 34].

6. What are the key principles in managing women with artificial valves?

Search Strategy: MEDLINE: pregnancy AND mechanical valve.

When artificial valves function appropriately, pregnancy can be hemodynamically tolerated well, but there is a baseline risk of 1–4% maternal mortality. Valve thromboses can increase this mortality risk to 65%, and the type of valve material and anticoagulation regimen used play a significant role in predicting thrombosis risk. Compared to donor and bioprosthetic valves, mechanical valves are more frequently used due to their durability and longevity, but anticoagulation must be used concomitantly due to the high propensity of thrombosis. Risk of hemorrhage, obstetric complications, and fetal teratogenicity in addition to valve thrombosis and the potential sequelae raise concern for pregnant women [2].

There are no randomized controlled trials to evaluate methods of anticoagulation, but smaller cohort studies and systematic reviews provide data for recommendations. Most recent reports suggest that warfarin used throughout the pregnancy elicits a 2% risk for thrombosis and also maternal mortality compared to substitution of unfractionated heparin (UFH) during the first trimester (6–12 weeks gestation), which carries a 10% risk for thrombosis and 4% risk for maternal mortality [58]. UFH used exclusively throughout the pregnancy conveys a 33% risk for thrombosis and 15% risk for maternal mortality [59]. Undoubtedly, warfarin seems to be the ideal anticoagulant; however, risks of embryopathy limit its use in the first trimester. Warfarin crosses the placenta and can create effects such as a depressed nasal bridge, bone stippling, congenital cardiac disease, growth restriction, developmental delay, and seizures, which describe the fetal warfarin syndrome. When doses <5 mg are used, the risks of embryopathy remain similar to that of the general population for congenital anomalies (2.5%); conversely, doses >5 mg can increase this risk up to 10% [59–64]. Use beyond the first trimester still carries a risk of central nervous system abnormalities and fetal hemorrhage given the immature liver enzymes and low levels of vitamin K dependent clotting factors in the fetus [2]. At delivery, fetal intracranial bleeding is a risk if a mother has a vaginal delivery while concurrently taking warfarin; therefore, transition to UFH nearing delivery is ideal or cesarean is necessary [2, 63].

If doses of warfarin remain <5 mg, then continuation throughout pregnancy is recommended. Alternatively, intravenous (IV) or IM UFH can be used 6–12 weeks gestation to avoid the risks of embryopathy if warfarin dose rises above 5 mg, but the increased risk of thrombosis must be accepted. UFH does not cross the placenta, but the risks of thrombocytopenia and osteoporosis do exist [65, 66]. Although low molecular weight heparin (LMWH) has fewer side effects and seems more convenient for home administration, use in pregnancy with mechanical valves is controversial due to the lack of supporting data regarding frequency of dosing, timing and goals of anti-Xa levels, and outcomes compared to warfarin and heparin. Small studies have reported thrombosis risks of 4% and 9% when LMWH was used only in the first trimester and throughout the pregnancy, respectively [58, 67–69]. Therapeutic dosing should begin at 1 mg kg^{-1} twice daily, and multiple studies have shown that fixed dosing compared to dose adjustments throughout pregnancy has a significantly higher risk for thrombosis [66, 70]. Increased renal clearance and volume of distribution as pregnancy progresses necessitates continued titration to a peak goal of 0.8–1.2 U ml^{-1} (four to six hours following dose). Some suggest that even three times daily dosing might be advantageous [38]. Currently, there is no official approval for LMWH use in pregnant women with mechanical heart valves, and it should be used judiciously.

Anticoagulation certainly helps protect against the risk for thrombosis in mechanical valves, but any regimen still carries obstetric and neonatal risks. Women must be counseled regarding the risk for miscarriage and retro-placental hemorrhage, which can precipitate preterm birth and fetal death [2, 59, 61–63, 70]. After appropriate counseling, a regimen must be devised for monitoring goals and frequency. The American College of Cardiology (ACC), American Heart Association (AHA), and ESC suggest warfarin be continued until pregnancy is achieved. Either continuing warfarin or transitioning to UFH from 6 to 12 weeks gestation is appropriate, with resumption of warfarin in the second and third trimesters. The AHA and ESC endorse the use of LMWH from 6 to 12 weeks gestation if peak anti-Xa level can be maintained 0.7–1.2 U ml^{-1}. International normalized ratio (INR) and activated partial thromboplastin time (aPTT) must be kept twice the control level, and weekly monitoring is suggested for any regimen [34, 71].

7. What are the fetal and neonatal risks associated with valvular lesions in pregnancy?

Search Strategy: MEDLINE: pregnancy AND valve disease AND maternal AND risks.

Among all the acquired cardiac and valvular lesions, common risks of fetal growth restriction, stillbirth, and preterm birth are observed and related to the severity of the disease and cardiac complications that arise, such as heart failure and arrhythmias. Women with stenotic lesions who are symptomatic or who have moderate to severe disease have a 5–25% risk for fetal growth restriction, 1–3% risk for stillbirth, and 30% risk for preterm birth [27, 29, 46]. Regurgitant lesions are better tolerated in pregnancy, but the overall risk for fetal growth restriction, stillbirth, and preterm birth are still slightly increased [13]. Beyond the baseline risks associated with decompensation of cardiac disease in pregnancy, medical therapy adds a trivial amount of increased risk to the fetus. Surgery can increase fetal mortality risk up to 30% depending on the type performed; percutaneous procedures are preferred over open heart surgery for valve replacement [2, 57].

8. During labor and delivery, what is the preferred mode of delivery, anesthesia method, and intrapartum monitoring for women with acquired or valvular lesions?

Search Strategy: *MEDLINE*: pregnancy AND valve disease AND delivery.

In general, women with acquired and valvular lesions should attempt a vaginal delivery with regional anesthesia whenever possible. Vaginal delivery has less risk of bleeding, infection, and venous thromboembolism, which can significantly impact a woman with cardiac disease [72]. There is limited data comparing outcomes following vaginal and cesarean delivery, but small studies have reported vaginal delivery success in women that even have moderate to severe disease. Those women with mild disease or repaired valvular lesions should undergo management similar to normal pregnant women. In most women with cardiac disease, spontaneous labor is preferred, and decision for induction of labor should take into account a woman's Bishop score, fetal status, maternal functional status, and timing of anticoagulation [1, 21, 30].

Short and pain-free labor is ideal to avoid hemodynamic changes associated with pain, contractions, and pushing. In women with stenotic lesions, caution with regional anesthesia to avoid a substantial drop in SVR and sufficient IV fluids to maintain adequate preload is urged. Volume should be carefully balanced in women with regurgitant lesions to avoid pulmonary edema and volume overload. Continuous monitoring of oxygen saturation, blood pressure, ECG, and arterial pressure in isolated cases are warranted during the labor and delivery course along with fetal monitoring that will display a direct reflection of placental perfusion and oxygenation. An assisted second stage is recommended to minimize pushing effort and expedite delivery. In isolated situations of severe stenosis with significant symptoms or pulmonary hypertension, it is reasonable to perform a cesarean under general anesthesia. Otherwise, cesarean is reserved for obstetric indications [1, 21, 30]. Delivery of all high-risk women with moderate to severe disease or significant symptoms should be performed in a tertiary care center with collaborative management by skilled obstetricians, cardiologists, and anesthesiologists [71, 73].

9. Is antibiotic prophylaxis necessary for pregnant women with cardiac disease?

Search Strategy: *MEDLINE*: pregnancy AND heart disease AND endocarditis.

IE in pregnancy is extremely rare with an incidence of 1/100 000 pregnancies (0.006%) [74], and there is just a slight increase for women with valvular or congenital cardiac disease [75]. Drug addiction, prosthetic valves, prior endocarditis, and untreated cyanotic heart disease are factors that place patients in the highest risk categories, but recommendations for antibiotic prophylaxis during pregnancy and invasive procedures for even the highest risk patients have evolved since early 2000 [76].

Previous recommendations for antibiotic prophylaxis were developed from a multitude of case reports and animal models that revealed transient bacteremia following invasive procedures. Nevertheless, the principle that antibiotic prophylaxis should decrease bacteremia, attachment of bacteria to the endocardium and subsequent IE has only been proven in animal models, and efficacy in humans is controversial [77–79]. Very few studies have correlated IE with invasive procedures, such as dental, which provokes the theory that the risk for IE is more likely to occur from cumulative low-grade bacteremia from daily activities, such as tooth-brushing or flossing, than from isolated high-grade bacteremia following dental procedures [80]. Furthermore, antibiotic use has been shown to be cost-ineffective, to intensify the emergence of resistant microorganisms, and to transmit a risk of anaphylaxis [77–79]. Beginning in 2002, restriction of antibiotic prophylaxis to the highest risk patients during dental procedures was propagated by the AHA, ACC, ESC, and National Institute for Health and Care Excellence (NICE), and no increase in IE has been observed [81–84]. Pregnant women with cardiac disease do not require antibiotic prophylaxis during labor and delivery, regardless of vaginal or cesarean mode. If these women have a high-risk characteristic, then the ESC supports considering prophylaxis during dental procedures [76, 85].

10. What care should be employed in the postpartum period for women with valvular lesions?

Search Strategy: *MEDLINE*: pregnancy AND valve disease AND delivery.

The largest hemodynamic changes and fluid shifts occur within 12–24 hours following delivery, so hemodynamic monitoring should persist for 24 hours. Fluid balance and monitoring for heart failure symptoms are important in this immediate postpartum time period. Following delivery, IV oxytocin infusion should ensue to prevent postpartum hemorrhage, and it has minimal effect on SVR. If additional uterotonics are necessary, then prostaglandin F analogues can be used. Misoprostol is supported as well, but there is a small increased risk of coronary vasospasm and arrhythmia. Methylergonovine is contra-indicated due to the 10% risk for vasoconstriction and hypertension [21, 86, 87]. Breastfeeding is recommended unless women are extremely symptomatic and critically ill.

Graded recommendations for the management of acquired valvular cardiac disease in pregnancy [175]:

- Prepregnancy counseling and risk assessment is indicated in all women with known or suspected congenital or acquired cardiovascular disease (I-C).
- High-risk women with cardiac disease should be cared for by a multidisciplinary team involving an obstetrician, cardiologist, and anesthesiologist, and delivery should occur at a specialized center (I-C).
- Cardiology follow-up should be outlined at the beginning of pregnancy; typical schedules range from twice to monthly (I-C).
- Echocardiography should be performed in any pregnant woman with new or unexplained cardiovascular signs or symptoms (I-C).
- Pregnant women with mechanical valves should utilize anticoagulation throughout pregnancy (I-C).
- Vaginal delivery with regional anesthesia is recommended as first choice for most women with cardiac disease (I-C).
- Management to prevent IE in pregnancy is the same as that for non-pregnant patients (I-C).
- In women undergoing a vaginal delivery, regional anesthesia and an elective operative delivery should be considered (IIa-C).

- Cesarean delivery should be considered for women with severe aortic stenosis, continued oral anticoagulation at time of delivery or severe symptomatic heart failure (IIa-C).
- If gestational age is >28 weeks, then delivery prior to cardiac surgery should be considered (IIa-C).
- Valvular or reparative cardiac surgery may be considered when conservative therapy has failed, a mother's life is threatened, and percutaneous treatment is not an option (IIb-C).
- Antibiotic therapy for the prevention of IE is not recommended during delivery (III-C).

Congenital cardiac disease

CASE SCENARIO

A 29-year-old gravida one presents to her initial prenatal visit in hopes of determining her due date along with identifying goals for care due to her diagnosis of Marfan syndrome. Crown rump length establishes a gestational age of eight weeks and three days, and further discussion regarding the patient's medical history unfolds. She reports that she routinely receives care with an internist and did see a cardiologist one year ago. Echocardiography at that time was obtained and reports an aortic root diameter of 3.7 cm^2, normal LV function (EF 55%) and normal chamber morphology. Her vitals at the current visit are normal with a blood pressure of 115/60, and she reports no complications in her medical health despite her diagnosis. Her paternal grandmother, father, and only brother are also affected with Marfan syndrome, and her grandmother passed away from an aortic dissection at 62 years. Her other family members are healthy. This pregnancy was unplanned, and she most desires knowing what the risks are to her and the fetus. If safe, she strongly desires to keep the pregnancy. She is also concerned that her child might be affected with Marfan due to the large number of affected family members, and she asks what the chance is of this occurring.

Clinical questions and critical review of the literature

1. What is the appropriate antepartum management for a woman with a congenital cardiac lesion?

Search Strategy: *MEDLINE*: pregnancy AND congenital heart disease AND management.

Women with congenital cardiac disease should receive routine prenatal care along with periodic cardiology assessment. Focus should be aimed on genetic counseling if not performed pre-conception, serial fetal growth assessment, and fetal surveillance testing if lesions are uncorrected, maternal cyanosis is present, or functional status is compromised. Cardiology evaluation with an echocardiogram to assess cardiac structure and function should occur every four to eight weeks or more frequently if there is greater disease severity or complications [2].

Attention to symptoms of heart failure, arrhythmias, and volume overload in women with congenital cardiac disease is warranted, but these are frequently confused with symptoms related to the physiologic changes of pregnancy. Echocardiography is a crucial imaging tool that can differentiate routine pregnancy symptoms from decompensation of cardiac disease [7]. It is also an important diagnostic tool when congenital cardiac lesions have not been previously identified and symptoms are precipitated by the hemodynamic changes of pregnancy [20]. Other imaging can be useful in conjunction or when echocardiography is unavailable, such as chest X-ray and ECG [7].

2. What are the recurrence risks for various congenital cardiac lesions to affect a subsequent child?

Search Strategy: MEDLINE: pregnancy AND congenital heart disease AND offspring.

Overall, studies have evaluated the presence of cardiac lesions in the offspring of parents with congenital cardiac disease, and a range of 3–7% recurrence risk is described. From a literature review of 6640 pregnancies in which a parent or sibling had congenital cardiac disease, 3% of the fetuses were affected with cardiac disease and one-third were congruent lesions [88]. In the prospective CARPREG study, 7% of fetuses were affected in the 432 live births that occurred among women with congenital cardiac disease [13]. If the same cardiac defect is propagated to the offspring, then VSDs, hypoplastic left heart syndrome, and aortic coarctation are the most common defects to recur among family members [88].

While overall recurrence risk for congenital cardiac lesions is reported as 3–7%, recurrence of specific lesions has been studied as well in a systematic literature review. Particularly looking at women with atrioventricular septal defects (AVSDs) in 88 pregnancies, 7 (8%) of the offspring were affected with some form of cardiac disease. In the same literature review, 68 women with unrepaired or palliated congenital cyanotic cardiac disease (TOF, transposition of the great vessels, tricuspid atresia, pulmonary atresia, single ventricle lesions, and Ebstein's) had a 7% incidence of offspring affected with cardiac disease. Of 121 pregnancies in women with congenital bicuspid aortic valve, 4% of offspring were found to have congenital cardiac disease [89].

Cardiac disease can also be inherited as part of a genetic syndrome, which have varying degrees of inheritance and penetrance. Marfan syndrome has an autosomal dominant inheritance pattern, so an affected parent will elicit a 50% risk for the fetus to be affected and possibly develop aortopathy and aneurysms [2, 23]. Congenital cardiac disease is also part of genetic syndromes such as 22q11 deletion, Noonan, Holt–Oram, Alagille, or Williams–Beuren syndrome. If a parent is affected with any of these, genetic counseling will help to provide risks for inheritance, but most of these conditions will develop from de novo mutations with variable penetrance [90].

3. What are the maternal risks associated with congenital cardiac lesions in pregnancy?

Search Strategy: *MEDLINE*: pregnancy AND congenital heart disease AND maternal AND risks.

Each congenital cardiac lesion poses unique risks and challenges that will be explored separately. ASDs are the most common maternal congenital lesions in pregnancy, and they are generally well tolerated in pregnancy, regardless if they are repaired. If repaired, then only a small risk (0.8% in a study of 123 women) of tachyarrhythmia exists for the mother [89], which occurs more frequently as age of repair increases [89, 91]. Women with unrepaired ASDs have a 5% risk for thromboembolic complications; paradoxical emboli from the lower extremity veins can be propagated to the right heart through the ASD and into systemic circulation [89]. Increased ambulation, compression stockings, and avoidance of IVC compression from lying supine will help avoid venous stasis, which can propagate emboli. Anticoagulation is recommended if prolonged immobility is warranted in pregnancy. IV filters should be utilized during labor and delivery to minimize risk of venous air emboli [92]. Additionally, caution should be taken to avoid hemorrhage and, if it occurs, volume status should be replaced immediately to avoid right-to-left shunting caused by a decreased preload and increased afterload. Closure of an ASD should be performed prior to pregnancy, and the only indication for closure during pregnancy is significant maternal deterioration. Catheter device closure can be performed under guidance of transesophageal or intracardiac echocardiography [93]. If concomitant pulmonary hypertension or Eisenmenger syndrome exists with an ASD, then pregnancy is contra-indicated, and discussion of effective contraception or early termination should occur [91].

Women with small or repaired VSDs with preserved LV function, normal pulmonary pressures, and a shunt ratio <1.7 will tolerate pregnancy with minimal risk to the mother or fetus. On the contrary, women with larger shunts and history of arrhythmias, LV dysfunction, or pulmonary hypertension have a much higher risk for cardiac complications to occur during pregnancy, showing a predominance of arrhythmias and heart failure [13, 73]. In a literature review from 1985 to 2007, there were no reports of arrhythmia or heart failure and one case of a cardiovascular event (myocardial infarction, stroke, cardiovascular mortality) among 83 women with a VSD, both repaired and unrepaired [89]. If Eisenmenger syndrome develops, pregnancy is contra-indicated [13].

Most women with congenital cyanotic heart disease have had reparative surgery upon reaching the reproductive years, but there are several with inoperable lesions who have survived with palliative care. Regardless of repair, this category of women has an overall risk of 30% for cardiac complications, mostly heart failure, arrhythmias, thromboembolic events, or deterioration of status [14, 89, 94–96]. Activity restriction, supplemental oxygen, iron therapy, and prophylactic anticoagulation are common therapies employed for women with cyanotic heart disease [97].

TOF is the most common congenital cyanotic lesion found in pregnancy. Several earlier studies reported pregnancies affected specifically by repaired TOF as uncomplicated with no adverse maternal effects. However, the sample size was extremely small, and limited hemodynamic parameters were evaluated [98–100]. More recent and larger studies have reported overall cardiac event rates of 7–8% during pregnancy for women with TOF. Consistent risk factors for cardiac events among women with congenital cyanotic heart disease include the presence of pulmonary hypertension, ventricular dysfunction, prepregnancy use of cardiac medications or NYHA class >2 [101, 102], and, most importantly, oxygen saturation <85% [94]. Corrective surgery or palliative valve replacement if significant regurgitant lesions are present should be performed prior to pregnancy. If symptoms onset during pregnancy, then diuretics and decreased physical activity can be advised; transcatheter valve replacement is reserved for women with symptoms refractory to medical therapy [28].

D-transposition of the great arteries involves interchanging of the pulmonary arteries and aorta while the ventricles remain in the correct anatomic location. Arterial switch (Jatene) or older less utilized atrial switch procedures (Mustard or Senning), can alleviate this disruption in blood flow to improve systemic oxygenation. Congenitally corrected L-transposition of the great arteries (atrioventricular and ventriculo-arterial discordance) is characterized by inversion of the ventricles in addition to transposition of the great arteries, which allows normal blood circulation through morphologically reversed ventricles. L-transposition and even D-transposition following an atrial switch procedure pose risk for arrhythmias (10%), significant heart block and heart failure (4–15%). There is a 10% risk for developing irreversible right ventricular decline [89, 103–105]. Very few reports of pregnancy following arterial switch procedures have been described, but optimal functional status prior to pregnancy seems to be a predictor of good outcome [106]. Those with ventricular dysfunction (EF <40%), NYHA class III–IV status, or severe tricuspid regurgitation should be counseled against pregnancy.

A spectrum of congenital lesions involves the pulmonic valve and bilateral ventricles. Isolated pulmonic stenosis can be well tolerated in pregnancy. If severe stenosis (peak Doppler gradient >64 mmHg) is present, then treatment with balloon valvuloplasty prior to pregnancy is ideal. Likewise, women with severe pulmonary regurgitation causing right ventricular dysfunction and symptoms of heart failure should undergo valve replacement prior to pregnancy

[28, 107]. Overall, risks during pregnancy for women with pulmonary valve stenosis include right ventricular heart failure and arrhythmias [28, 97, 108]. Only a few case reports discuss pregnancy outcomes of women with congenital lesions that exhibit a single ventricle (hypoplastic ventricle, atrioventricular valve atresia, double inlet ventricle, or unbalanced atrioventricular canal) that remain unrepaired, but there is an overwhelming concern for maternal morbidity and mortality with the onset of pulmonary vascular disease and the susceptibility to develop Eisenmenger syndrome [109–112].

The Fontan procedure is the procedure of choice to repair single ventricle physiology, as it relieves cyanosis and ventricular volume overload through application of a conduit that connects the right atrium to the pulmonary arteries [1, 2]. The Fontan circulation predisposes to right atrial hypertrophy, which can be exacerbated in pregnancy, increasing the risks for arrhythmias (25%), heart failure (5%), and a decline in functional capacity (15%) [2, 113, 114]. Echocardiography prior to pregnancy to assess ventricular function, vascular anatomy, and exclude atrial thrombi should be performed. Anticoagulation during pregnancy is recommended due to the increased risk of arrhythmias and thrombus formation with a dilated right atrium [1]. Pregnancy should be avoided in those with resting oxygen saturation <85%, severe ventricular dysfunction, moderate to severe atrioventricular valve regurgitation, or protein-losing enteropathy.

Aortopathies encompass several congenital cardiac lesions, such as coarctation, congenital bicuspid aortic valve and aortic stenosis, and aortic disease associated with Marfan or Turner syndrome. Concern for rupture of aortic and cerebral artery aneurysms exists for patients with all these conditions, and hypertension is more common collectively, which increases the risk for rupture. Coarctation should be repaired prior to pregnancy, and women with unrepaired or residual coarcts, uncontrolled hypertension or aneurysms are at significant risk for aortic rupture [115]. A retrospective review of 30 pregnancies complicated by coarctation (24 repaired) identified that aortic diameter <12 mm was significantly associated with cardiovascular events and hypertensive complications [116]. A total of 50% of women with congenital bicuspid aortic valve have dilation of the ascending aorta [117], which can be difficult to visualize with echocardiography, and computed tomography (CT) or magnetic resonance imaging (MRI) is suggested. Risk of aortic dissection and rupture remains smaller than women with Marfan syndrome, but outcomes data is rare [118]. Those with aortic roots >50 mm should be advised to avoid pregnancy until repaired [28].

Women with Marfan syndrome and normal aortic roots have a 1% risk for dissection in pregnancy, and more than half of these occur in the third trimester [119]. Pregnant women have a five times greater risk for dissection than those who are not pregnant, but this risk seems to be transient and not associated with an increased cumulative lifetime risk for complications [120]. Most studies report rare incidence of dissection with an aortic root <40 mm; however, there is no safe value for pregnancy [121]. While data is limited for pregnancy outcomes with aortic root diameter >45 mm, it is believed that this is the threshold to avoid pregnancy until repair can be performed. Even following aortic root replacement, risk for dissection remains in the residual aorta [121]. Counseling toward pregnancy and risks for dissection in women with aortic diameters 40–45 mm will depend on factors such as family history of dissection and recent rapid growth [122]. Women with Turner syndrome will have a 25–50% risk for cardiovascular malformations. In these women or others of small stature with aortic dilation, there is a 2% risk for dissection, and this can occur with much smaller aortic diameters. Therefore, an aortic root diameter >27 mm should be surgically corrected prior to pregnancy [123].

4. What are the obstetric, fetal and neonatal risks associated with congenital cardiac lesions?

Search Strategy: *MEDLINE*: pregnancy AND congenital heart disease AND maternal AND risks.

Apart from maternal cardiovascular risks that can occur during pregnancy, congenital cardiac lesions are associated with obstetric, fetal, and neonatal risks as well. Repaired ASDs seem to have no adverse effect on pregnancy or neonates, but women with unrepaired ASD lesions or a VSD have an increased risk for pre-eclampsia and to give birth to infants that are small for gestational age. Fetal mortality has been shown to increase for only those with AVSD, and this is reported as 6%. This is likely due to the complex nature of most cardiac lesions that typically involve an AVSD [15, 91].

Oxygen saturation is the most important predictive factor when assessing obstetric and fetal risks in women with cyanotic heart disease. Maintaining levels >90% can decrease fetal mortality to <10%, but women with persistent oxygen saturation <85% have only a 12% chance for delivering a live infant [94]. Given the compromised placental oxygen transfer, fetal growth restriction and preterm birth are increased in this population [93]. Specifically among women with TOF, fetal mortality risk has been reported up to 12% and preterm birth risk up to 45% [89].

Congenitally corrected L-transposition of the great arteries is associated with a more favorable risk profile than D-transposition (unrepaired and following atrial switch repair). Preterm birth and fetal death rates for L-transposition have been described as 9% and 1%, respectively, while D-transposition is associated with preterm birth and fetal death rates of 34% and 3%, respectively. Although many women are living to reproductive ages following newer arterial switch procedures, there are few reports of pregnancy outcomes in these individuals, but they remain promising [124].

With regards to pulmonic valve lesions, pulmonary regurgitation severity is a predictor of maternal cardiovascular events, while pulmonary stenosis severity is correlated to obstetric and neonatal complications. Women with pulmonary stenosis have a much higher risk for hypertensive disorders, fetal growth restriction and preterm birth [125]. Those with regurgitant lesions have shown no increased obstetric or neonatal risk. Women with unrepaired single ventricles will typically develop pulmonic stenosis or pulmonary vascular disease over time, with the propensity to develop Eisenmenger syndrome. Once this develops maternal mortality approaches 30–50%, and fetal mortality can reach up to 90% [94]. The Fontan circulation is now used to palliate a single ventricle, but very few pregnancies have been reported following this procedure. Improvement in obstetric and neonatal outcomes is expected, and a small series of 25 pregnancies reported seven preterm births (28%), one perinatal death, and no maternal deaths [89].

Congenital aortic disease encompasses a variety of lesions that increase risks for hypertensive disorders, preterm birth, and maternal and fetal mortality during pregnancy alongside the high susceptibility for aortic dissection. Among women with repaired aortic coarctation, improved long-term survival and a decrease in the onset of hypertensive disease is associated with earlier age of repair. During pregnancy, the risk for hypertensive disorders increases with a later age of repair; although the overall risk is doubled from baseline [89, 115]. Aggressive treatment of blood pressure is necessary, and percutaneous interventions during pregnancy are an option if hypertension persists despite medical therapy. Surgical procedures should be performed prior to pregnancy if possible because the risk for aortic dissection is increased following repair during pregnancy than if performed in a woman who is not pregnant [115, 126]. Risk for maternal mortality has been reported as 2.5%, and preterm birth risk has been described as 8% [115].

Pregnancies involving women with Marfan syndrome have been described to have a threefold increased risk for obstetric complications, mostly postpartum hemorrhage likely due to abnormal vasculature and connective tissue associated with the condition [127]. Additionally, there has been a twofold increase in preterm birth and fetal growth restriction described [127, 128]. Maternal and fetal mortality is associated with the incidence of aortic dissection, which begins to significantly rise with an aortic root diameter >40 mm [121]. A study of 11 women undergoing aortic valve replacement surgery in pregnancy reported no maternal deaths, but three fetal deaths occurred [129]. Women with Turner syndrome have an increased risk for underlying hypertension, and pre-eclampsia is increased in pregnancy. Aggressive control of blood pressure is warranted to avoid the risks of aortic dissection, which increases at a much smaller aortic root diameter (>27 mm) given the small stature of these women [130].

5. During labor and delivery, what is the preferred mode of delivery, anesthesia method, and intrapartum monitoring for women with congenital cardiac lesions?

Search Strategy: *MEDLINE*: pregnancy AND congenital heart disease AND delivery.

The same principles of labor and delivery apply to women with congenital cardiac lesions as those of valvular disease discussed earlier, and, unfortunately, there are no randomized studies to evaluate optimal delivery methods. Vaginal delivery is preferred in most scenarios to minimize risks of bleeding, infection, and thromboembolic events [72]. Hemodynamic changes during labor and delivery heighten due to contractions, increased sympathetic tone from pain and stress, and auto-transfusion of uterine blood flow following delivery. Early epidural placement can reduce pain and the sympathetic response associated, which can help ease cardiac workload. A shortened second stage can reduce the amount of valsalva utilized with pushing, which can alter hemodynamics, and this can be accomplished with an elective operative delivery. Women with repaired ASDs, cyanotic heart disease, or coarctation with normal functional status should proceed with labor and delivery in a routine fashion. Routine intrapartum monitoring should be employed, regional anesthesia is suggested, and cesarean can be reserved for obstetric indications.

Delivery at a tertiary center for NYHA class III–IV status or the highest risk cardiac lesions (WHO class III–IV) is recommended, and this includes pulmonary hypertension, Eisenmenger syndrome, unrepaired cyanotic heart disease, severe LV outflow obstruction, single ventricle physiology with or without repair, aortic dilation >40 mm, and mechanical valves [73, 89, 94]. Vaginal delivery with regional anesthesia remains ideal, but cesarean can be performed if maternal or fetal deterioration occurs. Occasionally, women with transposition of the great arteries or single ventricle physiology (repaired or unrepaired) will exhibit ventricular dysfunction or significant regurgitant lesions, which should prompt discussion of cesarean [131]. Additionally, women with severe stenotic lesions (pulmonary and aortic) and NYHA class III–IV status might better tolerate delivery via cesarean. In these situations with severe stenotic lesions or right-to-left shunts, such as Eisenmenger syndrome, general anesthesia might be indicated to avoid the potential of profound hypotension and decrease in preload that the systemic circulation is dependent upon in these women [132]. Aortic dilation >40 mm, and particularly >45 mm, in women with bicuspid aortic valves, Marfan or Turner syndrome merits discussion of cesarean to avoid the risk of aortic dissection that might occur with valsalva during labor [133]. Routine intrapartum fetal monitoring in addition to continuous monitoring of oxygen saturation, blood pressure, and ECG is warranted; arterial pressure monitoring might be indicated with severe lesions or with advanced symptoms.

6. What care should be employed in the postpartum period for women with congenital cardiac lesions?

Search Strategy: *MEDLINE*: pregnancy AND congenital heart disease AND delivery.

Routine postpartum care with some additional measures should be employed following delivery in a woman with congenital cardiac disease. Prevention of postpartum hemorrhage is crucial, and standard techniques of uterine massage and administration of oxytocin is recommended. Due to the theoretical risk of coronary vasospasm and arrhythmia associated with misoprostol and hypertension associated with methylergonovine, prostaglandin F analogues can be considered if further uterotonics are necessary. Large volume shifts during the delivery process create the greatest hemodynamic changes within the first 24 hours postpartum, so fluid status and signs and symptoms of heart failure and arrhythmia should be monitored closely [40, 86, 87]. Early ambulation and sequential compression devices are necessary with anticoagulation used for those with high risk indications, such as mechanical valves. Anticoagulation in women with cyanotic cardiac lesions can exacerbate intrinsic coagulation defects and precipitate hemorrhage and death [134]. Breastfeeding is recommended if the mother is well enough to engage in this activity. Women should be counseled regarding contraception and family planning with regards to their functional status and specific congenital lesion. Caution should be utilized with estrogen-containing options for women with increased thromboembolic risk, and Depo-Provera should be used carefully in women with heart failure due to fluid retention; otherwise, most methods, including the progestin implant, intrauterine device (IUD), and sterilization are safe for women with congenital cardiac disease [135].

Graded recommendations for the management of congenital cardiac disease in pregnancy [175]*:*

- Women with Marfan syndrome or any aortic disease should have imaging (CT/MRI) of the entire aorta prior to pregnancy (I-C).
- Women with aortic dilation should undergo echocardiography every four to eight weeks in pregnancy (I-C).
- Surgery should be performed prior to pregnancy in women with Marfan syndrome and ascending aortic dilation >45 mm (I-C).
- Women with cyanotic heart disease should be treated prior to pregnancy or advised against pregnancy (I-C).
- Vaginal delivery is preferred in women with ascending aortic diameter <40 mm (I-C).
- Cesarean delivery should be considered for women with ascending aortic dilation >45 mm, Eisenmenger syndrome or severe symptomatic heart failure (I-C).
- Vaginal delivery should be considered in women with ascending aortic diameter 40–45 mm (IIa-C).
- Women with a Fontan circulation should utilize anticoagulation throughout pregnancy (IIa-C).
- Surgery should be performed prior to pregnancy in women with congenital bicuspid aortic valve and ascending aortic diameter >50 mm (IIa-C).
- Women with resting oxygen saturation <85% should be advised against pregnancy (IIa-C).
- Women with transposition of the great arteries (TGA) and a systemic right ventricle with severe RV dysfunction or severe Tricuspid regurgitation (TR) should be advised against pregnancy (III-C).
- Women who have a Fontan circulation and severe AV valve regurgitation, cyanosis, or protein-losing enteropathy should be advised against pregnancy (III-C).

Cardiomyopathy

CASE SCENARIO

A 25-year-old gravida one, para one African-American woman awakens postpartum day two with complaints of epigastric pain, dyspnea, and increased swelling. She was induced at 37 weeks gestation for severe pre-eclampsia and underwent a successful vagina delivery. Blood pressures normalized following delivery, and labs were significant for liver function tests (LFTs) in the 1970s that are down-trending. Vitals are currently normal and oxygen saturation is 93%. Brain natriuretic peptide (BNP) is elevated at 2500. CXR indicates moderate pulmonary edema, and pulmonary angiography is negative for pulmonary embolus. Echocardiography reveals global hypokinesia and severe LV systolic dysfunction (EF 15%). She is alert but anxious, and her husband reports that she is normally healthy. Their newborn infant is healthy and resting in the bassinet at the bedside.

Clinical questions and critical review of the literature

1. How is peripartum cardiomyopathy defined and what are the risk factors for development?

Search Strategy: MEDLINE: pregnancy AND peripartum cardiomyopathy AND risks.

Peripartum cardiomyopathy (PPCM) is an idiopathic presentation of heart failure at the end of pregnancy or the subsequent months following delivery, which is secondary to LV systolic dysfunction. Potential etiologies of a compromised LV systolic function, such as myocardial infarction, valve disease, pulmonary hypertension, kidney, liver, or thyroid dysfunction, must be ruled out to elicit this diagnosis of exclusion [136]. PPCM is defined by the following criteria: onset within one month prior to delivery or five months following delivery, absence of an identifiable etiology, and no recognizable heart disease preceding the current event [137]. Evidence of cardiomegaly on CXR was classically used as a marker for diagnosis, but after 2000, The National Heart, Blood, and Lung Institute incorporated echocardiography to report LV systolic dysfunction (EF <45%) or fractional shortening (<30%) as a more specific characteristic [136]. Frequently, LV dilation (LV end diastolic dimension >2.7 cm m^{-2} body surface area) occurs and resembles dilated cardiomyopathy, but this is not a diagnostic criteria [14].

There have been many attempts to determine possible etiologies for PPCM, but no studies have been able to overwhelmingly support any particular pathophysiology. A literature review in 2007 evaluated risk factors and etiologies for PPCM based on a variety of small observational studies. Viral myocarditis, abnormal immune responses in pregnancy, cytokine-induced inflammation, malnutrition, increased adrenergic tone, and genetic factors were common proposals for contributing factors to PPCM [138]. A study that specifically evaluated inflammatory pathology that might lead to myocarditis and myocardial dysfunction reported a wide range of myocarditis (9–80%) based on endomyocardial biopsies. Along with these findings, inflammatory cytokines, such as interleukin-1, interleukin-6, and tumor necrosis factor (TNF) were also thought to play a role in myocardial damage [136]. Another prediction is that PPCM develops from oxidative stress leading to proteolytic cleavage of prolactin into pro-apoptotic fragments and angiostatic factors [139]. Without large, multi-center epidemiologic studies, the pathophysiology of PPCM will largely remain unknown.

Even without much understanding of the etiology of PPCM, there is evidence to support risk factors for developing the condition. The literature review stated above identified characteristics such as non-Caucasian ethnicity, advanced maternal age, multiparity, multiple gestation, prolonged tocolysis, and poor socioeconomic status as risks for the onset of PPCM [138]. A retrospective study of 535 women with PPCM reported African-American women as having the highest risk with Caucasian and Hispanic women having much lower but equal risks [140]. The average age of those affected with PPCM is 30 years in many studies, which lends to advanced maternal age as being a risk factor [137, 140, 141]. Other medical conditions, such as chronic hypertension and pre-gestational diabetes, have been reported as risk factors, but pregnancy-related hypertensive or diabetic conditions are less associated with PPCM [137, 141]. A review of 34 000 women with PPCM across the United States from 2004 to 2011 revealed that there has been an increasing risk among primiparous patients, all ethnic groups, and women with chronic hypertension and pre-gestational diabetes over time. The mean age of onset remained 30 years, and there was a decline in the rate of women with multiple gestation affected with PPCM [137].

2. What are common presenting features of peripartum cardiomyopathy, and what should be included in the diagnostic evaluation?

Search Strategy: *MEDLINE*: pregnancy AND peripartum cardiomyopathy AND evaluation.

Typical presenting symptoms of cardiomyopathy include those of any cardiac disease: dyspnea, fatigue, palpitations, and chest pain. Frequently peripheral edema, dilated neck veins, or pulmonary rales are identified also. Any of these signs or symptoms should prompt a thorough history of medication use, prior cardiac disease, family history, drug use, and determination of NYHA functional class status. A cardiac exam with evaluation of overall level of consciousness, vitals, oxygen saturation, and ECG can provide basic information that might raise concern for a cardiac condition. However, echocardiography should be performed if any suspicion arises, as this will evaluate chamber morphology, valve function and gradients, and LV systolic function to provide a much more accurate diagnosis of cardiomyopathy [142, 143].

3. How does peripartum cardiomyopathy differ from traditional forms of cardiomyopathy?

Search Strategy: MEDLINE: pregnancy AND cardiomyopathy AND management.

The classical pathophysiology of cardiomyopathy has been described as one of three types: hypertrophic, restrictive, or dilated. PPCM has many overlapping characteristics, but the most prominent difference is the underlying idiopathic etiology. The incidence of PPCM is unknown due to single site studies that have not been able to provide a general overall representation. Predictions range from 1/1000–1/4000 [137, 144, 145].

HCM is the most common type of cardiomyopathy that has an incidence of 1/500. This condition is primarily a myocardial disease with asymmetric hypertrophy of the interventricular basal septum that alters the mitral valve structure and creates mitral regurgitation and obstruction of the LV outflow tract [142]. There is a strong familial occurrence with 90% of cases inherited in an autosomal dominant pattern [146]. With a variable clinical course, HCM can go unnoticed for many years with no symptoms or can be associated with heart failure and sudden cardiac death among a wide age range [147]. Pregnancy can precipitate symptoms and initial diagnosis, but, even if identified prior, prepregnancy functional status and evidence of any outflow obstruction can predict risk of cardiac events during pregnancy [148]. Arrhythmias and heart failure are the most common concerns, and a β-receptor antagonist can be initiated empirically to help alleviate myocardial workload [149].

One of the most rare forms of cardiomyopathy is the restrictive type, which is an inherited condition characterized by restrictive physiology that prevents proper ventricular filling. Systolic function is typically preserved, but prognosis is poor [150]. There is little data to guide clinical management overall, so specific recommendations for pregnancy are lacking. Optimizing blood pressure, heart rate, blood volume, and myocardial ischemia with anti-hypertensive medications, diuretics, and β-receptor antagonists seems reasonable, as these factors will impact ventricular relaxation. Given the overall poor prognosis and little data on pregnancy outcomes, some recommend avoiding pregnancy due to the excess strain that pregnancy physiology can have on a woman with this condition [151].

Dilated cardiomyopathy has several common features with PPCM. Myocardial dysfunction in addition to one or both dilated ventricles and ventricular systolic dysfunction characterizes this condition, and symptoms onset later in disease progression [142]. The incidence has been reported as 1/2500 with 35% familial occurrence in an autosomal dominant inheritance pattern. Some identified etiologies include hypertension, viral infection, alcohol abuse, medication toxicity, and ischemic heart disease, but more than half of cases are idiopathic. Similar to hypertrophic types, poor prepregnancy functional class can increase the risk for cardiac events and deterioration in pregnancy. There is a higher propensity for decompensation in pregnancy with dilated cardiomyopathy types due to the strain increased blood volume creates for baseline dilated ventricles and suboptimal LV function [152]. There are variable outcomes in pregnancy with some reports of no change in EF throughout pregnancy [161]. Other studies describe cardiac events and mortality up to 40% and 10%, respectively, and this is correlated with a lower prepregnancy EF [8, 75, 153].

4. What are the risks associated with cardiomyopathy in pregnancy?

Search Strategy: *MEDLINE*: pregnancy AND cardiomyopathy AND outcomes.

Maternal morbidity and mortality can be amplified significantly with the onset of PPCM. Consistent across multiple studies, the rate of maternal adverse events (MAEs) has been reported as 13%, which encompasses acute pulmonary edema, thromboembolism, cardiogenic shock requiring mechanical circulatory support, heart transplant, implantable cardioverter defibrillator/permanent pacemaker implantation, and cardiac arrest [137, 143, 154]. Maternal mortality rates have varied over decades, but a large study from 2001 reports 9%, which reflects current therapeutic modalities [143]. A total of 50% of deaths occur within six weeks postpartum [155]. From the prospective clinical outcomes of 100 women in the Investigations of Pregnancy-Associated Cardiomyopathy (IPAC) initiated in 2009 by the National Heart, Lung, and Blood Institute, 13% had major adverse events and persistent severe cardiomyopathy (EF <35%) at 12 months. Predictive factors for MAE, persistent LV dysfunction, and mortality were African-American race (six-fold higher risk), initial EF <35%, left ventricular diameter (LVEDD) >6 cm, and presentation >six weeks postpartum [154, 155]. If diagnosed in pregnancy, risks to the fetus directly correlate with the severity of PPCM, but growth restriction, preterm birth, stillbirth, and perinatal mortality are all of concern [138, 156, 157].

Following an initial episode of PPCM, the risks related to a subsequent pregnancy need to be discussed. If EF on initial diagnosis is <25% or declines and persists at this level 6–12 months postpartum, then there is a 60% risk for end-stage cardiac disease and need for heart transplant. Women with persistent LV dysfunction have a significant risk for deterioration and mortality in a subsequent pregnancy, and they should be counseled to avoid pregnancy [158]. Regardless of recovery, studies report trends of LV function decline in subsequent pregnancies of any woman who has experienced PPCM prior, and varied reports indicate that EF <40–55% at the onset of a subsequent pregnancy increases the risk for deterioration [159, 160]. Overall, there is a 30–50% risk for recurrence of PPCM in a subsequent pregnancy. Additionally, the risks for MAE doubles, maternal mortality has been reported up to 20%, and risks of preterm birth and neonatal morbidity increases threefold [143]. Even if LV function improves, the risks for recurrence and morbidity and mortality associated should be discussed before a woman decides if a subsequent pregnancy is an appropriate decision.

Similar to PPCM, the classical types of cardiomyopathy also have increased maternal, fetal, and neonatal risks, but there is much less data describing these pregnancy outcomes. Those with HCM have been reported to have favorable outcomes, and adverse events and complications are related to prepregnancy LV function and symptoms [148]. Women with dilated cardiomyopathy can have a much more difficult time adapting to the physiologic changes of pregnancy given the baseline LV dilation and dysfunction. Maternal, obstetric, and fetal risks have been reported as higher than those with PPCM, but pregnancy does not seem to pose long-term risk for further complications [161, 162]. Given the lack of data regarding pregnancy in women with restrictive cardiomyopathy and the overall poor prognosis, some suggest avoiding pregnancy [151].

5. What is the treatment for peripartum and other forms of traditional cardiomyopathy in pregnancy?

Search Strategy: MEDLINE: pregnancy AND cardiomyopathy AND treatment.

Routine guidelines for management of acute and chronic heart failure in pregnancy apply to situations in which cardiomyopathy is the underlying etiology [163]. During pregnancy, afterload reduction can be achieved with hydralazine or nitrates, but angiotensin-converting enzyme (ACE) inhibitors, angiotensin II receptor blocker (ARB), and renin inhibitors are preferred in women who are postpartum. The latter medications are avoided in pregnancy due to fetotoxicity, but they are safe postpartum, even while breastfeeding. However, captopril, benazepril, or enalapril are favored [164, 165]. β-receptor antagonists, specifically β1-selective drugs such as metoprolol, should be used in all patients with heart failure [166]. Atenolol should not be used [167]. Diuretics can be administered if pulmonary congestion occurs, but these must always be used with caution to avoid placental hypoperfusion. Hydrochlorothiazide and furosemide are recommended [141]. Anticoagulation is indicated for women with heart failure or arrhythmias given the high risk for intra-cardiac thrombus. LMWH, heparin, or warfarin can be administered according to the stage of pregnancy or postpartum period [35, 163, 168]. A small study of 12 patients evaluated the effects of bromocriptine in addition to traditional heart failure medications in PPCM, and results indicated an improved EF with possible prevention of relapse in subsequent pregnancies [139, 169].

If inotropic agents are necessary, dopamine and levosimendan can be used, although there is no survival benefit associated with these [143, 166]. Once a patient is dependent on inotropes, though, she should be transferred to a facility that can evaluate for need of an intra-aortic balloon pump, ventricular assist device, or heart transplant. PPCM prognosis is much different from chronic traditional cardiomyopathy subtypes and has up to a 50% rate of spontaneous recovery within six months [160]. In women who have persistent PPCM despite medication therapy for greater than six months or those with chronic worsening cardiomyopathy, cardiac resynchronization therapy or implantable cardioverter-defibrillator (ICD) treatment is advised. If mechanical circulatory support is unavailable or does not allow recovery after 6–12 months of use, then cardiac transplant is typically discussed. All patients with cardiomyopathy, including PPCM and chronic traditional subtypes, have similar prognoses following transplants [170].

6. What type of delivery and monitoring is necessary in women with cardiomyopathy?

Search Strategy: MEDLINE: *pregnancy* AND cardiomyopathy AND delivery.

Women with cardiomyopathy should be followed by a multidisciplinary team of obstetricians, cardiologists, and anesthesiologists, and delivery should occur at a specialized care center if heart failure or progressive decline in functional status or LV function occurs. Vaginal delivery is preferred, and cesarean is reserved for obstetrical indications and significant hemodynamic instability due to the risks of higher blood loss and hemodynamic shifts, decreased oxygen delivery, and thromboembolism [142]. If a woman is tolerating heart failure well with medical therapy, then delivery 37–39 weeks is appropriate, but progressive functional decline or LV dysfunction might necessitate preterm delivery less than 37 weeks [171]. Regional anesthesia is preferred, but this should be used with caution in those with HCM due to LV outflow tract obstruction. Systemic vasodilation can be exacerbated and cause a decrease in afterload and preload, but slow infusion can help minimize this. Additionally, volume overload should be avoided due to LV systolic dysfunction. Routine intrapartum fetal monitoring in addition to continuous monitoring of oxygen saturation, blood pressure, and ECG is warranted; arterial pressure monitoring might be indicated with significant hemodynamic instability [172, 173].

7. What care should be employed in the postpartum period for women with cardiomyopathy?

Search Strategy: *MEDLINE*: pregnancy AND cardiomyopathy AND management.

Women should continue heart failure therapy and anticoagulation in the postpartum period with the addition of an ACE inhibitor. Breastfeeding is safe, even with an ACE inhibitor, but monitoring fetal weight during the first four weeks of life is important to identify the onset of renal dysfunction. Breastfeeding can prompt high metabolic demands and preclude cardiac improvement, so discussion with women who have heart failure is necessary to explain the risks and benefits [169]. Contraception is imperative, and pregnancy is contra-indicated in women with heart failure or in women with whom normalization of LV function occurred less than 12 months prior. Progestin methods have been reported to be the most efficacious, and any method with estrogen is contra-indicated in women with heart failure due to the exaggerated risks of thromboembolism [166].

Routine cardiology evaluation and echocardiogram should be continued until normal LV systolic function returns. Once normalized, there is no definitive data to support recommendations for when to stop therapy, but continuing β-receptor antagonist and ACE inhibitor for one year after a normal echocardiogram is reasonable [174]. If heart failure persists beyond 6–12 months from initiating therapy, then evaluation for mechanical assist devices or transplant can be implemented [170].

Graded recommendations for the management of cardiomyopathy in pregnancy [175]:

- Pregnant women with heart failure (HF) should be treated with the same guidelines as non-pregnant patients, with the exception of medications that are contra-indicated in pregnancy (I-B).
- Anticoagulation should be utilized in women with atrial fibrillation or HF (I-C).
- A β-receptor antagonist should be utilized in women with HCM (IIa-C).
- Vaginal delivery is preferred in women with cardiomyopathy (IIa-C).
- Cesarean delivery should be considered in women with cardiomyopathy and severe symptomatic LV dysfunction (IIa-C).
- Women with persistent LV dysfunction following PPCM should be advised against pregnancy (III-C).

Conclusion

Cardiac disease in pregnancy comprises a multitude of conditions, each with unique physiology, risks, and treatments. Appropriate evaluation and counseling prior to conception should occur for every woman, and, risk assessment scores can be applied to predict cardiac events in pregnancy. Once pregnant, women should receive care from a multidisciplinary care team that includes skilled obstetricians, cardiologists, and anesthesiologists. Ongoing assessment of symptoms and cardiac structure and function will allow early intervention if deterioration occurs. Medical therapy is preferred if intervention is necessary, and surgery should be avoided if at all possible to minimize morbidity and mortality to the mother and fetus. In most cases, vaginal delivery is preferred and tolerated well. However, cesarean is reserved for obstetric indications in addition to isolated cardiac conditions. Above all, care and delivery should be performed at a specialized center equipped to evaluate, treat, and monitor a woman with a high-risk cardiac condition.

References

1 Vitarelli, A. and Capotosto, L. (2011). Role of echocardiography in the assessment and management of adult congenital heart disease in pregnancy. *Int. J. Cardiovasc. Imaging* **27**: 843–857.

2 Hatton, R., Colman, J.M., Sermer, M. et al. (2012). Cardiac risks and management of complications in pregnant women with congenital heart disease. *Future Cardiol.* **8** (**2**): 315–327.

3 Cutforth, R. and MacDonald, C.B. (1966). Heart sounds and murmurs in pregnancy. *Am. Heart J.* **71**: 741–747.

4 Schwartz, D.B. and Schamroth, L. (1979). The effect of pregnancy on the frontal plane QRS axis. *J. Electrocardiol.* **12**: 279–281.

5 Boyle, D.M. and Lloyd-Jones, R.L. (1966). The electrocardiographic ST segment in pregnancy. *J. Obstet. Gynaecol. Br. Commonw.* **73**: 986–987.

6 Tsiaras, S. and Poppas, A. (2010). Cardiac disease in pregnancy: value of echocardiography. *Curr. Cardiol. Rep.* **12**: 250–256.

7 Naidoo, D.P. and Moodley, J. (2001). Management of the critically ill cardiac patient. *Best Prac. Res. Clin. Obstet. Gynaecol.* **15** (**4**): 523–544.

8 Henriquez, D.D., Roos-Hesselink, J.W., Schalij, M.J. et al. (2011). Treatment of valvular heart disease during pregnancy for improving maternal and neonatal outcome. *Cochrane Database Syst Rev* (**5**): CD008128. doi: 10.1002/14651858.CD008128.pub2.

9 Fretts, R.C., Schmittdiel, J., McLean, F.H. et al. (1995). Increased maternal age and the risk of fetal death. *N. Engl. J. Med.* **333**: 953.

10 Wanderer, J.P., Leffert, L.R., Mhyre, J.M. et al. (2013). Epidemiology of obstetric-related ICU admissions in Marylan. *Crit. Care Med.* **41** (**8**): 1844–1852.

11 The Criteria Committee for the New York Heart Association (1994). *Nomenclature and Criteria for Diagnosis of Diseases of the Heart and Great Vessels*, 9e, 253–255. Little Brown and Company.

12 Siu, S.C., Sermer, M., Harrison, D.A. et al. (1997). Risk and predictors for pregnancy-related complications in women with heart disease. *Circulation* **96**: 2789.

13 Siu, S.C., Sermer, M., Colman, J.M. et al. (2001). Prospective multicenter study of pregnancy outcomes in women with heart disease. *Circulation* **104**: 515–521.

14 Khairy, P., Ouyang, D.W., Fernandes, S.M. et al. (2006). Pregnancy outcomes in women with congenital heart disease. *Circulation* **113**: 517–527.

15 Drenthen, W., Boersma, E., Balci, A. et al. (2010). Predictors of pregnancy complications in women with congenital heart disease. *Eur. Heart J.* **31**: 2124–2132.

16 Ruys, P.T.E., Hall, R., Johnson, M.R. et al. (2012). WHO classification as a risk predictor in pregnancy and heart disease. *J. Am. Coll. Cardiol.* **29**: E843.

17 European Society of Gynecology (ESG), Association for European Paediatric Cardiology (AEPC), German Society for Gender Medicine (DGesGM) et al. (2011). ESC guidelines on the management of cardiovascular diseases during pregnancy: the Task Force on the Management of Cardiovascular Diseases during Pregnancy of the European Society of Cardiology (ESC). *Eur. Heart J.* **32**: 2147–3197.

18 Balci, A., Sollie-Szarynska, K.M., van der Bijl, A.G. et al. (2014). Prospective validation and assessment of cardiovascular and offspring risk models for pregnant women with congenital heart disease. *Heart* **100**: 1373.

19 Lu, C.W., Shih, J.C., Chen, S.Y. et al. (2015). Comparison of 3 risk estimation methods for predicting cardiac outcomes in pregnant women with congenital heart disease. *Circ. J.* **79**: 1609–1620.

20 Windram, J.D., Colman, J.M., Wald, R.M. et al. (2014). Valvular heart disease in pregnancy. *Best Prac. Res. Clin. Obstet. Gynaecol.* **28**: 507–518.

21 Elkayam, U. and Bitar, F. (2005). Valvular heart disease and pregnancy part I: native valves. *J. Am. Coll. Cardiol.* **46**: 223–230.

22 Royal College of Obstetricians and Gynaecologists (2011). *Good Practice Guidelines for the Management of Cardiac Disease and Pregnancy*. London, UK: The Royal College of Obstetricians and Gynaecologists.

23 Burn, J., Brennan, P., Little, J. et al. (1998). Recurrence risks in offspring of adults with major heart defects: results from first cohort of British collaborative study. *Lancet* **351**: 311–316.

24 Aggarwal, N., Suri, V., Goyal, A. et al. (2005). Closed mitral valvotomy in pregnancy and labor. *Int. J. Gynaecol. Obstet.* **88**: 118–121.

25 Demir, I., Yilmaz, H., Basarici, I. et al. (2002). Prognostic factors of mitral stenosis during pregnancy. *Anadolu Kardiyol. Derg.* **2**: 213–217.

26 Hameed, A., Karaalp, I.S., Tummala, P.P. et al. (2001). The effect of valvular heart disease on maternal and fetal outcome of pregnancy. *J. Am. Coll. Cardiol.* **37**: 893–899.

27 Silversides, C.K., Colman, J.M., Sermer, M., and Siu, S.C. (2003). Cardiac risk in pregnant women with rheumatic mitral stenosis. *Am. J. Cardiol.* **91**: 1382–1385.

28 Baumgartner, H., Bonhoeffer, P., DeGroot, N.M. et al. (2010). ESC guidelines for the management of grown-up congenital heart disease. *Eur. Heart J.* **31**: 2915–2957.

29 Yap, S.C., Drenthen, W., Pieper, P.G. et al. (2008). Risk of complications during pregnancy in women with congenital aortic stenosis. *Int. J. Cardiol.* **126**: 240–246.

30 Silversides, C.K., Colman, J.M., Sermer, M. et al. (2003). Early and intermediate-term outcomes of pregnancy with congenital aortic stenosis. *Am. J. Cardiol.* **91**: 1386–1389.

31 Balint, O.H., Siu, S.C., Mason, J. et al. (2010). Cardiac outcomes after pregnancy in women with congenital heart disease. *Heart* **96**: 1656–1661.

32 Lesniak-Sobelga, A., Tracz, W., KostKiewicz, M. et al. (2004). Clinical and echocardiographic assessment of pregnant women with valvular heart diseases—maternal and fetal outcomes. *Int. J. Cardiol.* **94**: 15–23.

33 Doig, J.C., McComb, J.M., and Reid, D.S. (1992). Incessant atrial tachycardia accelerated by pregnancy. *Br. Heart J.* **67**: 266–268.

34 Vahanian, A., Baumgartner, H., Bax, J. et al. (2007). Guidelines on the management of valvular heart disease: the Task Force on the Management of Valvular Heart Disease of the European Society of Cardiology. *Eur. Heart J.* **28**: 230–268.

35 Camm, A.J., Kirchhof, P., Lip, G.Y. et al. (2010). Guidelines for the management of atrial fibrillation: the Task Force for the Management of Atrial Fibrillation of the European Society of Cardiology (ESC). *Eur. Heart J.* **31**: 2369–2429.

36 Chen, C.R. and Cheng, T.O. (1995). Percutaneous balloon mitral valvuloplasty by the Inoue technique: a multicenter study of 4832 patients in China. *Am. Heart J.* **129** (**6**): 1197–1203.

37 Rahimtoola, S.H., Durairaj, A., Mehra, A., and Nuno, I. (2002). Current evaluation and management of patients with mitral stenosis. *Circulation* **106**: 1183–1188.

38 Pieper, P.G., Balci, A., and Van Dijk, A.P. (2008). Pregnancy in women with prosthetic heart valves. *Netherlands Heart J.* **16**: 406–411.

39 Visser, A.A., Coetzee, E.J., Grobler, C.J.F., and Cronje, H.S. (1996). Cardiac disease. In: *Obstetrics in Southern Africa*, 229. Pretoria: JL van Schaik.

40 Elkayam, U. and Gleicher, N. (1990). Haemodynamics and cardiac function during normal pregnancy and the puerperium. In: *Cardiac Problems in Pregnancy: Diagnosis and Management of Maternal and Fetus Disease*, 2e, 5–24. New York: Liss.

41 Iung, B., Garbarz, E., Michaud, P. et al. (1999). Late results of percutaneous mitral commissurotomy in a series of 1024 patients. Analysis of late clinical deterioration: frequency, anatomic findings, and predictive factors. *Circulation* **99**: 3272–3278.

42 Orrange, S.E., Kawanishi, D.T., Lopez, B.M. et al. (1997). Actuarial outcome after catheter balloon commissurotomy in patients with mitral stenosis. *Circulation* **95**: 382–389.

43 Palacios, I.F., Sanchez, P.L., Harrell, L.C. et al. (2002). Which patients benefit from percutaneous mitral balloon valvuloplasty? Prevalvuloplasty and postvalvuloplasty variables that predict longterm outcome. *Circulation* **105**: 1465–1471.

44 Ben Farhat, M., Gamra, H., Betbout, F. et al. (1997). Percutaneous balloon mitral commissurotomy during pregnancy. *Heart* **77**: 564–567.

45 Routray, S.N., Mishra, T.K., Swain, S. et al. (2004). Balloon mitral valvuloplasty during pregnancy. *Int. J. Gynaecol. Obstet.* **85**: 18–23.

46 Hameed, A., Karaalp, I.S., Tummala, P.P. et al. (2001). The effect of valvular heart disease on maternal and fetal outcome during pregnancy. *J. Am. Coll. Cardiol.* **37**: 893–899.

47 Malhotra, M., Sharma, J.B., Tripathii, P., and Arora, R. (2004). Maternal and fetal outcome in valvular heart disease. *Int. J. Gynaecol. Obstet.* **84**: 11–16.

48 Esteves, C.A., Munoz, J.S., Braga, S. et al. (2006). Immediate and long-term follow-up of percutaneous balloon mitral valvuloplasty in pregnant patients with rheumatic mitral stenosis. *Am. J. Cardiol.* **98**: 812–816.

49 Sivadasanpillai, H., Srinivasan, A., Sivasubramoniam, S. et al. (2005). Long-term outcome of patients undergoing balloon mitral valvotomy in pregnancy. *Am. J. Cardiol.* **95**: 1504–1506.

50 Patel, J.J., Mitha, A.S., Hassen, F. et al. (1993). Percutaneous balloon mitral valvotomy in pregnant patients with tight pliable mitral stenosis. *Am. Heart J.* **125**: 1106–1109.

51 Safian, R.D., Berman, A.D., Sachs, B. et al. (1988). Percutaneous balloon mitral valvuloplasty in pregnant women with mitral stenosis. *Catheter. Cardiovasc. Diagn.* **15**: 103–108.

52 Fawzi, M.E., Kinsara, A.J., Stefadouros, M. et al. (2001). Long-term outcome of mitral balloon valvotomy in pregnant women. *J. Heart Valve Dis.* **10**: 153–157.

53 de Souza, J.A., Martinez, E.E. Jr., Ambrose, J.A. et al. (2001). Percutaneous balloon mitral valvuloplasty in comparison with open mitral valve commissurotomy for mitral stenosis during pregnancy. *J. Am. Coll. Cardiol.* **37**: 900–903.

54 Weiss, B.M., von Segesser, L.K., Alon, E. et al. (1998). Outcome of cardiovascular surgery and pregnancy: a systematic review of the period 1984–1996. *Am. J. Obstet. Gynecol.* **179**: 1643–1653.

55 Vahanian, A. and Palacios, I.F. (2004). Percutaneous approaches to valvular disease. *Circulation* **109**: 1572–1579.

56 Cheng, T.O. (2002). Percutaneous mitral valvuloplasty by the Inoue balloon technique to the ideal procedure for treatment of significant mitral stenosis in pregnant women. *Catheter. Cardiovasc. Interv.* **57**: 323–324.

57 Bhargava, B., Agarwal, R., Yadav, R. et al. (1998). Percutaneous balloon aortic valvuloplasty during pregnancy: use of the Inoue balloon and the physiologic antegrade approach. *Catheter. Cardiovasc. Diagn.* **45**: 422–425.

58 Abildgaard, U., Sandset, P.M., Hammerstron, J. et al. (2009). Management of pregnant women with mechanical heart valve prosthesis: thromboprophylaxis with low molecular weight heparin. *Thromb. Res.* **124**: 262–267.

59 Chan, W.S., Anand, S., and Ginsberg, J.S. (2000). Anticoagulation of pregnant women with mechanical heart valves: a systematic review of the literature. *Arch. Intern. Med.* **160**: 191–196.

60 Sillesen, M., Hjortdal, V., Vejlstrup, N., and Sorensen, K. (2001). Pregnancy with prosthetic heart valves—30 years' nationwide experience in Denmark. *Eur. J. Cardiothorac. Surg.* **40**: 448–454.

61 Schaefer, C., Hannemann, D., Meister, R. et al. (2006). Vitamin K antagonists and pregnancy outcome. A multicentre prospective study. *Thromb. Haemost.* **95**: 949–957.

62 Vitale, N., De Feo, M., De Santo, L.S. et al. (1999). Dose-dependent fetal complications of warfarin in pregnant women with mechanical heart valves. *J. Am. Coll. Cardiol.* **33**: 1637–1641.

63 Van Driel, D., Wesseling, J., Sauer, P.J. et al. (2002). Teratogen update: fetal effects after *in utero* exposure to coumarins overview of cases, follow-up findings, and pathogenesis. *Teratology* **66**: 127–140.

64 Cotrufo, M., De Feo, M., De Santo, L.S. et al. (2002). Risk of warfain during pregnancy with mechanical valve prostheses. *Obstet. Gynecol.* **99**: 35–40.

65 Elkayam, U. and Bitar, F. (2005). Valvular heart disease and pregnancy: part II: prosthetic valves. *J. Am. Coll. Cardiol.* **46**: 403–410.

66 Oran, B., Lee-Parritz, A., and Ansell, J. (2004). Low molecular weight heparin for the prophylaxis of thromboembolism in women with prosthetic mechanical heart valves during pregnancy. *Thromb. Haemost.* **92**: 747–751.

67 McLintock, C., McCowan, L.M., and North, R.A. (2009). Maternal complications and pregnancy outcome in women with mechanical prosthetic heart valves treated with enoxaparin. *BJOG* **116**: 1585–1592.

68 Quinn, J., Von Klemperer, K., Brooks, R. et al. (2009). Use of high intensity adjusted dose low molecular weight heparin in women with mechanical heart valves during pregnancy: a single-center experience. *Haematologica* **94**: 1608–1612.

69 Yinon, Y., Siu, S.C., Warshafsky, C. et al. (2009). Use of low molecular weight heparin in women with mechanical heart valves. *Am. J. Cardiol.* **104**: 1259–1263.

70 Elkayam, U., Singh, H., Irani, A., and Akhter, M.W. (2004). Anticoagulation in pregnant women with prosthetic heart valves. *J. Cardiovasc. Pharmacol. Ther.* **9**: 107–115.

71 Bonow, R.O., Carabello, B.A., Chatterjee, K. et al. 2006 Writing Committee Members: American College of Cardiology/American Heart Association Task Force(2008). 2008 Focused update incorporated into the ACC/AHA 2006 guidelines for the management of patients with valvular heart disease: endorsed by the Society of Cardiovascular Anesthesiologists, 2008 endorsed by the Society of Cardiovascular Anesthesiologists, Society for Cardiovascular Angiography and Interventions, and Society of Thoracic Surgeons. *Circulation* **118**: 523–661.

72 Bonanno, C. and Gaddipati, S. (2008). Mechanisms of hemostasis at cesarean delivery. *Clin. Perinatol.* **35**: 531–547.

73 Warnes, C.A., Williams, R.G., Bashore, T.M. et al. (2008). ACC/AHA 2008 guidelines for the management of adults with congenital heart disease: executive summary: a report of the American College of Cardiology/American Heart Association Task Force on Practice Guidelines. *Circulation* **118**: 2395–2451.

74 Montoya, M., Karnath, B.M., and Ahmad, M. (2003). Endocarditis during pregnancy. *South Med. J.* **96**: 1156–1171.

75 Avila, W.S., Rossi, E.G., Ramires, J.A. et al. (2003). Pregnancy in patients with heart disease: experience with 1,000 cases. *Clin. Cardiol.* **26**: 135–142.

76 The Task Force for the Management of Infective Endocarditis of the European Society of Cardiology (ESC) endorsed by: European Association for Cardio-Thoracic Surgery (EACTS), the European Association of Nuclear Medicine (EANM) (2015). 2015 ESC guidelines for the management of infective endocarditis. *Eur. Heart J.*

77 Duval, X. and Leport, C. (2008). Prophylaxis of infective endocarditis: current tendencies, continuing controversies. *Lancet Infect. Dis.* **8**: 225–232.

78 Duval, X., Alla, F., Hoen, B. et al. (2006). Estimated risk of endocarditis in adults with predisposing cardiac conditions undergoing dental procedures with or without antibiotic prophylaxis. *Clin. Infect. Dis.* **42**: e102–e107.

79 Lee, P. and Shanson, D. (2007). Results of a UK survey of fatal anaphylaxis after oral amoxicillin. *J. Antimicrob. Chemother.* **60**: 1172–1173.

80 Lockhart, P.B., Brennan, M.T., Sasser, H.C. et al. (2008). Bacteremia associated with toothbrushing and dental extraction. *Circulation* **117**: 3118–3125.

81 Thornhill, M., Dayer, M., Forde, J. et al. (2011). Impact of the NICE guideline recommending cessation of antibiotic prophylaxis for prevention of infective endocarditis: before and after study. *BMJ* **342**: d2392.

82 Dayer, M.J., Chambers, J.B., Prendergast, B. et al. (2013). NICE guidance on antibiotic prophylaxis to prevent infective endocarditis: a survey of clinicians' attitudes. *QJM* **106**: 237–243.

83 Desimone, D.C., Tleyjeh, I.M., Correa de Sa, D.D. et al. (2012). Incidence of infective endocarditis caused by viridans group streptococci before and after publication of the 2007 American Heart Association's endocarditis prevention guidelines. *Circulation* **126**: 60–64.

84 Pasquali, S.K., He, X., Mohamad, Z. et al. (2012). Trends in endocarditis hospitalizations at US children's hospitals: impact of the 2007 American Heart Association Antibiotic Prophylaxis Guidelines. *Am. Heart J.* **163**: 894–899.

85 Nishimura, R.A., Otto, C.M., Bonow, R.O. et al. (2014, 2014). AHA/ACC guideline for the management of patients with valvular heart disease: a report of the American College of Cardiology/American Heart Association Task Force on Practice Guidelines. *J. Am. Coll. Cardiol.* **63**: e57–e185.

86 De Labriolle, A., Genee, O., Heggs, L.M., and Fauchier, L. (2009). Acute myocardial infarction following oral methyl-ergometrine intake. *Cardiovasc. Toxicol.* **9**: 46–48.

87 Svanstrom, M.C., Biber, B., Hanes, M. et al. (2008). Signs of myocardial ischaemia after injection of oxytocin: a randomized double-blind comparison of oxytocin and methylergometrine during caesarean section. *Br. J. Anaesth.* **100**: 683–689.

88 Gill, H.K., Splitt, M., Sharland, G.K., and Simpson, J.M. (2003). Patterns of recurrence of congenital heart disease: an analysis of 6,640 consecutive pregnancies evaluated by detailed fetal echocardiography. *J. Am. Coll. Cardiol.* **42**: 923.

89 Drenthen, W., Pieper, P.G., Roos-Hesselink, J.W. et al. (2007). Outcome of pregnancy in women with congenital heart disease: a literature review. *J. Am. Coll. Cardiol.* **49**: 2303–2311.

90 Pierpont, M.E., Basson, C.T., Benson, D.W. Jr. et al. (2007). Genetic basis for congenital heart defects: current knowledge: a scientific statement from the American Heart Association Congenital Cardiac Defects Committee, Council on Cardiovascular Disease in the Young: endorsed by the American Academy of Pediatrics. *Circulation* **115**: 3015–3038.

91 Yap, S.C., Drenthen, W., Meijboom, F.J. et al. (2009). Comparison of pregnancy outcomes in women with repaired versus unrepaired atrial septal defect. *BJOG* **116**: 1593–1601.

92 Sacco, R.L., Adams, R., Albers, G. et al. (2006). Guidelines for prevention of stroke in patients with ischemic stroke or transient ischemic attack: a statement for healthcare professionals from the American Heart Association/American Stroke Association Council on Stroke: co-sponsored by the Council on Cardiovascular Radiology and Intervention: the American Academy of Neurology affirms the value of this guideline. *Circulation* **113**: e409–e449.

93 Roche-Kelly, E. and Nelson-Piercy, C. (2014). Managing cardiovascular disease during pregnancy: best practice to optimize outcomes. *Future Cardiol.* **10**: 421–433.

94 Presbitero, P., Somerville, J., Stone, S. et al. (1994). Pregnancy in cyanotic congenital heart disease: outcome of mother and fetus. *Circulation* **89**: 2673.

95 Aggarwal, N., Suri, V., Kaur, H. et al. (2009). Retrospective analysis of outcome of pregnancy in women with congenital heart disease: single-centre experience from North India. *Aust. N. Z. J. Obstet. Gynaecol.* **49**: 376–381.

96 Zuber, M., Gautschi, N., Oechslin, E. et al. (1999). Outcome of pregnancy in women with congenital shunt lesions. *Heart* **81**: 271–275.

97 Warnes, C.A., Williams, R.G., Bashore, T.M. et al. (2008). ACC/AHA 2008 guidelines for the management of adults with congenital heart disease: a report of the American College of Cardiology/American Heart Association Task Force on Practice Guidelines. Developed in collaboration with the American Society of Echocardiography, Heart Rhythm Society, International Society for Adult Congenital Heart Disease, Society for Cardiovascular Angiography and Interventions, and Society of Thoracic Surgeons. *J. Am. Coll. Cardiol.* **52**: e1–e121.

98 Torres-Gomez, L.G., Inigo-Riesgo, C.A., Espinoza-Ortegon, M.A. et al. (2010). Pregnancy and tetralogy of Fallot with and without surgical correction. *Ginecol. Obstet. Mex.* **78**: 309–315.

99 Singh, H., Bolton, P.J., and Oakley, C.M. (1982). Pregnancy after surgical correction of tetralogy of Fallot. *Br. Med. J.* **285**: 168–170.

100 Nissenkorn, A., Friedman, S., Schonfeld, A., and Ovadia, J. (1984). Fetomaternal outcome in pregnancies after total correction of the tetralogy of Fallot. *Int. Surg.* **69**: 125–128.

101 Balci, A., Drenthen, W., Mulder, B.J. et al. (2011). Pregnancy in women with corrected tetralogy of Fallot: occurrence and predictors of adverse events. *Am. Heart J.* **161**: 307–313.

102 Veldtman, G.R., Connolly, H.M., Grogan, M. et al. (2004). Outcomes of pregnancy in women with tetralogy of Fallot. *J. Am. Coll. Cardiol.* **44**: 174–180.

103 Therrien, J., Barnes, I., and Somerville, J. (1999). Outcome of pregnancy in patients with congenitally corrected transposition of the great arteries. *Am. J. Cardiol.* **84**: 820–824.

104 Hornung, T.S., Bernard, E.J., Celermajer, D.S. et al. (1999). Right ventricular dysfunction in congenitally corrected transposition of the great arteries. *Am. J. Cardiol.* **84**: 1116–1119.

105 Drenthen, W., Pieper, P.G., Ploeg, M. et al. (2005). Risk of complications during pregnancy after Senning or Mustard (atrial) repair of complete transposition of the great arteries. *Eur. Heart J.* **26**: 2588–2595.

106 Tobler, D., Fernandes, S.M., Wald, R.M. et al. (2010). Pregnancy outcomes in women with transposition of the great arteries and arterial switch operation. *Am. J. Cardiol.* **106**: 417–420.

107 Greutmann, M., Von Klemperer, K., Brooks, R. et al. (2010). Pregnancy outcome in women with congenital heart disease and residual haemodynamic lesions of the right ventricular outflow tract. *Eur. Heart J.* **31**: 1764–1770.

108 Hayes, C.J., Gersony, W.M., Driscoll, D.J. et al. (1993). Second natural history study of congenital heart defects: results of treatment of patients with pulmonary valvular stenosis. *Circulation* **87**: 128–137.

109 Sumner, D., Melville, C., Smith, C.D. et al. (1992). Successful pregnancy in a patient with a single ventricle. *Eur. J. Obstet. Gynecol. Reprod. Biol.* **44**: 239.

110 Baumann, H., Schneider, H., Drack, G. et al. (1987). Pregnancy and delivery by caesarean section in a patient with transposition of the great arteries and single ventricle. *Br. J. Obstet. Gynaecol.* **94**: 704.

111 Leibbrandt, G., Munch, U., and Gander, M. (1982). Two successful pregnancies in a patient with single ventricle and transposition of the great arteries. *Int. J. Cardiol.* **1**: 257.

112 Fong, J., Druzin, M., Gimbel, A.A., and Fisher, J. (1990). Epidural anaesthesia for labour and caesarean section in a parturient with a single ventricle and transposition of the great arteries. *Can. J. Anaesth.* **37**: 680.

113 Drenthen, W., Pieper, P.G., Roos-Hesselink, J.W. et al. (2006). Pregnancy and delivery in women after Fontan palliation. *Heart* **92**: 1290–1294.

114 Canobbio, M.M., Mair, D.D., van der Velde, M., and Koos, B.J. (1996). Pregnancy outcomes after the Fontan repair. *J. Am. Cardiol.* **28**: 763–767.

115 Vriend, J.W., Drenthen, W., Pieper, P.G. et al. (2005). Outcome of pregnancy in patients after repair of aortic coarctation. *Eur. Heart J.* **26**: 2173–2178.

116 Jimenez-Juan, L., Krieger, E.V., Valente, A.M. et al. (2014). Cardiovascular magnetic resonance imaging predictors of pregnancy outcomes in women with coarctation of the aorta. *Eur. Heart J. Cardiovasc. Imaging* **15**: 299–306.

117 Fedak, P.W., Verma, S., David, T.E. et al. (2002). Clinical and pathophysiological implications of a bicuspid aortic valve. *Circulation* **106**: 900.

118 Immer, F.F., Bansi, A.G., Immer-Bansi, A.S. et al. (2003). Aortic dissection in pregnancy: analysis of risk factors and outcome. *Ann. Thorac. Surg.* **76**: 309–314.

119 Pyeritz, R.E. (1981). Maternal and fetal complications of pregnancy in the Marfan syndrome. *Am. J. Med.* **71**: 784–790.

120 Pacini, L., Digne, F., Boumendil, A. et al. (2009). Maternal complication of pregnancy in Marfan syndrome. *Int. J. Cardiol.* **136**: 156–161.

121 Therrien, J., Gatzoulis, M., Graham, T. et al. (2001). Canadian Cardiovascular Society Consensus Conference 2001 Update: recommendations for the management of adults with congenital heart disease—part II. *Can. J. Cardiol.* **17**: 10229–11050.

122 Meijboom, L.J., Vos, F.E., Timmermans, J. et al. (2005). Pregnancy and aortic root growth in the Marfan syndrome: a prospective study. *Eur. Heart J.* **26**: 914–920.

123 Wong, S.C., Cheung, M., and Zacharin, M. (2014). Aortic dilation and dissection in Turner syndrome: what we know, what we are unclear about and what we should do in clinical practice? *Int. J. Adolesc. Med. Health* **26**: 469–488.

124 Pleog, M., Drenthen, W., van Dijk, A., and Pieper, P.G. (2006). Successful pregnancy after an arterial switch procedure for transposition of the great arteries. *BJOG* **113**: 243.

125 Drenthen, W., Pieper, P.G., Roos-Hesselink, J.W. et al. (2006). Non-cardiac complications during pregnancy in women with isolated congenital pulmonary valvular stenosis. *Heart* **92**: 1838–1843.

126 Beauchesne, L.M., Connolly, H.M., Ammash, N.M., and Warnes, C.A. (2001). Coarctation of the aorta: outcome of pregnancy. *J. Am. Coll. Cardiol.* **38**: 1728–1733.

127 Curry, R.A., Gelson, E., Swan, L. et al. (2014). Marfan syndrome and pregnancy: maternal and neonatal outcomes. *BJOG* **121**: 610–617.

128 Hassan, N., Patenaude, V., Oddy, L., and Abenhaim, H. (2015). Pregnancy outcomes in Marfan syndrome: a retrospective cohort study. *Am. J. Perinatol.* **32**: 123–130.

129 Yates, M.T., Soppa, G., Smelt, J. et al. (2015). Perioperative management and outcomes of aortic surgery during pregnancy. *J. Thorac. Cardiovasc. Surg.* **149**: 607–610.

130 Matura, L.A., Ho, V.B., Rosin, D.R., and Bondy, C.A. (2007). Aortic dilation and dissection in Turner syndrome. *Circulation* **116**: 1663–1670.

131 Guedes, A., Mercier, L.A., Leduc, L. et al. (2004). Impact of pregnancy on the systemic right ventricle after a Mustard operation for transposition of the great arteries. *J. Am. Coll. Cardiol.* **44**: 433–437.

132 Leighton, B.L. and Halpern, S.H. (2002). The effects of epidural analgesia on labor, maternal, and neonatal outcomes: a systematic review. *Am. J. Obstet. Gynecol.* **186**: S69.

133 Gordon, C.F. 3rd and Johnson, M.D. (1993). Anesthetic management of the pregnant patient with Marfan syndrome. *J. Clin. Anesth.* **5**: 248–251.

134 Bates, S.M., Greer, I.A., Middeldorp, S. et al. (2012). VTE, thrombophilia, antithrombotic therapy, and pregnancy: antithrombotic therapy and prevention of thrombosis, 9th ed: American College of Chest Physicians Evidence-Based Clinical Practice Guidelines. *Chest* **141**: e691S–e736S.

135 Sciscione, A.C. and Callan, N.A. (1993). Congenital heart disease in adolescents and adults: pregnancy and contraception. *Cardiol. Clin.* **11**: 701–709.

136 Pearson, G.D., Veille, J.C., Rahimtoola, S. et al. (2000). Peripartum cardiomyopathy: National Heart, Lung and Blood Institute and Office of rare Diseases. (National Institute of Heart). Workshop recommendations and review. *JAMA* **283**: 1183–1188.

137 Kolte, D., Khera, S., Aronow, W.S. et al. (2014). Temporal trends in incidence and outcomes of peripartum cardiomyopathy in the United States: a nationwide population-based study. *JAHA* **114**: 1–13.

138 Ntusi, N.B. and Mayosi, B.M. (2009). Aetiology and risk factors of peripartum cardiomyopathy: a systematic review. *Int. J. Cardiol.* **131**: 168–179.

139 Hilfiker-Kleiner, D., Haghikia, A., Nonhoff, J., and Bauersachs, J. (2015). Peripartum cardiomyopathy: current management and future perspectives. *Eur. Heart J.* **36**: 1090–1097.

140 Kao, D.P., Hsich, E., and Lindenfeld, J. (2013). Characteristics, adverse events, and racial differences among delivering mothers with peripartum cardiomyopathy. *JACC* **1**: 409–416.

141 Sliwa, K., Fett, J., and Elkayam, U. (2006). Peripartum cardiomyopathy. *Lancet* **368**: 687–693.

142 Troiano, N.H. (2015). Cardiomyopathy during pregnancy. *J. Perinat. Neonatal. Nurs.* **29**: 222–228.

143 Elkayam, U., Tummala, P.P., Rao, K. et al. (2001). Maternal and fetal outcomes of subsequent pregnancies in women with peripartum cardiomyopathy. *NEJM* **344**: 1567–1571.

144 Krul, S.P., van der Smagt, J.J., van den Berg, M.P. et al. (2011). Systematic review of pregnancy in women with inherited cardiomyopathies. *Eur. J. Heart Fail.* **13**: 584–594.

145 Pyatt, J.R. and Dubey, G. (2011). Peripartum cardiomyopathy: current understanding, comprehensive management review and new developments. *Postgrad. Med. J.* **87**: 34–39.

146 Hershberger, R.E., Cowan, J., Morales, A., and Siegfried, J.D. (2009). Progress with genetic cardiomyopathies: screening, counseling, and testing in dilated, hypertrophic, and arrhythmogenic right ventricular dysplasia/cardiomyopathy. *Circ. Heart Fail.* **2**: 253–261.

147 Maron, B.J., Tajik, A.J., Ruttenberg, H.D. et al. (1982). Hypertrophic cardiomyopathy in infants: clinical features and natural history. *Circulation* **65**: 7.

148 Oakley, G.D.G., McGarry, K., Limb, D.G., and Oakley, C.M. (1997). Management of pregnancy in patients with hypertrophic cardiomyopathy. *NEJM* **336**: 775–785.

149 Ray, P., Murphy, G.J., and Shutt, L.E. (2004). Recognition and management of maternal cardiac disease in pregnancy. *Br. J. Anaesth.* **93**: 428–429.

150 Mogensen, J. and Arbustini, E. (2009). Restrictive cardiomyopathy. *Curr. Opin. Cardiol.* **24**: 214–220.

151 Jessup, M., Abraham, W.T., Casey, D.E. et al. (2009). 2009 focused update: ACCF/AHA guidelines for the diagnosis and management of heart failure in adults: a report of the American College of Cardiology Foundation/American Heart Association Task Force on Practice Guidelines: developed in collaboration with the International Society for Heart and Lung Transplantation. *Circulation* **119**: 1977–2016.

152 Felker, G.M., Thompson, R.E., Hare, J.M. et al. (2000). Underlying causes and long-term survival in patients with initially unexplained cardiomyopathy. *NEJM* **342**: 1077–1084.

153 Grewal, J., Siu, S.C., Ross, H.J. et al. (2009). Pregnancy outcomes in women with dilated cardiomyopathy. *J. Am. Coll. Cardiol.* **55**: 45–52.

154 McNamara, D.M., Elkayam, U., Alharethi, R. et al. (2015). Clinical outcomes for peripartum cardiomyopathy in North America: results of the IPAC (Investigations of Pregnancy-Associated Cardiomyopathy) study. *J. Am. Coll. Cardiol.* **66**: 905–914.

155 Whitehead, S.J., Berg, C.J., and Chang, J. (2003). Pregnancy-related mortality due to cardiomyopathy: United States, 1991–1997. *Obstet. Gynecol.* **106**: 1326–1331.

156 Hasan, J.A., Qureshi, A., Ramejo, B.B., and Kamran, A. (2010). Peripartum cardiomyopathy characteristics and outcome in a tertiary care hospital. *J. Pak. Med. Assoc.* **60**: 377–380.

157 Mandal, D., Mandal, S., Mukherjee, D. et al. (2011). Pregnancy and subsequent pregnancy outcomes in peripartum cardiomyopathy. *J. Obstet. Gynaecol. Res.* **37**: 222–227.

158 Witlin, A.G., Mabie, W.C., and Sibai, B.M. (1997). Peripartum cardiomyopathy: an ominous diagnosis. *Am. J. Obstet. Gynecol.* **176**: 182–188.

159 Fett, J.D., Fristoe, K.L., and Welsh, S.N. (2010). Risk of heart failure relapse in subsequent pregnancy among peripartum cardiomyopathy mothers. *Int. J. Gynaecol. Obstet.* **109**: 34–36.

160 Habli, M., O'Brien, T., Nowack, E. et al. (2008). Peripartum cardiomyopathy: prognostic factors for long-term maternal outcome. *Am. J. Obstet. Gynecol.* **199**: 415.

161 Avila, W.S., de Carvalho, M.E., Tschaen, C.K. et al. (2002). Pregnancy and peripartum cardiomyopathy: a comparative and prospective study. *Arg. Bras. Cardiol.* **79**: 484–493.

162 Thorne, S.A., Nelson-Piercy, C., MacGregor, A. et al. (2008). Pregnancy and contraception in heart disease and pulmonary arterial hypertension. *J. Fam. Plann. Reprod. Health Care* **32**: 78–81.

163 Dickstein, K., Cohen-Solal, A., Filippatos, G. et al. (2008). ESC guidelines for the diagnosis and treatment of acute and chronic heart failure 2008 of the European Society of Cardiology. Developed in collaboration with the Heart Failure Association of the ESC (HFA) and endorsed by the European Society of Intensive Care Medicine (ESICM). *Eur. J. Heart Fail.* **10**: 933–989.

164 Schaefer, C. (2003). Angiotensin II-receptor-antagonists: further evidence of fetotoxicity but not teratogenicity. *Birth Defects Res. A Clin. Mol. Teratol.* **67**: 591–594.

165 Cooper, W.O., Hernandez-Diaz, S., Arbogast, P.G. et al. (2006). Major congenital malformations after first-trimester exposure to ACE-inhibitors. *NEJM* **354**: 2443–2451.

166 Task force on the management of cardiovascular diseases during pregnancy of the European Society of Cardiology (2003). Expert consensus document on the management of the cardiovascular disease during pregnancy. *Eur. Heart J.* **24**: 761–781.

167 Lydakis, C., Gy, L., Beevers, M., and Beevers, D.G. (1999). Atenolol and fetal growth in pregnancies complicated by hypertension. *Am. J. Hypertens.* **12**: 541–547.

168 Fuster, V., Ryden, L.E., Cannom, D.S. et al. (2006). ACC/AHA/ESC 2006 guidelines for the management of patients with atrial fibrillation-executive summary: a report of the American College of Cardiology/American Heart Association Task Force no Practice Guidelines and the European Society of Cardiology Committee for Practice Guidelines. *Eur. Heart J.* **27**: 1979–2030.

169 Sliwa, K., Blauwet, L., Tibazarwa, K. et al. (2010). Evaluation of bromocriptine in the treatment of acute severe peripartum cardiomyopathy: a proof-of-concept pilot study. *Circulation* **121**: 1465–1473.

170 Rasmusson, K.D., Stehlik, J., Brown, R.N. et al. (2007). Long-term outcomes of cardiac transplantation for peri-partum cardiomyopathy: a multiinstitutional analysis. *J. Heart Lung Transplant.* **26**: 1097–1104.

171 Velickovic, I.A. and Leicht, C.H. (2004). Peripartum cardiomyopathy and cesarean section: report of two cases and literature review. *Arch. Gynecol. Obstet.* **270**: 307–310.

172 De Beus, E., van Mook, W.N., Ramsay, G. et al. (2003). Peripartum cardiomyopathy: a condition intensivists should be aware of. *Intensive Care Med.* **29**: 167–174.

173 Tomlinson, M. (2006). Cardiac diseases. In: *High Risk Pregnancy. Management Options*, 3e (ed. D.K. James, P.J. Steer, C.P. Weiner, et al.), 798–827. Philadelphia: Elsevier Saunders.

174 Goland, S., Modi, K., Bitar, F. et al. (2009). Clinical profile and predictors of complications in peripartum cardiomyopathy. *J. Card. Fail.* **15**: 645–650.

175 The Task Force on the Management of Cardiovascular Diseases during Pregnancy of the European Society of Cardiology (ESC) endorsed by the European Society of Gynecology (ESG), the Association of European Paediatric Cardiology (AEPC), and the German Society for Gender Medicine (DgesGM) (2011). ESC guidelines on the management of cardiovascular diseases during pregnancy. *Eur. Heart J.* **32**: 3147–3197.

27

CHAPTER 27
Renal disease

Arun Jeyabalan
Division of Maternal-Fetal Medicine, Department of Obstetrics, Gynecology and Reproductive Sciences, University of Pittsburgh School of Medicine, Magee-Women's Hospital, Pittsburgh, PA, USA

CLINICAL VIGNETTE

A 28-year-old primigravid woman at seven weeks of gestation is referred to you for chronic kidney disease secondary to acute glomerulonephritis at age 18. This is an unplanned but desired pregnancy. Her baseline serum creatinine has been stable at 1.2 mg dl^{-1} over that past 10 years. She is followed by a nephrologist. She does not have hypertension. She has been on lisinopril (angiotensin-converting-enzyme [ACE] inhibitor) for renal protection. How would you counsel, evaluate, and manage this patient?

Introduction

Chronic kidney disease (CKD) is estimated to affect up to 3% of all pregnancies [1, 2]. The prevalence is often underestimated since renal disease is frequently unrecognized prior to pregnancy and may be masked by the normal maternal physiological changes. Historically, CKD in pregnancy has been associated with significant perinatal morbidity and mortality. A 1975 editorial in the Lancet noted "children of women with renal disease used to be born dangerously or not at all, if their doctors had their way" [3]. Fortunately, a better understanding of CKD as well as advances in perinatal and neonatal care has led to improved pregnancy outcomes. A multi-disciplinary approach often including obstetricians, Maternal-Fetal Medicine specialists, nephrologists, neonatologists, and critical care medicine teams is necessary to optimize the health and well-being of both patients: the mother and her baby.

Renal adaptations during pregnancy

A fundamental appreciation of maternal renal and cardiovascular adaptations is a prerequisite to complete understanding, proper diagnosis, and management of kidney disease during pregnancy. Physiologic changes occur as early as the first trimester and include anatomic, hemodynamic, substrate handling and acid-base alterations [4, 5]. (See reference [5] for a detailed review on the topic.)

Anatomic changes: The size and volume of the kidneys increase due to the increase in blood volume and capacity of the collecting system. Dilation of the collecting system with hydronephrosis and hydroureter occurs in 80% of women by mid-pregnancy, likely secondary to hormonal effects resulting in smooth muscle relaxation [6, 7]. Right-sided ureteral dilation is greater than the left because of compression by the enlarged and dextro-rotated uterus as well as the ovarian vascular plexus at the level of the pelvic brim.

Hemodynamic adaptations: The increase in renal blood flow and glomerular filtration rate (GFR) is one of the earliest and most dramatic changes in pregnancy. By the third trimester, renal plasma flow is 50–85% above non-pregnant levels with a slight decline toward the very end of gestation. Secondarily, GFR also increases by 40–65%. In addition, there is marked reduction of systemic vascular resistance as well as an increase in cardiac output and plasma volume by approximately 50% and 40% above the non-pregnant baseline, respectively [4]. Progesterone, relaxin, and other luteal/placental hormones are likely responsible for these hemodynamic changes. These renal adaptations affect the normal ranges for standard laboratory parameters and have practical implications for the care of the pregnant woman (Table 27.1). For example, a serum creatinine of 0.9–1.0 mg dl^{-1} considered to be normal for an adult would be abnormal in a healthy pregnant woman.

Substrate handling: Some degree of proteinuria (<300 mg per 24 hours) is normal in advancing gestation and generally does not indicate renal compromise. This is likely due to increased GFR along with reduced resorption at the level of the proximal tubule [4]. Alteration in the glomerular membrane charge also allows for membrane permeability to negatively charged proteins. Women with baseline proteinuria generally have a progressive increase in total protein

Evidence-Based Obstetrics and Gynecology, First Edition. Edited by Errol R. Norwitz, Carolyn M. Zelop, David A. Miller, and David L. Keefe.

Table 27.1 Normal laboratory parameters in pregnancy

Variable	Change compared to non-pregnant values	Approximate normal value in pregnancy
Creatinine	↓	0.5 mg dl^{-1}
Blood urea nitrogen (BUN)	↓	9.0 mg dl^{-1}
Glomerular filtration rate (GFR)	↑	↑ ~40–65% above baseline
Creatinine clearance	↑	↑ ~25% above baseline
Sodium retention over pregnancy	↑	900–950 mEq
Plasma osmolality	↓	↓ ~10 mOsm kg^{-1} H_2O
Uric acid	↓	2.0–3.0 mg dl^{-1}
Urinary protein excretion	Variable to ↑	<300 mg per 24 hours
Urinary albumin excretion	Variable to ↑	<20 mg per 24 hours
Urinary glucose excretion	Variable to ↑	Variable
pCO_2	↓	↓ ~10 mmHg below baseline
Serum bicarbonate	↓	18–20 mEq l^{-1}

excretion with advancing gestation; however, the precise amount is inconsistent. Glucosuria is also not uncommon in pregnancy and does not necessarily indicate diabetes. Normally, glucose is freely filtered at the glomerulus and reabsorbed in the proximal tubule. The increased GFR and reduced proximal tubular reabsorption often results in glucose in the urine. Despite this marked increase in GFR, there is net sodium retention of 900–950 mEq over the course of pregnancy due to tubular reabsorption and total body water increases by 6–8 l.

Acid-base homeostasis: The kidney also plays an important role in acid-base homeostasis. Increased minute ventilation of pregnancy results in a respiratory alkalosis (pCO_2 is reduced by ~10 mmHg). A partial compensatory metabolic acidosis occurs via increased renal bicarbonate excretion. The resulting increase in CO_2 gradient across the placenta facilitates gas exchange and is beneficial for the fetus; however, it reduces the maternal capacity to buffer acids. These physiologic acid-base changes are important in the care of the pregnant woman, particularly in the Intensive care unit (ICU) setting [5].

Chronic kidney disease and pregnancy

As with other medical disorders of pregnancy, major considerations are (i) the effect of renal disease on pregnancy outcomes; and (ii) the impact of pregnancy on the course of renal disease. In taking an evidence-based approach to this topic, it is critical to understand the limitations of the published literature. Most studies have small numbers and are retrospective, often based in a single institution and lacking a comparison group. Importantly, preconception counseling, antenatal care, and follow-up are not standardized. With larger studies often spanning many years, changes in perinatal care such as administration of steroids for prematurity have improved but confounded comparison of outcomes. Furthermore, classification of kidney disease as well as the definition of outcomes has been inconsistent across the published literature. For example, premature delivery may be defined as less than 34 weeks' in some studies and less than 37 weeks' in others.

Classification: The standardized classification of CKD includes five stages based on progressively worsening GFR. Stage 1 CKD represents renal damage with normal to increased GFR and stage 5 is end-stage renal disease (ESRD) including dialysis (Table 27.2) [8]. Preconception classification is ideal, since standard formulas for GFR such as the Modification of Diet in Renal Disease equation may not accurately represent renal function in pregnancy [9]. If pre-pregnancy staging is not available, first trimester serum creatinine is most commonly used for classification. Earlier publications used a three-tiered classification system

Table 27.2 Stages of chronic kidney disease and *approximate correlation* with earlier pregnancy classifications

Stages of chronic kidney disease[a]			Earlier pregnancy classifications by baseline creatinine (mg dl^{-1})
Stage	Description	GFR (ml min^{-1}/1.73 m^2)	
1	Slight kidney damage with normal or increased GFR	≥90	Mild (serum creatinine <1.5)
2	Kidney damage with mildly decreased GFR	60–89	
3	Moderately decreased GFR	30–59	Moderate (serum creatinine 1.5–2.5)
4	Severely decreased GFR	15–29	Severe (serum creatinine >2.5)
5	Kidney failure	<15 or dialysis	End stage renal disease/dialysis

[a]Chronic kidney disease is defined as either kidney damage or GFR <60 ml min^{-1}/1.73 m^2 for ≥3 months. Kidney damage is defined as pathologic abnormalities or markers of damage including abnormalities in the composition of blood or urine tests or abnormalities on imaging studies. From the National Kidney Foundation, 2002 [8].

during pregnancy with mild (serum creatinine less than 1.4 mg dl^{-1}), moderate (serum creatinine 1.4–2.4 mg dl^{-1}), and severe (serum creatinine greater than or equal to 2.5 mg dl^{-1}) renal disease. Stages 3–5 CKD correspond to moderate and severe renal disease. Based on the existing data, pre-pregnancy renal function and hypertension have consistently emerged as the best predictors of adverse perinatal outcomes; thus, appropriate classification impacts counseling.

Impact of CKD on pregnancy outcomes: Adverse pregnancy outcomes associated with CKD include pre-eclampsia, fetal growth restriction, indicated preterm delivery, and perinatal death. With mild renal impairment, the frequency of live-births is greater than 90–95% [10–14]. Pregnancy outcomes are progressively worse with higher stages of CKD and hypertension. In Table 27.3a, we provide evidence-based estimates of adverse outcomes by degree of CKD adapted from reviews [1, 2, 4, 10, 15–18] and including a number of original studies [14, 19–26]. Pre-eclampsia is the most common adverse maternal outcome in women with pre-existing renal disease. In a 2011 systematic review of 13 cohort studies, women with CKD were more likely to develop gestational hypertension, pre-eclampsia, eclampsia or to die compared to women without CKD (12% versus 2%) [17]. In a recent systematic review, the odds ratio of pre-eclampsia in women with CKD (stages 1–3) was 10.36 (95% confidence interval, 6.28–17.09) compared to women without CKD [18]. Both reviews are limited by the quality of the individual studies, many of which had a small sample of CKD cases. Importantly, diagnosing pre-eclampsia is particularly challenging in women with baseline proteinuria and/or pre-existing hypertension associated with CKD since progression of proteinuria and higher blood pressures are not uncommon in the third trimester. A sudden escalation of blood pressure or proteinuria, new onset of pre-eclampsia symptoms (headache, visual changes, right upper quadrant, or epigastric pain), or other evidence end-organ dysfunction (thrombocytopenia or elevated liver transaminases) supports the diagnosis of pre-eclampsia. Renal biopsy is not indicated for the diagnosis of pre-eclampsia. Emerging data indicate that circulating angiogenic factors may be used to differentiate between pre-eclampsia and the benign third trimester progression of hypertension and/or proteinuria with CKD. Soluble Flt-1 (sFlt-1), a soluble receptor for vascular endothelial growth factor and placental growth factor (PlGF), is elevated weeks prior to and during pre-eclampsia. Conversely, PlGF is reduced [27]. These alterations are more pronounced when pre-eclampsia is of early-onset, severe, or associated with fetal growth restriction [28]. The PlGF as well as the ratio of sFlt-1/PlGF has been shown to predict pre-eclampsia in a number of studies [28]. A few studies, albeit with small numbers, indicate that PlGF, and/or the sFlt/PlGF ratio may be helpful in the differential diagnosis

Table 27.3a Pregnancy outcome based on pre-pregnancy renal function in women with chronic kidney disease[a]

Pre-pregnancy serum creatinine	Fetal growth restriction (%)	Preterm delivery (%)	Pre-eclampsia (%)	Live birth (%)
<1.4 mg dl^{-1}	5–26	13–24	6–29	>90–95%
1.4–2.5	31–64	30–79	~40	~90%
>2.5[b]	22–65	50–95	~60–80	Inadequately reported

[a]This category is limited by small numbers.
[b]Ranges are from selected studies 1984–2015 (see text), with pregnancies attaining ≥24 weeks when possible. Not all the studies included provide information in each of these categories. Modified and updated from refs [5, 15] includes data from refs [1, 2, 10, 15–18].

of pre-eclampsia and other high risk conditions including worsening CKD [29–34].

Adverse fetal/neonatal outcomes are also higher in pregnancies complicated by CKD (Table 27.3a). In the 2011 systematic review, preterm birth was significantly higher 13% compared to 6%; while higher but nonsignificant rates were noted for fetal growth restriction (5% vs 0%), small for gestational age (14% versus 8%), and stillbirth (5% versus 2%) [17]. Higher odds of preterm birth (5.7, 95% confidence interval of 3.3–10.0) and small for gestational age/low birth weight infants (4.9; CI, 3.0–7.8) were reported in the more recent systematic review [18]. As acknowledged by the both sets of authors, the quality of the primary studies inherently limits some of the conclusions and many had very small sample size. The incidence of fetal growth restriction is higher in women with CKD even in the absence of pre-eclampsia. Preterm delivery associated with CKD is most often indicated based on pre-eclampsia, fetal growth restriction, or progression of renal disease. Unfortunately, there is marked variability in the criteria for delivery and patient management such that comparison across studies is problematic. High risk obstetricians and neonatologists should be involved in the decision-making regarding timing of delivery and optimization of fetal/newborn care. (See Section 27.4).

Impact of pregnancy on CKD: High glomerular pressure and hyperfiltration contribute to progressive decline in GFR [35]. However, the precise effect of pregnancy-induced hyperfiltration on underlying CKD is incompletely understood. Using animal models, Baylis and colleagues demonstrated that glomerular capillary pressure is not increased during pregnancy [36, 37]. Extrapolating from these data, hyperfiltration of pregnancy is likely secondary to increased renal blood flow along with vasodilation of both efferent and afferent arterioles; thus, without marked increase in intra-glomerular pressure. This supports the lack of progressive, long-term decline of renal function in healthy women due to pregnancy. In pregnant women with CKD, however, it is common to observe worsening proteinuria (approximately 50%) and the development or worsening of hypertension (approximately 25%) which have potential to further damage the kidney [15]. In most cases, these changes resolve after delivery. Therefore, it is important to differentiate between temporary changes and long-term renal decline secondary to pregnancy.

Among women with mild CKD (stages 1 and 2), permanent decline in renal function occurs in 0–10% due to pregnancy which is comparable to the non-pregnant population. Jungers et al. studied 360 women with glomerulonephritis of whom 171 conceived and observed no difference in long-term renal function over 25 years in women who became pregnant compared to those who did not conceive [38]. A consistent and reassuring finding across this and a number of other studies is that women with mild CKD do not have long-term, permanent renal decline due to pregnancy (Table 27.3b) [11, 38–40]. With moderate and severe CKD, the findings are more complex. Early, small studies reported that greater than 50% of women with moderate CKD had permanent renal decline after pregnancy. In 1986, Imbasciati et al. reported that progression of renal disease was lower than earlier reports and found that one third of women with moderate CKD prior to pregnancy had long-term had decline in their renal function [20]. In a landmark paper on the topic, Jones and Hayslett reported on 82 pregnancies in 67 women with moderate to severe renal disease [21]. Among women with a baseline serum creatinine of 1.5–1.9 $mg\,dl^{-1}$, 40% had a decline of renal function during pregnancy and 2% had accelerated decline in GFR within six months post-delivery. If serum creatinine was greater than 2.0 $mg\,dl^{-1}$, 65% of women had decline in renal function in the third trimester and 33% had accelerated decline in renal function by six months postpartum. Eight women from the entire group progressed to end-stage renal failure within one year of pregnancy. A more recent study of women with stage 3–5 CKD assessed progression of renal disease before, during, and after pregnancy [22]. Women with a pre-pregnancy GFR of less than 40 $ml\,min^{-1}/1.73\,m^2$ and 24-hour protein excretion of greater than 1 g, but not either factor alone, had accelerated decline in renal function after pregnancy compared to before pregnancy. Together, these data may allow for more nuanced counseling in women with moderate CKD. With severe renal impairment (serum creatinine >3 $mg\,dl^{-1}$), women are less likely to ovulate, conceive spontaneously, and carry a pregnancy to full term [1]. Thus, the data are fewer in this group. However, it is likely that the same principle applies, that the higher stage of renal impairment the worse the outcomes.

Table 27.3b Estimated impact of pregnancy on maternal renal function in women with chronic kidney disease[a]

	Decline in renal function		
Pre-pregnancy serum creatinine	**During pregnancy (%)**	**Persisting post-delivery up to 6 weeks (%)**	**Accelerated renal dysfunction at 6–12 months (%)**
< 1.4 $mg\,dl^{-1}$	2	0	0
1.4–2.0	40	20	2
>2.0	65	50	33

[a]Modified and updated from refs [5, 15]; includes data from refs [11, 17, 18, 20–22, 38–40].

Management of pregnancy in women with CKD

These pregnancies should be managed by or with a Maternal-Fetal Medicine specialist in close cooperation with the multi-disciplinary team including nephrologists. Preconception counseling is paramount for all reproductive age women with renal disease. Effective contraception is recommended until renal function is stable and any systemic disease is well-controlled (e.g. systemic lupus erythematosus [SLE], diabetes). Pre-pregnancy renal function and hypertension have consistently emerged as the best predictors of adverse perinatal outcomes. Baseline laboratory tests should include a careful assessment of renal function (serum blood urea nitrogen ([BUN], creatinine, electrolytes including calcium and phosphorus as well as urine for microscopic evaluation, proteinuria, and 24-hour collection for creatinine clearance and total protein excretion). Although the 24-hour urine collection is fraught with problems including compliance, it can be useful along with the protein to creatinine ratio to assess baseline and changes in urine protein excretion across gestation including sudden increases that may indicate pre-eclampsia [41, 42]. Baseline liver transaminases and a complete blood count including platelets are useful as these parameters can be altered by pre-eclampsia later in the pregnancy. Blood pressure should be assessed and treated with medications considered safe in pregnancy (methyldopa, labetalol, calcium channel blockers such as nifedipine) [41]. In general, one agent is maximized before a second agent is added, partly to minimize fetal exposure to multiple medications. ACE inhibitors and angiotensin II receptor blockers (ARBs) should be avoided during pregnancy due to their association with birth defects in the first trimester and oligohydramnios and fetal renal failure in the third trimester [43, 44]. Diuretics tend not to be used in pregnancy due to their effect of reducing intravascular volume and potentially blood flow to the uterus. The target blood pressure goals for CKD in pregnancy are not well-defined based on the current evidence. The current recommendations for non-pregnant patients with CKD are to lower blood pressure below 130/80 to avoid progressive renal damage. This must be balanced against the blood pressure alterations that occur as a part of the normal pregnancy adaptations and the risk of reducing utero-placental perfusion. It is reassuring that "tight" blood pressure control in a randomized controlled trial of pregnant women with hypertension was found to be safe [45]. Low dose aspirin (81 mg daily) after the first trimester should be initiated for pre-eclampsia risk reduction based on individual patient data meta-analyses [46] and the favorable benefit to risk balance in this high risk group.

Anemia is common in pregnancy and if diagnosed, additional studies with appropriate iron, folate, and/or B12 supplementation should be instituted. If the anemia is secondary to renal dysfunction, most commonly with normocytic and normochromic red blood cell indices, then erythropoietin therapy is indicated [47]. In addition to routine prenatal care, renal function should be evaluated approximately once a month. Visits should occur every two to three weeks and then every one to two weeks after 28–30 weeks to monitor for the development of pre-eclampsia. Home blood pressure monitoring and self-monitoring for symptoms of pre-eclampsia are useful. Fetal surveillance should include an early ultrasound to establish accurate gestational age, detailed anatomic ultrasound survey between 18 and 20 weeks' gestation, and serial ultrasounds to monitor fetal growth. These are usually initiated at 24–26 weeks and then performed every three to four weeks thereafter. The frequency should be increased if there is evidence of fetal growth restriction. Doppler interrogation of the umbilical arteries can also be useful in the setting of suspected growth restriction. Fetal kick counts should be monitored daily by the mother starting at 28 weeks of pregnancy. Antenatal testing should be initiated between 28 and 32 weeks; this may include nonstress tests one to two times per week and/or biophysical profile testing each week. The frequency of testing may be increased if there are any concerns about fetal well-being. Antenatal glucocorticoids should be administered and neonatology team consulted if preterm delivery is anticipated [48, 49]. If both mother and baby are doing well, delivery at 39 weeks' is recommended. Vaginal route is the preferred mode of delivery with cesarean section reserved for the usual obstetric indications. Postpartum care should include close monitoring of blood pressure, optimization of medications and attention to renal function. Physiologic changes of pregnancy generally resolve by 10–12 weeks post-delivery. Breast feeding is encouraged in women with CKD. Rarely, breastfeeding may be contraindicated based on safety of particular medications.

For the patient in our clinical vignette with mild CKD (pre-pregnancy creatinine of $1.2\,\mathrm{mg\,dl^{-1}}$), we can reassure her that we do not anticipate pregnancy to permanently affect her renal function. The likelihood of live birth is greater than 90–95% but she is at increased risk for pre-eclampsia, fetal growth restriction, and preterm delivery. ACE inhibitors should be discontinued. If needed, anti-hypertensive medications that are safe in pregnancy may be initiated. She does not have a known hypertension history which is favorable for pregnancy. Low dose aspirin should be initiated after the first trimester. Multidisciplinary management approach with close maternal and fetal surveillance is as outlined above.

Specific renal disorders in pregnancy

For most types of CKD, pregnancy outcome and long-term renal function are largely dependent on baseline renal function (serum creatinine) and the presence or absence of hypertension. SLE and diabetes, common conditions in reproductive age women, warrant additional discussion. Due to space limitations, only key considerations as they apply to pregnancy and renal function will be reviewed.

Diabetic nephropathy – Renal deterioration secondary to diabetes follows a predictable progression to ESRD if untreated. Rigorous metabolic control, blood pressure treatment, and renal protection with ACE inhibitors or ARBs are all strategies to prevent the progression of diabetic nephropathy. Women with long standing diabetes often have renal impairment during their reproductive years. Pregnancy does not appear to accelerate renal decline in women with mild renal impairment (serum creatinine $<1.5\,\mathrm{mg\,dl^{-1}}$) [50]. As with CKD, the data for women with moderate and severe baseline renal disease are more controversial. One report suggested a 40% higher chance of renal deterioration attributable to pregnancy [51]. Although these women had good glycemic control, this study suffered from the lack of a control group. Worsening blood pressure over the course of pregnancy, particularly in the third trimester may contribute to the decline in renal function [52]. Larger, well controlled studies are needed to resolve this issue. To avoid potential renal decline, good glycemic, and blood pressure control are recommended during pregnancy. ACE inhibitors and ARBs should not be used in pregnancy secondary to association with fetal anomalies [43, 44].

SLE – SLE, an autoimmune condition that can affect multiple organs and to varying degrees, disproportionately affects women and tends to occur during the child-bearing years. Adverse pregnancy outcomes with SLE include pre-eclampsia, fetal growth restriction, preterm delivery, and stillbirth. Active lupus flares, renal involvement, antiphospholipid antibodies and anti-Ro(SSA) and La(SSB) antibodies confer additional risk [53]. A multi-disciplinary team is recommended for pregnancy care. A history of lupus nephritis or active lupus nephritis is associated with a higher rate of maternal and fetal complications [54, 55]; adverse outcomes are significantly lower when lupus nephritis is in remission [56]. Therefore, women are encouraged to delay pregnancy until disease is inactive or as stable as possible for 6–12 months.

Table 27.4 Clinical features that may help differentiate pre-eclampsia and acute glomerulonephritis[a]

	Pre-eclampsia	Acute glomerulonephritis
Gestational age	Onset usually in the third trimester (by definition after 20 weeks)	Any
Hypertension	Present	Often present
Systemic manifestations (may or may not be present)	• neurologic (headache, scotomata, visual disturbances, seizures) • hematologic (low platelets) • hepatic involvement (elevated transaminases)	• Collagen-vascular disease (e.g. systemic lupus erythematosus with associated symptoms such as fatigue, arthralgias, rash, fevers) • preceding infection (e.g. streptococcal infection)
Urine sediment	Isolated proteinuria Urine microscopy generally bland, may have findings of acute tubular necrosis (brown granular casts, renal tubular cells)	• Hematuria, red blood cell, oval fat bodies
Proteinuria	>300 mg/24	>2 g per 24 hours
Complement levels	↔	↓
ANA	↔	↑
Antistreptolysin-O titers	↔	↑
Other autoantibodies	↔	↑

[a]The diagnosis may be confusing. Presence or absence of above features is not absolute, but may assist in the diagnosis.

Active lupus nephritis and glomerulonephritis during pregnancy can be difficult to distinguish from pre-eclampsia particularly during the third trimester [4]. Clinical and laboratory features that can be used to differentiate between the two conditions are listed in Table 27.4. Treatment options for active lupus nephritis during pregnancy include high dose steroids and azathioprine. In contrast, the mainstay of pre-eclampsia treatment is delivery, particularly if severe. Therefore, accurate diagnosis is very important. Careful postpartum follow is also warranted given the risk of lupus flares and difficulty in differentiating between an SLE exacerbation and common postpartum symptoms such as fatigue.

Renal biopsy in pregnancy – Renal biopsy is often helpful in determining precise histologic diagnosis and guiding therapy in the setting of unexplained acute or chronic renal failure. The rate of serious complications in the non-pregnant population is low (<1%) [57]. Renal biopsy during pregnancy is associated with higher morbidity, possibly due to the increased renal blood flow and physiologic changes, and therefore warrants careful consideration. Accurate assessment of risk is limited by small case series' which are mostly retrospective. In a recent systematic review reporting on renal biopsies performed during pregnancy or postpartum, the risk of major complications including bleeding was significantly higher during pregnancy than postpartum (7% versus 1%) [58]. Bleeding requiring transfusion was the most frequent major complication. The complication rate was higher at 23–26 weeks compared to earlier in the pregnancy or post-delivery. Renal biopsy is not indicated for the diagnosis of pre-eclampsia; however, may be useful in selected situations wherein treatment options other than delivery would be considered based on the histologic diagnosis. Experts have suggested that renal biopsy be limited to sudden, unexplained deterioration of renal function prior to 32 weeks' given the higher procedure-related risks [59]. The gestational age limits at which to consider biopsy may need to be re-evaluated given the improved neonatal outcomes at 28–30 weeks' with antenatal glucocorticoid use and improved neonatal intensive care. Empiric medical therapy such as high dose steroids should be strongly considered before proceeding to renal biopsy during pregnancy if a particular diagnosis seems most likely. We recommend a multidisciplinary team approach to the decision-making with maternal-fetal medicine, nephrology, and neonatology specialists.

Dialysis

There have been substantial improvements in both fertility and pregnancy rates in women with ESRD and dialysis. The incidence of pregnancy among women on dialysis is estimated to be 0.3–1.5% per year [60, 61]. However, pregnancy in women on dialysis is associated with significant perinatal morbidity and mortality. Much of the evidence comes from case reports, case series, surveys, and registries. The first case report of a successful conception and pregnancy while on dialysis was published in 1971 [62]. Based on data from the 1980s and early 1990s and after exclusion of therapeutic abortions, the likelihood of fetal survival was reported to be 40–50% [63]. In 1994, Hou and colleague reported on 1281 women undergoing maintenance dialysis and since 1990, 52% of pregnancies resulted in surviving infants [64]. Based on two large surveys in Belgium (1472 women) and the United States (6230), the percentage of pregnancies resulting in a surviving infant was 52% and 40%, respectively [65, 66]. Data from the Australian and New Zealand Dialysis and Transplant registry indicate a live birth frequency of 73% among 77 pregnancies between 2000 and 2011 [67]. This was higher for women who conceived before starting dialysis compared to those who conceived while on maintenance dialysis (91% versus 63%). In a recent Canadian cohort of 22 pregnancies, live birth frequency was 86% with a more intensive dialysis protocol [68]. Morbidity is high with complications including preterm delivery (85%), fetal growth restriction (up to 90%), polyhydramnios (33–62%), and hypertensive disorders including pre-eclampsia (42–80%) based on estimates from the studies discussed above. Polyhydramnios is thought to be secondary to maternal uremia resulting in increased delivery of urea to the fetus. The high solute load leads to fetal diuresis, increased urine production and high amniotic fluid volume. Polyhydramnios and fluid shifts during dialysis are also associated with preterm premature rupture of membranes and preterm labor.

Perinatal outcomes are improved with a more intensive dialysis regimen along with close attention to the physiologic changes of pregnancy [69, 70]. Salient points include increasing dialysis time and frequency (20 or more hours per week), targeting a lower maternal BUN level (less than 45–50 mg dl^{-1}), as well as minimizing fluid shift and hypotension. Weight gain should be monitored closely and pregnancy associated weight gains must be taken into account when considering fluid management. Anemia should be managed aggressively with erythropoietin. Blood pressure control may be achieved with pharmacologic therapy and by removing excess intravascular fluid. Vigilant pregnancy management is essential and is similar to that outlined in the previous section on women with CKD. A special consideration is the fetal monitoring prior to and post-dialysis, particularly in the third trimester, as hypotension and increased contractions associated with dialysis may adversely affect fetal well-being and cause preterm labor. Given the overall poor prognosis for pregnancy, contraception should be addressed in sexually active women on dialysis and preconception consultation is essential. Pregnancy after renal transplant should be a consideration since outcomes are much better. Of note, it may be difficult to diagnose pregnancy in women with ESRD since beta human chorionic gonadotropin (βhCG) may be elevated in the non-pregnant state due to production by somatic cells and inadequate excretion by kidneys. Ultrasonography should be used to verify pregnancy and gestational age.

There are fewer data on peritoneal dialysis in pregnancy. Features of peritoneal dialysis that may have theoretical benefit in pregnancy include the lack of abrupt hypotension and fluid shifts, a more constant fluid and electrolyte environment for the fetus, and overall improved blood pressure control. Abdominal fullness and catheter drainage difficulties may affect adequacy of dialysis. Peritonitis, a potential complication of peritoneal dialysis, may pose a diagnostic problem during pregnancy, since chorioamnionitis and even labor can present with abdominal pain. Overall, there does not appear to be a difference in pregnancy outcomes based on mode of renal replacement therapy [66, 71].

Renal transplant

Fertility generally returns, and often rapidly, after renal transplantation. More than 90% of pregnancies that progress beyond the first trimester are successful [72–74]. With stable renal allograft function, renal function prior to pregnancy is a major predictor of outcome. As with CKD, pre-eclampsia, fetal growth restriction and preterm delivery are more frequent. Other factors such as time since transplant, origin of transplant, hypertension, and dosage and type of immunosuppressive therapy may affect prognosis [75]. Most of the data are from case series and transplant registries [16, 76–80]. The long-term effect of pregnancy on renal allograft function has been a major questions with somewhat conflicting results. The vast majority of studies indicate that pregnancy does not accelerate the decline of renal allograft function [81–83]. Rahamimov et al. evaluated long-term outcomes in 39 women with functioning renal allograft who became pregnant and compared them to three matched controls who were not pregnant [83]. Renal function and overall survival was similar at 1, 5, and 10 years post-transplant between the two groups. At the end of the 15-year follow-up period renal function was similar in both groups (72% in pregnant women versus 69% in control subjects).

Preconception and contraceptive counseling is recommended prior to transplant surgery and preferably in the early planning stages. Current recommendations based on consensus conferences of the American Transplant Society and other experts include the following [75, 80]:

1. Waiting at least one year after transplant before attempting pregnancy to ensure stability of graft function and to avoid complications related to rejection. This time frame must be individualized and balanced against the age and fertility of the patient.
2. Stable doses of immunosuppressive therapy that are considered safe for pregnancy. Ideally, prednisone $\leq$ 15 mg per day, azathioprine $\leq$ 2 mg kg^{-1} per day, cyclosporine $\leq$ 5 mg kg^{-1} per day, and tacrolimus $\leq$ 0.1–0.2 mg kg^{-1} per day.
3. No evidence of graft rejection.
4. Optimal and adequate allograft function (preferably serum creatinine <1.5 mg dl^{-1} and proteinuria of less than 500 mg per day.
5. Well-controlled blood pressure.

Immunosuppressive medications should not be stopped abruptly during pregnancy since these are important for preventing allograft rejection, maternal health, and the success of the pregnancy. Safety in pregnancy should be considered in the choice of agent(s). Prednisone, azathioprine, cyclosporine, and tacrolimus are the most commonly used immunosuppressive agents in pregnancy. Newer immunosuppressive drugs should be avoided until adequate data are accrued to support their safety in pregnancy.

Pregnancy care is similar to that outlined previously for women with CKD except for a few special considerations [4]. The dosage of immunosuppressive drugs may need to be adjusted during pregnancy due to the marked volume changes and enhanced hepatic metabolism. In general, if graft function is stable on prednisone and/or azathioprine then dosage can be maintained throughout pregnancy. Adjustment of cyclosporine and tacrolimus dose may be needed to achieve therapeutic blood concentrations. With respect to allograft function and rejection, frequent monitoring is recommended as with CKD. Rejection must be kept in the differential diagnosis of abdominal pain, fevers, and leukocytosis [84]. Given the immunosuppression, close monitoring for infections with appropriate therapy is recommended. Viral and parasitic infections that could affect pregnancy should also be considered including cytomegalovirus, herpes simplex virus and toxoplasmosis. Primary infections as well as reactivations are more common in women taking immunosuppressive drugs; therefore, serologic assessment is recommended prior to and/or during pregnancy. Appropriate counseling and therapy should be instituted if primary infection or reactivation is suspected. Although unusual, obstruction of the ureter has been reported secondary to the enlarging uterus. Vaginal delivery is recommended except for the usual obstetric indications. Location of the transplanted kidney should be confirmed by the operative report and clearly outlined in the prenatal chart. If cesarean section is required, then care must be taken to avoid trauma to the renal allograft. Breastfeeding should be encouraged; however, the safety of some of the immunosuppressive medications remains unclear and recommendations should be made accordingly.

In summary, adverse perinatal outcomes are higher in women with renal disorders. Preconception counseling and pregnancy care can be challenging. Multi-disciplinary management with appropriate specialists is important to optimize maternal and fetal well-being.

References

1 Davison, J.M. and Lindheimer, M.D. (2011). Pregnancy and chronic kidney disease. *Seminars in Nephrology* **31** (**1**): 86–99.

2 Cabiddu, G., Castellino, S., Gernone, G. et al. (2016). A best practice position statement on pregnancy in chronic kidney disease: the Italian Study Group on Kidney and Pregnancy. *Journal of Nephrology* **29** (**3**): 277–303.

3 Anonymous (1975). Pregnancy and renal disease. *Lancet* **2**: 801–802.

4 Jeyabalan, A. and Conrad, K.P. (2010). Renal physiology and pathophysiology in pregnancy. In: *Renal and Electrolyte Disorders*, 7e (ed. R.W. Schrier), 462–518. Philadelphia: Lippincott Williams & Wilkins.

5 Gammill, H.S. and Jeyabalan, A. (2005). Acute renal failure in pregnancy. *Critical Care Medicine* **33** (**10 Suppl**): S372–S384.

6 Cietak, K. and Newton, J. (1985). Serial qualitative maternal nephrosonography in pregnancy. *British Journal of Radiology* **58**: 399.

7 Conrad, K. (1992). Renal changes in pregnancy. *Urology Annals* **6**: 313–340.

8 National Kidney Foundation (2002). K/DOQI clinical practice guidelines for chronic kidney disease: evaluation, classification, and stratification. *American Journal of Kidney Diseases* **39** (**2 Suppl 1**): S1–S266.

9 Smith, M.C., Moran, P., Ward, M.K., and Davison, J.M. (2008). Assessment of glomerular filtration rate during pregnancy using the MDRD formula. *BJOG: An International Journal of Obstetrics & Gynaecology* **115** (**1**): 109–112.

10 Fischer, M.J. (2007). Chronic kidney disease and pregnancy: maternal and fetal outcomes. *Advances in Chronic Kidney Disease* **14** (**2**): 132–145.

11 Hou, S. (1985). Pregnancy in women with chronic renal disease. *New England Journal of Medicine* **312** (**13**): 836–839.

12 Hayslett, J.P. (1999). Kidney disease and pregnancy. *Kidney International* **25**: 579.

13 Packham, D.K., North, R.A., Fairley, K.F. et al. (1989). Primary glomerulonephritis and pregnancy. *Quarterly Journal of Medicine* **71** (**266**): 537–553.

14 Jungers, P., Chauveau, D., Choukroun, G. et al. (1997). Pregnancy in women with impaired renal function. *Clinical Nephrology* **47** (**5**): 281–288.

15 Williams, D.J., Davison, J.M., and Disorders, R. (2009). *Creasy and Resnik's Maternal-Fetal Medicine Principles and. Practice*, 6e (ed. R.K. Creasy, R. Resnik, J.D. Iams, et al.), 905–926. Philadelphia: Elsevier.

16 Vidaeff, A.C., Yeomans, E.R., and Ramin, S.M. (2008). Pregnancy in women with renal disease. Part I: general principles. *American Journal of Perinatology* **25** (**7**): 385–397.

17 Nevis, I.F., Reitsma, A., Dominic, A. et al. (2011). Pregnancy outcomes in women with chronic kidney disease: a systematic review. *Clinical Journal of the American Society of Nephrology* **6** (**11**): 2587–2598.

18 Zhang, J.J., Ma, X.X., Hao, L. et al. (2015). A systematic review and meta-analysis of outcomes of pregnancy in CKD and CKD outcomes in pregnancy. *Clinical Journal of the American Society of Nephrology* **10** (**11**): 1964–1978.

19 Fischer, M.J., Lehnerz, S.D., Hebert, J.R., and Parikh, C.R. (2004). Kidney disease is an independent risk factor for adverse

fetal and maternal outcomes in pregnancy. *American Journal of Kidney Diseases* **43** (**3**): 415–423.

20 Imbasciati, E., Pardi, G., Capetta, P. et al. (1986). Pregnancy in women with chronic renal failure. *American Journal of Nephrology* **6** (**3**): 193–198.

21 Jones, D.C. and Hayslett, J.P. (1996). Outcome of pregnancy in women with moderate or severe renal insufficiency. *The New England Journal of Medicine* **335** (**4**): 226–232.

22 Imbasciati, E., Gregorini, G., Cabiddu, G. et al. (2007). Pregnancy in CKD stages 3 to 5: fetal and maternal outcomes. *American Journal of Kidney Diseases* **49** (**6**): 753–762.

23 Jungers, P., Houillier, P., Chauveau, D. et al. (1996). Pregnancy in women with reflux nephropathy. *Kidney International* **50** (**2**): 593–599.

24 Trevisan, G., Ramos, J.G., Martins-Costa, S., and Barros, E.J. (2004). Pregnancy in patients with chronic renal insufficiency at Hospital de Clinicas of Porto Alegre, Brazil. *Renal Failure* **26** (**1**): 29–34.

25 Abe, S. (1994). The influence of pregnancy on the long-term renal prognosis of IgA nephropathy. *Clinical Nephrology* **41** (**2**): 61–64.

26 Bar, J., Ben-Rafael, Z., Padoa, A. et al. (2000). Prediction of pregnancy outcome in subgroups of women with renal disease. *Clinical Nephrology* **53** (**6**): 437–444.

27 Levine, R.J., Maynard, S.E., Qian, C. et al. (2004). Circulating angiogenic factors and the risk of pre-eclampsia. *New England Journal of Medicine* **350** (**7**): 672–683.

28 Staff, A.C. (2011). Circulating predictive biomarkers in pre-eclampsia. *Pregnancy Hypertens* **1** (**1**): 28–42.

29 Rana, S., Powe, C.E., Salahuddin, S. et al. (2012). Angiogenic factors and the risk of adverse outcomes in women with suspected pre-eclampsia. *Circulation* **125** (**7**): 911–919.

30 Moore Simas, T.A., Crawford, S.L., Solitro, M.J. et al. (2007). Angiogenic factors for the prediction of pre-eclampsia in high-risk women. *American Journal of Obstetrics and Gynecology* **197** (**3**): 244.e1–244.e8.

31 Duhig, K.E., Chappell, L.C., and Shennan, A.H. (2014). How placental growth factor detection might improve diagnosis and management of pre-eclampsia. *Expert Review of Molecular Diagnostics* **14** (**4**): 403–406.

32 Verlohren, S., Herraiz, I., Lapaire, O. et al. (2012). The sFlt-1/PlGF ratio in different types of hypertensive pregnancy disorders and its prognostic potential in preeclamptic patients. *American Journal of Obstetrics and Gynecology* **206** (**1**): 58 e1–58 e8.

33 Powers, R.W., Jeyabalan, A., Clifton, R.G. et al. (2010). Soluble fms-Like tyrosine kinase 1 (sFlt1), endoglin and placental growth factor (PlGF) in pre-eclampsia among high risk pregnancies. *PLoS One* **5** (**10**): e13263.

34 Masuyama, H., Nobumoto, E., Okimoto, N. et al. (2012). Superimposed pre-eclampsia in women with chronic kidney disease. *Gynecologic and Obstetric Investigation* **74** (**4**): 274–281.

35 Brenner, B.M., Meyer, T.W., and Hostetter, T.H. (1982). Dietary protein intake and the progressive nature of kidney disease: the role of hemodynamically mediated glomerular injury in the pathogenesis of progressive glomerular sclerosis in aging, renal ablation, and intrinsic renal disease. *New England Journal of Medicine* **307** (**11**): 652–659.

36 Baylis, C. (1980). The mechanism of the increase in glomerular filtration rate in the twelve-day pregnant rat. *Journal of Physiology* **305**: 405–414.

37 Baylis, C. (2003). Impact of pregnancy on underlying renal disease. *Advances in Renal Replacement Therapy* **10** (**1**): 31–39.

38 Jungers, P., Houillier, P., Forget, D. et al. (1995). Influence of pregnancy on the course of primary chronic glomerulonephritis. *Lancet* **346** (**8983**): 1122–1124.

39 Hayslett, J.P. (1984). Interaction of renal disease and pregnancy. *Kidney International* **25** (**3**): 579–587.

40 Surian, M., Imbasciati, E., Cosci, P. et al. (1984). Glomerular disease and pregnancy. A study of 123 pregnancies in patients with primary and secondary glomerular diseases. *Nephron* **36** (**2**): 101–105.

41 Roberts, J.M., August, P.A., Bakris, G. et al. (2013). Hypertension in pregnancy. Report of the American College of Obstetricians and Gynecologists' Task Force on Hypertension in Pregnancy. *Obstetrics and Gynecology* **122** (**5**): 1122–1131.

42 Lindheimer, M.D. and Kanter, D. (2010). Interpreting abnormal proteinuria in pregnancy: the need for a more pathophysiological approach. *Obstetrics and Gynecology* **115** (**2 Pt 1**): 365–375.

43 Laube, G.F., Kemper, M.J., Schubiger, G., and Neuhaus, T.J. (2007). Angiotensin-converting enzyme inhibitor fetopathy: long-term outcome. *Archives of Disease in Childhood. Fetal and Neonatal Edition* **92** (**5**): F402–F403.

44 Cooper, W.O., Hernandez-Diaz, S., Arbogast, P.G. et al. (2006). Major congenital malformations after first-trimester exposure to ACE inhibitors. *New England Journal of Medicine* **354** (**23**): 2443–2451.

45 Magee, L.A., von Dadelszen, P., Rey, E. et al. (2015). Less-tight versus tight control of hypertension in pregnancy. *The New England Journal of Medicine* **372** (**5**): 407–417.

46 Askie, L.M., Duley, L., Henderson-Smart, D.J. et al. (2007). Antiplatelet agents for prevention of pre-eclampsia: a meta-analysis of individual patient data. *Lancet* **369** (**9575**): 1791–1798.

47 Sienas, L., Wong, T., Collins, R., and Smith, J. (2013). Contemporary uses of erythropoietin in pregnancy: a literature review. *Obstetrical & Gynecological Survey* **68** (**8**): 594–602.

48 (1994). The effect of antenatal steroids for fetal maturation on perinatal outcomes. *NIH Consensus Statement* **12** (**2**): 1–24.

49 Gyamfi-Bannerman, C., Thom, E.A., Blackwell, S.C. et al. (2016). Antenatal betamethasone for women at risk for late preterm delivery. *The New England Journal of Medicine* **374** (**14**): 1311–1320.

50 Combs, C.A. and Kitzmiller, J.L. (1991). Diabetic nephropathy and pregnancy. *Clinical Obstetrics and Gynecology* **34** (**3**): 505–515.

51 Purdy, L.P., Hantsch, C.E., Molitch, M.E. et al. (1996). Effect of pregnancy on renal function in patients with moderate-to-severe diabetic renal insufficiency. *Diabetes Care* **19** (**10**): 1067–1074.

52 Gordon, M., Landon, M.B., Samuels, P. et al. (1996). Perinatal outcome and long-term follow-up associated with modern management of diabetic nephropathy. *Obstetrics & Gynecology* **87** (**3**): 401–409.

53 Lateef, A. and Petri, M. (2012). Management of pregnancy in systemic lupus erythematosus. *Nature Reviews Rheumatology* **8** (**12**): 710–718.

54 Gladman, D.D., Tandon, A., Ibanez, D., and Urowitz, M.B. (2010). The effect of lupus nephritis on pregnancy outcome and fetal and maternal complications. *The Journal of Rheumatology* **37** (**4**): 754–758.

55 Saavedra, M.A., Cruz-Reyes, C., Vera-Lastra, O. et al. (2012). Impact of previous lupus nephritis on maternal and fetal outcomes during pregnancy. *Clinical Rheumatology* **31** (**5**): 813–819.

56 Wagner, S.J., Craici, I., Reed, D. et al. (2009). Maternal and foetal outcomes in pregnant patients with active lupus nephritis. *Lupus* **18** (**4**): 342–347.

57 Parrish, A. (1992). Complications of percutaneous renal biopsy: a review of 37 years' experience. *Clinical Nephrology* **38**: 135–141.

58 Piccoli, G.B., Daidola, G., Attini, R. et al. (2013). Kidney biopsy in pregnancy: evidence for counselling? A systematic narrative review. *BJOG* **120** (**4**): 412–427.

59 Lindheimer, M.D. and Davison, J.M. (1987). Renal biopsy during pregnancy: 'to b … or not to b … ? *British Journal of Obstetrics and Gynaecology* **94** (**10**): 932–934.

60 Hou, S. (1999). Pregnancy in chronic renal insufficiency and end-stage renal disease. *American Journal of Kidney Diseases* **33** (**2**): 235–252.

61 Jungers, P., Houillier, P., Forget, D., and Henry-Amar, M. (1991). Specific controversies concerning the natural history of renal disease in pregnancy. *American Journal of Kidney Diseases* **17** (**2**): 116–122.

62 Confortini, P., Galanti, G., Ancona, G. et al. (1971). Full term pregnancy and successful delivery in a patient on chronic haemodialysis. *Proceedings of the European Dialysis and Transplant Association* **8**: 74–78.

63 Hou, S.H. (1994). Pregnancy in women on haemodialysis and peritoneal dialysis. *Baillieres Clinical Obstetrics and Gynaecology* **8** (**2**): 481–500.

64 Hou, S.H. (1994). Frequency and outcome of pregnancy in women on dialysis. *American Journal of Kidney Diseases* **23** (**1**): 60–63.

65 Bagon, J.A., Vernaeve, H., De Muylder, X. et al. (1998). Pregnancy and dialysis. *American Journal of Kidney Diseases* **31** (**5**): 756–765.

66 Okundaye, I., Abrinko, P., and Hou, S. (1998). Registry of pregnancy in dialysis patients. *American Journal of Kidney Diseases* **31** (**5**): 766–773.

67 Jesudason, S., Grace, B.S., and McDonald, S.P. (2014). Pregnancy outcomes according to dialysis commencing before or after conception in women with ESRD. *Clinical Journal of the American Society of Nephrology* **9** (**1**): 143–149.

68 Hladunewich, M.A., Hou, S., Odutayo, A. et al. (2014). Intensive hemodialysis associates with improved pregnancy outcomes: a Canadian and United States cohort comparison. *Journal of the American Society of Nephrology* **25** (**5**): 1103–1109.

69 Alkhunaizi, A., Melamed, N., and Hladunewich, M.A. (2015). Pregnancy in advanced chronic kidney disease and end-stage renal disease. *Current Opinion in Nephrology and Hypertension* **24** (**3**): 252–259.

70 Hou, S. (2002). Modification of dialysis regimens for pregnancy. *International Journal of Artificial Organs* **25** (**9**): 823–826.

71 Okundaye, I. and Hou, S. (1996). Management of pregnancy in women undergoing continuous ambulatory peritoneal dialysis. *Advances in Peritoneal Dialysis* **12**: 151–155.

72 Davison, J.M. (1991). Dialysis, transplantation, and pregnancy. *American Journal of Kidney Diseases* **17** (**2**): 127–132.

73 Muirhead, N., Sabharwal, A.R., Rieder, M.J. et al. (1992). The outcome of pregnancy following renal transplantation--the experience of a single center. *Transplantation* **54** (**3**): 429–432.

74 McKay, D.B. and Josephson, M.A. (2006). Pregnancy in recipients of solid organs--effects on mother and child. *New England Journal of Medicine* **354** (**12**): 1281–1293.

75 Josephson, M.A. and McKay, D.B. (2007). Considerations in the medical management of pregnancy in transplant recipients. *Advances in Chronic Kidney Disease* **14** (**2**): 156–167.

76 Coscia, L.A., Constantinescu, S., Moritz, M.J. et al. (2007). Report from the National Transplantation Pregnancy Registry (NTPR): outcomes of pregnancy after transplantation. *Clinical Transplants* 29–42.

77 Morris, P.J., Johnson, R.J., Fuggle, S.V. et al. (1999). Analysis of factors that affect outcome of primary cadaveric renal transplantation in the UK. HLA task force of the kidney advisory Group of the United Kingdom Transplant Support Service Authority (UKTSSA). *Lancet* **354** (**9185**): 1147–1152.

78 Briggs, J.D. and Jager, K. (2001). The first year of the new ERA-EDTA registry. *Nephrology, Dialysis, Transplantation* **16** (**6**): 1130–1131.

79 Bramham, K., Nelson-Piercy, C., Gao, H. et al. (2013). Pregnancy in renal transplant recipients: a UK national cohort study. *Clinical Journal of the American Society of Nephrology* **8** (**2**): 290–298.

80 Deshpande, N.A., James, N.T., Kucirka, L.M. et al. (2011). Pregnancy outcomes in kidney transplant recipients: a systematic review and meta-analysis. *American Journal of Transplantation* **11** (**11**): 2388–2404.

81 Sturgiss, S.N. and Davison, J.M. (1995). Effect of pregnancy on the long-term function of renal allografts: an update. *American Journal of Kidney Diseases* **26** (**1**): 54–56.

82 Salmela, K.T., Kyllonen, L.E., Holmberg, C., and Gronhagen-Riska, C. (1993). Impaired renal function after pregnancy in renal transplant recipients. *Transplantation* **56** (**6**): 1372–1375.

83 Rahamimov, R., Ben-Haroush, A., Wittenberg, C. et al. (2006). Pregnancy in renal transplant recipients: long-term effect on patient and graft survival. A single-center experience. *Transplantation* **81** (**5**): 660–664.

84 Josephson, M.A. (2011). Monitoring and managing graft health in the kidney transplant recipient. *Clinical Journal of the American Society of Nephrology* **6** (**7**): 1774–1780.

28 CHAPTER 28

Diabetes mellitus

Margaret Dziadosz and Ashley S. Roman

Department of Obstetrics and Gynecology, NYU School of Medicine, New York University, New York, NY, USA

CLINICAL SCENARIO

32-year-old G2P0010 at 14 weeks gestation presents for initial prenatal visit.

She has had limited medical care to date. On examination, you note that she is obese with a body mass index BMI of 45 kg m^{-2}. Doppler assessment of fetal heart rate (FHR) is 140 bpm. You decide to evaluate her glucose tolerance in addition to routine prenatal labs. Her one-hour glucose challenge test (50 g oral glucose load) returns 201 mg dl^{-1}.

Clinical questions

1. What are the different types of diabetes that may occur in pregnancy?

2. What causes gestational diabetes?

3. In pregnant patients, what are the best strategies for screening for diabetes?

4. What are the potential effects of diabetes on the fetus and how should the fetus be monitored?

5. In pregnancy, what are the blood sugar targets and how should diabetes be treated?

6. In pregnant women with diabetes, are there recommendations for delivery?

7. How should maternal blood glucose be monitored controlled during labor and delivery?

8. How should women be monitored in the post-partum period?

1. What are different types of diabetes that may occur in pregnancy?

Diabetes mellitus (DM) complicates approximately 6–7% of all pregnancies in the United States. The American Diabetes Association has classified glucose intolerance into three different types (Table 28.1). Gestational diabetes mellitus (GDM), or carbohydrate intolerance with onset or recognition during pregnancy, represents 90% of cases [1]. The White classification is another system for classifying diabetes in pregnancy (Table 28.2). White classification class A1 diabetes (GDMA1) represents pregnant women with gestational diabetes mellitus who are able to maintain glucose control with exercise and diet alterations. White classification class A2 diabetes (GDMA2) represents pregnant women with gestational diabetes who require medication therapy in order to maintain adequate glucose control.

The remaining 10% include both Type 1 and Type 2 diabetes mellitus. This cohort accounts for over eight million women in the US alone at any given time. Type 1 pregestational DM (DM1) occurs as the result of an autoimmune process that destroys pancreatic B cells, leading to a need for insulin therapy [2]. Type 2 pregestational DM (DM2) is characterized by peripheral insulin resistance and insufficiency. The rising epidemic of DM2 is associated with the increasing rate of obesity and metabolic syndrome.

2. What causes gestational diabetes?

Insulin resistance increase in pregnancy is largely related to an increase in placental hormones such as human placental lactogen (promotes lipolysis and decreased glucose uptake), prolactin, cortisol (insulin antagonist), tumor necrosis factor α, leptin, and placental growth hormone. Estrogen and progesterone further disrupt mechanisms of glucose and insulin [3]. Insulin sensitivity is greatest at the end of the first trimester, with the greatest risk of maternal hypoglycemia, and lowest insulin sensitivity in the third trimester, the time of greatest insulin requirement. A decrease in maternal exercise and an increase in caloric intake and altered adipose deposition compound glucose intolerance in pregnancy.

3. In pregnant patients, what are the best strategies for screening for diabetes?

All pregnant women who do not have a diagnosis of pregestational diabetes should be routinely screened for gestational diabetes at 24–28 weeks gestation. However, some debate exists over the optimal screening approach. The International Association of Diabetes and Pregnancy Study Groups (IADPSGs) recommend a one-step testing approach

Evidence-Based Obstetrics and Gynecology, First Edition. Edited by Errol R. Norwitz, Carolyn M. Zelop, David A. Miller, and David L. Keefe.

Table 28.1 American Diabetes Association three types of glucose intolerance

Classification	Mechanism of disease	No insulin required	Insulin required	Insulin required for survival
Type I diabetes mellitus	Immunologic destruction of pancreas	⟶	⟶	⟶
Type II diabetes mellitus	Resistance of pancreatic cells	⟶	⟶	
Gestational diabetes mellitus	Glucose intolerance not present prior to pregnancy	⟶	⟶	

Table 28.2 White classification for diabetes in pregnancy

Gestational diabetes mellitus (GDM)	
GDM A1	Controlled by diet, exercise
GDM A2	Requires medicotherapy
Pregestational diabetes mellitus	
A	Abnormal glucose tolerance at any age or duration treated only by nutritional therapy
B	Onset age ≥ 20 years and duration <10 years
C	Onset age 10–19 years and duration 10–19 years
D	Onset <10 years, duration >20 years, benign retinopathy, or hypertension (not pre-eclampsia)
D1	Onset <10 years
D2	Duration >20 years
D3	Benign retinopathy (microvascular)
D4	Hypertension (not pre-eclampsia)
R	Proliferative retinopathy or vitreous hemorrhage
F	Renal nephropathy and >500 mg dl^{-1} proteinuria
RF	Criteria met for both Type R and F
G	Multiple pregnancy failures
H	Evidence of arteriosclerotic heart disease
T	Prior renal transplantation

using the 75 g two-hour oral glucose tolerance test (GTT). A positive test results occurs if any single threshold is abnormal: fasting value 92 mg ml^{-1}, one-hour value 180 mg dl^{-1}, two-hour value 152 mg dl^{-1}.

The American College of Obstetricians and Gynecologists (ACOG) recommends the two-step approach. This involves a 50 g oral glucose challenge test (GCT), followed by a 100-g three-hour oral GTT in screen positive women (Table 28.3). A threshold of ≥130 mg dl^{-1} (7.5 mmol l^{-1}) to ≥140 mg dl^{-1} (7.8 mmol l^{-1}) may be used to determine candidates for the 3-hour oral GTT dependent on institutional preference [2]. If a patient has a value of ≥200 mg dl^{-1}, they do not require the 3-hour test for confirmation and are diagnosed with GDM.

For women at high risk of pregestational diabetes but who do not carry this diagnosis upon initiation of prenatal care, consideration should be given to screening for diabetes in the first trimester. Women with risk factors including obesity, known impaired glucose tolerance or a past history of GDM are candidates for early screening [4].

Early screening may include A1C analysis. A value >6.5% (>48 mmol mol^{-1}) is diagnostic of T2DM. In addition, a fasting glucose of >126 mg dl^{-1} or a GCT of >200 mg dl^{-1} are also diagnostic of T2DM [5].

4. What are the potential adverse effects of diabetes on the fetus and how should the fetus be monitored?

Adverse outcomes associated with DM in pregnancy include pre-eclampsia, hydramnios, macrosomia, or large for gestational age infant, maternal or infant birth trauma, operative delivery, neonatal respiratory problems, and metabolic complications such as hypoglycemia, hyperbilirubinemia, hypocalcemia, and erythremia, and fetal demise. In addition, if a mother is hyperglycemic during organogenesis, there is significantly increased risk of miscarriage and congenital anomalies [6–8].

Women with DM1, DM2, or GDM should be monitored more frequently during pregnancy. Visits are typically scheduled every two weeks until 28 weeks' gestation, after which it is common to monitor patients on a weekly basis. The goal of these visits is to assess glycemic control and adjust medications or diet as indicated.

Antepartum testing is recommended for all patients with DM in pregnancy.

Ultrasound examination in early gestation is recommended in cases of Type1 DM and Type2 DM to confirm viability and to assess for congenital anomalies. An additional ultrasound is recommended at 18–20 weeks for assessment of cardiac structure and normal organ development. Fetal echocardiogram should be considered in cases of Type1 DM and Type2 DM, as well as in any cases of suspected cardiac defects on routine ultrasonography [9–11].

Initiation of more frequent testing, including serial growth evaluation and nonstress test or biophysical profile should be considered at 32–34 weeks for women with pregestational DM [12]. Daily fetal movement counting is recommended for all women with DM in pregnancy. For women with poorly controlled GDM or women on medication treatment for GDM, fetal surveillance may be beneficial [13].

Table 28.3 Diagnostic criteria for three-hour 100 g oral GTT

	Glucose level			
	Carpenter and Coustan criteria		National Diabetes Data Group criteria	
	mg dl^{-1}	mmol l^{-1}	mg dl^{-1}	mmol l^{-1}
Fasting	95	5.3	105	5.8
One hour	180	10	190	10.6
Two hours	155	8.6	165	9.2
Three hours	140	7.8	145	8

5. In pregnancy, what are the blood sugar targets and how should diabetes be treated?

Target capillary glucose levels in pregnancy according to the American Diabetes Association and ACOG are listed below (Table 28.4). Glucose assessment should be performed at least fasting and three times daily in a postprandial pattern.

Continuous glucose monitoring has been considered for optimal glucose control in pregnancy and improved outcomes. Recent analysis shows higher mean glucose levels in the second and third trimester are associated with large-for-gestational-age (LGA) neonates during specific time periods in Type 1 DM. Continuous monitoring allows closer targeting of glucose control in order to prevent LGA neonates and macrosomia [14].

The mean goal of serum glucose levels is 100 mg dl^{-1}. The goal mean HgA1c as measured in pregnancy is 6.0%. HbA1c levels reflect glucose levels of the past two–three months, though this may vary in pregnancy due to changes in renal clearance and glomerular filtration rate (GFR). HbA1c 8% indicates mean glucose level of 180 mg dl^{-1}. Each 1% higher and lower than 8% reflect 30 mg dl^{-1} above or below 180 mg dl^{-1} [7]. With rising HbA1c, there is increased fetal anomalies, pre-eclampsia, preterm birth, LGA neonates, neonatal hypoglycemia, hyperbilirubinemia, birth trauma, neonatal intensive care unit (NICU) admission, and neonatal death. In Type 1 DM, HbA1c results are more related to adverse pregnancy outcomes than serial or continuous glucose monitoring [15].

Women require 1800–2500 kcal per day in pregnancy. This is approximately 300 kcal higher than in the non-pregnant state. Meal plans should include three meals daily and 2–4 snacks. Carbohydrates should make up 40% of daily intake, but 20% from proteins and 40% of remaining calories from fats (<10% unsaturated). Calories should be used at a rate of 10–20% for breakfast, 20–30% for lunch, 40–50% for dinner, and the remaining approximate 30% for snacks. Bedtime snacks prevent nighttime hypoglycemia and are recommended. Exercise can be of great value in pregnancy. It has shown to be safe and to lower glucose levels [16, 17].

Table 28.4 Target capillary glucose levels in pregnancy

Fasting	<90 mg dl^{-1}
Preprandial	<100 mg dl^{-1}
One hour postprandial	<140 mg dl^{-1}
Two hour postprandial	<120 mg dl^{-1}
2 a.m. – 6 a.m.	>60 mg dl^{-1}

Insulin is the standard drug for glucose management in pregnancy if nutritional therapy does not maintain normoglycemia [18]. It does not cross the placenta. The starting dose is typically 0.7–1.0 units kg^{-1} daily total, given in divided doses, with lower doses in the first trimester trending toward higher dose calculations for the third trimester. Needs in the first trimester average 0.7–0.8 U (kg/d)$^{-1}$ in the first trimester, which rise to 0.8–1 U (kg/d)$^{-1}$ in the second trimester, and 0.9–1.2 U (kg/d)$^{-1}$ in the third trimester.

Longer acting insulin such as neutral protamine hagedorn, or NPH (Humulin N, Novolin N), detemir (Levemir), glargine (Lantus) may be used once or twice daily in the morning or nighttime. Benefits of glargine include a steady state for 24 hours and no peak onset.

Short acting insulin such as lispro (HumaLog) and aspart (NovoLog) may be used at meal time due to rapid onset of action. Ideally, they should be administered immediately before eating, otherwise hypoglycemia should be cautioned. It is often paired with long acting insulin. Historically, regular insulin was used for day time control with meals, though its action of onset ranges between 30 and 60 minutes and it peak at 2–4 hours, which can be more difficult to utilize than more modern, rapid acting insulin options. It should be administered ½ hour prior to meals.

Continuous insulin infusion pumps may be used in DM1 or DM2 pregnant patients. They are helpful in detecting nocturnal glucose levels and decrease the need for serial insulin administration throughout the day.

Though insulin is the standard therapy for all diabetes mellitus in pregnancy, oral hypoglycemic agents are preferred by patients due to ease of administration, lower cost, and high acceptance rates. Glyburide use increased from 7.4% in 2000 to 64.5% in 2011 among pregnant patients.

Glyburide is a sulfonylurea that binds to pancreatic B cell receptors in increase insulin secretion and sensitivity in tissues. Metformin is a biguanide that inhibits hepatic gluconeogenesis and glucose absorption and stimulates glucose uptake in peripheral tissues [13, 18].

A meta-analysis of five randomized controlled trials comparing metformin to insulin showed less maternal weight gain, less pregnancy induced hypertension (PIH) with metformin use, but less preterm birth with insulin use [19]. A meta-analysis comparing glyburide to insulin use showed less maternal hypoglycemia with glyburide treatment, but less LGA, macrosomia, and neonatal hypoglycemia with insulin use [20].

In 2015, a 15 study systematic review and meta-analysis [18] evaluated treatment of gestational diabetes with either glibenclamide (glyburide), metformin, and insulin. Maternal outcomes considered included HbA1c levels, maternal hypoglycemia, pre-eclampsia, weight gain, mode of delivery, treatment failure of oral hypoglycemic medications, glucose measurements, PIH, and induction of labor. Fetal outcomes evaluated included gestational age at delivery, preterm birth, fetal birth weight, macrosomia, LGA, small-for-gestational-age (SGA), neonatal hypoglycemia, neonatal mortality, APGAR scores, obstetrical trauma, hyperbilirubinemia, need for respiratory support, stillbirth, and NICU admission.

When glyburide was compared with insulin, there was an increase in neonatal birth weight (pooled mean difference 109 g), macrosomia (Relative risk [RR] 2.62) and neonatal hypoglycemia (RR 2.02). Metformin treatment led to lower weight gain in pregnancy, less pregnancy related hypertension (RR 0.52), lower post prandial blood glucose measures, an increase in preterm birth (RR 1.5) and less severe neonatal hypoglycemia (RR 0.62) when compared to insulin treatment. When oral medications were compared, glyburide led to higher maternal weight gain during pregnancy, more macrosomia, and more LGA neonates. Glyburide had less treatment failure with need of insulin (23.5%) compared to metformin (26.8%). Maternal to fetal transfer of glyburide is the most likely reason for higher birth weights, risks of macrosomia and neonatal hypoglycemia. When considering outcomes, metformin is preferable to glyburide. Insulin remains the first choice agent due to the less macrosomia and preterm birth.

6. In pregnant women with diabetes, what are the recommendations for timing and mode delivery?

Though elective delivery prior to 39 weeks is discouraged by ACOG, late preterm (34 0/7–36 6/7 weeks of gestation) and early-term (37 0/7–38 6/7 weeks of gestation) birth may be considered in patients with DM. Women with GDM and good glucose control with either diet or medications can be managed expectantly. Poorly controlled GDM may be considered for late preterm or early term birth in an individualized manner. Women with pregestational DM that is well controlled are not candidates for early birth, however it is recommended to delivery prior to or at the estimated due date of 40 weeks of gestation. Women with pregestational DM and either vascular complications or poorly controlled disease are candidates for early term delivery and in rare, severe cases for late preterm delivery, though care should again be individualized [21, 22].

For women with macrosomia and estimated fetal weight > 4500 g, it is acceptable to offer primary cesarean delivery due to increased risk of shoulder dystocia and brachial plexus injury [23].

7. How should maternal blood glucose be monitored controlled during labor and delivery?

Maternal intrapartum hyperglycemia should be avoided in order to prevent neonatal hypoglycemia which can cause significant morbidity in early-life. The goal blood glucose level at the time of delivery is between 70 and 126 mg dl^{-1} [2, 24, 25]. Women with Type1 or Type2 DM and women with GDM treated with medications should have glucose level evaluated every 2–4 hours during the latent phase of labor. Glucose levels should be measured every one to two hours during the active phase and every hour during insulin infusion (Table 28.5). Women with GDM, controlled without medication may have blood glucose levels measured upon presentation and then every 4–6 hours [24].

An intravenous regular insulin infusion is recommended during induction of labor or active labor. Patients who use a continuous insulin pump may continue their basal rate during the intrapartum period.

Diabetic ketoacidosis is most commonly observed in DM1, though there is higher incidence in all women with DM during pregnancy at lower blood glucose levels of hyperglycemia and especially blood glucose levels >200 mg dl^{-1}, though may occur even with normoglycemia. Pregnant women are at increased risk in settings of infection, antenatal corticosteroid administration, poor medication compliance and insulin pump failure or non-compliance. Patient presentation ranges from normal complaints of pregnancy such as nausea and vomiting to altered mental status. It is important to realize that FHR deteriorations including decreased variability and late decelerations will improve with maternal treatment. Diagnosis includes pH <7.3, bicarbonate

Table 28.5 Regular insulin intrapartum infusion

Maternal glucose (mg dl^{-1})	Regular insulin (units per hour)	Intravenous solution
≤120	0	5% dextrose 0.45% NS
121–140	1.0	
141–160	2.0	0.45% NS
161–180	3.0	
181–200	4.0	
≥200	4.0 units subcutaneously; add short-acting or regular insulin IV push 2 units and titrate up	

level < 15 mEq l^{-1}, ketonuria, positive serum ketones, and an elevated anion gap.

Treatment includes vigorous intravenous hydration with isotonic NaCl, replacing 4–6 l in the first 12 hours (1 l first hour followed by 500 ml–1 l per hour for 2–4 hours, followed by 250 ml per hour thereafter). Insulin should be loaded at 0.2–0.4 U kg^{-1} and then maintained at 2–10 U per hour. Glucose replacement should be initiated with 5% dextrose in normal saline if or once glucose levels reach 250 mg dl^{-1}. It is important to monitor Potassium levels due to risk of hypokalemia and to start replacement with 20–30 mEq l^{-1} at normal serum levels. Bicarbonate levels may also needs to be replenished. It is recommended to add one ampule, or 44 mEq, to each l of saline if the pH is <7.1 [2]. Maternal morbidity is rare, though fetal morbidity rates are 10%.

8. How should women be monitored in the post-partum period?

Carbohydrate intolerance commonly resolves after delivery in cases of GDM. However, up to 1/3 of women with GDM will have impaired glucose tolerance six weeks post-partum and up to 50% will develop Type 2 DM in life [26–28]. Post-partum screening is recommended 6–12 weeks after delivery with GDM. Either a fasting glucose or a 75 g 2-hour oral GTT is recommended (Fasting 92 mg dl^{-1}, one hour 180 mg dl^{-1}, two hour 153 mg dl^{-1}). If normal, it is recommended to assess glycemic status every three years thereafter.

Post-partum testing has historically low completion rates. Point of care testing with HbA1c, random glucose or fasting glucose demonstrate higher completion rates and may be beneficial to consider in the post-partum period in addition to the oral GTT [29].

References

1 Wier, L.M., Witt, E., Burgess, J., and Elixhauser, A. (2006). *Hospitalizations Related to Diabetes in Pregnancy, 2008: Statistical Brief #102*. Healthcare Cost and Utilization Project (HCUP) Statistical Briefs. Rockville (MD): Agency for Health Care Policy and Research (US).

2 American College of Obstetricians and Gynecologists. ACOG Practice Bulletin. Pregestational Diabetes Mellitus No. 60. 2014.

3 Gilmartin, A.B., Ural, S.H., and Repke, J.T. (2008). Gestational diabetes mellitus. *Reviews in Obstetrics & Gynecology* **1** (**3**): 129–134.

4 American Diabetes Association (2011). Standards of medical care in diabetes – 2011. *Diabetes Care* **34** (**Suppl 1**): S11–S61.

5 Feldman, R.K., Tieu, R.S., and Yasumura, L. (2016). Gestational diabetes screening: The International Association of the Diabetes and Pregnancy Study Groups Compared with Carpenter-Coustan Screening. *Obstetrics and Gynecology* **127** (**1**): 10–17.

6 HAPO Study Cooperative Research Group (2009). Hyperglycemia and Adverse Pregnancy Outcome (HAPO) Study: associations with neonatal anthropometrics. *Diabetes* **58** (**2**): 453–459.

7 Landon, M.B., Mele, L., Spong, C.Y. et al. (2011). The relationship between maternal glycemia and perinatal outcome. *Obstetrics and Gynecology* **117**: 218–224.

8 Landon, M.B., Rice, M.M., Varner, M.W. et al. (2015). Mild gestational diabetes mellitus and long-term child health. *Diabetes Care* **38** (**3**): 445–452.

9 Nassr, A.A., El-Nashar, S.A., Shazly, S.A. et al. (2016). Expected probability of congenital heart disease and clinical utility of fetal echocardiography in pregnancies with pre-gestational diabetes. *European Journal of Obstetrics, Gynecology, and Reproductive Biology* **201**: 121–125.

10 Gabbay-Benziv, R., Reece, E.A., Wang, F., and Yang, P. (2015). Birth defects in pregestational diabetes: defect range, glycemic threshold and pathogenesis. *World Journal of Diabetes* **6** (**3**): 481–488.

11 Garg, S., Sharma, P., Sharma, D. et al. (2014). Use of fetal echocardiography for characterization of fetal cardiac structure in women with normal pregnancies and gestational diabetes mellitus. *Journal of Ultrasound in Medicine* **33** (**8**): 1365–1369.

12 Lalonde, A.B. (2005). Guidelines for vaginal birth after previous caesarean birth. *International Journal of Gynecology & Obstetrics*. **89** (**3**): 319–331.

13 American College of Obstetricians and Gynecologists (2001). ACOG practice bulletin. Clinical management guidelines for obstetrician-gynecologists. Number 30 September 2001 (replaces technical bulletin number 200, December 1994). Gestational diabetes. *Obstetrics and Gynecology* **98** (**3**): 525–538.

14 Law, G.R., Ellison, G.T., Secher, A.L. et al. (2015). Analysis of continuous glucose monitoring in pregnant women with diabetes: distinct temporal patterns of glucose associated with large-for-gestational-age infants. *Diabetes Care* **38** (**7**): 1319–1325.

15 Maresh, M.J., Holmes, V.A., Patterson, C.C. et al. (2015). Glycemic targets in the second and third trimester of pregnancy for women with type 1 diabetes. *Diabetes Care* **38** (**1**): 34–42.

16 American College of Obstetricians and Gynecologists (2015). ACOG Committee Opinion No. 650: physical activity and exercise during pregnancy and the postpartum period. *Obstetrics and Gynecology* **126** (**6**): e135–e142.

17 Taghiof, H., Rezai, S., and Henderson, C.E. (2015). Effect of an exercise intervention on gestational diabetes mellitus: a randomized controlled trial. *Obstetrics and Gynecology* **126** (**3**): 676.

18 Balsells, M., Garcia-Patterson, A., Sola, I. et al. (2015). Glibenclamide, metformin, and insulin for the treatment of gestational diabetes: a systematic review and meta-analysis. *BMJ (Clinical research ed)*. **h102**: 350.

19 Gui, J., Liu, Q., and Feng, L. (2013). Metformin vs insulin in the management of gestational diabetes: a meta-analysis. *PLoS One* **8** (**5**): e64585.

20 Zeng, Y.C., Li, M.J., Chen, Y. et al. (2014). The use of glyburide in the management of gestational diabetes mellitus: a meta-analysis. *Advances in Medical Sciences* **59** (**1**): 95–101.

21 American College of Obstetricians and Gynecologists (2013). ACOG Committee Opinion No. 560: Medically indicated late-preterm and early-term deliveries. *Obstetrics and Gynecology* **121** (**4**): 908–910.

22 Spong, C.Y., Mercer, B.M., D'Alton, M. et al. (2011). Timing of indicated late-preterm and early-term birth. *Obstetrics and Gynecology* **118** (**2 Pt 1**): 323–333.

23 Garabedian, C. and Deruelle, P. (2010). Delivery (timing, route, peripartum glycemic control) in women with gestational diabetes mellitus. *Diabetes & Metabolism* **36** (**6 Pt 2**): 515–521.

24 American Diabetes Association (2014). Standards of medical care in diabetes – 2014. *Diabetes Care* **37** (**Suppl 1**): S14–S80.

25 Blumer, I., Hadar, E., Hadden, D.R. et al. (2013). Diabetes and pregnancy: an endocrine society clinical practice guideline. *The Journal of Clinical Endocrinology and Metabolism* **98** (**11**): 4227–4249.

26 American College of Obstetricians and Gynecologists (2009). ACOG Committee Opinion No. 435: post-partum screening for abnormal glucose tolerance in women who had gestational diabetes mellitus. *Obstetrics and Gynecology* **113** (**6**): 1419–1421.

27 Russell, M.A., Phipps, M.G., Olson, C.L. et al. (2006). Rates of post-partum glucose testing after gestational diabetes mellitus. *Obstetrics and Gynecology* **108** (**6**): 1456–1462.

28 Bellamy, L., Casas, J.P., Hingorani, A.D., and Williams, D. (2009). Type 2 diabetes mellitus after gestational diabetes: a systematic review and meta-analysis. *Lancet* **373** (**9677**): 1773–1779.

29 Carson, M.P., Morgan, B., Gussman, D. et al. (2015). SUGAR: spotting undiagnosed glucose abnormal results – a new protocol to increase post-partum testing among women with gestational diabetes mellitus. *American Journal of Perinatology* **32** (**3**): 299–306.

29

CHAPTER 29
Thyroid disease

Sarah J. Kilpatrick

Department of Obstetrics and Gynecology, Cedars-Sinai Medical Center, Los Angeles, CA, USA

CLINICAL SCENARIO 1

A 29-year-old G2P0010 woman presents to your office for prenatal care at 12 weeks' gestation. She had a first trimester miscarriage two years ago. Her only medical problem that she is aware of is hypothyroidism for which she is on 75 mcg of synthroid per day. She has been experiencing significant nausea and some vomiting. She confirms she is taking her synthroid, but she also notes that she cannot tolerate her prenatal vitamins. She appears well, her current weight is 127 lbs and she reports that her pre-pregnancy weight was 130 lbs. Her BP is 110/66, HR 70, and urine dip is negative for protein, ketones, leukocytes, and esterase. Fetal heart tones are heard with the Doppler. The remainder of her physical exam is normal.

Background

Thyroid disease is the second most common endocrine disease encountered in pregnancy. Clinical hypothyroid disease, defined as elevated thyroid stimulating hormone (TSH) with suppressed free thyroid hormone (FT4) affects approximately 0.3–0.5% of pregnant women while it is likely that more than 1% of women come to pregnancy with a diagnosis of hypothyroid disease on T4 and are clinically euthyroid [1–3]. See Table 29.1 for the laboratory diagnostic criteria for thyroid diseases. The most common causes of hypothyroid disease in the US are Hashimoto's thyroiditis and treated Graves' disease. In contrast, worldwide the most common cause of hypothyroid disease is iodine deficiency. Subclinical hypothyroid disease, defined as an elevated TSH but normal FT4, is more prevalent in approximately 2% of pregnant women, and its impact on pregnancy is more controversial [1, 2]. Hyperthyroidism, largely Graves' disease, affects approximately 0.2% of pregnant women [1, 2, 4]. Uncontrolled hyper- or hypothyroid disease in pregnancy is associated with multiple adverse perinatal outcomes such as low birth weight, pre-eclampsia, and possibly fetal loss [5–7]. However, all of these are small, retrospective reports and certainly there will never be randomized trials comparing treated to untreated women with thyroid disease in pregnancy because it is well known that untreated clinical hyper- or hypothyroid disease in the nonpregnant individual leads to significant morbidity. Withholding appropriate treatment from pregnant women would be unacceptable. Hence clinical thyroid disease should be appropriately diagnosed and treated in pregnancy to achieve the best maternal and perinatal outcomes. Consistent with the concept that treatment of clinical thyroid disease optimizes outcome, women with treated clinical hypothyroid disease had no increase in adverse maternal or neonatal outcomes compared to women without thyroid disease in a large retrospective case-control study [3].

Understanding the effect of pregnancy on thyroid function is imperative to managing thyroid disease in the pregnant woman. Thyroid hormone production increases in pregnancy as does thyroid hormone binding globulin (TBG) beginning in early pregnancy because of the increase in estrogen and consequently the total (thyroxine (T4) and total triiodothyronine (T3) increase [8].Therefore unless one uses trimester specific norms, the typical laboratory norms are not relevant to pregnancy, although some have advocated to simply multiply the normal nonpregnant range of TT4 by 1.5 to adjust for pregnancy [9]. Free T4 and free T3 do not increase in pregnancy and may actually decrease slightly because of the increase in TBG. Traditionally, it has been thought that the normative range of TSH does not change in pregnancy. However, because human chorionic gonadotropin (HCG) is homologous to TSH with identical alpha subunits and similar beta subunits, as HCG rises in the first trimester it stimulates the TSH receptor which can result in transient increase in FT4 and suppression of TSH, particularly between 8 and 14 weeks' gestation. This normal suppression of TSH has led experts to suggest that in the

Evidence-Based Obstetrics and Gynecology, First Edition. Edited by Errol R. Norwitz, Carolyn M. Zelop, David A. Miller, and David L. Keefe.

Table 29.1 Thyroid dysfunction and TSH and FT4 Levels

Disorder	TSH	FT4
Clinical or Overt hypothyroidism	Elevated	Reduced
Subclinical hypothyroidism	Elevated	Normal
Hypothyroxinemia	Normal	Reduced
Clinical or Overt hyperthyroidism	Suppressed	Elevated
Subclinical hyperthyroidism	Suppressed	Normal
Hyperthyroxinemia	Normal	Elevated

Table 29.2 TSH trimester specific norms[a]

	TSH ($mIU\,l^{-1}$)
First trimester	0.1–2.5
Second trimester	0.2–3.0
Third trimester	0.3–3.0

[a]De Groot et al. 2012 [10] and Stagnaro-Green et al. 2011 [12].

first trimester the upper limit of normal TSH should be lowered to as low as 2.5–3.5 $mIU\,l^{-1}$ and several laboratories have adopted trimester specific norms for TSH [10–12]. See Table 29.2 for trimester specific norms for TSH and FT4. Suppression of TSH is more common in multiple gestations due to the increased placental mass, and occurred in 18% pregnancies in the first trimester; 10% of these women exhibited transient symptomatic thyrotoxicosis [13]. All of the women with symptomatic thyrotoxicosis had spontaneous remission within eight weeks [13]. Therefore, checking TSH in the first trimester should be reserved for the woman in whom one is concerned about clinical hyperthyroid or hypothyroid disease. Suppressed TSH in the first trimester is not diagnostic of hyperthyroidism.

Iodine clearance is significantly increased in pregnancy in part due to increased renal clearance from the increase in renal blood flow in pregnancy. This increase results in lower plasma iodide levels and in some women a small increase in thyroid gland size [14, 15]. In addition, there is significant transfer of maternal iodine to the fetus as the fetal thyroid gland becomes functional which makes maternal iodine supplementation important. The World Health Organization (WHO), The Institute of Medicine (IOM), the American Thyroid Association (ATA), and the Endocrine Society recommend that pregnant women receive a total of 220–250 μg of daily iodine [10, 16, 17]. Prenatal vitamins should have at least 150 μg per pill [18]. Potassium iodide is the preferred iodine source in pregnancy because it is a more consistent iodine source than kelp [17].

The fetal thyroid begins to use iodine by 10–12 weeks' gestation with subsequent production of T4 by 12–14 weeks' gestation [14]. T4 increases from approximately 18 week until 36 weeks when adult levels are reached [19]. Maternal T4 does cross the placenta in the first trimester and there is a correlation between fetal and maternal T4 levels [20]. Before 10–12 weeks' gestation, maternal T4 is the only source of T4 for the fetus and is important for brain development [21–23]. The most dramatic evidence of this is the resulting cretinism in neonates of mothers with severe iodine deficiency and subsequent severe untreated hypothyroidism during pregnancy [22]. Data in rats suggest that reduced maternal T4 in early pregnancy was associated with permanent abnormal brain development in fetuses [21]. Clearly clinical hypothyroidism should be avoided in pregnancy. Although TSH does not cross the placenta, thyrotropin-releasing hormone and TSH receptor immunoglobulins (thyroid stimulating immunoglobulin (TSI), thyroid-stimulating hormone-binding inhibitory immunoglobulin (TBII)) do cross the placenta.

Hypothyroid disease

Clinical questions

1. In pregnant women with hypothyroidism how should the dose of T4 be adjusted?

In a prospective series of women with primary hypothyroidism planning pregnancy, thyroid function was measured before and during pregnancy [24]. In 85% of the women it was necessary to increase the levothyroxine dose to offset the rise in TSH observed as early as five weeks' gestation. The authors recommended increasing the T4 dose by 30% by eight weeks gestation corresponding to their findings. The increased T4 requirement peaked at approximately 16 weeks' gestation with a mean 47% increase by that time. In another paper, only 38% of women with hypothyroid disease before pregnancy required an increase in their thyroid replacement. The only difference between the women requiring an increase and those not requiring one is that those women requiring an increase in dose had had a recent change in their medication dose before pregnancy [25]. Based on these two papers it seems reasonable to check a TSH in the first prenatal visit in women with hypothyroid disease and treat them appropriately. Alternatively, raising the replacement dose by 20–30% and repeating TSH in four weeks is acceptable.

2. In pregnant women being treated for hypothyroid disease what thyroid function and antibody tests should be performed? How frequently should they be repeated?

In general, it is sufficient to measure only TSH in women who come to pregnancy with a diagnosis of clinical hypothyroid disease. The goal during pregnancy is to maintain the TSH in the normal or pregnancy specific range throughout the entire pregnancy. As noted above many women will need an increase in their T4 replacement early in pregnancy. Once a change in dose has occurred it takes four to six weeks to see the maximum effect of the dose change. Therefore, there is no need to repeat the TSH until four weeks after a dose change. Once the TSH is in the desired range, then most obstetric experts recommend checking the TSH every trimester although endocrinologists recommend more frequent testing at every four to six weeks [11]. It is important to remember to reduce the dose of T4 postpartum if it was increased during pregnancy.

3. What are the implications of having thyroid peroxidase antibodies (TPOAb) present in pregnancy?

Approximately 5–10% of women are TPOAb positive in pregnancy [26–28]. The presence of TPOAb in pregnancy is associated with the development of postpartum thyroid dysfunction and the progression years later to hypothyroid disease [28, 29]. By seven years postpartum 46% of women positive for TPOAb in pregnancy developed thyroid dysfunction compared to only 1% of women without TPOAb during pregnancy [29]. However, how this should be managed in the pregnant patient is still unclear [28, 30]. For example, in a randomized controlled trial 55% of TPOAb positive women developed postpartum thyroid dysfunction, but that incidence was not significantly affected by prenatal iodine supplementation [28].

The relationship of prenatal TPOAb positivity and acute perinatal outcomes is not clear with multiple conflicting findings. A study from Finland reported a weak association between first trimester maternal TPOAb positivity and low birth weight (OR 1.7 (1.01–3.0)) but no association with preterm delivery (PTD) or small for gestational age [31]. They also found a significant increase in perinatal mortality with TPOAb positivity but no association between maternal clinical hypothyroid or subclinical hypothyroid disease and perinatal outcomes. Another study found no difference in perinatal outcomes between TPOAb positive, whether treated or not with T4, and TPOAb negative women [32]. TPOAb positivity in pregnancy has been associated with an increased risk in abruption [26, 33]; TPOAb positivity in the second but not first trimester of pregnancy was significantly associated with an increased risk for abruption, (OR 2.14; 0.18–3.89) although the percentage abruption was only 1.78% and 0.82% in the TPOAb positive and TPOAb negative women, respectively [33]. However, there are no reports evaluating the effect of any treatment to reduce this increased risk of abruption in TPOAb positive women. In other studies, no difference in PTD, hypertensive disorders, diabetes or preterm rupture of membranes was noted between TPOAb positive and negative women [26, 32, 34]. Although TPOAb cross the placenta there is no evidence that these antibodies affect fetal thyroid development [35].

TPOAb positivity has also been associated with a significant increase in the risk of miscarriage [36]. In a meta-analysis of case-control and cohort studies performed between 1991 and 2011, the OR was 3.90 (2.48–6.12) in cohort studies, and 1.80 (1.25–2.60) in case-control studies for miscarriage [36]. There are only two randomized controlled trials comparing treatment with thyroid hormone replacement to placebo in women with TPOAb [37, 38]. In one study over 900 pregnant women were screened for TPOAb, and the 115 women (11.7%) that were found to be positive for TPOAb were randomized to either supplemental T4 or no treatment [37]. Women were excluded for overt thyroid disease, so all women were euthyroid at the time of randomization. These two groups of women were then compared to TPOAb negative women. Untreated TPOAb positive women had significantly higher TSH and lower T4 by delivery than treated TPOAb positive or TPOAb negative women. Untreated TPOAb positive women had a significantly higher miscarriage rate than untreated or control women (13.8%, 3.5%, and 2.4%, respectively; $p < 0.05$). However, the Cochrane review disputes that this effect was significant (risk ratio of 0.25 (0.05, 1.15)) [39]. Preterm deliveries were significantly higher in untreated compared to treated and control women (22%, 7%, and 8% respectively; $p < 0.05$). Although 19% of the untreated women had an abnormally high TSH by the time of delivery, it is not clear how many developed clinical hypothyroid disease. The same investigators randomized women positive for TPOAb undergoing fertility treatment to levothyroxine or placebo and then compared these women to TPOAb negative women [38]. Pregnancy rates were similar between these groups. Although miscarriage was significantly higher in the TPOAb positive women compared to TPOAb negative women, oddly, they did not compare miscarriage rates between levothyroxine treated and placebo treated women, perhaps because the number in each group was so small. However, the 2011 meta-analysis concluded after analysis of the cohort, case-control and randomized control trials (RCTs), that presence of TPOAbs is associated with increased risk of miscarriage and, "there is evidence that treatment with levothyroxine can attenuate the risks" [36].

In a cohort study of 293 pregnant women, children's ability testing and IQ testing were compared in five-year-old children between those whose mothers who had TPOAb in pregnancy versus the mothers without TPOAb [30]. Even after controlling for maternal depression and current thyroid dysfunction, lower scores on the General Cognitive Scale remained significantly associated with TPOAb positivity during pregnancy, raising the concern that TPOAb positivity in pregnancy could be associated with impaired cognitive development in children [30]. There are no treatment trials as of 2016 testing whether treatment of TPOAb positive women during pregnancy impacts childhood outcomes.

4. Is subclinical hypothyroidism or hypothyroxinemia associated with poor perinatal or childhood outcomes?

In nonpregnant women subclinical hypothyroidism has been associated with eventual development of overt hypothyroidism, but data supporting associations with other morbidities such as development of abnormal lipids or cardiac disease are poor [40]. In addition, there are no data that support benefits of treatment with T4 in nonpregnant individuals with subclinical hypothyroidism [40]. Thus the interest in potential maternal effects of subclinical hypothyroidism has been focused on the fetal/neonatal effects. There are numerous conflicting retrospective and prospective series evaluating the potential associations of maternal subclinical hypothyroidism and perinatal and childhood outcomes [2, 41–45]. In a paper utilizing second trimester serum, 2.2% of the over 10 000 women screened were found to have elevated TSH [2]. These women were compared to those women with normal TSH and FT4 and there was no difference in miscarriage, hypertensive disease, diabetes, or PTD. In contrast, in screening over 17 000 pregnant women, those women with subclinical hypothyroidism had significantly higher rates of delivery less than 34 weeks (4% vs. 2.5%; $p = 0.01$), and abruption (1% vs. 0.3%; $p = 0.03$) compared to women with normal TSH [42]. In a case-control study comparing 11–13 week thyroid functions between 102 women who delivered before 34 weeks to 4318 women with a term delivery, no difference was reported in TPO antibody positivity, TSH or FT4 [41]. Utilizing the Swedish Medical Birth Register, a comparison of 8669 women reporting use of T4 during pregnancy to over 800 000 women who did not report use of T4, reported that pre-eclampsia was significantly higher in those women using T4 (1.32; 1.19–1.47) [46]. However, PTD was only marginally greater in the T4 treated women (OR 1.13; 1.03–1.25) and, neither small for gestational age, or birth weight <2500 g were significantly different between the groups. Subclinical hypothyroidism was not associated with development of gestational diabetes, but was associated with a significant increase in severe pre-eclampsia [44, 45]. Maternal hypothyroxinemia (FT4 subnormal but normal TSH) has not been shown to be associated with poor perinatal outcomes [47]. At a mean of 12 weeks, 1.3% of over 17 000 women had hypothyroxinemia and there was no difference in hypertensive disease, diabetes, PTD, or birth weight compared to women with normal thyroid function tests. In this same study women with subclinical hypothyroidism did have significantly higher PTD <34 weeks (4.3%) compared to women with normal thyroid function (2.5%) ($p = 0.005$). Thus the association between maternal elevated TSH or T4 treatment, with PTD or other obstetric complications appears to be negative or at least inconsistent.

Based on nonrandomized trial data the relationship between maternal subclinical hypothyroidism or hypothyroxinemia and childhood outcomes is even more unclear. A widely publicized study by Haddow reported that elevated maternal TSH in second trimester stored serum from 62 women was significantly associated with cognitive dysfunction in seven-year-old offspring [42]. Although the mean IQs were not significantly different, the children of the mothers with elevated TSH did significantly worse on 2/14 neurocognitive tests. In contrast, a much larger population based cohort study of over 2700 mothers and children reported no relationship between maternal TSH level and 18 or 30 month expressive language or nonverbal or verbal functioning [48]. In this study women with hypothyroidism were excluded. There is one prospective case-control study of 108 neonates whose mothers had FT4 in <10th percentile in the first trimester compared to controls with FT4 in the 50–90th percentiles [49]. The case neonates at three weeks of age had significantly worse score on only one variable (orientation) of a 7 variable neonatal behavioral assessment scale compared to the control neonates [49]. Severe hypothyroxinemia (FT4 <5th percentile in women with normal TSH) was significantly associated with expressive language delay and cognitive delay at 18 and 30 months [48]. A criticism of this paper is that all the childhood cognitive assessments were made by parents which could bias the results. However, if there is a significant relationship between reduced maternal thyroid function it makes more sense that low FT4 rather than elevated TSH would be the important variable because only T4 crosses the placenta [22]. These data are provocative and illustrate the need for randomized trials to test whether maternal treatment of either subclinical hypothyroidism or hypothyroxinemia would ameliorate childhood cognitive adverse outcomes.

Finally in 2017 the first large treatment trial of pregnant women with subclinical hypothyroidism was published [50]. Out of 97 226 pregnant women who were screened, 3.1% were identified with subclinical hypothyroidism. The 677 women who met inclusion criteria (singleton, <20 weeks gestation) were then randomized to placebo or levothyroxine and developmental testing was performed on their children annually until age 5. There was no difference in median IQ scores at five years of age between the placebo (94) and levothyroxine (97) exposed children. The results of this large randomized controlled trial that there was no difference in five-year-old IQ scores between those children of mothers with subclinical hypothyroidism treated with placebo compared to those treated with levothyroxine supports the current American College of Obstetricians and Gynecologists (ACOG) recommendation not to routinely screen pregnant women for subclinical hypothyroidism [51]. Of note, these investigators also screened for maternal hypothyroxinemia and randomized these woman to placebo versus levothyroxine and found no difference in five year old IQ scores in these children [50].

5. Is maternal subclinical hypothyroidism associated with later development of thyroid disease in women?

There are at least two reports that maternal subclinical hypothyroidism is associated with subsequent development of clinical hypothyroidism [43, 52]. There was an increase in the development of clinical hypothyroidism seven years after birth in a small study of 62 women who had subclinical hypothyroidism in pregnancy compared to controls with normal thyroid function (64% vs. 4%) [43]. A much larger study of over 5000 women followed for 20 years, found that overt hypothyroidism, subclinical hypothyroidism, and TPO antibody positivity in pregnancy were all significantly associated with development of thyroid disease [52]. These data suggest that if any of these diagnoses are made, the patient should be informed that she is at risk for later develop thyroid disease.

6. Should routine screening for hypothyroidism or subclinical hypothyroidism be offered in pregnancy?

The short answer is no, however it is illustrative to appreciate the historical debate on this question. Since the 1999 publication of the US paper suggesting an association between maternal low TSH and childhood cognitive impairment described above [43], routine screening of pregnant women for subclinical hypothyroid disease has been heavily debated [53]. This debate largely revolved around disparate view on two questions: (i) Are the data convincing that subclinical hypothyroidism in pregnancy is associated with poor cognitive childhood outcomes; and (ii) Is the fact that there are no trials showing any efficacy of treatment in pregnancy important before routine screening is implemented. Despite the publication of several national guidelines advocating for screening of only high-risk women, a high proportion of obstetric providers persist in screening low-risk women [16, 40, 51, 54, 55]. Any screening test should at least meet the following two criteria: it must address a common problem and there must be evidence that treatment ameliorates the problem. Between 2000 and 2011 there was no clear evidence that treatment of women with subclinical hypothyroidism with T4 had any positive effect on perinatal or neonatal morbidity. However, in 2012 the first randomized controlled trial comparing screening and then treating women with elevated TSH or low T4, to untreated women reported no difference in any outcomes including PTD or IQs in the three-year-old children [56]. Women were randomized to screen or control groups at initial prenatal visit. The women in the screened group were screened and if positive were treated with 150 mcg levothyroxine at a median gestational age of 13 3/7 weeks. The control women were screened, but the results were not reviewed until delivery and hence no treatment was provided. Five percent of over 20 000 women were screen positive. As of 2016 there are now clear data from a large randomized trial that show that treatment of either subclinical hypothyroidism or hypothyroxinemia does not affect childhood cognitive outcomes [50]. These findings definitively support existing guidelines by ACOG to not perform routine screening for hypothyroid disease in pregnancy [51, 54]. Not only is it still unclear if there are untoward effects on childhood cognitive outcomes of mothers with elevated TSH, there are now data to show that levothyroxine treatment does not affect childhood cognitive outcomes. To further illustrate the ambivalence over this question of routine screening of all pregnant women for thyroid disease, two recent guidelines written by endocrinologists for the Endocrine Society and the American Thyroid Association reflect different opinions [10, 12]. The ATA states that there are insufficient evidence to recommend for or against routine screening and the Endocrine Society states that they could not reach agreement on this topic with five authors for routine screening and eight authors with no recommendation [10–12].

Targeted screening for hypothyroid disease in pregnancy has been advocated by ACOG, The Endocrine Society and others [12, 16, 54]. Women that should be screened for hypothyroid disease include those women with a personal or strong family history of thyroid disease, a history of autoimmune disease such as Type 1 diabetes, have known positive TPO antibodies, goiter, or history of neck irradiation. Several studies have evaluated the efficacy of selected screening in pregnancy [27, 57]. In a prospective cohort study, pregnant women were screened for thyroid function and antibodies in the first trimester [57]. These results were compared between women with no high-risk history for thyroid disease and those women who were high-risk for thyroid disease. A total of 413 women (25%) were classified as high-risk. As expected significantly more high-risk women had elevated TSH (6.8% vs 1.0% $p<0.0001$). Although this validates the approach of screening only high-risk women, the authors pointed out that they would have missed the 0.3% of women in the low-risk group who had clinical hypothyroidism. Also of interest is that 23% of the women known to be on T4 were undertreated based on their elevated TSH. In a randomized controlled trial, over 4000 women in their first trimester were randomized to universal screening with TSH, FT4, and TPO antibodies versus testing only those women who were high-risk for thyroid disease [27]. In each group approximately 20% (21.1% and 19.9%) of women met criteria for being high-risk for thyroid disease and there was no difference in the percent of women who were euthyroid (approximately 97%) in each group. Hypothyroid was defined as TSH $>2.5\,\text{mIU}\,\text{l}^{-1}$ in TPOAb antibody positive women and these women were treated with levothyroxine. There were no women without TPOAb who had TSH $>5.9\,\text{mIU}\,\text{l}^{-1}$. There was no difference in perinatal adverse outcomes (including pre-eclampsia, miscarriage, gestational diabetes, and PTD) between the universal screen group and the test case finding group. However, the authors argue that screening the low-risk women picked up 2.8% with thyroid disease who were treated which might warrant screening low-risk women even if there is no difference in adverse perinatal outcomes.

7. Should women who are known to have subclinical hypothyroidism in pregnancy be treated with T4?

It is unclear whether treatment of women with subclinical hypothyroidism in pregnancy is warranted [10, 12]. The recent ATA guidelines concluded that there are insufficient data to recommend for or against treatment in women with subclinical hypothyroidism and negative TPO-ab but they do recommend treatment if TPO-ab are positive and a diagnosis of subclinical hypothyroidism has been made [12]. In contrast, the recent Society of Endocrinology guidelines recommend treatment regardless of presence of TPO-Ab although they acknowledge that the evidence to treat subclinical hypothyroidism in pregnancy when the TPO-Ab are negative is poor [10].

8. What is postpartum thyroiditis (PPT) and what are its predictors?

PPT can present as new onset of hypothyroidism or hyperthyroidism within the first year after delivery and occurs in approximately 7% of women living in iodine sufficient areas [16, 58]. The majority of women with PPT are TPOAb positive and 40% of women with TPOAb develop PPT [59, 60]. Therefore, the strongest predictor for PPT is the presence of TPOAb. PPT is typically transient. The hyperthyroid symptoms of PPT often present at approximately three months postpartum, are generally mild and last only a couple of months which distinguishes PPT from new onset Graves' disease. About 30% of women with PPT experience only hyperthyroid symptoms. Some women will exhibit hypothyroid symptoms after the initial hyperthyroidism while others exhibit only hypothyroid symptoms. The hypothyroid phase usually lasts only four to six months [61]. There are no trials that direct treatment of PPT. However, expert opinion suggests consideration of treatment of the hypothyroid phase if the TSH is >10 mIU l^{-1}, and consideration of propranolol for women with hyperthyroid symptoms [58]. If the woman is trying to conceive then treatment with synthroid is recommended for a TSH >4 mIU l^{-1} [58].

Conclusions

- Untreated clinical thyroid disease in pregnancy is associated with adverse perinatal and neonatal outcomes. Level of evidence: C; Class of recommendation: I.
- Whether subclinical hypothyroidism or hypothyroxinemia is associated with adverse neonatal or childhood outcomes is not clear. Level of evidence: B. Class of recommendation: II.
- Routine screening of all pregnant women for thyroid disease is not warranted because treatment trials show no effect of treatment. Level of evidence: A; Class of recommendation: I.

CLINICAL SCENARIO 2

A 37-year-old G2P1 woman is referred to you from her endocrinologist for prenatal care at 15 weeks' gestation. She has Grave's disease and is currently on propothiouricil (PTU) 100 mg three times per day. She has had Graves' disease for about a year and that she thinks it is controlled. She said her endocrinologist is uncomfortable managing her while she is pregnant and suggested that she might need to stop her PTU because of risks to the fetus. She already had her first trimester screening and her dates were consistent with the first trimester ultrasound. She appears well, her current weight is 145 lbs and she reports that her pre-pregnancy weight was 141 lbs. Her BP is 118/66, HR 90, and urine dip is negative for protein, ketones, leukocytes, and esterase. Fetal heart tones are 160 bpm heard with the Doppler. The remainder of her physical exam is normal. She has no other medical problems. She is very concerned about her Graves' disease and the risk to her fetus and wants to know if she should stop her PTU.

Background

Hyperthyroid disease also called thyrotoxicosis occurs in approximately 1–2/2000 pregnancies and the most common etiology is Graves' disease accounting for 95% of cases [35, 62]. Transient gestational hyperthyroidism can occur in the first and second trimester, but resolves without treatment as discussed earlier. Other rarer causes of hyperthyroid disease include toxic multinodular goiter, single toxic adenoma, subacute thyroiditis, and iodide induced hyperthyroidism. Most women who present in pregnancy with hyperthyroid disease will have already been diagnosed. The incidence of newly diagnosed Graves' disease in pregnancy is only 0.05% [42]. The management of Graves' disease in pregnancy is complicated by the fact that the antibodies causing the maternal disease cross the placenta and consequently may affect fetal thyroid function. There are two types of antibodies: TSI, also called thyroid receptor stimulating antibodies (TRAb), and TSH inhibitory immunoglobulins. TSI typically have the more predominant effect and their half-life is 21 days and 1–17% fetuses of mothers with Graves' disease may develop fetal or neonatal Graves' disease due to transplacental antibody transfer [35, 63–65]. Subclinical hyperthyroid disease as mentioned above has no known deleterious effects on perinatal outcomes [42].

Clinical questions

1. What are the risks to the fetus and the pregnancy with inadequately treated hyperthyroidism or Graves' disease?

Inadequately controlled hyperthyroidism during pregnancy has only been studied with retrospective case series and likely will never be subject to randomized trials. Small series have reported an increased association of uncontrolled maternal hyperthyroid disease with pre-eclampsia, PTD, intrauterine growth restriction (IUGR), maternal heart failure, thyroid storm, and fetal demise [5, 7, 66]. Heart failure occurred in 9% of untreated women [66]. In a large obstetric service in over 27 years only 13 women were identified with thyrotoxicosis and heart failure [66]. Of interest, 85% of them had an identified instigating event such as sepsis, pre-eclampsia or hemorrhage, and the heart failure resolved in all women after treatment. Women with thyrotoxicosis should be adequately treated during pregnancy. Significantly elevated maternal thyroid hormone also appears to be deleterious to the fetus with a high rate of miscarriage found in women with thyroid hormone resistance [67].

2. What are the treatment options for a pregnant woman with Graves' disease?

As of 2016 there are no randomized trials evaluating treatment of hyperthyroid disease in pregnant women [68]. Therefore the following discussion is based on small series and expert opinion. There are three treatment options for Graves' disease: radioactive iodine, thyroidectomy, or medical antithyroid therapy. Radioactive iodine is contraindicated in pregnancy because the iodine crosses the placenta and destroys the fetal thyroid. Medical treatment is the first line therapy in pregnancy [16]. All three thioamides (PTU, methimazole (MMI), and carbimazole) can been used in pregnancy and although similar, each has its particular risks. Carbimazole is not available in the United States. See Table 29.3 for review of the thioamides. Thyroidectomy can be done in pregnancy, but is generally reserved for the woman who has failed medical treatment.

PTU and MMI inhibit thyroid hormone synthesis of T4 and T3 by blocking the organification of iodine and have been shown to have similar effect on fetal thyroid function based on cord blood analysis at delivery [69, 70]. Normalization of maternal thyroid function occurred in seven to eight weeks after starting either drug [71]. All thioamides cross the placenta and hence can cause the fetus to become hypothyroid. Because of the risk of fetal hypothyroidism, the goal of medical treatment is to only suppress maternal FT4 to the upper limits of normal to minimize the amount of drug to which the fetus is exposed [16, 69]. Both drugs are excreted in breast milk although in low concentrations with PTU at 0.025–0.077% and MMI at 0.47% [33]. All three thioamides are approved for breastfeeding by the American Association of Pediatrics [72, 73]. Because MMI and carbimazole have a small association with fetal aplasia cutis and choanal atresia, PTU has traditionally been the preferred medical treatment of Graves' disease in pregnancy [69, 74, 75]. The choanal atresia risk has been estimated to have an odds ratio of 18 in one case-control study [74], while the aplasia cutis risk of 0.03% is very low and not likely different than the general population risk of aplasia cutis [75]. However, recently the Food and Drug Administration (FDA) released an alert that noted that the risk of hepatotoxicity resulting in death and liver transplant was associated more strongly with PTU than with MMI [76]. The estimated frequency of severe liver failure associated with PTU is 0.1% [77]. Based on the hepatotoxicity of PTU but the increased teratogenicity of MMI, the FDA and others recommended in 2010 that MMI be the preferred drug in pregnancy but consider PTU in the first trimester [77, 78]. Follow-up of children of mothers treated with MMI during pregnancy and while breastfeeding as long as 74 months after birth did not find any negative effects on thyroid function or intellectual development [79]. Occasionally, propranolol is indicated to control the acute symptoms of hyperthyroidism in pregnancy. Short-term use of propranolol is acceptable.

3. Which thyroid function and antibody tests should be followed to manage her Graves' disease in pregnancy?

In a patient with hyperthyroid symptoms who has not previously been diagnosed with Graves' disease the following should be measured: TSH, FT4, thyroid receptor antibodies to confirm the diagnosis of Graves' disease. The presence of antibodies will help to distinguish Graves' disease from gestational transient hyperthyroid disease. Dosing of MMI or PTU should be titrated to maintain the FT4 in the high range of normal adjusting the dose q four to six weeks as needed. Once a diagnosis of Graves' disease has been made, the need to follow maternal TSI is controversial. Clearly level of TSI correlates to risk of fetal or neonatal Graves' disease, but it is not clear that there is a level below which the fetal risk is eliminated [63, 64]. In a review of 230 pregnancies of women with Graves' disease, although maternal level

Table 29.3 Thioamides

Drug	Mode of action	Dose	Adverse effects
Propylthiouracil	Inhibits thyroxine synthesis; inhibits peripheral conversion of thyroxine to triiodothyronine	Starting: 300–600 mg per day total in q 8 hr. dosing; maintenance: 50–100 mg per day total in q 8 hr. dosing	Rash, fever, agranulocytosis, hepatic failure (higher for PTU than other thioamides)
Carbimazole	Inhibits thyroxine synthesis	Starting: 20–60 mg per day total in q 6–8 hr. dosing; maintenance: 5–20 mg per day total in q 6–8 hr. dosing	Rash, fever, agranulocytosis, hepatic failure, aplasia cutis and methimazole embryopathy
Methimazole	Inhibits thyroxine synthesis	Starting: 15–60 mg per day total in q 8 hr. dosing; maintenance: 5–15 mg per day total in q 8 hr. dosing	Rash, fever, agranulocytosis, hepatic failure, aplasia cutis and methimazole embryopathy

of TSI was significantly associated with risk of neonatal thyroid dysfunction, most of the neonates with IUGR and one third of the neonates with overt thyrotoxicosis occurred in mothers with low TSI [63]. In a retrospective review of 35 live births from 29 women with Graves' disease, there were six neonates with Graves' disease. Using a TSI Index units of >5 (normal was IU ≤ 1.3) there was 100% sensitivity, 76% specificity, 40% positive predictive value, and 100% negative predictive value for neonatal thyrotoxicosis [64]. Of interest five of the six neonates had fetal tachycardia and the fetus that did not have tachycardia had a mother with a prior neonate with thyrotoxicosis. These authors recommended that all women with Graves' disease have TSI measured and that if greater than 5 IU, neonatology be informed. Because of the increased risk of fetal Graves' with elevated TSI, Endocrine Society guidelines recommend checking TRAb prior to pregnancy or by the end of the second trimester in women with Graves' disease or a history of treated Graves' disease, or with a prior neonate with Graves' disease [10, 16]. Others have argued that any history of maternal Graves' disease should be communicated to the pediatric or neonatal service independent of what the level of TRAb is during the pregnancy, and that all such pregnancies should be followed closely for signs of fetal thyroid disease, and therefore if diagnosis of Graves' is confirmed there is no need to routinely check TSI [4]. Rather, TSI should be reserved for those women at highest risk for fetal thyrotoxicosis (history of previous baby with thyrotoxicosis) or those women who we may forget are at risk (Graves' disease treated with surgery or radioactive iodine). Women with prior treatment for Graves' disease who are on no antithyroid therapy during pregnancy may be at higher risk for having a fetus with thyrotoxicosis because of the exposure of the fetus to TSI not mitigated by antithyroid medication [80].

4. How should the fetus be followed in the woman with Graves' disease?

There is a risk of fetal or neonatal Graves' disease due to the transplacental passage of TSI, and a risk of fetal hypothyroidism due to the transplacental passage of thioamides if used. Fetal or neonatal thyrotoxicosis has been reported to occur in 1–17% of pregnancies in women with Graves' disease [63–65]. There was 13% incidence of neonatal hyperthyroid disease and 3% neonatal hypothyroidism in babies of mothers with Graves' disease [63]. Therefore, antenatal testing should be aimed at identification of possible fetal hyper- or hypothyroid disease. Markers of fetal thyrotoxicosis include IUGR, hydrops due to cardiac failure, and tachycardia. Goiter can also be a sign of either fetal hypothyroidism due to overtreatment with thioamides or fetal thyrotoxicosis from the TSI. Fetal goiter occurred in two of 26 pregnancies and one was associated with fetal hypothyroidism and the other with fetal hyperthyroidism [80]. Signs of neonatal thyrotoxicosis are similar and also include tremulousness, excessive appetite, cardiomegaly, and heart failure. There are no randomized trials to direct the appropriate antenatal evaluation of pregnancy in the woman with Graves' disease. In general ultrasound should be used at appropriate intervals to document fetal growth and assess the fetal neck for any evidence of goiter. The best intervals are not clear although one series performed ultrasound monthly to fetal growth, fetal neck, and fetal heart rate [80].

5. How would you diagnosis and treat fetal thyroid disease in pregnancy?

If fetal tachycardia, IUGR, or hydrops occur, then fetal thyrotoxicosis must be considered. In the presence of the fetal goiter, fetal hyperthyroidism and fetal hypothyroidism must be ruled out. Depending on the gestational age at which these signs occur the options include delivery, fetal cordocentesis, or empiric treatment. There are several case reports using fetal cordocentesis to obtain fetal T4 to both confirm fetal thyrotoxicosis and to direct maternal treatment with PTU to control the fetal thyrotoxicosis [80–82]. The largest series reported on 26 fetuses of 18 women with Graves' disease [80]. Their protocol called for offering umbilical cord blood sampling on any pregnancy that had elevated TSI, fetal tachycardia, fetal goiter, IUGR, or hydrops. Twelve pregnancies (12/26) had none of these abnormalities, while 14 met at least one of the criteria. No fetus had IUGR or hydrops. Only nine women of the 14 agreed to umbilical cord blood sampling. Four fetuses had normal thyroid functions, two were hyperthyroid and three were hypothyroid. There were two goiters and one fetus had thyrotoxicosis and the other had hypothyroid disease. These authors treated the three hypothyroid fetuses by reducing or stopping the maternal PTU and at least one of the mothers was clearly over treated with PTU so this complication could have been avoided. Both hyperthyroid fetuses had mothers who had had definitive treatment of their Graves' disease before pregnancy and were on synthroid only. For these women the authors started PTU. All of the fetuses requiring treatment had subsequent umbilical cord blood sampling to manage the treatment. All fetuses improved with treatment and goiters resolved before delivery [80].

6. Is hyperemesis gravidarum associated with hyperthyroidism?

Multiple reports have documented transient hyperthyroidism in women with hyperemesis [83–85]. Evidence of hyperthyroidism may occur in 70% of women with hyperemesis [84] and in women without hyperemesis as well. In all reports this hyperthyroidism resolved without treatment typically by 18–20 weeks gestation [83]. Transient hyperthyroidism of pregnancy, which occurs only in the first and second trimester, appears to be due to the elevated HCG which because of its homology to TSH acts to stimulate the TSH receptor in the thyroid resulting in hyperthyroidism. This does not require treatment and may be distinguished from true hyperthyroidism by: no evidence of prepregnancy hyperthyroidism, absence of any physical signs of hyperthyroidism, and negative thyroid antibodies [83]. However, because this is a benign condition with resolves on its own, routine thyroid function testing in women with hyperemesis is not indicated because no intervention is warranted. Despite this Endocrine Society guidelines suggest testing all women with hyperemesis for thyroid disease [16].

7. How would you assess a thyroid nodule in pregnancy?

In areas of iodine deficiency thyroid nodules have been reported to have an incidence as high as 15% and may increase in size during the pregnancy [86]. Less is known about incidence in iodine sufficient areas. Less than 20% of thyroid nodules in nonpregnant women are malignant but 39–50% of nodules were found in pregnancy to be malignant [87, 88]. However, data suggest that outcomes of thyroid cancer in pregnancy are no different than those in nonpregnant women [89]. A reasonable approach to assessment of a thyroid nodule was presented by Stagnaro-Green, 2011 [12]. Thyroid functions should be sent and a neck ultrasound should be followed by a fine needle aspirate and biopsy (FNAB) which has not been shown to have any increased risks in pregnancy. Depending on the results of the FNAB and in consultation with endocrinology and or surgery the appropriate management plan can be made which could include thyroid suppression, partial or total thyroidectomy during the pregnancy or postpartum depending on gestational age at diagnosis and type of thyroid cancer.

If a cancer is diagnosed, the decision to treat in pregnancy vs. wait until postpartum vs. terminate pregnancy to begin cancer treatments soon is based on balancing gestational age, cancer type, and the woman's choice.

Conclusions

• Hyperthyroid disease which is usually Graves' disease should be appropriately treated in pregnancy and medical treatment is preferred in pregnancy. Level of evidence: B; Class of recommendation: I.

• TSI cross the placenta and neonates of mothers with Graves' disease are at risk for thyroid dysfunction. Level of evidence: A. Class of recommendation: I.

• If Graves' disease is being treated with antithyroid medication the goal is to minimize the fetus to exposure from such medications because PTU and MMI cross the placenta and affect fetal thyroid function. Therefore maternal FT4 levels should be maintained in the high normal range. Level of evidence: B; Class of recommendation: I.

• High levels of maternal TSI increase the risk of fetal or neonatal Graves' disease. Level of evidence: A; Class of recommendation: I.

• The pediatric or neonatal care team should always be informed of maternal hyperthyroid disease. Level of evidence: C. Class of recommendation: IIa.

References

1 Casey, B.M., Dashe, J.S., Wells, C.E. et al. (2005). Subclinical hypothyroidism and pregnancy outcomes. *Obstet. Gynecol.* **105**: 239–245.

2 Cleary-Goldman, J., Malone, F.D., Lambert-Messerlian, G. et al. (2008). Maternal thyroid hypofunction and pregnancy outcome. *Obstet. Gynecol.* **112**: 85–92.

3 Tan, T.O., Cheng, Y.W., and Caughey, A.B. (2006). Are women who are treated for hypothyroidism at risk for pregnancy complications. *Am. J. Obstet. Gynecol.* **194**: e1–e3.

4 Ecker, J.L. and Musci, T.J. (1997). Treatment of thyroid disease in pregnancy. *Obstet. Gynecol. Clin. North Am.* **24**: 575–589.

5 Davis, L.E., Lucas, M.J., Hankins, G.D. et al. (1989). Thyrotoxicosis complicating pregnancy. *Am. J. Obstet. Gynecol.* **160**: 63–70.

6 Leung, A.S., Millar, L.K., Koonings, P.P. et al. (1993). Perinatal outcome in hypothyroid pregnancies. *Obstet. Gynecol.* **81**: 349–353.

7 Millar, L.K., Wing, D.A., Leung, A.S. et al. (1994). Low birth weight and pre-eclampsia in pregnancies complicated by hyperthyroidism. *Obstet. Gynecol.* **84**: 946–949.

8 Glinoer, D. (1999). What happens to the normal thyroid during pregnancy. *Thyroid* **9**: 631–635.

9 LeBeau, S.O. and Mandel, S.J. (2006). Thyroid disorders during pregnancy. *Endocrinol. Metab. Clin. North Am.* **35**: 117–136.

10 De Groot, L., Abalovich, M., Alexander, E.K. et al. (2012). Management of thyroid dysfunction during pregnancy and postpartum: an Endocrine Society Clinical Practice Guideline. *J. Clin. Endocrinol. Metab.* **97**: 2543–2565.

11 Lazarus, J.H. (2011). Thyroid function in pregnancy. *Br. Med. Bull.* **97**: 137–148.

12 Stagnaro-Green, A., Abalovich, M., Alexander, E. et al. (2011). Guidelines of the American Thyroid Association for the diagnosis and management of thyroid disease during pregnancy and postpartum. *Thyroid* **21**: 1081–1125.

13 Glinoer, D., De Nayer, P., Robyn, C. et al. (1993). Serum levels of intact human chorionic gonadotropin (HCG) and its free alpha and beta subunits, in relation to maternal thyroid stimulation during normal pregnancy. *J. Endocrinol. Invest.* **16**: 881–888.

14 Burrow, G.N., Fisher, D.A., and Larsen, P.R. (1994). Maternal and fetal thyroid function. *N. Engl. J. Med.* **331**: 1072–1078.

15 Rasmussen, N.G., Hornnes, P.J., and Hegedus, L. (1989). Ultrasonographically determined thyroid size in pregnancy and post partum: the goitrogenic effect of pregnancy. *Am. J. Obstet. Gynecol.* **160**: 1216–1220.

16 Abalovich, M., Amino, N., Barbour, L.A. et al. (2007). Management of thyroid dysfunction during pregnancy and postpartum: an endocrine society clinical practice guideline. *J. Clin. Endocrinol. Metab.* **92**: S1–S47.

17 Leung, A.M., Pearce, E.N., and Braverman, L.E. (2009). Iodine content of prenatal multivitamins in the United States. *N. Engl. J. Med.* **360**: 939–940.

18 American Thyroid Association Public Health CommitteeBecker, D.V., Braverman, L.E., Delange, F. et al. (2006). Iodine supplementation for pregnancy and lactation-United States and Canada: recommendations of the American Thyroid Association. *Thyroid* **16**: 949–951.

19 Radunovic, N., Dumez, Y., Nastic, D. et al. (1991). Thyroid function in fetus and mother during the second half of normal pregnancy. *Biol. Neonate* **59**: 139–148.

20 Calvo, R.M., Jauniaux, E., Gulbis, B. et al. (2002). Fetal tissues are exposed to biologically relevant free thyroxine concentrations during early phases of development. *J. Clin. Endocrinol. Metab.* **87**: 1768–1777.

21 Auso, E., Lavado-Autric, R., Cuevas, E. et al. (2004). A moderate and transient deficiency of maternal thyroid function at the beginning of fetal neocorticogenesis alters neuronal migration. *Endocrinology* **145**: 4037–4047.

22 Morreale de Escobar, G., Obregón, M.J., and Escobar del Rey, F. (2000). Is neuropsychological development related to maternal hypothyroidism or to maternal hypothyroxinemia. *J. Clin. Endocrinol. Metab.* **85**: 3975–3987.

23 Vulsma, T., Gons, M.H., and de Vijlder, J.J. (1989). Maternal-fetal transfer of thyroxine in congenital hypothyroidism due to a total organification defect or thyroid agenesis. *N. Engl. J. Med.* **321**: 13–16.

24 Alexander, E.K., Marqusee, E., Lawrence, J. et al. (2004). Timing and magnitude of increases in levothyroxine requirements during pregnancy in women with hypothyroidism. *N. Engl. J. Med.* **351**: 241–249.

25 Kothari, A. and Girling, J. (2008). Hypothyroidism in pregnancy pre-pregnancy thyroid status influences gestational thyroxine requirements. *BJOG* **115**: 1704–1708.

26 Abbassi-Ghanavati, M., Casey, B.M., Spong, C.Y. et al. (2010). Pregnancy outcomes in women with thyroid peroxidase antibodies. *Obstet. Gynecol.* **116**: 381–386.

27 Negro, R., Schwartz, A., Gismondi, R. et al. (2010). Universal screening versus case finding for detection and treatment of thyroid hormonal dysfunction during pregnancy. *J. Clin. Endocrinol. Metab.* **95**: 1699–1707.

28 Nohr, S.B., Jorgensen, A., Pedersen, K.M., and Laurberg, P. (2000). Postpartum thyroid dysfunction in pregnant thyroid peroxidase antibody-positive women living in an area with mild to moderate iodine deficiency: is iodine supplementation safe. *J. Clin. Endocrinol. Metab.* **85**: 3191–3198.

29 Premawardhana, L.D., Parkes, A.B., Ammari, F. et al. (2000). Postpartum thyroiditis and long-term thyroid status: prognostic influence of thyroid peroxidase antibodies and ultrasound echogenicity. *J. Clin. Endocrinol. Metab.* **85**: 71–75.

30 Pop, V.J., de Vries, E., van Baar, A.L. et al. (1995). Maternal thyroid peroxidase antibodies during pregnancy: a marker of impaired child development. *J. Clin. Endocrinol. Metab.* **80**: 3561–3566.

31 Mannisto, T., Vaarasmaki, M., Pouta, A. et al. (2009). Perinatal outcome of children born to mothers with thyroid dysfunction or antibodies: a prospective population-based cohort study. *J. Clin. Endocrinol. Metab.* **94**: 772–779.

32 Debieve, F., Duliere, S., Bernard, P. et al. (2009). To treat or not to treat euthyroid autoimmune disorder during pregnancy. *Gynecol. Obstet. Invest.* **67**: 178–182.

33 Haddow, J.E., McClain, M.R., Palomaki, G.E. et al. (2011). Thyroperoxidase and thyroglobulin antibodies in early pregnancy and placental abruption. *Obstet. Gynecol.* **117**: 287–292.

34 Haddow, J.E., Cleary-Goldman, J., McClain, M.R. et al. (2010). Thyroperoxidase and thyroglobulin antibodies in early pregnancy and preterm delivery. *Obstet. Gynecol.* **116**: 58–62.

35 Girling, J.C. (2006). Thyroid disorders in pregnancy. *Curr. Obstet. Gynaecol.* **16**: 47–53.

36 Thangaratinam, S., Tan, A., Knox, E. et al. (2011). Association between thyroid autoantibodies and miscarriage and preterm birth: meta-analysis of evidence. *BMJ* **342**: d2616.

37 Negro, R., Formoso, G., Mangieri, T. et al. (2006). Levothyroxine treatment in euthyroid pregnant women with autoimmune thyroid disease effects on obstetrical complications. *J. Clin. Endocrinol. Metab.* **91**: 2587–2591.

38 Negro, R., Mangieri, T., Coppola, L. et al. (2005). Levothyroxine treatment in thyroid peroxidase antibody-positive women undergoing assisted reproduction technologies: a prospective study. *Hum. Reprod.* **20**: 1529–1533.

39 Reid, S.M., Middleton, P., Cossich, M.C., and Crowther, C.A. (2010). Interventions for clinical and subclinical hypothyroidism in pregnancy. *Cochrane Database Syst. Rev.* (**7**): CD007752. doi: 10.1002/14651858.CD007752.pub3.

40 Surks, M.I., Ortiz, E., Daniels, G.H. et al. (2004). Subclinical thyroid disease: scientific review and guidelines for diagnosis and management. *JAMA* **291**: 228–238.

41 Ashoor, G., Maiz, N., Rotas, M. et al. (2011). Maternal thyroid function at 11–13 weeks of gestation and spontaneous preterm delivery. *Obstet. Gynecol.* **117**: 293–298.

42 Casey, B.M., Dashe, J.S., Wells, C.E. et al. (2006). Subclinical hyperthyroidism and pregnancy outcomes. *Obstet. Gynecol.* **107**: 337–341.

43 Haddow, J.E., Palomaki, G.E., Allan, W.C. et al. (1999). Maternal thyroid deficiency during pregnancy and subsequent neuropsychological development of the child. *N. Engl. J. Med.* **341**: 549–555.

44 Tudela, C.M., Casey, B.M., McIntire, D.D., and Cunningham, F.G. (2012). Relationship of subclinical thyroid disease to the incidence of gestational diabetes. *Obstet. Gynecol.* **119**: 983–988.

45 Wilson, K.L., Casey, B.M., McIntire, D.D. et al. (2012). Subclinical thyroid disease and the incidence of hypertension in pregnancy. *Obstet. Gynecol.* **119**: 315–320.

46 Wikner, B.N., Sparre, L.S., Stiller, C.O. et al. (2008). Maternal use of thyroid hormones in pregnancy and neonatal outcome. *Acta Obstet. Gynecol. Scand.* **87**: 617–627.

47 Casey, B.M., Dashe, J.S., Spong, C.Y. et al. (2007). Perinatal significance of isolated maternal hypothyroxinemia identified in the first half of pregnancy. *Obstet. Gynecol.* **109**: 1129–1135.

48 Henrichs, J., Bongers-Schokking, J.J., Schenk, J.J. et al. (2010). Maternal thyroid function during early pregnancy and cognitive

functioning in early childhood: the generation R study. *J. Clin. Endocrinol. Metab.* **95**: 4227–4234.

49 Kooistra, L., Crawford, S., van Baar, A.L. et al. (2006). Neonatal effects of maternal hypothyroxinemia during early pregnancy. *Pediatrics* **117**: 161–167.

50 Casey, B.M., Thom, E.A., Peaceman, A.M. et al. (2017). Treatment of subclinical hypothyroidism or hypothyroxinemia in pregnancy. *New Eng. J. Med.* **376**: 815–825.

51 American College of Obstetrics and Gynecologists (2015). ACOG Practice Bulletin 148. Thyroid disease in pregnancy. *Obstet. Gynecol.* **125**: 996–1005.

52 Mannisto, T., Vaarasmaki, M., Pouta, A. et al. (2010). Thyroid dysfunction and autoantibodies during pregnancy as predictive factors of pregnancy complications and maternal morbidity in later life. *J. Clin. Endocrinol. Metab.* **95**: 1084–1094.

53 Gyamfi, C., Wapner, R.J., and D'Alton, M.E. (2009). Thyroid dysfunction in pregnancy the basic science and clinical evidence surrounding the controversy in management. *Obstet. Gynecol.* **113**: 702–707.

54 American College of Obstetrics and Gynecologists (2007). ACOG committee opinion no. 381: subclinical hypothyroidism in pregnancy. *Obstet. Gynecol.* **110**: 959–960.

55 Haddow, J.E., McClain, M.R., Palomaki, G.E. et al. (2006). Screening for thyroid disorders during pregnancy: results of a survey in Maine. *Am. J. Obstet. Gynecol.* **194**: 471–474.

56 Lazarus, J.H., Bestwick, J.P., Channon, S. et al. (2012). Antenatal thyroid screening and childhood cognitive function. *N. Engl. J. Med.* **366**: 493–501.

57 Vaidya, B., Anthony, S., Bilous, M. et al. (2007). Detection of thyroid dysfunction in early pregnancy universal screening or targeted high-risk case finding. *J. Clin. Endocrinol. Metab.* **92**: 203–207.

58 Stagnaro-Green, A. (2002). Clinical review 152 postpartum thyroiditis. *J. Clin. Endocrinol. Metab.* **87**: 4042–4047.

59 Amino, N., Mori, H., Iwatani, Y. et al. (1982). High prevalence of transient post-partum thyrotoxicosis and hypothyroidism. *N. Engl. J. Med.* **306**: 849–852.

60 Premawardhana, L.D., Parkes, A.B., John, R. et al. (2004). Thyroid peroxidase antibodies in early pregnancy utility for prediction of postpartum thyroid dysfunction and implications for screening. *Thyroid* **14**: 610–615.

61 Stagnaro-Green, A. (2004). Postpartum thyroiditis. *Best Pract. Res. Clin. Endocrinol. Metab.* **18**: 303–316.

62 Marx, H., Amin, P., and Lazarus, J.H. (2008). Hyperthyroidism and pregnancy. *BMJ* **336**: 663–667.

63 Mitsuda, N., Tamaki, H., Amino, N. et al. (1992). Risk factors for developmental disorders in infants born to women with Graves' disease. *Obstet. Gynecol.* **80**: 359–364.

64 Peleg, D., Cada, S., Peleg, A., and Ben-Ami, M. (2002). The relationship between maternal serum thyroid-stimulating immunoglobulin and fetal and neonatal thyrotoxicosis. *Obstet. Gynecol.* **99**: 1040–1043.

65 Weetman, A.P. (2000). Graves' disease. *N. Engl. J. Med.* **343**: 1236–1248.

66 Sheffield, J.S. and Cunningham, F.G. (2004). Thyrotoxicosis and heart failure that complicate pregnancy. *Am. J. Obstet. Gynecol.* **190**: 211–217.

67 Anselmo, J., Cao, D., Karrison, T. et al. (2004). Fetal loss associated with excess thyroid hormone exposure. *JAMA* **292**: 691–695.

68 Earl, R., Crowther, C.A., and Middleton, P. (2010). Interventions for preventing and treating hyperthyroidism in pregnancy. *Cochrane Database Syst. Rev.* (**9**): CD008633. doi: 10.1002/14651858.CD008633.pub2.

69 Mandel, S.J., Brent, G.A., and Larsen, P.R. (1994). Review of antithyroid drug use during pregnancy and report of a case of aplasia cutis. *Thyroid* **4**: 129–133.

70 Momotani, N., Noh, J.Y., Ishikawa, N., and Ito, K. (1997). Effects of propylthiouracil and methimazole on fetal thyroid status in mothers with Graves' hyperthyroidism. *J. Clin. Endocrinol. Metab.* **82**: 3633–3636.

71 Wing, D.A., Millar, L.K., Koonings, P.P. et al. (1994). A comparison of propylthiouracil versus methimazole in the treatment of hyperthyroidism in pregnancy. *Am. J. Obstet. Gynecol.* **170**: 90–95.

72 American Academy of Pediatrics Committee on Drugs (2001). Transfer of drugs and other chemicals into human milk. *Pediatrics* **108**: 776–789.

73 Azizi, F. (1996). Effect of methimazole treatment of maternal thyrotoxicosis on thyroid function in breast-feeding infants. *J. Pediatr.* **128**: 855–858.

74 Barbero, P., Valdez, R., Rodríguez, H. et al. (2008). Choanal atresia associated with maternal hyperthyroidism treated with methimazole a case-control study. *Am. J. Med. Genet. A* **146A**: 2390–2395.

75 Van Dijke, C.P., Heydendael, R.J., and De Kleine, M.J. (1987). Methimazole, carbimazole, and congenital skin defects. *Ann. Intern. Med.* **106**: 60–61.

76 U.S. Food and Drug Administration (2010. Available from: http://www.fda.gov/Drugs/DrugSafety/PostmarketDrugSafety InformationforPatientsandProviders/DrugSafetyInformationfor HeathcareProfessionals/ucm162701.htm). *Information for Healthcare Professionals – Propylthiouracil-Induced Liver Failure*. Rockville, MD: FDA.

77 Cooper, D.S. and Rivkees, S.A. (2009). Putting propylthiouracil in perspective. *J. Clin. Endocrinol. Metab.* **94**: 1881–1882.

78 Food, U.S. and Administration, D. (2010. Available from: http://www.fda.gov/Drugs/DrugSafety/PostmarketDrugSafety InformationforPatientsandProviders/ucm209023.htm). *FDA Drug Safety Communication: New Boxed Warning on Severe Liver Injury with Propylthiouracil*. Rockville, MD: FDA.

79 Azizi, F., Khoshniat, M., Bahrainian, M., and Hedayati, M. (2000). Thyroid function and intellectual development of infants nursed by mothers taking methimazole. *J. Clin. Endocrinol. Metab.* **85**: 3233–3238.

80 Nachum, Z., Rakover, Y., Weiner, E., and Shalev, E. (2003). Graves' disease in pregnancy prospective evaluation of a selective invasive treatment protocol. *Am. J. Obstet. Gynecol.* **189**: 159–165.

81 Porreco, R.P. and Bloch, C.A. (1990). Fetal blood sampling in the management of intrauterine thyrotoxicosis. *Obstet. Gynecol.* **76**: 509–512.

82 Wenstrom, K.D., Weiner, C.P., Williamson, R.A., and Grant, S.S. (1990). Prenatal diagnosis of fetal hyperthyroidism using funipuncture. *Obstet. Gynecol.* **76**: 513–517.

83 Caffrey, T.J. (2000). Transient hyperthyroidism of hyperemesis gravidarum: a sheep in wolf's clothing. *J. Am. Board Fam. Pract.* **13**: 35–38.

84 Goodwin, T.M., Montoro, M., and Mestman, J.H. (1992). Transient hyperthyroidism and hyperemesis gravidarum: clinical aspects. *Am. J. Obstet. Gynecol.* **167**: 648–652.

85 Goodwin, T.M. and Hershman, J.M. (1997). Hyperthyroidism due to inappropriate production of human chorionic gonadotropin. *Clin. Obstet. Gynecol.* **40**: 32–44.

86 Kung, A.W., Chau, M.T., Lao, T.T. et al. (2002). The effect of pregnancy on thyroid nodule formation. *J. Clin. Endrocrinol. Metab.* **87**: 1010–1014.

87 Doherty, C., Shindo, M., Rice, D. et al. (1995). Management of thyroid nodules during pregnancy. *Laryngoscope J.* **105**: 251–255.

88 Rosen, I.B., Korman, M., and Walfish, P.G. (1997). Thyroid nodular disease in pregnancy current diagnosis and management. *Clin. Obstet. Gynecol.* **40**: 81–89.

89 Herzon, F., Morris, D., and Siegel, M. (1994). Coexistent thyroid cancer in pregnancy. *Arch. Otolaryngol. Head Neck Surg.* **120**: 1191–1193.

30 CHAPTER 30

Neurologic disease

Peter W. Kaplan, Emily L. Johnson, and Payam Mohassel

Johns Hopkins Bayview Medical Center, Department of Neurology, Johns Hopkins University School of Medicine, Baltimore, MD, USA

Introduction

Neurologic disease is common, affecting at least 1 in 200 pregnancies; the physiologic changes of pregnancy may also temporarily alter the course of chronic neurologic disease. Some of the most widespread neurologic disorders include epilepsy, stroke, multiple sclerosis (MS), and myasthenia gravis (MG). We present a case-based approach to these common neurologic problems seen in pregnancy.

Epilepsy is a chronic neurologic condition, affecting approximately one million women of childbearing age in the United States alone, and 3–5 pregnancies out of 1000 [1]. Much progress has been made over the last decades in our understanding of the risks related to antiepileptic drugs (AEDs), and women with epilepsy are no longer routinely counseled against having children.

Ischemic or hemorrhagic strokes are rising in frequency over the past decades; stroke-related hospitalizations have increased from 3 per 10 000 hospitalizations during pregnancy in 1994–1995, to 4.8 per 10 000 hospitalizations during pregnancy in 2010–2011 [2].

MS is often diagnosed in the childbearing years, and affects women nearly twice as frequently as men, which makes starting a family a significant concern of many MS patients. Twenty years ago, women with MS were told to avoid having children due to a belief that pregnancy would worsen the disease course [3]; this is now known to be untrue.

MG is the most common disorder of the neuromuscular junction, affecting about 1 in 5000 people; as with MS and other autoimmune neurological disorders, the childbearing years are a frequent time of onset, and women are affected at a higher rate than men.

Cooperation between the obstetrician and the neurologist is essential, including preconception counseling in cases of chronic neurologic disease whenever possible. With proper planning, good outcomes for pregnant patients with chronic neurologic disease are highly likely.

CASE SCENARIO: EPILEPSY

A 28-year-old woman eight weeks into her first trimester of pregnancy, presented to the emergency room with a seizure. She had a history of epilepsy, which had been previously well-controlled. Her seizure was similar to her prior seizures, with a generalized convulsion followed by a 20–30 minute period of confusion that had then resolved. She has been having difficulty with nausea and vomiting but is able to keep her medications down over the past few days. Recently, she has not been able to sleep properly, especially over the past two days. She has no fevers, chills, or other symptoms of infection. She reports complete compliance with her medications.

On examination, she is in no distress and her vital signs are normal. Her abdomen is soft and her lungs are clear to auscultation. Neurological exam shows a normal mental status and no abnormalities.

She would like to know what she can do to prevent further seizures, and wants advice on the safety of AEDs when taken during pregnancy.

Background

Epilepsy is one of the most frequent neurological conditions. It may also complicate pregnancy. Seizures occur in 0.3–0.6% of all pregnancies [4–7]. Obstetric complications are increased in women with epilepsy, and include preterm delivery, pre-eclampsia, placental abruption, hyperemesis gravidarum, and increased perinatal mortality. However, most women with epilepsy have good outcomes [8–10]. The aim of therapy during pregnancy should be to control convulsions with a single agent, using the lowest possible dose [11, 12]. The European Pregnancy Study Group using the International Registry of Antiepileptic Drugs and Pregnancy (EURAP) revealed that occasional partial seizures posed

Evidence-Based Obstetrics and Gynecology, First Edition. Edited by Errol R. Norwitz, Carolyn M. Zelop, David A. Miller, and David L. Keefe.

little risk to the mother and fetus; repeated convulsions on occasion could lead to fetal loss. Status epilepticus rarely caused maternal or fetal death, although clearly was to be avoided [13].

Clinical questions

1. What are the most common behavioral or non-pharmacologic causes of breakthrough seizures during pregnancy in women with epilepsy?

The most common causes of breakthrough seizures in pregnancy in women with epilepsy are similar to those seen in women who are not pregnant. The majority of women with epilepsy have similar seizure control during pregnancy, while approximately 20–30% experience more frequent or more severe seizures [13–15]. Mood changes and emotional stressors during pregnancy may have a major impact on seizure control [16]. Women may stop taking AEDs in pregnancy because of the fear of fetal malformations, thus emphasizing the need for an open dialogue between physician and patient regarding the relative safety of AEDs versus the risks of seizures [17]. Intractable nausea and vomiting during early pregnancy may decrease the amount of AED absorbed and hence adequacy of seizure control. Sleep deprivation may add to these physical and emotional stressors, leading to increased seizure frequency.

Several factors, such as stress, pain, sleep deprivation, over-breathing, and dehydration, may increase the risk of breakthrough seizures in the puerperium. While most women with epilepsy will have an uneventful labor and normal vaginal delivery, between 3.5% and 5% may have tonic-clonic seizures or even status epilepticus during puerperium [13]. In one recent study, seizures occurred in four of 32 (12.5%) patients with primary generalized epilepsy during labor as compared to 0 of 57 women with partial epilepsy [18]. Therefore, women at risk for seizures should be followed closely around the time of delivery.

2. What changes in AED pharmacokinetics occur during pregnancy and is therapeutic drug monitoring of value?

Several factors can change the blood level of AEDs during pregnancy. Increased plasma volume may affect the "loading dose", but not the daily dose. Reduced serum albumin concentrations, increased renal blood flow, and glomerular filtration rate, all may reduce the serum concentrations of AEDs [14, 19]. Different AEDs will be differently affected. The most pronounced decrease in AED concentration is reported with lamotrigine and oxcarbazepine (declines of up to 50%; increased clearance of up to 300%), likely due to their mode of elimination by glucuronidation [20–25]. Levetiracetam plasma concentrations may decline by 50% in the third trimester [26] and similar alterations are reported with almost all AEDs. Only the free level of valproate (not usually a drug of choice) may rise. Based on these observations, many experts advocate measuring maternal drug levels during pregnancy [27, 28], possibly monthly. In this way, AED blood levels can be titrated to drug dosage. Drug levels should also be obtained before pregnancy to document the patient's individual AED target zone.

3. Do breakthrough seizures affect fetal outcomes?

The literature contains little Grade 1–2 evidence, and mostly includes case series, case reports, reviews, and expert opinions. In addition, outcome data are confounded by several factors including lack of control for other confounding factors known to affect fetal outcomes (such as drug use, smoking, diet, and maternal age), and concurrent use of multiple AEDs during pregnancy.

Case studies report that partial seizures may affect fetal heart rate transiently with no known lasting effect. In the case of complex partial seizures, a few case reports showed prolonged uterine contraction or fetal heart rate deceleration [29, 30] but these are subject to publication bias toward adverse outcomes. The large prospective European and International Registry of Antiepileptic Drugs in Pregnancy (EURAP) study of 1956 pregnancies did not show any fetal loss due to non-convulsive seizures (partial or complex) or non-convulsive status epilepticus [13, 31]. Specifically, in this study, 406 of the women with known epilepsy developed non-convulsive seizures during pregnancy (approximately 25%); however, no miscarriages, fetal death, or any maternal morbidity was linked to single seizures.

Generalized tonic-clonic seizures have been reported to be associated with fetal abnormalities such as bradycardia, intracranial hemorrhage, cardiac slowing, or reduced beat-to-beat variability. However, the EURAP study showed no maternal deaths, miscarriages, or fetal loss due to isolated tonic clonic seizures. EURAP revealed that 2% of all pregnancies were complicated by status epilepticus and only one-third of these were convulsive status epilepticus with one stillbirth and no maternal mortality [13]. These studies suggest that the morbidity of status epilepticus in pregnancy is probably less than previously reported though controlled studies are lacking [31].

4. Which AEDs raise concerns during pregnancy?

In principle women with epilepsy should continue the AED that was needed to control seizures, particularly if other agents were unsuccessful. The challenges come with the use of valproate which poses significant risks for both fetal malformations and for developmental delay. In 2009, the American Academy of Neurology and American Epilepsy Society (AAN/AES) released practice parameters for management women with epilepsy during pregnancy [32]. They reported an increased risk of major congenital malformations with AED exposure in the first trimester (which was clearly demonstrated with valproate and phenobarbital). AED polytherapy probably contributes to an increased rate of major congenital malformations as compared with monotherapy [33]. Carbamazepine and lamotrigine yielded much more reassuring levels of teratogenesis in several national and international registries.

Switching AEDs during pregnancy carries the risk of break-through seizures, but occasionally has been attempted if valproate is not essential for seizure control, or for example, has been used for migraine prophylaxis. If valproate or phenobarbital can be discontinued or switched prior to pregnancy, this should be considered.

As noted above, AED use during pregnancy should be based on the given clinical situation [34]. Lamotrigine and carbamazepine are two of the most well-studied AEDs in pregnancy. The Lamotrigine Pregnancy Registry did not detect an appreciable increase in major congenital malformation in patients treated with lamotrigine as monotherapy during their first trimester in over 1500 pregnancies [35].

While there are limited data, levetiracetam may have a low rate of malformations if used during pregnancy but this remains to be established [36]. In the Australian registry of pregnancies, levetiracetam was associated with no major congenital malformations [37].

In conclusion, therapeutic drug monitoring of serum AED levels should be considered during pregnancy as levels may change significantly, especially those of lamotrigine and oxcarbazepine (Class IIa, Level B). Valproate and phenobarbital have an increased risk of major congenital malformations, and if these drugs can be safely replaced or discontinued prior to pregnancy, this should be considered (Class III, Level B for risk of teratogenesis). Lamotrigine and levetiracetam have relatively low rates of associated major congenital malformations, and may be preferred in women who are planning pregnancy (Class I, Level B).

Search strategy for each question

1. Search strategy: pregnancy AND epilepsy AND seizure control AND (behavior OR behaviour) AND search filters for systematic review. In addition, hand searched references of the search results.

2. Search strategy: pregnancy AND epilepsy AND seizure control AND anticonvulsants (MeSH) and search filters for systematic review. In addition, hand searched references of the search results.

3. Search strategy: pregnancy AND seizure AND fetal outcome and search filters for systematic review. In addition, hand searched references of the search results.

4. Search strategy: pregnancy AND anticonvulsants (MesH) and fetal AND outcome and search filters for systematic review. In addition, hand searched references of the search results.

Grading of evidence

Studies were reviewed and graded according to the American College of Cardiology (ACC) and the American Heart Association (AHA) clinical practice guidelines (available at www.acc.org and www.aha.org):

- Level of evidence A: recommendation based on evidence from multiple randomized trials or meta-analyses
- Level of evidence B: recommendation based on evidence from a single randomized trial or nonrandomized studies
- Level of evidence C: recommendation based on expert opinion, case studies, or standards of care.

Recommendation class was assigned based on the consensus (or lack thereof) and relative risks and benefits in the studies cited, classified as:

- Class I: conditions for which there is evidence and/or general agreement that a given procedure or treatment is useful and effective.
- Class II: conditions for which there is conflicting evidence and/or a divergence of opinion about the usefulness/efficacy of a procedure or treatment.
- Class IIa: weight of evidence/opinion is in favor of usefulness/efficacy.
- Class IIb: usefulness/efficacy is less well established by evidence/opinion.
- Class III: conditions for which there is evidence and/or general agreement that the procedure/treatment is not useful/effective and in some cases may be harmful.

CASE SCENARIO: ISCHEMIC STROKE

A 32-year-old woman with a past medical history of diabetes, hypertension, obesity, and hyperlipidemia who was two weeks postpartum after an uncomplicated full term pregnancy presented with an acute onset of aphasia, and right face and upper extremity weakness. She had been in her usual state of health until the night prior to presentation and woke up with these symptoms. She is unable to communicate.

She had a brain magnetic resonance imaging (MRI) that showed a large left middle cerebral artery (MCA) territory stroke involving the territory of the superior division of the MCA. On magnetic resonance angiography (MRA) imaging, she had evidence of decreased flow through the left MCA with drop-out of signal. Her echocardiogram showed no abnormalities and no evidence of cardiomyopathy or patent foramen ovale (PFO). Ultrasound of the neck showed no hemodynamically significant stenosis of the carotid arteries. Imaging of the brain showed evidence of intracranial atherosclerotic disease.

Her HbA1C was 9.5% and low-density lipoprotein (LDL) was 160. She was admitted to the stroke service and treated supportively. Prior to her discharge a week later, her right arm strength improved. She continued to have difficulty with word finding and writing, but language comprehension was mostly unaffected.

Background

Stroke is the third most common cause of death in the United States and is a leading cause of disability. During pregnancy and in the early postpartum period, stroke complicates approximately 1 in 6000 pregnancies. While different studies arrive at different estimates for stroke prevalence during pregnancy and puerperium [38], it is reported that 12–35% of cerebrovascular disease in those aged 15–45 years occurred during pregnancy or in the puerperium [39, 40]. Stroke is responsible for approximately 5–10% of all pregnancy-related maternal deaths in the United States each year and the survivors of stroke routinely are left with a significant disability [41, 42]. As a result, diagnosis, prevention, and treatment of risk factors leading to stroke are of utmost importance. In addition, acute stroke management may reduce morbidity and mortality from strokes during pregnancy or the puerperium.

Strokes are broadly categorized into two major groups: ischemic stroke, which comprise about 85% of all strokes; and hemorrhagic stroke accounting for the remainder. Cerebral venous thrombosis (CVT) and subarachnoid hemorrhage also are relatively common cerebrovascular complications seen during pregnancy or puerperium.

Clinical questions

1. What are the risk factors for stroke during pregnancy or puerperium?

Risk factors associated with atherosclerosis and stroke in general (such as age, hypertension, smoking, diabetes, hyperlipidemia, valvular heart disease, and hypercoagulable states) are also highly relevant in pregnancy [43]. In addition, most of the effect is seen in the puerperium [39]. Hypertension alone, which can be pre-existing or associated with pregnancy, can increase the risk of stroke during pregnancy by a factor of 9 [44, 45].

In addition, several other pregnancy-specific risk factors may add to these factors (see Question 2).

2. What risk factors specific to pregnancy predispose to stroke?

Eclampsia or pre-eclampsia is the most frequent risk factor for stroke related to pregnancy or the puerperium. Pregnancies complicated by eclampsia or pre-eclampsia increase the risk of maternal strokes, both ischemic and hemorrhagic [45–47]. Some studies suggest that pre-eclampsia was present in a quarter of all cases of hemorrhagic or ischemic strokes related to pregnancy [48]. The mechanism is not entirely clear but hypertension, lower socio-economic class, and endothelial dysfunction are thought to play a role [44, 49]. Microthrombi formation and an activation of the coagulation cascades may also be another contributor [50].

CVT can commonly complicate pregnancies with an incidence of about 1 in 11 000 deliveries [51]. Furthermore, CVTs are more common in the postpartum period, especially the first week after delivery [43, 52]. Dehydration may be a risk factor. The major clinical symptoms of CVT include headache, focal neurological signs, papilledema, seizures, and altered sensorium. Headaches are sometimes the only symptom. An MRI of the brain and an MR venogram can help in diagnosis. Compared to other patients with CVTs, those in pregnancy generally occur in younger women and tend to have a better prognosis [53].

Cardioembolic disease: Cardioembolism due to peripartum cardiomyopathy is a relatively common cause of stroke in young women [54, 55]. In addition, paradoxical emboli can occur in the presence of a PFO and deep CVT may also occur, especially in the setting of decreased mobility and the relative hypercoagulable state seen in pregnancy [56]; however, given the high prevalence of PFOs in the general population, no causal relationship has clearly been established. Moreover, treatment of strokes associated with PFOs with closure of the defect do not seem to provide significant benefit compared to the use of aspirin alone [57].

Arterial dissections leading to stroke do not seem to occur with greater frequency during pregnancy, delivery, or the puerperium compared to the general population.

3. What are the acute therapies for stroke that are available during pregnancy?

Thrombolytic therapy with recombinant tissue plasminogen activator (rt-tPA) has been shown to improve outcomes and mortality from ischemic strokes in non-pregnant patients. However, no controlled trials are available that have evaluated the efficacy or safety of treatment with rt-tPA of stroke during pregnancy. Rt-tPA is a category C drug and its benefits should be weighed against the risk to both mother and fetus. Thrombolytics have been used during pregnancy relatively safely [58–62] with little risk to the mother or the fetus but randomized trials are needed to further establish whether thrombolytic therapy is relatively safe when used for acute ischemic stroke during pregnancy.

In addition, interventional procedures with intra-arterial tPA or mechanical clot retrieval may provide an alternative therapy for stroke during pregnancy while minimizing exposure to thrombolytic drugs. Experience with these interventions during pregnancy is also limited.

4. What therapies reduce the risk of stroke during pregnancy?

No randomized controlled trials have evaluated the efficacy of antiplatelet therapy for treatment or prevention of stroke in pregnancy. In general, it is thought that in patients with several risk factors, antiplatelet therapy may be helpful in preventing strokes. There is experience with low-dose aspirin and it can probably be safely used for primary and secondary stroke prevention during pregnancy, especially during the second and third trimester [63, 64].

The mainstay of stroke treatment during pregnancy is that of treatment of underlying risk factors. Atherosclerotic risk factors should be treated and hypertension and diabetes should be controlled. Dehydration should be avoided, and the preterm pregnancy monitored for signs of pre-eclampsia. In addition, in patients with hematologic disease with a known hypercoagulable state, systemic anticoagulation may be required. Heparin and low molecular heparin are classified as category C drugs and there is substantial experience with their use during pregnancy without untoward effect. Protracted use of heparin does predispose to osteoporosis and thrombocytopenia in the mother, but no teratogenic effects are known. Warfarin is a category X drug with known adverse effects on the fetus and is not recommended for treatment during pregnancy.

In conclusion, typical stroke risk factors including hypertension and diabetes should be In conclusion, typical stroke risk factors including hypertension and diabetes should be controlled (Class I, Level B). Dehydration should be avoided (Class I, Level C), and signs of pre-eclampsia documented (Class I, Level B). Antiplatelet therapy with aspirin may be helpful in preventing strokes in patients with multiple risk factors, and can probably safely be used during the second and third trimester (Class IIb, Level C). Treatment with warfarin during pregnancy should be avoided (Class III, Level B for risk of harm from warfarin). Experience with tPA in pregnancy is limited.

Search strategy for each question

1. Search strategy: stroke AND pregnancy AND risk factors AND search filters for systematic review. In addition, hand searched references of the search results.
2. Search strategy: same as number 1.
3. Search strategy: pregnancy AND stroke AND thrombolysis and search filters for systematic review. In addition, hand searched references of the search results.
4. Search strategy: pregnancy AND stroke AND treatment and search filters for systematic review. In addition, hand searched references of the search results.

Grading of evidence

Studies were reviewed and graded according to the ACC and the AHA clinical practice guidelines (available at www.acc.org and www.aha.org):

- Level of evidence A: recommendation based on evidence from multiple randomized trials or meta-analyses.
- Level of evidence B: recommendation based on evidence from a single randomized trial or nonrandomized studies.
- Level of evidence C: recommendation based on expert opinion, case studies, or standards of care.

Recommendation class was assigned based on the consensus (or lack thereof) and relative risks and benefits in the studies cited, classified as:

- Class I: conditions for which there is evidence and/or general agreement that a given procedure or treatment is useful and effective
- Class II: conditions for which there is conflicting evidence and/or a divergence of opinion about the usefulness/efficacy of a procedure or treatment.
- Class IIa: weight of evidence/opinion is in favor of usefulness/efficacy.
- Class IIb: usefulness/efficacy is less well established by evidence/opinion.
- Class III: conditions for which there is evidence and/or general agreement that the procedure/treatment is not useful/effective and in some cases may be harmful.

CASE SCENARIO: MULTIPLE SCLEROSIS

A 31-year-old woman with a known history of MS presents to the neurology clinic for regular follow-up. She was diagnosed at 24 years of age with relapsing remitting MS and has been treated with glatiramer acetate injections. Since then, she has had two clinical exacerbations that were treated with steroids. She is planning to start a family and wants to know what to expect.

She is concerned about the effect of pregnancy on MS disease activity, effects of MS and/or her MS medication on the pregnancy, and risks to the health and birth of her child.

Background

MS is a relatively common (1 in 800) major neurologic disease with a strong predominance in women, especially young adults. There are different clinical sub-classifications of MS based on the pattern of disease progression over time. Patients with episodes of disease exacerbations and near complete recovery are referred to as having relapsing–remitting MS whereas those with progressive decline without discrete episodes of exacerbation are said to have progressive MS. Those with progressive symptoms superimposed on exacerbations are classified as progressive relapsing MS.

The etiology of MS is unknown, but genetic factors as well as environmental factor are thought to play a role. MS is an immune-mediated disease characterized by focal areas of inflammation in the central nervous system. MS affects many women of childbearing age, making pregnancy a major concern for many MS patients.

Clinical questions

1. What are the effects of pregnancy on MS disease activity?

Until the early 1950s, it was thought that pregnancy would have a deleterious effect on MS and women with MS were advised against pregnancy. However, several studies have failed to show any such deleterious effect [65, 66]. In fact, pregnancy is thought to reduce the risk of relapse of MS patients in up to 70% (in the third trimester) based on the Pregnancy and Multiple Sclerosis (PRIMS) trial [67]. However, there was a corresponding increase in relapse rate in the postpartum period in the study. Predictors of postpartum relapse included high disease activity in the year prior to the pregnancy and a higher MS disability score prior to pregnancy [67, 68].

Long-term effects of pregnancy on MS are not clear. Earlier studies had suggested a delay in the need for the use of a wheelchair after MS diagnosis in patients who had been pregnant as compared to nulliparous women with MS (18.6 years vs 12.5 years) [69]. Another cross-sectional study also suggested a small benefit of pregnancy on long-term outcomes of patients with MS; those with children reached an Extended Disability Scale Score (EDSS) of 6 at a later time since diagnosis [70]. In contrast, other studies have reported no significant difference in long-term disease outcomes between MS patients who had a pregnancy compared to nulliparous women. The PRIMS study reported no significant difference in disease outcomes after two years [67]. Similarly, in a cohort of 277 women with MS, parity was not found to influence the risk of secondary progression [71].

Taken together, pregnancy may decrease the rate of disease activity during pregnancy, but may have a neutral effect on long-term disease outcomes.

2. What are the effects of MS and MS medication on pregnancy?

Patients with MS are usually treated with one of several agents referred to as disease-modifying therapy. These include interferon or glatiramer acetate injections, natalizumab infusions, or mitoxantrone. In addition fingolimod is recently approved as the only oral therapy for MS.

The National MS Society Disease Management Consensus Statement emphasizes that none of these therapies is approved for women who are pregnant. However, some data are available from patients exposed to MS disease modifying therapy during pregnancy. In a systematic review, 15 studies were identified in which pregnancy and fetal outcomes in patients exposed to MS therapies were analyzed. A total of 761 patients received interferon beta, 97 glatiramer acetate, and 35 were exposed to natalizumab [72]. Compared to MS patients off disease-modifying therapy, those with interferon beta exposure were associated with lower mean birth weight (but not less than 2500 g) and preterm labor (but no Cesarean delivery); and no congenital anomalies, malformations or miscarriages. In the case of glatiramer acetate or natalizumab, these agents did not appear to be associated with preterm labor, lower birth weight, congenital anomalies, malformations, or miscarriages [72]. In another study, 311 women with relapsing-remitting MS were followed. Approximately 21% of the births were in the setting of unintentional exposure to disease- modifying therapies (interferon beta or glatiramer acetate) which were subsequently stopped within two months of gestation. Exposure was associated with no difference in perinatal outcomes but only a trend toward a greater risk of assisted vaginal delivery (OR = 3.0; 95% CI: 1.0–9.2) [73]. Information about other MS drugs is not available. As a result, in most cases the decision to continue these medications prior to conception and/or during pregnancy should be done on a case-by-case basis (Class I, Level B).

Search strategy for each question

1. Search strategy: pregnancy AND multiple sclerosis AND (prognosis OR disease progression (MeSH) OR exacerbation) AND search filters for systematic review. In addition, hand searched references of the search results.

2. Search strategy: pregnancy AND multiple sclerosis AND (therapy OR drug) AND search filters for systematic review. In addition, hand searched references of the search results.

Grading of evidence

Studies were reviewed and graded according to the ACC and the AHA clinical practice guidelines (available at www.acc.org and www.aha.org):

- Level of evidence A: recommendation based on evidence from multiple randomized trials or meta-analyses.
- Level of evidence B: recommendation based on evidence from a single randomized trial or nonrandomized studies.
- Level of evidence C: recommendation based on expert opinion, case studies, or standards of care.

Recommendation class was assigned based on the consensus (or lack thereof) and relative risks and benefits in the studies cited, classified as:

- Class I: conditions for which there is evidence and/or general agreement that a given procedure or treatment is useful and effective.
- Class II: conditions for which there is conflicting evidence and/or a divergence of opinion about the usefulness/efficacy of a procedure or treatment.
- Class IIa: weight of evidence/opinion is in favor of usefulness/efficacy.
- Class IIb: usefulness/efficacy is less well established by evidence/opinion.
- Class III: conditions for which there is evidence and/or general agreement that the procedure/treatment is not useful/effective and in some cases may be harmful.

CASE SCENARIO: MYASTHENIA GRAVIS

A 28-year-old woman now nine weeks pregnant has no significant past medical history. She presents to the emergency room with progressive fatigue, ptosis, and double vision. She has also noted increasing shortness of breath, and reports worsening of her symptoms in the late hours of the afternoon, and variability during the day. Neurological consultation proceeded with evaluation for a neuromuscular junction disease and she was diagnosed with MG based on clinical presentation, exam findings, and confirmed with the presence of anti-acetylcholine receptor antibodies in the serum. Repetitive stimulation testing on electromyography indicated changes diagnostic of a myasthenic picture.

Background

MG is a rare autoimmune disease affecting the neuromuscular junction which is clinically characterized by weakness and fatigability of skeletal muscles. The pathophysiology of the disease affects the transmission of acetylcholine at the neuromuscular junction, mainly involving the nicotinic acetylcholine receptor. Hence, smooth muscles, including the myometrium, remain relatively unaffected. The majority of patients (~80–90%) with MG have circulating serum antibodies against acetylcholine receptors. A second antibody against muscle specific kinase (MuSK) is found in others (5–10%), while still others have no identifiable autoantibodies. The effect of MG on pregnancy is not predictable. With severe exacerbations, respiratory compromise can occur. This can be important during labor as fatigue of the skeletal muscles may lead to respiratory crisis with respiratory failure.

Clinical questions

1. What are the effects of pregnancy on MG disease activity?

One of the earliest studies of effects of pregnancy on MG was published in the 1950s [74]. In this study, 22 pregnant women with MG with a total of 33 pregnancies were followed. In one third, worsening of MG activity occurred, whereas in the other two thirds, the disease remained unchanged, or improved. The exacerbations usually occurred during the first trimester, while during the second and third trimesters MG severity remained relatively unchanged. In another retrospective study of pregnancies in the Medical Birth Registry of Norway (MBRN), 135 pregnancies in mothers with MG were identified [75]. MG exacerbation was reported in 13 (10%) of cases. In one case, MG exacerbation resulted in intubation of the mother and delivery while she was on a respirator.

In another study, 64 pregnancies in 47 women with MG were followed, with a relapse rate of 18%, the majority of which occurred in the first trimester [76]. Thirty-nine percent had improvement of their MG symptoms during the pregnancy. However, in the postpartum period, MG symptoms worsened in 28% of the pregnancies. In a more recent study, 69 pregnancies of patients with MG were followed [77]. Ten patients (14.5%) developed MG deterioration during pregnancy and 11 (15.9%) during the puerperium – a total of 21 (30.4%) exacerbations occurred. Thirty-one patients (22.3%) remained unchanged and 17 (24.6%) improved.

Based on these studies, the evidence suggests that approximately 20–30% of patients with MG may experience deterioration of their symptoms during pregnancy while the remaining 70–80% may see improvement of their symptoms, or no change at all.

2. What are the effects of MG on pregnancy, delivery, and fetal well-being?

In an epidemiologic study, pregnancy complications were more frequent in women with MG, with the most common complication being a preterm rupture of membranes (PROM) [78]. In the MBRN study, complications during delivery were reported in 40/135 (30%) pregnancies with the most frequent complication being protracted labor/fetal distress (26 deliveries) and the second most frequent complication being PROM (eight deliveries) [75].

MG in the mother does not appear to predispose to major congenital malformations except for an increased rate of *arthrogryposis multiplex congenita*, reported in up to 2.2% of pregnancies [79, 80]. Arthrogryposis is thought to be the result of fetal paralysis rather than teratogenesis, arising as a result of crossing of maternal antibodies through the placenta to the fetus causing muscle weakness, during pregnancy [81–83].

All infants born to myasthenic mothers should be carefully observed for the symptoms of transitory neonatal myasthenia gravis (TNMG). This complication tends to occur in ~10–30% of infants of mothers with MG, and can cause hypotonia, feeding difficulties, or respiratory compromise; however, these symptoms resolve with supportive therapy [75, 77, 78, 83].

In conclusion, MG patients can have a normal pregnancy and delivery but the course may be unpredictable. Pregnancy complications include prolonged labor or PROM and maternal fatigue may prompt cesarean delivery. Children of mothers with MG are at risk for developing TNMG and are at higher risk for developing *arthrogryposis multiplex congenita*.

3. What is the role of thymectomy in preventing complications of MG during pregnancy?

Newborns of thymectomized mothers generally have a lower rate of neonatal myasthenia compared to those of non-thymectomized women [75, 77]. Except for the incidence of neonatal MG, no other significant differences in pregnancy, delivery complications, or frequency of MG exacerbations during pregnancy were found in mothers after thymectomy compared to those without thymectomy [75]. In conclusion, for women with MG who plan to have children, thymectomy should be considered so as to decrease the risk of TNMG (Class I, Level B).

Search strategy for each question

1. Search strategy: pregnancy AND myasthenia gravis AND (disease progression (MeSH) OR exacerbation) AND search filters for systematic review. In addition, hand searched references of the search results.

2. Search strategy: myasthenia gravis AND pregnancy AND (outcome OR delivery) AND search filters for systematic review. In addition, hand searched references of the search results.

3. Search strategy: thymectomy and myasthenia gravis and pregnancy AND search filters for systematic review. In addition, hand searched references of the search results.

Grading of evidence

Studies were reviewed and graded according to the ACC and the AHA clinical practice guidelines (available at www.acc.org and www.aha.org):

- Level of evidence A: recommendation based on evidence from multiple randomized trials or meta-analyses.
- Level of evidence B: recommendation based on evidence from a single randomized trial or nonrandomized studies.
- Level of evidence C: recommendation based on expert opinion, case studies, or standards of care.

Recommendation class was assigned based on the consensus (or lack thereof) and relative risks and benefits in the studies cited, classified as:

- Class I: conditions for which there is evidence and/or general agreement that a given procedure or treatment is useful and effective.
- Class II: conditions for which there is conflicting evidence and/or a divergence of opinion about the usefulness/efficacy of a procedure or treatment.
- Class IIa: weight of evidence/opinion is in favor of usefulness/efficacy.
- Class IIb: usefulness/efficacy is less well established by evidence/opinion.
- Class III: conditions for which there is evidence and/or general agreement that the procedure/treatment is not useful/effective and in some cases may be harmful.

References

Introduction

1 Yerby, M.S. (2000). Quality of life, epilepsy advances, and the evolving role of anticonvulsants in women with epilepsy. *Neurology* **55**: S21–S31.

2 Leffert, L.R., Clancy, C.R., Bateman, B.T. et al. (2015). Hypertensive disorders and pregnancy-related stroke. *Obstet. Gynecol.* **125**: 124–131.

3 Vukusic, S. and Marignier, R. (2015). Multiple sclerosis and pregnancy in the 'treatment era. *Nat. Rev. Neurol.* **11**: 280–289.

Case scenario: epilepsy

4 Nelson, K.B. and Ellenberg, J.H. (1982). Maternal seizure disorder, outcome of pregnancy, and neurologic abnormalities in the children. *Neurology* **32** (**11**): 1247–1254.

5 Thomas, S.V., Sindhu, K., Ajaykumar, B. et al. (2009). Maternal and obstetric outcome of women with epilepsy. *Seizure* **18** (**3**): 163–166.

6 Viinikainen, K., Heinonen, S., Eriksson, K., and Kalviainen, R. (2006). Community-based, prospective, controlled study of obstetric and neonatal outcome of 179 pregnancies in women with epilepsy. *Epilepsia* **47** (**1**): 186–192.

7 Yerby, M., Koepsell, T., and Daling, J. (1985). Pregnancy complications and outcomes in a cohort of women with epilepsy. *Epilepsia* **26** (**6**): 631–635.

8 Borthen, I., Eide, M.G., Daltveit, A.K., and Gilhus, N.E. (2011). Obstetric outcome in women with epilepsy: a hospital-based, retrospective study. *BJOG* **118** (**8**): 956–965.

9 Hiilesmaa, V.K., Bardy, A., and Teramo, K. (1985). Obstetric outcome in women with epilepsy. *Am. J. Obstet. Gynecol.* **152** (**5**): 499–504.

10 Pschirrer, E.R. (2004). Seizure disorders in pregnancy. *Obstet. Gynecol. Clin. North Am.* **31** (**2**): 373–384, vii.

11 Delgado-Escueta, A.V. and Janz, D. (1992). Consensus guidelines: preconception counseling, management, and care of the pregnant woman with epilepsy. *Neurology* **42** (**4**, **Suppl 5**): 149–160.

12 Holmes, L.B., Harvey, E.A., Coull, B.A. et al. (2001). The teratogenicity of anticonvulsant drugs. *N. Engl. J. Med.* **344** (**15**): 1132–1138.

13 Eurap Study Group (2006). Seizure control and treatment in pregnancy: observations from the EURAP epilepsy pregnancy registry. *Neurology* **66** (**3**): 354–360.

14 Brodtkorb, E. and Reimers, A. (2008). Seizure control and pharmacokinetics of antiepileptic drugs in pregnant women with epilepsy. *Seizure* **17** (**2**): 160–165.

15 Schmidt, D., Canger, R., Avanzini, G. et al. (1983). Change of seizure frequency in pregnant epileptic women. *J. Neurol. Neurosurg. Psychiatry* **46** (**8**): 751–755.

16 Fenwick, P. (1994). The behavioral treatment of epilepsy generation and inhibition of seizures. *Neurol. Clin.* **12** (**1**): 175–202.

17 Williams, J., Myson, V., Steward, S. et al. (2002). Self-discontinuation of antiepileptic medication in pregnancy: detection by hair analysis. *Epilepsia* **43** (**8**): 824–831.

18 Katz, J.M. and Devinsky, O. (2003). Primary generalized epilepsy: a risk factor for seizures in labor and delivery? *Seizure* **12** (**4**): 217–219.

19 Anderson, G.D. (2005). Pregnancy-induced changes in pharmacokinetics: a mechanistic-based approach. *Clin. Pharmacokinet.* **44** (**10**): 989–1008.

20 Pennell, P.B., Newport, D.J., Stowe, Z.N. et al. (2004). The impact of pregnancy and childbirth on the metabolism of lamotrigine. *Neurology* **62** (**2**): 292–295.

21 Pennell, P.B., Peng, L., Newport, D.J. et al. (2008). Lamotrigine in pregnancy: clearance, therapeutic drug monitoring, and seizure frequency. *Neurology* **70** (**22 Pt 2**): 2130–2136.

22 Reimers, A., Helde, G., Brathen, G., and Brodtkorb, E. (2011). Lamotrigine and its N2-glucuronide during pregnancy: the significance of renal clearance and estradiol. *Epilepsy Res.*

23 Tran, T.A., Leppik, I.E., Blesi, K. et al. (2002). Lamotrigine clearance during pregnancy. *Neurology* **59** (**2**): 251–255.

24 Mazzucchelli, I., Onat, F.Y., Ozkara, C. et al. (2006). Changes in the disposition of oxcarbazepine and its metabolites during pregnancy and the puerperium. *Epilepsia* **47** (**3**): 504–509.

25 Christensen, J., Sabers, A., and Sidenius, P. (2006). Oxcarbazepine concentrations during pregnancy: a retrospective study in patients with epilepsy. *Neurology* **67** (**8**): 1497–1499.

26 Tomson, T., Palm, R., Kallen, K. et al. (2007). Pharmacokinetics of levetiracetam during pregnancy, delivery, in the neonatal period, and lactation. *Epilepsia* **48** (**6**): 1111–1116.

27 Tomson, T. and Battino, D. (2007). Pharmacokinetics and therapeutic drug monitoring of newer antiepileptic drugs during pregnancy and the puerperium. *Clin. Pharmacokinet.* **46** (**3**): 209–219.

28 Burakgazi, E., Pollard, J., and Harden, C. (2011). The effect of pregnancy on seizure control and antiepileptic drugs in women with epilepsy. *Rev. Neurol. Dis.* **8** (**1–2**): 16–22.

29 Sahoo, S. and Klein, P. (2005). Maternal complex partial seizure associated with fetal distress. *Arch. Neurol.* **62** (**8**): 1304–1305.

30 Nei, M., Daly, S., and Liporace, J. (1998). A maternal complex partial seizure in labor can affect fetal heart rate. *Neurology* **51** (**3**): 904–906.

31 Kaplan, P.W., Norwitz, E.R., Ben-Menachem, E. et al. (2007). Obstetric risks for women with epilepsy during pregnancy. *Epilepsy Behav.* **11** (**3**): 283–291.

32 The American Academy of Neurology, Harden, C.L., Hopp, J. et al. (2009). Practice parameter update: management issues for women with epilepsy--focus on pregnancy (an evidence-based review): obstetrical complications and change in seizure frequency: report of the Quality Standards Subcommittee and Therapeutics and Technology Assessment Subcommittee of the American Academy of Neurology and American Epilepsy Society. *Neurology* **73** (**2**): 126–132.

33 Banach, R., Boskovic, R., Einarson, T., and Koren, G. (2010). Long-term developmental outcome of children of women with epilepsy, unexposed or exposed prenatally to antiepileptic drugs: a meta-analysis of cohort studies. *Drug Saf.* **33** (**1**): 73–79.

34 Klein, A.M. (2011). Epilepsy cases in pregnant and postpartum women: a practical approach. *Semin. Neurol.* **31** (**4**): 392–396.

35 Cunnington, M.C., Weil, J.G., Messenheimer, J.A. et al. (2011). Final results from 18 years of the International Lamotrigine Pregnancy Registry. *Neurology* **76** (**21**): 1817–1823.

36 Patsalos, P.N. (2000). Pharmacokinetic profile of levetiracetam: toward ideal characteristics. *Pharmacol. Ther.* **85** (**2**): 77–85.

37 Vajda, F.J., Graham, J., Roten, A. et al. (2012). Teratogenicity of the newer antiepileptic drugs – the Australian experience. *J. Clin. Neurosci.* **19** (**1**): 57–59.

Case scenario: ischemic stroke

38 Tate, J. and Bushnell, C. (2011). Pregnancy and stroke risk in women. *Womens Health (Lond)* **7** (**3**): 363–374.

39 Kittner, S.J., Stern, B.J., Feeser, B.R. et al. (1996). Pregnancy and the risk of stroke. *N. Engl. J. Med.* **335** (**11**): 768–774.

40 Liang, C.C., Chang, S.D., Lai, S.L. et al. (2006). Stroke complicating pregnancy and the puerperium. *Eur. J. Neurol.* **13** (**11**): 1256–1260.

41 Kaunitz, A.M., Hughes, J.M., Grimes, D.A. et al. (1985). Causes of maternal mortality in the United States. *Obstet. Gynecol.* **65** (**5**): 605–612.

42 Rochat, R.W., Koonin, L.M., Atrash, H.K., and Jewett, J.F. (1988). Maternal mortality in the United States: report from the Maternal Mortality Collaborative. *Obstet. Gynecol.* **72** (**1**): 91–97.

43 Lanska, D.J. and Kryscio, R.J. (2000). Risk factors for peripartum and postpartum stroke and intracranial venous thrombosis. *Stroke* **31** (**6**): 1274–1282.

44 Treadwell, S.D., Thanvi, B., and Robinson, T.G. (2008). Stroke in pregnancy and the puerperium. *Postgrad. Med. J.* **84** (**991**): 238–245.

45 James, A.H., Bushnell, C.D., Jamison, M.G., and Myers, E.R. (2005). Incidence and risk factors for stroke in pregnancy and the puerperium. *Obstet. Gynecol.* **106** (**3**): 509–516.

46 Sharshar, T., Lamy, C., and Mas, J.L. (1995). Incidence and causes of strokes associated with pregnancy and puerperium. A study in public hospitals of Ile de France. Stroke in Pregnancy Study Group. *Stroke* **26** (**6**): 930–936.

47 Wilson, B.J., Watson, M.S., Prescott, G.J. et al. (2003). Hypertensive diseases of pregnancy and risk of hypertension and stroke in later life: results from cohort study. *BMJ* **326** (**7394**): 845.

48 Ros, H.S., Lichtenstein, P., Bellocco, R. et al. (2002). Pulmonary embolism and stroke in relation to pregnancy: how can high-risk women be identified? *Am. J. Obstet. Gynecol.* **186** (**2**): 198–203.

49 Roberts, J.M. (1998). Endothelial dysfunction in pre-eclampsia. *Semin. Reprod. Endocrinol.* **16** (**1**): 5–15.

50 Roberts, J.M. and Cooper, D.W. (2001). Pathogenesis and genetics of pre-eclampsia. *Lancet* **357** (**9249**): 53–56.

51 Lanska, D.J. and Kryscio, R.J. (1997). Peripartum stroke and intracranial venous thrombosis in the National Hospital Discharge Survey. *Obstet. Gynecol.* **89** (**3**): 413–418.

52 Jaigobin, C. and Silver, F.L. (2000). Stroke and pregnancy. *Stroke* **31** (**12**): 2948–2951.

53 Cantu, C. and Barinagarrementeria, F. (1993). Cerebral venous thrombosis associated with pregnancy and puerperium. Review of 67 cases. *Stroke* **24** (**12**): 1880–1884.

54 Kittner, S.J., Stern, B.J., Wozniak, M. et al. (1998). Cerebral infarction in young adults: the Baltimore-Washington Cooperative Young Stroke Study. *Neurology* **50** (**4**): 890–894.

55 Ladwig, P. and Fischer, E. (1997). Peripartum cardiomyopathy. *Aust. N. Z. J. Obstet. Gynaecol.* **37** (**2**): 156–160.

56 Giberti, L., Bino, G., and Tanganelli, P. (2005). Pregnancy, patent foramen ovale and stroke: a case of pseudoperipheral facial palsy. Neurological sciences: official journal of the Italian Neurological Society and of the Italian Society of. *Clin. Neurophysiol.* **26** (**1**): 43–45.

57 Furlan, A.J., Reisman, M., Massaro, J. et al. (2012). Closure or medical therapy for cryptogenic stroke with patent foramen ovale. *N. Engl. J. Med.* **366** (**11**): 991–999.

58 Turrentine, M.A., Braems, G., and Ramirez, M.M. (1995). Use of thrombolytics for the treatment of thromboembolic disease during pregnancy. *Obstet. Gynecol. Surv.* **50** (**7**): 534–541.

59 De Keyser, J., Gdovinova, Z., Uyttenboogaart, M. et al. (2007). Intravenous alteplase for stroke: beyond the guidelines and in particular clinical situations. *Stroke* **38** (**9**): 2612–2618.

60 Dapprich, M. and Boessenecker, W. (2002). Fibrinolysis with alteplase in a pregnant woman with stroke. *Cerebrovasc. Dis.* **13** (**4**): 290.

61 Li, Y., Margraf, J., Kluck, B. et al. (2012). Thrombolytic therapy for ischemic stroke secondary to paradoxical embolism in pregnancy: a case report and literature review. *The Neurologist* **18** (**1**): 44–48.

62 Tassi, R., Acampa, M., Marotta, G. et al. (2012). Systemic thrombolysis for stroke in pregnancy. *American Journal of Emergency Medicine* **31** (**2**): 488.

63 Imperiale, T.F. and Petrulis, A.S. (1991). A meta-analysis of low-dose aspirin for the prevention of pregnancy-induced hypertensive disease. *JAMA* **266** (**2**): 260–264.

64 (1995). Low dose aspirin in pregnancy and early childhood development: follow up of the collaborative low dose aspirin study in pregnancy. CLASP collaborative group. *Br. J. Obstet. Gynaecol.* **102** (**11**): 861–868.

Case scenario: multiple sclerosis

65 Lee, M. and O'Brien, P. (2008). Pregnancy and multiple sclerosis. *J. Neurol. Neurosurg. Psychiatry* **79** (**12**): 1308–1311.

66 Coyle, P.K. (2012). Pregnancy and multiple sclerosis. *Neurol. Clin.* **30** (**3**): 877–888.

67 Vukusic, S., Hutchinson, M., Hours, M. et al., The Pregnancy In Multiple Sclerosis G(2004). Pregnancy and multiple sclerosis (the PRIMS study): clinical predictors of post-partum relapse. *Brain* **127** (**Pt 6**): 1353–1360.

68 Tsui, A. and Lee, M.A. (2011). Multiple sclerosis and pregnancy. *Curr. Opin. Obstet. Gynecol.* **23** (**6**): 435–439.

69 Runmarker, B. and Andersen, O. (1995). Pregnancy is associated with a lower risk of onset and a better prognosis in multiple sclerosis. *Brain* **118** (**Pt 1**): 253–261.

70 D'Hooghe, M.B., Nagels, G., and Uitdehaag, B.M. (2010). Long-term effects of childbirth in MS. *J. Neurol. Neurosurg. Psychiatry* **81** (**1**): 38–41.

71 Koch, M., Uyttenboogaart, M., Heersema, D. et al. (2009). Parity and secondary progression in multiple sclerosis. *J. Neurol. Neurosurg. Psychiatry* **80** (**6**): 676–678.

72 Lu, E., Wang, B.W., Guimond, C. et al. (2012). Disease-modifying drugs for multiple sclerosis in pregnancy: a systematic review. *Neurology*.

73 Lu, E., Dahlgren, L., Sadovnick, A. et al. (2012). Perinatal outcomes in women with multiple sclerosis exposed to disease-modifying drugs. *Mult. Scler.* **18** (**4**): 460–467.

Case scenario: myasthenia gravis

74 Schlezinger, N.S. (1955). Pregnancy in myasthenia gravis and neonatal myasthenia gravis. *Am. J. Med.* **19** (**5**): 718–720.

75 Hoff, J.M., Daltveit, A.K., and Gilhus, N.E. (2007). Myasthenia gravis in pregnancy and birth: identifying risk factors, optimising care. *Eur. J. Neurol.* **14** (**1**): 38–43.

76 Batocchi, A.P., Majolini, L., Evoli, A. et al. (1999). Course and treatment of myasthenia gravis during pregnancy. *Neurology* **52** (**3**): 447–452.

77 Djelmis, J., Sostarko, M., Mayer, D., and Ivanisevic, M. (2002). Myasthenia gravis in pregnancy: report on 69 cases. *Eur. J. Obstet. Gynecol. Reprod. Biol.* **104** (**1**): 21–25.

78 Hoff, J.M., Daltveit, A.K., and Gilhus, N.E. (2003). Myasthenia gravis: consequences for pregnancy, delivery, and the newborn. *Neurology* **61** (**10**): 1362–1366.

79 Hoff, J.M., Loane, M., Gilhus, N.E. et al. (2011). Arthrogryposis multiplexa congenita: an epidemiologic study of nearly 9 million births in 24 EUROCAT registers. *Eur. J. Obstet. Gynecol. Reprod. Biol.* **159** (**2**): 347–350.

80 Hoff, J.M., Daltveit, A.K., and Gilhus, N.E. (2006). Artrogryposis multiplex congenita – a rare fetal condition caused by maternal myasthenia gravis. *Acta Neurol. Scand. Suppl.* **183**: 26–27.

81 Polizzi, A., Huson, S.M., and Vincent, A. (2000). Teratogen update: maternal myasthenia gravis as a cause of congenital arthrogryposis. *Teratology* **62** (**5**): 332–341.

82 Drachman, D.B. (1971). The syndrome of arthrogryposis multiplex congenita. *Birth Defects Orig. Artic. Ser.* **7** (**2**): 90–97.

83 Briemberg, H.R. (2007). Neuromuscular diseases in pregnancy. *Semin. Neurol.* **27** (**5**): 460–466.

31

CHAPTER 31

Diagnosis and management of antiphospholipid syndrome

Cara Heuser[1] and Ware Branch[2]

[1] *Division of Maternal-Fetal Medicine, Department of Obstetrics and Gynecology, University of Utah and Intermountain Medical Center, Murray, UT, USA*

[2] *Division of Maternal-Fetal Medicine, Department of Obstetrics and Gynecology, Medical Director of Women and Newborns Clinical Program for Intermountain Healthcare, Intermountain Medical Center, University of Utah, Murray, UT, USA*

Introduction

Antiphospholipid syndrome (APS) is an autoimmune disease characterized by venous or arterial thrombosis and/or adverse pregnancy outcomes. Recurrent miscarriage, fetal death, and early delivery for pre-eclampsia or placental insufficiency have all been associated with APS. The diagnosis depends upon one or more of the aforementioned clinical events, in addition to one or more repeatedly-positive circulating antiphospholipid antibodies (aPL). aPL are a group of autoantibodies against either negatively-charged phospholipids or glycoproteins bound to the phospholipids. Diagnostic criteria for APS were revised in 2006 [1] and the laboratory criteria require detection of one or more of the following on at least two occasions 12 weeks apart: lupus anticoagulant (LAC), medium-to-high positive IgG or IgM anticardiolipin antibodies (aCL), and/or IgG or IgM anti-B2-glycoprotein-1 (aB2-GP-1) antibodies in a titer >99th percentile for the assay and laboratory. Patients with confirmed APS are treated with a heparin agent during pregnancy to prevent maternal thrombosis and to possibly improve pregnancy outcome. Pregnancies also require close monitoring for growth restriction, fetal compromise, and pre-eclampsia. Experts recommend those with prior thrombosis be considered for long-term anticoagulation. Catastrophic APS is a rare but life-threatening event that requires prompt evaluation and treatment.

Clinical vignettes

1. Obstetric APS (real APS without thrombosis)

A 28-year-old G2P0110 seeks your advice regarding another pregnancy. Her first pregnancy ended in an early miscarriage at eight weeks gestation. In her second pregnancy, she developed severe pre-eclampsia at 21 weeks gestation. Fetal demise was diagnosed the day of admission for induction. The stillborn fetus was morphologically normal and was small-for-gestational age. Tests for LAC were positive on the day of admission for induction and again three months later. The IgG anticardiolipin was 62 units on admission and 47 units three months later. She has no other important past medical or surgical history.

2. Thrombotic APS (APS with thrombosis)

At 33-year-old nulligravida has a history of pulmonary embolism two years ago after taking combination oral contraceptives for several months. Her hematologist found her to be positive for LAC and high-titer IgG and IgM anticardiolipin and anti-β_2-glycoprotein 1 antibodies at the time of presentation with pulmonary embolism and on two other occasions since. She has been on long-term anticoagulation with warfarin since her thrombotic event. She would like to know the risks entailed in taking on a pregnancy and how you would manage her anticoagulation therapy during pregnancy.

3. Concerning for APS, but laboratory confirmation pending

You are consulted regarding the management of a 29-year-old secundigravida whose first pregnancy was delivered at 33 weeks because of worsening placental insufficiency characterized by fetal growth restriction and oligohydramnios. The infant was small-for-gestational age, but is currently alive and well at three years of age. Testing done at the time of her delivery found the patient to be negative for LAC. IgG and IgM anticardiolipin results were 36 units and 53 units, respectively. IgG and IgM anti-β_2-glycoprotein 1 results were 21 units and 33 units,

Evidence-Based Obstetrics and Gynecology, First Edition. Edited by Errol R. Norwitz, Carolyn M. Zelop, David A. Miller, and David L. Keefe.

respectively. These have not been repeated. The patient is now 12 weeks gestation.

4. Infertility and early miscarriage with atypical antiphospholipid laboratory test results

A 37-year-old G3P1021 infertility patient is seeking your advice regarding her recent diagnosis of antiphospholipid syndrome by her infertility specialist. After having an uncomplicated first pregnancy eight year ago, the patient has had an early miscarriage <10 weeks gestation 18 months ago. Her past medical history is unremarkable, though she has a BMI of 34. Because of not becoming pregnant within the last 8 months, she went to see an infertility specialist. Her evaluation included an "antiphospholipid panel." The results of this panel shows that she is "low positive" for IgM antiphosphatidylinositol and antiphosphatidylserine antibodies and "moderate positive" for IgM antiphosphatidylethanolamine antibody. She is negative for anticardiolipin and was apparently not tested for LAC or anti-β_2-glycoprotein 1 antibodies. Her infertility specialist has told her that she has antiphospholipid syndrome and must take a heparinoid during her next pregnancy.

Clinical questions

What are the clinical presentations of APS?

APS may be diagnosed as a primary condition or may occur in a patient with other autoimmune disease(s), including systemic lupus erythematosus (SLE). Although the exact incidence and prevalence are not known, expert opinion holds that primary APS is about half as common as SLE. Population studies of APS are complicated by the misdiagnosis of patients with non-diagnostic, low titer positive tests for one or more of the three well-recognized antiphospholipid antibodies (aPL). Up to 5% of healthy women [2, 3] and up to 40% of patients with SLE [4] will test "positive" for aPL, though in some cases these will be at titers below the international criteria threshold for diagnosis. In the absence of clinical criteria, the risks associated with an incidentally-discovered positive aPL test are unknown; a diagnosis of APS should not be made on the basis of such results.

The diagnosis of definite APS [1] requires one or more episodes of thrombosis (arterial or venous) or one or more of the following pregnancy complications:

- Three or more otherwise unexplained recurrent early miscarriages (REMs) (anembryonic or embryonic losses <10 weeks gestation),
- One or more otherwise unexplained fetal deaths (≥10 weeks gestation),
- One or more preterm births occurring at less than 34 weeks gestation secondary to severe pre-eclampsia or placental insufficiency.

- *Recurrent Early Miscarriage.* Although some studies suggest that up to 15% of women with REM test positive for aPL [5, 6], the studies are limited by poor standardization of assays, inclusion of women with other causes of REM (e.g. chromosome translocations or uterine anomalies), inconsistent definitions of aPL positivity and recurrent miscarriage (differing number of losses and gestational ages), variable selection of controls, and even different isotypes of aPL tested. That said, authorities generally agree that a woman with three or more otherwise unexplained REMs and a repeatedly positive aPL result according to the international criteria have APS. However, authorities disagree regarding the frequency of APS among women with REM, with some groups finding very few cases of REM meeting international laboratory criteria [7, 8]. Experts also disagree about whether or not a woman with REM and either non-criteria aPL (e.g. a single positive test or a low titer result) or a positive result in a non-standardized assay has APS or "non-criteria" APS. This debate certainly would apply to our clinical vignette #4 [9–11].
- *Fetal Death.* Several recent large studies have examined the relationship between APS and fetal death. The Stillbirth Collaborative Research Network (SCRN) was a multicenter, population-based case-control study of stillbirths and life births [12]. In women who suffered a fetal death at or beyond 20 weeks of gestation, the investigators identified aPL (aCL or aβ2-GP-I antibodies) in 9.6%. Six percent of women with live births tested positive. When other causes of fetal death were excluded (e.g. fetal anomalies) in a strictly-applied algorithm, positive aPL tests were associated with an increased risk of fetal death two to five times greater than controls. Specifically, IgG aCL, IgM aCL, and IgG aβ2-GP-I antibodies were associated with five-, two-, and threefold increased odds of fetal death, respectively. The authors concluded that about 14% of unexplained fetal deaths were likely secondary to APS. Though prospective in nature and detailed in terms of the evaluation of stillbirth, this study was flawed by the lack of repeat testing. The Nimes Obstetricians and Hematologists – Antiphospholipid Syndrome (NOH-APS) study [13] was a prospective study of women with well-characterized APS, including repeatedly positive aPL results. Despite standard treatment in a next pregnancy, women who had a history of a prior fetal death or REM suffered a 16% and 8% fetal loss rate, respectively.
- *Preterm Delivery for Pre-eclampsia or Placental Insufficiency.* In spite of it being one of the obstetric clinical criteria for the diagnosis of APS, the association between aPL and preterm delivery secondary to placental insufficiency or severe pre-eclampsia remains ill-defined, as studies have been limited by variable definitions of placental insufficiency and pre-eclampsia, possible selection bias, and poor standardization of laboratory tests. Despite these limitations, studies that have examined women with severe pre-eclampsia suggest that between 5% and 10% of these patients will

have positive tests of aPL, as compared to 0.5% of controls [14–17]. The prospective NOH-APS study found that 10% of women with APS developed severe pre-eclampsia, despite standard treatment during pregnancy [13]. The relationship between aPL and early delivery for placental insufficiency in the absence of pre-eclampsia is frankly uncertain. Against this background, most experts agree that the association of aPL with indicated preterm delivery secondary to pre-eclampsia or placental insufficiency needs further study [11].

• *Thrombosis*. Lower extremity venous thrombosis represents about two-thirds of thrombotic APS cases and is the most common thrombotic presentation [18]. Recent studies suggest that about 10% of deep vein thrombosis (DVTs) are secondary to APS [19], though this figure varies with the population studied. Stroke is the most common arterial thrombotic presentation, and aPL antibodies are found in up to 20% of ischemic stroke patients under 50-years-old [20]. Nephropathy may be the presenting finding in patients with small vessel thrombosis [21]. APS can manifest in diverse and unusual ways including intracranial venous or arterial thrombosis, hepatic venous thrombosis, and intra-abdominal venous or arterial thrombosis.

• *Catastrophic APS (CAPS)*. CAPS is a rare but serious presentation of APS. This condition is characterized by rapid-onset, often small vessel, thrombosis leading to multiple organ failure and has a high mortality rate.

• *Other Clinical Associations*. Although not sufficient to make the diagnosis, other clinical features that may be seen with APS include immune thrombocytopenia, autoimmune hemolytic anemia, cardiac valvular lesions (Libman-Sachs endocarditis), chronic skin ulcers, false positive rapid plasma reagin (RPR) results, and cognitive impairment [4].

• **How is the diagnosis of APS made?**

Definite APS

International guidelines require one clinical criterion and at least one the presence of at least one repeatedly positive aPL [1]. The clinical criteria for APS are relatively non-specific and may be due to other factors or etiologies. Thus, the final diagnosis of APS rests on laboratory criteria. The specific laboratory criteria for APS are detailed in Table 31.1. Persistently positive aPL results are required on at least two occasions, at least 12 weeks apart because aPL may be transiently induced by conditions such as infection. Also, misleading or false-positive results in the LAC assays can occur due to the presence of anticoagulants or poor plasma collection or handling. Experience has shown that aPL immunoassay results for aCL or aβ2-GP-I may vary widely. In particular, it is imperative for each laboratory to define an individual titer >99th percentile for aβ2-GP-I. Time-tested, standard calibrators and units for the aCL assay have established, with >40 IgG units ("GPL") or IgM units ("MPL") being medium- or high-titer. The clinical significance of IgA aPL antibodies is unclear, and positive titers IgA titers do not currently establish the diagnosis. Most experts avoid checking IgA titers during the clinical evaluation for APS, as their significance is not established and is currently under investigation.

Table 31.1 Revised classification criteria for the antiphospholipid syndrome (APS) (modified from reference [1])

Clinical criteria

Vascular thrombosis[a]

a. One or more clinical episodes of arterial, venous, or small-vessel thrombosis in any tissue or organ with thrombosis confirmed by objective, validated criteria (i.e. unequivocal findings of appropriate imaging studies or histopathology. For histopathologic confirmation, thrombosis should be present without significant evidence of inflammation in the vessel wall.

Pregnancy morbidity

a. One or more unexplained deaths of a morphologically normal fetus at or beyond the 10th week of gestation, with normal fetal morphology documented by ultrasound or by direct examination of the fetus, OR

b. One or more premature births of a morphologically normal neonate at or before the 34th week of gestation because of eclampsia or severe pre-eclampsia or placental insufficiency,[b] OR

c. Three or more unexplained consecutive spontaneous abortions before the 10th week of gestation, with maternal anatomic or hormonal abnormalities and paternal and maternal chromosomal causes excluded.

Laboratory criteria[c]

a. Lupus anticoagulant present in plasma, on 2 or more occasions at least 12 weeks apart, detected according to the guidelines of the International Society on Thrombosis and Hemostasism, OR

b. Anticardiolipin antibody of IgG and/or IgM isotype in blood, present in medium or high titer (i.e. >40 GPL or MPL, or > the 99th percentile), on at least 2 occasions at least 12 weeks apart, measured by standardized enzyme-linked immunosorbent assay, OR

c. Anti-β2 glycoprotein-I antibody of IgG and/or IgM isotype in serum or plasma (in titer > the 99th percentile), present in medium or high titer, on at least 2 occasions at least 12 weeks apart, measured by standardized enzyme-linked immunosorbent assay.

Note that Definite APS is diagnosed if at least one clinical and one laboratory criteria are met.

[a]Superficial venous thrombosis is not included in the clinical criteria.

[b]Generally accepted features of placental insufficiency include: (i) abnormal or non-reassuring fetal surveillance test(s), e.g. a non-reactive non-stress test, suggestive of fetal hypoxemia, (ii) abnormal Doppler flow velocimetry waveform analysis suggestive of fetal hypoxemia, e.g. absent end-diastolic flow in the umbilical artery, (iii) oligohydramnios, e.g. an amniotic fluid index of 5 cm or less, or (iv) a postnatal birth weight less than the 10th percentile for the gestational age.

[c]Investigators are strongly advised to classify APS patients in studies into one of the following categories: I, more than one laboratory criteria present (any combination); IIa, LA present alone; IIb, aCL antibody present alone; IIc, anti-β_2 glycoprotein-I antibody present alone.

The assay for LAC involves a series of coagulation-based tests evaluating in-vitro clotting times and, if prolonged, isolating aPL as the culprit. The final result is reported as "positive" or "negative." Positive LAC may portend a worse prognosis than other aPL, with recent studies suggesting that the presence of LAC is associated with worse pregnancy outcomes and a higher risk of thrombosis [19–22] compared to positive results for aCL or aβ2-GP-I antibodies (in the absence of LAC). Most expert agree, however, that even isolated high-titer of aCL or aβ2-GP-I is also associated with more severe manifestations than lower titers. Some experts emphasize that "triple aPL positive" patients may be at higher risk of severe disease than either single or double positive patients [23, 24].

Catastrophic APS (CAPS)

Although uncommon, CAPS may occur during pregnancy [25] and may initially mimic other severe disease processes including hemolytic uremic syndrome and thrombotic thrombocytopenic purpura. The international criteria for the diagnosis of CAPS are listed in Table 31.2. The diagnosis is made when a patient has thrombosis in at least three organs in less than one week, microthrombosis in at least one organ, and persistent aPL positivity [26]. Clinical presentation of microthorombosis can vary and includes biopsy-proven small vessel thrombosis as well as features more typical of microangiopathies with ischemia from occlusion of arterioles and capillaries. Clinicians need to maintain a high-index of suspicion for CAPS in these settings as initial presentation can be vague and non-specific.

Table 31.2 Preliminary classification criteria for catastrophic antiphospholipid syndrome (CAPS) (modified from reference [23])

Criteria:

1. Evidence of involvement of three or more organs, systems, and/or tissues.
2. Development of manifestations simultaneously or in less than a week.
3. Confirmation by histopathology of small-vessel occlusion.[a]
4. Laboratory confirmation of the presence of antiphospholipid antibodies according to international criteria.[b]

Definite CAPS

- All four criteria present.

Probable CAPS

- All four criteria, except only two organs, systems, and/or tissues involved.
- All four criteria, except for the absence of laboratory confirmation of antiphospholipid antibodies by repeat testing.
- Criteria 1, 2, and 4.
- Criteria 1, 3, and 4, with the development of a third event more than one week but within one month of presentation, despite anticoagulation.

[a]Vasculitis may coexist, but significant thrombosis must be present as well.
[b]Positive antiphospholipid antibodies 12 weeks apart.

Possible or probable APS and equivocal cases

In practice, clinicians may not have the luxury of waiting 12 weeks to confirm or refute the laboratory confirmation of APS before management decisions need to be made. Take for example the clinical vignette #3 above in which the patient presents at 12 weeks gestation with a history of early placental insufficiency and positive aPL testing on one occasion. This patient is a risk for pregnancy complications based on history alone, and may be at further increased risk of adverse pregnancy outcome or maternal thrombosis if she proves repeatedly positive for aPL. Thus, the clinician and patient will need to weigh the pros and cons of treating with a heparinoid while awaiting confirmatory aPL testing. Another example would be a previously healthy woman presenting in pregnancy with possible stroke and evidence of small vessel occlusion in hepatic and renal beds who is initially positive for aPL. Concern for CAPS should prompt consideration of anticoagulation and other treatments while awaiting the opportunity for repeat aPL testing.

Some patients may present with a clinical history concerning for APS but equivocal laboratory testing. One of the most common scenarios is the woman with REM and a single positive aPL test or repeated "low-positive" results (e.g. aCL 20–39 GPL or MPL). Such cases do not have APS, at least according to international criteria, and in such cases, the clinician and patient must contend with the decisions about management in the absence of an evidence-based approach.

What are the management options for patients with APS?

Treatment during pregnancy

The aim of treatment of APS during pregnancy is to ameliorate or eliminate the risk of thrombosis and pregnancy complications related to APS (i.e. miscarriage, fetal death, pre-eclampsia, placental insufficiency). Patients may be counseled that with current treatment regimens and high-risk obstetric management, the likelihood of a successful pregnancy outcome, defined as the delivery of a viable infant, is greater than 70% [23, 27].

Low-dose aspirin (75–100 mg daily) (LDA) combined with a heparin agent is the currently recommended treatment for APS during pregnancy. This regimen provides venous thromboembolism (VTE) prophylaxis and may improve pregnancy outcomes. Many experts recommend that LDA be started prior to conception to maximize the possible beneficial effect on early implantation. The heparin agent (either unfractionated heparin (UFH) or low molecular weight heparin (LMWH)) is generally initiated after a viable pregnancy is established. Since patients with APS are at higher risk of immune thrombocytopenia, we recommend baseline evaluation of platelet count before starting aspirin or a heparin agent.

Patients on long-term anticoagulation require transition from their long-term anticoagulation agent, usually warfarin, to a heparin agent either prior to conception or in very early pregnancy. These patients, who generally meet clinical criteria for APS based on a prior thrombosis, should be on therapeutic dose anticoagulation (also sometimes called treatment dose, weight-based, or adjusted dose). One common regimen is enoxaparin at $1\,\mathrm{mg\,kg^{-1}}$ twice daily, though UFH or other LMWH agents may be used. Many experts periodically monitor anti-Xa levels, with a goal of $0.5–1.2\,\mathrm{IU\,ml^{-1}}$ (the reference range may vary by laboratory) drawn four to six hours after a dose.

Women who meet clinical criteria based on obstetric criteria and who have not had a previous thrombosis fall into two groups: (i) patients with REM prior to 10 weeks and (ii) patients with either a previous fetal death (after 10 weeks) or a history of early delivery for severe pre-eclampsia or placental insufficiency. Most experts recommend a prophylactic-dose heparin regimen for these patients. Commonly used regimens are UFH 7500 units twice daily or enoxaparin 40 mg daily.

Controversy exists regarding the impact of heparin treatment on obstetric outcomes. Trial results are available from four trials, primarily in women with REM [28–31]. In two studies, the addition of UFH to LDA [28, 29] improved the proportion of successful pregnancies. The other two trials showed no benefit with the addition of LMWH to LDA, although the live birth rates in the aspirin-only patients were actually quite good (70–75%). Studies of UFH versus LMWH in patients with primarily REM [32, 33] found no difference in outcomes. Other investigators have reported successful pregnancies in over 70% of APS patients with primarily REM using LDA alone [34, 35]. No heparin trials have included enough patients with either prior fetal death or a history of early delivery for pre-eclampsia or placental insufficiency to enable credible conclusions with regard to pregnancy outcomes.

Against this background, a Cochrane systematic review concluded that although the quality of studies was not high, "combined unfractionated heparin and aspirin may reduce pregnancy loss by 54% in women with APS and recurrent [early] miscarriage" [36]. Guidelines from the American College of Chest Physicians also advocate for heparin use. The ACCP guidelines state that "we recommend antepartum administration of prophylactic or intermediate-dose unfractionated heparin or prophylactic LMWH combined with low-dose aspirin" [37]. The American College of Obstetricians and Gynecologist allows for surveillance or prophylactic heparin in the antepartum period but recommends consideration of the latter [38]. Because the prevention of adverse pregnancy outcomes in women with APS who have suffered a fetal death or early delivery secondary to pre-eclampsia or placental insufficiency has not been evaluated by well-designed trials, professional societies have avoided unequivocal recommendations regarding the use of heparin agents to ameliorate these risks. In 2014, the International Congress on Antiphospholipid Antibodies noted the lack of evidence for preventing subsequent adverse pregnancy outcomes in women with APS diagnosed because of prior second or third trimester adverse outcomes, but acknowledged that such trials were unlikely to be performed.

Despite the uncertainty regarding the efficacy of heparin agents to improve pregnancy outcomes, there are several points on which there is wide expert consensus. First, in APS patients with a prior thrombosis, anticoagulation during pregnancy and the postpartum period is indicated [36, 37]. Second, in women with well-documented APS based on obstetric criteria without prior thrombosis, prophylactic dose anticoagulation should be strongly considered during pregnancy and postpartum as these patients are at risk for thrombosis [39]. Furthermore, even in the absence of solid scientific evidence that anticoagulation improves pregnancy outcomes, most patients and clinicians will choose "treatment" over no treatment when the intervention is thought to be associated with a low risk of harm. Prophylactic doses of UFH or LMWH are thought to be relatively safe and the risk for significant side effects is low [40–42].

After delivery, women with a history of thrombosis may restart their long-term anticoagulation regimen with vitamin K antagonists. Women with APS but without a prior thrombosis should be counseled that the benefits of prophylactic anticoagulation in the postpartum period likely outweigh the risks. Furthermore, a recent meta-analysis found that long-term aspirin therapy might decrease the risk of thrombosis [43]. Both warfarin and heparin products are compatible with breastfeeding.

Although some case series and small trials have suggested that glucocorticoid treatment may achieve similar pregnancy outcomes to those achieved with heparin [44, 45], the adverse effects of glucocorticoids have limited their use. Well-designed trials do not support the use of intravenous immune globulin (IVIG) either alone or in addition to heparin [46–48].

"Refractory obstetric APS"

Patients with "refractory obstetric APS" pose a unique challenge and scant data exist to guide management. These are patients who have suffered a recurrent fetal death or early delivery for severe pre-eclampsia or placental insufficiency despite standard treatment with aspirin and a heparin agent. One case series of 18 women with refractory obstetric APS showed a 60% pregnancy success rate when 10 mg of prednisolone daily through 14 weeks was added to the usual regimen of aspirin and heparin [49]. Animal and laboratory models have suggested that inflammation contributes to

APS related adverse pregnancy outcomes and, thus, agents that modulate excess inflammation may have some benefit.

Anecdotally, agents such as hydroxychloroquine and IVIG have shown promise in refractory obstetric APS (in addition to standard treatment). Fluvastatin has been shown to reduce proinflammatory and prothrombotic biomarkers in patients with APS [50]. Agents that inhibit complement activation, including eculizumab or pexelizumab, and tumor necrosis factor-alpha have shown promise in a laboratory setting but information regarding these drugs in pregnancy is extremely limited, important side effects exist, and the cost is often prohibitive. Statin agents have recently shown promise in preventing recurrent pre-eclampsia [51] and trials are in progress (e.g. NCT01717586).

We believe that women with refractory obstetric APS are at a much higher risk of periviable birth and grave maternal complications and should receive counseling to that effect. After such consultation, if the patient chooses to attempt a subsequent pregnancy, some of the aforementioned agents may be used in an attempt to maximize chance of successful outcome. Clinicians and patients must be clear on the lack of safety information and reasonable regimens may include hydroxychloroquine, low-dose prednisolone, or pravastatin.

Catastrophic APS

Although the optimal treatment of CAPS is uncertain, this condition with a high morbidity and mortality rate should be managed in conjunction with hematologic, rheumatologic, and critical-care specialists. In addition to supportive care, empiric treatments include anticoagulation with intravenous heparin, high-dose steroids, and plasma exchange [52]. IVIG may be of particular use in cases related to infection. Rituximab has shown promise, especially in patients with thrombocytopenia [53] and case reports have suggested that eculizumab may be helpful [54].

Pregnancy considerations

By definition, the risk for adverse pregnancy outcomes in women with APS in increased. Some case series have suggested a risk of 20% of hypertensive disorders or placental insufficiency in these patients [44]. The recent PROMISSSE study was a prospective observational assessment of pregnancy outcomes in 144 women with aPL, APS, or SLE [23]. Despite standard management, 20% of these patients suffered "adverse obstetric outcome". Specifically, 8% had a fetal death after 12 weeks and 8% required preterm delivery prior to 34 weeks for pre-eclampsia. Women with positive LAC, history of SLE, or prior thrombosis were at particular risk. The risk for composite adverse outcome was almost 40% in women with repeatedly positive LAC and over 50% in women with aPL and a history of thrombosis. The prospective NOH-APS study [13] evaluated outcomes in 500 women with APS who were diagnosed based on obstetric criteria (patients with prior thrombosis were excluded). Although all women received standard management, the iatrogenic preterm birth rate was significantly increased in cases compared to controls, occurring in 25% and 12%, respectively. The overall live birth rate was similar at about 70% in both groups but the risk of abruptions was significantly increased in the APS patients. After 20 weeks, APS patients had a 25% risk of pre-eclampsia, fetal growth restriction, abruption, or a combination of these, as compared to a 17.5% risk in the control population. In women with a prior fetal death and APS, 15% developed severe pre-eclampsia. In contrast, women who meet criteria for APS based on REM do not appear to be at higher risk of thrombosis, fetal death, pre-eclampsia, or placental insufficiency [28–31] and only 3% of these women developed severe pre-eclampsia.

The optimal surveillance strategy for patients with APS has not been defined and likely varies depending on the reason for APS diagnosis and other clinical factors. In an otherwise healthy woman, one reasonable approach is serial growth assessment with sonography beginning at 16–20 weeks and initiation of antenatal testing at 32 weeks. If other indications arise (e.g. fetal growth restriction, placental insufficiency, maternal hypertension), fetal surveillance should be initiated earlier.

Evidence

Diagnosis-Level B

The diagnosis of APS should be made on the basis of clinical criteria in addition to persistently positive aPL, as detailed in Table 31.1.

Treatment-Level B

Women with APS and a history of thrombosis should receive therapeutic-dose anticoagulation with UFH or LMWH in addition to LDA throughout pregnancy. Long-term oral anticoagulation agents may be resumed after delivery.

Women with APS and no history of thrombosis should be treated with LDA. The benefits of prophylactic dose UFH or LMWH likely outweigh the risks during pregnancy and postpartum.

Treatment-Level C

For woman with "refractory obstetric APS," providers may discuss the option of unproven but biologically-plausible empiric medications.

CAPS should be managed with a team approach. The optimal medical regimen has not been defined.

Surveillance-Level C

Allowing room for individualization, serial assessment of fetal growth and fetal well-being is recommended.

Returning to our clinical vignettes, the first two patients meet diagnostic criteria for APS. The patient in clinical vignette #1 has APS based on an obstetric clinical criterion, but has no history of thrombosis. She is also repeatedly positive for LAC as well as medium-to-high titer aCL. Once through early pregnancy, she will be at high risk for either fetal death or pre-eclampsia or placental insufficiency requiring preterm delivery. It is likely that the risk of thrombosis during pregnancy is also elevated. If she chooses to undertake another pregnancy, most experts would treat with LDA and thromboprophylactic-dose UFH or LMWH through pregnancy and postpartum. Careful attention should be paid to fetal growth, and antenatal testing should be initiated by 32 weeks or earlier if other indications arise.

The patient in clinical vignette #2, who has APS with a prior thrombotic event and is repeatedly positive for LAC and high titer aCL and aβ2-GP-I antibodies, is also at increased risk of the aforementioned pregnancy complications and fetal surveillance is indicated. She is also at risk for recurrent thrombosis and, in addition to LDA therapy, should be transitioned from her warfarin to a therapeutic dose of UFH or LMWH before six weeks gestation. She may resume warfarin postpartum.

Clinical vignette #3 represents the relatively common clinical scenario in which a patient does not meet laboratory criteria for APS but presents at such a time that clinical decision making must proceed before her repeat aPL testing is complete. There are several reasonable approaches in these circumstances. One approach would be to retest aPL promptly and base treatment decisions on results. Alternatively, the clinician might choose to treat presumptively while awaiting aPL results. The patient's history calls for careful attention to fetal growth and maternal status.

In our experience, the patient in clinical vignette #4 is all-to-common. She meets neither clinical nor laboratory criteria for APS. Her history of infertility, as well as her recent early miscarriage, are most likely related to her age, and maybe related to her BMI. Many such patients are convinced that they have APS or something like APS that would respond to treatment with UFH or LMWH, but in her case, treatment with UFH or LMWH to prevent miscarriage would be inappropriate. Although the clinician may be tempted to complete the laboratory evaluation, we recommend against it since the patient does not have a clinical history sufficient for diagnosis.

References

1 Miyakis, S., Lockshin, M.D., Atsumi, T. et al. (2006). International consensus statement on an update of the classification criteria for definite antiphospholipid syndrome (APS). *J. Thromb. Haemost.* **4**: 295–306.

2 Lockwood, C.J., Romero, R., Feinberg, R.F. et al. (1989). The prevalence and biologic significance of lupus anticoagulant and anticardiolipin antibodies in a general obstetric population. *Am. J. Obstet. Gynecol.* **161**: 369–373.

3 Harris, E.N. and Spinnato, J.A. (1991). Should anticardiolipin tests be performed in otherwise healthy pregnant women? *Am. J. Obstet. Gynecol.* **165**: 1272–1277.

4 Ruiz-Irastorza, G., Crowther, M., Branch, W., and Khamashta, M.A. (2010). Antiphospholipid syndrome. *Lancet* **376**: 1498–1509.

5 Branch, D.W., Gibson, M., and Silver, R.M. (2010). Clinical practice. Recurrent miscarriage. *N. Engl. J. Med.* **28** (**363**): 1740–1747.

6 Opatrny, L., David, M., Kahn, S.R. et al. (2006). Association between antiphospholipid antibodies and recurrent fetal loss in women without autoimmune disease: a metaanalysis. *J. Rheumatol.* **33**: 2214–2221.

7 Clark, C.A., Laskin, C.A., and Spitzer, K.A. (2012). Anticardiolipin antibodies and recurrent early pregnancy loss: a century of equivocal evidence. *Hum. Reprod. Update* **18**: 474–484.

8 Bowman, Z.S., Wunsche, V., Porter, T.F. et al. (2015). Prevalence of antiphospholipid antibodies and risk of subsequent adverse outcomes in women with prior pregnancy loss. *J. Rep. Immun.* **107**: 59–63.

9 Arachchillage, D.R., Machin, S.J., Mackie, I.J., and Cohen, H. (2015). Diagnosis and management of non-criteria obstetric antiphospholipid syndrome. *Thromb. Haemost.* **113** (**1**): 13–19.

10 Ramires de Jesús, G., Levy, R.A., Porter, T.F., and Branch, D.W. (2015 31). Limited evidence for diagnosing and treating "non-criteria obstetric antiphospholipid syndrome". *Thromb. Haemost.* **114** (**3**): 651–652. doi: 10.1160/TH15-02-0156.

11 de Jesus, G.R., Agmon-Levin, N., Andrade, C.A. et al. (2014). 14th international congress on antiphospholipid antibodies task force report on obstetric antiphospholipid syndrome. *Autoimmun. Rev.* **13**: 795–813.

12 Silver, R.M., Parker, C.B., Reddy, U.M. et al. (2013). Antiphospholipid antibodies in stillbirth. *Obstet. Gynecol.* **122**: 1–18.

13 Bouvier, S., Cochery-Nouvellon, E., Lavigne-Lissalde, G. et al. (2014). Comparative incidence of pregnancy outcomes in treated obstetric antiphospholipid syndrome: the NOH-APS observational study. *Blood* **123**: 404–413.

14 Branch, D.W., Andres, R., Digre, K.B. et al. (1989). The association of antiphospholipid antibodies with severe pre-eclampsia. *Obstet. Gynecol.* **73**: 541–545.

15 Kupferminc, M.J., Fait, G., Many, A. et al. (2000). Severe pre-eclampsia and high frequency of genetic thrombophilic mutations. *Obstet. Gynecol.* **96**: 45–49.

16 Lee, R.M., Brown, M.A., Branch, D.W. et al. (2003). Anticardiolipin and antibeta2-glycoprotein-I antibodies in pre-eclampsia. *Obstet. Gynecol.* **102** (**2**): 294–300.

17 Mello, G., Parretti, E., Marozio, L. et al. (2005). Thrombophilia is significantly associated with severe pre-eclampsia: results of a large-scale, case-controlled study. *Hypertension* **46**: 1270–1274.

18 Cerevera, R., Piette, U.C., Font, J. et al. (2002). Antiphospholipid syndrome. Clinical and immunologic manifestations and patterns of disease expression in a cohort of 1,000 patients. *Arthritis Rheum.* **46**: 1019–1027.

19 Andreoli, L., Chighizola, C.B., Banzato, A. et al. (2013). The estimated frequency of antiphospholipid antibodies in patients with pregnancy morbidity, stroke, myocardial infarction, and deep vein thrombosis. *Arthritis Care Res. (Hoboken)* **65**: 1869–1873.

20 Bushnell, C.D. and Goldstein, L.B. (2000). Diagnostic testing for coagulopathies in patients with ischemic stroke. *Stroke* **31**: 3067–3078.

21 Tektonidou, M., Sotsiou, F., Nakopoulou, L. et al. (2004). Antiphospholipid syndrome nephropathy in patients with systemic lupus erythematosus and antiphospholipid antibodies: prevalence, clinical associations, and long-term outcome. *Arthritis Rheum.* **50**: 2569–2579.

22 Galli, M., Luciani, D., Bertolini, G., and Barbui, T. (2003). Lupus anticoagulants are stronger risk factors for thrombosis than anticardiolipin antibodies in the antiphospholipid syndrome: a systematic review of the literature. *Blood* **101**: 1827–1832.

23 Lockshin, M.D., Kim, M., Laskin, C.A. et al. (2012). Prediction of adverse pregnancy outcome by the presence of lupus anticoagulant, but not anticardiolipin antibody, in patients with antiphospholipid antibodies. *Arthritis Rheum.* **64**: 2311–2318.

24 Pengo, V., Ruffatti, A., Legnani, C. et al. (2001). Incidence of a first thromboembolic event in asymptomatic carriers of high-risk antiphospholipid antibody profile: a multicenter prospective study. *Blood* **118**: 4714–4718.

25 Hanouna, G., Morel, N., Le Thi Huong, D. et al. (2013). Catastrophic antiphospholipid syndrome and pregnancy: an experience of 13 cases. *Rheumatology (Oxford)* **52**: 1635–1641.

26 Asherson, R., Cervera, R., de Groot, P. et al. (2003). Catastrophic antiphospholipid syndrome: international consensus statement on classification criteria and treatment guidelines. *Lupus* **12**: 530–534.

27 Bramham, K., Hunt, B.J., Germain, S. et al. (2010). Pregnancy outcome in different clinical phenotypes of antiphospholipid syndrome. *Lupus* **19**: 58–64.

28 Kutteh, W.H. (1996). Antiphospholipid antibody-associated recurrent pregnancy loss: treatment with heparin and low-dose aspirin is superior to low-dose aspirin alone. *Am. J. Obstet. Gynecol.* **174**: 1584.

29 Rai, R., Cohen, H., Dave, M. et al. (1997). Randomised controlled trial of aspirin and aspirin plus heparin in pregnant women with recurrent miscarriage associated with phospholipid antibodies (or antiphospholipid antibodies). *BMJ* **314**: 253.

30 Farquharson, R.G., Quenby, S., and Greaves, M. (2002). Antiphospholipid syndrome in pregnancy: a randomized, controlled trial of treatment. *Obstet. Gynecol.* **100**: 408.

31 Laskin, C.A., Spitzer, K.A., Clark, C.A. et al. (2009). Low molecular weight heparin and aspirin for recurrent pregnancy loss: results from the randomized, controlled hep/ASA trial. *J. Rheumatol.* **36**: 279–287.

32 Stephenson, M.D., Ballem, P.J., Tsang, P. et al. (2004). Treatment of antiphospholipid antibody syndrome (APS) in pregnancy: a randomized pilot trial comparing low molecular weight heparin to unfractionated heparin. *J. Obstet. Gynaecol. Can.* **26**: 729–734.

33 Noble, L.S., Kutteh, W.H., Lashey, N. et al. (2005). Antiphospholipid antibodies associated with recurrent pregnancy loss: prospective, multicenter, controlled pilot study comparing treatment with low-molecular- weight heparin versus unfractionated heparin. *Fertil. Steril.* **83**: 684–690.

34 Silver, R.K., MacGregor, S.N., Sholl, J.S. et al. (1993). Comparative trial of prednisone plus aspirin versus aspirin alone in the treatment of anticardiolipin antibody-positive obstetric patients. *Am. J. Obstet. Gynecol.* **169**: 1411–1417.

35 Pattison, N.S., Chamley, L.W., Birdsall, M. et al. (2000). Does aspirin have a role in improving pregnancy outcome for women with the antiphospholipid syndrome? A randomized controlled trial. *Am. J. Obstet. Gynecol.* **183**: 1008–1012.

36 Empson, M.B., Lassere, M., Craig, J.C., and Scott, J.R. Prevention of recurrent miscarriage for women with antiphospholipid antibody or lupus anticoagulant. *Cochrane Database Syst. Rev.* **205**, 2 (Art. No.: CD002859): doi: 10.1002/14651858.CD002859.pub2.

37 Bates, S.M., Greer, I.A., Middeldorp, S. et al. (2012). VTE, thrombophilia, antithrombotic therapy, and pregnancy. Antithrombotic therapy and prevention of thrombosis, 9th ed: American College of Chest Physicians Evidence-Based Clinical Practice Guidelines. *Chest* **141** (**2** (Suppl)): e691S–e736S.

38 (2012). Antiphospholipid syndrome. Practice bulletin no. 132. American College of Obstetricians and Gynecologists. *Obstet. Gynecol.* **120**: 1514–1521.

39 Lefèvre, G., Lambert, M., Bacri, J.L. et al. (2011). Thrombotic events during long-term follow-up of obstetric antiphospholipid syndrome patients. *Lupus* **20**: 861–865.

40 Rodger, M.A., Kahn, S.R., Cranney, A. et al. (2007). Long-term dalteparin in pregnancy not associated with a decrease in bone mineral density: substudy of a randomized controlled trial. *J. Thromb. Haemost.* **5**: 1600–1606.

41 Ruiz-Irastorza, G., Khamashta, M.A., and Hughes, G.R. (2002). Heparin and osteoporosis during pregnancy: 2002 update. *Lupus* **11** (**10**): 680–682.

42 Fausett, M.B., Vogtlander, M., Lee, R.M. et al. (2001). Heparin-induced thrombocytopenia is rare in pregnancy. *Am. J. Obstet. Gynecol.* **185**: 148–152.

43 Arnaud, L., Mathian, A., Ruffatti, A. et al. (2014). Efficacy of aspirin for the primary prevention of thrombosis in patients with antiphospholipid antibodies: an international and collaborative meta-analysis. *Autoimmun. Rev.* **13**: 281–291.

44 Branch, D.W. et al. (1992). Outcome of treated pregnancies in women with antiphospholipid syndrome: an update of the Utah experience. *Obstet. Gynecol.* **80**: 614–620.

45 Cowchock, F.S., Reece, E.A., Balaban, D. et al. (1992). Repeated fetal losses associated with antiphospholipid antibodies: a collaborative randomized trial comparing prednisone with low-dose heparin treatment. *Am. J. Obstet. Gynecol.* **166**: 1318–1323.

46 Triolo, G., Ferrante, A., Ciccia, F. et al. (2003). Randomized study of subcutaneous low molecular weight heparin plus aspirin versus intravenous immunoglobulin in the treatment of recurrent fetal loss associated with antiphospholipid antibodies. *Arthritis Rheum.* **48**: 728–731.

47 Branch, D.W., Peaceman, A.M., Druzin, M. et al. (2000). A multicenter, placebo-controlled pilot study of intravenous immune globulin treatment of antiphospholipid syndrome during pregnancy. The Pregnancy Loss Study Group. *Am. J. Obstet. Gynecol.* **182**: 122–127.

48 Vaquero, E., Lazzarin, N., Valensise, H. et al. (2001). Pregnancy outcome in recurrent spontaneous abortion associated with antiphospholipid antibodies: a comparative study of intravenous immunoglobulin versus prednisone plus low-dose aspirin. *Am. J. Reprod. Immunol.* **45**: 174–179.

49 Bramham, K., Thomas, M., Nelson-Piercy et al. (2011). First-trimester low-dose prednisolone in refractory antiphospholipid antibody-related pregnancy loss. *Blood* **117**: 6948–6951.

50 Costantine, M.M., Cleary, K., and Kennedy, E. (2013). Shriver National Institute of Child Health and Human Development Obstetric-Fetal Pharmacology Research Units Network. Pravastatin for the prevention of pre-eclampsia in high-risk pregnant women. *Obstet Gynecol* **121**: 349–353.

51 Erkan, D., Willis, R., Murthy, V.L. et al. (2014). A prospective open-label pilot study of fluvastatin on proinflammatory and prothrombotic biomarkers in antiphospholipid antibody positive patients. *Ann. Rheum. Dis.* **73**: 1176–1180.

52 Sciascia, S., Lopez-Pedrera, C., Roccatello, D., and Cuadrado, M.J. (2012). Catastrophic antiphospholipid syndrome (CAPS). *Best Prac. Res. Clin. Rheumatol.* **26**: 535–541.

53 Berman, H., Rodríguez-Pintó, I., Cervera, R. et al. (2013). Catastrophic Antiphospholipid Syndrome (CAPS) Registry Project Group (European Forum on Antiphospholipid Antibodies). Rituximab use in the catastrophic antiphospholipid syndrome: descriptive analysis of the CAPS registry patients receiving rituximab. *Autoimmun. Rev.* **12**: 1085–1090.

54 Lonze, B.E., Singer, A.L., and Montgomery, R.A. (2010). Eculizumab and renal transplantation in a patient with CAPS. *N. Engl. J. Med.* **362**: 1744–1745.

32 CHAPTER 32
Hematologic disease

Peter W. Marks
Center for Biologics Evaluation and Research, U.S. Food and Drug Administration, Silver Spring, MD, USA

CLINICAL VIGNETTE

A 26-year-old woman, G1P0, who is 16 weeks pregnant is noted to have a hematocrit of 28% and mean corpuscular volume (MCV) of 74 fl on routine laboratory studies. She has no significant past medical history and is taking no medications except a prenatal vitamin. Her family history is also unremarkable. Additional laboratory testing reveals a ferritin of 3 $\mu g\,l^{-1}$. A peripheral blood smear reveals hypochromic microcytic erythrocytes with no other significant abnormalities. Therapy with iron sulfate 325 mg orally twice daily is initiated. Eight weeks later her hematocrit is noted to have increased to 32%. She later presents when 36 weeks pregnant noting increasing ankle swelling. Her blood pressure is noted to be 170/95. Pitting edema is noted at the ankles. Urine dipstick is 2+ positive for protein. Laboratory studies are notable for a hematocrit of 27%, MCV of 80 fl, platelets of 60 000/μl, creatinine of 1.5 mg dl, alanine aminotransferase (ALT) of 210 $U\,l^{-1}$, lactate dehydrogenase (LDH) of 700 $IU\,l^{-1}$, total bilirubin of 1.3 mg dl. Coagulation tests are normal. The peripheral blood smear reveals 5–6 schistocytes per high power field. Hydralazine is administered for blood pressure control and magnesium sulfate is also administered. Labor is induced shortly thereafter with oxytocin and a healthy infant is born through an uncomplicated vaginal delivery. Two days following delivery the hematocrit is 25%, schistocytes are no longer seen on the peripheral blood smear, and liver function tests have normalized. She is continued on twice daily oral iron replacement therapy post-partum for three months, at which time her hematocrit is noted to be 36%.

Background

Hematologic issues of particular relevance to the field of obstetrics and gynecology include iron deficiency anemia, von Willebrand disease, immune thrombocytopenic purpura (ITP), and certain types of microangiopathic hemolytic anemia. Iron deficiency and iron deficiency anemia are common in women due to menstruation and pregnancy. In addition, some of the more common bleeding disorders such as von Willebrand disease require consideration when evaluating women for the cause of menorrhagia. Other disorders potentially associated with bleeding, such as ITP, are also encountered in women of child-bearing age. Normal pregnancy itself is associated with a number of hematologic changes including a decrease in hematocrit, modest thrombocytopenia, and increased von Willebrand, fibrinogen, and D-dimer levels [1]. This evidence-based review of the literature focuses on responding to six scenarios commonly encountered in clinical practice.

Clinical questions

1. How should blood loss anemia be managed in otherwise healthy women?
2. What is the appropriate approach to management of hemoglobin disorders that may be encountered during pregnancy, and what are the implications for the fetus?
3. What diagnostic evaluation should be performed in the evaluation of vaginal bleeding once gynecologic causes are investigated?
4. What represents optimal management of the different types of von Willebrand disease when bleeding is present?

Evidence-Based Obstetrics and Gynecology, First Edition. Edited by Errol R. Norwitz, Carolyn M. Zelop, David A. Miller, and David L. Keefe.

5. How should thrombocytopenia be evaluated and managed during pregnancy?
6. What is the appropriate diagnostic evaluation and management of microangiopathic disorders identified during pregnancy?

Critical appraisal of the literature

1. How should blood loss anemia be managed in otherwise healthy women?

- Medline: iron deficiency anemia AND women AND review and a separate search for iron deficiency treatment AND oral iron preparations OR intravenous iron preparations
- Hand-searching reference lists were used to identify additional articles of interest.
- Inclusion: References providing information relevant to the management of blood loss anemia published in the English language were included.

The first principle in the management of anemia due to iron deficiency resulting from blood loss is to identify the source of the bleeding with reasonable certainty. This may be determined simply by the history and physical examination and attributed to menstrual bleeding or blood loss associated with delivery in the case of menstruating women and those who are pregnant or postpartum. However, further diagnostic testing to unambiguously identify the source of bleeding is indicated in postmenopausal women, as otherwise there is a risk of missing sources of gastrointestinal blood loss, including colorectal malignancies.

Evidence indicates that in otherwise healthy women with a hemoglobin level below the normal range of 12–15.5 g dl^{-1}, a low serum ferritin level is the most reliable indicator of iron deficiency [2]. A low serum iron and elevated total iron binding capacity (TIBC) or serum transferrin level is also consistent with the diagnosis. Significant iron deficiency is associated with a hypochromic, microcytic anemia and decreased absolute reticulocyte count [3]. Additional tests that have been evaluated for the diagnosis of iron deficiency, such as the soluble transferrin receptor (sTf) or sTF/ferritin ratio, appear to contribute only modestly to the accurate diagnosis of iron deficiency [4].

Once iron deficiency or iron deficiency anemia is diagnosed, treatment with oral iron replacement is generally indicated. There are a variety of different iron salts available for oral use including ferrous sulfate, ferrous gluconate, ferrous fumarate, and ferrous carbonate. Although different preparations may have a different content of elemental iron and there are anecdotal claims that one preparation may be better tolerated than another, there is no clear benefit to the use of any one preparation in terms of safety or efficacy [5] (Table 32.1). For those women who cannot tolerate oral iron replacement therapy, and for those with symptomatic anemia, consideration can be given to the administration of intravenous iron. The potential benefits of this therapy,

Table 32.1 Some available iron preparations

Oral	Intravenous
Carboxyl iron	Ferric carboxymaltose
Ferric citrate	Ferric gluconate
Ferrous ascorbate	Ferumoxytol
Ferrous fumarate	High-molecular weight iron dextran[a]
Ferrous gluconate	Iron isomaltoside
Ferrous sulfate	Iron sucrose
Polysaccharide-iron complex	Low-molecular weight iron dextran

[a]Associated with the highest incidence of anaphylactic reactions among the intravenous iron preparations [6].

including more rapid resolution of anemia, must be balanced against the potential risks. Since a significant percentage of women (estimated at 15–25%) have difficulty tolerating oral iron, the availability of newer parenteral iron preparations with lower risk of anaphylaxis has provoked reevaluation of the potential benefits of parenteral iron [7]. As for oral iron preparations, there is little evidence in the literature to recommend use of one parenteral iron preparation over another, except that use of high molecular weight iron dextran, which has been associated with a relatively high number of anaphylactic reactions, has fallen out of favor. It has even been removed from the market in some countries. Low molecular weight dextran and other intravenous iron preparations associated with a lower incidence of this complication are preferred [6].

2. What is the appropriate approach to identification and management of hemoglobin disorders that may be encountered during pregnancy, and what are the implications for the fetus?

- Medline: hemoglobin disorders AND pregnancy and a separate search for sickle cell disease (SCD) OR thalassemia AND pregnancy AND transfusion.
- Hand-searching reference lists were used to identify additional articles of interest.
- Inclusion: References providing information relevant to the management of hemoglobin disorders during pregnancy published in the English language were included.

Women with hemoglobin disorders, including thalassemia and SCD, require appropriate management during pregnancy in order to help ensure the most optimal maternal and fetal outcomes. In addition, clinicians need to be aware that some previously undiagnosed women with hemoglobin disorders such as hemoglobin SC-sickle cell disease may first present during pregnancy with symptoms related to their underlying hemoglobinopathy [8]. Another important aspect relevant to overall management of women with hemoglobin disorders is providing appropriate genetic counseling, so that individuals can make informed choices before they become pregnant. The importance of appropriate genetic counseling prior to pregnancy is highlighted when there is a history of α-thalassemia. Each human chromosome 16 has two genes encoding α-globin. The form of α-thalassemia trait that is most common in Asian populations involves deletion of both genes from one chromosome. If such women conceive with partners who also carry this same trait, a quarter of the pregnancies will result in fetuses affected by absence of any functional α-globin genes, resulting in severe pre-eclampsia, hydrops fetalis and fetal demise in the absence of intrauterine exchange transfusions. Thus, identification, proper counseling, and intervention, if indicated, in such individuals are important.

Pregnancy is considered to be relatively safe, and favorable outcomes have been reported in patients with β-thalassemia major and β-thalassemia intermedia. However, these women are at risk for a variety of different maternal complications during pregnancy, including cardiac failure and thrombosis [9] (Table 32.2). Because these individuals may receive regular transfusions, they may be on iron chelation therapy, which generally should be discontinued. Regular transfusion therapy during pregnancy for individuals with β-thalassemia major, along with close monitoring is recommended.

Women with SCD, particularly those with sickle cell anemia (homozygous for hemoglobin S [HbS]), have an increased incidence of fetal loss, increased maternal mortality, and experience an increased number of complications, including vaso-occlusive crises and thrombosis during and immediately following pregnancy [13] (Table 32.2). The use of prophylactic blood transfusion in patients with SCD remains controversial [14]. Though some studies have shown some evidence of benefit, most of these trials have been relatively small and have had potential methodological issues.

Table 32.2 Pregnancy outcomes in some of the more common hemoglobin disorders

Disorder	Outcomes	Reference
Hemoglobin H disease (HbH, α-thalassemia with three deleted genes) N = 120 pregnancies compared with controls	Pre-eclampsia 9.2% in HbH versus 4.6% in controls (RR 1.36) Preterm delivery 24.9% in HbH versus 15.4% in controls (RR 1.42) Perinatal death 4.2% in HbH versus 1.3% in controls (RR 1.91)	[10]
β-thalassemia intermedia and major, including seven patients with HbH N = 129 pregnancies, no comparison group	Total live births 91 (70.5%) Premature births 10 (7.8%)	[11]
Sickle cell disease (SCD) (Included hemoglobin S disease and sickle cell disease unspecified) N = 344 SCD pregnancies compared with controls	Pre-eclampsia 10.2% in SCD versus 3.0% in controls (AOR 2.03) Severe pre-eclampsia 5.3% in SCD versus 0.9% in controls (AOR 3.75) Preterm delivery <32 weeks 7.0% in SCD versus 1.3% in controls (AOR 2.99) Neonatal demise 0.6% in SCD versus 0.2% in controls (AOR 2.10)	[12]

AOR, adjusted odds ratio; RR, relative risk.

3. What diagnostic evaluation should be performed in the evaluation of vaginal bleeding once gynecologic causes are investigated?

- Medline: women AND bleeding disorder AND diagnostic evaluation
- Hand-searching reference lists were used to identify additional articles of interest.
- Inclusion: References providing information relevant to the evaluation of hematologic causes of vaginal bleeding published in the English language were included.

The decision whether or not to initiate a diagnostic evaluation for a medical cause underlying menorrhagia depends on whether or not a gynecologic cause of bleeding is felt to be present or not. Thus, once a detailed personal and family history is obtained concentrating on factors that might contribute to bleeding, it is important to rule out anatomic causes in both adolescents and adults [15].

Following gynecologic evaluation, a careful medical and family history, along with history of any medications taken or dietary supplements consumed should be obtained. These historical features may help facilitate diagnosis of a disorder associated with excessive mucosal bleeding in individuals without a family history of a bleeding disorder who otherwise appear to be healthy (Table 32.3). In the absence of an established diagnosis, recommendations have been published recommending testing for the most common disorder associated with mucosal bleeding, von Willebrand disease [16].

To evaluate for von Willebrand disease, a panel three of tests consisting of the ristocetin cofactor assay (which evaluates von Willebrand factor activity), the von Willebrand antigen level, and the factor VIII level is usually obtained [17]. However, for screening purposes, it may be cost-effective to simply obtain a ristocetin cofactor level. This is associated with a relatively high sensitivity and specificity for the diagnosis of most forms of von Willebrand disease [18].

Table 32.3 Disorders associated with excessive mucosal bleeding in apparently healthy individuals

Acquired causes	*Decreased platelet number*
	Immune thrombocytopenic purpura (generally when platelets <30 000 μl^{-1})
	Impaired platelet function
	Aspirin
	Non-steroidal anti-inflammatory drugs (non-selective COX-1 and COX-2 inhibitors)
Congenital causes	*Hemostatic abnormalities*
	von Willebrand disorder
	Platelet function abnormalities
	Vascular abnormalities
	Hereditary hemorrhagic telangiectasia

If von Willebrand testing is normal and there is a reasonable suspicion for an underlying bleeding disorder, consideration should be given to evaluation of platelet function using platelet aggregation studies. Though use of platelet function analyzer testing (PFA-100) is more sensitive and specific than the traditional bleeding time for predicting the presence of a bleeding disorder, it is only about 50% sensitive for the most commonly encountered disorders [19]. Therefore, consideration may need to be given to obtaining platelet aggregation studies, which are more logistically challenging and technically difficult to perform than the PFA-100 test. If both von Willebrand and platelet function testing are unrevealing for a potential diagnosis, consideration may then need to be given to some of the less common diagnostic entities [20].

4. What represents optimal management of the different types of von Willebrand disease when bleeding is present?

- Medline: von Willebrand disease AND management AND review.
- Hand-searching reference lists were used to identify additional articles of interest.
- Inclusion: References providing information relevant to the management of bleeding in von Willebrand disease published in the English language were included.

A basic understand of the different types of von Willebrand disease and the physiologic changes in von Willebrand factor levels that occur in individuals is required for appropriate diagnosis and management of these disorders. This is particularly the case in obstetrics, as von Willebrand levels change markedly during the course of pregnancy and parturition.

There are three major types of von Willebrand deficiency [21] (Table 32.4). Type 1, which accounts for about 80–85% of von Willebrand disease, is a quantitative deficiency in which levels are generally 30–50% of normal. These individuals may present for evaluation of mucosal bleeding such as menometrorrhagia or may be entirely asymptomatic. Type 3 deficiency, which is rare, is also a quantitative deficiency. However, it is associated with complete or near complete absence of von Willebrand factor. These individuals are generally symptomatic from early childhood on. There are several different forms of Type 2 deficiency, all of which are at least in part qualitative in nature. The manifestation of the different Type 2 von Willebrand deficiencies depends on the nature of the underlying defects.

Table 32.4 Major types of von Willebrand disease and suggested management options

Type	Nature of defect	Treatments for bleeding
Type 1	Quantitative – Mild to moderate decrease in levels	Desmopressin (ddAVP) Antifibrinolytic agents Aminocaproic acid Tranexamic acid Appropriately labeled plasma-derived factor VIII concentrate or recombinant von Willebrand factor
Type 2A	Qualitative – Decreased high molecular weight multimers due to loss of function	Desmopressin (ddAVP) Antifibrinolytic agents Aminocaproic acid Tranexamic acid Appropriately labeled plasma-derived factor VIII concentrate or recombinant von Willebrand factor
Type 2B	Qualitative – Decreased high molecular weight multimers due to gain of function	Appropriately labeled plasma-derived factor VIII concentrate or recombinant von Willebrand factor
Type 2M	Qualitative – Decreased platelet binding with normal multimer distribution	desmopressin (ddAVP) Antifibrinolytic agents Aminocaproic acid Tranexamic acid Appropriately labeled plasma-derived factor VIII concentrate or recombinant von Willebrand factor
Type 2N	Qualitative – Decreased factor VIII binding due to abnormal factor VIII binding site	Appropriately labeled plasma-derived factor VIII concentrate
Type 3	Quantitative – Absence or severe decrease in levels	Appropriately labeled plasma-derived factor VIII concentrate

Optimal interpretation of whether or not von Willebrand factor levels are normal requires knowledge of the individual's blood type. There is a linkage between ABO blood groups and von Willebrand levels. Normally, levels are lowest in blood group O (about 70%), intermediate in blood groups A and B (about 100%), and highest in blood group AB (about 120%), with all values relative to a normal value of 100%. In addition, von Willebrand levels in the blood are affected by a number of different factors including stress and exercise.

Relevant to pregnancy, levels increase toward plateau by the second trimester and then decline rapidly following delivery [22]. Thus, individuals with Type 1 deficiency often do well through pregnancy and delivery, though they may experience increased postpartum bleeding. Various sources therefore suggest obtaining a von Willebrand panel to check levels during pregnancy, and if they are normal, managing these patients expectantly without administration of desmopressin or factor concentrates prior to delivery. If levels are low, desmopressin or factor concentrates may be indicated [23].

In contrast, due to the underlying nature of the qualitative defects, the management of delivery in patients with Type 2 and 3 von Willebrand disease may require the administration of factor concentrates (Table 32.4). Note that the use of desmopressin versus an appropriately labeled plasma-derived factor VIII concentrate or recombinant von Willebrand factor may depend on multiple factors, including the severity of the individual's von Willebrand disease and the nature of the bleeding episode or planned procedure.

5. How should thrombocytopenia be evaluated and managed during pregnancy?

Search Strategy

- Medline: pregnancy AND thrombocytopenia AND evaluation OR management
- Hand-searching reference lists were used to identify additional articles of interest.
- Inclusion: References providing information relevant to the evaluation or management of blood thrombocytopenia during pregnancy published in the English language were included.

Next to anemia, thrombocytopenia is the second most common hematologic abnormality observed during pregnancy, occurring in about 7–11% of pregnancies [24]. Appropriately ascertaining the most likely etiology is important, as certain conditions, such as gestational thrombocytopenia, are benign and need no treatment, whereas others, such as thrombotic thrombocytopenic purpura (TTP) require urgent intervention.

The most common causes of thrombocytopenia during pregnancy are gestational thrombocytopenia, severe pre-eclampsia or hemolysis or elevated liver function tests and low platelets (HELLP) syndrome, and ITP (Table 32.5). TTP is much less common that these other entities during pregnancy. When any of these disorders are under consideration, there is general agreement that during pregnancy appropriate laboratory evaluation of thrombocytopenia includes a complete blood count, review of a peripheral blood smear, serum chemistry and liver function tests, and a urinalysis [28].

Table 32.5 Common causes of thrombocytopenia during pregnancy

Disorder	Approximate incidence during pregnancy	Reference
Gestational thrombocytopenia	5%	[25]
Severe pre-eclampsia and HELLP syndrome	1%	[26]
Immune thrombocytopenic purpura (ITP)	0.1–0.01%	[27]

HELLP, hemolysis elevated liver function tests, low platelets.

The mechanism underlying gestational thrombocytopenia is not well defined. It is potentially thought to result in a shift in the normal range of the platelet count during pregnancy [29]. Unlike ITP, which can be associated with neonatal thrombocytopenia, gestational thrombocytopenia is generally not associated with a low platelet count in the neonate.

ITP also occurs in women during their childbearing years, and though it is not really more common during pregnancy, it is the most common cause of isolated thrombocytopenia during the first and second trimesters because it is a relatively common cause of isolated thrombocytopenia in women between 20 and 40 years of age [30]. Distinguishing ITP from gestational thrombocytopenia, however, can be challenging, particularly when the observed platelet count is in the range of 80 000100 000/μl. In practice, once other conditions are eliminated from the differential diagnosis, often the only way to make this distinction is by exclusion of other conditions and by following the platelet count over time in order to see if over time it falls to less than 80 000/μl, in which case in the absence of an alternative explanation a diagnosis of ITP may be established.

Gestational thrombocytopenia does not require intervention, nor does ITP, provided that the platelet count remains in a range that is appropriate for the anticipated method of delivery and accompanying interventions, such as placement of an epidural catheter. If no interventions for pain control and a normal vaginal delivery are planned, maternal platelet counts as low as 50 000/μl are considered acceptable for delivery, although there are reports in the literature of uncomplicated delivery with maternal platelet counts as low as 20 000/μl [31]. However, because there is not a good correlation between the maternal and fetal platelet counts, the neonate should be screened for thrombocytopenia [32]. Regarding placement of epidural catheters and the need for Caesarean section, in the absence of other complicating factors, a platelet count of between 80 000 and 100 000/μl is generally considered by obstetric anesthesiologists to be acceptable [33].

If a diagnosis of ITP is established, and it is felt to be desirable to increase the platelet count prior to delivery, aiming for the range of 70 000–100 000/μl is reasonable.

There is evidence for the effectiveness of both corticosteroids and intravenous immune globulin infusion in this setting [34]. Which therapy to use depends largely on provider and patient preference, as major differences in efficacy have not been reported.

The appropriate diagnostic evaluation and management for severe pre-eclampsia and HELLP syndrome is covered in Question 6 below.

6. What is the appropriate diagnostic evaluation and management of microangiopathic disorders identified during pregnancy?

- Medline: HELLP OR thrombotic microangiopathy AND pregnancy AND review.
- Hand-searching reference lists were used to identify additional articles of interest.
- Inclusion: References providing information relevant to the diagnostic evaluation and/or management of these disorders published in the English language were included.

A broad spectrum of microangiopathic disorders may present during pregnancy and the puerperium (Table 32.6). Though HELLP syndrome is specific to pregnancy, the other disorders are not. However, their incidence during pregnancy is increased relative to the general population.

Once a microangiopathic disorder is identified by the findings of red blood cell fragmentation associated with hemolysis, identifying the correct diagnosis rests upon correlating historical features and findings on the physical examination with appropriate laboratory diagnostic testing [39]. The complete blood count and peripheral blood smear should be reviewed for other relevant findings, such as thrombocytopenia. Coagulation testing, including at a minimum a prothrombin time (PT) and partial thromboplastin time (PTT) are indicated. If these coagulation tests are abnormal, a fibrinogen level should be obtained, because very low levels of fibrinogen may be associated with disseminated intravascular coagulation (DIC) due to amniotic fluid embolism during pregnancy [40]. Serum creatinine, liver function, and LDH tests should also be obtained.

Table 32.6 Incidence of microangiopathic disorders during pregnancy

Disorder	Frequency
Hemolysis, elevated liver function tests, and low platelets (HELLP) syndrome	1 in 200 to 1 in 120 pregnancies, including 10–20% of those with severe pre-eclampsia [35]
Thrombotic thrombocytopenic purpura (TTP)	1 in 25 000 pregnancies [36]
Atypical hemolytic uremic syndrome (aHUS)	1 in 25 000 pregnancies [37]
Disseminated intravascular coagulation (DIC)	3 in 10 000 deliveries [38]

Definitive diagnosis of the cause of a microangiopathic disorder can be challenging during pregnancy [41]. In individuals who are not pregnant, abnormal coagulation tests are generally indicative of DIC rather than other microangiopathic disorders such as TTP or atypical hemolytic uremic syndrome (aHUS). However, during pregnancy, about 15% of cases of HELLP syndrome are associated with DIC [38]. In general, such concomitant HELLP syndrome and DIC are associated with increased morbidity and mortality [42].

Management of severe pre-eclampsia and HELLP syndrome depends upon gestational age. Immediate delivery is recommended for severe pre-eclampsia after 34 weeks of gestation and for HELLP syndrome [43]. However, prior to 34 weeks of gestation, severe pre-eclampsia may be managed expectantly in some cases, although certain conditions may necessitate delivery, such as eclampsia, DIC, or abnormal fetal testing [44]. If expectant management is chosen, close monitoring is appropriate. Corticosteroids do not appear to be effective in the management of HELLP syndrome [45].

Acknowledgment

The opinions expressed in this manuscript are those of the author and do not represent the official position of the Food and Drug Administration or the government of the United States.

References

1 Rodger, M., Sheppard, D., Gándara, E., and Tinmouth, A. (2015). Haematological problems in obstetrics. *Best Pract. Res. Clin. Obstet. Gynaecol.* **29** (**5**): 671–684.

2 Peyrin-Biroulet, L., Williet, N., and Cacoub, P. (2015). Guidelines on the diagnosis and treatment of iron deficiency across indications: a systematic review. *Am. J. Nutr.* **102** (**6**): 1585–1594.

3 DeLoughery, T.G. (2014). Microcytic Anemia. *N. Engl. J. Med.* **371** (**14**): 1324–1331.

4 Lopez, A., Cacoub, P., Macdougall, I.C., and Peyrin-Biroulet, L. (2016). Iron deficiency anemia. *Lancet* **387** (**10021**): 907–916.

5 Auerbach, M. and Adamson, J.W. (2016). How we diagnose and treat iron deficiency anemia. *Am. J. Hematol.* **91** (**1**): 31–38.

6 Auerbach, M. and Ballard, H. (2010). Clinical use of intravenous iron: administration, efficacy, and safety. *Hematol. Am. Soc. Hematol. Educ. Program.* **2010**: 338–347.

7 Nielsen, O.H., Coskun, M., and Weiss, G. (2016). Iron replacement therapy: do we need new guidelines? *Curr. Opin. Gastroenterol.* **32** (**2**): 128–135.

8 Gualandro, S.F., Fonseca, H.H., Yokomizo, I.K. et al. (2015). Cohort study of adult patients with haemoglobin SC disease: clinical characteristics and predictors of mortality. *Br. J. Haematol.* **171** (**4**): 631–637.

9 Leung, T.Y. and Lao, T.T. (2012). Thalassaemia in pregnancy. *Best Pract. Res. Clin. Obstet. Gynaecol.* **26** (**1**): 37–51.

10 Tongsong, T., Srisupundit, K., and Luewan, S. (2009). Outcomes of pregnancies affected by hemoglobin H disease. *Int. J. Gynaecol. Obstet.* **104** (**3**): 206–208.

11 Thompson, A.A., Kim, H.-Y., Singer, S.T. et al. (2013). Pregnancy outcomes in women with thalassemia in North America and the UK. *Am. J. Hematol.* **88** (**9**): 771–773.

12 Kuo, K. and Caughey, A.B. (2016). Contemporary outcomes of sickle cell disease in pregnancy. *Am. J. Obstet. Gynecol.* doi: 10.1016/j.acog.2016.05.032.

13 Oteng-Ntim, E., Meeks, D., Seed, P.T. et al. (2015). Adverse maternal and perinatal outcomes in pregnant women with sickle cell disease: systematic review and meta-analysis. *Blood* **125** (**21**): 3316–3325.

14 Boga, C. and Ozdogu, H. (2016). Pregnancy and sickle cell disease: a review of the current literature. *Crit. Rev. Oncol. Hematol.* **98**: 364–374.

15 Bennett, A.R. and Gray, S.H. (2014). What to do when she's bleeding through: the recognition, evaluation, and management of abnormal uterine bleeding in adolescents. *Curr. Opin. Pediatr.* **26** (**4**): 413–419.

16 Committee on Adolescent Health Care; Committee on Gynecologic Practice (2013). Committee Opinion No. 580: von Willebrand disease in women. *Obstet. Gynecol.* **122** (**6**): 1368–1373.

17 Favaloro, E.J., Pasalic, L., and Curnow, J. (2016). Laboratory tests used to help diagnose von Willebrand disease: an update. *Pathology* **48** (**4**): 303–318.

18 Bucciarelli, P., Siboni, S.M., Stufano, F. et al. (2015). Predictors of von Willebrand disease diagnosis in individuals with borderline von Willebrand factor plasma levels. *J. Thromb. Haemost.* **13** (**2**): 228–236.

19 Sokkary, N.A., Venkateswaran, L., Dietrich, J.E., and Teruya, J. (2012). Platelet function disorders and menorrhagia in adolescents: a review of laboratory diagnosis. *J. Pediatr. Adolesc. Gynecol.* **25** (**4**): 233–237.

20 Boender, J., Kruip, M.J., and Leebeek, F.W. (2016). A diagnostic approach to mild bleeding disorders. *J. Thomb. Haemost.* doi: 10.1111/jth.13368.

21 Ng, C., Motto, D.G., and Di Paola, J. (2015). Diagnostic approach to von Willebrand disease. *Blood* **125** (**13**): 2029–2037.

22 Castaman, G., Goodeve, A., Eikenboom, J., and European Group on von Willebrand Disease (2013). Principles of care for the diagnosis and treatment of von Willebrand disease. *Haematologica* **98** (**5**): 667–674.

23 Lipe, B.C., Dumas, M.A., and Ornstein, D.L. (2011). Von Willebrand disease in pregnancy. *Hematol. Oncol. Clin. N. Am.* **25** (**2**): 335–358.

24 Bergmann, F. and Rath, W. (2015). The differential diagnosis of thrombocytopenia in pregnancy. *Dtsch. Arztebl. Int.* **112** (**47**): 795–802.

25 Crowther, M.A., Burrows, R.F., Ginsberg, J., and Kelton, J.G. (1996). Thrombocytopenia in pregnancy: diagnosis, pathogenesis and management. *Blood Rev.* **10** (**1**): 8–16.

26 Onisâi, M., Vlădăreanu, A.M., Delcea, C. et al. (2012). Perinatal outcome for pregnancies complicated with thrombocytopenia. *J. Matern. Fetal Neonatal. Med.* **25** (**9**): 1622–1626.

27 Gill, K.K. and Kelton, J.G. (2000). Management of idiopathic thrombocytopenic purpura in pregnancy. *Semin. Hematol.* **37** (**3**): 275–289.

28 Gernsheimer, T.B. (2012). Thrombocytopenia in pregnancy: is this immune thrombocytopenia or...? *Hematol. Am. Soc. Hematol. Educ. Program.* **2012**: 198–202.

29 Shehata, N., Burrows, R., and Kelton, J.G. (1999). Gestational thrombocytopenia. *Clin. Obstet. Gynecol.* **42** (**2**): 327–334.

30 Stavrou, E. and McCrae, K.R. (2009). Immune thrombocytopenia in pregnancy. *Hematol. Oncol. Clin. N. Am.* **23** (**6**): 1299–1316.

31 Gernsheimer, T., James, A.H., and Stasi, R. (2013). How I treat thrombocytopenia in pregnancy. *Blood* **121** (**1**): 38–47.

32 Sainio, S., Jarvenpaa, A.L., and Renlund, M. (2000). Thrombocytopenia in term infants: a population-based study. *Obstet. Gynecol.* **95** (**3**): 441–446.

33 Bernstein, J., Hua, B., Kahana, M. et al. (2016). Neuraxial anesthesia in parturients with low platelet counts. *Anesth. Analg.* **123** (**1**): 165–167.

34 (1997). Diagnosis and treatment of idiopathic thrombocytopenic purpura: recommendations of the American Society of Hematology. The American Society of Hematology ITP Practice Guideline Panel. *Ann Intern Med* **126** (**4**): 319–326.

35 Kirkpatrick, C.A. (2010). The HELLP syndrome. *Acta Clin.* **65** (**2**): 91–97.

36 Dashe, J.S., Ramin, S.M., and Cunningham, F.G. (1998). The long-term consequences of thrombotic microangiopathy (thrombotic thrombocytopenic purpura and hemolytic uremic syndrome) in pregnancy. *Obstet. Gynecol.* **91** (**5 Pt 1**): 662–668.

37 Fakhouri, F., Roumenina, L., Provot, F. et al. (2010). Pregnancy-associated hemolytic uremic syndrome revisited in the era of complement gene mutations. *J. Am. Soc. Nephrol.* **21** (**5**): 859–867.

38 Rattray, D.D., O'Connell, C.M., and Baskett, T.F. (2012). Acute disseminated intravascular coagulation in obstetrics: a tertiary centre population review (1980 to 2009). *J. Obstet. Gynaecol. Can.* **34** (**4**): 341–347.

39 Myers, B. (2012). Diagnosis and management of maternal thrombocytopenia in pregnancy. *Br. J. Haematol.* **158** (**1**): 3–15.

40 Sultan, P., Seligman, K., and Carvalho, B. (2016). Amniotic fluid embolism: update and review. *Curr. Opin. Anaethesiol.* **29** (**3**): 288–296.

41 Pels, S.G. and Paidas, M.J. (2011). Microangiopathic disorders in pregnancy. *Hematol. Oncol. Clin. N. Am.* **25** (**2**): 311–322.

42 Letsky, E.A. (2010). Disseminated intravascular coagulation. *Best Pract. Res. Clin. Obstet. Gynaecol.* **15** (**4**): 623–644.

43 Diagnosis, S., B.M. (2004). Controversies, and management of the syndrome of hemolysis, elevated liver enzymes, and low platelet count. *Obstet. Gynecol.* **103** (**5 Pt 1**): 981–991.

44 Publications Committee, Society for Maternal-Fetal Medicine and Sibai, B.M. (2011). Evaluation and management of severe pre-eclampsia before 34 weeks' gestation. *Am. J. Obstet. Gynecol.* **205** (**3**): 191–198.

45 Woudstra, D.M., Chandra, S., Hofmeyr, G.J., and Dowswell, T. (2010; 9 (Art. NO.: CD008148)). Corticosteroids for HELLP (hemolysis, elevated liver enzymes, low platelets) syndrome in pregnancy. *Cochrane Database Syst. Rev.* doi: 10.1002/14651858.CD008148.pub2.

33

CHAPTER 33

Infections in pregnancy

Jennifer Amorosa[1], Jane Goldman[2], and Rhoda Sperling[1,3]
[1]*Department of Obstetrics, Gynecology and Reproductive Sciences, Icahn School of Medicine, Mt Sinai Hospital, New York, NY, USA*
[2]*Division of Maternal-Fetal Medicine, Department of Obstetrics and Gynecology, The Valley Hospital, Ridgewood, NJ, USA*
[3]*Medicine, Infectious Diseases, Icahn School of Medicine, Mt Sinai Hospital, New York, NY, USA*

Cytomegalovirus

CLINICAL VIGNETTE

A thirty-one-year-old G2P1 daycare worker at 13 weeks presents with vague flu like symptoms. Cytomegalovirus titers IgG and IgM positive, suggesting a possible primary infection. She presents for counseling regarding the management of primary cytomegalovirus (CMV) infection in pregnancy.

A primary CMV diagnosis in pregnancy is complicated for both the patient and the physician. The outcomes are variable, so counseling the patient about short and long-term risks to the developing fetus is difficult. The timing of the infection impacts the risk of vertical transmission to the fetus as well as the long-term outcomes of the affected neonate. Current methods of diagnosis cannot accurately predict if a fetus will be affected and what the long-term consequences may be. Additionally, there is no proven in utero treatment for infected fetuses.

CMV is a double stranded DNA herpes virus. Infection can be primary or nonprimary. Primary CMV infection is the initial acquisition of the virus. Nonprimary infection results from reactivation of latent virus or reinfection with a different CMV strain. Transmission occurs by person to person contact with infected bodily secretions such as blood, urine, and saliva. Health care workers and those in contact with young children are at greatest risk. Seroprevalence increases with age and varies by geographic area and socioeconomic background.

The incubation period ranges from 28 to 60 days. Viremia can be detected two to three weeks after primary infection [1]. In pregnancy, rates of primary infection range from 1% to 7% [2]. Sometimes, primary CMV causes a mild febrile illness; however, 90% of women are asymptomatic, making the diagnosis difficult. A history of pre-existing maternal CMV seropositivity decreases, but does not eliminate, the risk of fetal infection because maternal antibodies to CMV cannot prevent reactivation or reinfection. Secondary infection in pregnancy may occur in up to 13% of patients [1].

While viral culture or polymerase chain reaction (PCR) of infected body fluids can be used to diagnose CMV, infection in adults is usually established by serologic testing. Maternal primary infection can be diagnosed by comparing anti-CMV IgG levels drawn three to four weeks apart. Seroconversion from negative to positive or greater than a fourfold increase in the anti-CMV IgG titers indicates infection. CMV avidity testing can also be used to aid in determining recent from prior CMV infections. High index values indicate that the infection occurred more than three months prior to testing, making avidity testing in the first trimester particularly helpful in excluding a diagnosis of an acute CMV infection post-conception.

CMV is the most common congenital infection, occurring in up to 2% of all neonates [3, 4]. The risk for severe fetal infection is higher after primary infection than after recurrent infection. Primary CMV is associated with 30–50% risk of mother-to-child transmission with a spectrum of disease that encompasses severe multi-organ disease, neurological impairments, and sensorineural hearing loss (SNHL). Chronic (latent) CMV has been associated with a lower overall risk of vertical transmission (1–3%) and infrequent severe multi-organ disease. SNHL is the most frequent sequelae [1].

At birth, the majority of infected newborns born to women with primary CMV will be asymptomatic; however, 12–18% will have clinical signs and symptoms of CMV and up to 25% will have neurological sequelae [1, 3]. Thirty percent of severely infected infants die, and 65–80% will have neurologic sequelae [1, 5]. Asymptomatic infants have a lower risk of developing long-term neurologic problems which include

Evidence-Based Obstetrics and Gynecology, First Edition. Edited by Errol R. Norwitz, Carolyn M. Zelop, David A. Miller, and David L. Keefe.

Table 33.1 Risk of fetal transmission based on timing of maternal CMV infection

Preconception	Periconception	First trimester	Second trimester	Third trimester
1–10 weeks before conception	One week before last menstrual period to 4–six weeks pregnant			
17%	35%	34–42%	43–44%	64–73%

Source: Adapted from Enders et al. [6].

progressive hearing and/or visual loss as well as cognitive impairment.

Vertical transmission occurs transplacentally. The timing of infection affects transmission rates in maternal primary infection (Table 33.1). Enders et al. evaluated 248 pregnancies with primary CMV infection. The mean rate of intrauterine transmission was approximately 38%. Transmission was significantly higher in the third trimester when compared to the first trimester. However, more serious sequelae occur after first trimester infection compared to other trimesters [6]. The neonate can also be infected by exposure to infected breast milk and cervical secretions. In contrast to infections acquired in-utero, infections acquired post-natally are often asymptomatic and are generally not associated with long-term adverse sequelae.

Prenatal diagnosis is an option for patients with a known primary infection or with ultrasound findings suggestive of CMV infection such as echogenic bowel, cerebral ventriculomegaly and calcifications and IUGR (Figures 33.1–33.4). Amniocentesis has a greater sensitivity after 21 weeks gestation and should be performed at least six to eight weeks after onset of maternal infection to perform PCR for CMV DNA. An earlier negative amniocentesis may provide false reassurance so a follow-up amniocentesis should be considered after 21 weeks gestation. Serial ultrasound assessment can also detect stigmata suggestive of fetal sequelae (Tables 33.2 and 33.3).

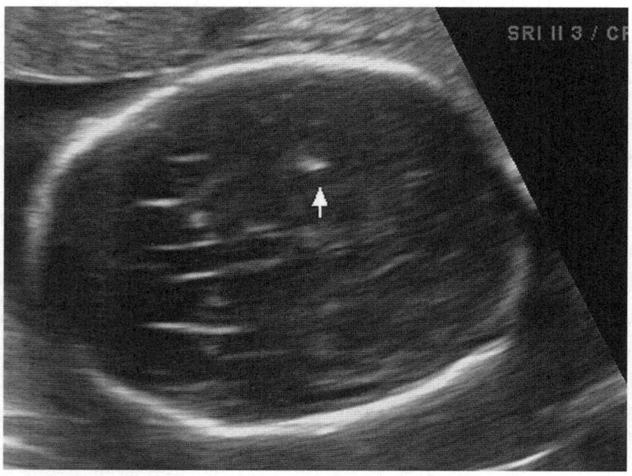

Figure 33.1 Intracerebral calcification.

Although fetal infection can be detected by PCR (sensitivity 78–98%), fetal prognosis is difficult to predict. Quantitative determination of viral load in amniotic fluid may help to predict fetal outcome. An abnormal ultrasound examination suggests a poor prognosis, while a normal ultrasound examination does not exclude the possibility of a symptomatic neonate or long-term neurologic morbidity. A negative result from prenatal diagnosis after primary infection in early pregnancy is associated with favorable outcomes [6].

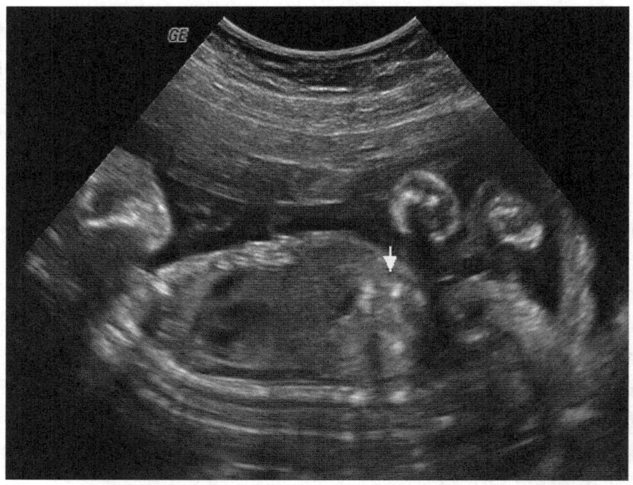

Figure 33.2 Echogenic bowel.

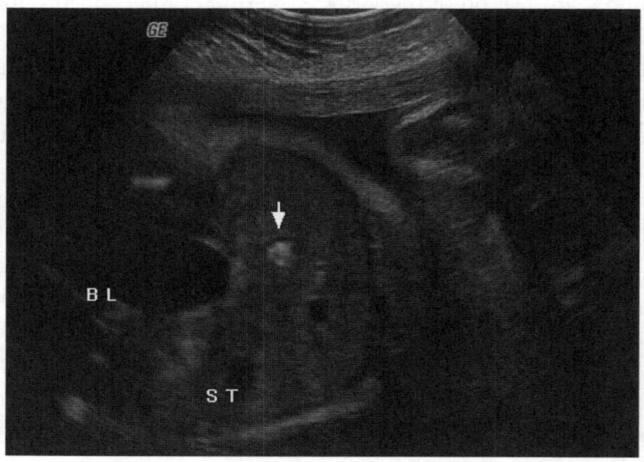

Figure 33.3 Abdominal calcification.

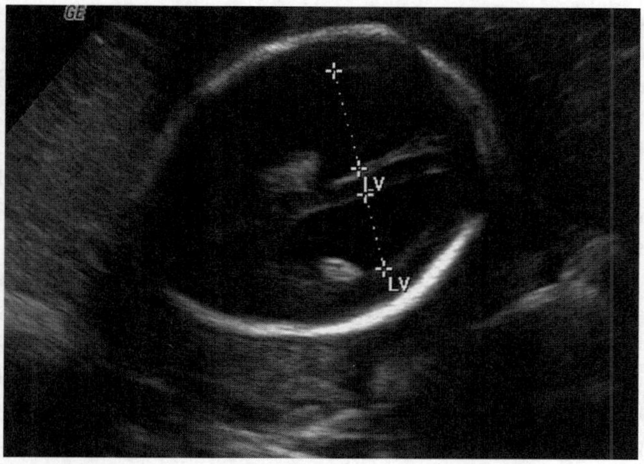

Figure 33.4 Ventriculomegaly.

Table 33.2 Possible ultrasound findings in fetuses affected with CMV

Abdominal and liver calcifications
Echogenic bowel
Echogenic kidneys
Intracranial calcifications
Cerebral ventriculomegaly
Ascites
Intrauterine growth restriction
Microcephaly
Hydrops
Enlarged placenta
Intrauterine fetal demise

Table 33.3 Potential results of serum testing after expose and management guidelines

IgM Result	IgG Result	Interpretation and management
Negative	Negative	Susceptible, repeat testing in four weeks
Negative	Positive	Immune, not at risk of transplacental transmission
Positive	Negative	Acute maternal infection, monitor for signs of fetal infection
Positive	Positive	Subacute maternal infection, monitor for signs of fetal infection

During pregnancy, there is no proven treatment to prevent fetal disease or reduce the risk of sequelae [7]. Antiviral drugs have not been well-studied during pregnancy for the prevention of mother-to-child transmission and CMV specific hyperimmunoglobulin therapy to reduce symptomatic infection in fetuses and neonates is still investigational. In three prospective studies, CMV-specific hyperimmune globulin administered to pregnant women with primary CMV infection was associated with decreased transmission and decreased severity of infection [8–10]. However, a recent randomized placebo-controlled double blind study of 124 pregnant women with primary CMV at 5–26 weeks did not demonstrate improved outcomes [11]. Rates of congenital infection and symptomatic neonates were similar in both the treatment and placebo group (30% versus 44%, 30% versus 24%). Additionally, there were more adverse obstetrical events in the hyperimmune globulin group than in the placebo group (13% versus 2%), including preterm delivery, preeclampsia, and intrauterine growth restriction.

Universal screening for CMV during pregnancy has not been recommended by ACOG as there are no efficacious treatments for CMV in pregnancy nor is there a CMV vaccine. However, this is an active area of research investigation. Good personal hygiene prevention strategies such as hand washing are recommended to prevent primary infection [1].

Parvovirus

> **CLINICAL VIGNETTE**
>
> A 27-year-old G2P1 at 14 weeks calls your office because her four-year-old daughter has a bright red rash on her cheeks. The child had a fever several days ago. The patient is concerned about her risk of infection and the implications for her pregnancy.

Parvovirus B19 is a single stranded DNA virus that is transmitted by respiratory secretions or hand to mouth contact. Most often it is a childhood illness. About 35–65% of pregnant women are immune [12–14]. The incidence of acute B19 infection in pregnancy is approximately 3.5% [12] and the risk of vertical transmission is 25% [15]. The risk of maternal parvovirus infection varies by level of exposure to the infected individual. Exposure to infected household members confers the highest risk [14, 16].

Virema from B19 begins roughly six days after exposure and continues for approximately one week [17]. By the time a patient is symptomatic, she is rarely contagious. Children develop a "slapped cheek" appearance and a "lace-like" rash on the extremities and trunk. Adults often develop a rash on the trunk, preceded by arthropathy of the hands, wrists, knees and ankles. Some patients are asymptomatic [18, 19]. Patients with an underlying chronic anemia, such as sickle cell anemia, may experience a transient aplastic crisis.

Intrauterine B19 infection can spontaneously resolve with no adverse sequelae or it can lead to severe fetal anemia resulting in fetal loss or hydrops fetalis. The overall rate of fetal loss reported in the literature ranges from 5% to 9%. The risk is highest if infection occurs during the first half of pregnancy [13, 19–21]. A prospective observational study of 1018 women with acute B19 infection found a fetal death rate of 6.3%. In all cases, maternal infection occurred before 20 weeks gestation. A total of 80% of the fetal deaths occurred within four weeks of maternal infection. Stillbirth, defined as a fetal death at or greater than 22 weeks gestational age, occurred in 0.6% of the pregnancies [19]. A Swedish study examined the etiology of intrauterine fetal deaths occurring at 28 weeks gestation or greater. During the seven-year study period, data was collected on 33 759 women, 93 of whom had an intrauterine fetal demise (IUFD) (0.3%). Parvovirus B19 was associated with 7 (7.5%) of the fetal deaths in this group making the overall rate 0.02% [22]. None of the seven fetuses were hydropic.

In addition to fetal loss, B19 can lead to hydrops fetalis. This risk is highest if the mother is infected in the first half of pregnancy [19, 23]. Enders et al. demonstrated that pregnancies affected by B19 had a 3.9% risk of developing hydrops fetalis; however, that rate increased to 7.1% if parvovirus B19 was acquired between weeks 13–20 of gestation. The risk decreased to less than 1% if the infection occurred after 32 weeks gestational age [19]. In a later study, the same group found a similar overall rate of hydrops (4.2%). Approximately 11% of fetuses infected between 9 and 20 weeks developed hydrops [23]. Mild hydrops may spontaneously resolved and be associated with favorable perinatal outcomes. On the other hand, severe hydrops can rapidly lead to fetal death if no intervention is undertaken. In fetuses that develop severe hydrops, fetal transfusion helps prevent fetal death. In a prospective study by Enders et al., 85% of fetuses who developed severe hydrops and were transfused survived. All of the fetuses with severe hydrops who were not transfused, died [19]. Fetuses with hydrops may be severely thrombocytopenic so exsanguination at time of transfusion is a concern [24, 25]. Platelet counts should be determined and platelets available at the time of any fetal procedure.

While several case reports have described congenital anomalies in infants affected by parvovirus infection, most intrauterine parvovirus infections are not associated with anomalies [12, 20, 21, 26–30].

IgM antibodies to parvovirus are detectable approximately 10 days after exposure and persist for at least three months. IgG antibodies are detectable several days after IgM and typically persist for years. Enzyme-linked immunosorbent assays (ELISA) and enzyme immunoassays (EIA) are 80–100% sensitive in diagnosing maternal B19 infection. IgM negative patients with significant exposure history, PCR testing may be used to detect disease when the patient's IgM levels are below the detection limit of ELISA [31, 32]. PCR is the best method for fetal diagnosis because it can detect small amounts of B19 DNA from amniotic fluid [15].

ACOG recommends that pregnant women who are exposed to Parvovirus B19 undergo serum screening as soon as possible after exposure to determine if further monitoring is needed. Women who are IgM negative and IgG positive are immune and are not at risk of transplacental transmission. Women who are IgM positive need to be monitored for potential fetal infection no matter what their IgG status. Women who are both IgM and IgG negative are susceptible to B19 infection and should have repeat testing performed in four weeks. If either IgM or IgG becomes positive, these women should be followed for potential fetal infection [1].

Pregnant women who become infected with parvovirus should be monitored with ultrasound every 1 to 2 weeks for 8 to 12 weeks following exposure to assess for developing anemia. The ultrasound exam should look for signs of hydrops such as ascites and placentomegaly and intrauterine growth restriction. Additionally, fetal middle cerebral artery Doppler assessment should be performed as this can reliably predict fetal anemia [33, 34]. Severely hydropic fetuses have a poor prognosis. If hydrops fetalis or severe fetal anemia is suspected, fetal blood sampling should be performed and intrauterine transfusion considered if the fetus is severely anemic [1, 35–37].

ACOG does not recommend routine screening for parvovirus in pregnancy given the low rate of seroconversion during pregnancy as well the variable rate of fetal transmission and range of potential sequelae. Instead testing should be performed on symptomatic patients and patients with exposure to suspected or confirmed cases [1].

Varicella zoster

CLINICAL VIGNETTE

A 35-year-old G2P1at 15 weeks calls your office because her unvaccinated seven-year-old nephew who recently visited developed a fever and vesicular rash that looks like chickenpox. The patient does not recall having chickenpox as child nor being vaccinated. The patient calls your office to discuss the risk to her pregnancy.

Varicella zoster virus (VZV) is a highly contagious DNA herpes virus that is transmitted by respiratory droplets, direct contact, or rarely airborne spread. Primary infection causes a diffuse vesicular rash commonly known as chickenpox. Children are most often affected; less than 5% of reported cases occur in adults older than 20 [38]. Since most US adults have immunity to VZV, varicella during pregnancy is rare with an incidence of 1–5 cases per 10 000 pregnancies [39]. Maternal infection during pregnancy can have serious maternal, fetal and neonatal consequences.

Besides the characteristic rash, pregnant women infected with varicella are at an increased risk of varicella pneumonia which can progress to hypoxia and respiratory failure. Before the introduction of antiretroviral treatment, reports estimated the incidence of VZV pneumonia in pregnancy as 10–20% [40] with mortality rates of up to

Table 33.4 Characteristic findings of congenital varicella syndrome

Limb hypoplasia
Ocular abnormalities
Neurologic abnormalities
Fetal growth restriction
Gastrointestinal abnormalities
Skin lesions

Table 33.5 Ultrasound findings suggestive of congenital varicella syndrome

Hyperechoic foci in the liver, heart, brain and bowl	Limb deformities and contractures
Hydrops	Cardiac malformations
Fetal growth restriction	Ventriculormegaly
Porencephaly	Microcephaly
Polyhydramnios	

40% [41]. Recently, Zhang et al. studied a cohort of nearly 1000 pregnancies from the Healthcare Cost and Utilization Project – Nationwide Inpatient Sample (HCUP-NIS) admitted with VZV infection. The incidence of VZV pneumonia was 2.5% (95% CI, 1.6–3.7) [39]. No maternal deaths were attributable to VZV pneumonia.

Varicella infection between weeks 8–20 of gestation puts the fetus at risk of developing congenital varicella syndrome [42], a rare syndrome is associated with multiple abnormalities (chorioretinitis, congenital cataracts, cerebral cortical atrophy as well as variable degrees of limb atrophy and skin scarring) (Table 33.4). Mortality rates have been reported to be as high as 30%. A total of 15% of cases develop herpes zoster by age four [43, 44].

In infected mothers, multiple cohort studies have reported that about 1% of fetuses will develop congenital varicella syndrome [45–55]. The risk appears to be slightly higher (2%) if the patient is infected between 13 and 20 weeks [53].

Infants delivered within two weeks of maternal varicella infection are at risk of developing severe varicella infections. The highest risk (17–30%) occurs between five days prior to and two days after delivery as the infant is born without having acquired antibody from the mother [56]. The clinical course of neonatal varicella varies depending on the timing of exposure and can range from a mild rash and fever to a disseminated infection. Neonatal varicella that occurs in the first 1–12 days of life is most likely caused by transplacental transmission of VZV, whereas an infant who becomes infected between 12 and 28 days after birth most likely acquired VZV postnatally [57].

The diagnosis of varicella is usually clinical. Laboratory confirmation can be obtained by detecting viral DNA by PCR testing of skin scrapings from the base of a vesicle or through immunofluorescence detection of VZV antigen. Vesicular fluid can also be cultured; however the process is slow and less sensitive than direct detection techniques. Prenatal diagnosis can be made via PCR of amniotic fluid and/or ultrasound diagnosis [58–63]. To avoid false negative results, amniocentesis should not be performed until one month after maternal infection [64]. Two studies have looked at laboratory prenatal diagnosis of varicella [46, 65]. Mouly et al. examined PCR testing of amniotic fluid in 107 fetuses and demonstrated an 8.4% transmission rate. Not all of the PCR positive infants had clinical manifestations at birth. Importantly, none of the infants who had a negative PCR went on to develop congenital varicella syndrome [46]. Similar results were reported by Kustermann et al. [65] supporting the idea that a negative PCR is reassuring.

At least five weeks should lapse between maternal infection and fetal ultrasound as imaging performed sooner has failed to detect deformities [60, 66, 67]. If associated anomalies are seen in the setting of a maternal infection, risk of fetal infection is high (Table 33.5). Pretorius et al. published a case series that described 37 maternal VZV infections. Five infants were diagnosed with congenital varicella syndrome, all of whom had sonographic abnormalities. The other 32 were unaffected and other than an isolated case of polyhydramnios, no other abnormalities were found [60].

Postnatally, the diagnosis of congenital varicella requires a history of first or second trimester maternal varicella infection, fetal abnormalities consistent with congenital varicella, and evidence of intrauterine VZV infection. Intrauterine VZV infection can be demonstrated by detection of VZV DNA in the newborn, the presence of VZV IgM antibodies in cord blood, the appearance of clinical zoster early in infancy, and/or the persistence of VZV IgG for more than seven months after birth [44].

Non-immune pregnant women who have been exposed to varicella should be treated with VariZIG, a purified immune globulin preparation made from human plasma containing high levels of anti-VZV antibodies (immunoglobulin G). It should be administered within 4–10 days of exposure [68]. Early administration (within four days) may produce milder symptoms in those who go on to develop varicella [69, 70]. Prior to the use of immune globulins, rates of infection were approximately 70–89%. A Phase III, multi-centered, three-arm randomized, active controlled study of non-immune pregnant patients who were treated either with VariZIG or its predecessor VZIG found that 29% of patients treated with VariZIG developed varicella – a significant reduction when compared to historical data [57, 70]. Study VZ-009, an expanded access protocol that administered VariZIG to high-risk patients including pregnant women showed a reduction the number of patient with VZV who developed VZV pneumonia suggesting that VariZIG helps to reduce the severity of chickenpox in exposed patients [71].

A cohort study by Enders suggests that intravenous immunoglobulin (IVIG) given to exposed women may prevent congenital varicella syndrome. There were nine cases of congenital varicella in this prospective study of 1373 women. None occurred in the infants of 97 varicella infected women who received post-exposure prophylaxis with anti-varicella zoster immunoglobulin [53].

When started within 24 hours of initial rash development, oral acyclovir reduces constitutional symptoms, total lesions and duration of lesion formation. Two pregnancy registries have not demonstrated an increased rate of congenital malformations in pregnant women treated with acyclovir [72, 73] so oral acyclovir or its prodrug valacyclovir should be considered in pregnancy if chickenpox lesions develop. Acyclovir is slowly and incompletely absorbed with bioavailability of about 15–30%; valacyclovir is the orally administered prodrug of acyclovir that overcomes the problem of poor oral bioavailability and exhibits improved pharmacokinetic properties. Historically, mortality rates were as high as 40% in pregnant women who developed VZV pneumonia [41]. While no randomized controlled trials have been performed, case reports and case series have suggested that treatment with intravenous acyclovir may reduce maternal morbidity and mortality [74–76]. A review by Smego found a mortality rate of 14% in patients treated with intravenous acyclovir [75] and a recent NICHD/MFMU case–control analysis of 18 women with VZV pneumonia treated with acyclovir had no maternal deaths [77].

Intravenous acyclovir may also help prevent neonatal varicella. Huang et al. who showed that a combination of intravenous acyclovir and IVIG effectively prevented neonatal varicella in infants whose mothers had a varicella rash either seven days prior to or five days after delivery, whereas 50% of the infants receiving IVIG alone developed neonatal varicella [78].

Pre-pregnancy vaccination is the best way to prevent fetal varicella infection. Highly effective, the varicella vaccine is an attenuated live virus vaccine that prevents ~98% cases of varicella [79]. First approved in the US in 1995, between 2000 and 2010, varicella incidence declined by 82%. In the first 12 years that the vaccination was available, varicella-related deaths decreased by 88% [80, 81]. Australian surveillance data also showed a significant reduction in rates of congenital and neonatal varicella (0.8–0.19% and 5.8–2% respectively) after the introduction of the vaccine [45].

In women contemplating pregnancy, varicella history should be elicited. Those with no clear history of a two-dose vaccine or varicella infection should be vaccinated. It is recommended that women wait for one to three months post-vaccination to conceive [82–84]. Varicella vaccination should be deferred until the postpartum period in non-immune patients as the vaccine is a live-attenuated virus vaccine and there are theoretical concerns that transplacental viremia could result in fetal infection and congenital varicella syndrome. That said, post-marketing surveillance studies of Varivax (Varicella Virus vaccine live [Oka/Merck]) demonstrated no cases of congenital varicella syndrome to women who were inadvertently vaccinated during pregnancy or within three months prior to conception [85, 86].

Ideally, women should be screened for varicella immune status prior to pregnancy. Those who don't have a disease or vaccination history should be vaccinated prior to conception. Seronegative women who are exposed to varicella during pregnancy should be given VariZIG within 10 days of exposure. In women who develop varicella, oral acyclovir or oral valacyclovir are likely to reduce the severity of clinical disease. Pregnant women who develop varicella pneumonia should be given IV acyclovir. Additionally, in infants of women who had varicella around the time of delivery, consideration should be given to treating the newborn with both IVIG and IV acyclovir in order to prevent neonatal varicella syndrome. Finally, seronegative women should be vaccinated in the immediate postpartum period.

Listeria

CLINICAL VIGNETTE

A 32-year old G3P2 at 32 weeks presented to labor and delivery with fever and a "flu-like" illness for the past two days. Her flu swab was negative. She denied sick contacts but reported that she inadvertently ate unpasteurized cheese. On physical examination, the patient was febrile to 38.2°C. Chest X-ray and urinalysis were within normal limits. The patient's white blood cell count was 17 000 ml^{-1}. Blood cultures were performed and demonstrated Gram-positive bacilli suggestive of *Listeria monocytogenes*.

Knowledge about listeriosis is important for health care providers. Prompt diagnosis and treatment reduces the risk of serious sequelae for the fetus and neonate. *L. monocytogenes* is a Gram-positive bacillus that is both aerobic and facultative anaerobic and has an intracellular transmission pattern [87]. Consuming listeria-contaminated food can cause listeriosis. Foods that can be contaminated with listeria include raw vegetables, raw milk, poultry, meat and fish [88]. Both ACOG and the CDC recommend that pregnant women avoid high-risk foods such as paté, meat spreads, refrigerated smoked seafood, unpasteurized milk, and unpasteurized soft cheeses. Hot dogs, lunch meat, and cold cuts should be heated to an internal temperature of 74°C. Raw fruits and vegetables should be washed thoroughly in running tap water prior to eating, peeling or cutting [89, 90].

Table 33.6 Symptoms that can be associated with maternal listeria infection

High fever	Septic abortion
Flu-like illness	Non-reassuring fetal heart tracing
GI symptoms such as diarrhea	Asymptomatic
Preterm labor	

In 2012, the incidence of listeriosis in the United States was 0.23 cases per 100 000 people [91]. Pregnant women are among the most susceptible and the incidence of pregnancy-associated listeriosis is at least 13–20 fold higher than in the general population [92–94]. A CDC surveillance study found that 27% of listeria infections in the US occurred in pregnant patients [95]. Most cases occur in healthy pregnant women with no predisposing risk factors [96]. There is a higher incidence in Hispanic women when compared to non-Hispanic women [92].

Diagnosing listeria in pregnancy can be complicated as it is rare and patients may be asymptomatic. Those experiencing a symptomatic infection most often present with a high fever or flu-like illness, often preceded by gastrointestinal symptoms such as diarrhea [94, 97] (Table 33.6). Mylonakis' review of 222 patients with perinatal listeriosis found that 65% of patients presented with fever, 34% had a "flu-like" syndrome, and 31% were asymptomatic [97]. In Craig's series, 66% of the women presented with preterm labor and 33% reported an "influenza–like" illness [98]. In Elinav's report of 115 patients, those presenting in the second trimester often had a septic abortion or fever whereas those presenting in the third trimester had fever or non-reassuring fetal monitoring [96]. Invasive listeriosis, which can present in the form of sepsis, meningitis or encephalitis, is extremely rare in pregnancy.

The increased risk of listeriosis in the latter half of pregnancy is likely related to the immune adaptations that occur during normal pregnancy including a weakening of adaptive immunity [99]. In a recent series of 115 pregnancy-associated listeria cases in Israel, 40% and 56% presented in the second and third trimesters respectively [96]. First trimester cases have been reported; however first and second trimester incidence may be underreported because listeriosis may be associated with fetal loss and products of conception are rarely cultured [100–102].

Any pregnant women who presents with high fever of unknown origin should be ruled out for listeria. Diagnosis requires culture from a sterile site such as blood, cerebral spinal fluid, or joint fluid [88]. Fecal cultures are not helpful since individuals can be carriers without evidence of clinical disease. It is important to specify to the lab that listeria is the organism in question because listeria may look like diphtheroids [88]. If an amniocentesis is performed, gram positive rods and meconium staining are often present. At delivery, placental cultures should be obtained.

While maternal morbidity from listeriosis is rare, fetal and neonatal infections can be severe, resulting in pregnancy loss, preterm delivery, neonatal meningitis, sepsis and neonatal demise [89]. In its most fulminant form, the fetus may be stillborn or die within hours of life from granulomatosis infantiseptica, a disseminated form of listerial infection characterized by widespread granulomas and microabscesses. More commonly, neonatal listeria infection manifests either as an early onset sepsis syndrome in premature infants or as late onset meningitis in term infants [88].

Mylonakis et al. conducted a case series of 11 pregnant women along with a literature review of 222 cases and found that approximately 1 out of 5 pregnancies complicated by listeriosis resulted in stillbirth or spontaneous abortion. Approximately two thirds of infants born to mothers affected by listeriosis developed clinical neonatal listeriosis and were diagnosed with a combination of bacteremia, sepsis, pneumonia and/or meningitis. In the literature review, 63% of the infected neonates recovered completely, 25% died, and 12% had adverse long-term outcomes such as neurologic complications [97]. McLauchlin studied 248 pregnancies affected by listeria infection: 19% of the fetus died in utero, and 95% of the liveborn infants were diagnosed with neonatal infection [102]. A total of 35% of those infants born alive but diagnosed with listeria died. Other series have reported perinatal case mortality rates of 22–45% [94, 98, 103–105].

In women with a presumptive exposure to listeria, ACOG recommends the following management strategies [89]:

In asymptomatic patients. No testing or treatment is recommended for an asymptomatic woman who reports consumption of a product that was recalled or implicated during a listeria outbreak.

In febrile patients with or without other symptoms of listeria. Exposed pregnant women with a fever higher than 100.6°F and signs/symptoms of listeriosis and no other cause of illness should be simultaneously tested for and treated for presumptive listeriosis.

When diagnosed early and treated appropriately, pregnancies affected by listeriosis can result in a healthy, term infant [106, 107]. Pregnant patients with listeria should be treated with high dose ampicillin of at least 6 g per day for at least 14 days. Some authors recommend continuing the antibiotics for the duration of the pregnancy [87]. This dose allows for adequate intracellular penetration and also effectively crosses the placenta. Gentamicin is often added due to synergism. In women who are allergic to penicillin or ampicillin and in whom desensitization cannot be performed, trimethoprim with sulfamethoxazole should be considered [108]. Trimethoprim-sulfamethoxozole should be avoided in the first trimester because it can affect folic acid metabolism and it should be avoided in the last month of pregnancy to avoid fetal kernicterus. In these cases, vancomycin may be considered an acceptable alternative.

Level of Evidence

CMV

Screening:

Level B Evidence

Routine serologic screening for CMV is not recommended in pregnancy.

Treatment:

Level A/Class IIb

Treatment with antiviral drugs or hyperimmune globulin to prevent fetal transmission or reduce the risk of fetal sequelae is not recommended.

PARVOVIRUS

Diagnosis/Screening:

Level B Evidence

- Routine serologic screening for Parvovirus B19 is not recommended in pregnancy.
- Pregnant women who have been exposed to Parvovirus B19 should have serologic testing performed as soon after exposure as possible in order to determine if they need monitored for seroconversion.
- In the setting of parvovirus, if fetal anemia or hydrops is suspected, fetal blood sampling should be performed to determine the fetal hematocrit so that fetal transfusion can be performed if necessary.

VARICELLA

Diagnosis:

Level B Evidence

- Fetuses of mothers infected with varicella can be diagnosed prenatally via a combination of detection of VZV DNA by PCR in amniotic fluid and fetal blood as well as ultrasound diagnosis [58].

Treatment:

Level B Evidence

- Non-immune pregnant women who have been exposed to varicella should be treated with VariZIG to help reduce rates of infection and congenital varicella syndrome.
- Pregnant women with varicella pneumonia should be treated with IV acyclovir.
- IV acyclovir and IVIG should be given to newborns whose mothers developed varicella near the time of delivery.

Level C Evidence

- Oral acyclovir should be considered in pregnancy if chickenpox lesions develop in order to help lessen symptom severity and duration.

Vaccination:

Level B Evidence

- All non-pregnant women who are seronegative should be vaccinated for varicella prior to pregnancy or immediately postpartum.

LISTERIA

Diagnosis:

Level C Evidence

- Any pregnant woman who presents with a high fever (>38.1) of unknown origin should be ruled out for listeria.
- Diagnosis of listeria requires culture from a sterile site such as blood, joint fluid or cerebral spinal fluid.

Treatment:

Level C Evidence

- Pregnant patients with known or suspected listeria should be treated with a minimum dose of 6 g ampicillin daily for at least 14 days.

References

1 American College of Obstetricians and Gynecologists (2015). Practice bulletin no. 151: cytomegalovirus, parvovirus B19, varicella zoster, and toxoplasmosis in pregnancy. *Obstetrics and Gynecology* **125** (**6**): 1510–1525.

2 Hyde, T.B., Schmid, D.S., and Cannon, M.J. (2010). Cytomegalovirus seroconversion rates and risk factors: implications for congenital CMV. *Reviews in Medical Virology* **20** (**5**): 311–326.

3 Dollard, S.C., Grosse, S.D., and Ross, D.S. (2007). New estimates of the prevalence of neurological and sensory sequelae and mortality associated with congenital cytomegalovirus infection. *Reviews in Medical Virology* **17** (**5**): 355–363.

4 Kenneson, A. and Cannon, M.J. (2007). Review and meta-analysis of the epidemiology of congenital cytomegalovirus (CMV) infection. *Reviews in Medical Virology* **17** (**4**): 253–276.

5 Turner, K.M., Lee, H.C., Boppana, S.B. et al. (2014). Incidence and impact of CMV infection in very low birth weight infants. *Pediatrics* **133** (**3**): e609–e615.

6 Enders, G., Daiminger, A., Bader, U. et al. (2011). Intrauterine transmission and clinical outcome of 248 pregnancies with primary cytomegalovirus infection in relation to gestational age. *Journal of Clinical Virology* **52** (**3**): 244–246.

7 McCarthy, F.P., Giles, M.L., Rowlands, S. et al. (2011 . 3 (Art. No.: CD008371)). Antenatal interventions for preventing the transmission of cytomegalovirus (CMV) from the mother to fetus during pregnancy and adverse outcomes in the congenitally infected infant. *The Cochrane Database of Systematic Reviews* doi: 10.1002/14651858.CD008371.

8 Nigro, G., Adler, S.P., La Torre, R. et al. (2005). Passive immunization during pregnancy for congenital cytomegalovirus infection. *The New England Journal of Medicine* **353** (**13**): 1350–1362.

9 Nigro, G., Adler, S.P., Parruti, G. et al. (2012). Immunoglobulin therapy of fetal cytomegalovirus infection occurring in the

first half of pregnancy--a case-control study of the outcome in children. *The Journal of Infectious Diseases* **205** (**2**): 215–227.

10 Visentin, S., Manara, R., Milanese, L. et al. (2012). Early primary cytomegalovirus infection in pregnancy: maternal hyperimmunoglobulin therapy improves outcomes among infants at 1 year of age. *Clinical Infectious Diseases* **55** (**4**): 497–503.

11 Revello, M.G., Lazzarotto, T., Guerra, B. et al. (2014). A randomized trial of hyperimmune globulin to prevent congenital cytomegalovirus. *The New England Journal of Medicine* **370** (**14**): 1316–1326.

12 Gratacos, E., Torres, P.J., Vidal, J. et al. (1995). The incidence of human parvovirus B19 infection during pregnancy and its impact on perinatal outcome. *The Journal of Infectious Diseases* **171** (**5**): 1360–1363.

13 Rodis, J.F., Quinn, D.L., Gary, G.W. Jr. et al. (1990). Management and outcomes of pregnancies complicated by human B19 parvovirus infection: a prospective study. *American Journal of Obstetrics and Gynecology* **163** (**4 Pt 1**): 1168–1171.

14 Valeur-Jensen, A.K., Pedersen, C.B., Westergaard, T. et al. (1999). Risk factors for parvovirus B19 infection in pregnancy. *JAMA* **281** (**12**): 1099–1105.

15 Markenson, G.R. and Yancey, M.K. (1998). Parvovirus B19 infections in pregnancy. *Seminars in Perinatology* **22** (**4**): 309–317.

16 Harger, J.H., Adler, S.P., Koch, W.C., and Harger, G.F. (1998). Prospective evaluation of 618 pregnant women exposed to parvovirus B19: risks and symptoms. *Obstetrics and Gynecology* **91** (**3**): 413–420.

17 Anderson, M.J.H.P., Davis, L.R., Willman, J.S. et al. (1985). Experimental parvoviral infection in humans. *The Journal of Infectious Diseases* **152** (**2**): 257–265.

18 Young, N.S. and Brown, K.E. (2004). Parvovirus B19. *The New England Journal of Medicine* **350** (**6**): 586–597.

19 Enders, M., Weidner, A., Zoellner, I. et al. (2004). Fetal morbidity and mortality after acute human parvovirus B19 infection in pregnancy: prospective evaluation of 1018 cases. *Prenatal Diagnosis* **24** (**7**): 513–518.

20 (1990). Prospective study of human parvovirus (B19) infection in pregnancy. Public health laboratory service working party on fifth disease. *BMJ* **300** (**6733**): 1166–1170.

21 Miller, E., Fairley, C.K., Cohen, B.J., and Seng, C. (1998). Immediate and long-term outcome of human parvovirus B19 infection in pregnancy. *British Journal of Obstetrics and Gynaecology* **105** (**2**): 174–178.

22 Skjoldebrand-Sparre, L., Tolfvenstam, T., Papadogiannakis, N. et al. (2000). Parvovirus B19 infection: association with third-trimester intrauterine fetal death. *BJOG* **107** (**4**): 476–480.

23 Enders, M., Klingel, K., Weidner, A. et al. (2010). Risk of fetal hydrops and non-hydropic late intrauterine fetal death after gestational parvovirus B19 infection. *Journal of Clinical Virology* **49** (**3**): 163–168.

24 de Haan, T.R., van den Akker, E.S., Porcelijn, L. et al. (2008). Thrombocytopenia in hydropic fetuses with parvovirus B19 infection: incidence, treatment and correlation with fetal B19 viral load. *BJOG* **115** (**1**): 76–81.

25 Segata, M., Chaoui, R., Khalek, N. et al. (2007). Fetal thrombocytopenia secondary to parvovirus infection. *American Journal of Obstetrics and Gynecology* **196** (**1**): 61.e1–61.e4.

26 Bonvicini, F., Puccetti, C., Salfi, N.C. et al. (2011). Gestational and fetal outcomes in B19 maternal infection: a problem of diagnosis. *Journal of Clinical Microbiology* **49** (**10**): 3514–3518.

27 Courtier, J., Schauer, G.M., Parer, J.T. et al. (2012). Polymicrogyria in a fetus with human parvovirus B19 infection: a case with radiologic-pathologic correlation. *Ultrasound in Obstetrics & Gynecology* **40** (**5**): 604–606.

28 Weiland, H.T., Vermey-Keers, C., Salimans, M.M. et al. (1987). Parvovirus B19 associated with fetal abnormality. *Lancet* **1** (**8534**): 682–683.

29 Katz, V.L., McCoy, M.C., Kuller, J.A., and Hansen, W.F. (1996). An association between fetal parvovirus B19 infection and fetal anomalies: a report of two cases. *American Journal of Perinatology* **13** (**1**): 43–45.

30 Kinney, J.S., Anderson, L.J., Farrar, J. et al. (1988). Risk of adverse outcomes of pregnancy after human parvovirus B19 infection. *The Journal of Infectious Diseases* **157** (**4**): 663–667.

31 Enders, M., Helbig, S., Hunjet, A. et al. (2007). Comparative evaluation of two commercial enzyme immunoassays for serodiagnosis of human parvovirus B19 infection. *Journal of Virological Methods* **146** (**1–2**): 409–413.

32 Schwarz, T.F., Jager, G., and Gilch, S. (1997). Comparison of seven commercial tests for the detection of parvovirus B19-specific IgM. *Zentralblatt fur Bakteriologie* **285** (**4**): 525–530.

33 Cosmi, E., Mari, G., Delle Chiaie, L. et al. (2002). Noninvasive diagnosis by Doppler ultrasonography of fetal anemia resulting from parvovirus infection. *American Journal of Obstetrics and Gynecology* **187** (**5**): 1290–1293.

34 Delle Chiaie, L., Buck, G., Grab, D., and Terinde, R. (2001). Prediction of fetal anemia with Doppler measurement of the middle cerebral artery peak systolic velocity in pregnancies complicated by maternal blood group alloimmunization or parvovirus B19 infection. *Ultrasound in Obstetrics & Gynecology* **18** (**3**): 232–236.

35 Odibo, A.O., Campbell, W.A., Feldman, D. et al. (1998). Resolution of human parvovirus B19-induced nonimmune hydrops after intrauterine transfusion. *Journal of Ultrasound in Medicine* **17** (**9**): 547–550.

36 Rodis, J.F., Borgida, A.F., Wilson, M. et al. (1998). Management of parvovirus infection in pregnancy and outcomes of hydrops: a survey of members of the Society of Perinatal Obstetricians. *American Journal of Obstetrics and Gynecology* **179** (**4**): 985–988.

37 Nagel, H.T., de Haan, T.R., Vandenbussche, F.P. et al. (2007). Long-term outcome after fetal transfusion for hydrops associated with parvovirus B19 infection. *Obstetrics and Gynecology* **109** (**1**): 42–47.

38 Marin, M.G.D., Chaves, S.S. et al. (2007). Prevention of varicella: recommendations of the advisory committee on

immunization practices (ACIP). *MMWR Recommondations and Reports* **56**: 1.

39 Zhang, H.J., Patenaude, V., and Abenhaim, H.A. (2015). Maternal outcomes in pregnancies affected by varicella zoster virus infections: population-based study on 7.7 million pregnancy admissions. *The Journal of Obstetrics and Gynaecology Research* **41** (**1**): 62–68.

40 Gardella, C. and Brown, Z.A. (2007). Managing varicella zoster infection in pregnancy. *Cleveland Clinic Journal of Medicine* **74** (**4**): 290–296.

41 Harris, R.E. and Rhoades, E.R. (1965). Varicella pneumonia complicating pregnancy. Report of a case and review of literature. *Obstetrics and Gynecology* **25**: 734–740.

42 Laforet, E.G. and Lynch, C.L. Jr. (1947). Multiple congenital defects following maternal varicella; report of a case. *The New England Journal of Medicine* **236** (**15**): 534–537.

43 Sanchez, M.A., Bello-Munoz, J.C., Cebrecos, I. et al. (2011). The prevalence of congenital varicella syndrome after a maternal infection, but before 20 weeks of pregnancy: a prospective cohort study. *The Journal of Maternal-Fetal & Neonatal Medicine* **24** (**2**): 341–347.

44 Lamont, R.F., Sobel, J.D., Carrington, D. et al. (2011). Varicella-zoster virus (chickenpox) infection in pregnancy. *BJOG* **118** (**10**): 1155–1162.

45 Khandaker, G., Marshall, H., Peadon, E. et al. (2011). Congenital and neonatal varicella: impact of the national varicella vaccination programme in Australia. *Archives of Disease in Childhood* **96** (**5**): 453–456.

46 Mouly, F., Mirlesse, V., Meritet, J.F. et al. (1997). Prenatal diagnosis of fetal varicella-zoster virus infection with polymerase chain reaction of amniotic fluid in 107 cases. *American Journal of Obstetrics and Gynecology* **177** (**4**): 894–898.

47 Figueroa-Damian, R. and Arredondo-Garcia, J.L. (1997). Perinatal outcome of pregnancies complicated with varicella infection during the first 20 weeks of gestation. *American Journal of Perinatology* **14** (**7**): 411–414.

48 Dufour, P., de Bievre, P., Vinatier, D. et al. (1996). Varicella and pregnancy. *European Journal of Obstetrics, Gynecology, and Reproductive Biology.* **66** (**2**): 119–123.

49 Balducci, J., Rodis, J.F., Rosengren, S. et al. (1992). Pregnancy outcome following first-trimester varicella infection. *Obstetrics and Gynecology* **79** (**1**): 5–6.

50 Paryani, S.G. and Arvin, A.M. (1986). Intrauterine infection with varicella-zoster virus after maternal varicella. *The New England Journal of Medicine* **314** (**24**): 1542–1546.

51 Tan, M.P. and Koren, G. (2006). Chickenpox in pregnancy: revisited. *Reproductive Toxicology* **21** (**4**): 410–420.

52 Jones, K.L., Johnson, K.A., and Chambers, C.D. (1994). Offspring of women infected with varicella during pregnancy: a prospective study. *Teratology* **49** (**1**): 29–32.

53 Enders, G., Miller, E., Cradock-Watson, J. et al. (1994). Consequences of varicella and herpes zoster in pregnancy: prospective study of 1739 cases. *Lancet* **343** (**8912**): 1548–1551.

54 Harger, J.H., Ernest, J.M., Thurnau, G.R. et al. (2002). Frequency of congenital varicella syndrome in a prospective cohort of 347 pregnant women. *Obstetrics and Gynecology.* **100** (**2**): 260–265.

55 Pastuszak, A.L., Levy, M., Schick, B. et al. (1994). Outcome after maternal varicella infection in the first 20 weeks of pregnancy. *The New England Journal of Medicine* **330** (**13**): 901–905.

56 Miller, E., Cradock-Watson, J.E., and Ridehalgh, M.K. (1989). Outcome in newborn babies given anti-varicella-zoster immunoglobulin after perinatal maternal infection with varicella-zoster virus. *Lancet* **2** (**8659**): 371–373.

57 Bapat, P. and Koren, G. (2013). The role of VariZIG in pregnancy. *Expert Review of Vaccines* **12** (**11**): 1243–1248.

58 Meyberg-Solomayer, G.C., Fehm, T., Muller-Hansen, I. et al. (2006). Prenatal ultrasound diagnosis, follow-up, and outcome of congenital varicella syndrome. *Fetal Diagnosis and Therapy* **21** (**3**): 296–301.

59 Tongsong, T., Srisupundit, K., and Traisrisilp, K. (2012). Prenatal sonographic diagnosis of congenital varicella syndrome. *Journal of Clinical Ultrasound* **40** (**3**): 176–178.

60 Pretorius, D.H., Hayward, I., Jones, K.L., and Stamm, E. (1992). Sonographic evaluation of pregnancies with maternal varicella infection. *Journal of Ultrasound in Medicine* **11** (**9**): 459–463.

61 Mirlesse, V., Duguy, N., Cynober, E. et al. (2004). Alphafoetoprotein and acetylcholinesterase in amniotic fluid as a factor suggesting fetal skin and nerve lesions in a case of congenital varicella syndrome. *Prenatal Diagnosis* **24** (**7**): 498–500.

62 Hartung, J., Enders, G., Chaoui, R. et al. (1999). Prenatal diagnosis of congenital varicella syndrome and detection of varicella-zoster virus in the fetus: a case report. *Prenatal Diagnosis* **19** (**2**): 163–166.

63 Hofmeyr, G.J., Moolla, S., and Lawrie, T. (1996). Prenatal sonographic diagnosis of congenital varicella infection--a case report. *Prenatal Diagnosis* **16** (**12**): 1148–1151.

64 Mandelbrot, L. (2012). Fetal varicella - diagnosis, management, and outcome. *Prenatal Diagnosis* **32** (**6**): 511–518.

65 Kustermann, A., Zoppini, C., Tassis, B. et al. (1996). Prenatal diagnosis of congenital varicella infection. *Prenatal Diagnosis.* **16** (**1**): 71–74.

66 Harding, B. and Baumer, J.A. (1988). Congenital varicella-zoster. A serologically proven case with necrotizing encephalitis and malformation. *Acta Neuropathologica* **76** (**3**): 311–315.

67 Scharf, A., Scherr, O., Enders, G., and Helftenbein, E. (1990). Virus detection in the fetal tissue of a premature delivery with a congenital varicella syndrome. A case report. *Journal of Perinatal Medicine* **18** (**4**): 317–322.

68 Centers for Disease Control and Prevention (CDC) (2013). Updated recommendations for use of VariZIG – United States, 2013. *MMWR* **62** (**28**): 574–576.

69 Enders, G. (1985). Management of varicella-zoster contact and infection in pregnancy using a standardized varicella-zoster ELISA test. *Postgrad Medical Journal* **61** (**Suppl 4**): 23–30.

70 Koren, G., Money, D., Boucher, M. et al. (2002). Serum concentrations, efficacy, and safety of a new, intravenously administered varicella zoster immune globulin in pregnant women. *Journal of Clinical Pharmacology* **42** (**3**): 267–274.

71 US Food and Drug Administration (FDA). Summary Basis for regulatory Action – VariZIG. 2012.

72 Stone, K.M., Reiff-Eldridge, R., White, A.D. et al. (2004). Pregnancy outcomes following systemic prenatal acyclovir exposure: conclusions from the international acyclovir pregnancy registry, 1984-1999. *Birth Defects Research. Part A, Clinical and Molecular Teratology.* **70** (**4**): 201–207.

73 Pasternak, B. and Hviid, A. (2010). Use of acyclovir, valacyclovir, and famciclovir in the first trimester of pregnancy and the risk of birth defects. *JAMA* **304** (**8**): 859–866.

74 Broussard, R.C., Payne, D.K., and George, R.B. (1991). Treatment with acyclovir of varicella pneumonia in pregnancy. *Chest* **99** (**4**): 1045–1047.

75 Smego, R.A. and Asperilla, M.O. (1991). Use of acyclovir for varicella pneumonia during pregnancy. *Obstetrics and Gynecology* **78** (**6**): 1112–1116.

76 Eder, S.E., Apuzzio, J.J., and Weiss, G. (1988). Varicella pneumonia during pregnancy. Treatment of two cases with acyclovir. *American Journal of Perinatology* **5** (**1**): 16–18.

77 Harger, J.H., Ernest, J.M., Thurnau, G.R. et al. (2002). Risk factors and outcome of varicella-zoster virus pneumonia in pregnant women. *The Journal of Infectious Diseases* **185** (**4**): 422–427.

78 Huang, Y.C., Lin, T.Y., Lin, Y.J. et al. (2001). Prophylaxis of intravenous immunoglobulin and acyclovir in perinatal varicella. *European Journal of Pediatrics* **160** (**2**): 91–94.

79 Centers for Disease Control and Prevention (CDC) (2015). *Chickenpox (Varicella).* Atlanta, GA: US Department of Health & Human Services.

80 Marin, M., Zhang, J.X., and Seward, J.F. (2011). Near elimination of varicella deaths in the US after implementation of the vaccination program. *Pediatrics* **128** (**2**): 214–220.

81 Centers for Disease Control and Prevention (CDC) (2015). *Monitoring the Impact of the Varicella Vaccination*. Atlanta, GA: US Department of Health & Human Services.

82 Merck. Varivax Prescribing Information. Obtainable from MerckVaccines.com. Revised 2018.

83 Pediatrics AAo. Chickenpox Vaccine: What You Need to Know (VIS). 11/21/2015.

84 Prevention CfDCa. Vaccines and Immunizations: Who Should Not Get Chickenpox Vaccine. 2012.

85 Wilson, E., Goss, M.A., Marin, M. et al. (2008). Varicella vaccine exposure during pregnancy: data from 10 years of the pregnancy registry. *The Journal of Infectious Diseases* **197** (**Suppl 2**): S178–S184.

86 Shields, K.E., Galil, K., Seward, J. et al. (2001). Varicella vaccine exposure during pregnancy: data from the first 5 years of the pregnancy registry. *Obstetrics and Gynecology* **98** (**1**): 14–19.

87 Janakiraman, V. (2008). Listeriosis in pregnancy: diagnosis, treatment, and prevention. *Reviews in Obstetrics & Gynecology* **1** (**4**): 179–185.

88 Lorber, B. (1997). Listeriosis. *Clinical Infectious Diseases* **24** (**1**): 1–9; quiz 10–11.

89 Committee on Obstetric Practice ACoO, Gynecologists (2014). Committee opinion no. 614: management of pregnant women with presumptive exposure to listeria monocytogenes. *Obstetrics and Gynecology* **124** (**6**): 1241–1244.

90 Prevention CfDCa. Listeria. 2013.

91 Adams, D.A., Jajosky, R.A., Ajani, U. et al. (2014). Summary of notifiable diseases–United States, 2012. *MMWR. Morbidity and Mortality Weekly Report* **61** (**53**): 1–121.

92 Silk, B.J., Date, K.A., Jackson, K.A. et al. (2012). Invasive listeriosis in the foodborne diseases active surveillance network (FoodNet), 2004–2009: further targeted prevention needed for higher-risk groups. *Clinical Infectious Diseases* **54** (**Suppl 5**): S396–S404.

93 Temple, M.E. and Nahata, M.C. (2000). Treatment of listeriosis. *The Annals of Pharmacotherapy* **34** (**5**): 656–661.

94 Jackson, K.A., Iwamoto, M., and Swerdlow, D. (2010). Pregnancy-associated listeriosis. *Epidemiology and Infection* **138** (**10**): 1503–1509.

95 Ciesielski, C.A., Hightower, A.W., Parsons, S.K., and Broome, C.V. (1988). Listeriosis in the United States: 1980–1982. *Archives of Internal Medicine* **148** (**6**): 1416–1419.

96 Elinav, H., Hershko-Klement, A., Valinsky, L. et al. (2014). Pregnancy-associated listeriosis: clinical characteristics and geospatial analysis of a 10-year period in Israel. *Clinical Infectious Diseases* **59** (**7**): 953–961.

97 Mylonakis, E., Paliou, M., Hohmann, E.L. et al. (2002). Listeriosis during pregnancy: a case series and review of 222 cases. *Medicine* **81** (**4**): 260–269.

98 Craig, S., Permezel, M., Doyle, L. et al. (1996). Perinatal infection with listeria monocytogenes. *The Australian & New Zealand Journal of Obstetrics & Gynaecology* **36** (**3**): 286–290.

99 Pazos, M., Sperling, R.S., Moran, T.M., and Kraus, T.A. (2012). The influence of pregnancy on systemic immunity. *Immunologic Research* **54** (**1–3**): 254–261.

100 Pezeshkian, R., Fernando, N., Carne, C.A., and Simanowitz, M.D. (1984). Listeriosis in mother and fetus during the first trimester of pregnancy. Case report. *British Journal of Obstetrics and Gynaecology* **91** (**1**): 85–86.

101 Lamont, R.F., Sobel, J., Mazaki-Tovi, S. et al. (2011). Listeriosis in human pregnancy: a systematic review. *Journal of Perinatal Medicine* **39** (**3**): 227–236.

102 McLauchlin, J. (1990). Human listeriosis in Britain, 1967-85, a summary of 722 cases. 1. Listeriosis during pregnancy and in the newborn. *Epidemiology and Infection* **104** (**2**): 181–189.

103 Benshushan, A., Tsafrir, A., Arbel, R. et al. (2002). Listeria infection during pregnancy: a 10 year experience. *The Israel Medical Association journal* **4** (**10**): 776–780.

104 Siegman-Igra, Y., Levin, R., Weinberger, M. et al. (2002). Listeria monocytogenes infection in Israel and review of cases worldwide. *Emerging Infectious Diseases* **8** (**3**): 305–310.

105 Gellin, B.G., Broome, C.V., Bibb, W.F. et al. (1991). The epidemiology of listeriosis in the United States–1986. Listeriosis Study Group. *American Journal of Epidemiology* **133** (**4**): 392–401.

106 Evans, J.R., Allen, A.C., Stinson, D.A. et al. (1985). Perinatal listeriosis: report of an outbreak. *Pediatric Infectious Disease* **4** (**3**): 237–241.

107 Fuchs, S., Hochner-Celnikier, D., and Shalev, O. (1994). First trimester listeriosis with normal fetal outcome. *European Journal of Clinical Microbiology & Infectious Diseases* **13** (**8**): 656–658.

108 Silver, H.M. (1998). Listeriosis during pregnancy. *Obstetrical & Gynecological Survey* **53** (**12**): 737–740.

34 CHAPTER 34
Venous thromboembolic disease

B. Ryan Ball and Michael J. Paidas
Department of Obstetrics, Gynecology and Reproductive Sciences, Yale School of Medicine, Section of Maternal-Fetal Medicine, New Haven, CN, USA

CLINICAL VIGNETTE

A 28-year-old G3P1011 presents for initial prenatal care. Her previous pregnancy was uncomplicated. Since her last delivery her father had an unprovoked deep vein thrombosis (DVT). During his evaluation he was found to be a carrier of a factor V Leiden gene mutation. She asks if this will affect her pregnancy in any way.

Introduction

Venous thromboembolism (VTE) comprises deep vein thrombosis (DVT) as well as pulmonary embolism (PE) and is regularly encountered in obstetrics. PE is one of the leading causes of maternal mortality in the United States. According to the CDC, in 2011–2012 it was the sixth most common cause of maternal mortality, accounting for 9.0% of maternal deaths [1]. Studies demonstrate an incidence of VTE varying between 0.6 and 2 per 1000 pregnancies. Most VTE events occur in the antepartum period [2–5], but in light of the shorter duration of the puerperium relative to the antepartum period, the incidence is actually higher in the puerperium [6]. Jacobsen, et al. found the incidence of VTE to be similar between the antepartum and postpartum periods, but DVT was more common in the antepartum period whereas PE was more common postpartum [7]. Virkus and colleagues [8] found the risk of VTE increases throughout the pregnancy with a marked rise at term, when pregnancy VTE risk was compared to non-contracepting women. The absolute risk per 10 000 pregnant woman years increased from 4.1 in weeks 1–11 to 59.3 in the 40th week. The risk decreased following birth to 21.5 in the first week to 3.8 in weeks 4–6 and returned to the baseline seven weeks after delivery.

The clinical diagnosis of VTE in pregnancy is frequently difficult due to the overlapping symptoms of normal pregnancy and VTE [9].

Clinical questions

1. What factors increase risk of VTE during pregnancy?
2. What is the best method of diagnosing VTE in pregnancy?
3. How should VTE in pregnancy be treated?
4. What can be done to effectively prevent VTE in pregnancy?

Risk factors

1. What factors increase risk of VTE during pregnancy?

Virchow's triad of hemostasis, endothelial injury, and hypercoagulability has long been recognized as risk factors for VTE. All of these elements are present in pregnancy.

Venous stasis begins as early as the first trimester and progressively increases throughout the pregnancy. Causes of the increased stasis include progesterone-induced venodilation, venous compression by the gravid uterus, and pulsatile compression of the left iliac vein by the right iliac artery [10]. Vascular injury occurs during the birth process and may be exacerbated by operative vaginal delivery.

Pregnancy is a time of significant physiologic changes in the maternal coagulation status. Activated protein C resistance increases and protein S activity is decreased. These changes and the elevated concentrations of fibrinogen and factors V, VIII, IX, and X all lead to increased thrombin production [11]. Concurrently, fibrinolysis is decreased by increased activity of plasminogen activator inhibitors type 1 and type 2 as well as decreased activity of tissue plasminogen activator [12].

Many factors have been shown to increase the risk of VTE in pregnancy (Table 34.1) [13]. The greatest risk for VTE in pregnancy is a personal history of prior VTE. In fact, 15–25% of VTEs in pregnancy are recurrences [14]. Thrombophilias are the next largest risk group accounting for 20–50% of VTEs occurring in pregnancy [15–17]. Other risk factors include increased parity, infection, operative vaginal delivery, cesarean delivery, smoking, obesity, cancer, and surgery [7, 16, 18–22].

Evidence-Based Obstetrics and Gynecology, First Edition. Edited by Errol R. Norwitz, Carolyn M. Zelop, David A. Miller, and David L. Keefe.

Table 34.1 American College of Chest Physicians risk factors for venous thromboembolism

Major risk factors
Immobility (strict bed rest for ≥1 wk in the antepartum period)
Post-partum hemorrhage ≥1000 ml with surgery
Previous VTE
Pre-eclampsia with fetal growth restriction
Thrombophilia
Antithrombin
Factor V Leiden (homozygous or heterozygous)
Prothrombin G20210A (homozygous or heterozygous
Medical conditions
Systemic lupus erythematosus
Heart disease
Sickle cell disease
Blood transfusion
Post-partum infection
Minor risk factors
BMI > 30 kg m^{-2}
Multiple gestation
Post-partum hemorrhage >1 l
Smoking >10 cigarettes d^{-1}
Fetal growth restriction
Thrombophilia
Protein C deficiency
Protein S deficiency
Pre-eclampsia

A number of inherited thrombophilias increase the risk of developing VTE during pregnancy (Table 34.2) [23]. The American College of Chest Physicians (ACCP) considers Factor V Leiden (FVL), Prothrombin G20210A, and antithrombin deficiency (ATD) major risk factors while Protein C and S deficiencies are minor risk factors for VTE in pregnancy.

FVL is the thrombophilia most commonly encountered by obstetricians. Its prevalence is highest in Caucasians of European decent with carrier frequencies estimated at 5–9% and is less common among those of Asian and African descent [24]. Only about 1% of women with FVL mutations are homozygous and they tend have to have a higher incidence of VTE [25, 26]. Retrospective data demonstrates heterozygous carriers of FVL have a 5–10-fold relative risk for VTE during pregnancy, and it is present in 43% of pregnant women with their first thrombotic event [27–30]. Among heterozygotes without a family or personal history of thrombosis, the risk of VTE is only 0.25%. For patients with a family or personal history of VTE, the risk may be as high as 10% [28]. One large multicenter prospective National Institute of Child Health and Human Development (NICHD) study looked at 4885 gravid patients without a personal history of thrombotic event. Of the 134 FVL carriers, there was no increased risk of VTE [31].

The second most prevalent inherited thrombophilia is Prothrombin G20210A (PGM), which leads to elevated prothrombin levels. Among European Caucasians the carrier prevalence is 2–4%. Similar to FVL, PGM is less common in those of Asian and African descent [24, 25]. Studies have shown a wide range in the carrier frequency among women having their first VTE during pregnancy with rates ranging from 3.8% to 31% [27, 30]. Women who are carriers of PGM without a personal or family history of VTE appear to have a low risk (0.37%) of VTE during pregnancy; however, that risk increases to over 10% for those with prior VTE or for family history of VTE. The probability appears to be higher for those who are homozygous for PGM mutation, but the available data is limited [30]. Even without a prior history of VTE FVL and PGM compound heterozygotes have a much higher risk (4.6%) of a VTE during pregnancy and puerperium even without a prior history [27].

Less common but more thrombogenic than FVL or PGM is ATD. Many mutations have been identified at the antithrombin gene loci, which lead to a wide spectrum of phenotypes. Type I disease is a quantitative disorder while type II is a qualitative dysfunction. Type I is less common, comprising only 12% of the cases of ATD, but it is much more thrombogenic, accounting for 80% of symptomatic cases. In contrast to FVL and PGM the prevalence of ATD in highest in Asian populations with some groups having a prevalence of up to 2–5%, while among Caucasian Europeans it is estimated at 0.02–1.15% [24, 32]. The risk of VTE in pregnancy can be high with ATD, but there is large variability among phenotypes. Robertson reported an OR 4.69 for VTE in pregnancy [26]. Retrospective studies have estimated the odds ratio for the more thrombogenic type 1 disease to be 282 compared to a much smaller risk with type II disease (OR 28) [13, 33]. It is estimated that the lifetime risk of VTE in those with type I disease is 50% [34]. One case series of 63 untreated women with type 1 ATD who went through pregnancy without anticoagulation found 18% had a thrombotic complication during pregnancy and additional 33% had a VTE postpartum [35].

Protein C is an anticoagulant responsible for the deactivation of factor Va and factor VIIIa thereby inhibiting clot formation [25]. Deficiencies in protein C synthesis or function are found in 0.2–0.3% of those with European ancestry and is more common in those of Asian and African descent [24]. Protein C deficiency is moderately pro-thrombogenic during pregnancy. The risk is likely proportional to the deficiency of substrate and/or function. Zotz et al. found the relative risk of a first VTE in pregnancy to be RR 3.0 if using <73% of normal protein C activity as the cutoff and RR 13.0 if using <50% as the cutoff in a case control study [28]. A review of available retrospective case controlled studies showed a modest risk of VTE (OR 4.76) in patients with hereditary protein C deficiency [26].

Table 34.2 The risk of venous thromboembolism in pregnant patient with selected thrombophilias

Condition	Prevalence in European populations	Prevalence in patients with VTE in pregnancy	Risk of VTE without prior history	Risk of VTE with prior history
Factor V Leiden (FVL)				
Heterozygous	5.3%	44	0.26%	>10%
Homozygous	0.07%	<1	1.50%	>10%
Prothrombin mutation (PGM)				
Heterozygous	2.90%	17	0.37–0.5%	>10%
Homozygous	0.02%	<1	2.8	>10%
Compound FVL/PGM	0.17%	<1		4.70%
Protein C deficiency	0.2–0.3%	<14	0.8–1.7%	
Protein S deficiency	0.03–0.13%	12	<1–6.6%	
Antithrombin deficiency	0.02–1.1%	1	3–7.2%	11–40%

Source: Adapted from: Han CS, Paidas MJ, Lockwood CJ. Clotting disorders. In: High Risk Pregnancy: Management Options, 4th edition. Edited by David K. James, Philip J. Steer, Carl P. Weiner, Bernard Gonik, Caroline A. Crowther, and Stephen Robson, 2010. Elsevier, Philadelphia, PA.

Protein S accelerates activated protein C's disruption of factors Va and VIIIa, ultimately suppressing thrombin formation. It is a less common than protein C deficiency with a prevalence of 0.03–0.13% in the Caucasian European population. Due to the infrequency of protein S deficiency there are limited studies regarding its risks during pregnancy. Robertson's review of available case controlled studies showed an OR 3.19 of VTE and pregnancy [26]. Conard et al.'s evaluation of 44 pregnancies in 17 patients with congenital protein S deficiency showed no thrombosis during pregnancies without anticoagulation, but had five post-partum thrombotic events (17%) [35].

Diagnosis

2. What is the best method of diagnosing VTE in pregnancy?

DVT

Clinical symptoms

The typical presentation of a patient with DVT is erythema, edema, warmth, and pain in the affected area. A palpable venous cord or Homan's sign may be present. These findings, however, are nonspecific and studies show them present in only about 50% of patients with confirmed DVT.

D dimer

Laboratory assays for D-dimer (a fibrin degradation product) levels are commonly used to rule out venous thrombosis in non-pregnant patients. When D-dimer levels are low, the chance of DVT is low. These tests are not usually helpful in pregnancy because the physiologic increases in D-dimer levels in pregnancy exceed normal values in 78% of second trimester and 100% of third trimester patients [36]. Chan, et al. found that D-dimer values were elevated throughout pregnancy and were further increased in pregnant women diagnosed with DVT. By increasing the threshold value they were able to improve the specificity without a significant decrease in sensitivity [37]. Prospective trials are needed to further evaluate the use of the increased threshold values in the management of DVT during pregnancy.

Imaging

The gold standard test for diagnosis of DVT is a venogram with IV contrast. However, because of the invasive nature of the test and other good alternatives, it is rarely used today.

The most common test for diagnosis is Doppler venous ultrasound. This is done by insonating the veins of the leg and serially compressing them with the ultrasound transducer. A non-compressible vein is indicative of venous thrombosis. The sensitivity and specificity of venous ultrasound in proximal thrombosis is 90–100% but is lower for distal veins [38]. Goodacre et al. found that in non-pregnant patients the sensitivity in proximal DVT was 96.4% and 75.2% in distal DVTs [39].

PE

Clinical symptoms

Symptoms of PE include shortness of breath, chest pain, hypoxia, tachycardia, cough, tachypnea, hemoptysis, hypotension, and syncope [40, 41]. Among 38 pregnant women diagnosed with acute PE the most common findings were tachycardia (65%), dyspnea (63%), tachypnea (57%), pleuritic chest pain (55%), cough (24%), and sweating (18%) [42].

Imaging

Diagnostic testing for PE has changed over the years. Originally, pulmonary angiography was considered the gold standard. The ventilation-perfusion scan replaced pulmonary angiography because of the invasive nature of

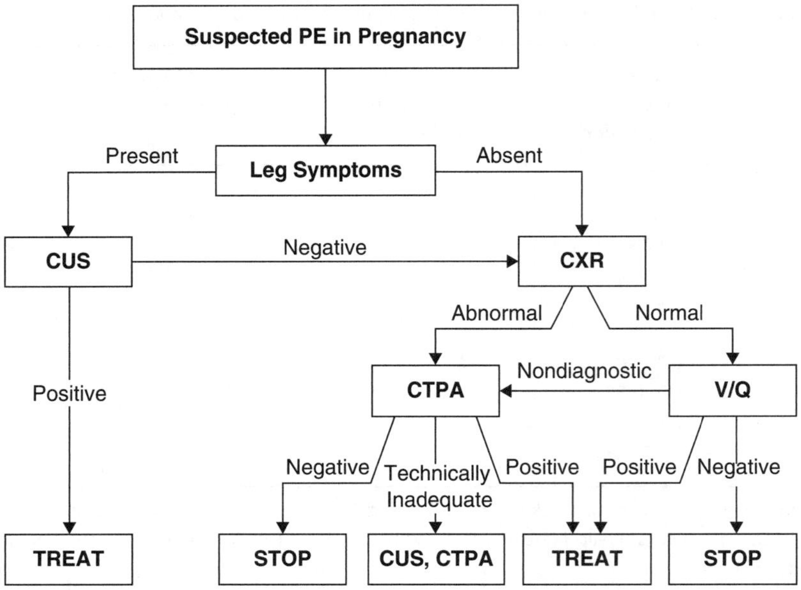

Figure 34.1 Diagnostic algorithm for suspected PE in pregnancy. Source: Reprinted with permission of the American Thoracic Society. Copyright © 2016 American Thoracic Society. Published in: Leung AN, Bull TM Jaeschke R, Lockwood CJ, Boiselle PM, Hurwitz LM, James AH, McCullough LB, Menda Y, Paidas MJ, Royal HD, Tapson VF, Winer-Muram HT, Chervenak FA, Cody DD, McNitt-Gray MF, Stave CD, Tuttle BD; *Am J Respir Crit Care Med* 2011, 184, 1200–1208. The *American Journal of Respiratory and Critical Care Medicine* is an official journal of the American Thoracic Society.

the test and associated complications. In more recent years, CT pulmonary angiography has become more common and outside of pregnancy is usually the diagnostic test of choice.

Historically pulmonary angiography was considered the diagnostic gold standard for PE. The sensitivity is lower with more peripheral lesions, decreasing from 98% for lobar emboli to 90% for segmental emboli, and 66% for subsegmental emboli [43]. The complications of pulmonary angiography include a mortality risk of 0.5% and respiratory failure, renal failure, or hematoma requiring transfusion occurred in 0.8% of patients [44]. Because of these risks and the availability of good alternatives pulmonary angiography is rarely used today.

Ventilation-perfusion scanning involves the comparison of the distribution of radiolabeled aerosols and intravenously injected radiolabeled isotopes. Diagnostic results (high probability, very low probability, and normal) occur in 75–94% of scans. The 94% value was obtained in patients with normal CXR and no previous history of asthma or chronic obstructive pulmonary disease (COPD) [41, 45–47].

Spiral CT angiography is performed by injecting IV radiographic contrast while scanning the lung fields to evaluate for filling defects in the pulmonary vasculature. It is less useful for subsegmental lesions or in PE of the right middle lobe as the vessels are oriented horizontally. CT scanning does have the advantage of being able to concurrently evaluate for other pulmonary pathology. Among patients being evaluated for PE 12–13% had significant radiographic findings on CT. The most common were pneumonia (5–7%) and pulmonary edema (2–6%) [46, 47]. Among pregnant patients the rates of non-diagnostic CT angiography are increased over threefold [48]. Others have shown rates of non-diagnostic studies from 6 to 36% [40, 47, 49].

Suggested diagnostic algorithm

The American Thoracic Society and Society of Thoracic Radiology published a clinical practice guideline for the diagnosis of PE in pregnancy in 2011 that is illustrated in Figure 34.1 [50]. It has also been endorsed by the American College of Obstetricians and Gynecologists. If symptoms of DVT are present in the legs, venous US should be done first and treatment initiated if DVT is present. No further evaluation is necessary as the treatment for DVT and PE are identical. If there are no leg symptoms or the venous US in normal, then a CXR should be performed. If the CXR is abnormal then CT angiography should be performed, otherwise a V/Q scan is preferred.

Treatment

3. How should VTE in pregnancy be treated?

Patients diagnosed with VTE during pregnancy must be anticoagulated with a therapeutic regimen for the duration of the pregnancy and puerperium or 20 weeks, whichever is longer. Anticoagulation can be initiated in the outpatient setting, but inpatient may be more appropriate for large clots, hemodynamic instability, or maternal comorbidities [51].

Unfractionated heparin (UFH) is an injectable or intravenous anticoagulant commonly used in the obstetrical population. UFH binds to antithrombin, resulting in deactivation of coagulation factors IIa and Xa. Because it does not cross the placenta, it is not teratogenic. Its effects can be reversed with protamine sulfate. Side effects may include hemorrhage, bone loss, and heparin-induced thrombocytopenia (HIT). None of these are commonly seen with prophylactic dosing. Calcium supplementation and periodic platelet monitoring is recommended for women receiving UFH.

UFH is usually started as in IV infusion. The dose is titrated until activated partial thromboplastin time (aPTT) levels of 1.5–2.5 times control is obtained four to six hours after the heparin dose. Once adequate aPTT levels are consistently obtained the patient can be transitioned to subcutaneous injections every 8–12 hours with the goal to keep the aPTT (six hours after injection) 1.5–2 times control [51].

Low molecular weight heparins (LMWHs) are a similar group of injectable anticoagulants also commonly used during pregnancy. LMWH is not teratogenic as it does not cross the placenta. One disadvantage of LMWH is that protamine is less effective in reversing its effects. Because they are more easily used and have fewer side effects, such as HIT, they are often the preferred over heparin. Patients are typically transition to UFH at 36 weeks of gestation or earlier if there is a high risk of preterm delivery. This conversion is typically performed to decrease the risk of neuraxial anesthesia and bleeding complications around the time of delivery. However, a recent recommendation suggests continuation of LMWH until delivery [52].

Therapeutic LMWH dosing is started at $1\,mg\,kg^{-1}$ twice daily. Dosages should be titrated until an anti-factor Xa level of $0.6–1\,U\,ml^{-1}$ is achieved four to six hours after the LMWH injection.

Fondaparinux is a synthetic pentasaccharide that binds antithrombin, effectively inhibiting Factor Xa. Though its use in pregnancy is limited, some small patient series have been completed showing its use safely pregnancy [53]. It may be an alternative for patients with heparin hypersensitivity or a history of HIT. Fondaparinux does cross the placenta causing small but measurable amounts of anti-factor Xa activity in umbilical cord blood samples [54]. More studies are needed to thoroughly evaluate its safety in pregnancy, but its use is appropriate in carefully selected patients, especially those patients with heparin induced thrombocytopenia [13, 55].

The decision to use warfarin in pregnancy is more complicated. Warfarin is an oral vitamin K antagonist frequently used for anticoagulation in the general population. Use during embryogenesis is known to be teratogenic. For patients who conceive on warfarin, conversion to another anticoagulant (typically LMWH) should occur as early as possible once pregnancy is documented, around five weeks of gestation. Another option is to convert patients from warfarin to LMWH prior to attempting conception. Warfarin use during embryogenesis causes malformations including nasal and mid-face hypoplasia, CNS abnormalities, and skeletal malformations. Warfarin is also usually avoided later in pregnancy because it places the fetus at risk of bleeding complications. The exception is in women with mechanical heart valves, where it is suggested warfarin is superior in preventing thrombotic complications.

Prevention

4. What can be done to effectively prevent VTE in pregnancy?

Because VTE is a major cause of maternal mortality worldwide its prevention has the opportunity to significantly decrease maternal morbidity. Major organizations, including the American Congress of Obstetricians and Gynecologists, the ACCP, and the Royal College of Obstetricians and Gynecologists, have all developed guidelines to prevent VTE in pregnancy [13, 51, 56]. There is, however, wide variation in their recommendations. Unfortunately, there are not adequate randomized trials upon which to base recommendations [57]. The National Partnership for Maternal Safety (NPMS) of the Council on Patient Safety in Women's Healthcare convened a workgroup to review the different professional organizations' current guidelines and research evidence and make VTE prophylaxis recommendations [58].

The Joint Commission requires the assessment of thromboembolic risk for hospitalized patients, but has exempted the obstetric patients [59]. The NPMS working group recommends assessing thromboembolic risk for pregnant and postpartum patients at the initial prenatal visit, during antepartum admissions, following delivery, and prior to discharge after delivery. The Caprini [60] and Padua [61] scoring systems are widely used in non-obstetric populations and were modified by the NPMS to include the risks most commonly found in obstetric patients.

ACOG recommendations

ACOG's guidelines recommend anticoagulation for women at risk of VTE during pregnancy and the puerperium. Specific recommendations are made for women with a history of VTE or high-risk thrombophilia, but no recommendations are made for women with other risk factors. ACOG recommends the use of pneumatic compression devices for all patients having a cesarean delivery. The addition of pharmacologic thromboprophylaxis is recommended for patients with additional risk factors, but does not make recommendations for what additional risk factors warrant pharmacologic treatment [51].

ACCP recommendations

The ACCP recommends thromboprophylaxis with LMWH or UFH for hospitalized non-surgical patients with a Padua score of ≥4. For uncomplicated cesarean deliveries they recommend early ambulation with the addition of pneumatic compression devices or pharmacologic prophylaxis if the patient has one major or two minor risk factors for VTE.

Table 34.3 National Partnership for Maternal Safety recommendations for antepartum outpatient prophylaxis

Clinical history	Anticoagulation
Multiple prior venous thromboembolism episodes Prior venous thromboembolism with high-risk thrombophilia Prior venous thromboembolism with acquired thrombophilia	Treatment-dose LMW heparin or UFH
Idiopathic prior venous thromboembolism Prior venous thromboembolism with pregnancy or oral contraceptive Prior venous thromboembolism with low-risk thrombophilia Family history of venous thromboembolism with high-risk thrombophilia High-risk thrombophilia (including acquired)	Prophylactic-dose LMW heparin or UFH
Low-risk thrombophilia Prior venous thromboembolism provoked Low-risk thrombophilia and family history of venous thromboembolism	No treatment

LMW, low-molecular-weight; UFH, unfractionated heparin.
Source: I went looking for the original source and found it today at:https://www.acog.org/-/media/Districts/District-II/Public/SMI/v2/VTESlideSetNov2015Update052317.pdf?dmc=1&ts=20180723T1801489170
Modified from Safe Motherhood Initiative. Maternal Safety Bundle for Venous Thromboembolism. Available at: https://www.acog.org/-/media/Districts/District-II/Public/SMI/v2/VTESlideSetNov2015Update052317.pdf?dmc=1&ts=20180723T1801489170
The sources cited with this table in the Safe Motherhood Initiative publication are: Thromboembolism in Pregnancy. Practice Bulletin No. 123. American College of Obstetricians and Gynecologists. Obstet Gynecol 2011;118 : 718–29 and Bates SM, Greer IA, Middeldorp S, Veenstra DL, Prabulos AM, Vandvik PO, et al. VTE, thrombophilia, antithrombotic therapy, and pregnancy: Antithrombotic Therapy and Prevention of Thrombosis, 9th edn. American College of Chest Physicians Evidence-Based Clinical Practice Guidelines. Chest 2012;141:e691S–736S; Used with permission. D'Alton ME, Friedman AM, Smiley RM, Montgomery DM, Paidas MJ, D'Oria R, Frost JL, Hameed AB, Karsnitz D, Levy BS, Clark SL. National Partnership for Maternal Safety: Consensus Bundle on Venous Thromboembolism. Obstet Gynecol 2016.

Table 34.4 National Partnership for Maternal Safety recommendations for postpartum prophylaxis after hospitalization for childbirth

Clinical history	Anticoagulation
Multiple prior venous thromboembolism episodes Prior venous thromboembolism with high-risk thrombophilia Prior venous thromboembolism with acquired thrombophilia	6 wk treatment-dose LMW heparin or UFH
Idiopathic prior venous thromboembolism Prior venous thromboembolism with pregnancy or oral contraceptive Prior venous thromboembolism with low-risk thrombophilia Family history of venous thromboembolism with high-risk thrombophilia High-risk thrombophilia (including acquired) Prior venous thromboembolism provoked[a] Low-risk thrombophilia and family history of venous thromboembolism[a]	6 wk prophylactic-dose LMW heparin or UFH
Low-risk thrombophilia	No treatment

LMW, low-molecular-weight; UFH, unfractionated heparin.
[a]Changes from initial assessment.
Source: Modified from Safe Motherhood Initiative. Maternal Safety Bundle for Venous Thromboembolism. Available at: https://www.acog.org/-/media/Districts/District-II/Public/SMI/v2/VTESlideSetNov2015Update052317.pdf?dmc=1&ts=20180723T1801489170
The sources cited with this table in the Safe Motherhood Initiative publication are: Thromboembolism in Pregnancy. Practice Bulletin No. 123. American College of Obstetricians and Gynecologists. Obstet Gynecol 2011;118:718–29 and Bates SM, Greer IA, Middeldorp S, Veenstra DL, Prabulos AM, Vandvik PO, et al. VTE, thrombophilia, antithrombotic therapy, and pregnancy: Antithrombotic Therapy and Prevention of Thrombosis, 9th edn: American College of Chest Physicians Evidence-Based Clinical Practice Guidelines. Chest 2012;141:e691S–736S; Used with permission. D'Alton ME, Friedman AM, Smiley RM, Montgomery DM, Paidas MJ, D'Oria R, Frost JL, Hameed AB, Karsnitz D, Levy BS, Clark SL. National Partnership for Maternal Safety: Consensus Bundle on Venous Thromboembolism. Obstet Gynecol 2016.

Those patients at highest risk should be treated with both pneumatic compression and prophylactic LMWH [13].

RCOG recommendations

The RCOG is more aggressive in recommending pharmacologic thromboprophylaxis than ACOG or the ACCP. They use a scoring system that includes risk factors such as smoking, age > 35 years, BMI > 30 kg m^{-2}, and multiple gestations to calculate risk and the need for antepartum and postpartum prophylaxis. Unless otherwise contraindicated, they recommend prophylaxis for all antepartum admissions. For cesarean deliveries they recommend at least 10 days of prophylactic anticoagulation [56].

NPMS recommendations

NPMS recommends that a risk assessment be performed during the first prenatal visit. Similar to the ACOG [16] and ACCP [13] recommendations, patients with a high risk of VTE due to personal or family history of VTE or thrombophilia should receive anticoagulation (Table 34.3) [58]. Additionally, women taking aspirin for prevention of preeclampsia should discontinue the aspirin at 35–36 weeks.

For antepartum hospital admissions expected to be three days or longer they recommend prophylaxis with daily LMWH or twice daily UFH unless there is a high risk or bleeding or imminent delivery. Patients already receiving LMWH or UFH as an outpatient should have it continued during their hospitalization. Those with a high risk of bleeding or delivery should be treated with pneumatic compression devices or prophylactic UFH.

During labor women with a history of VTE or thrombophilia should use pneumatic compression devices and should be receive postpartum LMWH or UFH. While not recommended, pharmacologic prophylaxis may be considered for women with multiple risk factors by the modified Caprini, modified Padua, or RCOG criteria.

All women having a cesarean delivery should have pneumatic compression devices during the procedure and postoperatively until they are fully ambulatory if they are not receiving pharmacologic prophylaxis. NPMS recommends the use of LMWH or UFH postoperatively in women with risk factors. The guidelines also allow hospitals the option to treat all patients having cesarean deliveries with prophylactic LMWH or UFH as is recommended by the RCOG [56].

Anticoagulation in the puerperium is recommended for those women with a personal or family history of VTE or thrombophilias and is based on the recommendation of ACOG and the ACCP (Table 34.4) [13, 51, 62].

References

1 Centers for Disease Control and Prevention. Pregnancy Mortality Surveillance System 2016 [updated 1/21/2016. Available from: http://www.cdc.gov/reproductivehealth/maternalinfanthealth/pmss.html.

2 Ginsberg, J.S., Brill-Edwards, P., Burrows, R.F. et al. (1992). Venous thrombosis during pregnancy: leg and trimester of presentation. *Thromb. Haemost.* **67** (**5**): 519–520.

3 Bergqvist, A., Bergqvist, D., and Hallbook, T. (1983). Deep vein thrombosis during pregnancy. A prospective study. *Acta Obstet. Gynecol. Scand.* **62** (**5**): 443–448.

4 Bergqvist, D. and Hedner, U. (1983). Pregnancy and venous thrombo-embolism. *Acta Obstet. Gynecol. Scand.* **62** (**5**): 449–453.

5 Macklon, N.S. and Greer, I.A. (1996). Venous thromboembolic disease in obstetrics and gynaecology: the Scottish experience. *Scott. Med. J.* **41** (**3**): 83–86.

6 McColl, M., Ramsay, J., Tait, R. et al. (1997). Risk factors for pregnancy associated venous thromboembolism. *Thromb. Haemost.* **78** (**4**): 1183–1188.

7 Jacobsen, A.F., Skjeldestad, F.E., and Sandset, P.M. (2008). Incidence and risk patterns of venous thromboembolism in pregnancy and puerperium – a register-based case-control study. *Am. J. Obstet. Gynecol.* **198** (**2**): 233 e1–233 e7.

8 Virkus, R.A., Løkkegaard, E.C.L., Bergholt, T. et al. (2011). Venous thromboembolism in pregnant and puerperal women in Denmark 1995–2005. *Thromb. Haemost.* **106** (**2**): 304–309.

9 Marik, P.E. and Plante, L.A. (2008). Venous thromboembolic disease and pregnancy. *N. Engl. J. Med.* **359** (**19**): 2025–2033.

10 Macklon, N.S., Greer, I.A., and Bowman, A.W. (1997). An ultrasound study of gestational and postural changes in the deep venous system of the leg in pregnancy. *Br. J. Obstet. Gynaecol.* **104** (**2**): 191–197.

11 Clark, P., Brennand, J., Conkie, J.A. et al. (1998). Activated protein C sensitivity, protein C, protein S and coagulation in normal pregnancy. *Thromb. Haemost.* **79** (**6**): 1166–1170.

12 Rosenkranz, A., Hiden, M., Leschnik, B. et al. (2008). Calibrated automated thrombin generation in normal uncomplicated pregnancy. *Thromb. Haemost.* **99** (**2**): 331–337.

13 Bates, S.M., Greer, I.A., Middeldorp, S. et al. (2012). VTE, thrombophilia, antithrombotic therapy, and pregnancy: antithrombotic therapy and prevention of thrombosis: American College of Chest Physicians evidence-based clinical practice guidelines. *CHEST J.* **141** (**2_suppl**): e691S–e736S.

14 Pabinger, I., Grafenhofer, H., Kyrle, P.A. et al. (2002). Temporary increase in the risk for recurrence during pregnancy in women with a history of venous thromboembolism. *Blood* **100** (**3**): 1060–1062.

15 James, A.H. (2009). Venous thromboembolism in pregnancy. *Arterioscler. Thromb. Vasc. Biol.* **29** (**3**): 326–331.

16 James, A.H., Jamison, M.G., Brancazio, L.R., and Myers, E.R. (2006). Venous thromboembolism during pregnancy and the postpartum period: incidence, risk factors, and mortality. *Am. J. Obstet. Gynecol.* **194** (**5**): 1311–1315.

17 James, A.H., Tapson, V.F., and Goldhaber, S.Z. (2005). Thrombosis during pregnancy and the postpartum period. *Am. J. Obstet. Gynecol.* **193** (**1**): 216–219.

18 Danilenko-Dixon, D.R., Heit, J.A., Silverstein, M.D. et al. (2001). Risk factors for deep vein thrombosis and pulmonary embolism during pregnancy or post partum: a

population-based, case-control study. *Am. J. Obstet. Gynecol.* **184** (**2**): 104–110.

19 Ukoss, K.M. (2008). Antenatal pulmonary embolism: risk factors, management and outcomes. *BJOG* **115** (**4**): 453–461.

20 Larsen, T.B., Sorensen, H.T., Gislum, M., and Johnsen, S.P. (2007). Maternal smoking, obesity, and risk of venous thromboembolism during pregnancy and the puerperium: a population-based nested case-control study. *Thromb. Res.* **120** (**4**): 505–509.

21 Lindqvist, P., Dahlback, B., and Marsal, K. (1999). Thrombotic risk during pregnancy: a population study. *Obstet. Gynecol.* **94** (**4**): 595–599.

22 Simpson, E.L., Lawrenson, R.A., Nightingale, A.L., and Farmer, R.D. (2001). Venous thromboembolism in pregnancy and the puerperium: incidence and additional risk factors from a London perinatal database. *BJOG* **108** (**1**): 56–60.

23 Han, C.S., Paidas, M.J., and Lockwood, C.J. (2010). Clotting disorders. In: *High Risk Pregnancy: Management Options-Expert Consult* (ed. D.K. James, P.J. Steer, C.P. Weiner and B. Gonik). Elsevier Health Sciences, Fourth edition: 739–752.

24 Margaglione, M. and Grandone, E. (2011). Population genetics of venous thromboembolism. A narrative review. *Thromb. Haemost.* **105** (**2**): 221–231.

25 Franco, R.F. and Reitsma, P.H. (2001). Genetic risk factors of venous thrombosis. *Hum. Genet.* **109** (**4**): 369–384.

26 Robertson, L., Wu, O., Langhorne, P. et al. (2006). Thrombophilia in pregnancy: a systematic review. *Br. J. Haematol.* **132** (**2**): 171–196.

27 Gerhardt, A., Scharf, R.E., Beckmann, M.W. et al. (2000). Prothrombin and factor V mutations in women with a history of thrombosis during pregnancy and the puerperium. *N. Engl. J. Med.* **342** (**6**): 374–380.

28 Zotz, R.B., Gerhardt, A., and Scharf, R.E. (2003). Inherited thrombophilia and gestational venous thromboembolism. *Best Pract. Res. Clin. Haematol.* **16** (**2**): 243–259.

29 Martinelli, I., De Stefano, V., Taioli, E. et al. (2002). Inherited thrombophilia and first venous thromboembolism during pregnancy and puerperium. *Thromb. Haemost.* **87** (**5**): 791–795.

30 Jacobsen, A., Dahm, A., Bergrem, A. et al. (2010). Risk of venous thrombosis in pregnancy among carriers of the factor V Leiden and the prothrombin gene G20210A polymorphisms. *J. Thromb. Haemost.* **8** (**11**): 2443–2449.

31 Dizon-Townson, D., Miller, C., Sibai, B. et al. (2012). The relationship of the factor V Leiden mutation and pregnancy outcomes for mother and fetus. *Am. J. Perinatol.* **29** (**3**): 225.

32 Patnaik, M. and Moll, S. (2008). Inherited antithrombin deficiency: a review. *Haemophilia* **14** (**6**): 1229–1239.

33 McColl, M., Ellison, J., Reid, F. et al. (2000). Prothrombin 20210 G→ a, MTHFR C677T mutations in women with venous thromboembolism associated with pregnancy. *BJOG: Int. J. Obstet. Gynaecol.* **107** (**4**): 565–569.

34 Duhl, A.J., Paidas, M.J., Ural, S.H. et al. (2007). Antithrombotic therapy and pregnancy: consensus report and recommendations for prevention and treatment of venous thromboembolism and adverse pregnancy outcomes. *Am. J. Obstet. Gynecol.* **197** (**5**): 457.e1–457.e21.

35 Conard, J., Horellou, M., Van Dreden, P. et al. (1990). Thrombosis and pregnancy in congenital deficiencies in AT III, protein C or protein S: study of 78 women. *Thromb. Haemost.* **63** (**2**): 319–320.

36 Kline, J.A., Williams, G.W., and Hernandez-Nino, J. (2005). D-dimer concentrations in normal pregnancy: new diagnostic thresholds are needed. *Clin. Chem.* **51** (**5**): 825–829.

37 Chan, W.S., Lee, A., Spencer, F.A. et al. (2010). D-dimer testing in pregnant patients: towards determining the next 'level' in the diagnosis of deep vein thrombosis. *J. Thromb. Haemost.* **8** (**5**): 1004–1011.

38 Kassai, B., Boissel, J.P., Cucherat, M. et al. (2004). A systematic review of the accuracy of ultrasound in the diagnosis of deep venous thrombosis in asymptomatic patients. *Thromb. Haemost.* **91** (**4**): 655–666.

39 Goodacre, S., Sampson, F., Thomas, S. et al. (2005). Systematic review and meta-analysis of the diagnostic accuracy of ultrasonography for deep vein thrombosis. *BMC Med. Imaging* **5**: 6.

40 Cahill, A.G., Stout, M.J., Macones, G.A., and Bhalla, S. (2009). Diagnosing pulmonary embolism in pregnancy using computed-tomographic angiography or ventilation-perfusion. *Obstet. Gynecol.* **114** (**1**): 124–129.

41 Chan, W.S., Ray, J.G., Murray, S. et al. (2002). Suspected pulmonary embolism in pregnancy: clinical presentation, results of lung scanning, and subsequent maternal and pediatric outcomes. *Arch. Intern. Med.* **162** (**10**): 1170–1175.

42 Gherman, R.B., Goodwin, T.M., Leung, B. et al. (1999). Incidence, clinical characteristics, and timing of objectively diagnosed venous thromboembolism during pregnancy. *Obstet. Gynecol.* **94** (**5, Part 1**): 730–734.

43 Stein, P.D., Terrin, M.L., Gottschalk, A. et al. (1992). Value of ventilation/perfusion scans versus perfusion scans alone in acute pulmonary embolism. *Am. J. Cardiol.* **69** (**14**): 1239–1241.

44 Fedullo, P.F. and Tapson, V.F. (2003). Clinical practice. The evaluation of suspected pulmonary embolism. *N. Engl. J. Med.* **349** (**13**): 1247–1256.

45 Scarsbrook, A.F., Bradley, K.M., and Gleeson, F.V. (2007). Perfusion scintigraphy: diagnostic utility in pregnant women with suspected pulmonary embolic disease. *Eur. Radiol.* **17** (**10**): 2554–2560.

46 Shahir, K., Goodman, L.R., Tali, A. et al. (2010). Pulmonary embolism in pregnancy: CT pulmonary angiography versus perfusion scanning. *AJR Am. J. Roentgenol.* **195** (**3**): W214–W220.

47 Revel, M.P., Cohen, S., Sanchez, O. et al. (2011). Pulmonary embolism during pregnancy: diagnosis with lung scintigraphy or CT angiography? *Radiology* **258** (**2**): 590–598.

48 UK-I, J.M., Freeman, S.J., Boylan, T., and Cheow, H.K. (2008). Quality of CT pulmonary angiography for suspected pulmonary embolus in pregnancy. *Eur. Radiol.* **18** (**12**): 2709–2715.

49 Ridge, C.A., McDermott, S., Freyne, B.J. et al. (2009). Pulmonary embolism in pregnancy: comparison of pulmonary CT angiography and lung scintigraphy. *AJR Am. J. Roentgenol.* **193** (**5**): 1223–1227.

50 Leung, A.N., Bull, T.M., Jaeschke, R. et al. (2011). An official American Thoracic Society/Society of Thoracic Radiology clinical practice guideline: evaluation of suspected pulmonary embolism in pregnancy. *Am. J. Respir. Crit. Care Med.* **184** (**10**): 1200–1208.

51 James, A.A. (2011). Practice bulletin no. 123: thromboembolism in pregnancy. *Obstet. Gynecol.* **118** (**3**): 718–729.

52 Solomon, C.G. and Greer, I.A. (2015). Pregnancy complicated by venous thrombosis. *N. Engl. J. Med.* **373** (**6**): 540–547.

53 Knol, H.M., Schultinge, L., Erwich, J.J., and Meijer, K. (2010). Fondaparinux as an alternative anticoagulant therapy during pregnancy. *J. Thromb. Haemost.* **8** (**8**): 1876–1879.

54 Dempfle, C.E. (2004). Minor transplacental passage of fondaparinux in vivo. *N. Engl. J. Med.* **350** (**18**): 1914–1915.

55 De Carolis, M.P., Salvi, S., Botta, A. et al. (2015). Cerebral sinovenous thrombosis in neonatal antiphospholipid syndrome: a new entity? *Lupus* **24** (**3**): 231–234.

56 The Royal College of Obstetricians and Gynaecologists (2015). *Reducing the Risk of Venous Thromboembolism during Pregnancy and the Puerperium. Green-Top Guideline No. 37a.* RCOG.

57 Bain, E., Wilson, A., Tooher, R. et al. (2014). Prophylaxis for venous thromboembolic disease in pregnancy and the early postnatal period. *Cochrane Database Syst. Rev.* **2**: CD001689. doi: 10.1002/14651858.CD001689.pub3.

58 D'Alton, M.E., Friedman, A.M., Smiley, R.M. et al. (2016). National Partnership for maternal safety: consensus bundle on venous thromboembolism. *Obstet. Gynecol.* **128** (**6**): 1450.

59 The Joint Commission (2009). Approved: more options for hospital core measures. *Joint Commission perspectives Joint Commission on Accreditation of Healthcare Organizations* **29** (**4**): 4–6.

60 Bahl, V., Hu, H.M., Henke, P.K. et al. (2010). A validation study of a retrospective venous thromboembolism risk scoring method. *Ann. Surg.* **251** (**2**): 344–350.

61 Barbar, S., Noventa, F., Rossetto, V. et al. (2010). A risk assessment model for the identification of hospitalized medical patients at risk for venous thromboembolism: the Padua prediction score. *J. Thromb. Haemost.* **8** (**11**): 2450–2457.

62 Practice Bulletin No. 138 (2013). Inherited Thrombophilias in pregnancy. *Obstet. Gynecol.* **122** (**3**): 706–716.

35 CHAPTER 35
Gastrointestinal disorders

Shivani R. Patel and Richard H. Lee
Division of Maternal-Fetal Medicine, Department of Obstetrics and Gynecology, University of Southern California, Keck School of Medicine, Los Angeles, CA, USA

This chapter will focus on cholelithiasis, pancreatitis, intrahepatic cholestasis of pregnancy, inflammatory bowel diseases, and appendicitis.

Cholelithiasis

Background

Pregnant women who present with nausea/vomiting, heartburn, and/or right upper quadrant/epigastric pain can be challenging as these symptoms can be normal in pregnancy or may be related to either obstetric or non-obstetric gastrointestinal conditions. In the setting of these symptoms clinicians must consider either cholelithiasis or cholecystitis as an etiology. Symptomatic cholelithiasis is a common non-obstetric gastrointestinal condition encountered in pregnancy complicating 1–3% of pregnancies [1]. Acute cholecystitis is less common affecting only 0.1% of pregnancies [1]. Pregnancy increases the risk of gallstone formation due to increased levels of estrogen and progesterone [1]. Additionally the elevated progesterone levels are a risk factor for acute cholecystitis [1]. Cholelithiasis can lead to acute cholecystitis, which can lead to adverse maternal and fetal consequences. In the setting of pregnancy the treatment of cholelithiasis can be challenging, and inadequate treatment can lead to acute cholecystitis.

Clinical questions

1. In pregnant patients with abdominal pain and/or nausea and vomiting (population) what is the diagnostic value (diagnostic test characteristics) of various symptoms and physical examination findings (tests) in the diagnosis of symptomatic cholelithiasis (outcome)?

2. In pregnant patients with symptoms (population) are the classic findings of acute cholecystitis (diagnostic test characteristics) on ultrasound (test) reliable in diagnosing acute cholecystitis (outcome)?

3. In pregnant patients treated with conservative management for cholecystitis (population) what are the maternal and fetal risks (assessment/outcomes) compared to those who underwent definitive surgical management (control)?

4. In pregnant patients treated with laparoscopic cholecystectomy (LAC) (population) what are the maternal and fetal risks (assessment/outcomes) compared to those who underwent open cholecystectomy (OC) (control)?

Critical appraisal of the literature

1. In pregnant patients with abdominal pain and/or nausea and vomiting (population) what is the diagnostic value (diagnostic test characteristics) of various symptoms and physical examination findings (tests) in the diagnosis of symptomatic cholelithiasis (outcome)?

Patients with symptomatic cholelithiasis frequently present with symptoms of right upper quadrant (RUQ) pain, epigastric pain, nausea, and vomiting. In pregnant individuals these symptoms can represent normal changes of pregnancy such as nausea/vomiting of pregnancy or gastritis. Symptomatic cholelithiasis can also be associated with laboratory abnormalities such as leukocytosis and elevated transaminases. Similar to the symptoms described above, mild leukocytosis is a normal physiologic change of pregnancy that can make diagnosis difficult. Many studies have looked at symptomatic cholelithiasis in pregnancy to clarify if the classic symptoms of cholelithiasis along with fever, leukocytosis, and physical exam findings remain reliable in pregnancy. In a retrospective review done by Lu et al. RUQ pain was required for diagnosis of symptomatic cholelithiasis, and of these patients, 52% also reported vomiting [2]. Swisher et al. reported that 96% of cases of symptomatic cholelithiasis in pregnancy presented with complaints of pain and 77.8% of cases reported vomiting [3]. On laboratory evaluation a mild leukocytosis up to 16 900/mm^3 can be the result of the normal physiology of pregnancy [4]. It has been shown that symptomatic cholelithiasis in pregnancy is similarly associated with a mild leukocytosis. Swisher et al. found that the mean white blood cell (WBC) count in the confirmed cases

Evidence-Based Obstetrics and Gynecology, First Edition. Edited by Errol R. Norwitz, Carolyn M. Zelop, David A. Miller, and David L. Keefe.

of symptomatic cholelithiasis was 10–17.5 × $10^3/\mu l$ while those with acute cholecystitis had a mean WBC count at the upper end of this range at 17.5 × $10^3/\mu l$ [3]. In the study done by Lu et al., the WBC count ranged from 9–12 × $10^3/\mu l$ in patients with symptomatic cholelithiasis, and again acute cholecystitis was associated with a higher WBC (12 × $10^3/\mu l$) [2]. Frequently transaminases are elevated in patients with acute cholecystitis and can help in making the diagnosis. Lu et al. found them to be mildly elevated at an average of 49 U/l [2]. Similarly, alanine aminotransferase (ALT) values were elevated at 45 U/l [2]. The finding of fever is rare in cases of acute cholecystitis with only 10% of patients having a temperature greater than 38.5°C [2].

In summary, the classic symptoms of symptomatic cholelithiasis are still applicable in the setting of pregnancy. The literature shows that the majority of cases of acute cholecystitis during pregnancy present with some constellation of the symptoms of right upper quadrant pain, nausea, and vomiting. These patients might also have a mild leukocytosis that may be undifferentiable from the normal elevation in WBC count in pregnancy. However, fever is not a reliable marker to diagnose acute cholecystitis in pregnancy. Thus if a pregnant patient presents with any of these signs or symptoms, the medical literature supports that acute cholecystitis must be included in the differential and excluded.

2. In pregnant patients with symptoms (population) are the classic findings of acute cholecystitis (diagnostic test characteristics) on ultrasound (test) reliable in diagnosing acute cholecystitis (outcome)?

Classic ultrasound findings of acute cholecystitis cluster around findings consistent with inflammation of the gallbladder. These findings include gallbladder wall edema defined by a thickness >3 mm, pericholecystic fluid, calculi, and a sonographic Murphy's sign [5]. Lu et al. reported that 95% of patients with acute cholecystitis had gallstones present on ultrasound [2]. They also found that a thickened gallbladder wall was present in 40% of cases and pericholecystic fluid was found in 15% [2]. Similarly Swisher et al. found that on ultrasound cholelithiasis was present in 100% of cases of acute cholecystitis and 56% concurrently had gallbladder wall thickening [3].

In the literature the diagnostic value of ultrasound in the setting of acute cholecystitis is clearly reliable if a constellation of findings is used. It appears that when gallstones are visible it is a reliable method for diagnosing acute cholecystitis in pregnancy. Additionally the findings of gallbladder wall thickening and pericholecystic fluid can further bolster ones diagnosis. Thus, in pregnancy, ultrasound can aid in making the diagnosis when physical exam and laboratory findings are suggestive of acute cholecystitis.

3. In pregnant patients treated with conservative management for cholecystitis (population) what are the maternal and fetal risks (assessment/outcomes) compared to those who underwent definitive surgical management (control)?

The treatment options of acute cholecystitis include both nonsurgical conservative management and cholecystectomy. Nonsurgical management consists of bowel rest, intravenous hydration, intravenous antibiotics, and analgesia for pain [5]. In the setting of pregnancy conservative management can pose risks to both the mother and the fetus. Maternal risks include treatment failure, recurrent episodes, need for emergency surgery, and longer hospital stay. The risks of treatment failure include gangrenous cholecystitis, gallbladder perforation, cholecystoenteric fistulas, choledocholithiasis, and ascending cholangitis [1, 3, 5]. Fetal risks include spontaneous abortion, intrauterine fetal demise, and premature birth. Swisher et al. reviewed maternal and fetal outcomes in patients with acute cholecystitis compared to those with biliary colic [3]. They found that 44% of patients with acute cholecystitis fail initial conservative therapy [3]. The relapse rate requiring hospitalization during pregnancy with conservative management is 22–58% [2, 3, 6]. Muench et al. describe a series in which delay in operative management resulted in multiple admissions for recurrent episodes [7]. As the number of episodes of recurrence increase, the number of additional hospital days increases by 2–11 days [2, 3]. Rates of relapse appear to be higher in patients who present earlier in pregnancy; 65% in the first and second trimesters compared 35% in the third trimester [2]. Swisher et al. found that the rate of relapse was highest in the first trimester and lowest if they presented in the third trimester [3]. Preterm contractions are experienced by 28% of patients managed conservatively compared to 31% who underwent cholecystectomy [2]. There is a higher rate of preterm delivery in patients managed nonoperatively (17% vs. 0%) [2]. There is also a higher rate of induction of labor (7–10%) in patients conservatively to aid in alleviation of symptoms [2, 3, 6]. Dixon et al. reported that spontaneous abortion occurred in 12% of patients with symptomatic cholelithiasis [6]. Maternal and fetal mortality are rare events with no studies describing maternal mortality and only one study finding a fetal mortality rate of 4.7% [2, 3].

Conservative management remains the initial treatment of choice in the pregnant population. However, given the increased risks to both the mother and fetus consideration should be given to operative management, especially when the patient's initial presentation is early in pregnancy.

4. In pregnant patients treated with laparoscopic cholecystectomy (population) what are the maternal and fetal risks (assessment/outcomes) compared to those who underwent open cholecystectomy (control)?

Cholecystectomy is the definitive treatment for acute cholecystitis. It is well known that definitive treatment prevents maternal and fetal morbidity and mortality associated with conservative management. In the era of minimally invasive surgery laparoscopy is increasingly being used in the pregnant population.

Barone et al. found that patients undergoing lupus anticoagulant (LAC) are more likely to be earlier in gestation (16 weeks) compared to those undergoing OC (23 weeks) [8]. They reported one maternal death (5%) two weeks after surgery in the LAC group secondary to intra-abdominal hemorrhage and one spontaneous abortion five weeks after surgery [8]. Barone et al. also reported that 30% of patients in the OC group required treatment for preterm contractions with 3.8% experiencing preterm delivery. This was compared to 5% in the LAC group receiving treatment for preterm contractions and 0% delivering prematurely [8]. In the same paper a review of studies showed only 1/61 patients experienced a spontaneous abortion after LAC [8]. Similarly Cosenza et al. found that there was no difference in fetal loss when comparing LAC to OC, and also found no difference in operative time and blood loss [9]. In a small series comparing LAC to OC, those who underwent LAC were able to tolerate regular diet faster compared to OC (0.3 vs. 0.6 days) [2]. They found no increased risk of preterm delivery or preterm contractions in the LAC group [2]. Affleck et al. also reported no difference in preterm delivery rates between a laparoscopic approach versus an open approach, and Gouldman et al. reported no preterm births in their study of patients undergoing LAC [10, 11]. Muench et al. determined that LAC was safe in pregnancy with favorable short-term and long-term fetal outcomes, including no spontaneous abortions or preterm births [7].

LAC is safe in pregnancy and can provide more favorable maternal and fetal outcomes than an open approach. Given the above evidence, a LAC should be considered in patients with acute cholecystitis.

Pancreatitis

Background

Pancreatitis has an incidence of approximately 1 per 1000–10 000 pregnancies [12, 13]. It is most commonly caused by cholelithiasis [14]. It is associated with an increased risk for preterm birth and maternal/fetal morbidity and mortality [15]. Treatment for pancreatitis revolves around treating the cause. The mainstay of treatment for biliary pancreatitis includes conservative management, LAC, or endoscopic retrograde cholangiopancreatography. If left untreated, biliary pancreatitis has a high risk of recurrence during the pregnancy and puerperium [16, 17].

Clinical questions

1. In pregnant patients with acute pancreatitis what is the diagnostic value of physical symptoms and laboratory tests such as serum lipase.

2. In pregnant patients with acute pancreatitis what imaging modalities should be considered first choice in making a diagnosis?

3. What are the treatment options for acute pancreatitis in pregnancy?

Critical appraisal of the literature

1. In pregnant patients with acute pancreatitis what is the diagnostic value of physical symptoms and laboratory tests such as serum lipase.

The symptoms of acute pancreatitis are non-specific and can mimic other diseases seen in pregnancy. The differential diagnosis of acute pancreatitis includes preeclampsia, acute fatty liver of pregnancy, HELLP syndrome, appendicitis, gastritis, peptic ulcer disease, ovarian torsion, cholelithiasis, bowel obstruction, chorioamnionitis, and placental abruption. There is a third trimester prominence in incidence although it can occur at any time during pregnancy [12, 18]. The majority of cases of acute pancreatitis in pregnancy are caused by choledocholithiasis and less likely from alcohol abuse, hypertriglyceridemia, idiopathic, and medications [13, 14].

Symptoms of acute pancreatitis include nausea and vomiting, severe upper abdominal pain, and fever. Signs can include fever, jaundice, upper abdominal tenderness to palpation, and guarding. Laboratory findings that may be elevated include: WBC count, amylase, lipase, serum transaminases, glucose, lactate dehydrogenase, blood urea nitrogen, and base deficit. Findings that may be decreased include: serum calcium and partial pressure of oxygen. The serum lipase has a sensitivity of 94% and specificity of 96% for acute pancreatitis [19]. Ranson's criteria which is used to assess disease severity and risk for mortality from pancreatitis has not be subjugated to validation in pregnancy [20].

2. In pregnant patients with acute pancreatitis what imaging modalities should be considered first choice in making a diagnosis?

Upper abdominal ultrasound is a safe and sensitive method of diagnosing cholelithiasis in the setting of acute pancreatitis. When the diagnosis is uncertain consideration should be made for magnetic resonance imaging (MRI) of the abdomen. MRI can also provide further detail on the pancreas such as the presence of pseudocysts or hemorrhage within the pancreas [21–24].

3. What are the treatment options for acute pancreatitis in pregnancy?

The management of patients with pancreatitis involves restricting oral intake, providing pain control and nutritional support. Antibiotics are no longer recommended. Definitive treatment for pancreatitis is dependent on the cause. If pancreatitis is caused by choledocholithiasis (i.e. biliary pancreatitis) the mainstays of treatment have included conservative management, OC, LAC, and endoscopic-retrograde cholangiopancreatography (ERCP). Data are limited to retrospective case–control studies or small case series. Conservative management may be associated with an increased risk for fetal mortality (8.0 vs. 2.6%, $P = 0.28$) [25]. There is no evidence to suggest superiority of cholecystectomy over ERCP [25]. Data regarding the recurrence of symptoms and hospitalizations is largely extrapolated from patients with cholelithiasis. Conservative management is associated with an increased risk of recurrence on the order of 70%. Intervention with either ERCP or cholecystectomy has been shown to reduce the risk of subsequent hospitalization and recurrent symptoms. One small case-series of seven pregnant patients showed successful treatment of biliary pancreatitis with the use of magnetic resonance cholangiopancreatography, ERCP and sphincterotomy, then LAC [26]. Treatment ultimately depends on a combination of disease severity, maternal/fetal status, gestational age, and the experience of the surgeon or gastroenterologist. Ducarme et al. suggest the following: conservative treatment in the first trimester and LAC in the second trimester; in the second trimester, LAC; in the third trimester, conservative treatment or ERCP with biliary endoscopic sphincterotomy, and LAC postpartum [19]. For the treatment of pancreatitis in pregnancy induced by hypertriglyceridemia, there are limited data to provide recommendations. Options in this setting include treatments used for non-pregnant patients which include fat restriction, nutritional supplements, plasma exchange, heparin, and insulin. Pseudocysts rarely develop but if they do, the majority can be observed as spontaneous resolution is on the order of 30–40%. Laparoscopic, endoscopic, and percutaneous drainage of pseudocysts have been reported. The prognosis for spontaneous resolution is greater if the pseudocyst is asymptomatic, <6 cm, and has been present for less than six weeks [27].

Intrahepatic cholestasis of pregnancy

Background

Intrahepatic cholestasis of pregnancy (ICP) has a prevalence of approximately 1% [28]. The clinical manifestation of ICP is pruritus in the absence of rash. The pruritus has been described as total-body itching with a predilection for the palms of the hands and soles of the feet. Laboratory values that are associated with ICP include elevated total serum bile acid concentration, transaminitis, hyperbilirubinemia, or alterations in the bile acid ratios. Maternal outcome is generally good, but there is an association with sudden fetal death.

Clinical questions

1. What are the risks to the fetus?
2. Is there a critical bile acid concentration threshold at which adverse perinatal outcomes are avoided?
3. What medical therapy should be given in ICP?
4. Is there any way to reduce the risk of fetal death from ICP?

Critical appraisal of the literature

1. What are the risks to the fetus?

The most concerning aspect of ICP is its association with adverse perinatal outcome [28]. Although maternal complications from ICP are rare, there are several adverse fetal effects including preterm labor, meconium aspiration, and fetal death [29]. Reid et al. analyzed complications in 56 pregnancies with ICP and reported an astonishingly high rate of adverse outcomes (e.g. perinatal mortality rate 11%, meconium staining 27%, abnormal antepartum fetal heart rate pattern 14%, preterm delivery rate 36%) [30]. Similarly, Fisk et al. reported a 45% incidence of meconium staining, 44% incidence of preterm labor, 22% incidence intrapartum fetal distress, and a 3.5% perinatal mortality rate. The most important observations noted by Fisk et al. were twofold. Firstly, given the absence of growth restriction in cases with fetal deaths, chronic uteroplacental insufficiency was believed to be less likely a cause for this complication in ICP. Secondly, the lower perinatal mortality rate compared to previous reports was attributed to closer surveillance during pregnancy with induction of labor by 37 weeks or earlier if there were any signs of fetal distress [31]. Williamson et al. reported an overall intrauterine death rate of 7% with 90% (18/20) of the deaths occurring after 37 weeks gestation [32]. To date, the exact mechanism of fetal death is unknown.

2. Is there a critical bile acid concentration threshold at which adverse perinatal outcomes are avoided?

Glantz et al. demonstrated bile acid concentrations $\geq 40\,\mu mol\,l^{-1}$ to be associated with an increased risk for adverse complications (i.e. preterm delivery, asphyxial events, meconium staining) [33]. Alternatively, there are reports of fetal death occurring with lower or normalized bile acid concentrations [34, 35].

3. What medical therapy should be given in ICP?

Ursodeoxycholic acid (UDCA) is the main treatment given for ICP. It has been superior to other agents in reducing pruritus, lowering the bile acid concentration, and improving liver transaminase profiles (e.g. S-adenosyl-L-methionine, cholestyramine, dexamethasone) [36–45].

4. Is there any way to reduce the risk of fetal death from ICP?

There are no randomized controlled trials addressing this. Some experts recommend delivery at or around 36 weeks of gestation based on increased observation of fetal and neonatal deaths to those fetuses delivered after 36 weeks gestation [46]. Fetal deaths attributed to ICP do occur prior to 36 weeks gestation; however, the risk of prematurity vs. the risk of stillbirth need to be weighed when making delivery plans. To date, there are no antepartum testing measures to predict or reduce the risk of stillbirth from ICP.

Inflammatory bowel disease

Background

Inflammatory bowel disease (IBD) in pregnancy consists of Crohn's disease and ulcerative colitis. The majority of patients with IBD are diagnosed before 35 years of age and will therefore affect women of reproductive age. Crohn's disease is characterized by transmural, granulomatous inflammation anywhere along the gastrointestinal tract. Ulcerative colitis involves mucosal inflammation primarily of the rectum but can extend to the rest of the colon.

Clinical questions

1. What is the effect of IBD on pregnancy?
2. How does pregnancy affect IBD?
3. What is the recommended mode of delivery?
4. What medications can be used IBD in pregnancy?

Critical appraisal of the literature

1. What is the effect of IBD on pregnancy?

Retrospective nature of studies investigating pregnancy outcomes in IBD, many data are conflicting. Nevertheless, the effect of IBD on pregnancy depends primarily on disease activity at the time of conception. Women with quiescent disease that is well-controlled appear to have similar pregnancy outcomes as the general population [47, 48]. However, if there is active disease at conception there are some data to suggest an increased risk for spontaneous abortion, late preterm birth and low birth weight [49–53]. Patient's with IBD can be reassured there does not appear to be an increased risk stillbirth or congenital anomalies [54].

2. How does pregnancy affect IBD?

The rate of disease flare appears to be similar or slightly less in pregnancy as the non-pregnant state; however, it is uncertain if this may be an effect of smoking cessation with pregnancy [55]. Again, if there is disease activity at conception is portends a worse prognosis [56]. Whether or not there is a trimester-specific predilection for a flare is uncertain as it may be affected by discontinuation of medication in the post-partum period, physiologic alterations in the immune system, or during the time of breast-feeding.

3. What is the recommended mode of delivery?

Based on limited data, Cesarean delivery should be reserved for patients with active perianal disease. In the absence of perianal disease, Cesarean delivery should be reserved for standard obstetrical indications. If vaginal delivery is attempted, episiotomy should be avoided because of an increased risk for perineal disease in women with Crohn's disease [57, 58].

4. What medications can be used IBD in pregnancy?

Aminosalicylates. 5-ASA compounds include sulfasalazine and mesalamine and are considered safe in pregnancy and breast feeding. Because of a possible antifolate effect, patients taking sulfasalazine should take 2 mg of folic acid daily before conception and during the pregnancy [59–61].

Corticosteroids. These are generally considered low risk in pregnancy. There may be a small increased risk for cleft palate. Glucocorticoids are associated with an increased risk for gestational diabetes, hypertension, and premature rupture of membranes [62].

Azathioprine/6-mercaptopurine. These medications have not been associated with congenital anomalies. These medications may be associated with an increased risk for preterm birth. In general, these medications are considered low risk in pregnancy, and patients who conceive while taking these medications should continue them throughout the pregnancy. Breastfeeding is considered generally considered safe with these medications [63–69].

Cyclosporine. This is used in ulcerative colitis that is refractory to steroid treatment. It has not been found to increase the risk of congenital malformations. Some data suggests an increased risk for preterm birth. Breastfeeding is not recommended because therapeutic levels have been found in breastfed infants and the risk for immunosuppression in the infant [70–72].

Infliximab. This is a tumor necrosis factor inhibitor used in the treatment of IBD. It appears to be low risk for the use in pregnancy and does not appear to increase the risk of congenital anomalies. That said, Infliximab does cross the placenta and it is recommended to avoid treatment 10 weeks for delivery. Based on case reports, Infliximab may be safe to use during breastfeeding [73–76].

Adalimubab. Case reports suggest adalimubab is safe to use in the first two trimesters of pregnancy. Similar to infliximab, it is suggested discontinue this medication 10 weeks before delivery. The safety of breast-feeding with this medication is less known [77, 78].

Certolizumab. Only limited data exists on this use of this medication in pregnancy. Reports have demonstrated only limited transfer of this medication across the placenta [79].

Natalizumab. Limited data exists on the safety of the use of this medication in pregnancy [80].

Metronidazole. Is generally considered safe in pregnancy but should be limited to short courses [81].

Ciprofloxacin is not recommended in pregnancy as quinolones have been associated with arthropathy in animal studies [80, 82]

Methotrexate. Is contraindicated in pregnancy. Discontinuation of methotrexate is recommended three to six months before attempting conception [80, 83].

Appendicitis

Background

Pregnant women who present with abdominal pain, nausea/vomiting, and/or anorexia can be a diagnostic enigma as these symptoms are common to both pregnancy and non-obstetric gastrointestinal conditions. However every clinician must have a high suspicion for appendicitis in any pregnant woman who presents with any or all of these symptoms, irrespective of the trimester of pregnancy. Appendicitis is one of the most common non-obstetric gastrointestinal conditions encountered during pregnancy and complicates about 1/1500 pregnancies [84]. An acute appendicitis normally leads to a dilated and inflamed appendix that, if not treated adequately, can rupture and lead to adverse maternal and fetal consequences. Both maternal and fetal outcomes are dependent on a timely diagnosis and proper treatment. In the setting of pregnancy the diagnosis of appendicitis can be challenging given that the symptoms of appendicitis can be normal physiologic changes associated with pregnancy, and it can be difficult to visualize the appendix on imaging secondary to an enlarged gravid uterus.

Clinical questions

1. In pregnant patients with abdominal pain and/or nausea and vomiting (population) what is the diagnostic value (diagnostic test characteristics) of various symptoms and physical examination findings (tests) in the diagnosis of acute appendicitis (outcome)?
2. In pregnant patients with symptoms (population) what is the sensitivity and specificity (diagnostic test characteristics) of ultrasound (test) in diagnosing appendicitis (outcome)?
3. In pregnant patients with a nondiagnostic ultrasound (population) what is the sensitivity and specificity (diagnostic test criteria) of CT and MRI (test) in diagnosing appendicitis (outcome)?
4. In pregnant patients with possible appendicitis (population) what is the negative appendectomy rate (NAR) (diagnostic test criteria) of exploratory surgery (test) compared to the general population?
5. In pregnant patients with a delay in treatment of appendicitis (population) what are the maternal and fetal risks (assessment/outcomes) compared to those treated in a timely manner (control)?

Critical appraisal of the literature

1. In pregnant patients with abdominal pain and/or nausea and vomiting (population) what is the diagnostic value (diagnostic test characteristics) of various symptoms, physical examination findings, and laboratory tests (tests) in the diagnosis of acute appendicitis (outcome)?

Patients with acute appendicitis frequently present with the classic symptoms of right lower quadrant (RLQ) pain, nausea, vomiting, and anorexia. Some patients however may not complain of all these symptoms, and in pregnant individuals these symptoms can represent normal signs of pregnancy. Acute appendicitis can also be associated with a fever and, on laboratory evaluation, a mild leukocytosis. Similar to the symptoms described above, mild leukocytosis is a normal physiologic change of pregnancy which can further confuse the picture.

A number of studies have looked at appendicitis in pregnancy to clarify if the classic symptoms of appendicitis along with fever, leukocytosis, and physical exam findings remain reliable in pregnancy. In a retrospective review done by Cunningham et al. [84] they found that 88% of patients with appendicitis complained of RLQ pain, nausea with or without vomiting was present in 97.1% of cases, and 75% of patients reported anorexia. Mahmoodian [85] reported that 85.7% of cases of appendicitis in pregnancy presented with complaints of RLQ pain, 42.8% of cases complained of anorexia, 71.4% of patients reported vomiting, and 100% of cases reported nausea. A few other studies have confirmed these findings indicating that the classic symptoms of RLQ pain, nausea, emesis, and anorexia are consistent findings of appendicitis during pregnancy (Table 35.1). On physical exam direct abdominal tenderness and the presence of rebound tenderness are not normal findings of pregnancy and thus can aide in the diagnosis of appendicitis. One study found that 83% of pregnancy patients with appendicitis had direct abdominal tenderness on exam and 70% had rebound tenderness [86]. Weingold et al. [87] showed that 92% of patients had direct abdominal tenderness with 58% experiencing rebound

Table 35.1 Summary of studies examining symptoms and physical exam findings in appendicitis in pregnancy

	Percentage of cases of appendicitis during pregnancy				
	Cunningham et al. [84]	Mahmoodian [85]	Babaknia et al. [86]	Weingold [87]	Mourad et al. [88]
Symptom					
RLQ pain	88%	85.7%%	70%	79.2%	83–85%
Nausea/Vomiting	97.1%	71.4%	77%	58.2%	
Anorexia	75%	42.8%	66%	70.8%	
Physical exam					
Direct abdominal tenderness	94%		83%	92%	
Rebound tenderness	75%		70%	58%	
Leukocytosis (>10 000/mm^3)	76.5%	85.6%	75%		

tenderness. Similarly another study [84] described that 94% of patients had direct abdominal tenderness with rebound tenderness being present in 75% of patients. On laboratory evaluation a mild leukocytosis up to 16 900 mm^s can be the result of the normal physiology of pregnancy [4]. It has been shown that appendicitis in pregnancy is similarly associated with a mild leukocytosis. Mourad et al. [88] found that the mean WBC count in the confirmed cases of appendicitis was $16.4 \times 10^9\ l^{-1}$ (range $8–27 \times 10^9\ l^{-1}$) while those without appendicitis had a mean WBC count of $14.0 \times 10^9\ l^{-1}$ (range $6–25 \times 10^9\ l^{-}$). In the study done by Babaknia et al. [86], a WBC count >15 000/mm^3 was found in only 25% of cases and 50% of cases had a WBC count between 10 000 and 15 000/mm^3. A third study [85] showed that 42.8% of cases had a WBC count ≥16 000/mm^3 and 42.8% had a WBC count between 10 000 and 16 000/mm^3. Cunningham et al. [84] showed that 76.5% of patients with appendicitis during pregnancy had a WBC >11 000/mm^3 (Table 35.1). The finding of fever may or may not be present in cases of appendicitis and is not a normal finding in pregnancy. Four studies in the literature evaluated the temperature findings associate with appendicitis in the setting of pregnancy. Mourad et al. [88] found no difference in mean maximal temperature between the patients with appendicitis (37.6, 35.5–39.5°C) and those found not to have appendicitis (37.8, 36.7–38.9°C). Similarly, Babaknia et al. [86] found that only 18% of patients had a temperature >100.2°F. Cunningham et al. [84] reported that fever was present in 85% of patients with 75% of them having a temperature ≤100.8°F and Weingold et al. [87] also found that 66.7% of cases had a temperature <38°C.

In summary, the classic symptoms of appendicitis are still applicable in the setting of pregnancy. The literature shows that the majority of cases of appendicitis during pregnancy present with some constellation of the symptoms of RLQ pain, nausea, vomiting, and anorexia. These patients also have a mild leukocytosis that may be undifferentiable from the normal elevation in WBC count in pregnancy. Additionally, fever is not a reliable marker to diagnose appendicitis in pregnancy. Thus if a pregnant patient presents with any of these signs or symptoms, the medical literature supports that appendicitis must be included in the differential and excluded.

2. In pregnant patients with symptoms (population) what is the sensitivity and specificity (diagnostic test characteristics) of ultrasound (test) in diagnosing appendicitis (outcome)?

Appendicitis in the nonpregnant population is usually diagnosed with the aide of computed tomography (CT) imaging. However, appendicitis during pregnancy has classically been diagnosed with the use of ultrasound in an effort to prevent fetal exposure to ionizing radiation. Real-time high resolution ultrasound with graded-compression technique is used to locate a non-compressible appendix and diagnose appendicitis. In the setting of pregnancy this can be challenging given the enlarged gravid uterus and possible changes in the position of the appendix. Four studies in the literature have examined the ability to diagnose appendicitis with the use of ultrasound with graded-compression technique. Lim et al. [89] found that when the appendix was visualized in pregnant patients suspected of having appendicitis, ultrasound using graded-compression had a sensitivity of 100%, specificity of 96%, positive predictive value (PPV) of 94%, and negative predictive value (NPV) of 100%. They found that ultrasound was non-diagnostic in 7% of cases secondary to inability to visualize the appendix. Similarly Israel et al. [90] looked at the ability of graded-compression ultrasound to diagnose appendicitis in the setting of pregnancy. They reported that when the appendix was visualized the sensitivity was 50%, the specificity was 100%, the PPV was 100%, and the NPV was 66%. It was also found that ultrasound did not identify the appendix in 88% of cases making it non-diagnostic in these cases. A retrospective review [91] showed similar results with ultrasound having 66% sensitivity, 95% specificity, a PPV of 66%, a NPV of 95%, and a non-diagnostic rate of 0%. On the other hand Mullins et al. [92] described a sensitivity of 100%, specificity of 83.3%, PPV of 50%, and NPV of 100%, and a non-diagnostic rate of 75.9% (Table 35.2).

Table 35.2 Summary of studies examining the ability of ultrasound, CT, and MRI to diagnose appendicitis in pregnancy

	Sensitivity and specificity					
	Ultrasound		CT		MRI	
	Sensitivity	Specificity	Sensitivity	Specificity	Sensitivity	Specificity
Lim et al. [89]	100%	96%				
Israel et al. [90]	50%	100%			100%	100%
Barloon et al. [91]	66%	95%				
Mullins et al. [92]	100%	83.3%	100%	100%		
Ames Castro et al. [93]	100%	100%	100%	100%		
Lazarus et al. [94]			92%	99%		
Pedrosa et al. [95]					100%	94%

In the literature the diagnostic value of ultrasound using graded-compression technique to diagnose appendicitis in pregnancy is clearly variable. It appears that when the appendix is visible it is a reliable method for diagnosing appendicitis in pregnancy. However, the variability makes it an unreliable tool. The variability is mainly due to an inability to identify the appendix in many cases and thus the ability to diagnose appendicitis in pregnancy on ultrasound is operator dependent.

3. In pregnant patients with a nondiagnostic ultrasound (population) what is the sensitivity and specificity (diagnostic test criteria) of CT and MRI (test) in diagnosing appendicitis (outcome)?

Given the high non-diagnostic rate of ultrasound in the setting of suspected appendicitis in pregnancy, CT and MRI imaging have become more popular. While CT scans with contrast are the gold standard by which appendicitis is diagnosed in the general population, CT scans done in pregnancy are traditionally done without contrast to avoid exposure to the fetus. Although the sample size was small, in the first study done evaluating the use of CT in pregnancy to evaluate for appendicitis, Ames Castro et al. [93] showed a sensitivity and specificity of 100% and a nondiagnostic rate of 0%. In the study described above regarding ultrasound in pregnancy, Mullins et al. [92] compared ultrasound to CT and found that in the 10 patients evaluated using CT imaging there was 100% sensitivity, specificity, PPV, and NPV with a 0% indeterminate rate. Lazarus et al. [94] described the sensitivity of CT imaging for diagnosing appendicitis in pregnancy to be 92% and the specificity to be 99% (Table 35.2). In a systematic review by Basaran et al. [96] the pooled sensitivity of CT was 85.7% and the pooled specificity was 97.4%.

In order to avoid ionizing radiation exposure to the fetus, MRI is increasingly being used to aide in the diagnosis of appendicitis in pregnancy. Israel et al. [90] compared ultrasound to MRI in diagnosing appendicitis in pregnancy and found that when the appendix was identified the sensitivity, specificity, PPV, and NPV were 100%. The nondiagnostic rate due to inability to visualize the appendix was 48%. Another study [95] looked at MRI in cases where ultrasound was nondiagnostic and found that in these cases MRI has a sensitivity of 100%, a specificity of 94%, a PPV of 1.4%, and a NPV of 100%. MRI was nondiagnostic in 6% of cases. Basaran et al. [96] also found that for MRI the pooled sensitivity of diagnosing appendicitis during pregnancy was 80% and the pooled specificity was 99%. Similar to ultrasound, it appears that the nondiagnostic rate of MRI is not 0% as it was in the above studies regarding CT scans, and is dependent on the ability to visualize the appendix. The inability to visualize the appendix in MRI however is not operator dependent and is likely related more to the size and position of the appendix.

In summary the literature shows that CT continues to be a reliable method to diagnose appendicitis, even in the setting of pregnancy. MRI also appears to be reliable, but only when the appendix is visualized which seems to be a problem with MRI, similar to ultrasound. It seems that when appendicitis is suspected in a pregnant woman it is reasonable to start with ultrasound, and if indeterminate then proceed with CT or MRI.

4. In pregnant patients with possible appendicitis (population) what is the negative appendectomy rate (diagnostic test criteria) of exploratory surgery (test) compared to the general population?

Evidenced by the above discussion diagnosing appendicitis in pregnancy can be difficult, and many times neither a diagnosis confirming appendicitis nor a diagnosis excluding it able to be made. In these cases a clinical judgment must be made as to whether or not to proceed with an exploratory surgery. Many times these operations end with the finding of a normal appendix on pathology and these cases are classified in the literature as a "negative appendectomy rate" (NAR). A number of studies have looked at the NAR in pregnancy. Ito et al. [97] compared pregnant to nonpregnant women and found that the NAR was higher in pregnant woman (36% vs 14%, $p < 0.001$). Another study showed that the NAR in pregnant woman is 37% compared to 25% in the general population [98]. A retrospective review looking at 10 patients who underwent exploration for suspected appendicitis yielded a 20% NAR [99]. And one final study looking at over 3000 pregnant women undergoing appendectomy found that 23% had a NAR compared to 18% of nonpregnant women [100].

Clearly, compared to the general population, the NAR during pregnancy is higher. This is due mainly to the inability to accurately make the diagnosis prior to surgery. The confusing history and physical exam findings coupled with possibly unreliable laboratory findings, and lastly the inability for imaging studies to definitely visualize the appendix make appendicitis in pregnancy a difficult diagnosis.

5. In pregnant patients with a delay in treatment of appendicitis (population) what are the maternal and fetal risks (assessment/outcomes) compared to those treated in a timely manner (control)?

In the setting of pregnancy the risks of an untreated appendicitis include both maternal and fetal adverse outcomes. Maternal risks include appendiceal rupture, sepsis, preterm labor, and death. Fetal risks include spontaneous abortion, intrauterine fetal demise, and premature birth. Each of these risks increases with a delay in diagnosis and treatment and with rupture or perforation of the appendix. Tamir et al. [101] compared delay of operative treatment of more than 24 hours. They found that 100% of perforations occurred after ≥24 hours and perforations lead to a doubling in hospital stay from6 days to 12 days. Maternal mortality is rare from appendicitis, but can increase to 4% in cases of a ruptured appendix [102]. It has been reported that the fetal loss rate increases from 1.5–9% to 36–43% with perforation [86, 99, 103]. Preterm birth occurred in 33%

of cases of ruptured appendicitis compared to 0% in simple acute appendicitis in one series [99]. Based on the literature it is clear that a delay in the treatment of appendicitis leads to adverse maternal and fetal outcomes. While the NAR is higher in pregnant women, the risks of delay in treatment in cases when the diagnosis is still in question are substantial to both the mother and fetus. These risks must be taken into account when considering whether or not to proceed with surgery in cases where the diagnosis may still be in question.

Recommendations

1. Ultrasound is a reliable method of diagnosing cholelithiasis and cholecystitis in pregnancy. (I)
2. Initial treatment of symptomatic cholelithiasis is conservative. However, there is a high rate of relapse during pregnancy. Surgery should be considered if there is recurrent presentation (2C) Surgical treatment should be considered in pregnant patients with cholecystitis (2B).
3. Laparoscopic surgery may be used to treat cholethiasis or cholecystitis (during pregnancy (2B).
4. Ultrasound can be used to diagnose acute pancreatitis in pregnancy. When the diagnosis is uncertain MRI may be used in pregnancy (2C).
5. Patients with intrahepatic cholestasis should be started on UDCA (IA).
6. Delivery for patients with intrahepatic cholestasis should occur at approximately 36 weeks of gestation (2B).
7. In patients with inflammatory bowel disease, Cesarean delivery should be reserved for patients with active perianal disease (1C).
8. When appendicitis is suspected in a pregnant woman, it is reasonable to start imaging with ultrasound, and if indeterminate then proceed with CT or MRI (2B).

References

Cholelithiasis

1 Gilo, N.B., Amini, D., and Landy, H.J. (2009). Appendicitis and cholecystitis in pregnancy. *Clin. Obstet. Gynecol.* **52** (**4**): 586–596.

2 Lu, E.J., Curet, M.J., El-Sayed, Y.Y., and Kirkwood, K.S. (2004). Medical versus surgical management of biliary tract disease in pregnancy. *Am. J. Surg.* **188** (**6**): 755–759.

3 Swisher, S.G., Schmit, P.J., Hunt, K.K. et al. (1994). Biliary disease during pregnancy. *Am. J. Surg.* **168** (**6**): 576–579.

4 Abassi-Ghanavati, M., Greer, L., and Cunningham, F.G. (2009). Pregnancy and laboratory studies: a reference table for clinicians. *Obstet. Gynecol.* **114** (**6**): 1326–1331.

5 Dietrich, C.S. 3rd, Hill, C.C., and Hueman, M. (2008). Surgical diseases presenting in pregnancy. *Surg. Clin. N. Am.* **88** (**2**): 403–419.

6 Dixon, N.P., Faddis, D.M., and Silberman, H. (1987). Aggressive management of cholecystitis during pregnancy. *Am. J. Surg.* **154** (**3**): 292–294.

7 Muench, J., Albrink, M., Serafini, F. et al. (2001). Delay in treatment of biliary disease during pregnancy increases morbidity and can be avoided with safe laparoscopic cholecystectomy. *Am. Surg.* **67** (**6**): 539–542.

8 Barone, J.E., Bears, S., Chen, S. et al. (1999). Outcome study of cholecystectomy during pregnancy. *Am. J. Surg.* **177** (**3**): 232–236.

9 Cosenza, C.A., Saffari, B., Jabbour, N. et al. (1999). Surgical management of biliary gallstone disease during pregnancy. *Am. J. Surg.* **178** (**6**): 545–548.

10 Affleck, D.G., Handrahan, D.L., Egger, M.J., and Price, R.R. (1999). The laparoscopic management of appendicitis and cholelithiasis during pregnancy. *Am. J. Surg.* **178** (**6**): 523–529.

11 Gouldman, J.W., Sticca, R.P., Rippon, M.B., and McAlhany, J.C. Jr. (1998). Laparoscopic cholecystectomy in pregnancy. *Am. Surg.* **64** (**1**): 93–97.

Pancreatitis

12 Igbinosa, O., Poddar, S., and Pitchumoni, C. (2013). Pregnancy associated pancreatitis revisited. *Clin. Res. Hepatol. Gastroenterol.* **37** (**2**): 177–181.

13 Eddy, J.J., Gideonsen, M.D., Song, J.Y. et al. (2008). Pancreatitis in pregnancy. *Obstet. Gynecol.* **112** (**5**): 1075–1081.

14 Papadakis, E.P., Sarigianni, M., Mikhailidis, D.P. et al. (2011). Acute pancreatitis in pregnancy: an overview. *Eur. J. Obstet. Gynecol. Reprod. Biol.* **159** (**2**): 261–266.

15 Hernandez, A., Petrov, M.S., Brooks, D.C. et al. (2007). Acute pancreatitis and pregnancy: a 10-year single center experience. *J. Gastroint.l Surg.* **11** (**12**): 1623–1627.

16 Wilkinson, E.J. (1973). Acute pancreatitis in pregnancy: a review of 98 cases and a report of 8 new cases. *Obstet. Gynecol. Surv.* **28** (**5**): 281–303.

17 Swisher, S.G., Hunt, K.K., Schmit, P.J. et al. (1994). Management of pancreatitis complicating pregnancy. *Am. Surg.* **60** (**10**): 759–762.

18 Ramin, K.D., Ramin, S.M., Richey, S.D., and Cunningham, F.G. (1995). Acute pancreatitis in pregnancy. *Am. J. obstet. gynecol.* **173** (**1**): 187–191.

19 Ducarme, G., Maire, F., Chatel, P. et al. (2014). Acute pancreatitis during pregnancy: a review. *J. Perinatol.* **34** (**2**): 87–94.

20 Ranson, J.H. (1982). Etiological and prognostic factors in human acute pancreatitis: a review. *Am. J. Gastroenterol.* **77** (**9**): 633–638.

21 Roumieu, F., Ponchon, T., Audra, P., and Gaucherand, P. (2008). Acute pancreatitis in pregnancy: place of the different explorations (magnetic resonance cholangiopancreatography, endoscopic ultrasonography) and their therapeutic consequences. *Eur. J. Obstet. Gynecol. Reprod. Biol.* **140** (**1**): 141–142.

22 Birchard, K.R., Brown, M.A., Hyslop, W.B., and Firat, Z. (2005). Semelka RC. MRI of acute abdominal and pelvic pain in pregnant patients. *Am. J. Roentgenol.* **184** (**2**): 452–458.

23 Jabbour, N., Brenner, M., Gagandeep, S. et al. (2005). Major hepatobiliary surgery during pregnancy: safety and timing. *Am. Surg.* **71** (**4**): 354–358.

24 Tuech, J.J., Binelli, C., Aube, C. et al. (2000). Management of choledocholithiasis during pregnancy by magnetic resonance cholangiography and laparoscopic common bile duct stone extraction. *Surg. Laparosc. Endosc. Percutan Tech.* **10** (**5**): 323–325.

25 Date, R.S., Kaushal, M., and Ramesh, A. (2008). A review of the management of gallstone disease and its complications in pregnancy. *Am. J. Surg.* **196** (**4**): 599–608.

26 Polydorou, A., Karapanos, K., Vezakis, A. et al. (2012). A multimodal approach to acute biliary pancreatitis during pregnancy: a case series. *Surg. Laparosc. Endosc. Percutan. Tech.* **22** (**5**): 429–432.

27 Bansal, V.K., Misra, M.C., Goswami, A. et al. (2012). Laparoscopic management of pseudocyst of the pancreas in a pregnant patient. *Surg. Laparosc. Endosc. Percutan. Tech.* **22** (**1**): e37–e38.

Intrahepatic cholestasis of pregnancy

28 Abedin, P., Weaver, J.B., and Egginton, E. (1999). Intrahepatic cholestasis of pregnancy: prevalence and ethnic distribution. *Ethn. Health* **4** (**1–2**): 35–37.

29 Alsulyman, O.M., Ouzounian, J.G., Ames-Castro, M., and Goodwin, T.M. (1996). Intrahepatic cholestasis of pregnancy: perinatal outcome associated with expectant management. *Am. J. Obstet. Gynecol.* **175** (**4 Pt 1**): 957–960.

30 Reid, R., Ivey, K.J., Rencoret, R.H., and Storey, B. (1976). Fetal complications of obstetric cholestasis. *Br. Med. J.* **1** (**6014**): 870–872.

31 Fisk, N.M. and Storey, G.N. (1988). Fetal outcome in obstetric cholestasis. *Br. J. Obstet. Gynaecol.* **95** (**11**): 1137–1143.

32 Williamson, C., Hems, L.M., Goulis, D.G. et al. (2004). Clinical outcome in a series of cases of obstetric cholestasis identified via a patient support group. *BJOG* **111** (**7**): 676–681.

33 Glantz, A., Marschall, H.U., and Mattsson, L.A. (2004). Intrahepatic cholestasis of pregnancy: relationships between bile acid levels and fetal complication rates. *Hepatology* **40** (**2**): 467–474.

34 Lee, R.H., Incerpi, M.H., Miller, D.A. et al. (2009). Sudden fetal death in intrahepatic cholestasis of pregnancy. *Obstet. Gynecol.* **113** (**2 Pt 2**): 528–531.

35 Sentilhes, L., Verspyck, E., Pia, P., and Marpeau, L. (2006). Fetal death in a patient with intrahepatic cholestasis of pregnancy. *Obstet. Gynecol.* **107** (**2 Pt 2**): 458–460.

36 Bacq, Y., Sentilhes, L., Reyes, H.B. et al. (2012). Efficacy of ursodeoxycholic acid in treating intrahepatic cholestasis of pregnancy: a meta-analysis. *Gastroenterology* **143** (**6**): 1492–1501.

37 Burrows, R.F., Clavisi, O., and Burrows, E. (2001). Interventions for treating cholestasis in pregnancy. *Cochrane Database Syst. Rev.* 4 (Art. No.: CD000493).

38 Floreani, A., Paternoster, D., Melis, A., and Grella, P.V. (1996). S-adenosylmethionine versus ursodeoxycholic acid in the treatment of intrahepatic cholestasis of pregnancy: preliminary results of a controlled trial. *Eur. J. Obstet. Gynecol. Reprod. Biol.* **67** (**2**): 109–113.

39 Kondrackiene, J., Beuers, U., and Kupcinskas, L. (2005). Efficacy and safety of ursodeoxycholic acid versus cholestyramine in intrahepatic cholestasis of pregnancy. *Gastroenterology* **129** (**3**): 894–901.

40 Mazzella, G., Rizzo, N., Azzaroli, F. et al. (2001). Ursodeoxycholic acid administration in patients with cholestasis of pregnancy: effects on primary bile acids in babies and mothers. *Hepatology* **33** (**3**): 504–508.

41 Nicastri, P.L., Diaferia, A., Tartagni, M., and Loizzi, P. (1998). Fanelli M. A randomised placebo-controlled trial of ursodeoxycholic acid and S-adenosylmethionine in the treatment of intrahepatic cholestasis of pregnancy. *Br. J. Obstet. Gynaecol.* **105** (**11**): 1205–1207.

42 Palma, J., Reyes, H., Ribalta, J. et al. (1997). Ursodeoxycholic acid in the treatment of cholestasis of pregnancy: a randomized, double-blind study controlled with placebo. *J. Hepatol.* **27** (**6**): 1022–1028.

43 Roncaglia, N., Locatelli, A., Arreghini, A. et al. (2004). A randomised controlled trial of ursodeoxycholic acid and S-adenosyl-l-methionine in the treatment of gestational cholestasis. *BJOG* **111** (**1**): 17–21.

44 Zapata, R., Sandoval, L., Palma, J. et al. (2005). Ursodeoxycholic acid in the treatment of intrahepatic cholestasis of pregnancy. A 12-year experience. *Liver Int.* **25** (**3**): 548–554.

45 Gurung, V., Middleton, P., Milan, S.J. et al. (2013). Interventions for treating cholestasis in pregnancy. *Cochrane Database Syst. Rev.* 6 (Art. No.: CD0004930).

46 Puljic, A., Kim, E., Page, J. et al. (2015 May). The risk of infant and fetal death by each additional week of expectant management in intrahepatic cholestasis of pregnancy by gestational age. *Am. J. Obstet. Gynecol.* **212** (**5**, **5**): 667.e1. doi: 10.1016/j.ajog.2015.02.012 Epub 2015 Feb 14.

Inflammatory bowel disease

47 Bush, M.C., Patel, S., Lapinski, R.H., and Stone, J.L. (2004). Perinatal outcomes in inflammatory bowel disease. *J. Matern. Fetal Neonatal med.* **15** (**4**): 237–241.

48 Calderwood, A.H. and Kane, S.V. (2004). IBD and pregnancy. *MedGenMed* **6** (**4**): 14.

49 Elbaz, G., Fich, A., Levy, A. et al. (2005). Inflammatory bowel disease and preterm delivery. *Int. J. Gynaecol. Obstet.* **90** (**3**): 193–197.

50 Moser, M.A., Okun, N.B., Mayes, D.C., and Bailey, R.J. (2000). Crohn's disease, pregnancy, and birth weight. *Am. J. Gastroenterol.* **95** (**4**): 1021–1026.

51 Dominitz, J.A., Young, J.C., and Boyko, E.J. (2002). Outcomes of infants born to mothers with inflammatory bowel disease: a population-based cohort study. *Am. J. Gastroenterol.* **97** (**3**): 641–648.

52 Reddy, D., Murphy, S.J., Kane, S.V. et al. (2008). Relapses of inflammatory bowel disease during pregnancy: in-hospital management and birth outcomes. *Am. J. Gastroenterol.* **103** (**5**): 1203–1209.

53 Beniada, A., Benoist, G., Maurel, J., and Dreyfus, M. (2005). Inflammatory bowel disease and pregnancy: report of 76 cases and review of the literature. *J. Gynecol. Obstet. Biol. Reprod.* **34** (**6**): 581–588.

54 Cornish, J., Tan, E., Teare, J. et al. (2007). A meta-analysis on the influence of inflammatory bowel disease on pregnancy. *Gut* **56** (**6**): 830–837.

55 Agret, F., Cosnes, J., Hassani, Z. et al. (2005). Impact of pregnancy on the clinical activity of Crohn's disease. *Aliment Pharmacol. Therap.* **21** (**5**): 509–513.

56 Willoughby, C.P. and Truelove, S.C. (1980). Ulcerative colitis and pregnancy. *Gut* **21** (**6**): 469–474.

57 Ilnyckyji, A., Blanchard, J.F., Rawsthorne, P., and Bernstein, C.N. (1999). Perianal Crohn's disease and pregnancy: role of the mode of delivery. *Am. J. Gastroenterol.* **94** (**11**): 3274–3278.

58 Brandt, L.J., Estabrook, S.G., and Reinus, J.F. (1995). Results of a survey to evaluate whether vaginal delivery and episiotomy lead to perineal involvement in women with Crohn's disease. *Am. J. Gastroenterol.* **90** (**11**): 1918–1922.

59 Diav-Citrin, O., Park, Y.H., Veerasuntharam, G. et al. (1998). The safety of mesalamine in human pregnancy: a prospective controlled cohort study. *Gastroenterology* **114** (**1**): 23–28.

60 Norgard, B., Czeizel, A.E., Rockenbauer, M. et al. (2001). Population-based case control study of the safety of sulfasalazine use during pregnancy. *Aliment Pharmacol. Therap.* **15** (**4**): 483–486.

61 Rahimi, R., Nikfar, S., Rezaie, A., and Abdollahi, M. (2008). Pregnancy outcome in women with inflammatory bowel disease following exposure to 5-aminosalicylic acid drugs: a meta-analysis. *Reprod. Toxicol.* **25** (**2**): 271–275.

62 Park-Wyllie, L., Mazzotta, P., Pastuszak, A. et al. (2000). Birth defects after maternal exposure to corticosteroids: prospective cohort study and meta-analysis of epidemiological studies. *Teratology* **62** (**6**): 385–392.

63 Moretti, M.E., Verjee, Z., Ito, S., and Koren, G. (2006). Breast-feeding during maternal use of azathioprine. *Ann. Pharmacother.* **40** (**12**): 2269–2272.

64 Zlatanic, J., Korelitz, B.I., Rajapakse, R. et al. (2003). Complications of pregnancy and child development after cessation of treatment with 6-mercaptopurine for inflammatory bowel disease. *J. Clin. Gastroenterol.* **36** (**4**): 303–309.

65 Langagergaard, V., Pedersen, L., Gislum, M. et al. (2007). Birth outcome in women treated with azathioprine or mercaptopurine during pregnancy: a Danish nationwide cohort study. *Aliment Pharmacol. Therap.* **25** (**1**): 73–81.

66 Polifka, J.E. and Friedman, J.M. (2002). Teratogen update: azathioprine and 6-mercaptopurine. *Teratology* **65** (**5**): 240–261.

67 Moskovitz, D.N., Bodian, C., Chapman, M.L. et al. (2004). The effect on the fetus of medications used to treat pregnant inflammatory bowel-disease patients. *Am. J. Gastroenterol.* **99** (**4**): 656–661.

68 Francella, A., Dyan, A., Bodian, C. et al. (2003). The safety of 6-mercaptopurine for childbearing patients with inflammatory bowel disease: a retrospective cohort study. *Gastroenterology* **124** (**1**): 9–17.

69 Pearson, D.C., May, G.R., Fick, G., and Sutherland, L.R. (2000). Azathioprine for maintaining remission of Crohn's disease. *Cochrane Database Syst. Rev.* 2 (Art. No.: CD000067).

70 Bar Oz, B., Hackman, R., Einarson, T., and Koren, G. (2001). Pregnancy outcome after cyclosporine therapy during pregnancy: a meta-analysis. *Transplantation* **71** (**8**): 1051–1055.

71 Armenti, V.T., Radomski, J.S., Moritz, M.J. et al. (2005). Report from the National Transplantation Pregnancy Registry (NTPR): outcomes of pregnancy after transplantation. *Clin. Transpl.* 69–83.

72 Armenti, V.T., Ahlswede, K.M., Ahlswede, B.A. et al. (1994). National transplantation pregnancy registry--outcomes of 154 pregnancies in cyclosporine-treated female kidney transplant recipients. *Transplantation* **57** (**4**): 502–506.

73 Vasiliauskas, E.A., Church, J.A., Silverman, N. et al. (2006). Case report: evidence for transplacental transfer of maternally administered infliximab to the newborn. *Clin. Gastroenterol. Hepatol.* **4** (**10**): 1255–1258.

74 Zelinkova, Z., de Haar, C., de Ridder, L. et al. (2011). High intra-uterine exposure to infliximab following maternal anti-TNF treatment during pregnancy. *Aliment Pharmacol. Therap.* **33** (**9**): 1053–1058.

75 Katz, J.A., Antoni, C., Keenan, G.F. et al. (2004). Outcome of pregnancy in women receiving infliximab for the treatment of Crohn's disease and rheumatoid arthritis. *Am. J. Gastroenterol.* **99** (**12**): 2385–2392.

76 Mahadevan, U., Kane, S., Sandborn, W.J. et al. (2005). Intentional infliximab use during pregnancy for induction or maintenance of remission in Crohn's disease. *Aliment Pharmacol. Therap.* **21** (**6**): 733–738.

77 Mishkin, D.S., Van Deinse, W., Becker, J.M., and Farraye, F.A. (2006). Successful use of adalimumab (Humira) for Crohn's disease in pregnancy. *Inflamm. Bowel Dis.* **12** (**8**): 827–828.

78 Vesga, L., Terdiman, J.P., and Mahadevan, U. (2005). Adalimumab use in pregnancy. *Gut* **54** (**6**): 890.

79 Mahadevan, U., Cucchiara, S., Hyams, J.S. et al. (2011 Feb). The London position statement of the world congress of gastroenterology on biological therapy for IBD with the European Crohn's and colitis organisation: pregnancy and pediatrics. *Am. J. Gastroenterol.* **106** (**2**): 214–223; quiz 24.

80 Nielsen, O.H., Maxwell, C., and Hendel, J. (2014). IBD medications during pregnancy and lactation. *Nat. Rev. Gastroenterol. Hepatol.* **11** (**2**): 116–127.

81 Czeizel, A.E. and Rockenbauer, M. (1998). A population based case-control teratologic study of oral metronidazole treatment during pregnancy. *Br. J. Obstet. Gynaecol.* **105** (**3**): 322–327.

82 Loebstein, R., Addis, A., Ho, E. et al. (1998). Pregnancy outcome following gestational exposure to fluoroquinolones: a multicenter prospective controlled study. *Antimicrob. Agents Chemother.* **42** (**6**): 1336–1339.

83 Chakravarty, E.F., Sanchez-Yamamoto, D., and Bush, T.M. (2003). The use of disease modifying antirheumatic drugs in women with rheumatoid arthritis of childbearing age: a survey of practice patterns and pregnancy outcomes. *J. Rheumatol.* **30** (**2**): 241–246.

Appendicitis

84 Cunningham, F.G. and McCubbin, J.M. (1975). Appendicitis complicating pregnancy. *Obstet. Gynecol.* **45**: 415–420.

85 Mahmoodian, S. (1992). Appendicitis complicating pregnancy. *South. Med. J.* **85**: 19–23.

86 Babaknia, A., Parsa, H., and Woodruff, J. (1977). Appendicitis in pregnancy. *Obstet. Gynecol.* **50** (**1**): 40–44.

87 Weingold, A.B. (1983). Appendicits in pregnancy. *Clin. Obstet. Gynecol.* **26** (**4**): 801–809.

88 Mourad, J., Eilliott, J., Erickson, L., and Lisboa, L. (2000). Appendicitis in pregnancy: new information that contradicts long-held clinical beliefs. *Am. J. Obstet. Gynecol.* **182** (**5**): 1027–1029.

89 Lim, H.K., Bae, S.H., and Seo, G.S. (1992). Diagnosis of acute appendicitis in pregnant women: value of Sonography. *AJR* 159.

90 Israel, G., Malguria, N., McCarthy, S. et al. (2008). MRI vs. ultrasound for suspected appendicitis during pregnancy. *J. Magn. Reson. Imaging* **28** (**2**): 428–433.

91 Barloon, T.J., Brown, B.P., Abu-Yousef, M.M. et al. (1995). Sonography of acute appendicitis in pregnancy. *Abdom. Imaging.* **20** (**2**): 149–151.

92 Mullins, M., Rhea, J., Greene, M., and Novelline, R.A. (2001). Diagnostic imaging of suspected appendicitis in pregnant women: comparison of CT to ultrasonography. *Emerg. Radiol.* **8**: 262–266.

93 Ames Castro, M., Shipp, T.D., Castro, E.E. et al. (2001). The use of helical computer tomography in pregnancy for the diagnosis of acute appendicitis. *Am. J. Obstet. Gynecol.* **184** (**5**): 954–957.

94 Lazarus, E., Mayo-Smith, W., Mainiero, M., and Spencer, P. (2007). CT in the evaluation of nontraumatic abdominal pain in pregnant women. *Radiology* **244** (**3**): 784–790.

95 Pedrosa, I., Levine, D., Eyvazzadeh, A. et al. (2006). MR imaging evaluation of acute appendicitis in pregnancy. *Radiology* **238** (**3**): 891–899.

96 Basaran, A. and Basaran, M. (2009). Diagnosis of acute appendicitis during pregnancy: a systematic review. *Obstet. Gynecol. Surv.* **64** (**7**): 481–488.

97 Ito, K., Ito, H., Whang, E., and Tavakkolizadeh, A. (2011). Appendectomy in pregnancy: evluation of the risks of a negative appendectomy. *Am. J. Surg.* [Epub ahead of print].

98 Wallace, C., Petrov, M., Soyvel, D. et al. (2008). Influence of imaging on the negative appendectomy rate in pregnancy. *J. Gastrointest. Surg.* **12**: 46–50.

99 Horowitz, M., Gomez, G., Santiesteban, R., and Burkett, G. (1985). Acute appendicitis during pregnancy. *Arch. Surg.* **120** (**12**): 1362–1367.

100 McGory, M., Zingmond, D., Tillou, A. et al. (2007). Negative appendectomy in pregnant women is associated with a substantial risk of fetal loss. *J. Am. Coll. Surg.* **205**: 534–540.

101 Tamir, I.L., Bongard, F.S., and Klein, S.R. (1990). Acute appendicitis in the pregnant patient. *Am. J. Surg.* **160** (**6**): 571–575.

102 Guttman, R., Goldman, R., and Koren, G. (2004). Appendicitis during pregnancy. *Can. Fam. Physician* **50**: 355–357.

103 Pastore, P., Loomis, D., and Sauret, J. (2006). Appendicitis in pregnancy. *J. Am. Board Fam. Med.* **19**: 621–626.

36

CHAPTER 36
Psychiatric disease

Michael K. Simoni and Kimberly Yonkers
Department of Psychiatry, Yale School of Medicine, Yale, New Haven, CN, USA

> **CLINICAL SCENARIO**
>
> A 26-year-old female presents to your office for her first prenatal visit at approximately eight weeks gestation. She is pregnant for the second time, and experienced postpartum depression after her first pregnancy. The pregnancy and postpartum course were otherwise unremarkable. She was recently diagnosed with a major depressive episode again, and began taking the antidepressant escitalopram (a serotonin reuptake inhibitor) a few months ago. She says the medication helped her tremendously. She has never been hospitalized for psychiatric reasons.
>
> Upon examination, she desires to keep the pregnancy and feels safe at home. She is currently experiencing fatigue and increases in her appetite, which are consistent with her current stage of pregnancy. She denies a depressed mood or thoughts of harming herself or others. The remainder of her exam is unremarkable.
>
> She has been seeing a psychotherapist, and she and her therapist are wondering if she can discontinue her medication for at least the beginning of the pregnancy. She has heard stories in the media that these medications may cause terrible problems to her baby such as heart problems. On the other hand, she is not sure she can remain emotionally well through pregnancy and wonders whether any particular antidepressant is safer than another and what you think the risks are if she needs to restart medication later in the pregnancy. She remembers her last postpartum episode and definitely does not want to feel like that again. However, she is also interested in breastfeeding since she was unable to do this with her last pregnancy.

Introduction

Depressive symptoms are common prior to, and during pregnancy. Estimates show between 14% and 18% of pregnant women will experience antenatal depressive symptoms. Among that group, 50–70% qualify as a major depressive episode [1, 2]. After pregnancy, postpartum mothers have been found to have a similar prevalence of depression as the general population [3]. Retrospective analyses demonstrate depression may be increasing in our society and around the world, getting more prevalent with each successive generation [4–6]. If so, more pregnant women will experience this mental health issue.

National survey data suggest the majority of these cases will go undiagnosed or untreated [7]. Untreated depression increases the risk of suicide, miscarriage, and other potential risks to the woman and her fetus [8]. However, patient concerns may lead women to discontinue medication treatment, as the idea of a potential effect on her child may influence her decision. In some instances this is justifiable – some women may be able to stay well during pregnancy without medication while other women may do well with psychotherapy alone. However, other women with a major depressive episode may require pharmacological treatment and awareness of risk factors, treatment options, and effects can lead to better outcomes for the mother–baby connection, as well as the individuals involved.

Clinical questions

1. In women with a history of a depressive disorder who wish to or have recently conceived, does discontinuing psychiatric medication (i) increase the risk of recurrence of illness; and (ii) does discontinuation promote poor maternal and fetal outcomes?

About 5–8% of women are receiving antidepressants at the time of fertilization [9]. The patient, psychiatrist, and obstetrician should collectively discuss whether to continue or discontinue antidepressant medication during pregnancy. Psychiatrists and obstetricians are concerned about both the health of the patient and offspring's health and hence would like to avoid a potential maternal relapse. Clinicians

Evidence-Based Obstetrics and Gynecology, First Edition. Edited by Errol R. Norwitz, Carolyn M. Zelop, David A. Miller, and David L. Keefe.

and patients may also have concerns about possible adverse effects of medication. These concerns should be discussed in a thorough and un-biased manner and clinicians should conduct a risk assessment.

Of those who discontinue treatment during pregnancy, depression history, illness severity, and treatment history are factors that may influence risk for recurrence of a depressive disorder. Characteristics of the course of illness, including greater number of previous depressive episodes, younger age of onset, and presence of concurrent psychiatric conditions, increase the likelihood that a pregnant woman will experience a recurrence during her prenatal period.

2. In pregnant patients with first trimester complaints of emotional symptoms, what are the sensitivity and specificity of various historical risk factors and symptoms in the diagnosis of major depressive disorder, or bipolar I disorder?

Symptoms for depressive disorders include depressed mood, anhedonia (loss of interest), significant weight loss or gain, sleep changes, psychomotor changes, fatigue, feelings of worthlessness or guilt, inability to concentrate, and thoughts of death or self-harm. A unipolar major depressive episode includes five of these symptoms, with one being either depressed mood or anhedonia, for at least two consecutive weeks. A minor depressive episode will include dysphoria or anhedonia, and one or two other symptoms, also during a continuous two-week period [2].

Women are often screened for antenatal depression with questionnaires and surveys such as the Center for Epidemiologic Studies Depression Scale (CES-D), Beck Depression Inventory (BDI), and Patient Health Questionnaire 9 (PHQ-9) [10]. However, diagnosing depression during pregnancy can be difficult for providers because of similarities between physiological changes of pregnancy and symptoms of a depressive episode. The Edinburgh Postnatal Depression Scale (EPDS) takes this into account by focusing on emotional symptoms [10]. The cut-off score in validity studies is 12/13 [11]. Using this threshold in postnatal women, the sensitivity for detected a woman with a major depressive episode was 0.75 and the positive predictive value as 0.24 [11]. A study of pregnant and postpartum women (n = 91) found that at a score of greater than 12, the sensitivity was 0.78, specificity 0.77, positive predictive value of 0.66, and negative predictive value of 0.86 [12].

A patient's social history before pregnancy can indicate risk for development of a major depressive episode during pregnancy. Marital status, relationship with partner, history of partner violence, and educational level completed, are predictive factors in multiple studies [13–15]. Age during pregnancy may have some relevance but studies vary on whether specific age groups, such as adolescence or advanced maternal age elevate risk [14, 16]. Pregnancy-related risk factors, such as fear of childbirth and unplanned pregnancy are associated with increased risk of developing a depressive disorder [14].

A thorough history and physical at the initial prenatal visit would be sufficient to identify past psychiatric, social, and pregnancy-related factors to evaluate for risk for antenatal depression. Patients who identify as high-risk for depression should be followed throughout their pregnancy for signs and symptoms for mood disorders. Given that typical physiologic changes of pregnancy can be confused for a depressive disorder, reliance on non-physiological symptoms can help, make a diagnosis.

3. In pregnant women with a major depressive episode, does treatment with antidepressants associate with an increased risk of adverse perinatal outcomes?

In the United States, it is estimated that 11–13% of pregnant women have been prescribed an antidepressant at some point in their pregnancy [17, 18]. Prevalence of antidepressant use during pregnancy has increased since the 1990s, but has been declining recently as warnings emerge of specific selective serotonin reuptake inhibitor (SSRI)-associated adverse outcomes during pregnancy [19, 20]. Many pregnant women discontinue medication on their own when they become pregnant; others do so with the recommendation or approval of their treating physician. Accordingly, studies find lower rates of antidepressant use in the third trimester of pregnancy compared to the first trimester [20].

Women may elect to cease treatment with just an intention to become pregnant. Despite earlier reports to the contrary, periconceptional use of antidepressants does not appear to be related to spontaneous abortion. In a clever analysis of 1 279 840 pregnancies, Anderson et al. found that women who were undergoing treatment with an SSRI had a higher rate of spontaneous abortion. However, when they looked at women who took the same medication but stopped treatment in the 3–12 months prior to pregnancy, the rate of spontaneous abortion was as high as in women who continued medication [21]. This study suggests that factors related to the need for antidepressant treatment, but not that treatment itself is linked with spontaneous miscarriage. These results were in line with an earlier study that found women who had a history of treatment with antidepressants had similar rates of spontaneous abortion as women who underwent antidepressant treatment in pregnancy [22].

Antidepressant use has not been shown to influence quantitative outcomes of *in vitro* fertilization (IVF) treatment. randomized control trials (RCTs) and retrospective reviews have not found a difference in serum estradiol levels, oocyte number, quality during retrieval and their subsequent maturation [23, 24]. However, there was a negative trend in pregnancy rates for SSRI users in two studies. In one study, overall the SSRI users had poorer pregnancy rates; per cycle started – 17.1% vs 28.9%; per embryo transfer – 23.3% vs 32.1%; live birth rate 14.6% vs 21.2%; the difference was not statistically significant – possibly due to the small number of subjects [24, 25]. Notably, cycle cancellation rates have been shown to be significantly higher among SSRI users (26.8% versus 10.0% in non-SSRI users) [25] due to a poor ovarian response to fertility treatment. The authors stated that while the direct impact of SSRI's on the canceled cycles was unclear, it is possible there was an interaction with the gonadal axis in some fashion [25].

Depression has already been linked to a higher incidence of preterm birth (PTB), but an additional increased risk of PTB has been associated with both mixed antidepressant and SSRI use [26–29], although there is some disagreement among studies [30]. A meta-analysis attributed a 1.74 relative risk increase of PTB in patients who have used SSRI's at any point during pregnancy [26]. Further analysis shows that a majority of these births are primarily late preterm (34–37 weeks) [29]. Additionally, there is limited evidence that spontaneous PTB, but not indicated PTB is associated with antidepressant use in pregnancy [31].

Researchers have also focused on associations between antenatal antidepressant use and various birth defects. Conclusions have been on both sides of an association due to difficulties comparing studies and cofounding factors [32–34]. Meta-analyses show that the rate of malformations associated with antidepressant use in pregnancy is a magnitude smaller than the rates that one sees with teratogens such as tretinoin [35].

A meta-analysis in 2010 established paroxetine use and cardiac defects had a prevalence odds ratio of 1.46, or one more case of a cardiac defect per 200 newborns exposed to paroxetine as a fetus [36]. GlaxoSmithKline themselves have acknowledged the risk, labeled the drug as Category D [37].

Other congenital birth defects have been associated with such as omphalocele and neural tube defects have also been cited in the literature, but studies have several limitations [38–42]. A recent study that used a large multi-site case-control study to replicate previous findings in the literature found associations between first trimester exposure to paroxetine and cardiac defects, anencephaly, gastroschisis and, omphalocele, as well as fluoxetine and right ventricular flow defects and craniosynostosis [43]. This lack of consistency has not further clarified risks and one is left assuming a small risk associated with a variety of the detected malformations.

Postnatal adaptation syndrome (PNAS) is a pattern of symptoms found in infants exposed to antidepressants at any time during gestation [44, 45]. The infant may suffer from symptoms such as tachypnea, hypothermia, hypoglycemia, and irritability for days to weeks – similar to those found in adult SSRI-discontinuation syndrome and serotonin syndrome [46]. Research estimates of PNAS in up to 30% of exposed infants, prompted the FDA to issue a statement in 2004 encouraging providers to adjust dosage during the third trimester of pregnancy [45–47]. The problem with this strategy is that it can increase the risk of relapse in mother as she approaches delivery. Furthermore, it is not clear whether this tact will decrease rates of PNAS.

Long-term developmental data regarding intrauterine exposure to antidepressants is limited, but studies are currently being conducted. Of note, several new case-control cohort studies found a significant increased risk of developmental disorders such as autism-spectrum disorder and attention-deficit hyperactive disorder if a depressed pregnant woman used antidepressants during their pregnancy [48–53]. Conversely, the largest population-based study did not find a significant association between SSRI use during pregnancy and risk of autism spectrum disorder [54]. A causal relationship is difficult to determine, but if there is one, the effect is small.

In conclusion, antidepressant use has been linked to a variety of maternal, fetal, and obstetrical complications. Studies on the topic have their limitations typically arising from confounding. Many women who take antidepressants are also undergoing treatment with other psychotropic and non-psychotropic medication that can cause adverse birth outcomes [55]. As well, women who require antidepressant treatment may also be engaging in unhealthy habits such as licit or illicit substance use. Observational data can control for these factors if information about confounders is accurately collected but many women are reluctant to disclose these problems. Several medications, most notably paroxetine, are associated with various congenital anomalies if used during organogenesis. PTB has a consistent association with antidepressant use, but most these agents appear to shorten gestation by only a few days. As research of antidepressant ages, more data will surface regarding its effect on fertilization and long-term sequelae, such as child development.

4. In pregnant women with a major depressive episode, are there non-pharmacological treatments that can reduce depressive symptoms significantly when compared to the antidepressants?

Management of depression during pregnancy primarily relies on severity of presenting symptoms [9, 56]. Patients with mild depression, or simply depressive symptoms, may be appropriate candidates to trial non-pharmacological management options or use them as adjunct therapy. Psychotherapy, such as cognitive behavioral therapy (CBT) or interpersonal psychotherapy (IPT), is by far used most often. In non-pregnant women, there is a significant amount of evidence that CBT may be equivalent to antidepressant medication for treatment of mild to moderate depressive symptoms, and have some efficacy for severe depression. Also, relapse rates may be lower for CBT than medication, providing support for CBT as a cost-effective, first-line treatment for many depressed patients. A pilot study randomized CBT for pregnant women and saw twice as many respondents improve in major depressive disorder (MDD) symptoms by 15-weeks than women receiving standard care [57]. A small, RCT comparing IPT to peer-education saw a significantly better improvement in depression scores and recovery rate in the IPT group by the end of 16 weekly treatments [58]. The relative convenience of IPT and CBT as a non-pharmacological treatment method led to the American Psychiatric Association and the American College of Obstetricians and Gynecologists (ACOG) to recommend psychotherapy as an alternative to antidepressants for pregnant women, as well as a first line treatment in certain circumstances, such as mild-to-moderate depression [56].

Other studied options for non-pharmacological methods include yoga, massage therapy, acupuncture, physical activity, and light therapy [59]. These studies are usually conducted on a volunteer basis or with small sample sizes. Although many have still managed to show significant improvement of depressive symptoms in these limited studies, varying intervention protocols, and depression scoring make hard to reach a consensus on recommendations for each intervention [59].

The use of any alternative method requires close monitoring of depressive symptom progression with proper follow-up. If improvement is minimal, the physician must consider antidepressant treatment. Antidepressants are typically the first line treatment for severe depression in pregnancy, but one or more non-pharmacological methods may be used as adjunct therapy. In any case, if the depression progresses with suicidal or homicidal thoughts, the patient should be referred immediately to an appropriate physician or directed to an emergency department for further evaluation.

5. In women who are breastfeeding and have a history of psychiatric illness, which medications are found in high concentrations in breastmilk and may cause adverse effects to the newborn?

Multiple professional organizations support breastfeeding as a priority for infant health. Breastmilk is the most nutritious diet possible for a newborn in that it includes various proteins (i.e. antibodies) to further develop physiologic systems after birth. The act of breastfeeding itself creates a mother–baby bond that provides psychosocial benefits to mother and baby individually, and as a unit.

Postpartum depression occurs at a rate similar to that of non-pregnant women, but the symptoms expressed during these and other psychiatric illnesses may interfere with lactation. The general consensus is that the benefits of breastfeeding outweigh the risks of adverse effects of most psychiatric medications [60–63]. The contraindications that have been issued by manufacturers, various international drug policy organizations, and professional organizations are based on scant data from small, underpopulated, underpowered studies with short-term follow-up or case reports [61, 62]. Unfortunately, much of the literature is based upon case reports and this needs to be considered when making recommendations.

Pharmacokinetics can help substantiate information provided by available reports, and promote evidence-based choices. In order for clinicians to best estimate which drugs may obtain a theoretical risk, characteristics such as half-life, time till peak maternal serum level. Percentage of drug bound to maternal protein predicts that a high affinity to proteins (>80%), and more likely to stay within plasma. Milk-to-plasma ratio is used to directly compare the concentration of each compartment but this may vary depending upon the portion of breastmilk assayed (e.g. foremilk or hindmilk). Finally, oral bioavailability predicts how much of the drug or its active metabolites will actually be absorbed by the infant. Individually, these characteristics point to different potential medication risks, but none reason enough to contraindicate use in a breastfeeding mother. Concentration levels of drug in infant serum may also be related to antidepressant use during the prenatal period.

A review by Fortinguerra et al. suggested that infant daily dosage (mg/kg/day) received through the breastmilk, relative to the maternal dose, can be used to distinguish at-risk medications [62]. In this scenario, sertraline, paroxetine, and fluvoxamine would be the safest antidepressants. Chlorpromazine and olanzapine would be safest antipsychotics. The threshold for concern is placed around a relative-infant dose (RID) of 10%. Studies find that citalopram and fluoxetine, followed by escitalopram are close to that threshold. Clozapine, lithium, and sulpiride (not used in the United States) would be contraindicated agents.

American Academy of Pediatrics (AAP) suggest that a provider counsel the patient about the potential risks of psychiatric medication use and lactation when a drug is found in infant serum concentrations that exceed 10% of maternal plasma concentration [60].

Breastfeeding while taking antidepressants is, overall, not considered harmful. It is estimated a fetus is exposed to less antidepressants during breastfeeding than if the mother was taking them during pregnancy. First-line therapy recommendations per psychiatric diagnoses are based on pharmacokinetics and reports of adverse events. Those considered first-line include sertraline, paroxetine, fluvoxamine, and nortriptyline [61, 62]. Mothers and physicians should monitor for typical symptoms of toxicity such as sedation, nausea, reduced suckling, or other signs that would be expected of the drugs. Reports of all such symptoms are low. There have been reports of SSRIs and an association with delay of lactation initiation [64]. However, this was insignificant by the fourth day of the postpartum period, and again by two-week postpartum check [64, 65]. The serotonin and norepinephrine reuptake inhibitors (SNRIs) venlafaxine and duloxetine are acceptable next-line against [61, 62]. Doxepin is contraindicated due to a reported episode of respiratory depression in a baby with elevated levels of doxepin and corresponding metabolites [63, 66].

Studies are limited for antipsychotic use during lactation. Available information indicates clozapine may be associated with agranulocytosis, and is thus contraindicated. Olanzapine has a favorable pharmacokinetic profile and is not contraindicated, but rare adverse events have been reported [62, 67]. Potential signs of toxicity include lethargy, sedation, and motor development (due to potential long-term use). This points to the need for clinician's to monitor the infant and not simply rely on serum levels of a medication.

Use of lithium during lactation has long been problematic by some, primarily based on older literature reporting adverse events and pharmacokinetics (high RID 69%) [61, 62]. As more research surfaces, this is being revisited, and it is widely held that earlier studies overestimated the risk of lithium use in pregnancy. While the concentration of lithium found in infant serum of treated mothers has shown to be low [68] it also needs to be acknowledged that lithium fully equilibrates with maternal serum levels in breast milk.

Benzodiazepines are safe for infants at low doses due to their milk-to-plasma ratio [63]. If given in high doses, or if an infant has a metabolic impairment, symptoms of lethargy, and poor feeding may occur. By design, neonatal hepatic metabolism is under-developed. Hence their metabolic activity and their lower renal clearance contribute to higher levels. Any changes in infant behavior should prompt re-consideration of benzodiazepine use during lactation.

Valproate, which is used to treat individuals with manic depressive illness, is found in breastmilk and infant serum in low levels. A case of thrombocytopenia and anemia has been reported, but use of this drug is supported by the World Health Organization experts who review medications for LactMed and the AAP [63]. If used, clinicians should monitor the infant for bruising and bleeding. Carbamazepine's profile results in high concentrations in breastmilk and infant serum [62]. Adverse events associated with its use include sedation, poor sucking, and withdrawal reactions. Three cases of hepatic dysfunction have been noted, but all were complicated by intrauterine exposure and concurrent drug therapy [62, 63]. Since monotherapy has shown no adverse effects, it is not contraindicated.

Official organizations such as AAP and ACOG have difficulty keeping up with the number of studies and the speed of new developments. Physicians and providers should consider consulting the government database LactMed (https://toxnet.nlm.nih.gov/newtoxnet/lactmed.htm) for the most current and comprehensive information. If needed, there are many options of psychiatric medications deemed safe for use during lactation. Research is unable to confidently conclude the safety of a select few, and there are even fewer that have established contraindications. When physicians are presented with a questionable scenario, the risks of an antidepressant should be compared to the risks of the psychiatric episode to the mother-baby relationship. More research is needed to validate many more possible medications.

6. What risk factors, symptoms, and tools have proven to be significant in assessing self-harm and suicidal ideation in the pregnant and postpartum women?

Pregnancy may provide some protection against self-harm and suicide ideation when compared to the general population [69]. However, women of reproductive age constitute those most at risk to act on suicide ideation [70]. Thus it should not come as surprise that national data indicate self-harm and suicide as leading causes of maternal morbidity and mortality [71]. Additionally, providers may be under-diagnosing the risk depending on the method of inquiry and on the patient to volunteer the information [72, 73].

There are no pregnancy-specific tools to screen for self-harm or suicide ideation during the gestational period and clinicians rely on depression measures. Both the PHQ-9 and the EPDS include a specific question for identifying those at risk for self-harm. These screens, as well as all other screens, are not meant to substitute a professional's clinical assessment. For any positive screening, the professional should proceed with further counseling and assessing the acuity of the situation by asking about a plan or access to means of harm [10]. This may merit referral to a psychiatric provider.

The level of severity of mental illness, as well as history of self-harm, is an indicator of risk of self-harm and suicide attempts in pregnant and postpartum women [72, 74, 75]. Additionally, unpartnered, non-Caucasian, less educated women are at an increased risk of responding positively to thoughts of self-harm on screening [72, 74, 76]. Women who are publicly-insured may also be at risk, raising the question of access or lower socioeconomic class as a risk factor [74, 76]. Standard of care involves screening women for thoughts of self-harm and suicide ideation during their postpartum visit, which occurs around 6-weeks postpartum. Patients with the risk factors outlined above, are still exhibiting an increased risk of self-harm and suicide ideation at one-year postpartum, raising the question of further monitoring for those at-risk [72].

Practice should include routine screening for evaluation of depressive symptoms, including self-harm and suicide ideation [10]. Given a positive response, the patient should be evaluated and provided proper resources for counseling and social services. Referral should be made to proper psychiatric care if warranted.

References

1 Gavin, N.I., Gaynes, B.N., Lohr, K.N. et al. (2005). Perinatal depression: a systematic review of prevalence and incidence. *Obstetrics and Gynecology* **106**: 1071–1083.

2 Yonkers, K.A., Vigod, S., and Ross, L.E. (2011). Diagnosis, pathophysiology, and management of mood disorders in pregnant and postpartum women. *Obstetrics and Gynecology* **117**: 961–977.

3 Gaynes, B.N., Gavin, N., Meltzer-Brody, S. et al. (2005). Perinatal depression: prevalence, screening accuracy, and screening outcomes. *Evidence Report/Technology Assessment (Summary)* 1–8.

4 Hidaka, B.H. (2012). Depression as a disease of modernity: explanations for increasing prevalence. *Journal of Affective Disorders* **140**: 205–214.

5 Kocher, M.S., Smith, J.T., Iversen, M.D. et al. (2011). Reliability, validity, and responsiveness of a modified international knee documentation committee subjective knee form (Pedi-IKDC) in children with knee disorders. *American Journal of Sports Medicine* **39**: 933–939.

6 Weissman, M.M., Wickramaratne, P., Greenwald, S. et al. (1992). The changing rate of major depression: cross-national comparisons. *JAMA* **268**: 3098–3105.

7 Ko, J.Y., Farr, S.L., Dietz, P.M., and Robbins, C.L. (2012). Depression and treatment among U.S. pregnant and nonpregnant women of reproductive age, 2005–2009. *Journal of Women's Health (Larchmt)* **21**: 830–836.

8 Stewart, D.E. (2011). Clinical practice. Depression during pregnancy. *The New England Journal of Medicine* **365**: 1605–1611.

9 Yonkers, K.A., Gotman, N., Smith, M.V. et al. (2011). Does antidepressant use attenuate the risk of a major depressive episode in pregnancy? *Epidemiology* **22**: 848–854.

10 Committee Opinion (2015). The American College of Obstetricians and Gynecologists Committee opinion no. 630. Screening for perinatal depression. *Obstetrics and Gynecology* **125**: 1268–1271.

11 Cox, J.L., Chapman, G., Murray, D., and Jones, P. (1996). Validation of the Edinburgh postnatal depression scale (EPDS) in non-postnatal women. *Journal of Affective Disorders* **39**: 185–189.

12 Grigoriadis, S., de Camps Meschino, D., Barrons, E. et al. (2011). Mood and anxiety disorders in a sample of Canadian perinatal women referred for psychiatric care. *Archives of Women's Mental Health* **14**: 325–333.

13 Martini, J., Petzoldt, J., Einsle, F. et al. (2015). Risk factors and course patterns of anxiety and depressive disorders during pregnancy and after delivery: a prospective-longitudinal study. *Journal of Affective Disorders* **175**: 385–395.

14 Raisanen, S., Lehto, S.M., Nielsen, H.S. et al. (2014). Risk factors for and perinatal outcomes of major depression during pregnancy: a population-based analysis during 2002–2010 in Finland. *BMJ Open* **4**: e004883.

15 Lydsdottir, L.B., Howard, L.M., Olafsdottir, H. et al. (2014). The mental health characteristics of pregnant women with depressive symptoms identified by the Edinburgh postnatal depression scale. *The Journal of Clinical Psychiatry* **75**: 393–398.

16 Melville, J.L., Gavin, A., Guo, Y. et al. (2010). Depressive disorders during pregnancy: prevalence and risk factors in a large urban sample. *Obstetrics and Gynecology* **116**: 1064–1070.

17 Cooper, W.O., Willy, M.E., Pont, S.J., and Ray, W.A. (2007). Increasing use of antidepressants in pregnancy. *American Journal of Obstetrics and Gynecology* **196**: 544 e1–544 e5.

18 Barber, C. (2008). The medicated Americans. *Scientific American Mind* **19**: 44–51.

19 Petersen, I., Gilbert, R.E., Evans, S.J. et al. (2011). Pregnancy as a major determinant for discontinuation of antidepressants: an analysis of data from the health improvement network. *The Journal of Clinical Psychiatry* **72**: 979–985.

20 Huybrechts, K.F., Palmsten, K., Mogun, H. et al. (2013). National trends in antidepressant medication treatment among publicly insured pregnant women. *General Hospital Psychiatry* **35**: 265–271.

21 Andersen, J.T., Andersen, N.L., Horwitz, H. et al. (2014). Exposure to selective serotonin reuptake inhibitors in early pregnancy and the risk of miscarriage. *Obstetrics and Gynecology* **124**: 655–661.

22 Ban, L., Tata, L.J., West, J. et al. (2012). Live and non-live pregnancy outcomes among women with depression and anxiety: a population-based study. *PLoS One* **7**: e43462.

23 Serafini, P., Lobo, D.S., Grosman, A. et al. (2009). Fluoxetine treatment for anxiety in women undergoing in vitro fertilization. *International Journal of Gynaecology and Obstetrics: the Official Organ of the International Federation of Gynaecology and Obstetrics* **105**: 136–139.

24 Klock, S.C., Sheinin, S., Kazer, R., and Zhang, X. (2004). A pilot study of the relationship between selective serotonin reuptake inhibitors and in vitro fertilization outcome. *Fertility and Sterility* **82**: 968–969.

25 Friedman, B.E., Rogers, J.L., Shahine, L.K. et al. (2009). Effect of selective serotonin reuptake inhibitors on in vitro fertilization outcome. *Fertility and Sterility* **92**: 1312–1314.

26 Huang, H., Coleman, S., Bridge, J.A. et al. (2013). A meta-analysis of the relationship between antidepressant use in pregnancy and the risk of preterm birth and low birth weight. *General Hospital Psychiatry* **36** (**1**): 13–18.

27 El Marroun, H., Jaddoe, V.W., Hudziak, J.J. et al. (2012). Maternal use of selective serotonin reuptake inhibitors, fetal growth, and risk of adverse birth outcomes. *Archives of General Psychiatry* **69**: 706–714.

28 Lund, N., Pedersen, L.H., and Henriksen, T.B. (2009). Selective serotonin reuptake inhibitor exposure in utero and pregnancy outcomes. *Archieve Pediatrics Adolescent Medicine* **163**: 949–954.

29 Wisner, K.L., Sit, D.K., Hanusa, B.H. et al. (2009). Major depression and antidepressant treatment: impact on pregnancy and neonatal outcomes. *The American Journal of Psychiatry* **166**: 557–566.

30 Malm, H., Sourander, A., Gissler, M. et al. (2015). Pregnancy complications following prenatal exposure to SSRIs or maternal psychiatric disorders: results from population-based national register data. *The American Journal of Psychiatry* **172**: 1224–1232.

31 Yonkers, K.A., Norwitz, E.R., Smith, M.V. et al. (2012). Depression and serotonin reuptake inhibitor treatment as risk factors for preterm birth. *Epidemiology* **23**: 677–685.

32 Hoffman, J.I. and Kaplan, S. (2002). The incidence of congenital heart disease. *Journal of the American College of Cardiology* **39**: 1890–1900.

33 Centers for Disease Control and Prevention (2008). Update on overall prevalence of major birth defects – Atlanta, Georgia, 1978–2005. *MMWR Morbidity and Mortality Weekly Report* **57**: 1–5.

34 Reller, M.D., Strickland, M.J., Riehle-Colarusso, T. et al. (2008). Prevalence of congenital heart defects in metropolitan Atlanta, 1998–2005. *The Journal of Pediatrics* **153**: 807–813.

35 Greene, M.F. (2007). Teratogenicity of SSRIs – serious concern or much ado about little? *The New England Journal of Medicine* **356**: 2732–2733.

36 Wurst, K.E., Poole, C., Ephross, S.A., and Olshan, A.F. (2010). First trimester paroxetine use and the prevalence of congenital, specifically cardiac, defects: a meta-analysis of epidemiological studies. *Birth Defects Research Part A, Clinical and Molecular Teratology* **88**: 159–170.

37 Food and Drug Administration (FDA) Antidepressant use in pregnancy. 2005. at http://www.fda.gov/downloads/Safety/MedWatch/SafetyInformation/SafetyAlertsforHumanMedicalProducts/UCM164865.pdf. Accessed 10 July 2018.

38 Bakker, M.K., De Walle, H.E., Wilffert, B., and de Jong-Van den Berg, L.T. (2010). Fluoxetine and infantile hypertrophic pylorus stenosis: a signal from a birth defects-drug exposure surveillance study. *Pharmacoepidemiology and Drug Safety* **19**: 808–813.

39 Yonkers, K.A., Blackwell, K.A., Glover, J., and Forray, A. (2014). Antidepressant use in pregnant and postpartum women. *Annual Review of Clinical Psychology* **10**: 369–392.

40 Louik, C., Lin, A.E., Werler, M.M. et al. (2007). First-trimester use of selective serotonin-reuptake inhibitors and the risk of birth defects. *The New England Journal of Medicine* **356**: 2675–2683.

41 Oberlander, T.F., Warburton, W., Misri, S. et al. (2008). Major congenital malformations following prenatal exposure to serotonin reuptake inhibitors and benzodiazepines using population-based health data. *Birth Defects Research Part B Developmental and Reproductive Toxicology* **83**: 68–76.

42 Pedersen, L.H., Henriksen, T.B., Vestergaard, M. et al. (2009). Selective serotonin reuptake inhibitors in pregnancy and congenital malformations: population based cohort study. *BMJ* **339**: b3569.

43 Reefhuis, J., Devine, O., Friedman, J.M. et al. (2015). National Birth Defects Prevention S. Specific SSRIs and birth defects: Bayesian analysis to interpret new data in the context of previous reports. *BMJ* **351**: h3190.

44 Byatt, N., Deligiannidis, K.M., and Freeman, M.P. (2013). Antidepressant use in pregnancy: a critical review focused on risks and controversies. *Acta Psychiatrica Scandinavica* **127**: 94–114.

45 Levinson-Castiel, R., Merlob, P., Linder, N. et al. (2006). Neonatal abstinence syndrome after in utero exposure to selective serotonin reuptake inhibitors in term infants. *Archives of Pediatrics & Adolescent Medicine* **160**: 173–176.

46 Chambers, C.D., Johnson, K.A., Dick, L.M. et al. (1996). Birth outcomes in pregnant women taking fluoxetine. *The New England Journal of Medicine* **335**: 1010–1015.

47 US Food and Drug Administration. Safety Alerts for Human Medical Products. 2004. (accessed 17 September 2018, at https://www.fda.gov/ScienceResearch/SpecialTopics/PediatricTherapeuticsResearch/ucm123229.htm.)

48 Rai, D., Lee, B.K., Dalman, C. et al. (2013). Parental depression, maternal antidepressant use during pregnancy, and risk of autism spectrum disorders: population based case-control study. *BMJ* **346**: f2059-f.

49 Croen, L.A., Grether, J.K., Yoshida, C.K. et al. (2011). Antidepressant use during pregnancy and childhood autism spectrum disorders. *Archives of General Psychiatry* **68**: 1104–1112.

50 Harrington, R.A., Lee, L.C., Crum, R.M. et al. (2014). Prenatal SSRI use and offspring with autism spectrum disorder or developmental delay. *Pediatrics* **133**: e1241–e1248.

51 Clements, C.C., Castro, V.M., Blumenthal, S.R. et al. (2015). Prenatal antidepressant exposure is associated with risk for attention-deficit hyperactivity disorder but not autism spectrum disorder in a large health system. *Molecular Psychiatry* **20**: 727–734.

52 Boukhris, T., Sheehy, O., Mottron, L., and Bérard, A. ANtidepressant use during pregnancy and the risk of autism spectrum disorder in children. *JAMA Pediatrics* **2015**: 1–8.

53 El Marroun, H., White, T.J., van der Knaap, N.J. et al. (2014). Prenatal exposure to selective serotonin reuptake inhibitors and social responsiveness symptoms of autism: population-based study of young children. *The British Journal of Psychiatry: the Journal of Mental Science* **205**: 95–102.

54 Hviid, A., Melbye, M., and Pasternak, B. (2013). Use of selective serotonin reuptake inhibitors during pregnancy and risk of autism. *The New England Journal of Medicine* **369**: 2406–2415.

55 Kallen, B., Nilsson, E., and Olausson, P.O. (2011). Antidepressant use during pregnancy: comparison of data obtained from a prescription register and from antenatal care records. *European Journal of Clinical Pharmacology* **67**: 839–845.

56 Yonkers, K.A., Wisner, K.L., Stewart, D.E. et al. (2009). The management of depression during pregnancy: a report from the American Psychiatric Association and the American College of Obstetricians and Gynecologists. *General Hospital Psychiatry* **31**: 403–413.

57 Burns, A., O'Mahen, H., Baxter, H. et al. (2013). A pilot randomised controlled trial of cognitive behavioural therapy for antenatal depression. *BMC Psychiatry* **13**: 33.

58 Spinelli, M.G. and Endicott, J. (2003). Controlled clinical trial of interpersonal psychotherapy versus parenting education program for depressed pregnant women. *The American Journal of Psychiatry* **160**: 555–562.

59 Dennis, C.L. and Dowswell, T. (2013). Interventions (other than pharmacological, psychosocial or psychological) for treating antenatal depression. *Cochrane Database of Systematic Review* **7**: CD006795. doi: 10.1002/14651858.CD006795.pub3.

60 Sachs, H.C. (2013). The transfer of drugs and therapeutics into human breast milk: an update on selected topics. *Pediatrics* **132**: e796–e809.

61 Davanzo, R., Copertino, M., De Cunto, A. et al. (2011). Antidepressant drugs and breastfeeding: a review of the literature. Breastfeeding medicine: the official journal of the academy of. *Breastfeeding Medicine* **6**: 89–98.

62 Fortinguerra, F., Clavenna, A., and Bonati, M. (2009). Psychotropic drug use during breastfeeding: a review of the evidence. *Pediatrics* **124**: e547–e556.

63 (2008). ACOG Practice Bulletin: clinical management guidelines for obstetrician-gynecologists number 92, April 2008 (replaces practice bulletin number 87, November 2007). Use of psychiatric medications during pregnancy and lactation. *Obstetrics and Gynecology* **111**: 1001–1020.

64 Marshall, A.M., Nommsen-Rivers, L.A., Hernandez, L.L. et al. (2010). Serotonin transport and metabolism in the mammary gland modulates secretory activation and involution. *The Journal of Clinical Endocrinology and Metabolism* **95**: 837–846.

65 Gorman, J.R., Kao, K., and Chambers, C.D. (2012). Breastfeeding among women exposed to antidepressants during pregnancy. *Journal of Human Lactation: Official Journal of International Lactation Consultant Association* **28**: 181–188.

66 Matheson, I., Pande, H., and Alertsen, A.R. (1985). Respiratory depression caused by N-desmethyldoxepin in breast milk. *Lancet (London, England)* **2**: 1124.

67 Gentile, S. (2008). Infant safety with antipsychotic therapy in breast-feeding: a systematic review. *The Journal of Clinical Psychiatry* **69**: 666–673.

68 Viguera, A.C., Newport, D.J., Ritchie, J. et al. (2007). Lithium in breast milk and nursing infants: clinical implications. *The American Journal of Psychiatry* **164**: 342–345.

69 Oates, M. (2003). Suicide: the leading cause of maternal death. *The British Journal of Psychiatry: the Journal of Mental Science* **183**: 279–281.

70 Kessler, R.C., Borges, G., and Walters, E.E. (1999). Prevalence of and risk factors for lifetime suicide attempts in the National Comorbidity Survey. *Archives of General Psychiatry* **56**: 617–626.

71 Palladino, C.L., Singh, V., Campbell, J. et al. (2011). Homicide and suicide during the perinatal period: findings from the National Violent Death Reporting System. *Obstetrics and Gynecology* **118**: 1056–1063.

72 Pope, C.J., Xie, B., Sharma, V., and Campbell, M.K. (2013). A prospective study of thoughts of self-harm and suicidal ideation during the postpartum period in women with mood disorders. *Archives of Women's Mental Health* **16**: 483–488.

73 Newport, D.J., Levey, L.C., Pennell, P.B. et al. (2007). Suicidal ideation in pregnancy: assessment and clinical implications. *Archives of Women's Mental Health* **10**: 181–187.

74 Kim, J.J., La Porte, L.M., Saleh, M.P. et al. (2015). Suicide risk among perinatal women who report thoughts of self-harm on depression screens. *Obstetrics and Gynecology* **125**: 885–893.

75 Castro, E.C.T., Brancaglion, M.Y., Cardoso, M.N. et al. (2015). Suicidality among pregnant women in Brazil: prevalence and risk factors. *Archives of Women's Mental Health* **19** (**2**): 343–348.

76 Wisner, K.L., Sit, D.K., McShea, M.C. et al. (2013). Onset timing, thoughts of self-harm, and diagnoses in postpartum women with screen-positive depression findings. *JAMA Psychiatry* **70**: 490–498.

37

CHAPTER 37
Preterm labor

Joses A. Jain and Cynthia Gyamfi-Bannerman
Columbia University Medical Center, New York, NY, USA

> **CLINICAL VIGNETTE 1**
>
> A 25-year-old Gravida 2 Para 0101 presents to the office at 12 weeks' gestation for a prenatal care visit. Her prior pregnancy was two years ago and resulted in a spontaneous vaginal delivery at 28 weeks' gestation after presenting to the hospital in labor. Her infant had a prolonged and complicated course in the neonatal intensive care unit. She is worried about a similar outcome occurring again, and asks you about her available options to prevent this in her current pregnancy.

> **CLINICAL VIGNETTE 2**
>
> A 25-year-old Gravida 1 Para 0 presents at 27 weeks' gestation with painful, regular contractions. Her cervix is dilated to 3 cm and 90% effaced, and the fetus is in cephalic presentation. The fetal heart tracing demonstrates a normal baseline with moderate variability and no decelerations, and she is contracting every three minutes on tocometry. She has no significant medical or surgical history and her pregnancy had previously been uncomplicated. She asks you to do everything that you can to provide the best outcome for her infant.

Background

Preterm birth is the leading cause of perinatal morbidity and mortality worldwide, the sequelae of which result in over one million infant deaths each year. Spontaneous preterm labor is the result of multiple pathophysiologic processes, and contributes to approximately 70% of all cases of preterm birth [1]. The resultant burden is the leading cause of neonatal morbidity and mortality, accounting for 36.5% of infant deaths and 25–50% of cases of long-term neurologic impairment in children [2]. The incidence of preterm-related complications is inversely proportional to the gestational age at the time of delivery [3]. Thus, both pharmacologic and non-pharmacologic strategies that have been developed to improve the outcomes in pregnancies complicated by preterm labor have targeted two goals: the prolongation of pregnancy and the optimization of the preterm neonate's transition to extrauterine life.

The diagnosis of spontaneous preterm labor has been given multiple definitions by various authors. The classic definition requires the clinical criteria of uterine contractions and documented cervical change (in dilatation, effacement, or both) with intact membranes at 20–36 6/7 weeks gestation. An alternative definition requires an initial presentation with regular contractions and cervical dilatation of at least 2 cm between 20 and 36 6/7 weeks gestation. With this definition, however, only 10% of women diagnosed with preterm labor actually deliver within seven days of presentation [4]. A more recently proposed definition consists of uterine contractions (more than 4 in 20 minutes or more than 8 in 60 minutes) with a transvaginal ultrasound-determined cervical length of less than 20 mm, or 20–29 mm with a positive fetal fibronectin (FFN) test, at 20–36 6/7 weeks gestation [5]. Regardless of the definition used, the identification of a woman who will actually deliver a premature infant remains a challenge.

This chapter will consider the quality of evidence pertaining to the diagnostic tools available in the identification and risk-stratification of a women at risk for having a preterm birth, including elements of clinical history, transvaginal ultrasound, and fetal fibronectin. The evidence in the literature regarding the management of these patients will then be evaluated. Historically proposed non-pharmacologic interventions such as bed rest, hydration, and relaxation techniques, in addition to pharmacologic interventions such as tocolysis, antibiotics, antenatal corticosteroids, and magnesium sulfate will also be examined.

Evidence-Based Obstetrics and Gynecology, First Edition. Edited by Errol R. Norwitz, Carolyn M. Zelop, David A. Miller, and David L. Keefe.

Clinical questions

1. What factors place a women at risk for having a spontaneous preterm birth?

Many potential risk factors can lead to multiple possible pathways that culminate in the end result of spontaneous preterm birth. Table 37.1 lists some of these risk factors with corresponding references to the literature. Although many of these have been identified, the inherent challenge in successful primary prevention is that many women who have a spontaneous preterm birth have no identifiable risk factors [25]. Of the risk factors that have been identified, a history of a prior preterm birth is the most significant, with subsequent preterm births often occurring at the same gestational age. In a large prospective study by Mercer et al. involving 1711 multiparous women with singleton gestations, those with a prior preterm delivery carried a 2.5-fold increase in the risk of spontaneous preterm delivery compared to those without a prior preterm delivery (21.7% vs. 8.8%, relative risk (RR) 2.5). An early prior spontaneous preterm delivery (23–27 weeks gestation) was most highly associated with early spontaneous preterm delivery less than 28 weeks gestation (RR 22.1) [26].

2. What diagnostic tests are available to identify patients who are at a high risk of having a spontaneous preterm delivery?

Transvaginal ultrasound

The finding of a shortened cervical length as measured by transvaginal ultrasound has been established as a known independent risk factor for preterm birth [4]. As a result, cervical length screening by transvaginal ultrasonography in women with a prior preterm birth has been shown to be a useful predictive tool for the risk of a subsequent preterm birth. In a blinded observational study by Owen et al., a cervical length assessment between 16 weeks and 18 weeks 6 days' gestation, augmented by serial evaluations up to 23 weeks 6 days' gestation, was able to predict spontaneous preterm birth prior to 35 weeks' gestation in women with a history of a prior spontaneous preterm birth

Table 37.1 Risk factors for spontaneous preterm birth with corresponding references to the literature

	Risk factor	Risk	References
Prior pregnancy history	Prior spontaneous preterm birth	RR 6.4 (95% CI 4.4–9.2)	Goldenberg et al. [6]
	Prior surgical uterine evacuation	OR 1.44 (95% CI 1.09–1.90)	Saccone et al. [7]
	Short interpregnancy interval (≤6 mo)	OR 3.6 (95% CI 1.41–8.98)	Rodrigues et al. [8]
Demographics	Non-hispanic black race	OR 1.78 (95% CI 1.59–2.00)	Srinivasjois et al. [9]
	Age ≥ 40 yr	OR 1.4 (95% CI 1.1–1.7)	Cleary-Goldman et al. [10]
Uterine factors	Congenital Mullerian anomalies	OR 5.9 (95% CI 4.3–8.1)	Hua et al. [11]
	Uterine fibroids (≥5–6 cm), or multiple fibroids	OR 1.5 (95% CI 1.3–1.7)	Klatsky et al. [12]
Cervical factors	Prior cervical conization	OR 4.7 (95% CI 2.22–7.10)	Klaritsch et al. [13]
		OR 1.99 (95% CI 1.81–2.20)	Jakobsson et al. [14]
	Prior LEEP	RR 2.61 (95% CI 2.02–3.20)	Jakobsson et al. [15]
		RR 1.61 (95% CI 1.35–1.92)	
			Connor et al. [16]
	Short cervix	RR inversely related to cervical length.	Iams et al. [17]
Assisted reproductive technology	In-vitro fertilization	OR 2.0 (95% CI 1.7–2.2)	Jackson et al. [18]
Infection	Periodontal disease	OR 2.83 (95% CI 1.95–4.10)	Vergnes et al. [19]
		OR 4.45 (95% CI 2.16–9.18)	
			Jeffcoat et al. [20]
	Asymptomatic bacteriuria	OR 2.08 (95% CI 1.45–3.03)	Klein et al. [21]
	Bacterial vaginosis before 16 wk	OR 7.55 (95% CI 1.8–31.7)	Klein et al. [21]
	Gonorrhea	OR 5.31 (95% CI 1.57–17.9)	Klein et al. [21]
	Chlamydia (at 24 wk)	OR 2.2 (95% CI 1.03–4.78)	Klein et al. [21]
	Trichomonas vaginalis	OR 1.3 (95% CI 1.1–1.4)	Klein et al. [21]
Behavioral factors	Smoking (>10 cigarettes/day)	OR 1.7 (95% CI 1.4–2.0)	Kyrklund-Blomberg et al. [22]
	Underweight	RR 1.32 (95% CI 1.10–1.57)	Han et al. [23]
	Maternal stress	OR 1.16 (95% CI 1.05–1.29)	Copper et al. [24]

[27]. Multiple studies have also demonstrated the predictive value of cervical length screening, including a systematic review by Crane and Hutchens in 2008 [28]. However, the utility of transvaginal ultrasound is limited in that it carries a sensitivity of approximately 70% with a 20% false-positive rate [27]. The optimal timing and identification of appropriate candidates for cervical length screening also remains a source of controversy. A Cochrane review from 2013 demonstrated insufficient evidence to recommend routine screening of asymptomatic or symptomatic pregnant women with transvaginal sonography, identifying a non-significant association between knowledge of cervical length result and a lower incidence of preterm birth [29]. On the other hand, limiting screening to women with historical risk factors for preterm birth would lead to approximately 40% of women with a short cervix being undiagnosed [30]. For this reason, economic analyses regarding universal screening have been published with results demonstrating that such an approach may be reasonable and cost-effective [31, 32]. As will be discussed later in this chapter, vaginal progesterone has been shown to be an effective intervention to decrease the risk of spontaneous preterm birth in women with a short cervix; this may add further justification to the concept of universal screening, as this intervention has been included in decision analysis studies [31, 32].

Fetal fibronectin (FFN)

The fetal fibronectin test is a commonly used diagnostic tool that detects the presence of the glycoprotein in vaginal and cervical secretions. This test has been incorporated into clinical practice as a stratification tool to identify those women who are at high risk of having a preterm birth after presenting with symptoms of preterm labor. A systematic review of five randomized controlled trials involving knowledge of FFN results versus no such knowledge in 474 pregnant women did not find enough evidence to support or refute the use of the fetal fibronectin test in the management of women with symptoms of preterm labor [33]. The review did find an association between the knowledge of FFN results and a lower incidence of preterm birth before 37 weeks. Another recent systematic review and meta-analysis by Berghella et al. demonstrated that fetal fibronectin testing in singleton gestations with threatened preterm labor is not associated with the prevention of spontaneous preterm birth or an improvement in perinatal outcome, but is associated with higher costs [34]. Based on the results of these reviews, there is currently insufficient evidence to recommend the routine use of fetal fibronectin as a secondary screening tool.

3. What is the role of progesterone in the prevention of spontaneous preterm birth?

Progesterone is a steroid hormone that is essential for early pregnancy maintenance and appears to have a role in maintaining uterine quiescence in the latter half of pregnancy. Progesterone also appears to possess anti-inflammatory properties that may protect against a precipitating elaboration of cytokines and matrix metalloproteinases that lead to preterm birth [35]. Two landmark studies published in 2003 by Meis et al. and da Fonseca et al. initially illustrated the utility of progesterone in the prevention of preterm birth. Meis et al. demonstrated the role of 17 alpha-hydroxyprogesterone caproate in the prevention of recurrent preterm birth in the Maternal Fetal Medicine Units (MFMU) network trial [36]. In this study, 459 women with a history of a spontaneous singleton preterm delivery at less than 37 weeks' gestation were randomly assigned to receive weekly intramuscular injections of hydroxyprogesterone caproate (250 mg) or placebo beginning at 16–20 weeks' gestation and continuing until either 36 weeks' gestation or until delivery if earlier. Women treated with progesterone had a reduced risk of delivery compared to women treated with placebo at all gestational ages studied: less than 37 weeks (RR 0.66, 95% CI 0.54–0.81), less than 35 weeks (RR 0.67, 95% CI 0.48–0.93), and less than 32 weeks (RR 0.58, 95% CI 0.37–0.91). Infants born to women who were treated with progesterone also experienced significant reductions in the rates of birth weight less than 2500 g, necrotizing enterocolitis, the need for supplemental oxygen, and intraventricular hemorrhage compared to infants born to women treated with placebo [36].

In the Brazilian trial by da Fonseca et al., 142 women at high risk for preterm delivery (based on at least one prior spontaneous preterm birth, prophylactic cervical cerclage, or uterine malformation) were randomized to receive daily progesterone vaginal suppositories (100 mg) or placebo from 24 through 34 weeks' gestation [37]. Women in the treatment group had a decreased risk of delivery at less than 37 weeks (14% vs. 29%) and less than 34 weeks (3% vs. 19%) when compared to women in the placebo group [37]. A subsequent multi-center, double-blinded, randomized controlled trial by Hassan et al. also demonstrated evidence to support the use of vaginal progesterone for the prevention of preterm birth in women with a sonographic short cervix [38].

A Cochrane meta-analysis from 2013 included 36 randomized controlled trials (8523 women and 12 515 infants) involving prenatal progesterone for the prevention of preterm birth. In women with a history of a prior preterm birth, progesterone administration was associated with a significant reduction in overall perinatal mortality (RR 0.5, 95% CI 0.33–0.75), preterm birth less than 34 weeks (RR 0.31, 95% CI 0.14–0.69), preterm birth less than 37 weeks (RR 0.55, 95% CI 0.42–0.74), infant birth weight less than 2500 g (RR 0.58, 95% CI 0.42–0.79), the use of assisted ventilation (RR 0.40, 95% CI 0.18–0.90), necrotizing enterocolitis (RR 0.30, 95% CI 0.10–0.89), neonatal death (RR 0.45, 95% CI 0.27–0.76), and admission to neonatal intensive care unit (NICU) (RR 0.24, 95% CI 0.14–0.40). Subgroup analyses did not identify a differential effect on the majority of outcomes examined when considering the route of administration (intramuscular vs. vaginal vs. oral) [39].

The above results contrast to those of the OPPTIMUM trial, which was published after the 2013 Cochrane meta-analysis. The OPPTIMUM trial was a double-blind, randomized, placebo-controlled trial of vaginal progesterone 200 mg taken daily beginning at 22–24 weeks gestation, and ending at 34 weeks gestation. The trial consisted of women at high risk of preterm birth due to a history of previous spontaneous birth at ≤34 weeks gestation, cervical length ≤ 25 mm, or a positive fetal fibronectin test combined with other clinical risk factors for preterm birth (any one of a history of preterm birth, second trimester loss, preterm premature fetal membrane rupture, or a history of a cervical procedure). Vaginal progesterone administration did not result in a significantly decreased incidence of the primary obstetric outcome (preterm birth before 34 weeks or fetal death), the primary neonatal outcome (a composite of neonatal death, brain injury, and bronchopulmonary dysplasia), or the primary childhood outcome (standardized cognitive score at two years of age) in comparison to placebo. However, there did appear to be a reduction in neonatal brain injury in the treatment group. Subgroup analysis indicated a possible treatment effect in women who had a history of a prior spontaneous preterm birth, but only for the composite neonatal outcome [40]. Although these results contrast the prior findings in the literature, it is important to note that the compliance rate in this study was 69%, far less than the 88.5% reported compliance rate in the study by Hassan et al. [38, 40]. Regardless, the OPPTIMUM study does raise new questions regarding the effectiveness of progesterone as an intervention for the prevention of preterm birth.

4. How should a patient who is at a high risk of having a spontaneous preterm birth be managed in the prenatal period?

Antenatal management of a woman with a history of a prior preterm birth is dependent on a number of factors involving both her prior pregnancy outcomes and her clinical status at the time of her assessment. A detailed history should be obtained, with attention paid to the circumstances and events surrounding the prior preterm delivery (i.e. bleeding, infection, contractions, ruptured membranes) any interventions employed, and the gestational age at delivery.

Cervical length surveillance, as discussed above, has an important role in screening for the presence of a short cervix in high-risk women; however the optimum timing and frequency of transvaginal sonography is not well established. Two randomized controlled trials have demonstrated that a measurement of cervical length at 18–24 weeks, followed by vaginal progesterone treatment of women in whom short cervix is identified, results in a 40% decrease in the incidence of preterm birth, and a significant reduction in composite neonatal morbidity and mortality [38, 41]. Although a systematic review demonstrated that changes in cervical length over two or more examinations were not more predictive of preterm birth than a single cervical length measurement at 18–24 weeks, several studies have demonstrated that in women with a short cervix, a change in cervical length on subsequent ultrasound examinations has been shown to impact the risk of preterm birth [42–44].

In a multi-center, randomized controlled trial involving 1014 women with a history of a prior preterm birth, 302 were randomized to either undergo a cerclage or not undergo a cerclage after transvaginal ultrasound screening identified a cervical length less than 25 mm [45]. There was no significant difference in the primary study outcome of preterm birth at less than 35 weeks' gestation. However, cerclage placement was associated with significant reductions in deliveries prior to 24 weeks' gestation (RR 0.44, 95% CI 0.21–0.92), deliveries prior to 37 weeks' gestation (RR 0.75, 95% CI 0.60–0.93), and in perinatal death (RR 0.54, 95% CI 0.29–0.99). In a secondary analysis of this study, cerclage placement for a cervical length of less than 15 mm was associated with a significant decrease in preterm birth at less than 35 weeks' gestation (RR 0.23, 95% CI 0.08–0.66) [45].

Based on the pooled results of five clinical trials, in a singleton pregnancy with prior spontaneous preterm birth at less than 34 weeks' gestation and cervical length less than 25 mm before 24 weeks' gestation, cerclage was associated with a 30% reduction in the risk of preterm birth at less than 35 weeks' gestation (RR 0.7, 95% CI 0.55–0.89) and a 36% reduction in composite perinatal mortality and morbidity (RR 0.64, 95% CI 0.45–0.91) [45–48].

There is currently insufficient evidence to support the notion of an additive effect of progesterone and cerclage together in reducing the risk of preterm birth. There is also currently no evidence to support the simultaneous use of multiple formulations of progesterone, or the changing of progesterone formulations (i.e. the addition of or changing to vaginal progesterone in a woman receiving intramuscular progesterone due to a history of a prior preterm birth, and in whom a short cervix is diagnosed).

Table 37.2 contains evidence-based management recommendations that are listed according to a patient's clinical history and ultrasound findings.

5. What are the available interventions to reduce neonatal morbidity and mortality from a preterm birth?

Antenatal corticosteroids

In the seminal article by Liggins and Howie in 1972, the world was first introduced to the concept of maternal betamethasone administration for the acceleration of functional fetal lung maturation [56]. In their randomized controlled trial involving 213 mothers in spontaneous preterm labor, they were able to demonstrate significant reductions in the rate and severity of respiratory distress

Table 37.2 Evidence-based management recommendations listed according to patient's clinical history and ultrasound findings

Clinical scenario	Suggested management	Evidence
Singleton gestation, prior spontaneous preterm birth, normal cervical length.	17-OH-progesterone caproate 250 mg intramuscular injection weekly beginning between 16 and 20 wk gestation and continued through 36 wk gestation or delivery. Progesterone vaginal suppositories may be a reasonable alternative.	Meis et al. [36] Dodd et al. [39]
Singleton gestation, prior spontaneous preterm birth, cervical length < 25 mm	17-OH-progesterone caproate 250 mg intramuscular injection weekly beginning between 16 and 20 wk gestation and continued through 36 wk gestation or delivery. An ultrasound-indicated cerclage may be considered prior to 24 wk (in the absence of signs of infection).	Iams et al. [43] Owen et al. [45]
Singleton gestation, no prior spontaneous preterm birth, cervical length < =20 mm	Progesterone vaginal suppository 90–200 mg each night from time of diagnosis through 36 wk gestation.	da Fonseca et al. [37] Hassan et al. [38] Dodd et al. [39] Fonseca et al. [41]
Multiple gestation, no prior spontaneous preterm birth, normal cervical length	No role for progesterone or cerclage.	Combs et al. [50] Norman et al. [51] Rouse et al. [52]
Twin gestation, prior spontaneous preterm birth	17-OH-progesterone caproate 250 mg intramuscular injection weekly beginning between 16 and 20 wk gestation and continued through 36 wk gestation or delivery. Progesterone vaginal suppositories may be a reasonable alternative.	Meis et al. [36]
Twin gestation, no prior spontaneous preterm birth, cervical length ≤ 20 mm	Vaginal progesterone may be an effective therapy. Cerclage is not recommended.	No current data available. A clinical trial evaluating the use of vaginal progesterone and pessary (PROSPECT) is currently underway. More information is available at: https://clinicaltrials.gov/ct2/show/NCT02518594
Preterm premature rupture of membranes	No role for progesterone or cerclage.	Briery et al. [53]
Positive fetal fibronectin	No role for progesterone or cerclage based on this test alone.	Berghella et al. [33]
Threatened preterm labor, undelivered	No role for progesterone or cerclage.	Rozenberg et al. [54]
Singleton pregnancy, prior midtrimester loss complicated by asymptomatic cervical dilatation	17-OH-progesterone caproate 250 mg intramuscular injection weekly beginning between 16 and 20 wk gestation and continued through 36 wk gestation or delivery. A history-indicated transcervical cerclage may be considered at 12 to 14 wk.	Iams et al. [49]
Singleton pregnancy, prior spontaneous preterm birth, asymptomatic cervical dilatation.	17-OH-progesterone caproate 250 mg intramuscular injection weekly beginning between 16 and 20 wk gestation and continued through 36 wk gestation or delivery. A physical examination-indicated transcervical cerclage may be considered prior to 24 wk (in the absence of signs of infection).	Meis et al. [36] Owen et al. [45] Iams et al. [49] Ehsanipoor et al. [55]

syndrome and the incidence of early neonatal mortality in mothers treated with betamethasone over controls. Since this time, a multitude of randomized trials examining the risks and benefits of antenatal corticosteroids have been performed, providing validation to the original study by Liggins and Howie. A Cochrane review from 2006 included 21 of these trials and demonstrated that treatment with antenatal corticosteroids is associated with an overall reduction in neonatal death (RR 0.69, 95% CI 0.58–0.81), respiratory distress syndrome (RR 0.66, 95% CI 0.59–0.73), interventricular hemorrhage (RR 0.54, 95% CI 0.43–0.69, necrotizing enterocolitis (RR 0.46, 95% CI 0.29–0.74), intensive care unit admissions (RR 0.80, 95% CI 0.65–0.99), and systemic infections in the first 48 hours of life (RR 0.56, 95% CI 0.38–0.85) [57].

The use of antenatal corticosteroids prior to 34 weeks' gestation has been the standard of care for women at high risk for delivery within seven days. In 2016, however, the results of the Antenatal Late Preterm Steroids (ALPS) trial, conducted by the Eunice Kennedy Shriver National Institute of Child Health and Human Development (NICHD), MFMU Network, brought new evidence to the benefit of this treatment in the late preterm period [58]. In this multi-center, double-blinded, placebo-controlled, randomized trial involving 2831 women with singleton gestations between 34 and 36 weeks five days' gestation, treatment with antenatal corticosteroids was associated with a significant decrease in the need for neonatal respiratory support within the first 72 hours of life (RR 0.80, 95% CI 0.66–0.97) compared to controls. There were also significant decreases the rates of severe respiratory morbidity (a composite outcome of continuous positive airway pressure or high-flow nasal cannula for at least 12 continuous hours, supplemental oxygen with a fraction of inspired oxygen of at least 0.30 for at least 24 continuous hours, extracorporeal membrane oxygenation or mechanical ventilation, stillbirth, or neonatal death within 72 hours after delivery), bronchopulmonary dysplasia, transient tachypnea of the newborn, the need for resuscitation at birth, and the need for postnatal surfactant [58, 59]. Importantly, the ALPS protocol did not attempt to change the standard clinical management of late preterm pregnancies apart from the administration of betamethasone; there were no attempts to delay delivery with tocolysis for preterm labor or expectant management for pre-eclampsia with severe features or premature rupture of membranes. Although this new evidence supports the administration of betamethasone for women at high risk of any preterm delivery (prior to 37 weeks), beyond 34 weeks there is currently no evidence to recommend efforts to delay delivery for the purpose of completing this treatment [59].

Repeat or rescue dosing of antenatal corticosteroids remains an area of controversy. The potential benefit of multiple courses of betamethasone was evaluated in the Australasian Collaborative Trial of Repeat Doses of Steroids (ACTORDS) in 2006 [60]. In this randomized controlled trial, 982 women were assigned to receive weekly betamethasone or placebo following an initial course of steroids prior to 32 weeks' gestation. Treatment was associated with a decreased incidence of respiratory distress syndrome (RR 0.82, 95% CI 0.71–0.95) and severe lung disease (RR 0.60, CI 0.46–0.79), in addition to a decreased need for oxygen therapy and a shorter duration of mechanical ventilation [60]. Repeat steroid dosing was also evaluated in a Cochrane systematic review in 2015. In 10 trials involving 4733 women and 5700 babies, repeat steroid administration in women at risk of preterm birth seven or more days after an initial course of prenatal steroids demonstrated reduced risks of respiratory distress syndrome (RR 0.83, 95% CI 0.75–0.91), and composite serious infant outcome (perinatal death, bronchopulmonary dysplasia, serious intraventricular hemorrhage, necrotizing enterocolitis, sepsis, periventricular leukomalacia, or retinopathy of prematurity) (RR 0.84, 95% CI 0.75–0.94), without any increase in maternal infectious morbidity, the likelihood of cesarean, or outcomes at early childhood follow-up [61]. However, the potential benefits of repeat steroid administration must be weighed against the risks. In a trial by the NICHD MFMU Network in 2006, fetuses exposed to multiple courses of antenatal steroids were at a significantly increased risk of growth restriction [62]. A dose–response relationship was also identified between the number of steroid courses and a decrease in fetal growth in a secondary analysis of the Multiple Courses of Antenatal Corticosteroids for Preterm Birth study [63]. The decision to repeat steroid administration in a woman who remains at high risk of preterm birth should involve careful consideration of the potential benefits and harms. Based on the above data, repeat steroids should be considered in those individuals at risk for preterm delivery prior to 34 weeks, and for whom at least seven days have elapsed since the initial course.

Magnesium sulfate

The protective benefit against cerebral palsy for preterm neonates exposed to magnesium sulfate in-utero has been established in several randomized controlled trials and meta-analyses. The NICHD-MFMU and the National Institute for Neurological Disorders and Stroke performed the Beneficial Effects of Antenatal Magnesium Sulfate (BEAM) trial, a multicenter placebo-controlled trial of magnesium sulfate, which was published in 2008 [64]. This study randomized 2241 women at risk for imminent delivery between 24 and 31 weeks' gestation to receive either magnesium sulfate (6 g loading dose followed by a $2\,g\,h^{-1}$ infusion) or placebo. The rate of moderate to severe cerebral palsy was significantly lower in the magnesium group (RR 0.55, 95% CI 0.32–0.95) compared to the placebo group; however the significant reduction was only evident in pregnancies randomized at less than 28 weeks' gestation [64].

A 2009 Cochrane review of five trials evaluating the protective benefit of antenatal magnesium sulfate therapy demonstrated significant reductions in the risk of any cerebral palsy (RR 0.68, 95% CI 0.54–0.87), moderate/severe cerebral palsy (RR 0.64; 95% CI 0.44–0.92), and gross motor dysfunction (RR 0.61, 95% CI 0.44–0.85) [65]. The number needed to treat to prevent one child from developing cerebral palsy was 63. There were no significant differences in maternal outcomes; however, many women in the magnesium group experienced side effects that led to the treatment being discontinued [65].

Two subsequent meta-analyses have since been published demonstrating similar findings, with no additional differences detected in the incidence of infant blindness, deafness, or developmental delay, Apgar scores, intraventricular hemorrhage, periventricular leukomalacia, neonatal seizures, or the need for ongoing respiratory support [66, 67]. One of these meta-analyses stratified trials into two groups according to the gestational age at randomization: less than 32–34 weeks, or less than 30 weeks. There were significant reductions in the risk of cerebral palsy in both groups (RR 0.7 and 0.69, respectively). The numbers needed to treat to prevent one child from developing cerebral palsy were 56 in the less than 32–34 weeks group, and 46 in the less than 30 weeks group [67].

Currently, the optimal gestational age at administration, dosing regimen, and timing and duration of therapy of magnesium sulfate in a woman at risk of an imminent preterm delivery remain unclear and require further investigation. Several guidelines exist based on the limited data available, with several institution-specific variations. Regardless, magnesium sulfate appears to be most effective in decreasing the risk of cerebral palsy and severe motor dysfunction in women prior to 32–34 weeks' gestation who are expected to have a preterm delivery within 24 hours, and therapy should be considered in candidates who fit this profile.

6. What is the role of tocolysis in patients presenting with preterm labor?

The interruption of uterine contractions has been the historical focus of preterm labor prevention, as preterm contractions are the most common clinical sign observed prior to a preterm birth. Although short-term pregnancy prolongation via tocolysis may have a role in the management of preterm labor (i.e. allowing for the administration of antenatal corticosteroids and magnesium sulfate), there is currently no evidence to suggest that tocolysis itself, or the resultant delay in delivery, has any significant benefit on neonatal outcomes. The current literature supports tocolysis with beta-adrenergic receptor agonists, calcium channel blockers, or non-steroidal anti-inflammatory drugs (NSAID's) for short-term pregnancy prolongation (up to 48 hours) in order to facilitate antenatal corticosteroid administration [68, 70].

Magnesium sulfate is ineffective in delaying or preventing preterm birth, as demonstrated in a systematic review of 37 trials consisting of 3571 women [71]. In its role as a tocolytic agent, magnesium sulfate was shown to have no significant advantages, and its use for this purpose may be associated with an increased risk of total fetal, neonatal, or infant mortality. Despite this, however, beneficial effects of magnesium were demonstrated when used in appropriate subsets of women, such as those who develop pre-eclampsia, and for infant neuroprotection when delivery occurs prior to 32–34 weeks' gestation. If magnesium sulfate is used in the setting of preterm labor for fetal neuroprotection, an alternative tocolytic agent may be considered for short-term therapy [71]. However, the simultaneous administration of magnesium sulfate and calcium channel blockers requires discretion due to potential serious maternal complications, such as the suppression of heart rate and contractility, decreased left ventricular systolic pressure, and neuromuscular blockade. Indomethacin, an NSAID, has been evaluated in several retrospective studies, and may be used in conjunction with magnesium sulfate; however, therapy should be restricted to women prior to 32 weeks' gestation due to the risks of in utero constriction of the ductus arteriosus.

There is currently no evidence to support the use of maintenance tocolysis (i.e. continued tocolysis beyond the initial acute period of threatened preterm labor) for the prevention of preterm birth and the improvement of neonatal outcomes. A Cochrane review comparing magnesium sulfate maintenance tocolysis to beta-adrenergic receptor agonists or placebo demonstrated no differences in adverse neonatal outcomes [71]. Similarly, a Cochrane review evaluating the use of terbutaline infusion pumps and oral beta-mimetics for maintenance tocolysis also demonstrated no significant benefit in comparison to saline placebo, and these interventions are not recommended for this purpose [72].

7. Should prophylactic antibiotics be used in the treatment preterm labor for women with intact membranes?

A systematic review from 2013 included 14 studies involving 7837 women in preterm labor at a mean gestational age of 30–32 weeks and compared routine administration of antibiotics before membrane rupture with placebo for women without signs of infection [73]. Although antibiotics reduced the number of women who developed infections, there was no difference in the outcomes of birth prior to 36 or 37 weeks, perinatal mortality, or NICU admission. Antibiotic therapy was also associated with an increase in neonatal deaths, functional impairment, and cerebral palsy at seven years of age. Based on the results of this review, routine antibiotic administration in cases of threatened preterm labor with intact membranes and no clear sign of infection is not recommended [73]. However, intrapartum antibiotic prophylaxis for the prevention of neonatal Group B Streptococcal infections is recommended for women in preterm labor who do not have a documented culture result.

8. What are the roles of non-pharmacologic strategies in the management of preterm labor?

Bed rest

The prescription of bed rest has, historically, been one of the first steps in management of threatened preterm labor and was supported by observational studies that identified an association between intense physical activity and preterm birth. One trial that randomized 1266 women to either bed rest, placebo, or no intervention, found no significant difference between groups with respect to the rate of spontaneous birth prior to 37 weeks [74]. However, due to lack of reporting, the study was at an unclear risk of bias for most domains [74, 75]. There is currently no evidence to definitively support or refute the use of bed rest as a preventive strategy for preterm labor. Given the potential adverse effects of bed rest including venous thromboembolism, deconditioning, and increased healthcare associated costs, women at risk of preterm birth should be counseled regarding both the potential benefits and the potential harms.

Hydration

Intravenous fluid hydration is often used in patients who present with symptoms of preterm labor in the hope that the extra fluid may have a tocolytic effect. A Cochrane review including two studies with 228 women found no evidence of a benefit in the routine use of hydration to prevent preterm labor, even in the period of evaluation soon after admission, except in women who were dehydrated [76–78]. Due to the paucity of data in this area, there is insufficient evidence to currently support the routine use of hydration as a specific treatment for women who present with preterm labor.

Relaxation therapy

The impact of a woman's psychological stress on pregnancy is unclear. Relaxation techniques such as meditation, prenatal massage, yoga, reflexology, breathing exercises, visualization, music therapy, and aromatherapy as treatment methods for preterm labor were evaluated in a Cochrane review that included 11 small randomized controlled trials [79]. The review included a total of 833 women; however, the findings were unable to be pooled into any meta-analyses as each study used different forms of relaxation in different comparisons with insufficient information. Although one study demonstrated that relaxation therapy was associated with reduced maternal stress, increased birthweight, and fewer cesarean deliveries compared with routine prenatal care for women not in preterm labor, there was no evidence of either benefit or harm for women in preterm labor [79]. Thus, there is no current evidence to either support or discourage the use of relaxation techniques in the management of preterm labor.

Conclusions and recommendations

- Progesterone supplementation should be offered to women with a singleton gestation and a history of a prior spontaneous preterm singleton birth, with administration beginning at 16–24 weeks' gestation and continuing until 36 weeks' gestation.
- Cervical length surveillance via transvaginal ultrasounds should be considered in women at high risk of preterm birth. Universal screening for all pregnant women may be a reasonable approach.
- Vaginal progesterone should be offered to women with a singleton gestation and no prior history of spontaneous preterm birth if a cervical length less than or equal to 20 mm is identified prior to 24 weeks' gestation.
- Antenatal corticosteroids should be administered for women who are between 24 and 37 weeks' gestation and are at risk of having a preterm delivery within seven days.
- Repeat corticosteroids may be considered in women who remain at high risk of a preterm delivery prior to 34 weeks, and for whom at least seven days have elapsed since the initial course.
- Magnesium sulfate reduces the risk of cerebral palsy in preterm neonates when delivery is anticipated prior to 32 weeks' gestation.
- Tocolysis with beta-adrenergic agents, calcium channel blockers, or NSAIDs should be restricted to short-term pregnancy prolongation (up to 48 hours) in order to facilitate the administration of antenatal corticosteroids.
- Antibiotics should not be used for the purpose of pregnancy prolongation in women with preterm labor and intact membranes.
- Bed rest, hydration, and relaxation techniques have not been shown to be effective for the prevention of preterm birth or the management of preterm labor, and there is insufficient evidence to recommend the routine use of these techniques.

References

1 Romero, R., Dey, S., and Fisher, S. (2014). Preterm labor: one syndrome, many causes. *Science* **345** (**6198**): 760–765.

2 MacDorman, M., Callaghan, W., Mathews, T. et al. (2006. Available at: http://www.cdc.gov/nchs/data/hestat/infantmort99-04/infantmort99-04.htm). *Trends in Preterm-Related Infant Mortality by Race and Ethnicity: United States, 1999–2004*. National Center for Health Statistics. accessed 1 May 2016.

3 Usher, R., Allen, A., and McLean, F. (1971). Risk of respiratory distress syndrome related to gestational age, route of delivery, and maternal diabetes. *Am. J. Obstet. Gynecol.* **111** (**6**): 826–832.

4 Fuchs, I., Henrich, W., Osthues, K. et al. (2004). Sonographic cervical length in singleton pregnancies with intact membranes presenting with threatened preterm labor. *Ultrasound Obstet. Gynecol.* **24**: 554–557.

5 Ness, A., Visintin, J., Ricci, E. et al. (2007). Does knowledge of cervical length and fetal fibronectin affect management of women with threatened preterm labor? A randomized trial. *Am. J. Obstet. Gynecol.* **197** (**4**): 426.e1–426.e7.

6 Goldenberg, R., Iams, J., Mercer, B. et al. (1998). The preterm prediction study: the value of new vs standard risk factors in predicting early and all spontaneous preterm births. *Am. J. Public. Health* **88**: 233–238.

7 Saccone, G., Perriera, L., and Berghella, V. (2016). Prior uterine evacuation of pregnancy as independent risk factor for preterm birth: a systematic review and metaanalysis. *Am. J. Obstet. Gynecol.* **214** (**5**): 572–591.

8 Rodrigues, T. and Barros, H. (2008). Short interpregnancy interval and risk of spontaneous preterm delivery. *Eur. J. Obstet. Gynecol. Reprod. Biol.* **136** (**2**): 184–188.

9 Srinivasjois, R., Shah, S., and Shah, P. (2012). Biracial couples and adverse birth outcomes: a systematic review and meta-analyses. *Acta Obstet. Gynecol. Scand.* **91** (**10**): 1134.

10 Cleary-Goldman, J., Malone, F., Vidaver, J. et al. (2005). Impact of maternal age on obstetric outcome. *Obstet. Gynecol.* **105** (**5**): 983–990.

11 Hua, M., Odibo, A., Longman, R. et al. (2011). Congenital uterine anomalies and adverse pregnancy outcomes. *Am. J. Obstet. Gynecol.* **205**: 558.e1–558.e5.

12 Klatsky, P., Tran, N., Caughey, A. et al. (2008). Fibroids and reproductive outcomes: a systematic literature review from conception to delivery. *Am. J. Obstet. Gynecol.* **198** (**4**): 357.

13 Klaritsch, P., Reich, O., Giuliani, A. et al. (2006). Delivery outcome after cold-knife coniation of the cervix. *Gynecol. Oncol.* **103** (**2**): 604–607.

14 Jakobsson, J., Gissler, M., Sainio, S. et al. (2007). Preterm delivery after surgical treatment for cervical intraepithelial Neoplasia. *Obstet. Gynecol.* **109** (**2**): 309–313.

15 Jakobsson, J., Gissler, M., Paavonen, J. et al. (2009). Loop electrosurgical excision procedure and the risk for preterm birth. *Obstet. Gynecol.* **114** (**3**): 504–510.

16 Connor, S., Frey, H., Cahill, A. et al. (2014). Loop electrosurgical excision procedure and risk of preterm birth: a systematic review and meta-analysis. *Obstet. Gynecol.* **123** (**4**): 752–761.

17 Iams, J., Goldenberg, R., Meis, P. et al. (1996). The length of the cervix and the risk of spontaneous premature delivery. National Institute of Child Health and Human Development maternal fetal medicine unit network. *N. Engl. J. Med.* **334** (**9**): 567–572.

18 Jackson, R., Gibson, K., Wu, Y. et al. (2004). Perinatal outcomes in singletons following in-vitro fertilization: a meta-analysis. *Obstet. Gynecol.* **103** (**3**): 551.

19 Vergnes, J. and Sixou, M. (2007). Preterm low birth weight and maternal periodontal status: a meta-analysis. *Am. J. Obstet. Gynecol.* **196** (**2**): 135.e1.

20 Jeffcoat, M., Geurs, N., Reddy, M. et al. (2001). Periodontal infection and preterm birth: results of a prospective study. *J. Am. Dent. Assoc.* **132** (**7**): 875–880.

21 Klein, L. and Gibbs, R. (2004). Use of microbial cultures and antibiotics in the prevention of infection-associated preterm birth. *Am. J. Obstet. Gynecol.* **190**: 1493.

22 Kyrklund-Blomberg, N. and Cnattingius, S. (1998). Preterm birth and maternal smoking: risks related to gestational age and onset of delivery. *Am. J. Obstet. Gynecol.* **179** (**4**): 1051.

23 Han, Z., Mulla, S., Beyene, J. et al. (2011). Maternal underweight and the risk of preterm birth and low birth weight: a systematic review and meta-analysis. *Int. J. Epidemiol.* **40** (**1**): 65–101.

24 Copper, R., Goldenberg, R., Das, A. et al. (1996). The preterm prediction study: maternal stress is associated with spontaneous preterm birth at less than thirty-five weeks gestation. *Am. J. Obstet. Gynecol.* **175** (**5**): 1286–1292.

25 Robinson JN, Norwitz E. Risk factors for preterm labor and delivery. UpToDate 2016. Available at: http://www.uptodate .com/contents/risk-factors-for-preterm-labor-and-delivery. accessed 10 July 2018.

26 Mercer, B., Goldenberg, R., Moawad, A. et al. (1999). The preterm prediction study: effect of gestational age and cause of preterm birth on subsequent obstetric outcome. National Institute of Child Health and Human Development maternal-fetal medicine units network. *Am. J. Obstet. Gynecol.* **181** (**5 Pt 1**): 1216.

27 Owen, J., Yost, N., Berghella, V. et al. (2001). Mid-trimester endovaginal sonography in women at high risk for spontaneous preterm birth. National Institute of Child Health and Human Development, maternal-fetal medicine units network. *JAMA* **286** (**11**): 1340.

28 Crane, J. and Hutchens, D. (2008). Transvaginal sonographic measurement of cervical length to predict preterm birth in asymptomatic women at increased risk: a systematic review. *Ultrasound Obstet. Gynecol.* **31** (**5**): 579.

29 Berghella, V., Baxter, J., and Hendrix, N. (2013). Cervical assessment by ultrasound for preventing preterm delivery. *Cochrane Database Syst. Rev.* **1**: CD007235.

30 Miller, E., Tita, A., and Grobman, W. (2015). Second-trimester cervical length screening among asymptomatic women: an evaluation of risk-based strategies. *Obstet. Gynecol.* **126** (**1**): 61.

31 Cahill, A., Odibo, A., Caughey, A. et al. (2010). Universal cervical length screening and treatmet with vaginal progesterone to prevent preterm birth: a decision and economic analysis. *Am. J. Obstet. Gynecol.* **202**: 548.e1–548.e8.

32 Werner, E., Han, C., Pettker, C. et al. (2011). Universal cervical-length screening to prevent preterm birth: a cost-effectiveness analysis. *Ultrasound Obstet. Gynecol.* **38**: 32–37.

33 Berghella, V., Hayes, E., Visintine, J. et al. (2008). Fetal fibronectin testing for reducing the risk of preterm birth. *Cochrane Database Syst. Rev.* (**4**): CD006843. doi: 10.1002/14651858.

34 Berghella, V. and Saccone, G. (2016. Published online. Available at: http://www.ajog.org/article/S0002-9378%2816%2930136-3/abstract). Fetal fibronectin testing for prevention of preterm birth in singleton pregnancies with threatened preterm labor: a systematic review and meta-analysis of randomized controlled trials. *Am. J. Obstet. Gynecol.*. accessed 5 May 2016.

35 Greene, M. (2003). Progesterone and preterm delivery – Déjà vu all over again. *N. Engl. J. Med.* **348**: 2453–2455.

36 Meis, P., Klebanoff, M., Thom, E. et al. (2003). Prevention of recurrent preterm delivery by 17 alpha-hydroxyprogesterone caproate. *N. Engl. J. Med.* **348**: 2379–2385.

37 da Fonseca, E., Bittar, R., Carvalho, M. et al. (2003). Prophylactic administration of progesterone by vaginal suppository to reduce the incidence of spontaneous preterm birth in women at increased risk: a randomized placebo-controlled double-blind study. *Am. J. Obstet. Gynecol.* **188** (**2**): 419–424.

38 Hassan, S., Romero, R., Vidyadhari, D. et al. (2011). Vaginal progesterone reduces the rate of preterm birth in women with a sonographic short cervix: a multicenter, randomized, double-blind, placebo-controlled trial. *Ultrasound Obstet. Gynecol.* **38**: 18–31.

39 Dodd, J., Jones, L., Flenady, V. et al. (2013). Prenatal administration of progesterone for preventing preterm birth in women considered to be at risk of preterm birth. *Cochrane Database Syst. Rev.* (**7**): CD004947. doi: 10.1002/14651858.

40 Norman, J., Marlow, N., Messow, C. et al. (2016. Published Online February 23, 2016. Available at: http://www.thelancet.com/journals/lancet/article/PIIS0140-6736%2816%2900350-0/fulltext). Vaginal progesterone prophylaxis for preterm birth (the OPPTIMUM study): a multicentre, randomised, double-blind trial. *Lancet*. accessed 10 July 2018.

41 Fonseca, E., Celik, E., Parra, M. et al. (2007). Progesterone and the risk of preterm birth among women with a short cervix. *N. Engl. J. Med.* **357** (**5**): 462.

42 Conde-Agudelo, A. and Romero, R. (2015). Predictive accuracy of changes in transvaginal sonographic cervical length over time for preterm birth: a systematic review and metaanalysis. *Am. J. Obstet. Gynecol.* **213** (**6**): 789.

43 Iams, J., Cebrik, D., Lynch, C. et al. (2011). The rate of cervical change and the phenotype of spontaneous preterm birth. *Am. J. Obstet. Gynecol.* **205** (**2**): 130.e1.

44 Moroz, L. and Simhan, H. (2012). Rate of sonographic cervical shortening and the risk of spontaneous preterm birth. *Am. J. Obstet. Gynecol.* **206** (**3**): 234.e1.

45 Owen, J., Hankins, G., Iams, J. et al. (2009). Multicenter randomized trial of cerclage for preterm birth prevention in high-risk women withs hortened midtrimester cervical length. *Am. J. Obstet. Gynecol.* **201**: 375.e1–375.e8.

46 Berghella, V., Odibo, A., To, M. et al. (2005). Cerclage for short cervix on ultrasonography: meta-analysis of trials using individual patient-level data. *Obstet. Gynecol.* **106**: 181–189.

47 Berghella, V., Rafael, T., Szychowski, J. et al. (2011). Cerclage for short cervix on ultrasonography in women with singleton gestations and previous preterm birth: a meta-analysis. *Obstet. Gynecol.* **117**: 663–671.

48 (2012). Prediction and Prevention of Preterm Birth. ACOG Practice Bulletin No. 130. *Obstet. Gynecol.* **120** (**4**): 964–973. Reaffirmed 2014.

49 Iams, J. and Berghella, V. (2010). Care for women with prior preterm birth. *Am. J. Obstet. Gynecol.* **203** (**2**): 89–100.

50 Combs, C., Garite, T., Maurel, K. et al. (2011). 17-hydroxyprogesterone caproate for twin pregnancy: a double-blind randomized clinical trial. *Am. J. Obstet. Gynecol.* **204** (**3**): 221.e1–e8.

51 Norman, J., Mackenzie, F., Owen, P. et al. (2009). Progesterone for the preventino of preterm birth in twin pregnancy (STOPPIT): a randomised, double-blind, placebo-controlled study and meta-analysis. *Lancet* **373** (**9680**): 2034–2040.

52 Rouse, D., Caritis, S., Peaceman, A. et al. (2007). A trial of 17 alpha-hydroxyprogesterone caproate to prevent prematurity in twins. *N. Engl. J. Med.* **357**: 454–461.

53 Briery, C., Veillon, E., Klauser, C. et al. (2011). Women with preterm premature rupture of membranes do not benefit from weekly progesterone. *Am. J. Obstet. Gynecol.* **204** (**1**): 54.e1–54.e5.

54 Rozenberg, P., Chauveaud, A., Deruelle, P. et al. (2012). Prevention of preterm delivery after successful tocolysis in preterm labor by 17 alpha-hydroxyprogesterone caproate: a randomized controlled trial. *Am. J. Obstet. Gynecol.* **206** (**3**): 206.e1–206.e9.

55 Ehsanipoor, R., Seligman, N., Saccone, G. et al. (2015). Physical examination-indicated cerclage: a systematic review and meta-analysis. *Obstet. Gynecol.* **126** (**1**): 125.

56 Liggins, G. and Howie, R. (1972). A controlled trial of antepartum glucocorticoid treatment for the prevention of the respiratory distress syndrome in premature infants. *Pediatrics* **50** (**4**).

57 Roberts, D. and Dalziel, S. (2006). Antenatal corticosteroids for accelerating fetal lung maturation for women at risk of preterm birth. *Cochrane Database Syst. Rev.* (**3**): CD004454. doi: 10.1002/14651858.CD004454.pub2.

58 Gyamfi-Bannerman, C., Thom, E., Blackwell, S. et al. (2016). Antenatal betamethasone for women at risk for late preterm delivery. *N. Engl. J. Med.* **374**: 1311–1320.

59 (2016). *Implementation of the Use of Antenatal Corticosteroids in the Late Preterm Birth Period in Women at Risk for Preterm Delivery*. Society for Maternal-Fetal Medicine (SMFM) Publications Committee http://www.ajog.org/article/S0002-9378%2816%2900475-0/pdf. accessed 30 April 2016.

60 Crowther, C., Haslam, R., Hiller, J. et al. (2006). Neonatal respiratory distress syndrome after repeat exposure to antenatal corticosteroids: a randomised controlled trial. *Lancet* **367** (**9526**): 1913.

61 Crowther, C., McKinlay, C., Middelton, P. et al. (2015). Repeat doses of prenatal corticosteroids for women at risk of preterm birth for improving health outcomes. *Cochrane Database Syst. Rev.* (**7**): CD003935. doi: 10.1002/14651858.CD003935.pub4.

62 Wapner, R., Sorokin, Y., Thom, E. et al. (2006). Single versus weekly courses of antenatal corticosteroids: evaluation of safety and efficacy. *Am. J. Obstet. Gynecol.* **195** (**3**): 633.

63 Murphy, K., Willan, A., Hannah, M. et al. (2012). Effect of antenatal corticosteroids on fetal growth and gestational age at birth. *Obstet. Gynecol.* **119** (**5**): 917–923.

64 Rouse, D., Hirtz, D., Thom, E. et al. (2008). A randomized trial of magnesium sulfate for the prevention of cerebral palsy. *N. Engl. J. Med.* **359**: 895–905.

65 Doyle, L., Crowther, C., Middletone, P. et al. (2009). Magnesium sulphate for women at risk of preterm birth for neuroprotection of the fetus. *Cochrane Database Syst. Rev.* (**1**): CD004661. doi: 10.1002/14651858.

66 Doyle, L., Crowther, C., Middleton, P. et al. (2009). Antenatal magnesium sulfate and neurologic outcome in preterm infants: a systematic review. *Obstet. Gynecol.* **113** (**6**): 1327.

67 Constantine, M. and Weiner, S. (2009). Effects of antenatal exposure to magnesium sulfate on neuroprotection and mortality in preterm infants: a meta-analysis. *Obstet. Gynecol.* **114** (**2 Pt 1**): 354–364.

68 Anotayanonth, S., Subhedar, N., Neilson, J. et al. (2004). Betamimetics for inhibiting preterm labour. *Cochrane Database Syst. Rev.* (**4**): CD004352. doi: 10.1002/14651858.CD004352.pub2.

69 King, J., Flenady, V., Papatsonis, D. et al. (2003). Calcium channel blockers for inhibiting preterm labour. *Cochrane Database Syst. Rev.* (**1**): CD002255. doi: 10.1002/14651858.CD002255.

70 King, J., Flenady, V., Cole, S. et al. (2005). Cyclo-oxygenase (COX) inhibitors for treating preterm labour. *Cochrane Database Syst. Rev.* (**2**): CD001992. doi: 10.1002/14651858.CD001992.pub2.

71 Crowther, C., Brown, J., McKinlay, C. et al. (2014). Magnesium sulphate for preventing preterm birth in threatened preterm labour. *Cochrane Database Syst. Rev.* (**8**): CD001060. doi: 10.1002/14651858.CD001060.

72 Chawanpaiboon, S., Laopaiboon, M., Lumbiganon, P. et al. (2014). Terbutaline pump maintenance therapy after threatened preterm labour for reducing adverse neonatal outcomes. *Cochrane Database Syst. Rev.* (**3**): CD010800. doi: 10.1002/14651858.CD010800.pub2.

73 Flenady, V., Hawley, G., and Stock, O. (2013). Prophylactic antibiotics for inhibiting preterm labour with intact membranes. *Cochrane Database Syst. Rev.* (**12**): CD000246. doi: 10.1002/14651858.CD000246.pub2.

74 Hobel, C., Ross, M., Bemis, R. et al. (1994). The West Los Angeles preterm birth prevention project: I. Program impact on high-risk women. *Am. J. Obstet. Gynecol.* **170**: 54–62.

75 Sosa, C., Althabe, F., Belizan, J. et al. (2007). Bed rest in singleton pregnancies for preventing preterm birth. *Cochrane Database Syst. Rev.* (**4**): CD003581. doi: 10.1002/14651858.CD003581.pub2.

76 Guinn, D., Goepfert, A., Owen, J. et al. (1997). Management options in women with preterm uterine contractions: a randomized clinical trial. *Am. J. Obstet. Gynecol.* **177**: 814–818.

77 Helfgott, A., Willis, D., Abuhamad, A. et al. (1991). Effect of hydration and/or sedation in threatened preterm labor. *Am. J. Obstet. Gynecol.* **164**: 310.

78 Stan, C., Boulvain, M., Pfister, R. et al. (2013). Hydration for treatment of preterm labour. *Cochrane Database Syst. Rev.* (**11**): CD003096. doi: 10.1002/14651858.CD003096.

79 Khianman, B., Pattanittum, P., Thinkhamrop, J. et al. (2012). Relaxation therapy for preventing and treating preterm labour. *Cochrane Database Syst. Rev.* (**8**): CD007426. doi: 10.1002/14651858.CD007426.pub2.

38

CHAPTER 38

Preterm premature rupture of membranes (PPROM)

George Graham and Stephanie Bakaysa

Department of Maternal-Fetal Medicine, Tufts Medical Center, Boston, MA, USA

CLINICAL VIGNETTE

A 29-year-old G1P0 at 29 3/7 weeks of gestation presented to Labor and Delivery after a gush of fluid at home. She denied contractions or vaginal bleeding. She felt normal fetal movement. Her past medical and surgical histories were uncomplicated, and this has been an uncomplicated pregnancy to date.

On examination, the patient appeared in no distress. Her temperature was 98.6°F, blood pressure 110/70 mmHg, heart rate 95 beats per minute, and respiratory rate 18 breaths per minute. Her abdomen was gravid, soft, and non-tender. On sterile speculum exam (SSE) there was clear fluid pooling in the posterior cul-de-sac. The cervix appeared closed with no bleeding. The fetal heart rate was 145 beats per minute with moderate variability and accelerations that increased by 10 beats per minute for 10 seconds without decelerations. There were no contractions on the tocodynamometer.

Background

Premature birth, defined as delivery <37 0/7 weeks of gestation, is a leading cause of perinatal morbidity and mortality in the United States, and creates a substantial economic burden [1, 2]. In 2013, 11% (448 875) of all births in the United States occurred prior to 37 0/7 weeks of gestation, and 3.3% (133 000) occurred prior to 34 0/7 weeks of gestation [3]. Preterm premature rupture of membranes (PPROMs) refers to rupture of membranes (ROMs) prior to 37 0/7 weeks of gestation and prior to the onset of labor. PPROM has been implicated in 30–40% of all preterm births, and complicates 2–4% of all singleton pregnancies and 7–20% of all twin pregnancies [4–8]. The diagnosis of PPROM can lead to additional medical care and a significant cost. This chapter will review the etiologies, complications, diagnosis, and management of PPROM.

Etiology of preterm premature rupture of membranes

The fetal membranes include the amnion, which lines the amniotic cavity, and the chorion, which is attached to the maternal decidua. The amnion and chorion are adherent to one another by an extracellular matrix composed of collagens. These membranes contain the amniotic fluid and provide a physical barrier to ascending infection. PPROM is a pathological condition and has been associated with many factors that overlap with risk factors for preterm birth. Intra-amniotic infection (IAI) is associated with PPROM, however the cause and effect relationship is not always certain [9]. Additional risk factors associated with PPROM include a history of PPROM, genital tract infection, vaginal bleeding in pregnancy, cigarette smoking, short cervical length, low body mass index, low socioeconomic status, and drug abuse [10–14]. However, the majority of cases of PPROM occur without an identifiable risk factor.

Complications of preterm premature rupture of membranes

PPROM has complications for both the mother and her fetus. The maternal complications include infection, sepsis, preterm labor, and placental abruption. Clinical IAI is diagnosed in 15–25% of patients with PPROM, while post-partum endometritis complicates 15–20% of PPROM [9, 15, 16]. Placental abruption occurs in 2–5% of women with PPROM [17, 18].

The fetal complications of PPROM include preterm delivery, a non-reassuring fetal heart rate, umbilical cord prolapse,

Evidence-Based Obstetrics and Gynecology, First Edition. Edited by Errol R. Norwitz, Carolyn M. Zelop, David A. Miller, and David L. Keefe.

and intrauterine fetal demise [10]. The risk of stillbirth in women with PPROM is 1–2%, with infection and umbilical cord accidents as contributing factors [19]. PPROM is associated with neonatal complications that vary depending on the gestational age at the time of membrane rupture and delivery, and can include respiratory distress syndrome, neonatal sepsis, intraventricular hemorrhage, necrotizing enterocolitis, and neurodevelopmental impairment [10].

Diagnosis

An accurate diagnosis of PPROM is essential, as failure to diagnose PPROM could result in withholding beneficial treatments for the mother and fetus, while an incorrect diagnosis could lead to unnecessary interventions and a costly hospital admission. The diagnosis of ROMs is generally a clinical diagnosis based on symptoms suggestive of ROM and exam findings.

The symptoms of ROM may include a gush of fluid from the vagina, vaginal bleeding, increased vaginal discharge, or a persistent leakage of a fluid. These symptoms need to be further evaluated as they could also be attributed to causes other than ROM, including urinary incontinence, physiological vaginal discharge, infection, or placental abruption.

A SSE is often the first step to look for pooling of fluid in the posterior cul-de-sac of the vagina and to obtain a fluid sample for pH testing and microscopy. The pH of amniotic fluid is between 7.1 and 7.3, which is more alkaline than normal vaginal fluid, which has a pH of 4.5–6.0. Nitrazine paper can be used to test for amniotic fluid, as nitrazine paper will turn blue when exposed to fluid with a pH above 6.0. When amniotic fluid dries on a glass slide, the salt content crystallizes and develops a characteristic appearance of ferning when viewed under a microscope. The presence of pooling, nitrazine paper turning blue, and ferning are suggestive, but not diagnostic, of ROM.

The nitrazine test has a 17% false positive and 10% false negative rate. Contaminants, such as blood, urine, semen, and discharge from certain vaginal and cervical infections, can increase the pH of vaginal fluid above 6.0 and result in a false positive nitrazine test. Ferning has a 6% false positive and 13% false negative rate. False positive ferning can result from the salt content in cervical mucus, semen, and fingerprints on the slide. False negative results for both nitrazine testing and ferning can result when an inadequate sample of amniotic fluid is obtained [20]. The combination of pooling and ferning has a sensitivity of 51–98% and a specificity of 70–88% [21–24]. Because of the low sensitivity of these tests, if the suspicion for ROM is high and the ferning and nitrazine tests are negative, then the exam could be repeated after a period with the patient in the supine position. Additionally, ultrasound may be useful in the evaluation of ROM, as a low amniotic fluid volume supports the diagnosis, while a normal or high amniotic fluid volume may make the diagnosis of ROMs less likely.

The gold standard for the diagnosis of ROM is an amniocentesis with intra-amniotic instillation of indigo carmine. ROM is diagnosed if blue dye is present on a vaginal tampon 20–30 minutes after the injection of indigo carmine into the amniotic cavity. Because of the risks associated with an amniocentesis, including placental abruption, infection, ROM, and fetal demise, this procedure is used selectively, and is currently limited by a shortage of indigo carmine. Fluorescein instillation into the amniotic cavity followed by a speculum exam and visualization of the cervix with an ultraviolet light 15–45 minutes after the injection has been used as an alternative to indigo carmine. However, the use fluorescein is not routine in clinical practice [25]. Methylene blue and toluidine blue are not appropriate substitutes for indigo carmine because these substances have been implicated in fetal small intestinal atresia, methemoglobinemia, and fetal death [26, 27].

Biochemical markers detected in the cervicovaginal fluid have been investigated to identify amniotic fluid in the vagina and aid in the noninvasive diagnosis of ROM. The AmniSure® ROM Test (Qiagen, Germantown, Maryland) detects placental alpha macroglobulin-1 (PAMG-1), a 34 kDa glycoprotein present in the amniotic fluid in significantly higher concentrations than maternal serum or secretions. AmniSure has been shown to be highly sensitive and specific for ROM when compared to conventional testing with a sensitivity and specificity of 96% and 100%, respectively. AmniSure is more likely to generate a false positive result with labor or advanced cervical dilation [28–31]. Another biochemical marker, Actim PROM (Cooper Surgical, Trumbull, Connecticut), detects insulin-like growth factor-binding protein 1 (IGFBP-1) and has been shown to be 89% sensitive and 83% specific, and superior to both nitrazine and ferning [32]. The diagnostic accuracy of the PAMG-1 and IGFBP-1 tests has been studied in a prospective study in women with vaginal bleeding and concern for ROM. PAMG-1 was less susceptible than IGFBP-2 to interference by blood, with a sensitivity for the identification of amniotic fluid of 99% versus 91%, and a specificity of 92% versus 75%, respectively [33]. Although comparative studies have shown that AmniSure is superior to Actim PROM for the diagnosis of ROM, a meta-analysis did not show a difference when the two products were compared in the same clinical scenario [34–36].

Additional biochemical markers that have been evaluated for the diagnosis of ROM include diamine oxidase, alpha-fetoprotein, soluble intercellular adhesion molecule-1, fibronectin, prolactin, beta subunit of human chorionic gonadotropin, creatinine, urea, lactate, and Axl receptor tyrosine kinase, however their clinical utility in the diagnosis of ROM is limited at this time [37–54]. There is ongoing research utilizing proteomics and mass spectrometry to identify potential biomarkers of ROM [55].

Management of PPROM

Further maternal and fetal evaluation is necessary after the diagnosis of PPROM. Foremost, an accurate gestational age and fetal viability must be established. In an executive summary by the Eunice Kennedy Schriver National Institute of Child Health and Human Development, Society for Maternal Fetal Medicine, American Academy of Pediatrics and the American Congress of Obstetricians and Gynecologists (ACOG), the fetal periviable period was defined as the gestational age between 20 0/7 weeks and 25 6/7 weeks of gestation [56]. The gestational age at which intervention on behalf of the fetus occurs is generally based on regional and local definitions of viability, as well as a discussion between the patient, obstetrician, and neonatologist. Survival estimates for the baby that take into consideration gestational age, estimated fetal weight, corticosteroid administration, plurality, and fetal sex can aid in this discussion.

Obstetric interventions are not recommended when PPROM occurs at a previable gestational age, and management of previable PPROM will be discussed separately. During the periviable period (20 0/7 weeks to 25 6/7 weeks gestation), certain obstetric interventions are not recommended, while some should be considered, and others are recommended depending on decisions regarding resuscitation and the family's preferences after appropriate counseling [57]. If a woman's fetus is of a viable gestational age or periviable and she is a candidate for intervention, then she should be admitted or transferred to a center that can provide both the obstetric and neonatal expertise to care for the mother and a preterm baby.

The initial evaluation of the periviable and viable fetus with suspected PPROM should include confirmation of the diagnosis, as well as an ultrasound determination of the fetal presentation, amniotic fluid volume, and estimated fetal weight. Fetal well-being should be evaluated by an external fetal heart rate monitor and the presence or absence of uterine contractions should be established by external monitoring. A culture for group B streptococcus (GBS) should be obtained prior to antibiotic administration. Unless the patient is in active labor, a visual assessment of the cervix with a SSE to determine dilation and effacement is preferred over a digital exam, as digital exams have been associated with an increased risk of infection [10].

Evaluation of maternal and fetal status is necessary to determine which patients are candidates for expectant management and those patients for whom delivery is indicated. The diagnoses of cord prolapse and significant placental abruption are obstetric emergencies which necessitate immediate delivery of the viable fetus. Similarly, advanced cervical dilation with fetal malpresentation may be an indication for cesarean delivery. Delivery should also be considered for IAI, labor, and a non-reassuring fetal heart rate tracing or biophysical profile. In the absence of the above indications for delivery, hospitalization, and expectant management are recommended for pregnancies complicated by PPROM at less than 34 0/7 weeks. During hospital admission, periodic evaluations to exclude IAI, labor, placental abruption, and non-reassuring fetal status are performed to determine if delivery is indicated. Antenatal testing is suggested to ensure fetal wellbeing, although the frequency and method of evaluation has not been established. At our institution we generally perform daily nonstress tests, weekly biophysical profiles to follow the amniotic fluid volume and fetal presentation, and assess the fetal growth every three to four weeks. More frequent testing may be performed in cases of anhydramnios or fetal growth restriction. Currently, outpatient management is not recommended for PPROM at a viable gestational age [10].

The latency period

In the absence of indications for delivery, expectant management is recommended to decrease the risks to the baby associated with prematurity. The latency period is defined as the time between ROMs and delivery, either spontaneous or indicated. At least 50% of women with ROM who undergo expectant management deliver within a week [58]. Factors associated with a shorter latency period include a later gestational age at the time of ROM, oligohydramnios, cervical dilation >1 cm, cervical length < 2 cm, fetal growth restriction, and nulliparity [19, 59, 60]. Re-accumulation of the amniotic fluid after PPROM has been associated with an increased latency and decreased perinatal morbidity and mortality [61]. Certain interventions, such as antenatal corticosteroids, magnesium sulfate for neuroprotection, and delivery at 34 0/7 weeks have been shown to improve neonatal outcomes, while latency antibiotics have been shown to prolong latency in women with PPROM.

Corticosteroids for prematurity

Antenatal corticosteroids have been shown to decrease neonatal mortality, respiratory distress syndrome, intraventricular hemorrhage, and necrotizing enterocolitis in infants born to women with PPROM [62, 63]. A single course of corticosteroids is recommended in cases of PPROM between 24 0/7 and 34 0/7 weeks of gestation, and may be considered as early as 23 0/7 weeks of gestation. Antenatal corticosteroids are not recommended prior to 23 0/7 weeks of gestation, as they have not been shown to decrease the risk of complications in infants born prior to 23 0/7 weeks of gestation [10, 57]. Betamethasone, 12 mg intramuscularly 24 hours apart times 2 doses, or alternatively dexamethasone, 6 mg intramuscularly every 6 hours times 4 doses, have been shown to provide benefits for infants born preterm without increasing the risk of infection in the mother or neonate [64]. While a repeat course of antenatal corticosteroids has not been shown to increase the rate of neonatal sepsis or maternal chorioamnionitis in PPROM compared to a single course, a clear benefit has not been demonstrated. Therefore, there is currently insufficient evidence to recommend for or against a repeat course of corticosteroids in the setting of PPROM [10, 65, 66].

Magnesium sulfate for fetal neuroprotection

Randomized control trials and meta-analyses have shown that magnesium sulfate given to women at risk for preterm delivery reduces the risk of a diagnosis of cerebral palsy in the infants [67–69]. In the largest randomized control trial evaluating the neuroprotective benefits of magnesium sulfate, 86% of the subjects were diagnosed with PPROM. In this trial composed primarily of patients with PPROM, magnesium sulfate was administered between 24 0/7 weeks and 31 6/7 weeks to women at risk for imminent delivery and decreased the risk of cerebral palsy in the infants [70]. Magnesium sulfate has been found to be both cost effective ($1462.60 vs $1607.50) and result in improved outcomes (56.7022 vs. 56.6972 quality-adjusted life years) when administered to women at risk for preterm birth due to PPROM less than 32 0/7 weeks of gestation [71]. The use of magnesium sulfate for fetal neuroprotection has not been shown to prolong latency in women with PPROM without labor between 24 0/7 and 32 0/7 weeks gestation [72]. The optimal dose and duration of magnesium sulfate has not been determined. At our institution we administer a 6 g intravenous bolus of magnesium sulfate, over 30 minutes, followed by a 2 g h^{-1} maintenance infusion if delivery is felt to be imminent.

Magnesium sulfate for fetal neuroprotection should be considered for women with PPROM at risk of imminent delivery after 23 0/7 weeks, and is recommended between 24 0/7 weeks and 32 0/7 weeks [12, 68, 70].

Prophylactic antibiotics in PPROM

Prophylactic antibiotics in the setting of PPROM under 34 0/7 weeks of gestation has been shown to increase the latency period, reduce infectious morbidity, and reduce gestational age-dependent morbidity [16, 73–75]. A retrospective study evaluated 17 877 pregnancies at a single institution in which PPROM occurred in 1.7% of patients. In the absence of any medical interventions, including prophylactic antibiotics and corticosteroids, greater than 90% of women entered spontaneous labor within 48 hours [76]. In contrast, another retrospective study with 66 775 patients, in which the rate of PPROM was 1.4%, patients were administered prophylactic antibiotics and corticosteroids, and only 26% of women delivered within 48 hours of ROM [60]. Similarly, a randomized trial by the National Institute of Child Health and Human Development Maternal Fetal Medicine Unit showed a significant prolongation in pregnancy in women with PPROM who were administered prophylactic antibiotics (6.1 versus 2.9 days, $p < 0.01$) [74].

The current recommendation from the ACOG is for a 7-day course of erythromycin and ampicillin or amoxicillin during expectant management [10]. This antibiotic regimen is based on the above study by the National Institute of Child Health and Human Development Maternal Fetal Medicine Unit which demonstrated that intravenous ampicillin (2 g every 6 hours) with intravenous erythromycin (250 mg every 6 hours) for 48 hours, followed by 5 days of oral amoxicillin (250 mg every 8 hours) and oral erythromycin (333 mg every 8 hours) resulted in a significant prolongation of pregnancy in with PPROM [74]. Due to the ease of administration and an improved side effect profile, some experts recommend a single oral or intravenous dose of azithromycin as a substitute for erythromycin [77]. A retrospective cohort study did not show a difference in the latency period, chorioamnionitis, cesarean delivery, Apgar scores, birth weight, neonatal death, neonatal sepsis, or neonatal respiratory distress syndrome between women with PPROM who received ampicillin and erythromycin as compared to ampicillin and azithromycin [78]. In women with PPROM and a penicillin allergy, ACOG currently recommends erythromycin as a single agent for prophylaxis [10]. Some experts recommend intravenous cefazolin (1 g every 8 hours for 48 hours) followed by oral cephalexin (500 mg every 6 hours for 5 days) for women with PPROM and a mild allergy to penicillin. While patients with a severe allergy to penicillin, defined as anaphylaxis, angioedema, respiratory distress, or urticaria within 30 minutes of drug administration, are treated with 48 hours of intravenous gentamicin (7 mg kg^{-1} ideal body weight) and clindamycin (900 mg every 8 hours) followed by 5 days of oral clindamycin (300 mg every 8 hours) [77].

Prophylactic antibiotics to prolong latency during expectant management of patients with PPROM could be considered between 20 0/7 and 23 6/7, and are recommended between 24 0/7 and 34 0/7 [57]. Regardless of the regimen or duration of prophylactic antibiotic treatment, candidates for intrapartum GBS prophylaxis should be treated during labor [10].

Tocolysis

Multiple studies have been performed to evaluate if tocolysis prolongs latency and improves neonatal outcomes in the setting of PPROM. A Cochrane review of eight randomized controlled trials in women with PPROM between 23 0/7 weeks and 36 6/7 weeks of gestation did not show sufficient evidence that tocolysis improved neonatal outcomes in PPROM. Although tocolysis was associated with an increase in the latency period (mean difference 73 hours, 95% CI 20–126 hours) and fewer births within 48 hours (average RR 0.55, 95% CI 0.32–0.95), there was an increase in chorioamnionitis in the group that received tocolytics, as well as a need for ventilation in the neonates (RR 2.46, 95% CI 1.14–5.34) and five minute Apgar scores <7 (RR 6.05, 95% CI 1.65–22.23) [79]. Importantly, women in these early studies on tocolysis in PPROM did not uniformly receive latency antibiotics or corticosteroids, which is in contrast to the current standard of care. Because tocolysis has not been shown to prolong latency or improve neonatal outcomes in women with PPROM who are in active labor, it is currently not recommended [10].

Timing of delivery in PPROM

Currently ACOG recommends expectant management for women with PPROM prior to 34 0/7 weeks, as long as there are no maternal or fetal complications, with delivery at 34 0/7 weeks. When PPROM occurs after 34 0/7 weeks, delivery is recommended [10]. A 2010 Cochrane review of seven randomized trials of women with PPROM between 24 0/7 and 37 0/7 weeks of gestation concluded that the data remained insufficient to recommend delayed or immediate delivery in the setting of PPROM [80]. Randomized controlled studies have evaluated the maternal and neonatal risks and benefits of increasing the gestational age at delivery in PPROM. Rates of neonatal sepsis, respiratory distress syndrome, and cesarean delivery did not differ between those women with PPROM randomized to induction of labor at 34 0/7 weeks or expectant management until 37 0/7 weeks of gestation. However, the women managed expectantly beyond 34 0/7 weeks had an increased rate of chorioamnionitis, which was associated with adverse neonatal outcomes even after controlling for steroids, gestational age at PPROM, and gestational age at delivery [81–83]. A randomized controlled trial comparing immediate delivery versus expectant management in women with PPROM between 34 0/7 weeks and 36 6/7 weeks of gestation found no difference in the primary outcome of neonatal sepsis (RR 0.8, CI 0.5–1.3). However, the neonates in the immediate delivery group had an increased rate of respiratory distress (RR 1.6, CI 1.1–2.3), need for mechanical ventilation (RR 1.4, CI 1–1.8), and intensive care unit stay (median stay of two versus four days, $P < 0.0001$). While the mothers in the immediate delivery group had a decrease in antepartum and intrapartum bleeding (RR 0.6, CI 0.4–0.9), fever (RR 0.4, CI 0.2–0.9), post-partum antibiotic administration (RR 0.8, CI 0.7–1.0), and length of hospital stay ($P < 0.001$), there was an increase in the cesarean delivery rate compared with women managed expectantly until 36 6/7 weeks (RR 1.4, CI 1.2–1.7) [84]. At this time, ACOG does not recommend prolonging pregnancy beyond 34 0/7 weeks of gestation in the setting of PPROM. If the patient desires expectant management beyond 34 0/7 weeks, then she should be thoroughly counseled about the maternal and fetal risks and benefits of prolonging pregnancy, and expectant management should not extend beyond 37 0/7 weeks [10].

Preterm premature rupture of membranes before fetal viability

Previable PPROM occurs in <1% of all deliveries and is associated with high rates of adverse maternal and neonatal outcomes, including previable delivery, delivery at extreme prematurity, pulmonary hypoplasia, and fetal deformations secondary to oligohydramnios, neonatal sepsis, placental abruption, retained placenta, chorioamnionitis, endometritis, and maternal sepsis [85]. Expectant management of women with previable PPROM has a 1% risk of maternal sepsis, which has led to isolated cases of death [10]. Risk factors for previable PPROM include tobacco use, cervical incompetence, previous second trimester delivery, previous termination <20 weeks of gestation, and a history of PPROM [86].

Previable PPROM requires a careful evaluation and counseling about management options, which include induction of labor and expectant management [51]. If a patient with previable PPROM elects for expectant management after counseling about the maternal and fetal risks, then antibiotics may be considered as early as 20 0/7 weeks, however GBS prophylaxis, corticosteroids, tocolysis, and magnesium sulfate for neuroprotection are not recommended until viability [10].

Women with previable PPROM and no evidence of abruption, chorioamnionitis, or labor after a period of observation can be managed as an outpatient until fetal viability is reached. Outpatient management of women with previable PPROM requires close follow-up for evidence of infection. Once viability is reached and the patient desires intervention, she should be admitted for expectant management with latency antibiotics, corticosteroids, and periodic fetal evaluations as outlined above. Even if the pregnancy reaches a viable gestational age, the risks of pulmonary hypoplasia, prematurity, and sepsis remain higher than controls matched for gestational age [87]. In an observational study of 61 women with PPROM between 18 0/7 weeks and 26 0/7 weeks of gestation, in which latency antibiotics but not corticosteroids were administered, the risk of stillbirth or miscarriage was 30%. Of those fetuses that survived to delivery, the outcome was poor with a 54% neonatal mortality rate. Birth weight was the only significant independent predictor of healthy survival [88]. While not standard of care, interventions have been investigated to prolong the latency period in periviable PPROM. A retrospective study in which women with PPROM at less than 23 0/7 weeks of gestation were given antibiotics, corticosteroids, tocolytics, a cervical cerclage, and a continuous amnio-infusion, had an average latency period of 24 days and a neonatal survival of 60%, with no cases of maternal sepsis [89].

Special circumstances

PPROM following an invasive procedure

Women with ROM after an amniocentesis have improved outcomes compared to women with spontaneous PPROM [90]. Membranes can reseal and the amniotic fluid volume can normalize, with an expected favorable outcome [10, 90]. There is ongoing research into techniques to reseal the fetal membranes after iatrogenic PPROM, however these are not yet clinically available.

Cervical cerclage

The management of PPROM can be complicated by the presence of a cervical cerclage. In a meta-analysis that included six studies with a total of 293 patients, cerclage retention did not significantly prolong the latency period, however pregnancy was prolonged for 48 hours for corticosteroid administration. Cerclage retention was not associated with an increased rate of neonatal sepsis or death, however there was a significant increase in chorioamnionitis [91]. In a trial of 56 patients randomized to cerclage retention or removal at the time of PPROM, there was no statistically significant difference in chorioamnionitis, pregnancy prolongation by one week, or the neonatal composite outcome [92]. Although cerclage retention may prolong pregnancy for steroid administration, it comes at the expense of an increased risk of chorioamnionitis. At this time the evidence is inconclusive that cerclage retention is beneficial in the setting of PPROM.

Herpes simplex virus (HSV)

If Herpes simplex virus (HSV) lesions are present in a woman with PPROM at a time when delivery is indicated, then the usual obstetric guidelines should be followed and a cesarean delivery should be recommended. However, in cases of PPROM without an indication for delivery, one must weigh the risks of prematurity versus the risk of an ascending fetal infection, which will depend on whether the HSV outbreak is recurrent or primary. In cases of PPROM with a recurrent lesion, expectant management with the addition of intravenous acyclovir ($5\,\mathrm{mg\,kg^{-1}}$ every eight hours) to decrease viral shedding and the duration of active lesions would be reasonable [10]. Given the increased risk of fetal transmission during a primary HSV infection, some experts recommend cesarean delivery for women with PPROM between 28 and 32 weeks. Patients with PPROM and a primary HSV infection less than 28–32 weeks gestation, should be managed expectantly with the addition of intravenous acyclovir.

Human immunodeficiency virus (HIV)

The management of PPROM can be further complicated in the Human immunodeficiency virus (HIV) positive woman. Early studies demonstrated increased rates of vertical transmission in women with CD4 counts less than 20% and ROMs greater than four hours [93]. In today's setting, vertical transmission rates differ significantly between women on antiretroviral therapy (ART) with low or undetectable viral loads and untreated woman. Newer data suggests that membrane rupture greater than four hours in women with low or undetectable viral loads on ART does not increase the perinatal transmission rate [94, 95]. Data is lacking in women with HIV and prolonged membrane rupture remote from delivery. In this situation, the management plan should be individualized and take into consideration gestational age, viral load, and whether or not the patient is on ART.

Conclusions

PPROM is a leading cause of preterm birth. An accurate diagnosis of PPROM is essential; however current tests for ROM are limited by a low sensitivity and specificity for the detection of amniotic fluid. Contemporary management of PPROM is based on the gestational age and attempts to balance the risks of prematurity versus the maternal and fetal risks of infection, as well as other complications. When PPROM occurs prior to 34 0/7 weeks, expectant management is recommended as long as there are no maternal or fetal contraindications. Expectant management of PPROM includes hospital admission, latency antibiotics, corticosteroids for fetal benefits, magnesium sulfate for fetal neuroprotection if less than 32 0/7 weeks of gestation, and delivery at 34 0/7 weeks. When PPROM occurs after 34 0/7 weeks, delivery is currently recommended. In certain clinical situations, the management of PPROM needs to be individualized and is often based on expert opinion, as data to guide management in some circumstances is limited. Research is ongoing regarding the optimal gestational age for delivery following PPROM and the identification of accurate noninvasive diagnostic tests for ROM.

References

1 Martin, J.A., Hamilton, B.E., Ventura, S.J. et al. (2012). Births: final data for 2010. *Natl. Vital. Stat. Rep.* **61** (**1**): 1–72.

2 Mathews, T.J. and MacDorman, M.F. (2010). Infant mortality statistics from the 2006 period linked birth/infant death data set. *Natl. Vital. Stat. Rep.* **58** (**17**): 1–31.

3 Martin, J.A., Hamilton, B.E., Osterman, M.J. et al. (2015). Births: final data for 2013. *Natl. Vital. Stat. Rep.* **64** (**1**): 1–65.

4 Mercer, B.M., Goldenberg, R.L., Meis, P.J. et al. (2000). The Preterm Prediction Study: prediction of preterm premature rupture of membranes through clinical findings and ancillary testing. The National Institute of Child Health and Human Development Maternal-Fetal Medicine Units Network. *Am. J. Obstet. Gynecol.* **183** (**3**): 738–745.

5 Ohlsson, A. (1989). Treatments of preterm premature rupture of the membranes: a meta-analysis. *Am. J. Obstet. Gynecol.* **160** (**4**): 890–906.

6 (1998). ACOG practice bulletin. Premature rupture of membranes. Clinical management guidelines for obstetrician-gynecologists. Number 1, June 1998. American College of Obstetricians and Gynecologists. *Int. J. Gynaecol. Obstet.* **63** (**1**): 75–84.

7 Parry, S. and Strauss, J.F. 3rd (1998). Premature rupture of the fetal membranes. *N. Engl. J. Med.* **338** (**10**): 663–670.

8 (2007). Practice Bulletin No. 80: premature rupture of membranes. Clinical management guidelines for obstetrician-gynecologists. *Obstet. Gynecol.* **109** (**4**): 1007–1019.

9 Garite, T.J. and Freeman, R.K. (1982). Chorioamnionitis in the preterm gestation. *Obstet. Gynecol.* **59** (**5**): 539–545.

10 (2016). Practice Bulletin No. 160 Summary: Premature Rupture of Membranes. *Obstet. Gynecol.* **127** (**1**): 192–194.

11 Asrat, T., Lewis, D.F., Garite, T.J. et al. (1991). Rate of recurrence of preterm premature rupture of membranes in consecutive pregnancies. *Am. J. Obstet. Gynecol.* **165** (**4 Pt 1**): 1111–1115.

12 (2013). Practice Bulletin No. 139: Premature Rupture of Membranes. *Obstet. Gynecol.* **122**: 918–930.

13 Harger, J.H., Hsing, A.W., Tuomala, R.E. et al. (1990). Risk factors for preterm premature rupture of fetal membranes: a multicenter case-control study. *Am. J. Obstet. Gynecol.* **163** (**1 Pt 1**): 130–137.

14 Mercer, B.M., Goldenberg, R.L., Moawad, A.H. et al. (1999). The preterm prediction study: effect of gestational age and cause of preterm birth on subsequent obstetric outcome. National Institute of Child Health and Human Development Maternal-Fetal Medicine Units Network. *Am. J. Obstet. Gynecol.* **181** (**5 Pt 1**): 1216–1221.

15 Beydoun, S.N. and Yasin, S.Y. (1986). Premature rupture of the membranes before 28 weeks: conservative management. *Am. J. Obstet. Gynecol.* **155** (**3**): 471–479.

16 Kenyon, S., Boulvain, M., and Neilson, J.P. (2010). Antibiotics for preterm rupture of membranes. *Cochrane Database Syst. Rev.* (**8**): CD001058. doi: 10.1002/14651858.CD001058.

17 Ananth, C.V., Oyelese, Y., Srinivas, N. et al. (2004). Preterm premature rupture of membranes, intrauterine infection, and oligohydramnios: risk factors for placental abruption. *Obstet. Gynecol.* **104** (**1**): 71–77.

18 Major, C.A., de Veciana, M., Lewis, D.F., and Morgan, M.A. (1995). Preterm premature rupture of membranes and abruptio placentae: is there an association between these pregnancy complications? *Am. J. Obstet. Gynecol.* **172** (**2 Pt 1**): 672–676.

19 Mercer, B.M., Rabello, Y.A., Thurnau, G.R. et al. (2006). The NICHD-MFMU antibiotic treatment of preterm PROM study: impact of initial amniotic fluid volume on pregnancy outcome. *Am. J. Obstet. Gynecol.* **194** (**2**): 438–445.

20 Friedman, M.L. and McElin, T.W. (1969). Diagnosis of ruptured fetal membranes. Clinical study and review of the literature. *Am. J. Obstet. Gynecol.* **104** (**4**): 544–550.

21 de Haan, H.H., Offermans, P.M., Smits, F. et al. (1994). Value of the fern test to confirm or reject the diagnosis of ruptured membranes is modest in nonlaboring women presenting with nonspecific vaginal fluid loss. *Am. J. Perinatol.* **11** (**1**): 46–50.

22 Gorodeski, I.G., Haimovitz, L., and Bahari, C.M. (1982). Reevaluation of the pH, ferning and nile blue sulphate staining methods in pregnant women with premature rupture of the fetal membranes. *J. Perinat. Med.* **10** (**6**): 286–292.

23 Reece, E.A., Chervenak, F.A., Moya, F.R., and Hobbins, J.C. (1984). Amniotic fluid arborization: effect of blood, meconium, and pH alterations. *Obstet. Gynecol.* **64** (**2**): 248–250.

24 Rosemond, R.L., Lombardi, S.J., and Boehm, F.H. (1990). Ferning of amniotic fluid contaminated with blood. *Obstet. Gynecol.* **75** (**3 Pt 1**): 338–340.

25 Smith, R.P. (1976). A technic for the detection of rupture of the membranes. A review and preliminary report. *Obstet. Gynecol.* **48** (**2**): 172–176.

26 McEnerney, J.K. and McEnerney, L.N. (1983). Unfavorable neonatal outcome after intraamniotic injection of methylene blue. *Obstet. Gynecol.* **61** (**3 Suppl**): 35S–37S.

27 Mehler, K., Oberthuer, A., Weisshaar, G. et al. (2013). Hemolytic anemia and methemoglobinemia in a preterm baby as a complication of antenatal intraamnial injection of toluidine blue. *Klin. Padiatr.* **225** (**5**): 263–265.

28 Cousins, L.M., Smok, D.P., Lovett, S.M., and Poeltler, D.M. (2005). AmniSure placental alpha microglobulin-1 rapid immunoassay versus standard diagnostic methods for detection of rupture of membranes. *Am. J. Perinatol.* **22** (**6**): 317–320.

29 Lee, S.E., Park, J.S., Norwitz, E.R. et al. (2007). Measurement of placental alpha-microglobulin-1 in cervicovaginal discharge to diagnose rupture of membranes. *Obstet. Gynecol.* **109** (**3**): 634–640.

30 Lee, S.M., Romero, R., Park, J.W. et al. (2012). The clinical significance of a positive Amnisure test in women with preterm labor and intact membranes. *J. Matern. Fetal Neonatal Med.* **25** (**9**): 1690–1698.

31 Ng, B.K., Lim, P.S., Shafiee, M.N. et al. (2013). Comparison between AmniSure placental alpha microglobulin-1 rapid immunoassay and standard diagnostic methods for detection of rupture of membranes. *Biomed. Res. Int.* **2013**: 587438.

32 Abdelazim, I.A. (2014). Insulin-like growth factor binding protein-1 (Actim PROM test) for detection of premature rupture of fetal membranes. *J. Obstet. Gynaecol. Res.* **40** (**4**): 961–967.

33 Ramsauer, B., Duwe, W., Schlehe, B. et al. (2015). Effect of blood on ROM diagnosis accuracy of PAMG-1 and IGFBP-1 detecting rapid tests. *J. Perinat. Med.* **43** (**4**): 417–422.

34 Palacio, M., Kuhnert, M., Berger, R. et al. (2014). Meta-analysis of studies on biochemical marker tests for the diagnosis of premature rupture of membranes: comparison of performance indexes. *BMC Pregnancy Childbirth* **14**: 183.

35 Pollet-Villard, M., Cartier, R., Gaucherand, P., and Doret, M. (2011). Detection of placental alpha microglobulin-1 versus insulin-like growth factor-binding protein-1 in amniotic fluid at term: a comparative study. *Am. J. Perinatol.* **28** (**6**): 489–494.

36 Ramsauer, B., Vidaeff, A.C., Hosli, I. et al. (2013). The diagnosis of rupture of fetal membranes (ROM): a meta-analysis. *J. Perinat. Med.* **41** (**3**): 233–240.

37 Abdelazim, I.A. (2013). Fetal fibronectin (Quick Check fFN test((R))) for detection of premature rupture of fetal membranes. *Arch. Gynecol. Obstet.* **287** (**2**): 205–210.

38 Abdelazim, I.A., Abdelrazak, K.M., Al-Kadi, M. et al. (2014). Fetal fibronectin (Quick Check fFN test) versus placental alpha microglobulin-1 (AmniSure test) for detection of premature rupture of fetal membranes. *Arch. Gynecol. Obstet.* **290** (**3**): 457–464.

39 Buyukbayrak, E.E., Turan, C., Unal, O. et al. (2004). Diagnostic power of the vaginal washing-fluid prolactin assay as an alternative method for the diagnosis of premature rupture of membranes. *J. Matern. Fetal Neonatal Med.* **15** (**2**): 120–125.

40 Esim, E., Turan, C., Unal, O. et al. (2003). Diagnosis of premature rupture of membranes by identification of beta-HCG in vaginal washing fluid. *Eur. J. Obstet. Gynecol. Reprod. Biol.* **107** (**1**): 37–40.

41 Gahl, W.A., Kozina, T.J., Fuhrmann, D.D., and Vale, A.M. (1982). Diamine oxidase in the diagnosis of ruptured fetal membranes. *Obstet. Gynecol.* **60** (**3**): 297–304.

42 Kafali, H. and Oksuzler, C. (2007). Vaginal fluid urea and creatinine in diagnosis of premature rupture of membranes. *Arch. Gynecol. Obstet.* **275** (**3**): 157–160.

43 Kim, Y.H., Park, Y.W., Kwon, H.S. et al. (2005). Vaginal fluid beta-human chorionic gonadotropin level in the diagnosis of premature rupture of membranes. *Acta Obstet. Gynecol. Scand.* **84** (**8**): 802–805.

44 Kishida, T., Yamada, H., Negishi, H. et al. (1996). Diagnosis of premature rupture of the membranes in preterm patients, using an improved AFP kit: comparison with ROM-check and/or nitrazine test. *Eur. J. Obstet. Gynecol. Reprod. Biol.* **69** (**2**): 77–82.

45 Koninckx, P.R., Trappeniers, H., and Van Assche, F.A. (1981). Prolactin concentration in vaginal fluid: a new method for diagnosing ruptured membranes. *Br. J. Obstet. Gynaecol.* **88** (**6**): 607–610.

46 Li, H.Y. and Chang, T.S. (2000). Vaginal fluid creatinine, human chorionic gonadotropin and alpha-fetoprotein levels for detecting premature rupture of membranes. *Zhonghua Yi Xue Za Zhi (Taipei)* **63** (**9**): 686–690.

47 Lockwood, C.J., Senyei, A.E., Dische, M.R. et al. (1991). Fetal fibronectin in cervical and vaginal secretions as a predictor of preterm delivery. *N. Engl. J. Med.* **325** (**10**): 669–674.

48 Mor, A., Tal, R., Haberman, S. et al. (2015). Alpha-fetoprotein as a tool to distinguish amniotic fluid from urine, vaginal discharge, and semen. *Obstet. Gynecol.* **125** (**2**): 448–452.

49 Sekhavat, L., Firouzabadi, R.D., and Mojiri, P. (2012). Practicability of vaginal washing fluid creatinine level in detecting premature rupture of membranes. *Arch. Gynecol. Obstet.* **286** (**1**): 25–28.

50 Shahin, M. and Raslan, H. (2007). Comparative study of three amniotic fluid markers in premature rupture of membranes: prolactin, beta subunit of human chorionic gonadotropin, and alpha-fetoprotein. *Gynecol. Obstet. Invest.* **63** (**4**): 195–199.

51 Thomasino, T., Levi, C., Draper, M., and Neubert, A.G. (2013). Diagnosing rupture of membranes using combination monoclonal/polyclonal immunologic protein detection. *J. Reprod. Med.* **58** (**5–6**): 187–194.

52 Wang, T., Zhou, R., Xiong, W. et al. (2013). Clinical evaluation of soluble intercellular adhesion molecule-1 and insulin like growth factor-binding protein-1-based rapid immunoassays for the diagnosis of prelabor rupture of membranes. *J. Perinat. Med.* **41** (**2**): 181–185.

53 Wiberg-Itzel, E., Cnattingius, S., and Nordstrom, L. (2005). Lactate determination in vaginal fluids: a new method in the diagnosis of prelabour rupture of membranes. *BJOG* **112** (**6**): 754–758.

54 Zanjani, M.S. and Haghighi, L. (2012). Vaginal fluid creatinine for the detection of premature rupture of membranes. *J. Obstet. Gynaecol. Res.* **38** (**3**): 505–508.

55 Consonni, S., Mainini, V., Pizzardi, A. et al. (2014). Non-invasively collected amniotic fluid as a source of possible biomarkers for premature rupture of membranes investigated by proteomic approach. *Arch. Gynecol. Obstet.* **289** (**2**): 299–306.

56 Raju, T.N., Mercer, B.M., Burchfield, D.J., and Joseph, G.F. Jr. (2014). Periviable birth: executive summary of a joint workshop by the Eunice Kennedy Shriver National Institute of Child Health and Human Development, Society for Maternal-Fetal Medicine, American Academy of Pediatrics, and American College of Obstetricians and Gynecologists. *Am. J. Obstet. Gynecol.* **210** (**5**): 406–417.

57 (2015). ACOG Obstetric Care Consensus No. 3 Summary: Periviable Birth. *Obstet. Gynecol.* **126** (**5**): 1123–1125.

58 Mercer, B.M. (2003). Preterm premature rupture of the membranes. *Obstet. Gynecol.* **101** (**1**): 178–193.

59 Mehra, S., Amon, E., Hopkins, S. et al. (2015). Transvaginal cervical length and amniotic fluid index: can it predict delivery latency following preterm premature rupture of membranes? *Am. J. Obstet. Gynecol.* **212** (**3**): 400 e1–400 e9.

60 Melamed, N., Hadar, E., Ben-Haroush, A. et al. (2009). Factors affecting the duration of the latency period in preterm premature rupture of membranes. *J. Matern. Fetal Neonatal Med.* **22** (**11**): 1051–1056.

61 Johnson, J.W., Egerman, R.S., and Moorhead, J. (1990). Cases with ruptured membranes that "reseal". *Am. J. Obstet. Gynecol.* **163** (**3**): 1024–1030. discussion 30-2.

62 Roberts, D. and Dalziel, S. (2006). Antenatal corticosteroids for accelerating fetal lung maturation for women at risk of preterm birth. *Cochrane Database Syst. Rev.* (**3**): CD004454. doi: 10.1002/14651858.CD004454.pub2.

63 Vidaeff, A.C., Ramin, S.M., and Gilstrap, L.C. 3rd (2001). Antenatal corticosteroids in women with preterm premature rupture of the membranes. *Clin. Perinatol.* **28** (**4**): 797–805.

64 Brownfoot, F.C., Gagliardi, D.I., Bain, E. et al. (2013). Different corticosteroids and regimens for accelerating fetal lung maturation for women at risk of preterm birth. *Cochrane Database Syst. Rev.* (**8**): CD006764. doi: 10.1002/14651858.CD006764.pub3.

65 Brookfield, K.F., El-Sayed, Y.Y., Chao, L. et al. (2015). Antenatal corticosteroids for preterm premature rupture of membranes: single or repeat course? *Am. J. Perinatol.* **32** (**6**): 537–544.

66 Gyamfi-Bannerman, C. and Son, M. (2014). Preterm premature rupture of membranes and the rate of neonatal sepsis after two courses of antenatal corticosteroids. *Obstet. Gynecol.* **124** (**5**): 999–1003.

67 Hirtz, D.G., Weiner, S.J., Bulas, D. et al. (2015). Antenatal magnesium and cerebral palsy in preterm infants. *J. Pediatr.* **167** (**4**): 834–9 e3.

68 Doyle, L.W., Crowther, C.A., Middleton, P. et al. (2009). Magnesium sulphate for women at risk of preterm birth for neuroprotection of the fetus. *Cochrane Database Syst. Rev.* (**1**): CD004661. doi: 10.1002/14651858.CD004661.pub3.

69 Costantine, M.M., Weiner, S.J., and Kennedy, E. (2009). Shriver National Institute of Child H, Human Development Maternal-Fetal Medicine Units N. Effects of antenatal exposure to magnesium sulfate on neuroprotection and mortality in preterm infants: a meta-analysis. *Obstet Gynecol.* **114** (**2 Pt 1**): 354–364.

70 Rouse, D.J., Hirtz, D.G., Thom, E. et al. (2008). A randomized, controlled trial of magnesium sulfate for the prevention of cerebral palsy. *N. Engl. J. Med.* **359** (**9**): 895–905.

71 Cahill, A.G., Odibo, A.O., Stout, M.J. et al. (2011). Magnesium sulfate therapy for the prevention of cerebral palsy in preterm infants: a decision-analytic and economic analysis. *Am. J. Obstet. Gynecol.* **205** (**6**): 542 e1–542 e7.

72 Horton, A.L., Lai, Y., Rouse, D.J. et al. (2015). Effect of magnesium sulfate administration for neuroprotection on latency in women with preterm premature rupture of membranes. *Am. J. Perinatol.* **32** (**4**): 387–392.

73 Kenyon, S., Boulvain, M., and Neilson, J.P. (2013). Antibiotics for preterm rupture of membranes. *Cochrane Database Syst. Rev.* (**12**): CD001058. doi: 10.1002/14651858.CD001058.

74 Mercer, B.M., Miodovnik, M., Thurnau, G.R. et al. (1997). Antibiotic therapy for reduction of infant morbidity after preterm premature rupture of the membranes. A randomized controlled trial. National Institute of Child Health and Human Development Maternal-Fetal Medicine Units Network. *JAMA* **278** (**12**): 989–995.

75 Kenyon, S.L., Taylor, D.J., Tarnow-Mordi, W., and Group OC (2001). Broad-spectrum antibiotics for preterm, prelabour rupture of fetal membranes: the ORACLE I randomised trial. ORACLE Collaborative Group. *Lancet* **357** (**9261**): 979–988.

76 Cox, S.M., Williams, M.L., and Leveno, K.J. (1988). The natural history of preterm ruptured membranes: what to expect of expectant management. *Obstet Gynecol.* **71** (**4**): 558–562.

77 Duff, P. (2016). *Preterm premature (prelabor) rupture of membranes.* Waltham, MA: Up To Date.

78 Pierson, R.C., Gordon, S.S., and Haas, D.M. (2014). A retrospective comparison of antibiotic regimens for preterm premature rupture of membranes. *Obstet. Gynecol.* **124** (**3**): 515–519.

79 Mackeen, A.D., Seibel-Seamon, J., Muhammad, J. et al. (2014). Tocolytics for preterm premature rupture of membranes. *Cochrane Database Syst. Rev.* (**2**): CD007062. doi: 10.1002/14651858.CD007062.pub2.

80 Buchanan, S.L., Crowther, C.A., Levett, K.M. et al. (2010). Planned early birth versus expectant management for women with preterm prelabour rupture of membranes prior to 37 weeks' gestation for improving pregnancy outcome. *Cochrane Database Syst. Rev.* (**3**): CD004735. doi: 10.1002/14651858.CD004735.pub4.

81 Lee, S.M., Park, J.W., Kim, B.J. et al. (2013). Acute histologic chorioamnionitis is a risk factor for adverse neonatal outcome in late preterm birth after preterm premature rupture of membranes. *PLoS One* **8** (**12**): e79941.

82 van der Ham, D.P., van der Heyden, J.L., Opmeer, B.C. et al. (2012). Management of late-preterm premature rupture of membranes: the PPROMEXIL-2 trial. *Am. J. Obstet. Gynecol.* **207** (**4**): 276 e1–276 e10.

83 van der Ham, D.P., Vijgen, S.M., Nijhuis, J.G. et al. (2012). Induction of labor versus expectant management in women with preterm prelabor rupture of membranes between 34 and 37 weeks: a randomized controlled trial. *PLoS Med.* **9** (**4**): e1001208.

84 Morris, J.M., Roberts, C.L., Bowen, J.R. et al. (2015). Immediate delivery compared with expectant management after preterm pre-labour rupture of the membranes close to term (PPROMT trial): a randomised controlled trial. *Lancet.*

85 Waters, T.P. and Mercer, B.M. (2009). The management of preterm premature rupture of the membranes near the limit of fetal viability. *Am. J. Obstet. Gynecol.* **201** (**3**): 230–240.

86 Kilpatrick, S.J., Patil, R., Connell, J. et al. (2006). Risk factors for previable premature rupture of membranes or advanced cervical dilation: a case control study. *Am. J. Obstet. Gynecol.* **194** (**4**): 1168–1174. discussion 74-5.

87 Soylu, H., Jefferies, A., Diambomba, Y. et al. (2010). Rupture of membranes before the age of viability and birth after the age of viability: comparison of outcomes in a matched cohort study. *J. Perinatol.* **30** (**10**): 645–649.

88 Esteves, J.S., de Sa, R.A., de Carvalho, P.R., and Coca Velarde, L.G. (2015). Neonatal outcome in women with preterm premature rupture of membranes (PPROM) between 18 and 26 weeks. *J. Matern. Fetal Neonatal Med.* 1–5.

89 Miyazaki, K., Furuhashi, M., Yoshida, K., and Ishikawa, K. (2012). Aggressive intervention of previable preterm premature rupture of membranes. *Acta Obstet. Gynecol. Scand.* **91** (**8**): 923–929.

90 Borgida, A.F., Mills, A.A., Feldman, D.M. et al. (2000). Outcome of pregnancies complicated by ruptured membranes after genetic amniocentesis. *Am. J. Obstet. Gynecol.* **183** (**4**): 937–939.

91 Pergialiotis, V., Gkioka, E., Bakoyiannis, I. et al. (2015). Retention of cervical cerclage after preterm premature rupture of the

membranes: a critical appraisal. *Arch. Gynecol. Obstet.* **291** (**4**): 745–753.

92 Galyean, A., Garite, T.J., Maurel, K. et al. (2014). Removal versus retention of cerclage in preterm premature rupture of membranes: a randomized controlled trial. *Am. J. Obstet. Gynecol.* **211** (**4**): 399 e1–399 e7.

93 Minkoff, H., Burns, D.N., Landesman, S. et al. (1995). The relationship of the duration of ruptured membranes to vertical transmission of human immunodeficiency virus. *Am. J. Obstet. Gynecol.* **173** (**2**): 585–589.

94 Cotter, A.M., Brookfield, K.F., Duthely, L.M. et al. (2012). Duration of membrane rupture and risk of perinatal transmission of HIV-1 in the era of combination antiretroviral therapy. *Am. J. Obstet. Gynecol.* **207** (**6**): 482 e1–482 e5.

95 Peters, H., Byrne, L., De Ruiter, A. et al. (2015). Duration of ruptured membranes and mother-to-child HIV transmission: a prospective population-based surveillance study. *BJOG*.

39

CHAPTER 39 Antepartum hemorrhage

Joanna Gibson[1], Nada Sabir[2], and James Neilson[3]
[1] *Obstetrics and Gynecology, Yorkshire and Humber, UK*
[2] *Obstetrics and Gynecology/Maternal Medicine, Bradford Teaching Hospitals NHS Foundation Trust, Bradford, UK*
[3] *Obstetrics and Gynecology, University of Liverpool, Liverpool, UK*

Background

Ante-partum hemorrhage (APH) is defined as bleeding from 24 weeks of pregnancy until birth arising from or in the genital tract [1]. 27.1% (CI 19.9–36.2) of maternal deaths between 2003 and 2009, are due to hemorrhage. Antepartum hemorrhage was the primary culprit in 6.5%, intrapartum in 0.9%, and postpartum hemorrhage in 19.7% [2].

Antepartum hemorrhage complicates 2–5% of all pregnancies and remains a cause of maternal and fetal morbidity and mortality [3]. Antepartum hemorrhage of unknown origin occurs in 50% cases [4] and carries an increased risk of induction of labor and preterm delivery [5]. These babies have increased risk of admission to neonatal intensive care unit (NICU), low birth weights and hyperbilirubinemia.

Placental insertion abnormalities including vasa previa, placenta previa, accreta, increta, and percreta are an important cause of ante-partum hemorrhage and may contribute to up to 50%. Other possible causes of antepartum hemorrhage include cervical ectropion, infection, genital tract malignancy, vulvo-vaginal varicosities, trauma, and hematological disorders. Antepartum hemorrhage is a known sequela from domestic violence.

Management

As antepartum hemorrhage can cause significant mortality and morbidity to both mother and fetus, timely assessment of maternal and fetal condition is essential. It is vital to manage significant hemorrhage promptly with maternal resuscitation to manage the subsequent hypovolemic shock. This can be complicated by severe anemia, acute kidney injury, disseminated intravascular consumptive coagulopathy, sepsis and complications from blood transfusions such as transfusion reactions and transfusion related lung injury. Antepartum hemorrhage is often followed by significant postpartum hemorrhage; therefore active measures should be taken to reduce this.

In the presence of antepartum hemorrhage, fetal mortality and morbidity is related to prematurity, intra-uterine growth restriction, anemia, and hypoxia.

A Kleihauer test can be carried out in Rhesus negative patient to quantify the feto-maternal hemorrhage. It is not a sensitive test to diagnose placental abruption [1].

CLINICAL SCENARIO 1

A 37-year-old woman at 26 weeks gestation in her fourth pregnancy presents with a history of painless vaginal bleeding after intercourse. Her previous pregnancy was complicated by a cesarean section for fetal distress three years previously. The other two pregnancies were uncomplicated vaginal deliveries.

She had a normal dating scan at 11 weeks followed by a structurally normal anomaly scan at 20 weeks. However, at this scan the placenta was reported to be anterior partially covering the internal cervical os.

On assessment her pulse rate was 78 bpm, blood pressure of 125/88 mmHg and she was afebrile. Abdominal examination revealed a gravid uterus with symphysis fundal height of 30 cm, a fetus in transverse lie, fetal heart activity was present and irregular uterine activity felt. Speculum examination revealed a closed cervical os with a small amount of fresh bleeding.

Clinical questions

1. What is the prevalence of placenta previa?

Placenta previa is diagnosed when the placenta is implanted into the lower segment of the uterus, close to (placenta previa minor) or covering the internal os of the cervix (placenta previa major), diagnosed on ultrasound.

Evidence-Based Obstetrics and Gynecology, First Edition. Edited by Errol R. Norwitz, Carolyn M. Zelop, David A. Miller, and David L. Keefe.

The overall prevalence rate of placenta previa was shown to be 4 per 1000 births [6]. Previous C-section as a consistently described risk factor for placenta previa, accreta, and abruption [7].

A retrospective cohort study between 2000 and 2009 showed a twofold increase in rates of placenta previa in first pregnancies delivered by C-section (8.7 per 1000 births) compared to women with vaginal first deliveries (4.4 per 1000 births). By adjusting for the effect of previous C-section and placenta previa rate in England, this meta-analysis showed that 359 primiparous deliveries by C-section would result in one additional case of placenta previa in subsequent pregnancies [8].

A systematic review and random-effects meta-analysis showed an overall worldwide prevalence of placenta previa of 5.2 per 1000 pregnancies (95% CI 4.5–5.9). Increased prevalence was seen in Asian studies (12.2 per 1000 pregnancies 95% CI 9.5–15.2) compared to, North America (2.9 per 100 pregnancies, 95% CI 2.3–3.5), European studies (3.6 per 1000 pregnancies, 95% CI 2.8–4.6) and Sub-Saharan Africa (2.7 per 1000 pregnancies; 95% CI: 0.3–11.0) suggesting some variation in prevalence by region but it is unclear if this is due to genetic or ethnic differences or other unknown factors [9].

2. What is the accuracy of ultrasound in the diagnosis of low lying placenta?

Traditionally placenta previa was diagnosed as a result of painless bleeding or fetal malpresentation in later pregnancy, however placental localization is now possible through routine ultrasound in the ante-natal period [10].

Concerns regarding the accuracy of transabdominal ultrasound (TAS) have been raised in cases of maternal obesity, overfilling of maternal bladder, difficulty identifying the lower edge of the [11]. Posterior placentas, under-filling the bladder and interference of the fetal head have also been cited as possible causes for inaccuracy on TAS [12].

Transvaginal ultrasound (TVS) has been shown to be superior to the transabdominal route [13, 14]. It is accurate for diagnosing a low-lying placenta but also can be used to measure the distance between the placental edge and cervical os in the second and third trimester. Therefore TVS can be used to assess the persistence of placenta previa at term [15].

The location of the placenta is identified at the routine anomaly scan (TAS) in the second trimester. If the placenta is found to be low lying, a TVS should be performed, as this may reclassify 26–60% of cases reducing the need for third trimester scanning [16].

Magnetic resonance imaging (MRI) has been shown to be useful to provide further information in cases of uncertainty when placenta accreta is suspected [17]. MRI may provide more detailed information in the degree of placenta previa when compared to ultrasound but there is no difference in placental localization [18].

3. How safe is trans-vaginal scan in the diagnosis of placenta previa?

Several studies have shown that trans-vaginal scanning has no increased risk of hemorrhage in cases of placenta previa [13, 19–22].

Several of these also showed trans-vaginal scanning to be superior to trans-abdominal scanning in correctly identifying placenta previa [13, 19] with one study showing the accuracy of diagnosis of 92.8% for the trans-vaginal route compared with 75.7% for trans-abdominal method [22].

Trans-vaginal scanning in the second trimester is deemed safe and important to gain more information about a low lying placenta [16].

4. What is a rising placenta?

The phenomenon of a "rising placenta" is due to the formation of the lower segment from around 28th week of pregnancy which displaces the placenta upwards. Thus, a low lying placenta may be diagnosed in about 5% of women at 16–18 weeks, but placenta previa is found at delivery in only 10% of the 5% (0.05% overall) as the placenta "rises" with the formation of the lower segment and growth of upper segment [10]. Recent evidence suggests that 96% of cases of low-lying placenta diagnosed between 16 and 24 weeks had resolved by 36 weeks [23]. However partial or total placenta previa is more likely to persist at term [24].

This phenomenon is more pronounced when the placenta is anterior compared to posterior due to the relative growth of the anterior lower segment. Placental migration has been reported to be less probable in cases of posterior placenta. A mean rate of migration with anterior placenta previa is 2.6 mm per week, compared to 1.6 mm per week in the posterior placenta previa [25].

Placental migration is also less probable in cases where it existed with a previous scar. A previous C-section delivery was an independent risk factor for persistent previa in women diagnosed with previa in the second trimester, $P < 0.05$ [26].

5. What happens if the placenta is covering the internal os at anomaly scan (18–24 weeks)?

Evidence suggests that if the placenta is found to be covering the internal os more than 2 cm at the anomaly scan, then adequate "migration" away from the os to enable a vaginal delivery is unlikely. Several studies have shown lower migration rates in these cases [26]. Follow up scans for placental position is therefore recommended.

It has been suggested that the initial position of placental edge relative to the internal os at 26 weeks along with rate of migration can be used to predict mode of delivery, with cases where the placental edge overlaps the internal os by more than 20 mm resulting in C-section [15]. However, it was also found that if the placenta covers the internal os by 10 mm or more when scanned between 15 and 24 weeks' gestation, those patients were at risk of placenta previa at delivery with 100% sensitivity and 85% specificity (positive predictive value 38), [27]. As placental migration is less likely in the presence of a uterine scar, therefore risk factors for placental invasion such as previous uterine surgery/trauma should be considered. In these cases, further imaging could be considered to identify possible placenta accreta/increta/percreta which would alter management of delivery. A large systematic review found ultrasound to have high specificity and sensitivity to diagnose invasion (sensitivity, 90.72 (95% CI, 87.2–93.6)%; specificity, 96.94 (95% CI, 96.3–97.5)%; especially when color Doppler is used (sensitivity, 90.74 (95% CI, 85.2–94.7)%; specificity, 87.68 (95% CI, 84.6–90.4)% [28].

There is inadequate data on which to base the most appropriate dates for follow up scanning in cases of low lying placenta. The Royal College of Obstetricians and Gynaecologist (RCOG) in the UK recommend follow up scanning at 32 weeks if major placenta previa or accreta is suspected at the 20/40 anomaly scan and the women remains asymptomatic. In cases of symptomatic placenta previa minor, a follow-up scan at 36 weeks will aid decisions on mode of delivery [16, 29]. However in cases of ante-partum hemorrhage, appropriate management should be based on the clinical situation.

Placental localization scans in women who have had a previous C-section of uterine surgery are recommended [30]. MRI can be used to further characterize placental implantation disorders, however sensitivity and specificity have been reported to be similar to ultrasound. MRI has been shown to have good predictive accuracy for diagnosis with high predictive accuracy for assessment of depth and topography, with no difference identified in diagnosis in sensitivity ($P = 0.24$) or the specificity ($P = 0.91$) between ultrasound and MRI was identified [31].

6. Is there a role of tocolysis in the management of bleeding placenta previa?

Tocolysis is when drugs are given in order to stop labor with the aim of prolonging pregnancy. There is a growing body of evidence for their use in bleeding placenta previa.

Significant uterine activity has been observed in cases with bleeding placenta previa. The process of lower segment growth and development is associated with potential placental separation and triggering uterine activity. It has been reported that 40% of cases of placenta previa were associated with spontaneous rupture of membranes, spontaneous labor or other problems leading to delivery before 37 weeks [32].

It is conventionally believed that uterine contractions may help containing the ongoing bleed, by compressing bleeding vessels at the placental bed. However, a number of reports suggested beneficial effect of tocolysis in management of bleeding placenta previa including prolongation of pregnancy.

The use of tocolysis in the management of bleeding placenta previa theoretically can be beneficial.

One of the potential benefits to prolong pregnancy is to allow time to give corticosteroids to enhance fetal lung maturity. Cochrane systematic review supports their use e to reduce potential problems related to prematurity including respiratory distress syndrome, intra-ventricular hemorrhage, necrotizing enterocolitis, and systemic infection [33].

In the only small randomized controlled trial of 60 patients with symptomatic placenta previa between 28 and 34 weeks of gestation, tocolysis with ritodrine for 7 days was compared to no treatment. Treatment was associated with prolongation of pregnancy (25.33 ± 17.7 days compared with 14.47 ± 20.33 days, $P < 0.05$) and an increased birth weight (2.27 ± 0.59 kg compared with 1.95 ± 0.55 kg). No difference in maternal complications were shown, and particularly no increased incidence of bleeding, no difference in total blood loss or number of blood transfusions found [34]. However ritodrine has known potential cardiovascular risks including tachycardia and palpitation and both are non-desirable with patients suffering from bleeding related hypotension.

Retrospective analysis shows that in preterm labor with placenta previa, tocolysis can reduce preterm delivery rates, improve birthweights, especially when long term maintenance drugs (terbutaline) compared to short term drugs (magnesium sulfate). There was no observed statistical difference in incidence of recurrent bleeding, interval from admission to first recurrent bleeding, and need for blood transfusion [35].

When tocolysis was used to prolong pregnancy in women with abruption and placenta previa, there were no adverse maternal or fetal effects reported, with no increase in fetal distress or need for transfusion [36].

Although there are no known added risks reported with the available studies there is no clear evidence on the benefit gained. Therefore, there is currently not enough good evidence to support the use of tocolytics to improve perinatal outcome in cases of bleeding placenta previa. A review of the evidence (one randomized control trial and two retrospective studies) in 2011 suggested that if tocolytics are used, their use should be restricted to 48 hours [37]. More studies and trials are needed to back up or refute the potential benefits of tocolytics in the management of placenta previa.

7. What is the place of home management in the care of women with major placenta previa?

Traditionally patients with major placenta previa were hospitalized until delivery [38] aiming to prolong pregnancy to 37 weeks and to manage complications in a timely fashion. More recently, long hospital admissions have been shown to have social, psychological, financial, and domestic implications on a woman and her family [3]. The notion of home care was brought to discussion following a retrospective analysis. The study involved 15 930 patients including 58 with placenta previa and concluded that "in the majority of cases with or without bleeding and irrespective of the degree of previa out-patient management would appear safe and effective" [39].

It has been shown that in cases of symptomatic placenta previa major early delivery, by C-section, of lower birth-weight babies requiring neonatal unit admission were more likely outcomes compared to those who were asymptomatic. Therefore out-patient management can be appropriate and the number of bleeds rather than the degree of placenta previa should be considered with more caution [40].

The Cochrane systematic review on interventions for suspected placenta previa included one randomized control trial showing reduction in hospital stay for those managed as out-patients with no difference in neonatal morbidity [41].

It may also be important to consider cost implications of inpatient treatment. A retrospective analysis showed no difference in maternal or fetal morbidity by reduced inpatient stay and therefore cost for mothers and mother–infant pairs [42].

In conclusion, home or hospital management can be appropriate and it may be best to consider each individual case. During outpatient management the patient should be able to directly access the hospital if they become symptomatic in any way. International opinion agrees on the recommendation that women at risk of major obstetric hemorrhage should remain close to a hospital able to manage this emergency for the third trimester of pregnancy [16].

8. At what gestation should delivery be planned, and at what gestation should it occur?

A large systematic review showed the preterm delivery rates for low-lying/marginal placenta (26.9%), placenta previa (43.5%), and increased risk for preterm delivery in patients with placenta previa (risk ratio [RR], 5.32; 95% confidence interval [CI], 4.39–6.45). This prematurity can lead to significant morbidity and mortality. This review also showed increased risk of NICU admissions (RR, 4.09; 95% CI, 2.80–5.97), neonatal death (RR, 5.44; 95% CI, 3.03–9.78), and perinatal death (RR, 3.01; 95% CI, 1.41–6.43) with placenta previa [43].

To reduce risk of respiratory distress and need for prolonged neonatal unit support, corticosteroids are routinely administered to those electively delivered before 38 weeks [33].

The care bundle working group [29] looked at over 1000 cases of placenta previa over 10 years and found that it is rare for delivery to be required prior to 32 weeks but around 40% will be delivered as an emergency before 38 weeks' gestation. This is in general agreement with previous data [39].

Individualized patient care is likely to be appropriate in those cases where prediction of onset of labor is difficult. In patients with uncomplicated placenta previa the general consensus is to aim for delivery between 38 and 39 weeks as a balance between neonatal respiratory morbidity and risks of heavy bleeding.

9. Can women with pregnancies complicated by placenta previa aim for a vaginal birth?

Currently there is not enough good quality data from large scale studies which consider mode of delivery with associated outcomes of maternal and neonatal morbidity where the placenta lies <20 mm away from the internal os, therefore this is the cut off which is generally used when counseling women regarding mode of delivery in placenta previa.

Women with placenta previa are at higher risk of post-partum hemorrhage, blood transfusion, and hysterectomy [44].

A vaginal birth can be considered when the placental edge – os distance is >2 cm and the placenta described as low lying, but delivery should be by elective C-section if the distance is <1 cm or less [45].

Various small studies looking at rate of vaginal delivery in cases where placenta-os distance of 11–20 mm concluded that the rate of vaginal birth varied between 36% and 76.5% [46–48].

It has been suggested that other factors such as the thickness of the lower edge of the placenta and the position (anterior or posterior) may also affect clinical outcome. A small study was the first to show that women with thicker leading edge (>1 cm) of placenta are more likely to have a cesarean section ($P = 0.02$), hysterectomy or severe hemorrhage than those with a thinner placental edge [49].

Therefore these factors may be considered, in addition to the clinical situation, maternal preferences and resources when deciding the optimal mode of delivery.

10. How would the management plan differ in cases of suspected placenta previa accreta, increta, or percreta?

A morbidly adherent placenta is a low lying placenta that invades into or through the myometrium. This is further defined by the depth of placental invasion: accreta invades the myometrium (80% of cases), increta invades deeply through the full thickness of the uterus (15%) and a percreta invades through the uterus to the serosal layer, sometimes with associated invasion into the bladder and other structures within the pelvis (5%).

It is most likely to occur when the decidua basalis is deficient, therefore predisposing factors include infection, previous surgery, including cesarean section.

It is the leading cause for intrapartum hysterectomy and often associated with significant morbidity. The risk of hysterectomy with placenta previa and uterine scar is 10% but with placenta previa accreta it is 66% [50]. There is an increased risk of preterm labor, and perinatal morbidity and mortality in those diagnosed with major placenta previa or accreta [51].

The management of placenta previa accreta incorporates pre-delivery planning, intrapartum multidisciplinary management and post-partum intensive care support. Establishing diagnosis early in pregnancy allows for adequate multidisciplinary based care and planning for delivery. There are no randomized controlled trials found on management of placenta previa accreta. Most studies are observational and of small numbers.

Raised index of suspicion with those at increased risk including advanced maternal age and previous scarring, may improve early detection rate. Antenatal diagnosis can reduce estimated blood loss and transfusion requirements [52].

Ultrasound was found to be highly accurate, especially when combined with color Doppler for diagnosis of invasive placentation in high-risk women [28].

MRI has also been found to be very accurate in diagnosing placental invasion for both depth and topography [31]. Both ultrasound and MRI have high specificity and sensitivity indicating that either mode of imaging can be appropriate in further characterization of placental site and invasion [31, 53].

A large prospective observation cohort study of 30 132 women undergoing C-section before labor (evidence level II) showed serious maternal morbidity (such as surgical complications, admission to intensive care unit (ICU) and hysterectomy) with increasing and subsequent deliveries by C-section. The risk of placenta accreta in placenta previa was 3%, 11%, 40%, 61%, and 67% for first, second, third, fourth, and fifth or more repeat cesarean deliveries, respectively. Hysterectomy was required in 0.65% first, 0.42% second, 0.90% third, 2.41% fourth, 3.49% fifth, and 8.99% sixth or more cesarean deliveries. Therefore it is suggested that counseling before a primary elective C-section includes discussion over future family planning/number of desired pregnancies [54].

In the UK, to optimize clinical management, a care bundle has been recommended and tested for placenta previa after previous cesarean section. This includes six main criteria: multidisciplinary involvement in preoperative planning; consultant obstetrician planning and directly supervising delivery; consultant anesthetist planning and directly supervising anesthetic at delivery; blood and blood products available on site; discussion and consent including possible intervention (hysterectomy, leaving the placenta in situ, cell salvage, and intervention radiology); and high dependency care availability [29].

This care bundle was tested in a pilot study and was found easy to use, whilst encouraging multi-disciplinary planning and prompting senior input [55].

The American College of Obstetricians and Gynaecologist (ACOG) also recommends individualized delivery planning including decisions regarding most appropriate surgical management. It generally recommends cesarean hysterectomy with placenta left in situ, but in individual cases where fertility preservation is preferred other options may be considered such as leaving the placenta in situ or partial resection of the placenta. However, further management, including hysterectomy may be required after the C-section, therefore this should be considered and discussed with the patient before delivery [56].

Conclusion

Clinical history and assessment suggests a diagnosis of placenta previa in the presence of ante-partum hemorrhage and uterine activity at 26 weeks gestation. Hemodynamic stability of the mother is imperative, followed by close monitoring of fetal heartbeat on the cardiotocograph. Preparations for delivery by C-section should be made including corticosteroids for fetal lung maturity and tocolysis could be considered after discussion with a senior obstetrician. However if bleeding and uterine activity settle and there is no fetal distress, a conservative approach can be considered with further imaging such as TVS or MRI at a later gestation.

CLINICAL SCENARIO 2

A 19-year-old primigravida presented at 36 weeks with sudden onset severe abdominal pain and mild vaginal bleeding.

She booked late in pregnancy with no early pregnancy dating ultrasound. No structural abnormality was identified at the 21-week anomaly scan, the placenta was reported to be anterior high and clear of the internal cervical os. Her hospital records revealed repeated concerns with domestic violence and history of cocaine misuse.

On assessment her pulse rate was 125 bpm, blood pressure of 105/58 mmHg and she was afebrile. Abdominal examination revealed a gravid uterus with SFH of 36 cm, fetal parts were difficult to palpate, fetal heart activity was absent, abdominal wall was tense and uterine activity felt. Ultrasound study to confirm absent fetal heart activity also revealed a suspicious looking placenta and skin overlying was very tender to touch. Speculum examination revealed a 2 cm dilated cervical os with fresh bleeding.

Clinical questions

1. How can placental abruption be predicted?

Placental abruption is premature separation of the placenta from the uterine wall, ranging from a marginal to complete abruption, before or during labor. Risk factors include smoking, advanced or young maternal age, drug misuse (especially cocaine and amphetamine) hypertension, pre-eclampsia, and preterm premature rupture of membranes [57].

However it has been reported that up to 70% of cases of abruption occur in low risk women and cannot be predicted from maternal reproductive risk factors [56]. Abruption may or may not be associated with vaginal bleeding as can be revealed or concealed. Therefore the extent of vaginal bleeding may not be directly in proportion to the extent of abruption. It is a critical diagnosis to consider if a woman presents with constant pain associated with a tense "woody" abdomen and with or without uterine activity. She may become hemodynamically unstable. It is likely there will be fetal distress.

Up to 1% of pregnancies are complicated by placental abruption, and it is an important cause of perinatal mortality and morbidity [57]. The etiology behind placental abruption is unclear, although most cases can be explained by vascular, inflammatory, or immunological factors [58]. A previous placental abruption is the most accurate predictor of a subsequent abruption; therefore such a history should be considered in future ante-natal care [58].

A large Norwegian study found that a woman has a 3.8% risk (adjusted OR = 11.5, 95% CI = 9.1–14.6) of a severe abruption in a subsequent pregnancy that follows one with a severe abruption, and severe abruption resulted in a twofold risk in sisters [59]. A meta-analysis showed that a subsequent placental abruption is 10 times more likely after a previous pregnancy with an abruption and is three times more likely when there is preterm rupture of membranes (PROM) or essential hypertension, [60]. Pre-eclampsia, major multiparity have been shown to be independent risk factors for placental abruption [61, 62] along with velamentous umbilical cord insertion, cigarette smoking, previous fetal death, maternal age of over 35 years, and previous miscarriage [61].

Association between cocaine abuse and placental associated syndromes such as placental abruption, infarction, and pre-eclampsia has been shown. These placental disorders are 58% more likely in those who abused cocaine, with the highest odds for placental abruption (OR = 2.79, 95% CI: 2.19, 3.55) [63].

Placental abruption is difficult to predict, with prediction models tested and shown to have poor sensitivity of 12% [64].

2. How can it be prevented?

Although the cause of placental abruption is often unclear, some lifestyle changes may contribute to its prevention such as those suggested in a Cochrane review including smoking cessation and preventing or avoiding drug misuse [65].

A large epidemiological study showed that smokers were twice as likely to have placental abruption than non-smokers (RR = 2.05, 95% CI 1.75–2.40) with no evidence of increasing likelihood of placental disorders with increasing number of cigarettes smoked. However there was no association of smoking and uterine bleeding of unknown cause [66].

It has been proposed that smoking causes placental problems due to vasoconstriction with resulting decrease in uterine blood flow but also carbon monoxide, nicotine, and cyanide accumulation which can be prevented by cessation of smoking [67].

Low dose aspirin has raised risk of harm with respect to placental abruption [68].

There is conflicting evidence over the use of low molecular weight heparin to reduce maternal morbidity related to placental abruption and other complications associated with the placenta.

Low molecular weight heparin may play a role in reducing placental abruption in addition to other placenta related outcomes such as pre-eclampsia, fetal growth restriction and stillbirth [69].

It may be especially useful in reducing placenta-mediated pregnancy complications in those who had experienced them before, making it a useful intervention in those who have already been identified as being at risk [70]. However, there is conflicting evidence which suggests it does not reduce complications [71]. Therefore, further evidence is needed in this area in order to guide practice appropriately.

3. When should delivery occur?

Placental abruption can range from a marginal bleed with a normal continuous cardiotocography (CTG) to a massive hemorrhage with an intrauterine death. The main principles of management include immediate resuscitation in order to achieve hemodynamic stability and active initiation of labor. Any delay in management may lead to further abruption, bleeding, and hemodynamic instability. This is because the accumulating clot can be a self-extending process causing more separation and more hemorrhage. In cases of extensive concealed abruption blood can infiltrate the myometrium.

There is no evidence from trials to demonstrate the best management in placental abruption, therefore management decisions must be based on knowledge derived from other sources [65].

Thus appropriate management depends on the clinical condition of the mother and fetus. If the mother is hemodynamically unstable then resuscitation of the mother should be priority. If the mother is stable but there is evidence of fetal distress (and good fetal outcome expected) then delivery should be expedited appropriately.

Abruption involving >50% of the placenta is often associated with intra-uterine death [58]. In cases of fetal death, in most cases it is more appropriate to aim for a vaginal delivery [1, 65] however if a woman has previously had a C-section the risks and benefits of induction of labor should be considered [72]. Vaginal birth may be appropriate if the mother is hemodynamically stable but C-section can be considered in where there is maternal compromise. There is increased risk of hemorrhage with placental abruption and this should be considered in the ante-natal, intrapartum, and post-partum period. In the presence of intra-uterine death, there is an increased risk of disseminated intravascular coagulation requiring vigorous management with appropriate blood components [57].

In cases of fetal death as a result of placental abruption, a decision regarding mode of delivery should be made on the clinical situation, the mother's previous history and her wishes.

4. What's the place of expectant management for indeterminate/unexplained ante-partum hemorrhage?

There may be a place for expectant management for unexplained ante-partum hemorrhage is the patient is hemodynamically stable with no signs of fetal distress. One advantage to expectant management could be to allow time for further investigation such as further imaging which may change management.

Ultrasound may be useful in cases when diagnosis is not certain, but only if this does not delay management [62].

In women who were scanned within 14 days of delivery, ultrasound has been shown to have low sensitivity (24%) but high specificity (96%) for placental abruption, with a positive predictive value of 88% and a negative predictive value of 53%. This suggests ultrasound is not sensitive for diagnosing placental abruption and diagnosis using ultrasound leads to more aggressive treatment and worse neonatal outcome [73].

MRI may become a helpful tool in aiding diagnosis of unexplained ante-partum hemorrhage [74] and can be superior to ultrasound [75].

However further studies are needed to further clarify the role of imaging in expectant management in unexplained ante-partum hemorrhage.

Conclusion

Placental abruption is difficult to predict and is largely unpreventable. The priority is to have high index of suspicion, address maternal hemodynamic instability, followed by appropriate delivery of the fetus, appropriate bereavement services and counseling for future pregnancy with the appropriate ante-natal care should be considered.

CLINICAL SCENARIO 3

A 28-year-old primigravida presented at 34 weeks with lower abdominal pain and mild watery vaginal loss. No structural abnormality was identified at 21-week anomaly scan, the placenta was reported to be anterior and low lying. At 34 weeks a TAS was carried out for suspected small for gestational age pregnancy. The fetal growth was on the 15th centile and the placenta was anterior and 25 mm away from the internal os, amniotic fluid volume lower than normal for gestation.

On assessment her pulse rate was 86 bpm, blood pressure of 110/78 mmHg and she was afebrile. Abdominal examination revealed a gravid uterus with SFH of 36 cm, fetal heart activity was present, irregular uterine activities were felt. Speculum examination was inconclusive. The history was strongly suggestive of spontaneous rupture of membranes. She was admitted and received a course of corticosteroids. The next day her vaginal loss increased and was becoming progressively blood stained. She was transferred to the delivery suite for induction of labor. Fetal heart monitoring was normal. Six hours into the induction process she was assessed and artificial rupture of membranes was carried out.

The vaginal loss was grossly blood stained, the fetal monitoring trace showed sinusoidal pattern, therefore the decision was made for immediate delivery by cesarean section.

Clinical questions

1. How can vasa previa be predicted?

Vasa previa is where fetal vessels which are unprotected by placenta or umbilical cord, run through the membranes over the internal cervical os, below the fetal presenting part [76–78].

Vasa previa conveys no major maternal risk but there is significant risk to the fetus. This is because the unprotected fetal vessels are at risk of disruption leading to fetal hemorrhage and subsequent demise. It has been suggested that fetal mortality rate is as high as at least 56% from fetal exsanguinations [78]. There is also an increased risk of preterm delivery (81.9%, RR, 3.36; 95% CI, 2.76–4.09) with an increased perinatal death rate (RR, 4.52; 95% CI, 2.77–7.39) [16].

Hemorrhage often occurs at the time of rupture of membranes, therefore a diagnosis of vasa previa should always be considered in cases of per vaginal bleeding with fetal distress after artificial or spontaneous rupture of membranes. The incidence of vasa previa is generally estimated to be between one in 2000 and one in 6000 pregnancies [78]. However, one prospective study of first trimester ultrasound findings showed the incidence to be as high as one in 365 pregnancies [78].

Reported risk factors also include *in vitro* fertilization, fetal abnormalities mainly renal tract abnormalities and spina bifida and a low lying placenta in the second trimester [79].

A multicenter study found that survival rates in vasa previa are much higher when diagnosis is made antenatally (97% compared to 44% in 61 cases, $P < 0.001$). Regression analysis showed that ante-natal diagnosis ($P < 0.001$) and gestational age ($P = 0.01$) were the only significant predictors of neonatal survival [80].

As the hemorrhage occurs after membrane rupture, delivery should be by planned elective C-section prior to labor, often after hospitalization after 32 weeks with administration of steroids for fetal lung maturity [12].

2. How can diagnosis be made?

The diagnosis is often a clinical one, and is often made after an episode of ante-partum hemorrhage after rupture of membranes although bleeding can occur without membrane rupture. However there may be signs of fetal distress requiring delivery by emergency C-section without hemorrhage likely due to compression of fetal vessel overlying the cervix after rupture of membranes [81]. Antenatal ultrasound can be used to diagnose vasa previa. The ultrasound appearance of vasa previa is of linear or circular echolucent structures near or overlying the cervix [82].

Although women routinely undergo identification of placental site on routine ultrasound screening for vasa previa is currently not recommended by the RCOG. This is due to lack of knowledge of the epidemiology and natural history, along with limitations of identification and issues surrounding TVS training in the UK [1]. However a guideline for the management of vasa previa has been published in Canada suggesting that further evaluation for placental cord insertion should be considered in those cases of low lying placenta as neonatal survival rates increase from 44% to 97% when diagnosed antenatally [12]. The case for screening for vasa previa has been presented on the basis of high fetal mortality when diagnosed, ability for and availability of appropriate antenatal ultrasound scan (USS) screening and diagnosis along with suitable management option of elective C-section [83].

A low lying placenta is a known risk factor for vasa previa. Vasa previa is known to be associated with velamentous cord insertion and or fetal vessels running between accessory lobes. It has been found that using ultrasound to confirm the position of placental cord insertion including velamentous cord and those in the lower uterine segment is a useful way to detect vasa previa [84].

A systematic review showed trans-vaginal ultrasound with color Doppler has high accuracy for the diagnosis of vasa previa [85].

It has been found that low insertion of the cord can be identified at 9–13 weeks gestation and may be a useful method of detecting vasa previa [86].

Therefore, if a low lying placenta is identified at the routine 20/40 anomaly scan, the position of cord insertion should be evaluated further which can be done safely with transvaginal scanning (with color Dopplers) [12].

It has been suggested that diagnosis of vasa previa is best considered during the second trimester scanning [87]. There may be a role of MRI in further characterizing placental structures where it is unclear on transvaginal ultrasound scan (TVUSS) [88].

Conclusion

Vasa previa is difficult to predict and diagnose. When a low lying placenta is seen during anomaly scanning, further trans-vaginal scanning should take place to further characterize the placenta. The diagnosis of vasa previa should be considered in any woman with bleeding with rupture of membranes, and once diagnosed, delivery should be expedited by emergency C-section.

References

1 Royal College of Obstetricians and Gynaecologists (2011). *Antepartum Haemorrhage. Green-Top Guideline No. 63*. London: RCOG.

2 Say, L., Chou, D., Gemmill, A. et al. (2014). Global causes of maternal death: a WHO systematic analysis. *The Lancet Global Health* **2** (**6**): e323–e333.

3 Sinha, P. and Kuruba, N. (2008). Ante-partum haemorrhage: an update. *Journal of Obstetrics and Gynaecology* **28** (**4**): 377–381.

4 Altvorst, M.E.W.A., Chan, E.H.Y., Taylor, R.S. et al. (2011). Antepartum haemorrhage of unknown origin and maternal cigarette smoking beyond the first trimester. *Australian and New Zealand Journal of Obstetrics and Gynaecology* **52** (**2**): 161–166.

5 Bhandari, S., Raja, E., Shetty, A., and Bhattacharya, S. (2013). Maternal and perinatal consequences of antepartum haemorrhage of unknown origin. *BJOG: An International Journal of Obstetrics and Gynaecology* **121** (**1**): 44–52.

6 Faiz, A.S. and Ananth, C.V. (2003). Etiology and risk factors for placenta previa: an overview and meta-analysis of observational studies. *The Journal of Maternal-Fetal and Neonatal Medicine* **13** (**3**): 175–190.

7 Klar, M. and Michels, K.B. (2014). Cesarean section and placental disorders in subsequent pregnancies – a meta-analysis. *Journal of Perinatal Medicine* **42** (**5**).

8 Gurol-Urganci, I., Cromwell, D.A., Edozien, L.C. et al. (2011). Risk of placenta previa in second birth after first birth cesarean section: a population-based study and meta-analysis. *BMC Pregnancy and Childbirth* **11**: 95.

9 Cresswell, J.A., Ronsmans, C., Calvert, C., and Filippi, V. (2013). Prevalence of placenta praevia by world region: a systematic review and meta-analysis. *Tropical Medicine and International Health* **18** (**6**): 712–724.

10 Neilson, J.P. (2003). Interventions for suspected placenta praevia. *Cochrane Database of Systematic Reviews* (**2**): CD001998. doi: 10.1002/14651858.CD001998.

11 Sunna, E. (1999). Transvaginal and transabdominal ultrasound for the diagnosis of placenta praevia. *Journal of Obstetrics and Gynaecology* **19** (**2**): 152–154.

12 Gagnon, R., Morin, L., Bly, S. et al. (2009). Guidelines for the management of vasa Previa. *Journal of Obstetrics and Gynaecology Canada* **31** (**8**): 748–753.

13 Farine, D., Fox, H.E., Jakobson, S., and Timor-Tritsch, I.E. (1988). Vaginal ultrasound for diagnosis of placenta previa. *American Journal of Obstetrics and Gynecology* [Internet]. Sep [cited 2016 Apr 26] **159** (**3**): 566–569.

14 Smith, R.S., Lauria, M.R., Comstock, C.H. et al. (1997). Transvaginal ultrasonography for all placentas that appear to be low-lying or over the internal cervical os. *Ultrasound in Obstetrics and Gynecology* **9** (**1**): 22–24.

15 Oppenheimer, L., Holmes, P., Simpson, N., and Dabrowski, A. (2001). Diagnosis of low-lying placenta: can migration in the

third trimester predict outcome? *Ultrasound in Obstetrics and Gynecology* **18** (**2**): 100–102.

16 Royal College of Obstetricians and Gynaecologists. Placenta Praevia, Placenta Praevia Accreta and Vasa Praevia: Diagnosis and Management). Greetntop Guideline No. 27.2011.

17 Maher, M.A., Abdelaziz, A., and Bazeed, M.F. (2013). Diagnostic accuracy of ultrasound and MRI in the prenatal diagnosis of placenta accreta. *Acta Obstetricia et Gynecologica Scandinavica* **92** (**9**): 1017–1022.

18 Powell, M.C., Buckley, J., Price, H. et al. (1986). Magnetic resonance imaging and placental previa. *American Journal of Obstetrics and Gynecology* **154** (**3**): 565–569.

19 Leerentveld, R.A., Gilberts, E.C.A.M., Arnold, M.J.C.W.J., and Wladimiroff, J.W. (1990). Accuracy and safety of transvaginal sonographic placental localization. *Obstetrics and Gynecology* **76** (**5**): 759–762.

20 Sherman, S.J., Carlson, D.E., Platt, L.D., and Medearis, A.L. (1992). Transvaginal ultrasound: does it help in the diagnosis of placenta previa? *Ultrasound in Obstetrics and Gynecology* **2** (**4**): 256–260.

21 Timor-Tritsch, I.E. and Yunis, R.A. (1993). Confirming the safety of transvaginal sonography in patients suspected of placenta previa. *Obstetrics and Gynecology* **81** (**5(Pt 1)**): 742–744.

22 Tan, N.H., Abu, M., Woo, J.L.S., and Tahir, H.M. (1995). The role of transvaginal sonography in the diagnosis of placenta praevia. *The Australian and New Zealand Journal of Obstetrics and Gynaecology* **35** (**1**): 42–45.

23 Heller, H.T., Mullen, K.M., Gordon, R.W. et al. (2014). Outcomes of pregnancies with a low-lying placenta diagnosed on second-trimester sonography. *Journal of Ultrasound in Medicine* **33** (**4**): 691–696.

24 Chama, C., Wanony, I.I., and Usman, J. (2004). From low-lying implantation to placenta praevia: a longitudinal ultrasonic assessment. *Journal of Obstetrics and Gynaecology* **24** (**5**): 516–518.

25 Cho, J.Y., Lee, Y.-H., Moon, M.H., and Lee, J.H. (2008). Difference in migration of placenta according to the location and type of placenta previa. *Journal of Clinical Ultrasound* **36** (**2**): 79–84.

26 Dashe, J.S., McIntire, D.D., Ramus, R.M. et al. (2002). Persistence of placenta previa according to gestational age at ultrasound detection. *Obstetrics and Gynecology* **99** (**5, Part 1**): 692–697.

27 Lauria, M.R., Smith, R.S., Treadwell, M.C. et al. (1996). The use of second-trimester transvaginal sonogmphy to predict placenta previa. *Ultrasound in Obstetrics and Gynecology* **8** (**5**): 337–340.

28 D'Antonio, F., Iacovella, C., and Bhide, A. (2013). Prenatal identification of invasive placentation using ultrasound: systematic review and meta-analysis. *Ultrasound in Obstetrics and Gynecology* **42** (**5**): 509–517.

29 RCOG and National Patient Safety Agency (2010). *Placenta Praevia After Caesarean Section Care Bundle: Background Information for Healthcare Professionals*. London: Royal College of Obstetricians and Gynecologists.

30 Lewis, G. (ed.) (2007). *Saving Mothers' Lives: reviewing maternal deaths to make motherhood safer – 2003–2005. The Seventh Report on Confidential Enquiries into Maternal Deaths in the United Kingdom. London*. CEMACH www.cmace.org.uk/Publications/CEMACH-Publications/Maternal-and-PerinatalHealth/Saving-Mothers--Lives-2003-2005_full.aspx. (accessed 10 July 2018).

31 D'Antonio, F., Iacovella, C., Palacios-Jaraquemada, J. et al. (2014). Prenatal identification of invasive placentation using magnetic resonance imaging: systematic review and meta-analysis. *Ultrasound in Obstetrics and Gynecology* **44** (**1**): 8–16.

32 Brenner, W.E., Edelman, D.A., and Hendricks, C.H. (1978). Characteristics of patients with placenta previa and results of 'expectant management'. *American Journal of Obstetrics and Gynecology* **132** (**2**): 180–191.

33 Roberts, D. and Dalziel, S.R. (2006). Antenatal corticosteroids for accelerating fetal lung maturation for women at risk of preterm birth. *Cochrane Database of Systematic Reviews* (**3**): CD004454. doi: 10.1002/14651858.CD004454.pub2.

34 Sharma, A., Suri, V., and Gupta, I. (2004). Tocolytic therapy in conservative management of symptomatic placenta previa. *International Journal of Gynecology and Obstetrics* **84** (**2**): 109–113.

35 Besinger, R.E., Moniak, C.W., Paskiewicz, L.S. et al. (1995). The effect of tocolytic use in the management of symptomatic placenta previa. *American Journal of Obstetrics and Gynecology* **172** (**6**): 1770–1778.

36 Towers, C.V., Pircon, R.A., and Heppard, M. (1999). Is tocolysis safe in the management of third-trimester bleeding? *American Journal of Obstetrics and Gynecology* **180** (**6**): 1572–1578.

37 Bose, D., Assel, B., Hill, J., and Chauhan, S. (2010). Maintenance tocolytics for preterm symptomatic placenta previa: a review. *American Journal of Perinatology* **28** (**01**): 045–050.

38 Macafee, C.H.G. (1945). Placenta praevia – a study of 174 cases. *BJOG: An International Journal of Obstetrics and Gynaecology* **52** (**4**): 313–324.

39 Love, C.D.B. and Wallace, E.M. (1996). Pregnancies complicated by placenta praevia: what is appropriate management? *BJOG : An International Journal of Obstetrics and Gynaecology* **103** (**9**): 864–867.

40 Love, C.D.B., Fernando, K.J., Sargent, L., and Hughes, R.G. (2004). Major placenta praevia should not preclude out-patient management. *European Journal of Obstetrics, Gynecology, and Reproductive Biology* **117** (**1**): 24–29.

41 Wing, D.A., Paul, R.H., and Millar, L.K. (1996). Management of the symptomatic placenta previa: a randomized, controlled trial of inpatient versus outpatient expectant management. *American Journal of Obstetrics and Gynecology* **175** (**4**): 806–811.

42 Droste, S. and Keil, K. (1994). Expectant management of placenta previa: cost-benefit analysis of outpatient treatment. *American Journal of Obstetrics and Gynecology* **170** (**5**): 1254–1257.

43 Vahanian, S.A., Lavery, J.A., Ananth, C.V., and Vintzileos, A. (2015). Placental implantation abnormalities and risk of preterm

delivery: a systematic review and metaanalysis. *American Journal of Obstetrics and Gynecology* **213** (**4**): S78–S90.

44 Onwere, C., Gurol-Urganci, I., Cromwell, D.A. et al. (2011). Maternal morbidity associated with placenta praevia among women who had elective caesarean section. *European Journal of Obstetrics, Gynecology, and Reproductive Biology* **159** (**1**): 62–66.

45 Bhide, A., Prefumo, F., Moore, J. et al. (2003). Placental edge to internal os distance in the late third trimester and mode of delivery in placenta praevia. *BJOG: An International Journal of Obstetrics and Gynaecology* **110** (**9**): 860–864.

46 Wortman, A.C., Twickler, D.M., McIntire, D.D., and Dashe, J.S. (2015). Bleeding complications in pregnancies with low-lying placenta. *The Journal of Maternal-Fetal and Neonatal Medicine* **29** (**9**): 1367–1371.

47 Al Wadi, K., Schneider, C., Burym, C. et al. (2014). Evaluating the safety of labour in women with a placental edge 11 to 20mm from the internal cervical os. *Journal of Obstetrics and Gynaecology Canada* **36** (**8**): 674–677.

48 Bronsteen, R., Valice, R., Lee, W. et al. (2009). Effect of a low-lying placenta on delivery outcome. *Ultrasound in Obstetrics and Gynecology* **33** (**2**): 204–208.

49 Ghourab, S. (2001). Third-trimester transvaginal ultrasonography in placenta previa: does the shape of the lower placental edge predict clinical outcome? *Ultrasound in Obstetrics and Gynecology* **18** (**2**): 103–108.

50 Chattopadhyay, S.K., Kharif, H., and Sherbeeni, M.M. (1993). Placenta praevia and accreta after previous caesarean section. *European Journal of Obstetrics, Gynecology, and Reproductive Biology* **52** (**3**): 151–156.

51 Zlatnik, M.G., Cheng, Y.W., Norton, M.E. et al. (2007). Placenta previa and the risk of preterm delivery. *The Journal of Maternal-Fetal and Neonatal Medicine* **20** (**10**): 719–723.

52 Tikkanen, M., Paavonen, J., Loukovaara, M., and Stefanovic, V. (2011). Antenatal diagnosis of placenta accreta leads to reduced blood loss. *Acta Obstetricia et Gynecologica Scandinavica* **90** (**10**): 1140–1146.

53 Meng, X., Xie, L., and Song, W. (2013). Comparing the diagnostic value of ultrasound and magnetic resonance imaging for placenta Accreta: a systematic review and meta-analysis. *Ultrasound in Medicine and Biology* **39** (**11**): 1958–1965.

54 Silver, R.M., Landon, M.B., Rouse, D.J. et al. (2006). Maternal morbidity associated with multiple repeat Cesarean deliveries. *Obstetrics and Gynecology* **107** (**6**): 1226–1232.

55 Paterson-Brown, S. and Singh, C. (2010). Developing a care bundle for the management of suspected placenta accreta. *The Obstetrician and Gynaecologist* **12** (**1**): 21–27.

56 The American College of Obstetricians and Gynaecologists (2012). Committee opinion no. 529. *Obstetrics and Gynecology* **120**: 207–211.

57 Oyelese, Y. and Ananth, C.V. (2006). Placental Abruption. *Obstetrics and Gynecology* **108** (**4**): 1005–1016.

58 Tikkanen, M. (2010). Etiology, clinical manifestations, and prediction of placental abruption. *Acta Obstetricia et Gynecologica Scandinavica* **89** (**6**): 732–740.

59 Rasmussen, S. and Irgens, L. (2009). Occurrence of placental abruption in relatives. *BJOG: An International Journal of Obstetrics and Gynaecology* **116** (**5**): 693–699.

60 Ananth, C., Savitz, D., and Williams, M. (1996). Placental abruption and its association with hypertension and prolonged rupture of membranes: a methodologic review and meta-analysis. *Obstetrics and Gynecology* **88** (**2**): 309–318.

61 Toivonen, S., Heinonen, S., Anttila, M. et al. (2002). Reproductive risk factors, Doppler findings, and outcome of affected births in placental abruption: a population-based analysis. *American Journal of Perinatology* **19** (**8**): 451–460.

62 Boisramé, T., Sananès, N., Fritz, G. et al. (2014). Placental abruption: risk factors, management and maternal–fetal prognosis. Cohort study over 10 years. *European Journal of Obstetrics, Gynecology, and Reproductive Biology* **179**: 100–104.

63 Mbah, A.K., Alio, A.P., Fombo, D.W. et al. (2012). Association between cocaine abuse in pregnancy and placenta-associated syndromes using propensity score matching approach. *Early Human Development* **88** (**6**): 333–337.

64 Odibo, A., Cahill, A., Stamilio, D. et al. (2007). Predicting placental abruption and Previa in women with a previous Cesarean delivery. *American Journal of Perinatology* **24** (**5**): 299–305.

65 Neilson, J.P. (2003). Interventions for treating placental abruption. *Cochrane Database of Systematic Reviews* (**1**): CD003247. doi: 10.1002/14651858.CD003247.

66 Ananth, C.V., Savitz, D.A., and Luther, E.R. (1996). Maternal cigarette smoking as a risk factor for placental abruption, placenta Previa, and uterine bleeding in pregnancy. *American Journal of Epidemiology* **144** (**9**): 881–889.

67 Phelan, S. (2014). Smoking cessation in pregnancy. *Obstetrics and Gynecology Clinics of North America* **41** (**2**): 255–266.

68 Xu, T., Zhou, F., Deng, C. et al. (2015). Low-dose aspirin for preventing preeclampsia and its complications: a meta-analysis. *The Journal of Clinical Hypertension* **17** (**7**): 567–573.

69 Duffett, L. and Rodger, M. (2014). LMWH to prevent placenta-mediated pregnancy complications: an update. *British Journal of Haematology* **168** (**5**): 619–638.

70 Rodger, M.A., Carrier, M., Le Gal, G. et al. (2013). Meta-analysis of low-molecular-weight heparin to prevent recurrent placenta-mediated pregnancy complications. *Blood* **123** (**6**): 822–828.

71 Rodger, M.A., Langlois, N.J., de Vries, J.I. et al. (2014). Low-molecular-weight heparin for prevention of placenta-mediated pregnancy complications: protocol for a systematic review and individual patient data meta-analysis (AFFIRM). *Systematic Reviews* **3** (**1**): 69.

72 Royal College of Obstetricians and Gynaecologists (2010). *Late Intrauterine Fetal Death and Stillbirth Green-Top Guideline No. 55.* London: RCOG.

73 Glantz, C. and Purnell, L. (2002). Clinical utility of Sonography in the diagnosis and treatment of placental abruption. *Journal of Ultrasound in Medicine* **21** (**8**): 837–840.

74 Masselli, G., Brunelli, R., Parasassi, T. et al. (2011). Magnetic resonance imaging of clinically stable late pregnancy bleeding: beyond ultrasound. *European Radiology* **21** (**9**): 1841–1849.

75 Masselli, G., Brunelli, R., Di Tola, M. et al. (2011). MR imaging in the evaluation of placental abruption: correlation with Sonographic findings. *Radiology* **259** (**1**): 222–230.

76 Oyelese, Y. and Smulian, J.C. (2006). Placenta Previa, Placenta Accreta, and vasa Previa. *Obstetrics and Gynecology* **108** (**3, Part 1**): 694.

77 Oyelese, K.O., Turner, M., Lees, C., and Campbell, S. (1999). Vasa Previa. *Obstetrical and Gynecological Survey* **54** (**2**): 138–145.

78 Hasegawa, J., Nakamura, M., Ichizuka, K. et al. (2012). Vasa previa is not infrequent. *The Journal of Maternal-Fetal and Neonatal Medicine* **25** (**12**): 2795–2796.

79 Baulies, S., Maiz, N., Muñoz, A. et al. (2007). Prenatal ultrasound diagnosis of vasa praevia and analysis of risk factors. *Prenatal Diagnosis* **27** (**7**): 595–599.

80 Oyelese, Y., Catanzarite, V., Prefumo, F. et al. (2004). Vasa previa: the impact of prenatal diagnosis on outcomes. *Obstetrics and Gynecology* **103** (**5, Part 1**): 937–942.

81 Cordero, D.R., Helfgott, A.W., Landy, H.J. et al. (1993). A non-hemorrhagic manifestation of vasa previa: a clinicopathologic case report. *Obstetrics and Gynecology* **82** (**4**): 698–700.

82 Lee, W., Lee, V.L., Kirk, J.S. et al. (2000). Vasa Previa. *Obstetrics and Gynecology* **95** (**4**): 572–576.

83 Atkinson, A. and Oyelese, Y. (2013). Vasa Previa: the case for routine screening. *Fetal and Maternal Medicine Review* **24** (**04**): 277–288.

84 Hasegawa, J., Farina, A., Nakamura, M. et al. (2010). Analysis of the ultrasonographic findings predictive of vasa previa. *Prenatal Diagnosis* **30** (**12–13**): 1121–1125.

85 Ruiter, L., Kok, N., Limpens, J. et al. (2015). Systematic review of accuracy of ultrasound in the diagnosis of vasa previa. *Ultrasound in Obstetrics and Gynecology* **45** (**5**): 516–522.

86 Hasegawa, J., Nakamura, M., Sekizawa, A. et al. (2011). Prediction of risk for vasa previa at 9–13 weeks' gestation. *Journal of Obstetrics and Gynaecology Research* **37** (**10**): 1346–1351.

87 Kanda, E., Matsuda, Y., Kamitomo, M. et al. (2011). Prenatal diagnosis and management of vasa previa: a 6-year review. *Journal of Obstetrics and Gynaecology Research* **37** (**10**): 1391–1396.

88 Kikuchi, A., Uemura, R., Serikawa, T. et al. (2010). Clinical significances of magnetic resonance imaging in prenatal diagnosis of vasa previa in a woman with bilobed placentas. *Journal of Obstetrics and Gynaecology Research* **37** (**1**): 75–78.

40 CHAPTER 40
Vaginal birth after cesarean delivery

Carolyn M. Zelop
Ultrasound and Perinatal Research, Division of MFM and Department of Obstetrics and Gynecology, The Valley Hospital, Ridgewood, NJ, USA
Department of Obstetrics and Gynecology, NYU School of Medicine, New York, NY, USA

Background

Controversy regarding the optimal mode of delivery has plagued the first decade of the new millennium. During this time period, the cesarean birth rate has skyrocketed to an unprecedented height close to 33%. Not only has the primary rate accelerated, but the repeat cesarean rate has risen while the vaginal birth after previous cesarean (VBAC) rate has plummeted to less than 10% [1].

New concerns regarding complications stemming from multiple uterine events mainly abnormal placentation leading to maternal hemorrhage and possible hysterectomy have rekindled an interest in Trial of Labor (TOL) after previous cesarean birth [1]. One major impediment to implementing a more liberal policy of TOL after previous cesarean is fear of uterine rupture. While this devastating complication occurs in roughly 1% of all TOL after previous cesarean birth, the maternal and neonatal morbidity and even mortality may be significant [2]. We now understand through clinical experience and epidemiological research that all TOLs are not alike. Ideally, the most appropriate candidates eligible for TOL after previous cesarean will have the highest chance of success and the lowest risk of uterine rupture. The purpose of this chapter is to explore the factors that have been suggested to alter the risk of uterine rupture during TOL after previous cesarean and analyze the quality of evidence surrounding each variable. When assessing the risk of uterine rupture during TOL after previous cesarean, factors to be considered include: obstetrical history, demographics, factors that impact the integrity of the scar, antepartum and intrapartum factors. Thorough evaluation of these risk factors will enable the patient and her provider to develop a care plan for choosing the optimal route of delivery given her history of prior cesarean birth.

Before considering the quality of evidence surrounding each factor, it is important to recognize that there are no randomized controlled trials comparing planned elective repeat cesarean versus planned TOL after previous cesarean birth. While the diversity and caliber of available literature is noteworthy, the limitations of non-randomized studies must be acknowledged since these studies cannot adjust for the inherent clinical insight required for each delivery plan formulated by the patient and her care provider. Additionally, studies that identify uterine rupture only by ICD-9/10 codes may be biased by misclassification of this important outcome variable and lead to overestimation of the association.

Embarking upon a discussion of uterine rupture requires a clarification of its definition since there have been some inconsistencies in the literature regarding uterine events. Uterine rupture as defined by the recent National Institute of Health (NIH) Consensus Development Conference entitled "Vaginal Birth After Cesarean: New Insights" is a complete anatomic separation of the uterine wall regardless of the presence of symptoms with or without extrusion of the fetal placental unit [3]. Another uterine event, uterine dehiscence is a partial or less severe variant with at least the serosa intact. While these entities should not be grouped together, some authorities view uterine dehiscence as a near miss. The true prevalence of uterine dehiscence is also difficult to ascertain since its asymptomatic nature may cause it to go unrecognized. In addition, uterine rupture, may not always involve the actual healed hysterotomy. Factors other than the integrity of the healed scar must also play a part in the mechanism of uterine rupture when the separation occurs in other locations remote from the previous hysterotomy.

Evidence-Based Obstetrics and Gynecology, First Edition. Edited by Errol R. Norwitz, Carolyn M. Zelop, David A. Miller, and David L. Keefe.

CLINICAL VIGNETTE

A 29-year-old Caucasian G3P2 presents for prenatal care in the first trimester. Her obstetrical history is remarkable for a term vaginal delivery followed by a cesarean birth two years later for a breech presentation after a failed version. She presents her operative report for your review which demonstrates a two layer closure of a low transverse vertical hysterotomy. She requests that you review with her at her next prenatal visit her delivery options including the possibility of TOL after previous cesarean birth. She particularly asks you address her risk of uterine rupture.

Critical review of the literature and clinical questions

1. What are the obstetrical history factors that influence uterine rupture?

Prior preterm cesarean birth

There are at least five studies [4–8] in the literature that assess the risk of uterine rupture associated with prior preterm cesarean birth and a subsequent TOL. Four are retrospective cohort or case control studies with variable sample sizes. The studies vary in the definition used for prior preterm delivery and the actual number of patients delivered at a particular prior preterm gestational age. The largest prospective observational study [8] controlling for multiple confounders affecting the rate of uterine rupture reported a minimally statistically significant increase risk for uterine rupture during a TOL with a prior preterm cesarean birth (Odds Ratio (OR) 1.6 95%CI (1.01–2.50); $p = 0.043$).

History of prior vaginal delivery

Two retrospective cohort studies [9, 10] in the literature focused upon the primary effect of previous vaginal delivery upon the risk of uterine rupture during a TOL after previous cesarean birth. Additionally, a large prospective observational trial [11] focused upon the effect of previous VBAC upon a subsequent TOL. De Lau et al. [12] performed a systematic review exploring the effect prior vaginal delivery upon this outcome, but they included data sets abstracted as subsets from manuscripts where prior vaginal delivery and uterine rupture were not the main thrust of the study. Their conclusion echoed the conclusions of the primary studies detailed here. Prior vaginal delivery significantly reduces the risk of uterine rupture even when it occurs prior to the index cesarean birth. Additionally, Mercer et al. [11] demonstrated that prior VBACs do not increase the risk of uterine rupture. In other words, the healed uterus does not appear to be more susceptible but rather less susceptible to subsequent pregnancies that test the integrity of the prior hysterotomy. Prior vaginal delivery, including VBAC also increases the success of TOL after previous cesarean.

2. What are the antepartum factors that influence the risk of uterine rupture?

Gestational age of current pregnancy

TOL beyond the estimated day of delivery (EDD)

The literature contains four retrospective cohort studies [13–16] that examine the effect of gestational age after the EDD and the risk of uterine rupture. All studies attempted to control for possible confounders that might affect the rate of uterine rupture during a TOL after previous cesarean especially for birth weight and induction of labor. The results are divergent; however, the studies vary by sample size. The two largest studies, Coassolo et al. [13] and Zelop et al. [14] do not demonstrate an increased rate of uterine rupture during a TOL after the EDD reporting a rate of 1.1–1.3 versus 0.8–1.0% in patients less than or equal to EDD. Post EDD TOL is less successful than a TOL prior to or at the EDD. Induction of labor, however, prior to or at the EDD does not improve the outcome.

Preterm TOL after previous cesarean

Survey of the literature reveals two retrospective cohort studies [16, 17] and one prospective observational study [18] in women with prior cesarean birth that demonstrate a decrease rate of uterine rupture and comparable or higher success rate of a TOL after previous cesarean during a preterm gestation in the current pregnancy.

Demographic variables

3. Does maternal age affect the risk of uterine rupture during a trial of labor after previous cesarean birth?

There are three retrospective cohort studies [19–21] that evaluate the association between maternal age and the risk of uterine rupture. The studies vary according to the manner in which patients are grouped in certain age strata. Shipp et al. [19] examines the association using a dichotomous categorization of less than 30 years of age and greater than or equal to 30 years of age while Bujold et al. [20] and Srinivas et al. [21] employed a three tiered approach. All three studies substantiate decrease success in TOL in older women. All studies attempted to control for possible confounders. Shipp et al. reported a threefold increased risk of uterine rupture among women at least 30 years of age. Bujold et al. did not confirm this increased risk, however, a smaller sample size may have led to a Type II error. Srinivas analyzed VBAC related complications which included uterine rupture and revealed an increased risk in women 35 years of age or older. The proposed mechanism of increased maternal age interfering with wound healing including hysterotomy is plausible. However, analysis of age at index cesarean would further substantiate the basis of this theory.

Maternal Body Mass Index (BMI)

Management of women with previous cesarean delivery and elevated BMI presents a true clinical dilemma. Repeat surgery has multiple risks, but is large maternal BMI associated with an elevated risk of uterine rupture during a TOL after previous cesarean. While there are several studies examining this question, the sample sizes are variable, some studies compare outcomes of women undergoing TOL after previous cesarean versus elective repeat cesarean delivery (ERCD) while others compare maternal outcomes stratified by increasing levels of maternal BMI attempting a TOL [22–26]. Some researchers have presented analyses of the same population using these two study designs [23, 25]. Hibbard et al. [22] employing the Maternal-Fetal Medicine (MFM) units of prospectively collected data provides the most comprehensive analysis and conclusions. Data was stratified across increasing categories of maternal BMI to examine the effect of maternal BMI on the risk of uterine rupture during TOL after prior cesarean. Uterine disruptive events increased in the morbidly obese (2.1% versus 0.9%; $p = 0.03$) compared with normal BMI women. Uterine rupture was elevated in morbidly obese women compared to women with normal BMI, but this rate was not statistically different (1.2% vs. 0.6%; $p = 0.12$). This study confirmed the decrease success associated with larger BMI compared to normal BMI in women undergoing TOL after prior cesarean. However, there is a lingering question whether a higher rate of induction in obese women with prior cesarean may bias these results [23].

Fetal size

4. Does a larger fetus increase the risk of rupture during TOL after previous cesarean?

Ideally, the impact of the estimated fetal weight (the passenger) upon the risk of uterine rupture is the variable of interest. However, birth weight has been utilized as a proxy for this assessment in the literature. Three retrospective cohort studies [27–29] which controlled for potential confounders including prior indication for previous cesarean analyzed the association between increasing birth weight and the risk of uterine rupture during a TOL after previous cesarean birth. Birth weight greater than or equal to 4000 g was associated with an increased risk of uterine rupture reaching statistical significance in two of the three studies and highest in those without a previous vaginal delivery (3.2–3.6%). Success of TOL after previous cesarean birth decreases with increasing birth weight. Overall rates of success have been affected by confounders with the lowest success rates (41%) observed in women undergoing labor induction with no prior vaginal delivery and birth weights greater than or equal to 4000 g. Using logistic regression and adjusting for potential confounders, Peaceman et al. reported the odds of success decreased by 3.8% for each increase of 100 g in birth weight in a TOL relative to the index cesarean birth weight employing the prospectively collected MFM unit's observational trial [30].

5. How do factors affecting the integrity of the scar influence the rate of uterine rupture?

The sonographic measurement of the thickness of the lower uterine segment (LUS) has been proposed as a method to assess the risk of uterine rupture during a TOL after previous cesarean birth [31, 32]. A systematic review performed by Jastrow et al. [33] examined the diagnostic accuracy of sonographic measurement of the LUS thickness near term in predicting LUS disruption. They concluded that sonographic LUS thickness correlated inversely with the risk of uterine rupture during a TOL after previous cesarean. However, lack of standardization of the measurement technique and the heterogeneity of the studies precludes the determination of an ideal cut-off value that is clinically useful. Since this publication, Martin et al. [34] have suggested that ultrasonographic measurement of the LUS muscular thickness transvaginally appears more reliable than a transabdominal full thickness measurement. Three- dimensional approach may offer promise for off-line analysis allowing patients to be evaluated from geographically remote areas. One of the difficulties that plagues this approach is that uterine rupture remote from the uterine scar cannot be predicted from this technique [35].

Greater than one previous hysterotomy

Three studies, two retrospective cohorts [36, 37] and one prospective observational study [38] analyze the influence of greater than one previous cesarean delivery upon the risk of uterine rupture during a TOL after prior cesarean birth. The prospective observational study patients were derived from patients managed from 1999 to 2002 whereas patients from the other two studies (Caughey et al. [36] and Macones et al. [37] were from older cohorts dating back to 1984 but published since 1998. The patients managed more recently may have benefited from knowledge regarding uterine rupture risk that may have influenced their ultimate planned mode of delivery. The two retrospective cohort studies demonstrate a 2–4.8 fold increase risk of uterine rupture in women during a TOL with an absolute rate of 1.8–3.7% risk of rupture. All three studies attempted to control for confounders through logistic regression analysis. While all three studies demonstrated a statistically increased risk of morbidity in those attempting VBAC with greater than one previous hysterotomy, absolute risks remained small and those with prior vaginal delivery had the lowest risk of uterine rupture (0.36 OR; 95% CI (0.08–0.88)).

Interdelivery interval

Four retrospective cohort studies [39–42] (two using similar databases from the same institutions using four more years of data) [40, 41] and one case control study [43] have evaluated the effect of interdelivery interval upon the risk of uterine rupture during a TOL after previous cesarean birth. The studies actually examined different intervals: interpregnancy and or interdelivery but attempted to control for confounders using multiple logistic regression. Consistently, a shorter interval was associated with an increased risk of uterine rupture. Shipp et al. [39] reported a threefold increase risk of uterine rupture associated with interdelivery interval of less than or equal to 18 months (95% CI 1.2, 7.2) after controlling for potential confounding.

One possible mechanism that might explain the increased risk of rupture with a short interdelivery interval is incomplete repair or healing of the uterine hysterotomy. The literature suggests that complete uterine involution and restoration of zonal anatomy may require at least six months or longer as evaluated by Magnetic resonance imaging (MRI) [39].

Uterine incision type

Most of the literature analyzes the risk of uterine rupture during a TOL of a prior low transverse hysterotomy or an unknown scar location presumed to be a low transverse incision based upon clinical context of the delivery. The largest cohort examined retrospectively by Shipp et al. [44] reported a similar rate of uterine rupture between women with prior low vertical (0.8%) versus low transverse (1.0%; $p > 0.999$). This study possessed an 80% power to detect an increase from 1 to 3%; comparable to uterine rupture risk with two prior cesarean births undergoing TOL.

Single versus double layer closure

Two retrospective cohort studies [45, 46] and one case control study [47] evaluated the risk of uterine rupture during a subsequent TOL after previous cesarean birth. The cohort studies reported conflicting results, but may be weakened by small sample sizes. The case control study does utilize multivariable analysis to control for confounders and reported a modest association (OR = 2.69; 95% CI 1.37–5.28) between uterine rupture and TOL after previous cesarean where a single closure was utilized. Factors such as postoperative infection complicating the index cesarean delivery, suture material and method of closure may also compromise the integrity of the hysterotomy scar.

6. How do intrapartum factors influence uterine rupture rates?

Labor induction and augmentation

The literature is complicated by the various inconsistencies of exposure among cohorts examined. Some patients received oxytocin as an induction and augmentation agent while others received prostaglandins for cervical ripening followed by oxytocin for further induction and augmentation. Mechanical cervical ripening was also utilized followed by oxytocin for further induction and augmentation. There are several prostaglandins studied with different dosages and preparations. All of these complicate the analysis of the association between uterine rupture and labor induction and labor augmentation. Smaller studies such as Rayburn et al. [48] in which 143 patients were randomized to receive weekly intracervical PGE2 starting at 39 weeks as outpatients while 151 patients were treated expectantly demonstrated no increased risk of uterine rupture associated with cervical ripening. Of note, this study was not placebo controlled or blinded and it was funded by a pharmaceutical company that was involved in the execution of the study. However, larger more recent studies have raised questions of safety which will be further discussed below.

There are 15 additional contemporary studies [49–63] (Table 40.1) in the literature with the main objective to evaluate the effect of induction and augmentation upon the risk of uterine rupture during a TOL after previous cesarean birth. Two retrospective cohort studies (Zelop et al. [49] and Ravasia et al. [50]) and two prospective observational studies (Grobman et al. [59] and Kwee et al. [60]) demonstrate an increase risk of uterine rupture in women undergoing labor induction compared to spontaneous labor (1.4–3.1%). Prior vaginal delivery appears protective while multiple sequential agents seem to result in the highest risks [64]. The use of cervical ripening agents and an unfavorable modified Bishop's score are associated with greater chance of uterine rupture and less chance of successful TOL after previous cesarean [54, 56, 60]. All ripening agents may not be equivalent in their effect upon the risk of uterine rupture. Mechanical ripening agents such as the Foley bulb technique, seem to be less associated with the chance of uterine rupture, but these results are inconsistent and some studies suggest that this method of induction is less efficacious [55, 56]. Misoprostol has been linked to some of the highest rates of uterine rupture [65]. However, even larger studies that rely on ICD-9/10 codes to identify cases are prone to misclassification leading to uncontrolled bias that compromise the interpretation of data. There are several observations that substantiate an association between stimulated labor and uterine rupture. Buhimschi et al. [35] have demonstrated that uterine rupture tends to occur at the site of prior hysterotomy instead of other remote sites when women are exposed to prostaglandins suggesting that biochemical changes of the collagen component compromised the integrity of hysterotomy scar. Additionally, Cahill et al. [58, 61] observed a dose response to oxytocin leading to uterine rupture reporting a fourfold or greater risk with doses greater that 20 $mU\,min^{-1}$. Harper et al. [63] in a nested case-control study also suggests that length of labor and an initial unfavorable cervical exam are responsible for the increase risk of uterine rupture during the induction process and not induction per se.

Augmentation of labor has been linked to an increased risk of uterine rupture, but inconsistently in the literature. Rates of uterine rupture ranging from 1.0 to 1.9% have been reported compared to spontaneous labor during a TOL after prior cesarean birth [49, 51, 60]. Again, it appears that maximal dose, rather than the overall time of exposure to oxytocin is associated with uterine rupture. These observations mandate a judicious use of oxytocin in women undergoing TOL after previous cesarean with particular attention to dosage going no higher than 20 $mU\,min^{-1}$ [58, 61].

Table 40.1 Augmentation and induction.

Author, year of publication	Study type	Cases	Controls	Exposure/intervention	Outcome/results
Zelop et al. 1999 [49]	Retrospective cohort study	Induced and or augmented labor with one prior cesarean and no other deliveries	Spontaneously laboring with one prior cesarean and no other deliveries	Induction with oxytocin and/or cervical ripening with PGE2 Augmentation with oxytocin	Rate of uterine rupture associated with induction was 2.3% in comparison to 0.7% with spontaneous labor ($p = 0.001$) In a logistic regression model controlling for confounders, induction of labor with oxytocin was associated with 4.6 fold increase risk of uterine rupture (95% CI, 1.5–14.1) Augmentation with oxytocin was associated with 2.3 fold increase risk of rupture (95% CI, 0.8–7.0)
Ravasia et al. 2000 [50]	Retrospective cohort study	Induced labor with different methods and prior cesarean birth	Spontaneously laboring with prior cesarean birth	Induction of labor with PGE2 cervical ripening with or without oxytocin Induction of labor with intracervical Foley bulb followed by oxytocin Induction not requiring cervical ripening	Rate of uterine rupture associated with induction was 1.4% compared with 0.45% with spontaneous labor; $P = 0.0004$ Uterine rupture associated with PGE2 = 2.9%; $p = 0.004$ Intracervical Foley bulb = 0.76%; $p = 0.47$ Labor induction without cervical ripening =0.74%; $p = 0.38$
Goetzl et al. 2001 [51]	Nested case control study	Uterine rupture during a trial of labor after one previous cesarean	Four controls undergoing trial of labor after a single previous cesarean birth matched for birthweight, year of birth, induction or augmentation	Oxytocin duration, maximal dose, mean total dose, and duration at maximal dose	Uterine rupture with exposure to oxytocin was associated with an episode of hyperstimulation $P = 0.05$ Positive predictive value of hyperstimulation for uterine rupture is 2.8%
Ben-Aroya et al. 2002 [52]	Retrospective cohort study	Induced labor with one prior cesarean	Non-induced labor with prior cesarean with or without augmentation	Uterine rupture and other outcomes in those induced with Foley catheter versus PGE2 versus non-induced labor	No difference in epidural usage and oxytocin augmentation Uterine rupture rate was 0% in induced and 0.1% in controls Foley catheter induction less successful (50.9% versus 64.8%; $P = <0.01$)

(*continued overleaf*)

Table 40.1 *(continued)*

Author, year of publication	Study type	Cases	Controls	Exposure/intervention	Outcome/results
Delaney et al. 2003 [53]	Retrospective cohort study	Induced labor with one prior cesarean	Spontaneous labor with one previous cesarean	Uterine rupture rates in cases versus controls	Non-statistically significant increased rate of uterine rupture in induced versus spontaneous (0.7% versus 0.3%; $p = 0.128$) PGE2 induction associated with non-statistically significant increase rate of uterine rupture (1.1% versus 0.6%; $p = 0.62$)
Bujold et al. 2004 [54]	Retrospective cohort study	Induced labor with one prior cesarean		Rate of uterine rupture and success stratified across four strata of bishop scores Those with unfavorable Bishop Score < 6 underwent cervical ripening with Foley bulb Multivariate regression analysis was performed to adjust for confounders	Rates of uterine rupture were inversely correlated with Bishop scores but not statistically different (2.1% for Bishop Score 0–2;1.8% for Bishop Score 3–5; 0.5% for Bishop Score 6–8 and 0.0% for 9–12; $p = 0.48$) Bishop Score ≥ 6 was associated with success OR = 2.07, 95% CI 1.28–3.35
Bujold et al. 2004 [55]	Retrospective cohort study	Induced labor after previous cesarean	Spontaneous labor after previous cesarean with or without oxytocin augmentation	Induction performed via amniotomy with or without oxytocin versus cervical ripening using transcervical Foley catheter Rates of uterine rupture and success were compared among the three groups PGE2 use was excluded Logistic regression analysis adjusted for confounding variables	Rates of rupture not statistically different across the three groups: spontaneous labor versus amniotomy with or without oxytocin versus ripening with transcervical Foley bulb (1.1% versus 1.2% versus 1.6%; $p = 0.81$) Modified Bishop Score ≤ 4 was associated with less success with an OR = 0.53 (95% CI 0.34–0.84) in logistic regression model
Hoffman et al. 2004 [56]	Retrospective observational study	TOL after previous cesarean with uterine rupture in a single institution	TOL after previous cesarean and no uterine rupture	Percent of induction, cervical ripening, oxytocin exposure and cervical status were compared between cases and controls	Preinduction cervical ripening was significantly associated with uterine rupture (OR = 3.92; 95% CI, 1.8–8.6) Less success (46.7% versus 76.9%; $p = <0.001$) Rupture associated with Foley catheter was (6.52%; 95% CI, 2.35–10.7). PGE2 gel =0.0% and Misoprostol was (25%; 95 CI, 0.0–63.7)

Yogev et al. 2004 [57]	Retrospective cohort design	Induced labor after prior cesarean	Spontaneous labor after previous cesarean	Rates of uterine rupture and success were compared in those induced with PGE2 versus spontaneous labor	No uterine ruptures in those induced versus 0.42% in the control group, (nonsignificant) Success was similar in both groups (36% versus 37.3%; P = 0.8)
Cahill et al. 2007 [58]	Retrospective cohort study design	TOL after previous cesarean with oxytocin exposure	TOL after previous cesarean without oxytocin exposure	Rates of uterine rupture were compared between those exposed and unexposed to oxytocin Stratified analysis in which rupture rates were compared over categories of maximum oxytocin dosages Logistic regression model controlled for confounders while assessing association between maximal dose ranges and uterine rupture	Rate of uterine rupture in those exposed to oxytocin was 1.4% versus 0.6% without oxytocin exposure Rate of uterine rupture increased incrementally with increasing maximal dose of oxytocin Ranging from 0.6% in those receiving no oxytocin to 2,1% in those receiving 21–30 mU min^{-1} (adjusted OR = 2.98; 95% CI 1.51–5.9; p = 0.002)
Grobman et al. 2007 [59]	Prospective observational study	Induced labor with prior cesarean birth with or without vaginal delivery	Spontaneous labor with prior cesarean birth with or without prior vaginal delivery	Rates of uterine rupture and success were compared between those laboring spontaneously or through induction Stratified by history of prior vaginal delivery Univariable and multivariable logistic regression to control for confounders was performed	Increased risk of uterine rupture only in those with no prior vaginal delivery (1.5% versus 0.8%; p = 0.02; and 0.6% versus 0.4%; p = 0.42) Unfavorable cervix at labor induction increased the risk of repeat cesarean birth
Kwee et al. 2007 [60]	Prospective observational multicenter study	Induced or augmented labor with previous cesarean birth	Labor without exposure to uterotonic agents with prior cesarean birth	Rates of uterine rupture were compared among those receiving no uterotonics versus oxytocin for augmentation versus oxytocin with or without prostaglandins	Rate of uterine rupture without uterotonics is 0.8% versus 1.9% for augmented labor ()R = 2.2; (95%CI, 1.04–5.0) and 3.1% for induced labor (OR = 3.8; 95 CI, 2.0–7.3)

(continued overleaf)

Table 40.1 *(continued)*

Author, year of publication	Study type	Cases	Controls	Exposure/intervention	Outcome/results
Cahill et al. 2008 [61]	Nested case control study	Cases of uterine rupture during a trial of labor after previous cesarean	Controls without evidence of uterine rupture during a trial of labor after previous cesarean birth	Both controls and cases were exposed to oxytocin Time to event analysis was performed to examine the effect of maximum oxytocin dose and duration of treatment upon the risk of uterine rupture	Maximum oxytocin ranges greater than 20 mU min^{-1} increased the risk of uterine rupture fourfold or greater(21–30 mU min^{-1}: HR = 3.92; 95%CI, 1.06–14.52; 31–40 mU min^{-1}: HR = 4.57; 95%CI, 1.0–20.82) Time as duration or labor or time as duration to oxytocin exposure did not reveal a significant increased risk association
Gomez et al. 2011 [62]	Retrospective cohort study	Inducted labor after previous cesarean	Induced labor after previous cesarean birth	Comparison of rates of success and uterine rupture in those induced with vaginal insert dinoprostone versus oxytocin	No differences in rate of cesarean (35.6% versus 34.1%; p = 0.71) Overall rate of uterine rupture was 1.7% (1.6% in the dinoprostone group versus 1.8% in the oxytocin group; p = 0.89)
Harper et al. 2011 [63]	Nested case control study	Uterine rupture sustained during labor after previous cesarean birth	Labor after previous cesarean without uterine rupture	Time to event analysis with subjects grouped according to induction of labor versus spontaneous labor A secondary analysis was performed to examine the effect of oxytocin for induction versus augmentation compared to no oxytocin Another secondary analysis was performed to examine the effect of cervical dilation at the initiation of oxytocin	When accounting for the length of labor, induction and spontaneous labor have similar rates of rupture(HR = 1.52; 95%CI, 0.97–2, 36) An initial unfavorable exam was associated with increased risk of uterine rupture (HR= 4.09; 95%CI, 1.82–9.17)

7. Can uterine rupture be predicted?

Contemporary models for the prediction of uterine rupture

Given the data presented above, is it possible to develop a prediction tool that has enough sensitivity to be clinically useful for optimizing the choice of candidates for a TOL after previous cesarean birth? Several models have been proposed and warrant further discussion. Shipp et al. [66] developed an assessment tool for the prediction of intrapartum uterine rupture based upon antepartum factors including maternal age, number of previous cesareans, interdelivery interval and history of previous vaginal delivery. Implementation of this scoring system based upon 4384 TOLs and analysis of 40 symptomatic uterine ruptures, permitted 81% of the cohort to undergo TOL while preventing 60% of uterine ruptures. In this model, 36 ERCD are required to prevent one symptomatic uterine rupture. While this model offers reliability based upon a robust sample size, the cohort was not large enough to facilitate a validation phase. Macones et al. [67] proposed another model incorporating both antepartum and early labor factors and using receiver operating curves. Based upon their calculations which yielded a 40% false positive rate, these researchers concluded that uterine rupture cannot be reliably predicted employing either individual or combinations of clinical factors. Lastly, Grobman et al. [68] employing the MFM units' data sought to construct a graphic nomogram that would be clinically useful to determine an individual patient's risk of uterine rupture. A subpopulation of the cohort would be used as a training set and the remainder as a testing set. Their optimal final prediction model, which was based upon induction and history of prior vaginal delivery had poor discriminating ability and did not allow the determination of a clinically useful estimate of an individual patient's risk of uterine rupture. In summary, the development of an accurate model for the prediction of an individual women's risk of uterine rupture remains a viable clinical research question.

Conclusions and recommendations

The optimal mode of delivery for women with previous cesarean has been intensely debated during the new millennium. Fueled by concerns regarding abnormal placentation and massive maternal hemorrhage, TOL after previous cesarean remains a viable option. The most perilous risk encountered during a TOL after previous cesarean is uterine rupture which can result in both maternal and fetal compromise. Review of the literature does not reveal any randomized controlled trials between TOL after previous cesarean and ERCD. However, further review of the literature reveals studies that examine the impact of antepartum and intrapartum factors that may influence the risk of uterine rupture for a particular patient. Returning to our clinical vignette, the patient appears to have clinical factors that lower her risk for uterine rupture during a TOL after previous cesarean especially if she presents in spontaneous labor. Development of an accurate model to predict an individual's unique risk for uterine rupture remains a viable clinical research question.

References

1 Curtain, S.C., Gregory, K.D., Korst, L.M. et al. (2015). Maternal morbidity for vaginal and cesarean deliveries, according to previous cesarean history: new data from the birth certificate, 2013. *NSVR* **64** (**4**): 1–14.

2 Chauhan, S.P., Martin, J.N., Henrichs, C.E. et al. (2003). Maternal and perinatal complications with uterine rupture in 142,075 patients who attempted vaginal birth after cesarean delivery: a review of the literature. *American Journal of Obstetrics and Gynecology* **189**: 408–417.

3 NIH Concensus Development Conference on vaginal Birth After Cesarean: New Insights. March 8–10, 2010. Bethesda, MD. available at: http://concensus.nih.gov/2010/images/vbac/vbac_statement.pdf. accessed 11 July 2018.

4 Harper, L.M., Cahill, A.G., Stamilio, D.M. et al. (2009). Effect of gestational age at the prior cesarean delivery on maternal morbidity in subsequent VBAC attempt. *American Journal of Obstetrics and Gynecology* **200** (**3**): 276 e1–276 e6. Epub 2009/01/27.

5 Estrade, S., Schmitz, T., Cabrol, D. et al. (2009). History of cesarean before 32 weeks' gestation and trial of labor: what is the risk of uterine rupture? *Acta Obstetricia et Gynecologica Scandinavica* **88** (**2**): 149–153. Epub 2008/10/28.

6 Rochelson, B., Pagano, M., Conetta, L. et al. (2005). Previous preterm cesarean delivery: identification of a new risk factor for uterine rupture in VBAC candidates. *The Journal of Maternal-Fetal & Neonatal Medicine: The Official Journal of the European Association of Perinatal Medicine, the Federation of Asia and Oceania Perinatal Societies, the International Society of Perinatal Obstet* **18** (**5**): 339–342. Epub 2006/01/05.

7 Kwee, A., Smink, M., Van Der Laar, R., and Bruinse, H.W. (2007). Outcome of subsequent delivery after a previous early preterm cesarean section. *The Journal of Maternal-Fetal & Neonatal Medicine: The Official Journal of the European Association of Perinatal Medicine, the Federation of Asia and Oceania Perinatal Societies, the International Society of Perinatal Obstet* **20** (**1**): 33–37. Epub 2007/04/18.

8 Sciscione, A.C., Landon, M.B., Leveno, K.J. et al. (2008). Previous preterm cesarean delivery and risk of subsequent uterine rupture. *Obstetrics and Gynecology* **111** (**3**): 648–653. Epub 2008/03/04.

9 Hendler, I. and Bujold, E. (2004). Effect of prior vaginal delivery or prior vaginal birth after cesarean delivery on obstetric outcomes in women undergoing trial of labor. *Obstetrics and Gynecology* **104** (**2**): 273–277. Epub 2004/08/05.

10 Zelop, C.M., Shipp, T.D., Repke, J.T. et al. (2000). Effect of previous vaginal delivery on the risk of uterine rupture during a subsequent trial of labor. *American Journal of Obstetrics and Gynecology* **183** (**5**): 1184–1186. Epub 2000/11/21.

11 Mercer, B.M., Gilbert, S., Landon, M.B. et al. (2008). Labor outcomes with increasing number of prior vaginal births after cesarean delivery. *Obstetrics and Gynecology* **111** (**2 Pt 1**): 285–291. Epub 2008/02/02.

12 de Lau, H., Gremmels, H., Schuitemaker, N.W., and Kwee, A. (2011). Risk of uterine rupture in women undergoing trial of labour with a history of both a caesarean section and a vaginal delivery. *Archives of Gynecology and Obstetrics* 1–6.

13 Coassolo, K.M., Stamilio, D.M., Pare, E. et al. (2005). Safety and efficacy of vaginal birth after cesarean attempts at or beyond 40 weeks of gestation. *Obstetrics and Gynecology* **106** (**4**): 700–706. Epub 2005/10/04.

14 Zelop, C.M., Shipp, T.D., Cohen, A. et al. (2001). Trial of labor after 40 weeks' gestation in women with prior cesarean. *Obstetrics and Gynecology* **97** (**3**): 391–393. Epub 2001/03/10.

15 Kiran, T.S., Chui, Y.K., Bethel, J., and Bhal, P.S. (2006). Is gestational age an independent variable affecting uterine scar rupture rates? *European Journal of Obstetrics, Gynecology, and Reproductive Biology* **126** (**1**): 68–71. Epub 2005/10/14.

16 Hammoud, A., Hendler, I., Gauthier, R.J. et al. (2004). The effect of gestational age on trial of labor after cesarean section. *The Journal of Maternal-Fetal & Neonatal Medicine: The Official Journal of the European Association of Perinatal Medicine, the Federation of Asia and Oceania Perinatal Societies, the International Society of Perinatal Obstet* **15** (**3**): 202–206. Epub 2004/07/29.

17 Quinones, J.N., Stamilio, D.M., Pare, E. et al. (2005). The effect of prematurity on vaginal birth after cesarean delivery: success and maternal morbidity. *Obstetrics and Gynecology* **105** (**3**): 519–524. Epub 2005/03/02.

18 Durnwald, C.P., Rouse, D.J., Leveno, K.J. et al. (2006). The maternal-fetal medicine units cesarean registry: safety and efficacy of a trial of labor in preterm pregnancy after a prior cesarean delivery. *American Journal of Obstetrics and Gynecology* **195** (**4**): 1119–1126. Epub 2006/09/27.

19 Shipp, T.D., Zelop, C., Repke, J.T. et al. (2002). The association of maternal age and symptomatic uterine rupture during a trial of labor after prior cesarean delivery. *Obstetrics and Gynecology* **99** (**4**): 585–588. Epub 2002/06/01.

20 Bujold, E., Hammoud, A.O., Hendler, I. et al. (2004). Trial of labor in patients with a previous cesarean section: does maternal age influence the outcome? *American Journal of Obstetrics and Gynecology* **190** (**4**): 1113–1118. Epub 2004/05/01.

21 Srinivas, S.K., Stamilio, D.M., Sammel, M.D. et al. (2007). Vaginal birth after caesarean delivery: does maternal age affect safety and success? *Paediatric and Perinatal Epidemiology* **21** (**2**): 114–120. Epub 2007/02/17.

22 Hibbard, J.U., Gilbert, S., Landon, M.B. et al. (2006). Trial of labor or repeat cesarean delivery in women with morbid obesity and previous cesarean delivery. *Obstetrics and Gynecology* **108** (**1**): 125–133. Epub 2006/07/04.

23 Chauhan, S.P., Magann, E.F., Carroll, C.S. et al. (2001). Mode of delivery for the morbidly obese with prior cesarean delivery: vaginal versus repeat cesarean section. *American Journal of Obstetrics and Gynecology* **185** (**2**): 349–354. Epub 2001/08/24.

24 Bujold, E., Hammoud, A., Schild, C. et al. (2005). The role of maternal body mass index in outcomes of vaginal births after cesarean. *American Journal of Obstetrics and Gynecology* **193** (**4**): 1517–1521. Epub 2005/10/06.

25 Carroll, C.S. Sr., Magann, E.F., Chauhan, S.P. et al. (2003). Vaginal birth after cesarean section versus elective repeat cesarean delivery: weight-based outcomes. *American Journal of Obstetrics and Gynecology* **188** (**6**): 1516–1520. discussion 20-2. Epub 2003/06/26.

26 Edwards, R.K., Harnsberger, D.S., Johnson, I.M. et al. (2003). Deciding on route of delivery for obese women with prior cesarean. *American Journal of Obstetrics and Gynecology* **189**: 385–389.

27 Jastrow, N., Roberge, S., Gauthier, R.J. et al. (2010). Effect of birth weight on adverse obstetric outcomes in vaginal birth after cesarean delivery. *Obstetrics and Gynecology* **115** (**2 Pt 1**): 338–343. Epub 2010/01/23.

28 Zelop, C.M., Shipp, T.D., Repke, J.T. et al. (2001). Outcomes of trial of labor following previous cesarean delivery among women with fetuses weighing >4000 g. *American Journal of Obstetrics and Gynecology* **185** (**4**): 903–905. Epub 2001/10/20.

29 Elkousy, M.A., Sammel, M., Stevens, E. et al. (2003). The effect of birth weight on vaginal birth after cesarean delivery success rates. *American Journal of Obstetrics and Gynecology* **188** (**3**): 824–830. Epub 2003/03/14.

30 Peaceman, A.M., Gersnoviez, R., Landon, M.B. et al. (2006). The MFMU cesarean registry: impact of fetal size on trial of labor success for patients with previous cesarean for dystocia. *American Journal of Obstetrics and Gynecology* **195** (**4**): 1127–1131. Epub 2006/09/27.

31 Bujold, E., Jastrow, N., Simoneau, J. et al. (2009). Prediction of complete uterine rupture by sonographic evaluation of the lower uterine segment. *American Journal of Obstetrics and Gynecology* **201** (**3**): 320 e1–320 e6. Epub 2009/09/08.

32 Kushtagi, P. and Garepalli, S. (2011). Sonographic assessment of lower uterine segment at term in women with previous cesarean delivery. *Archives of Gynecology and Obstetrics* **283** (**3**): 455–459. Epub 2010/02/11.

33 Jastrow, N., Chaillet, N., Roberge, S. et al. (2010). Sonographic lower uterine segment thickness and risk of uterine scar defect: a systematic review. *Journal of Obstetrics and Gynaecology Canada: JOGC = Journal D'obstetrique et Gynecologie du Canada : JOGC* **32** (**4**): 321–327. Epub 2010/05/27.

34 Martins, W.P., Barra, D.A., Gallarreta, C.O. et al. (2009). Lower uterine segment thickness measurement in pregnant women with previous cesarean section: reliability analysis using two- and three- dimensional transabdominal and transvaginal ultrasound. *Ultrasound in Obstetrics & Gynecology* **33**: 301–306.

35 Buhimschi, C.S., Buhimschi, I.A., Patel, S. et al. (2005). Rupture of the uterine scar during term labour: contractility or biochemistry? *BJOG: An International Journal of Obstetrics and Gynaecology* **112** (**1**): 38–42. Epub 2005/01/25.

36 Caughey, A.B., Shipp, T.D., Repke, J.T. et al. (1999). Rate of uterine rupture during a trial of labor in women with one or two prior cesarean deliveries. *American Journal of Obstetrics and Gynecology* **181** (**4**): 872–876. Epub 1999/10/16.

37 Macones, G.A., Cahill, A., Pare, E. et al. (2005). Obstetric outcomes in women with two prior cesarean deliveries: is vaginal birth after cesarean delivery a viable option? *American Journal of Obstetrics and Gynecology* **192** (**4**): 1223–1228; discussion 8-9. Epub 2005/04/23.

38 Landon, M.B., Spong, C.Y., Thom, E. et al. (2006). Risk of uterine rupture with a trial of labor in women with multiple and single prior cesarean delivery. *Obstetrics and Gynecology* **108** (**1**): 12–20. Epub 2006/07/04.

39 Shipp, T.D., Zelop, C.M., Repke, J.T. et al. (2001). Interdelivery interval and risk of symptomatic uterine rupture. *Obstetrics and Gynecology* **97** (**2**): 175–177. Epub 2001/02/13.

40 Bujold, E., Mehta, S.H., Bujold, C., and Gauthier, R.J. (2002). Interdelivery interval and uterine rupture. *American Journal of Obstetrics and Gynecology* **187** (**5**): 1199–1202. Epub 2002/11/20.

41 Bujold, E. and Gauthier, R.J. (2010). Risk of uterine rupture associated with an interdelivery interval between 18 and 24 months. *Obstetrics and Gynecology* **115** (**5**): 1003–1006. Epub 2010/04/23.

42 Stamilio, D.M., DeFranco, E., Pare, E. et al. (2007). Short interpregnancy interval: risk of uterine rupture and complications of vaginal birth after cesarean delivery. *Obstetrics and Gynecology* **110** (**5**): 1075–1082. Epub 2007/11/06.

43 Esposito, M.A., Menihan, C.A., and Malee, M.P. (2000). Association of interpregnancy interval with uterine scar failure in labor: a case-control study. *American Journal of Obstetrics and Gynecology* **183** (**5**): 1180–1183. Epub 2000/11/21.

44 Shipp, T.D., Zelop, C.M., Repke, J.T. et al. (1999). Intrapartum uterine rupture and dehiscence in patients with prior lower uterine segment vertical and transverse incisions. *Obstetrics and Gynecology* **94** (**5 Pt 1**): 735–740. Epub 1999/11/05.

45 Durnwald, C. and Mercer, B. (2003). Uterine rupture, perioperative and perinatal morbidity after single-layer and double-layer closure at cesarean delivery. *American Journal of Obstetrics and Gynecology* **189**: 925–929.

46 Gyamfi, C., Juhasz, G., Gyamfi, P. et al. (2006). Single- versus double-layer uterine incision closure and uterine rupture. *The Journal of Maternal-Fetal & Neonatal Medicine: The Official Journal of the European Association of Perinatal Medicine, the Federation of Asia and Oceania Perinatal Societies, the International Society of Perinatal Obstet* **19** (**10**): 639–643. Epub 2006/11/23.

47 Bujold, E., Goyet, M., Marcoux, S. et al. (2010). The role of uterine closure in the risk of uterine rupture. *Obstetrics and Gynecology* **116** (**1**): 43–50. Epub 2010/06/23.

48 Rayburn, W.F., Gittens, L.N., Lucas, M.J. et al. (1999). Weekly administration of prostaglandin E2 gel compared with expectant management in women with previous cesareans. Prepidil Gel Study Group. *Obstetrics and Gynecology* **94** (**2**): 250–254. Epub 1999/08/04.

49 Zelop, C.M., Shipp, T.D., Repke, J.T. et al. (1999). Uterine rupture during induced or augmented labor in gravid women with one prior cesarean delivery. *American Journal of Obstetrics and Gynecology* **181** (**4**): 882–886. Epub 1999/10/16.

50 Ravasia, D.J., Wood, S.L., and Pollard, J.K. (2000). Uterine rupture during induced trial of labor among women with previous cesarean delivery. *American Journal of Obstetrics and Gynecology* **183** (**5**): 1176–1179. Epub 2000/11/21.

51 Goetzl, L., Shipp, T.D., Cohen, A. et al. (2001). Oxytocin dose and the risk of uterine rupture in trial of labor after cesarean. *Obstetrics and Gynecology* **97** (**3**): 381–384. Epub 2001/03/10.

52 Ben-Aroya, Z., Hallak, M., Segal, D. et al. (2002). Ripening of the uterine cervix in a post-cesarean parturient: prostaglandin E2 versus foley catheter. *The Journal of Maternal-Fetal & Neonatal Medicine: The Official Journal of the European Association of Perinatal Medicine, the Federation of Asia and Oceania Perinatal Societies, the International Society of Perinatal Obstet* **12** (**1**): 42–45. Epub 2002/11/09.

53 Delaney, T. and Young, D.C. (2003). Spontaneous versus induced labor after a previous cesarean delivery. *Obstetrics and Gynecology* **102** (**1**): 39–44. Epub 2003/07/10.

54 Bujold, E., Blackwell, S.C., Hendler, I. et al. (2004). Modified Bishop's score and induction of labor in patients with a previous cesarean delivery. *American Journal of Obstetrics and Gynecology* **191** (**5**): 1644–1648. Epub 2004/11/18.

55 Bujold, E., Blackwell, S.C., and Gauthier, R.J. (2004). Cervical ripening with transcervical Foley catheter and the risk of uterine rupture. *Obstetrics and Gynecology* **103** (**1**): 18–23. Epub 2004/01/06.

56 Hoffman, M.K., Sciscione, A., Srinivasana, M. et al. (2004). Uterine rupture in patients with a prior cesarean delivery: the impact of cervical ripening. *American Journal of Perinatology* **21** (**4**): 217–222. Epub 2004/05/29.

57 Yogev, Y., Ben-Haroush, A., Lahav, E. et al. (2004). Induction of labor with prostaglandin E2 in women with previous cesarean section and unfavorable cervix. *European Journal of Obstetrics, Gynecology, and Reproductive Biology* **116** (**2**): 173–176. Epub 2004/09/11.

58 Cahill, A.G., Stamilio, D.M., Odibo, A.O. et al. (2007). Does a maximum dose of oxytocin affect risk for uterine rupture in candidates for vaginal birth after cesarean delivery? *American Journal of Obstetrics and Gynecology* **197** (**5**): 495 e1–495 e5. Epub 2007/08/24.

59 Grobman, W.A., Gilbert, S., Landon, M.B. et al. (2007). Outcomes of induction of labor after one prior cesarean. *Obstetrics and Gynecology* **109** (**2 Pt 1**): 262–269. Epub 2007/02/03.

60 Kwee, A., Bots, M.L., Visser, G.H., and Bruinse, H.W. (2007). Obstetric management and outcome of pregnancy in women with a history of caesarean section in the Netherlands. *European Journal of Obstetrics, Gynecology, and Reproductive Biology* **132** (**2**): 171–176. Epub 2006/08/15.

61 Cahill, A.G., Waterman, B.M., Stamilio, D.M. et al. (2008). Higher maximum doses of oxytocin are associated with an unacceptably high risk for uterine rupture in patients attempting vaginal birth after cesarean delivery. *American Journal of Obstetrics and Gynecology* **199** (**1**): 32 e1–32 e5. Epub 2008/05/06.

62 Gomez, L.R., Burgos, J., Cobos, P. et al. (2011). Oxytocin versus dinoprostone vaginal insert for induction of labor after previous cesarean section: a retrospective comparative study. *Journal of Perinatal Medicine* **39** (**4**): 397–402. Epub 2011/05/25.

63 Harper, L.M., Cahill, A.G., Boslaugh, S. et al. Association of induction of labor and uterine rupture in women attempting vaginal birth after cesarean: a survival analysis. *American Journal of Obstetrics and Gynecology* **2011**. Epub 2011/10/18.

64 Macones, G.A., Peipert, J., Nelson, D.B. et al. (2005). Maternal complications with vaginal birth after cesarean delivery: a multicenter study. *American Journal of Obstetrics and Gynecology* **193** (**5**): 1656–1662. Epub 2005/11/02.

65 Lydon-Rochelle, M., Holt, V.L., Easterling, T.R., and Martin, D.P. (2001). Risk of uterine rupture during labor among women with a prior cesarean delivery. *The New England Journal of Medicine* **345** (**1**): 3–8. Epub 2001/07/07.

66 Shipp, T.D., Zelop, C., and Lieberman, E. (2008). Assessment of the rate of uterine rupture at the first prenatal visit: a preliminary evaluation. *The Journal of Maternal-fetal & Neonatal Medicine : The Official Journal of the European Association of Perinatal Medicine, the Federation of Asia and Oceania Perinatal Societies, the International Society of Perinatal Obstet* **21** (**2**): 129–133. Epub 2008/02/02.

67 Macones, G.A., Cahill, A.G., Stamilio, D.M. et al. (2006). Can uterine rupture in patients attempting vaginal birth after cesarean delivery be predicted? *American Journal of Obstetrics and Gynecology* **195** (**4**): 1148–1152. Epub 2006/09/27.

68 Grobman, W.A., Lai, Y., Landon, M.B. et al. (2008). Prediction of uterine rupture associated with attempted vaginal birth after cesarean delivery. *American Journal of Obstetrics and Gynecology* **199** (**1**): 30 e1–30 e5. Epub 2008/04/29.

41

CHAPTER 41
Post-term pregnancy

John Smulian and Joanne Quinones
Department of Obstetrics and Gynecology, Maternal Fetal Medicine, Lehigh Valley Health Network, The Center for Advanced Perinatal Care, Allentown, PA, USA; University of South Florida-Morsani College of Medicine, Tampa, FL, USA

CASE SCENARIO

A 24-year-old married Latina female G1P0 at 40 weeks 1 day gestation has presented to the obstetrician's office for her weekly prenatal visit. Her pregnancy course gerhas been uncomplicated and her pre-pregnancy body mass index (BMI) is $28\,kg\,m^{-2}$. She was examined and found to be 2 cm dilated but is not in labor yet. She is asking about the next steps including timing and methods of her delivery since she is one day past her due date. She is advised about expectant management until she enters spontaneous labor and she enquires about the risks of continuing her pregnancy past her due date.

Introduction

The term pregnancy was conventionally defined as delivery occurring between 37 and 42 weeks gestation. Post-term pregnancy was thus defined as a pregnancy that has reached or extended past 42 + 0 weeks gestation from the last menstrual period.

Because fetal maturation is a continuum throughout fetal life including the six weeks of a "term" pregnancy, and neonatal outcomes differ along that continuum [1], a "Defining 'term' pregnancy" workgroup met and made recommendations for defining "term" pregnancy. The workshop defined births occurring between 37 weeks 0 days and 38 weeks 6 days as "early term", those between 39 weeks 0 days and 40 weeks 6 days as "full term" and those between 41 weeks 0 days and 41 weeks 6 days gestation as late term pregnancy [2]. Post-term pregnancy, defined as a pregnancy that extends to 42 weeks 0 days and beyond or a gestational length of 294 days or more, occurs in 5–10% of all births [3]. Such distinctions allow also for better counseling of women about neonatal outcomes. Post-term pregnancy has been associated with maternal and perinatal risks which will be reviewed in this chapter.

In order to address your patient's questions about her plan for labor and delivery if she is past her due date and has not delivered spontaneously, a literature review is performed to address the following questions.

Clinical questions

1. What are risk factors for post-term pregnancy?

When evaluating a patient's risk for a post-term pregnancy, it is necessary to confirm that pregnancy dating is indeed correct. The most common way of dating a pregnancy, last menstrual period, assumes that a woman has regular cycles with a 14 day follicular phase. With irregular cycles or a shorter/longer follicular phase, dating by ultrasound, not last menstrual period, is more reliable and decreases the risk of labor induction for post-term pregnancy [4, 5]. Literature has shown that the use of first trimester ultrasound screening is effective in reducing post-term labor induction rates [6].

Large epidemiologic studies have evaluated additional risk factors for post-term pregnancy in well-dated gestations. Using data from the Danish Birth Cohort, 53 392 participants with live-born singleton deliveries between 1998 and 2001 were interviewed at 12 and 30 weeks' gestation, and 6 and 18 months after delivery. In this study, increased BMI ($25–29\,kg\,m^{-2}$) and nulliparity were identified as risk factors for post-term pregnancy, with adjusted odds ratios (AORs) of 1.24 (95% CI 1.15–1.34) and 1.35 (95% CI 1.27–1.44), respectively [7]. The risk of being post-term increased by 37% with a BMI at $30–34\,kg\,m^{-2}$; at a BMI of $35\,kg\,m^{-2}$ or more the adjusted odds ratio (OR) was 1.52 (95% CI 1.28–1.82) [7]. A population-based observational study used data from the Cardiff Birth Survey to evaluate pregnancy outcomes according to BMI in otherwise uncomplicated singleton pregnancies [8]. In this study, women with a BMI > $30\,kg\,m^{-2}$ were at an increased risk of postdates pregnancy and more likely to require induction of labor because of prolonged pregnancy. A retrospective study of 9336

Evidence-Based Obstetrics and Gynecology, First Edition. Edited by Errol R. Norwitz, Carolyn M. Zelop, David A. Miller, and David L. Keefe.

term births in California evaluated the association between pre-pregnancy BMI and the length of pregnancy and found that higher pre-pregnancy BMI was associated with higher risk of progressing past 40 weeks [9]. In this study, 28.5% of obese women progressed to >41 weeks' gestation vs. 18.3% and 21.9% of underweight and normal weight women, respectively ($p < 0.001$). Interestingly, in logistic regression analysis with gestational age of >41 weeks as the outcome and BMI as a continuous predictor, an increase of 1 BMI unit was associated with an adjusted odds ratio of post-term pregnancy of 1.29 (95% CI, 1.21–1.38). The above studies suggest a potential influence of hormonal factors in the pathway to parturition.

A retrospective cohort study of term singleton pregnancies at a managed care organization found obesity, nulliparity, and maternal age 30–39 years and 40 years and older were also risk factors for prolonged and post-term pregnancy [10]. The mechanisms for these associations remain unclear.

Previous post-term pregnancy is another risk factor for a repeat post-term pregnancy. Using data from the Danish medical birth registry on a 5% random sample of women with two or more pregnancies between 1980 and 1992, the recurrence risk for post-term pregnancy was 19.8% [11]. The study also found a tendency for more post-term deliveries the longer the interpregnancy interval, suggesting both genetic and environmental predispositions to post-term delivery [11]. Studies have also found that women had a reduced risk of recurrent post-term pregnancy if they changed partners between pregnancies, suggesting that post-term delivery may be in part determined by paternal genes [12].

Rare conditions associated with prolonged pregnancy include anencephaly, placental sulfatase insufficiency, absence of the fetal pituitary, and fetal adrenal hypoplasia in the human fetus [13, 14]. Male sex has also been identified as a risk factor for post-term pregnancy [3]. One common finding among these conditions is the lack the high concentrations of estrogen that are usually seen in normal pregnancy.

2. What are the risks of post-term pregnancy to mother and fetus?

Maternal and fetal risks increase in post-term pregnancies [15]. A study using a 10 year cohort of Norwegian births found an increased risk of obstetric trauma and labor dysfunction, related to both large for gestational age size and post-term birth when compared to term births [16]. A cross-sectional study using records from the Danish Medical Birth Registry evaluated women who gave birth to a singleton liveborn infant at >42 weeks of gestation and compared them to a random sample of women delivered spontaneously at term. The study found an overall maternal complication rate of 30%, including postpartum hemorrhage (AOR 1.37 [95% CI 1.28–1.46]), cephalopelvic disproportion (AOR 1.91 [95% CI 1.77–2.07]), cervical rupture (AOR 1.45 [95% CI 1.26–1.67]), dystocia (AOR 1.71 [95% CI 1.30–2.25]), intrapartum fetal demise (AOR 3.14 [95% CI 1.11–8.90]), cesarean delivery (AOR 1.58 [95% CI 1.51–1.66]), and infection (AOR 1.21 [95% CI 1.03–1.41]) [17]. In this study, the risk of maternal injury was not related to neonatal birthweight. An increased risk of cesarean has not been uniformly reported in all studies. A study comparing induction of labor vs. serial monitoring in post-term pregnancy found a lower risk of cesarean delivery in induced post-term patients (21.2% vs. 24.5%, $p = 0.03$). Interestingly, the lower risk of cesarean delivery was mostly due to a lower number of cesareans performed for fetal heart rate abnormalities in the women induced and there was no difference in the rate of cesareans for failure to progress or failed induction between the groups [18]. A recent retrospective cohort study of low-risk term women evaluating the risk of perinatal complications by gestational age found that delivery at 41 weeks was associated with a higher overall febrile morbidity and cesarean delivery [19].

Fetal risks of post-term pregnancy include macrosomia, intrauterine growth restriction, oligohydramnios and intrauterine fetal demise. An earlier study using records from over 370 000 reported births between 1987 and 1989 in New York City evaluated the residual prospective risk of stillbirth as a function of gestational age [20]. By 40 weeks the risk of stillbirth was 1 in 475, rising progressively to one in 375 at 43 weeks [20]. A study from a 10 year cohort of Norwegian births found that in post-term births, risk factors for perinatal mortality included small for gestational age (adjusted relative risk 5.68; 95% CI 4.37, 7.38) and maternal age >35 years (adjusted relative risk 1.88; 95% CI 1.22, 2.89) [16]. Data from the Danish Medical Birth Registry found an increased risk of dystocia (AOR 1.71 [95% CI 1.30–2.25]) and intrapartum fetal demise (AOR 3.14 [95% CI 1.11–8.90]) in women who gave birth at >42 weeks of gestation [17]. A recent retrospective study of women delivered beyond 37 weeks gestation from 1992 to 2002 at a single community hospital found an increased risk of complications as gestational age advanced, with a significant increased rate of intrauterine fetal death beyond 41 weeks gestation [21]. The risk for intrauterine fetal demise was more than 2.5 times greater between 41 and 42 weeks of gestation as compared with before 40 weeks of gestation [21]. In another study comparing outcomes in term pregnancies by week of gestation, delivery at 41 weeks had a higher risk of birthweight greater than 4500 g (AOR 3.57 [95% CI 3.45–3.69]), neonatal injury (AOR 1.27 [95% CI 1.17–1.37]) and meconium aspiration (AOR 2.12 [95% CI 1.91–2.35]) when compared to deliveries at 39 weeks gestation [19]. See Table 41.1 for summary of risks.

3. What is the optimum timing for delivery in a post-term pregnancy?

There is persistent controversy about the optimal timing for delivery in pregnancy. Prior to the introduction of routine

Table 41.1 Perinatal risks of post-term pregnancy

Maternal	Fetal	Neonatal
Operative delivery	Macrosomia	Shoulder dystocia
Cesarean delivery	Meconium	Meconium aspiration syndrome
Perineal trauma	Intrauterine growth restriction	Intensive care unit admission
Postpartum hemorrhage	Oligohydramnios	Neonatal convulsions
Endomyometritis	Intrauterine fetal demise	Perinatal asphyxia

ultrasound for accurate dating, there was significant inaccuracy for assigning an estimated due date. This is due to the challenges in estimating conception timing when there are highly variable times of ovulation within variable menstrual cycles. Because of the inaccuracy in estimating true dates, pregnancies were often allowed to continue beyond 42 weeks as long as fetal surveillance was reassuring. This was acceptable since many of those pregnancies were not truly post-dates. In a study of over 44 000 women, the impact of different methods of dating a pregnancy on the incidence of pregnancies lasting beyond 42 weeks was assessed [22]. The rate of delivery beyond 42 weeks was 6.4% using only menstrual dating versus 1.9% when based on ultrasound only. First trimester ultrasound appears to have a greater effect on accurately dating a pregnancy than only second trimester dating [6]. Overall the risk for having an induction of labor for a post-term pregnancy is estimated to be reduced by 41% with the use of early ultrasound dating [23].

There is an increased risk for maternal complications as pregnancy progresses beyond 40 weeks including cesarean delivery, operative vaginal delivery, third and fourth degree lacerations, postpartum hemorrhage and febrile morbidity [17, 21, 24, 25]. There are also reported increased fetal and infant risks with advancing gestation such as stillbirth and perinatal death, abnormal acid-base status, birth trauma, sepsis, intracranial hemorrhage, meconium aspiration syndrome and respiratory distress [17, 21, 25–30]. Therefore, it is reasonable to establish a management plan that balances those increasing risks of prolonging a pregnancy with the risks for intervention through induction of labor. Research to assess the optimum timing of delivery has been challenging due to the difficulty in selecting the appropriate methodology to use for studies as well as the selection of appropriate outcomes.

A number of early studies that tried to assess the relative risks versus benefits of delivery interventions compared outcomes of women delivered with induction of labor versus spontaneous labor. Those studies relatively consistently demonstrated an increased risk for cesarean delivery with induction of labor [31–37]. Not surprisingly, there were greater maternal and infant complications in the induction groups. The difficulty with these earlier studies was inherent in their study designs. It is not fair to compare spontaneous labors to induced labors, since spontaneous labor would be expected to have an easier course with fewer complications. Induction of labor is a management intervention whereas spontaneous labor is an event. The better study design would be a comparison of labor induction versus expectant management at each week of gestation past 40 weeks. There are a number of trials that have employed this methodology. Gülmezoglu et al. performed a meta-analysis of trails comparing labor induction to expectant management at 41–42 weeks of gestation. Induction of labor at or beyond 41 completed weeks was associated with fewer perinatal deaths (Risk Ratio (RR) 0.3 95% CI 0.09, 0.99), with no evidence of a significant difference in the cesarean section rate for women in the induction group [38]. In a more recent meta-analysis of randomized-controlled trials comparing induction of labor versus expectant management for post-dates that included additional studies (total of 19), there was a 15% reduction in the cesarean delivery rate with an OR of 0.85 (95% CI: 0.76, 0.95) [39]. There were no differences in the risks for cesarean delivery for fetal distress, operative vaginal delivery, postpartum hemorrhage, and several neonatal outcome measures. The risk for perinatal death was 63% reduced with induction of labor although this was only borderline significant with an OR of 0.37 (95% CI of 0.14, 1.00).

Based on the available information, it appears that induction of labor once a person reaches 41 weeks confers a small advantage for a modestly lower cesarean rate without causing either maternal or fetal harm. There may be an advantage for decreasing stillbirths, but the absolute risk is very low. As a variety of societies have suggested, it is reasonable to consider induction of labor once a pregnancy reaches 41 0/7 weeks, but women can also elect expectant management with fetal surveillance at least twice weekly until 42 0/7 weeks, after which delivery should be encouraged [15, 40, 41] (Figure 41.1).

For women with prolonged pregnancies who enter labor spontaneously, there are no specific recommendations for changing labor management from standard obstetric procedures. For those who undergo an induction of labor, cervical ripening (prostaglandin agents or mechanical devices such as a balloon catheter) should be considered for an unfavorable cervix (Bishop's score of ≤ 6), with oxytocin reserved for those with a favorable cervix [42].

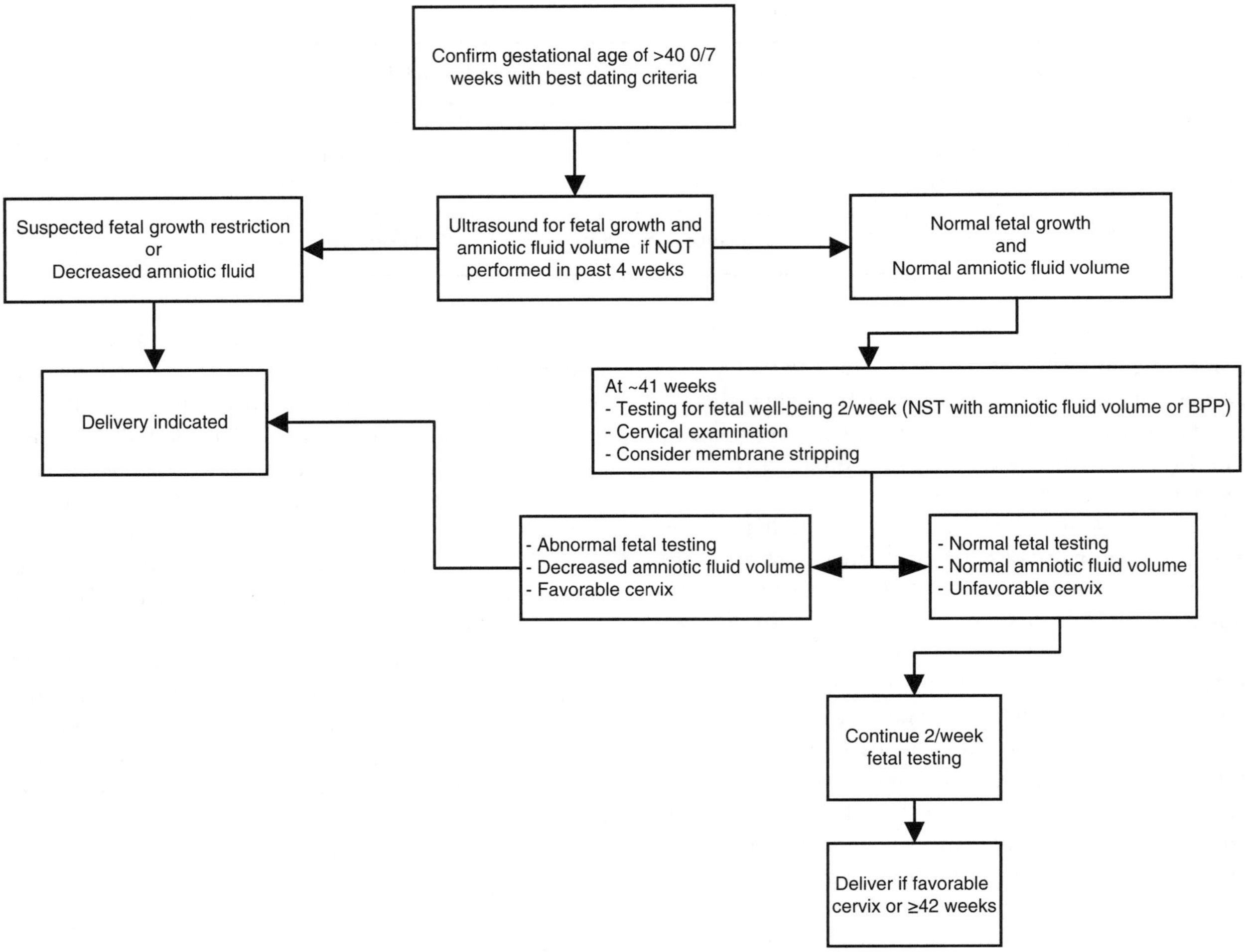

Figure 41.1 A suggested management algorithm for prolonged pregnancies.

In summary, fetal surveillance allows continuation of pregnancy beyond 40 weeks, but the ability of the various testing strategies to predict fetal compromise and prevent fetal death are limited for post-term pregnancies. Given the increase in perinatal morbidity and mortality that accelerates at 42 weeks and the increase in maternal complications as pregnancy progresses, it is reasonable to deliver otherwise uncomplicated pregnancies with normal fetal testing and normal amniotic fluid volumes (AFVs) between 41 0/7 and 41 6/7 weeks of gestation. Pregnancies can be allowed to go beyond 42 0/7 weeks, but only after thorough counseling of the mother with informed consent about the increasing risks and decreasing benefits for pregnancy continuation.

4. How should a prolonged pregnancy be evaluated?

The primary purpose of antenatal fetal surveillance is to prevent fetal death. However, an important secondary objective is to prevent fetal morbidity. In order to know whether any testing strategy is successful at either of these two objectives, one must know the baseline rates of the conditions that are to be prevented [43]. While the baseline rates of fetal death may have been known prior to the initiation of fetal testing strategies, medical care of prolonged pregnancies has changed significantly in the past 30 years. It is probably no longer possible to determine the true natural history risk for fetal death after 41 weeks in normal pregnancies in this era, due to the nearly universal strategy in developed nations of fetal surveillance for those gestations with interventions for abnormal testing and delivery by 42 weeks, even with normal testing [15, 40, 41]. Therefore, it is difficult to prove the benefit of fetal surveillance in the post-term period for prevention of fetal morbidity and mortality since most pregnancies are delivered before in utero problems develop.

5. What are the best tests for fetal well-being and how should testing be implemented?

There are a variety of methods that are used for assessing fetal well-being including fetal movement monitoring (kick counts), the non-stress test (NST), contraction stress test (CST), biophysical profile (BPP), AFV assessment, a modified BPP (NST with AFV), ultrasound for fetal size estimation, fetal vessel Doppler assessment, and fetal kick counts [44, 45]. Each of these has strengths and weaknesses. Importantly, no test works equally well in all circumstances.

Fetal kick counting is a non-specific patient-controlled surveillance technique that is designed as a low cost, low resource method for identifying fetuses that may have decreased activity levels due to developing hypoxia and acidemia. Because this method has not been consistently linked with reduced perinatal mortality, there is no clear consensus that it should be routinely utilized in pregnancies to avoid stillbirths, recognizing there may be other benefits for improved patient engagement with the pregnancy [44, 46]. Its role specific to prolonged pregnancies is largely unexplored.

The concept of "condition-specific testing" refers to the notion that the performance of a particular test is dependent on pathophysiologic condition that paces the fetus at risk [45]. Unlike severe preterm fetal growth restriction and pre-eclampsia, which are often associated with decreased uteroplacental blood flow, the pathophysiology of fetal compromise in a post-dates pregnancy is more likely to be decreased gas-exchange across the aging villi. Placentas from prolonged pregnancies often have increased syncytial knots and villous maturity abnormalities even though outcomes might be normal. However, some of these findings may increase the chance of compromised gas exchange rather than typical uteroplacental insufficiency [47, 48]. This makes it unlikely that umbilical artery Doppler studies would be helpful in prolonged pregnancies as has been demonstrated [48, 49]. Similarly, routine evaluation of the Doppler interrogation of the fetal middle cerebral artery does not appear to be useful with prolonged pregnancies, although there may be some brain sparing redistribution of blood flow when there is already oligohydramnios [50, 51].

The most useful tests for assessing the fetus in a prolonged pregnancy include accurate ultrasound dating in the first trimester (to reduce the rate of postdates pregnancy) [15, 40, 41], estimated weight by ultrasound to identify the growth restricted fetus [52], amniotic fluid assessment, the NST and the BPP [15, 40, 41, 44, 45]. Fetuses suspected to have growth restriction diagnosed by 36 weeks should be considered for delivery before the pregnancy becomes prolonged, since perinatal outcomes are similar whether there is delivery or expectant care. Delivery will prevent a fetal demise and continued surveillance can be expensive, using many resources without improving outcomes [53]. Fetal growth restriction in the prolonged pregnancy is an indication for delivery due to the higher rates of fetal and neonatal complications.

One common feature of any of the recommended testing scheme for monitoring a prolonged pregnancy includes AFV assessments as represented by the BPP or modified BPP. Amniotic fluid typically decreases progressively in late gestation [54]. Oligohydramnios in a post-term pregnancy is associated with poorer outcomes including fetal heart rate abnormalities, meconium stained fluid, fetal growth restriction, cesarean delivery and fetal demise [15, 40, 55–59]. There are several studies that suggest a lower false positive rate and lower intervention rates if the AFV is measured using a deepest vertical pocket of fluid method (normal of ≥2 × 2 cm) compared with an amniotic fluid index (amniotic fluid index (AFI) normal of ≥5 cm). Fetal and neonatal outcomes do not seem to differ significantly regardless of the fluid measurement methodology [60–62].

Several reasonably effective testing strategies have been proposed for evaluating the fetal condition in prolonged pregnancies. Importantly, no single strategy or test will prevent all fetal deaths. The optimum strategy has not been defined by randomized controlled trials, but most include some combination of the NST with AFV assessments and the BPP. Direct comparison of these tests is difficult due to the different ways each is used. However, there is a consensus that the testing should be performed at least twice weekly once the pregnancy reaches 41 weeks to reduce the false negative rate [15, 40, 41, 63]. Whether a BPP is performed along with the AFV assessment is often decided at an institutional level and depends on the patient population and facility resources. In many institutions, a complete BPP is used as a follow-up test to a non-reactive NST. Spontaneous decelerations on the NST should prompt a consideration for delivery. Regardless of the methodology used, the perinatal mortality rate for pregnancies undergoing regular testing is low. While the CST has a high negative predictive value, it is considered to have a high false positive rate and is a resource-intensive test to perform [64]. Importantly, the CST does not appear to hold any advantage over the NST with AFV assessments for prolonged pregnancies [65].

Most epidemiologic studies have shown an increased risk of perinatal mortality after 40 weeks when the risk is calculated for ongoing pregnancies [20, 28, 66]. At 40 weeks the risk of fetal death in women with prenatal care has been estimated to be 1 per 926, which increases to 1 in 826 at 41 weeks and 1 in 769 at 42 weeks [66]. The prospective risk for stillbirth for women receiving prenatal care is somewhat lower than for all women and the risks for these women decrease from approximately 1 in 1250 births at 41 weeks to 1 in 950 births at 42 weeks [45]. Since the risk for fetal death with a normal BPP (all indications) is about 1 in 1300, [67] it seems reasonable to start fetal testing by 41 weeks. This is supported by a number of society guidelines [15, 40, 41]. Continued testing after 42 weeks may not provide significant benefits over delivery, due to the false negative risks with the current fetal assessment tests when the risk of fetal death is primarily due to a gas-exchange issue [45]. Figure 41.1 shows a suggested management algorithm for prolonged pregnancies.

6. Are there complementary or alternative medicine approaches to the management of the post-term pregnancy?

There are few areas of pregnancy care that generate more opinions from the public than methods for shortening pregnancy duration and initiating labor. A number of herbal or manipulation strategies are often discussed as alternatives to the more standard approaches used by physicians in hospital settings, particularly in the setting of post-term gestations. These often have an appeal for pregnant women as seeming more natural and, therefore, safer. The most commonly discussed approaches include blue cohosh (*Caulophyllum thalictroides*), black cohosh (*Cimicifuga racemosa*), red raspberry leaf, castor oil, evening primrose oil, acupuncture, and Shiatsu massage [68–76].

In a national survey of 172 certified nurse midwives, 90 (52%) reported the use of herbal preparations to stimulate labor. Of these, 64% used blue cohosh, 45% used black cohosh, 63% used red raspberry leaf, 93% used castor oil, and 60% used evening primrose oil. Most of these midwives learned about these methods from other midwives and not from formal education programs [77]. Similarly, surveys from 139 California midwives indicated that of the 67% using herbs in pregnancy, approximately 70% used herbs for labor induction [78]. Unfortunately, very few of these methods have been rigorously studied for efficacy [79].

Blue cohosh has been associated with uterine hyperstimulation, fetal tachycardia, perinatal stroke, acute myocardial infarction with congestive heart failure and shock, and severe multi-organ hypoxic injury. There is also *in vitro* evidence that blue cohosh may have teratogenic, embryotoxic, and oxytoxic effects [68]. It also has been shown to significantly impair mitochondrial function, which may contribute to cytotoxicity and idiosyncratic organ damage [80]. There are no trials to assess induction of labor efficacy and its use is not recommended. Black cohosh has not been studied to determine its efficacy in induction of labor. However, it appears to have some hormonal biologic activity based in *in vitro* studies and its ability to treat menopausal symptoms, although it has unknown effects on pregnancy [69]. There are no clinical studies on the use of red raspberry leaf for initiating labor. However, *in vitro* studies suggest there is no direct effect on uterine contractility [70]. In a review of 3 studies involving 233 women examining the use of castor oil, there was no demonstrated reduction in cesarean rates, instrumented delivery, meconium-stained fluid or Apgar scores. All women using castor oil reported significant nausea [71]. There has been only one other small study of 103 women with intact membranes seen at 40–42 weeks for antepartum testing, 57.7% of 52 randomized to oral castor oil and 4.2% of 48 randomized to no treatment developed active labor within 24 hours, which does suggests the potential for a benefit with labor initiation [81]. There are limited data on the efficacy of evening primrose oil for shortening pregnancy duration. One small study suggested that evening primrose oil does not shorten gestation or labor and may be associated with increases in prolonged membrane rupture, oxytocin augmentation, arrest of descent and operative vaginal delivery [82].

There are limited high quality studies of acupuncture for induction of labor. However a Cochrane review of 14 studies from 2220 women suggested that there was no consistently demonstrated advantage for using acupuncture for most outcome of interest related to labor. The authors did note that there was one trial that suggested improved cervical ripening and one that suggested shorter labors [73]. There is one randomized controlled trial in 288 women examining Shiatsu massage techniques for postdate pregnancies that demonstrated a higher rate of spontaneous labor (56.9%) compared to a control group 8.3% [74]. This was consistent with results of one other retrospective study that also suggested a benefit [75].

Although not often considered an alternative or complementary medicine intervention, the commonly used method of stripping or sweeping membranes deserves mention. This technique involves the insertion of a finger through a dilated cervix and then "sweeping" the finger circumferentially to separate the chorionic membrane attachment of the gestational sac from the lower uterine segment around the internal os. Significant increases in phospholipase A2 activity and prostaglandin F2a (PGF2a) levels are found after membrane stripping [82]. In a review of 22 randomized-controlled trials of this technique, there was a reduced pregnancy duration, a 41% reduction in pregnancies continuing beyond 41 weeks and a 72% reduction in going beyond 42 weeks. There was no evidence in an increase in either maternal or neonatal infections, although other side-effects of discomfort, bleeding, and contractions were higher [83]. Therefore, membrane sweeping or stripping can be considered as a method for avoiding prolonged pregnancy and induction of labor.

In summary, none of the commonly used herbal interventions in pregnancy have been demonstrated to have efficacy for shortening gestation and many of them have reported significant side effects. These should not be used to treat post-term pregnancies. Likewise, acupuncture has not been shown to have benefit and is not recommended. Shiatsu massage has no known risk to pregnancy and there is limited information that suggests a possible benefit. This technique may be considered in women who are looking for alternative methods for shortening labor, although further study is needed to confirm efficacy. Finally, membrane stripping can be considered as an intervention to reduce the likelihood of prolonging the pregnancy and the need for induction of labor.

References

1 Tita, A.T., Landon, M.B., Spong, C.Y. et al. (2009). Eunice Kennedy Shriver NICHD maternal-Fetal medicine units network. Timing of elective repeat cesarean delivery at term and neonatal outcomes. *N. Engl. J. Med.* **360**: 111–120.

2 Spong, C.Y. (2013). Defining "term" pregnancy: recommendations from the defining "term" pregnancy workgroup. *JAMA* **309**: 2445.

3 Shea, K.M., Wilcox, A.J., and Little, R.E. (1998). Postterm delivery: a challenge for epidemiologic research. *Epidemiology* **9**: 199–204.

4 Goldenberg, R.L., Davis, R.O., Cutter, G.R. et al. (1989). Prematurity, postdates, and growth retardation: the influence of use of ultrasonography on reported gestational age. *Am. J. Obstet. Gynecol.* **160**: 462–470.

5 Savitz, D.A., Terry, J.W. Jr., Dole, N. et al. (2002). Comparison of pregnancy dating by last menstrual period, ultrasound scanning, and their combination. *Am. J. Obstet. Gynecol.* **187**: 1660–1666.

6 Bennett, K.A., Crane, J., O'Shea, P. et al. (2004). First trimester ultrasound screening is effective in reducing postterm labor induction rates: a randomized controlled trial. *Am. J. Obstet. Gynecol.* **190**: 1077–1081.

7 Olesen, A.W., Westergaard, J.G., and Olsen, J. (2006). Prenatal risk indicators of prolonged pregnancy. The Danish birth cohort 1998-2001. *Acta Obstet.Gynecol.* **85**: 1338–1341.

8 Usha Kiran, T.S., Hemmadi, S., Bethel, J., and Evans, J. (2005). Outcome of pregnancy in a woman with an increased body mass index. *BJOG* **112**: 768–772.

9 Stotland, N.E., Washington, A.E., and Caughey, A.B. (2007). Pre-pregnancy body mass index and length of gestation at term. *Am. J. Obstet. Gynecol.* **197**: 378.e1-5.

10 Caughey, A.B., Stotland, N.E., Washington, A.E., and Escobar, G.J. (2009). Who is at risk for prolonged and postterm pregnancy? *Am. J. Obstet. Gynecol.* **200**: 683.e1–683.e5.

11 Olesen, A.W., Basso, O., and Olsen, J. (1999). An estimate of the tendency to repeat postterm delivery. *Epidemiology* **10**: 468–469.

12 Olesen, A.W., Basso, O., and Olsen, J. (2003). Risk of recurrence of prolonged pregnancy. *BMJ* **326**: 476.

13 McDonald, P.C. and Siiteri, P.K. (1965). Origin of estrogen in women pregnant with an anencephalic fetus. *J. Clin. Invest.* **44**: 465–474.

14 Cunningham, F.G., Leveno, K.J., Bloom, S.L. et al. (eds.) (2014). *Williams Obstetrics*, 24e. Mc-Graw Hill Education.

15 American College of Obstetricians and Gynecologists (2014). Management of late-term and postterm pregnancies. Practice Bulletin No. 146. *Obstet. Gynecol.* **124**: 390–396.

16 Campbell, M.K., Østbye, T., and Irgens, L.M. (1997). Post-term birth: risk factors and outcomes in a 10-year cohort of Norwegian births. *Obstet. Gynecol.* **89**: 543–548.

17 Olesen, A.W., Westergaard, J.G., and Olsen, J. (2003). Perinatal and maternal complications related to postterm delivery: a national register-based study, 1978-1993. *Am. J. Obstet. Gynecol.* **189**: 222–227.

18 Hannah, M.E., Hannah, W.J., Hellman, J. et al. (1992). Induction of labor as compared with serial antenatal monitoring in post-term pregnancy – a randomized controlled trial. *N. Eng. J. Med.* **326**: 1587–1592.

19 Cheng, Y.W., Nicholson, J.M., Nakagawa, S. et al. (2008). Perinatal outcomes in low-risk term pregnancies: do they differ by week of gestation? *Am. J. Obstet. Gynecol.* **199**: 370.e1–370.e7.

20 Feldman, G.B. (1992). Prospective risk of stillbirth. *Obstet. Gynecol.* **79**: 547–553.

21 Caughey, A.B. and Musci, T.J. (2004). Complications of term pregnancies beyond 37 weeks of gestation. *Obstet. Gynecol.* **103**: 57–62.

22 Blondel, B., Morin, I., Platt, R.W. et al. (2002). Algorithms for combining menstrual and ultrasound estimates of gestational age: consequences for rates of preterm and postterm birth. *BJOG* **109**: 718–720.

23 Whitworth, M., Bricker, L., and Mullan, C. (2015). Ultrasound for fetal assessment in early pregnancy. *Cochrane Database Syst. Rev.* (**7**): CD007058. doi: 10.1002/14651858.

24 Caughey, A.B. and Bishop, J.T. (2006). Maternal complications of pregnancy increase beyond 40 weeks of gestation in low-risk women. *J. Perinatol.* **26**: 540–545.

25 Caughey, A.B., Stotland, N.E., Washington, A.E., and Escobar, G.J. (2007). Maternal and obstetric complications of pregnancy are associated with increasing gestational age at term. *Am. J. Obstet. Gynecol.* **196**: 155.e1-6.

26 Caughey, A.B., Washington, A.E., and Laros, R.K. Jr. (2005). Neonatal complications of term pregnancy: rates by gestational age increase in a continuous, not threshold, fashion. *Am. J. Obstet. Gynecol.* **192**: 185–190.

27 Smith, G.C. (2001). Life-table analysis of the risk of perinatal death at term and post-term in singleton pregnancies. *Am. J. Obstet. Gynecol.* **184**: 489–496.

28 Hilder, L., Costeloe, K., and Thilaganathan, B. (1998). Prolonged pregnancy: evaluating gestation-specific risks of fetal and infant mortality. *Br. J. Obstet. Gynaecol.* **105**: 169–173.

29 Heimstad, R., Romundstad, P.R., Eik-Nes, S.H., and Salvesen, K.A. (2006). Outcomes of pregnancy beyond 37 weeks of gestation. *Obstet. Gynecol.* **108**: 500–508.

30 Zhang, X. and Kramer, M.S. (2009). Variations in mortality and morbidity by gestational age among infants born at term. *J. Pediatr.* **154**: 358–362.

31 Cammu, H., Martens, G., Ruyssinck, G., and Amy, J.J. (2002). Outcome after elective labor induction in nulliparous women: a matched cohort study. *Am. J. Obstet. Gynecol.* **186**: 240–244.

32 Dublin, S., Lydon-Rochelle, M., Kaplan, R.C. et al. (2000). Maternal and neonatal outcomes after induction of labor without an identified indication. *Am. J. Obstet. Gynecol.* **183**: 986–994.

33 Maslow, A.S. and Sweeny, A.L. (2000). Elective induction of labor as a risk factor for cesarean delivery among low-risk women at term. *Obstet. Gynecol.* **95**: 917–922.

34 Seyb, S.T., Berka, R.J., Socol, M.L., and Dooley, S.L. (1999). Risk of cesarean delivery with elective induction of labor at term in nulliparous women. *Obstet. Gynecol.* **94**: 600–607.

35 Vrouenraets, F.P., Roumen, F.J., Dehing, C.J. et al. (2005). Bishop score and risk of cesarean delivery after induction of labor in nulliparous women. *Obstet. Gynecol.* **105**: 690–697.

36 Macer, J.A., Macer, C.L., and Chan, L.S. (1992). Elective induction versus spontaneous labor: a retrospective study of complications and outcome. *Am. J. Obstet. Gynecol.* **166**: 1690–1696; discussion 6–7.

37 Vahratian, A., Zhang, J., Troendle, J.F. et al. (2005). Labor progression and risk of cesarean delivery in electively induced nulliparas. *Obstet. Gynecol.* **105**: 698–704.

38 Gülmezoglu, A.M., Crowther, C.A., Middleton, P., and Heatley, E. (2012). Induction of labour for improving birth outcomes for women at or beyond term. *Cochrane Database Syst. Rev.* (**6**): CD004945. doi: 10.1002/14651858.

39 Wood, S., Cooper, S., and Ross, S. (2014). Does induction of labour increase the risk of caesarean section? A systematic review and meta-analysis of trials in women with intact membranes. *BJOG* **121**: 674–685.

40 Vayssière, C., Haumonte, J.B., Chantry, A. et al. (2013). French College of Gynecologists and Obstetricians (CNGOF). Prolonged and post-term pregnancies: guidelines for clinical practice from the French College of Gynecologists and Obstetricians (CNGOF). *Eur. J. Obstet. Gynecol. Reprod. Biol.* **169**: 10–16.

41 Clinical Practice Obstetrics Committee; Maternal Fetal Medicine Committee, Delaney, M., Roggensack, A. et al. (2008). Guidelines for the management of pregnancy at 41+0 to 42+0 weeks. *J. Obstet. Gynaecol. Can.* **30**: 800–823.

42 ACOG Committee on Practice Bulletins – Obstetrics (2009). ACOG practice bulletin no.107: induction of labor. *Obstet. Gynecol.* **114**: 386–397.

43 Ananth, C.V., Smulian, J.C., and Vintzileos, A.M. (1997). Epidemiology of antepartum fetal testing. *Curr. Opin. Obstet. Gynecol.* **9**: 101–106.

44 Signore, C., Freeman, R.K., and Spong, C.Y. (2009). Antenatal testing-a reevaluation: executive summary of a Eunice Kennedy Shriver National Institute of Child Health and Human Development workshop. *Obstet. Gynecol.* **113**: 687–701.

45 Kontopoulos, E.V. and Vintzileos, A.M. (2004). Condition-specific antepartum fetal testing. *Am. J. Obstet. Gynecol.* **191**: 1546–1551.

46 Mangesi, L., Hofmeyr, G.J., Smith, V., and Smyth, R.M. (2015). Fetal movement counting for assessment of fetal wellbeing. *Cochrane Database Syst. Rev.* (**10**): CD004909. doi: 10.1002/14651858.

47 Benirschke, K., Burton, G., and Baergen, R.N. (eds.) (2012). Histopathological approach to villous alterations. In: *Pathology of the Human Placenta*, 6the, 395–397. Berlin: Springer.

48 Guidetti, D.A., Divon, M.Y., Cavalieri, R.L. et al. (1987). Fetal umbilical artery flow velocimetry in postdate pregnancies. *Am. J. Obstet. Gynecol.* **157**: 1521–1523.

49 Zimmermann, P., Albäck, T., Koskinen, J. et al. (1995). Doppler flow velocimetry of the umbilical artery, uteroplacental arteries and fetal middle cerebral artery in prolonged pregnancy. *Ultrasound Obstet. Gynecol.* **5**: 189–197.

50 D'Antonio, F., Patel, D., Chandrasekharan, N. et al. (2013). Role of cerebroplacental ratio for fetal assessment in prolonged pregnancy. *Ultrasound Obstet. Gynecol.* **42**: 196–200.

51 Selam, B., Koksal, R., and Ozcan, T. (2000). Fetal arterial and venous Doppler parameters in the interpretation of oligohydramnios in postterm pregnancies. *Ultrasound Obstet. Gynecol.* **15**: 403–406.

52 O'Reilly-Green, C.P. and Divon, M.Y. (1999). Receiver operating characteristic curves of ultrasonographic estimates of fetal weight for prediction of fetal growth restriction in prolonged pregnancies. *Am. J. Obstet. Gynecol.* **181**: 1133–1138.

53 Boers, K.E., Vijgen, S.M., Bijlenga, D. et al. (2010). Scherjon SA; DIGITAT study group. Induction versus expectant monitoring for intrauterine growth restriction at term: randomised equivalence trial (DIGITAT). *BMJ* **341**: c7087.

54 Marks, A.D. and Divon, M.Y. (1992). Longitudinal study of the amniotic fluid index in post-dates pregnancy. *Obstet. Gynecol.* **79**: 229–233.

55 Phelan, J.P., Platt, L.D., Yeh, S.Y. et al. (1985). The role of ultrasound assessment of amniotic fluid volume in the management of the postdate pregnancy. *Am. J. Obstet. Gynecol.* **151**: 304–308.

56 Bochner, C.J., Medearis, A.L., Davis, J. et al. (1987). Antepartum predictors of fetal distress in postterm pregnancy. *Am. J. Obstet. Gynecol.* **157**: 353–358.

57 Chamberlain, P.F., Manning, F.A., Morrison, I. et al. (1984). Ultrasound evaluation of amniotic fluid volume. I. The relationship of marginal and decreased amniotic fluid volumes to perinatal outcome. *Am. J. Obstet. Gynecol.* **150**: 245–249.

58 Lam, H., Leung, W.C., Lee, C.P., and Lao, T.T. (2006). Amniotic fluid volume at 41 weeks and infant outcome. *J. Reprod. Med.* **51**: 484–488.

59 Morris, J.M., Thompson, K., Smithey, J. et al. (2003). The usefulness of ultrasound assessment of amniotic fluid in predicting adverse outcome in prolonged pregnancy: a prospective blinded observational study. *BJOG* **110**: 989–994.

60 Rosati, P., Guariglia, L., Cavaliere, A.F. et al. (2015). A comparison between amniotic fluid index and the single deepest vertical pocket technique in predicting adverse outcome in prolonged pregnancy. *J. Prenat. Med.* **9**: 12–15.

61 Nabhan, A.F. and Abdelmoula, Y.A. (2008). Amniotic fluid index versus single deepest vertical pocket as a screening test for preventing adverse pregnancy outcome. *Cochrane Database Syst. Rev.* (**3**): CD006593. doi: 10.1002/14651858.

62 Kehl, S., Schelkle, A., Thomas, A. et al. (2015). Single deepest vertical pocket or amniotic fluid index as evaluation test for preventing adverse pregnancy outcome (SAFE trial): a multicentre, open-label randomised controlled trial. *Ultrasound Obstet. Gynecol.* doi: 10.1002/uog.14924.

63 Boehm, F.H., Salyer, S., Shah, D.M., and Vaughn, W.K. (1986). Improved outcome of twice weekly nonstress testing. *Obstet. Gynecol.* **67**: 566–568.

64 Gauthier, R.J., Evertson, L.R., and Paul, R.H. (1979). Antepartum fetal heart rate testing. II. Intrapartum fetal heart rate observation and newborn outcome following a positive contraction stress test. *Am. J. Obstet. Gynecol.* **133**: 34–39.

65 Druzin, M.L., Karver, M.L., Wagner, W. et al. (1992). Prospective evaluation of the contraction stress and nonstress tests in the management of post-term pregnancy. *Surg. Gynecol. Obstet.* **174**: 507–512.

66 Cotzias, C.S., Paterson-Brown, S., and Fisk, N.M. (1999). Prospective risk of unexplained stillbirth in singleton pregnancies at term: population based analysis. *BMJ* **319**: 287–288.

67 Dayal, A.K., Manning, F.A., Berck, D.J. et al. (1999). Fetal death after normal biophysical profile score: an eighteen-year experience. *Am. J. Obstet. Gynecol.* **181**: 1231–1236.

68 Dugoua, J.J., Perri, D., Seely, D. et al. (2008). Safety and efficacy of blue cohosh (*Caulophyllum thalictroides*) during pregnancy and lactation. *Can. J. Clin. Pharmacol.* **15**: e66–e73.

69 Dugoua, J.J., Seely, D., Perri, D. et al. (2006). Safety and efficacy of black cohosh (*Cimicifuga racemosa*) during pregnancy and lactation. *Can. J. Clin. Pharmacol.* **13**: e257–e261.

70 Jing Zheng, P.M.J., Holloway, A.C., and Crankshaw, D.J. (2010). The effects of commercial preparations of red raspberry leaf on the contractility of the rat's uterus in vitro. *Reprod. Sci.* **17**: 494–501.

71 Kelly, A.J., Kavanagh, J., and Thomas, J. (2013). Castor oil, bath and/or enema for cervical priming and induction of labour. *Cochrane Database Syst. Rev.* (**7**): CD003099.

72 Dove, D. and Johnson, P. (1999). Oral evening primrose oil: its effect on length of pregnancy and selected intrapartum outcomes in low-risk nulliparous women. *J. Nurse Midwifery* **44**: 320–324.

73 Smith, C.A., Crowther, C.A., and Grant, S.J. (2013). Acupuncture for induction of labour. *Cochrane Database Syst. Rev.* (**8**): CD002962.

74 Teimoori, B., Rajabi, S., Navvabi-Rigi, S.D., and Arbabisarjou, A. (2014). Evaluation effect of shiatsu technique on labor induction in post-term pregnancy. *Glob. J. Health Sci.* **7**: 177–183.

75 Ingram, J., Domagala, C., and Yates, S. (2005). The effects of shiatsu on post-term pregnancy. *Complement Ther. Med.* **13**: 11–15.

76 Dante, G., Bellei, G., Neri, I., and Facchinetti, F. (2014). Herbal therapies in pregnancy: what works? *Curr. Opin. Obstet. Gynecol.* **26**: 83–91.

77 Mozurkewich, E.L., Chilimigras, J.L., Berman, D.R. et al. (2011). Methods of induction of labour: a systematic review. *BMC Pregnancy Childbirth.* **11**: 84.

78 McFarlin, B.L., Gibson, M.H., O'Rear, J., and Harman, P. (1999). A national survey of herbal preparation use by nurse-midwives for labor stimulation. Review of the literature and recommendations for practice. *J. Nurse Midwifery* **44**: 205–216.

79 Dennehy, C., Tsourounis, C., Bui, L., and King, T.L. (2010). The use of herbs by California midwives. *J. Obstet. Gynecol. Neonatal. Nurs.* **39**: 684–693.

80 Datta, S., Mahdi, F., Ali, Z. et al. (2014). Toxins in botanical dietary supplements: blue cohosh components disrupt cellular respiration and mitochondrial membrane potential. *J. Nat. Prod.* **77**: 111–117.

81 Garry, D., Figueroa, R., Guillaume, J., and Cucco, V. (2000). Use of castor oil in pregnancies at term. *Altern. Ther. Health Med.* **6**: 77–79.

82 McColgin, S.W., Bennett, W.A., Roach, H. et al. (1993). Parturitional factors associated with membrane stripping. *Am. J. Obstet. Gynecol.* **169**: 71–77.

83 Boulvain, M., Stan, C., and Irion, O. (2005). Membrane sweeping for induction of labour. *Cochrane Database Syst Rev.* (**1**): CD000451.

Fetal complications

42

CHAPTER 42
Disorders of amniotic fluid volume

Marie Beall and Michael Ross
Obstetrics and Gynecology, Harbor UCLA Medical Center, Torrance, CA, USA

CLINICAL SCENARIO

A 32-year-old female, gravida three para one at 32 weeks of gestational age, presents to the office complaining of progressive shortness of breath. She complains that for the past two weeks she has had increasing difficulty breathing. She is now unable to do her usual household activities without discomfort, and for the past three days she has slept in a chair, as she is not able to lie flat in bed. She reports that this is different from her first pregnancy, and that she also feels that her abdomen is bigger than in her first pregnancy. She reports normal fetal movement. She has recently relocated to the area and has not initiated prenatal care here; records from her prior prenatal care provider are not immediately available. She denies other medical problems, and provides an image from a first trimester ultrasound that corroborates her dating of 32 weeks.

On physical exam she is a slender woman with an obviously protuberant abdomen. Her respiratory rate is 24 per minute. Her abdomen is tense and nontender, with a fundal height of 42 cm. Fetal parts are difficult to palpate abdominally. Fetal heart tones are auscultated in the right lower quadrant at 140 bpm.

Background

Near term, the primary sources of amniotic fluid (AF) are fetal urine and liquid produced by the fetal lungs; the major routes for resorption of fluid are via fetal swallowing and the intramembranous pathway (from AF to the fetal circulation across the fetal membranes). Minor pathways for AF production and clearance include secretions from the fetal oral-nasal cavities and the transmembranous pathway (from AF to maternal circulation).

Estimates of the volume of fetal urine production vary widely [1, 2], however consensus best estimates of daily amniotic volume flows in the near term fetus are [3]:

Production:
- Fetal urine production – 800–1200 ml per day
- Fetal lung liquid secretion – 170 ml per day
- Oral–nasal secretions – 25 ml per day

Resorption:
- Fetal swallowing – 500–1000 ml per day
- Intramembranous flow – 200–400 ml per day
- Transmembranous flow – 10 ml per day

AF volume increases dramatically during the first two-thirds of human pregnancy, from 20 ml at 10 weeks to an average of 770 ml at 28 weeks. After 28 weeks, the AF volume changes little until term, although it may decrease after 39–40 weeks [4]. As these figures indicate, the fetus (on average) replaces the entire AF volume in less than 24 hours. Although the average AF volume in the third trimester is 700–800 ml, there is a wide range of normal fluids, and a normal fetus at 32 weeks may have more than 2000 ml, or less than 500 ml of AF. This wide range of normal compounds the problem of assessing the AF volume.

Polyhydramnios is the condition of excessive AF, occurring in 1–3% of pregnancies [5, 6]. Knowledge of AF dynamics informs our understanding of the underlying etiology of polyhydramnios. In general, polyhydramnios may be caused either by excess fetal urine flow, or by a defect in fetal swallowing or high gut obstructions that do not allow for AF resorption. These effects may be associated with a wide variety of factors, including genetic, environmental, toxic, infectious, and others.

Clinical questions

In order to address the issues of most relevance to your patient and to help in searching the literature for evidence

Evidence-Based Obstetrics and Gynecology, First Edition. Edited by Errol R. Norwitz, Carolyn M. Zelop, David A. Miller, and David L. Keefe.

regarding those issues, you choose the following clinical questions:

1. In pregnant patients in the third trimester (population) what is the sensitivity and specificity (diagnostic test characteristics) of ultrasound (test) for the diagnosis of amniotic fluid abnormalities associated with poor perinatal outcome (outcome)?

2. In pregnant patients with polyhydramnios (population) what is the diagnostic value (diagnostic test characteristics) of ultrasound and amniocentesis (tests) for the diagnosis of fetal anomalies (outcome)?

3. In pregnant patients with idiopathic polyhydramnios (population) what is the prognostic value (test characteristics) of antenatal testing by nonstress test or biophysical profile (tests) for the diagnosis of fetal wellbeing (outcome)?

4. In pregnant patients with polyhydramnios (population) what is the efficacy of amnioreduction (AR) (treatment) in relieving maternal symptoms and preventing preterm delivery (outcomes) compared to no treatment (control)?

5. In pregnant patients with polyhydramnios (population) what is the efficacy of indomethacin (treatment) in relieving maternal symptoms and preventing preterm delivery (outcomes) compared to no treatment (control)?

1. In pregnant patients in the third trimester (population) what is the sensitivity and specificity (diagnostic test characteristics) of ultrasound (test) for the diagnosis of amniotic fluid abnormalities associated with poor perinatal outcome (outcome)?

AF volume abnormalities, specifically polyhydramnios, are associated with an increased risk for poor perinatal outcome, making identification of abnormal AF volume a concern. A diagnosis of an AF volume abnormality may be suspected by physical exam, but the diagnosis is generally made by examination of the fluid. Although AF volume can be assessed by invasive means, such as dye dilution, these are not commonly used in clinical practice. Clinically, the amount of AF is most commonly evaluated using ultrasound. The most commonly used semi-quantitative techniques include amniotic fluid index (AFI) [7, 8], and the single deepest pocket (SDP) [9]:

1. In assessing the AFI, the sonographer measures the deepest AF pocket in each of the four quadrants of the maternal abdomen. The AFI is the sum of the four measurements.

2. The SDP is the single largest measurement obtained as for an AFI.

3. Other sonographic methods have included quantification of vertical and horizontal measurements of the AF pockets; such measurements have been found to be poorly reflective of AF volume [10].

4. Subjective assessment of amniotic fluid volume by an experienced ultrasound practitioner may be as accurate as semiquantitative methods in identifying normal AF volumes [11].

Commonly used definitions of AF abnormalities include an AFI of >24 cm (polyhydramnios) or <5 cm (oligohydramnios), or a SDP of >8 or <2 cm. Polyhydramnios is often categorized as mild, moderate, or severe; although these terms are not strictly defined, they correspond roughly to AFIs of 25–30, 30–35, and >35 cm [12] or SDPs of 8–10, 10–12, and >12 cm [13].

A recent systematic review compared the AFI to the SDP for predicting adverse antepartum, intrapartum, and perinatal outcome. The AFI was no better than the SDP for predicting an adverse outcome [14]. Significantly more fetuses were categorized as having oligohydramnios by AFI (Risk Ratio (RR) 2.3), leading to more obstetrical interventions without improving perinatal outcome.

In addition to outcome studies, there are studies in women with polyhydramnios comparing the various clinical methods of amniotic fluid assessment against a quantitative technique such as dye-dilution [15, 16]. Available studies are indicated in Table 42.1. Both AFI and SDP demonstrated poor sensitivity for the diagnosis of polyhydramnios, although the specificity was high. In a population at risk for the condition either of these methods may be of value in making the diagnosis in combination with other findings.

Level of Evidence: A

Strength of recommendation: Class IIa

2. In pregnant patients with polyhydramnios (population) what is the diagnostic value (diagnostic test characteristics) of ultrasound (test) for the diagnosis of fetal anomalies (outcome)?

The frequency of an anomalous infant increases with increasing amniotic fluid volume. One study found mild, moderate, and severe polyhydramnios associated with an 8%, 12%, and 31% risk, respectively [17]. Both fetal ultrasound and amniocentesis have been performed to evaluate this risk in the face of polyhydramnios.

Comprehensive fetal ultrasound has been advocated to evaluate the fetus for congenital anomalies. A number of descriptive studies address the success of ultrasound in detecting anomalies of the fetus in screening programs. After searching for studies, results were included if they reported total anomalies detected, and if they reported work

Table 42.1 Performance of various clinical measures of AF volume in the diagnosis of polyhydramnios (Polyhydramnios diagnosed by an objective method)

	N (polyhydramnios/total)	Sensitivity	Specificity	PPV	NPV	Reference
AFI	13/144	30	98	57	93	[10]
SDP	17/175	29	94	45	89	[14]

AFI, amniotic fluid index; SDP, single deepest pocket; PPV, positive predictive value; NPV, negative predictive value.

Table 42.2 Detection rate for total fetal anomalies by prenatal ultrasound. The overall detection rate (sensitivity) is 40% with a range of 35–71.4%

Year/ location	Total subjects	Abnormals	Detection rate	Reference
2010 – Spain	Not specified	812	56.3%	[18]
2009 – Italy	42 256	1050	55.05%	[19]
2004 – Europe	1 013 352	25 400	35%	[20]
1999 – Germany	11 172	297	53%	[21]
1998 – England	33 376	725	55%	[22]
1998 – US	901	28	71.4%	[23]
1998 – Europe	Not specified	3685	61.4%	[24]

performed (at least in part) after 1995, when there was a major change in ultrasound technology. Studies were excluded if they reported only data from first trimester exams, a population with limited relevance to investigation of polyhydramnios. Included studies are listed in Table 42.2. These studies are retrospective surveys, in some cases over many institutions and/or many years. Methods of ascertainment for total anomalies are not standardized. In two cases the total population from which the population of anomalies was derived was not specified. The overall detection rate of fetal anomalies in these studies is 40%. If the large study from Europe is excluded, as the scans in this case may have been performed by less-trained personnel, the detection rate (sensitivity) is 59%. The specificity of the test is not addressed by all studies, but in the studies that report it the specificity is universally above 99% (Table 42.3). One study specifically investigated the detection of fetal bowel atresia, an anatomic cause of polyhydramnios. In this retrospective study, the sensitivity and specificity of ultrasound in detecting fetal small bowel obstruction after 32 weeks of gestation were 67% and 71% respectively [25].

The data suggest that ultrasound has significant utility in detecting fetal anomalies associated with polyhydramnios, but that the absence of ultrasound findings may be associated with an appreciable risk of anomalies if the a priori risk is high. This result may explain the increase in the risk for aneuploidy with polyhydramnios, even in the

Table 42.3 False positive rate (FPR) for detection of fetal anomalies by prenatal ultrasound. Specificity (1-FPR) is above 99% in all cases

Year/ location	# Total	# Abnormals	# False positive	FPR	Reference
1998 – US	901	28	5	0.6%	[23]
2009 – Italy	42 256	1050	50	0.12%	[19]
1998 – England	33 376	725	174[a]	0.5%	[22]
			14[b]	0.04%	

[a]Includes "soft signs" of aneuploidy.
[b]Excludes "soft signs."

presence of a negative ultrasound for anomalies. Reported risks are 10% for fetal aneuploidy in polyhydramnios with fetal anomalies and 1% for fetal aneuploidy if anomalies are not seen [26], suggesting that amniocentesis be offered in either case, although the available data is of too poor a quality to guide care in the case of the patient without fetal anomalies and who is otherwise of low risk for fetal aneuploidy [27]. Another study suggests that chromosomal anomalies may be more likely if the polyhydramnios is associated with fetal growth restriction [16], although the number of chromosomal abnormalities is too small to state the increase in risk. In summary, available data supports detailed ultrasound for pregnancies complicated by polyhydramnios when another explanation is not apparent. In the presence of a fetal anomaly or fetal growth restriction, evaluation for fetal aneuploidy is appropriate. With an apparently normal fetus, the appropriateness of evaluation for fetal aneuploidy depends on other maternal risk factors, maternal preference, and the degree of polyhydramnios.

For ultrasound:
Level of evidence: B
Strength of recommendation: I

For amniocentesis
Level of evidence: C
Strength of recommendation: IIa

3. In pregnant patients with idiopathic polyhydramnios (population) what is the prognostic value (test characteristics) of antenatal testing by nonstress test or biophysical profile (tests) for the diagnosis of fetal wellbeing (outcome)?

Polyhydramnios is associated with an increased risk for various adverse pregnancy outcomes [28] and with an increased risk for perinatal mortality [29]. No randomized trials have evaluated whether pregnancies complicated by polyhydramnios benefit from any method of antenatal surveillance. Given the increased risk of adverse pregnancy outcomes, many experts recommend a regimen of antenatal testing in the third trimester in the patient with polyhydramnios. Several approaches have been suggested, including Doppler flow velocimetry of the middle cerebral artery, nonstress tests, biophysical profiles, and contraction stress tests [30]. Most centers routinely perform some form of testing with nonstress test or modified or complete biophysical profile, but there is no evidence for the efficacy of this approach.
Level of evidence: C
Strength of recommendation: IIb

4. In pregnant patients with polyhydramnios (population) what is the efficacy of AR (treatment) in relieving maternal symptoms and preventing preterm delivery (outcomes) compared to no treatment (control)?

The goal of symptomatic treatment in polyhydramnios is to relieve intolerable maternal symptoms, to avert preterm delivery and to relieve excessive intra-amniotic pressure that has been associated with impaired fetal oxygenation in some reports [31]. Mild and moderate polyhydramnios are therefore usually managed expectantly, and treatment reserved for symptomatic patients and for those with severe polyhydramnios. One approach is the removal of large amounts of AF by therapeutic amniocentesis, or AR. AR has been successful in alleviating the maternal symptoms of polyhydramnios [32]. The procedure has also been used to avert preterm delivery and to improve fetal oxygenation by reducing intraamniotic pressure [33], however there is no good evidence of efficacy for fetal indications [34] in singleton pregnancy. Studies limited to singletons suggest a delay in delivery of up to seven weeks; however the studies are of very limited size, and do not include control groups [32, 35, 36]. Two protocols have been used for AR: standard AR, in which fluid is removed at a rate of 45–90 ml min^{-1}, or aggressive AR, in which fluid is removed more rapidly; there is no evidence to suggest a difference in outcome between the techniques [37]. Standard AR is associated with a 4–12% risk of complications, including Preterm premature rupture of membrane (PPROM), infection, placental abruption and fetal death [37, 38]. Aggressive AR is reported to be associated with a 3–15% risk of similar complications [39]. It is not known whether some or all of these complications occurred as a part of the natural history of polyhydramnios, as none of the reported studies had an untreated control arm.

In summary, AR is appropriate for acute relief of maternal symptoms. Given the known circulation of AF, AR would not be expected to cause a long-term reduction in AF volume. If AR is elected, the approach may be either the standard or aggressive protocol.

For maternal symptoms:
Level of evidence: B
Strength of recommendation: I

For prevention of preterm labor
Level of Evidence: B
Strength of recommendation: III

5. In pregnant patients with polyhydramnios (population) what is the efficacy of indomethacin (treatment) in relieving maternal symptoms and preventing preterm delivery (outcomes) compared to no treatment (control)?

One possible treatment paradigm for polyhydramnios is to reduce fetal urine production. Although maternal dehydration should reduce maternal-to-fetal water flow, and thus urine production, manipulations of maternal plasma volume or osmolality, as with diuretics, are not generally used as this may also reduce placental blood flow and impair fetal oxygenation [40]. In contrast, fetal urine flow in polyhydramnios has been directly manipulated with the use of prostaglandin synthase inhibitors with good results. A number of case series and case reports have documented the use of indomethacin to treat polyhydramnios [41–47], although there are no randomized trials for this indication. The pertinent case series are summarized in Table 42.4. Indomethacin may act via an effect on the fetal membranes [5], but most likely it acts by increasing the resorption of water in the renal tubule via its inhibition of the effects of prostaglandin [5]. This reduces fetal urine production, with an associated fall in AF, especially in those with nonobstructive causes of polyhydramnios, and after 26 weeks gestation [48]. Indomethacin may also reduce the risk of preterm delivery with polyhydramnios via an anti-inflammatory effect, as preterm labor due to uterine overdistention may have an inflammatory etiology [49]. The most commonly-used dose of indomethacin is 25 mg every six hours [5], although some authors have used doses up to 200 mg per day [44, 47, 50]. In most reports, the dose is reduced or stopped if there is oligohydramnios or signs of constriction of the fetal ductus. Otherwise, if the treatment is successful in reducing the AF volume, the indomethacin is continued until a gestational age of 32–34 weeks. It may be possible to taper the dose and discontinue indomethacin treatment earlier if severe polyhydramnios does not recur, but published reports do not compare various strategies for stopping the medication.

Indomethacin use has been associated with a variety of undesirable fetal effects, including closure or constriction of

Table 42.4 Effect of indomethacin on maternal symptoms, fluid volume, and delivery timing. All studies are observational; all indicate an effect of indomethacin on AF volume and maternal symptoms. Delivery delay due to the drug is difficult to assess without a control group. One additional study concerned only twins and is omitted, the results were similar

Year/ location	# Patients Total	Dose	Maternal symptoms relieved	AF reduced	Average delivery delay (DD)/ duration of treatment (DOT)	Reference
2000 – India	12	2.2–3.0 mg kg^{-1} per day	11/12	10/12	DD 4.6 weeks	[47]
1993 – Spain	7	2.2–2.5 mg kg^{-1} per day	Not stated	6/7	DD 5.1 weeks	[46]
1990 – Greece	15	2.0–2.2 mg kg^{-1} per day	Not stated	15/15	DOT 3.3 weeks	[41]
1990 – US	8	25 mg q 6 h	7/8	6/8	DOT 25 days	[42]
1987 – US	8	2.2–3.0 mg kg^{-1} per day	8/8	8/8	DOT 2–11 weeks	[43]

the ductus arteriosus [46] and the development of oligohydramnios [51] and fetal renal damage [52, 53], although not all reports support these associations [54], and many reports find no association between complications of indomethacin and gestational age or duration of therapy [54]. Recommendations regarding appropriate fetal monitoring for indomethacin complications include periodic assessments of AF volume and ductal flow, although there is no consensus on the timing of these. Assessment of amniotic fluid volume has been proposed daily [55] to weekly [56]. The most common recommendation to assess for ductal closure is fetal echocardiography 24 hours after beginning the medication, and weekly thereafter [57].

In summary, indomethacin appears to be effective in reducing AF volume in most affected pregnancies, and in sustaining the reduction. In view of the potential for serious fetal complications, the dose and duration of therapy should be limited to the lowest effective. Good information is lacking regarding identification of patients at highest risk or the best monitoring strategy.

For reducing AF volume
Level of evidence: A
Strength of recommendation: II

Case conclusion

You order a brief ultrasound, which reveals an AFI of 45 cm. The fetus appears active; the bedside ultrasound does not reveal gross fetal anomalies. You request a consultation with the Maternal-Fetal Medicine specialist for further management. A detailed ultrasound reveals a "double bubble" suggestive of fetal duodenal atresia. The estimated fetal weight is 1790 g, 25th%ile for the gestational age of 32 weeks. Given the maternal respiratory embarrassment, the consultant performs a therapeutic amniocentesis, removing 1500 cm^3 of amniotic fluid. Given the apparent fetal anomaly, the suspicion for a chromosomal abnormality is high, and amniotic fluid is sent for fetal karyotype. The fetal karyotype is found to be 47, XX + 21 (a female fetus with Down syndrome). After the AR the mother is more comfortable and is able to perform her usual activities. In view of the obstructive etiology and the gestational age, the consultant chooses not to utilize indomethacin in this patient, understanding that the fluid would likely rapidly reaccumulate. The patient is followed, and requires two more ARs for intractable maternal symptoms, one four days after the first, and the second a week after that. At 34 weeks and three days of gestation the patient returns, again with severe shortness of breath. At this time the fetal heart rate pattern has changed, and suggests fetal hypoxemia. The patient is delivered by Cesarean due to a non-reassuring fetal heart rate pattern of a 2055 g female infant with Apgar scores of 6 at one minute and 7 at five minutes. The infant scores poorly for tone and respiratory effort; it is the opinion of the neonatologist that this is consistent with the diagnosis of Down syndrome. The mother's recovery from surgery is uneventful, and she is discharged on post-operative day three. The infant initially has mild respiratory symptoms, and is maintained on intravenous nutrition for several days until her pulmonary function stabilizes. She subsequently undergoes duodenoduodenostomy with a good functional result. Further workup does not reveal any cardiac abnormality or other physical anomalies, and she is discharged home at two weeks of life.

References

1 Lotgering, F.K. and Wallenburg, H.C. (1986). Mechanisms of production and clearance of amniotic fluid. *Semin. Perinatol.* **10** (**2**): 94–102.

2 Rabinowitz, R., Peters, M.T., Vyas, S. et al. (1989). Measurement of fetal urine production in normal pregnancy by real-time ultrasonography. *Am. J. Obstet. Gynecol.* **161** (**5**): 1264–1266.

3 Brace, R.A. and Ross, M.G. (1998). Amniotic fluid volume regulation. In: *Fetus and Neonate-Volume 4: Body Fluids and Kidney Function* (ed. R.A. Brace, M.A. Hansen and C.H. Rodeck), 88–105. Cambridge University Press.

4 Brace, R.A. and Wolf, E.J. (1989). Normal amniotic fluid volume changes throughout pregnancy. *Am. J. Obstet. Gynecol.* **161** (**2**): 382–388.

5 Moise, K.J. Jr. (1997). Polyhydramnios. *Clin. Obstet. Gynecol.* **40** (**2**): 266–279.

6 Volante, E., Gramellini, D., Moretti, S. et al. (2004). Alteration of the amniotic fluid and neonatal outcome. *Acta Biomed.* **75** (**Suppl 1**): 71–75.

7 Phelan, J.P., Smith, C.V., Broussard, P., and Small, M. (1987). Amniotic fluid volume assessment with the four-quadrant technique at 36–42 weeks' gestation. *J. Reprod. Med.* **32** (**7**): 540–542.

8 Phelan, J.P., Ahn, M.O., Smith, C.V. et al. (1987). Amniotic fluid index measurements during pregnancy. *J. Reprod. Med.* **32** (**8**): 601–604.

9 Chamberlain, P.F., Manning, F.A., Morrison, I. et al. (1984). Ultrasound evaluation of amniotic fluid volume. I. The relationship of marginal and decreased amniotic fluid volumes to perinatal outcome. *Am. J. Obstet. Gynecol.* **150** (**3**): 245–249.

10 Chauhan, S.P., Magann, E.F., Morrison, J.C. et al. (1997). Ultrasonographic assessment of amniotic fluid does not reflect actual amniotic fluid volume. *Am. J. Obstet. Gynecol.* **177** (**2**): 291–296.

11 Magann, E.F., Perry, K.G. Jr., Chauhan, S.P. et al. (1997). The accuracy of ultrasound evaluation of amniotic fluid volume in singleton pregnancies: the effect of operator experience and ultrasound interpretative technique. *J. Clin. Ultrasound* **25** (**5**): 249–253.

12 Lazebnik, N. and Many, A. (1999). The severity of polyhydramnios, estimated fetal weight and preterm delivery are independent risk factors for the presence of congenital malformations. *Gynecol. Obstet. Invest.* **48** (**1**): 28–32.

13 Hill, L.M., Breckle, R., Thomas, M.L., and Fries, J.K. (1987). Polyhydramnios: ultrasonically detected prevalence and neonatal outcome. *Obstet. Gynecol.* **69** (**1**): 21–25.

14 Nabhan, A.F. and Abdelmoula, Y.A. (2008). Amniotic fluid index versus single deepest vertical pocket as a screening test for preventing adverse pregnancy outcome. *Cochrane Database Syst. Rev.* (**3**): CD006593. doi: 10.1002/14651858.

15 Magann, E.F., Chauhan, S.P., Barrilleaux, P.S. et al. (2000). Amniotic fluid index and single deepest pocket: weak indicators of abnormal amniotic volumes. *Obstet. Gynecol.* **96** (**5 Pt 1**): 737–740.

16 Barnhard, Y., Bar-Hava, I., and Divon, M.Y. (1995). Is polyhydramnios in an ultrasonographically normal fetus an indication for genetic evaluation? *Am. J. Obstet. Gynecol.* **173** (**5**): 1523–1527.

17 Chamberlain, P.F., Manning, F.A., Morrison, I. et al. (1984). Ultrasound evaluation of amniotic fluid volume. II. The relationship of increased amniotic fluid volume to perinatal outcome. *Am. J. Obstet. Gynecol.* **150** (**3**): 250–254.

18 Campana, H., Ermini, M., Aiello, H.A. et al. (2010). Prenatal sonographic detection of birth defects in 18 hospitals from South America. *J. Ultrasound Med.* **29** (**2**): 203–212.

19 Fadda, G.M., Capobianco, G., Balata, A. et al. (2009). Routine second trimester ultrasound screening for prenatal detection of fetal malformations in Sassari University Hospital, Italy: 23 years of experience in 42, 256 pregnancies. *Eur. J. Obstet. Gynecol. Reprod. Biol.* **144** (**2**): 110–114.

20 Garne, E., Loane, M., de Vigan, C. et al. (2004). Prenatal diagnostic procedures used in pregnancies with congenital malformations in 14 regions of Europe. *Prenat Diagn.* **24** (**11**): 908–912.

21 Behrens, O., Steiner, C., Bohmer, S., and Muhlhaus, K. (1999). Efficacy of ultrasound screening in pregnancy. *Zentralbl. Gynakol.* **121** (**5**): 228–232.

22 Boyd, P.A., Chamberlain, P., and Hicks, N.R. (1998). 6-year experience of prenatal diagnosis in an unselected population in Oxford, UK. *Lancet* **352** (**9140**): 1577–1581.

23 Magriples, U. and Copel, J.A. (1998). Accurate detection of anomalies by routine ultrasonography in an indigent clinic population. *Am. J. Obstet. Gynecol.* **179** (**4**): 978–981.

24 Grandjean, H., Larroque, D., and Levi, S. (1998). Sensitivity of routine ultrasound screening of pregnancies in the Eurofetus database. *Ann. N. Y. Acad. Sci.* **847**: 118–124.

25 John, R., D'Antonio, F., Khalil, A. et al. (2015). Diagnostic accuracy of prenatal ultrasound in identifying Jejunal and Ileal Atresia. *Fetal Diagn Ther.* **38** (**2**): 142–146.

26 Dashe, J.S., McIntire, D.D., Ramus, R.M. et al. (2002). Hydramnios: anomaly prevalence and sonographic detection. *Obstet. Gynecol.* **100** (**1**): 134–139.

27 Sagi-Dain, L. and Sagi, S. (2015). Chromosomal aberrations in idiopathic polyhydramnios: a systematic review and meta-analysis. *Eur. J. Med. Genet.* **58** (**8**): 409–415.

28 Aviram, A., Salzer, L., Hiersch, L. et al. (2015). Association of isolated polyhydramnios at or beyond 34 weeks of gestation and pregnancy outcome. *Obstet. Gynecol.* **125** (**4**): 825–832.

29 Pilliod, R.A., Page, J.M., Burwick, R.M. et al. (2015). The risk of fetal death in nonanomalous pregnancies affected by polyhydramnios. *Am. J. Obstet. Gynecol.* **213** (**3**): 410–416.

30 Magann, E.F., Chauhan, S.P., Doherty, D.A. et al. (2007). Morrison JC, A review of idiopathic hydramnios and pregnancy outcomes. *Obstet. Gynecol. Surv.* **62** (**12**): 795–802.

31 Fisk, N.M., Vaughan, J., and Talbert, D. (1994). Impaired fetal blood gas status in polyhydramnios and its relation to raised amniotic pressure. *Fetal Diagn Ther.* **9** (**1**): 7–13.

32 Piantelli, G., Bedocchi, L., Cavicchioni, O. et al. (2004). Amnioreduction for treatment of severe polyhydramnios. *Acta Biomed.* **75** (**Suppl 1**): 56–58.

33 Bower, S.J., Flack, N.J., Sepulveda, W. et al. (1995). Uterine artery blood flow response to correction of amniotic fluid volume. *Am. J. Obstet. Gynecol.* **173** (**2**): 502–507.

34 Roberts, D., Gates, S., Kilby, M., and Neilson, J.P. (2008). Interventions for twin-twin transfusion syndrome: a Cochrane review. *Ultrasound Obstet. Gynecol.* **31** (**6**): 701–711.

35 Elliott, J.P., Sawyer, A.T., Radin, T.G., and Strong, R.E. (1994). Large-volume therapeutic amniocentesis in the treatment of hydramnios. *Obstet. Gynecol.* **84** (**6**): 1025–1027.

36 Dickinson, J.E., Tjioe, Y.Y., Jude, E. et al. (2014). Amnioreduction in the management of polyhydramnios complicating singleton pregnancies. *Am. J. Obstet. Gynecol.* **211** (**4**): 434–437.

37 Coviello, D., Bonati, F., Montefusco, S.M. et al. (2004). Amnioreduction. *Acta Biomed.* **75** (**Suppl 1**): 31–33.

38 Mari, G., Roberts, A., Detti, L. et al. (2001). Perinatal morbidity and mortality rates in severe twin–twin transfusion syndrome: results of the International Amnioreduction Registry. *Am. J. Obstet. Gynecol.* **185** (**3**): 708–715.

39 Leung, W.C., Jouannic, J.M., Hyett, J. et al. (2004). Procedure-related complications of rapid amniodrainage in the treatment of polyhydramnios. *Ultrasound Obstet. Gynecol.* **23** (**2**): 154–158.

40 Carr, D.B., Gavrila, D., Brateng, D., and Easterling, T.R. (2007). Maternal hemodynamic changes associated with furosemide treatment. *Hypertens Pregnancy* **26** (**2**): 173–178.

41 Mamopoulos, M., Assimakopoulos, E., Reece, E.A. et al. (1990). Maternal indomethacin therapy in the treatment of polyhydramnios. *Am. J. Obstet. Gynecol.* **162** (**5**): 1225–1229.

42 Kirshon, B., Mari, G., and Moise, K.J. Jr. (1990). Indomethacin therapy in the treatment of symptomatic polyhydramnios. *Obstet. Gynecol.* **75** (**2**): 202–205.

43 Cabrol, D., Landesman, R., Muller, J. et al. (1987). Treatment of polyhydramnios with prostaglandin synthetase inhibitor (indomethacin). *Am. J. Obstet. Gynecol.* **157** (**2**): 422–426.

44 Lange, I.R., Harman, C.R., Ash, K.M. et al. (1989). Twin with hydramnios: treating premature labor at source. *Am. J. Obstet. Gynecol.* **160** (**3**): 552–557.

45 Deeny, M. and Haxton, M.J. (1993). Indomethacin use to control gross polyhydramnios complicating triplet pregnancy. *Br. J. Obstet. Gynaecol.* **100** (**3**): 281–282.

46 Carmona, F., Martinez-Roman, S., Mortera, C. et al. (1993). Efficacy and safety of indomethacin therapy for polyhydramnios. *Eur. J. Obstet. Gynecol. Reprod. Biol.* **52** (**3**): 175–180.

47 Abhyankar, S. and Salvi, V.S. (2000). Indomethacin therapy in hydramnios. *J. Postgrad Med.* **46** (**3**): 176–178.

48 Harman, C.R. (2008). Amniotic fluid abnormalities. *Semin. Perinatol.* **32** (**4**): 288–294.

49 Adams Waldorf, K.M., Singh, N., Mohan, A.R. et al. (2015). Uterine overdistention induces preterm labor mediated by inflammation: observations in pregnant women and nonhuman primates. *Am. J. Obstet. Gynecol.*

50 Panting-Kemp, A., Nguyen, T., Chang, E. et al. (1999). Idiopathic polyhydramnios and perinatal outcome. *Am. J. Obstet. Gynecol.* **181** (**5 Pt 1**): 1079–1082.

51 Sawdy, R.J., Lye, S., Fisk, N.M., and Bennett, P.R. (2003). A double-blind randomized study of fetal side effects during and after the short-term maternal administration of indomethacin, sulindac, and nimesulide for the treatment of preterm labor. *Am. J. Obstet. Gynecol.* **188** (**4**): 1046–1051.

52 Cuzzolin, L., Dal, C.M., and Fanos, V. (2001). NSAID-induced nephrotoxicity from the fetus to the child. *Drug Saf.* **24** (**1**): 9–18.

53 Gloor, J.M., Muchant, D.G., and Norling, L.L. (1993). Prenatal maternal indomethacin use resulting in prolonged neonatal renal insufficiency. *J. Perinatol.* **13** (**6**): 425–427.

54 Savage, A.H., Anderson, B.L., and Simhan, H.N. (2007). The safety of prolonged indomethacin therapy. *Am. J. Perinatol.* **24** (**4**): 207–213.

55 Sandruck, J.C., Grobman, W.A., and Gerber, S.E. (2005). The effect of short-term indomethacin therapy on amniotic fluid volume. *Am. J. Obstet. Gynecol.* **192** (**5**): 1443–1445.

56 Moise, K.J. Jr. (1991). Indomethacin therapy in the treatment of symptomatic polyhydramnios. *Clin. Obstet. Gynecol.* **34** (**2**): 310–318.

57 Abou-Ghannam, G., Usta, I.M., and Nassar, A.H. (2012). Indomethacin in pregnancy: applications and safety. *Am. J. Perinatol.* **29** (**3**): 175–186.

43 CHAPTER 43
Disorders of fetal growth

Katherine R. Goetzinger[1] and Anthony O. Odibo[2]
[1] *Department of Obstetrics, Gynecology and Reproductive Sciences, University of Maryland School of Medicine, Baltimore, MD, USA*
[2] *Department of Obstetrics & Gynecology, University of South Florida, Tampa, FL, USA*

CLINICAL SCENARIOS

(a) A 32-year-old G2P1001 female has an ultrasound performed at 33 weeks gestation to assess fetal growth given that she is measuring small for dates clinically. Her obstetric history is significant for one previous full-term uncomplicated vaginal delivery. She has no significant past medical history. Her current medications include a prenatal vitamin and iron. Ultrasound demonstrates a fetus in vertex presentation. Estimated fetal weight (EFW) is 1640 g which is <10th percentile for gestational age. Amniotic fluid volume (AFI) is within normal limits. Umbilical artery (UA) Doppler studies are performed, and the pulsatility index (PI) measures >95th percentile for gestational age. Her blood pressure is measured to be 124/86 mmHg. She presents to her obstetrician with questions regarding what this new diagnosis of fetal growth restriction (FGR) will mean for her baby and how the remainder of her pregnancy should be managed.

(b) A 28-year-old G1P0 female has an ultrasound performed at 36 weeks gestation to assess fetal growth and amniotic fluid given that her fundal height is measuring 41 cm. She has no past medical history. Her pregnancy has been uncomplicated except for an elevated one-hour glucose challenge test and normal three-hour glucose tolerance test. Ultrasound demonstrates a fetus in vertex presentation. EFW is 3710 g which is >90th percentile for gestational age. She strongly wants to avoid a Cesarean delivery if possible. She asks her obstetrician when her labor can be induced to avoid her baby from growing too large.

Background

Disorders of fetal growth are commonly encountered in obstetrical practice. Although clinical estimation of fetal weight through symphysis-fundal height measurements may provide the first sign of aberrant fetal growth, ultrasound estimation of fetal weight remains the gold standard for diagnosing fetal growth disorders in developed countries. Ultrasound estimation of fetal weight is typically derived using polynomial equations which combine measurements of biparietal diameter, head circumference, abdominal circumference, and femur length. These estimates of fetal weight are then plotted on population-based growth curves by gestational age. Despite quality improvements in sonography over the years, there still remains a 6–15% margin of error in the sonographic prediction of fetal weight [1–3].

FGR has traditionally been defined as an EFW <10th percentile for gestational age; however, not all fetuses <10th percentile are pathologically small. In an attempt to identify fetuses who are pathologically growth-restricted, others have proposed definitions such as EFW <5th percentile, EFW<3rd percentile, EFW two standard deviations below the mean for gestational age, abdominal circumference <10th percentile for gestational age and EFW <10th percentile with Doppler abnormalities. While these more stringent definitions may have high positive predictive values, they also may miss a significant proportion of truly growth-restricted fetuses who do not necessarily meet such strict criteria [4]. Etiologies for FGR can be divided into extrinsic and intrinsic factors. The most common intrinsic etiologies include aneuploidy, congenital malformations, and congenital infection [5–7]. Extrinsic etiologies include chronic maternal hypoxia, maternal vascular disorders such as hypertension, diabetes, and pre-eclampsia, poor maternal weight gain, and exposure to tobacco, illicit drugs, or teratogens [8–10]. The majority of these disorders cause relative placental hypo-perfusion, thereby decreasing the flow of highly-oxygenated blood to the fetus. In the absence of an identifiable cause for FGR, it becomes virtually impossible to distinguish pathologic FGR and constitutional "smallness" in utero.

Large for gestational age (LGA) has traditionally been defined as EFW >90th percentile for gestational age; however, macrosomia is defined by absolute EFW >4000 g. Risk

Evidence-Based Obstetrics and Gynecology, First Edition. Edited by Errol R. Norwitz, Carolyn M. Zelop, David A. Miller, and David L. Keefe.

factors for macrosomia include maternal pre-gestational or gestational diabetes, obesity, gestational age >40 weeks, prior child with macrosomia, excessive pregnancy weight gain, hydrops fetalis, and an elevated 50 g glucose challenge test with a normal 100 g glucose tolerance test [11, 12]. Macrosomia is most associated with adverse maternal and fetal events at the time of delivery. Macrosomic fetuses are at an increased risk for shoulder dystocia and its related fetal injuries such as clavicular fractures, humeral fractures, and brachial plexus injuries. Maternal adverse events associated with macrosomia include increased risk for Cesarean section, postpartum hemorrhage, and third and fourth degree lacerations [4]. Despite heightened awareness of these adverse risks, approximately 50% of macrosomic fetuses are not diagnosed until the time of birth [13–15].

Clinical questions

In order to appropriately manage the patients in the above clinical scenarios, a critical appraisal of the literature was performed to address the following questions surrounding the management of pregnancies affected by fetal growth disorders.

1. Does the use of customized fetal growth curves improve the detection rate of FGR as well as improve subsequent neonatal outcomes?

2. Does antepartum surveillance with non-stress tests (NSTs) or biophysical profiles (BPPs) affect perinatal outcome in growth-restricted fetuses?

3. What is the predictive value of Doppler studies in identifying fetuses at risk for adverse pregnancy outcomes when performed on growth-restricted fetuses in the third trimester?

4. What is the optimal timing of delivery in growth-restricted fetuses?

5. Should supplementation with vitamins and antioxidants play a role in the prevention or treatment of FGR?

6. What is the association between FGR and both short-term and long-term neonatal health consequences?

7. In the setting of fetal macrosomia, does prophylactic induction of labor decrease the risk of Cesarean section?

8. At which threshold of EFW should Cesarean delivery be offered in order to prevent shoulder dystocia?

Critical appraisal of the literature

1. Does the use of customized fetal growth curves improve the detection rate of FGR as well as improve subsequent neonatal outcomes?

Using standardized population-based growth curves, approximately 10% of pregnancies will be diagnosed with small-for-gestational age (SGA) fetuses; however, not all of these fetuses will be pathologically growth-restricted. Additionally, some fetuses who measure greater than the 10th percentile for gestational age actually will be pathologically growth-restricted and will be missed using population-based growth curves. This has led to the concept of "individualized fetal growth potential." Using this concept, a predicted "term optimal weight" is calculated for each fetus adjusting for maternal physiologic or constitutional variables such as height, weight, parity, and ethnicity. A customized fetal growth curve is then created which is used to follow fetal growth throughout pregnancy [16, 17]. In the context of this conceptual model, a fetus who should measure in the 70th percentile for gestational age but is actually measuring in the 25th percentile may be at higher risk for perinatal morbidity and mortality than a fetus who measures in the 8th percentile who is born to constitutionally small parents.

To date, there are no randomized controlled trials (RCTs) comparing customized growth curves to population-based standards; however, there have been multiple, large observational studies evaluating the use of these customized growth curves in predicting perinatal morbidity in mortality. In 2009, Gardosi et al. retrospectively compared perinatal outcomes in pregnancies classified as SGA by both population-based and customized growth curves. In this study, 17.4% of babies who were classified as SGA by population-based standards were not SGA by customized standards. Additionally, 32.7% of babies who were classified as SGA by customized standards would not have met SGA criteria by population-based standards. This group of patients who were identified as SGA using the customized growth curve only had the highest risk of adverse perinatal outcomes including pre-eclampsia, stillbirth, and neonatal death [18]. Additionally, Odibo et al. have demonstrated that customized growth curves have a sensitivity and specificity of 32.7% and 95.1%, respectively, for predicting stillbirth compared to a sensitivity and specificity of 0.8% and 98.0% using population-based standards [19]. These particular studies derived their customized growth curves using norms from particular United States populations; however, similar results have been replicated both in other samplings of the US population as well as in other European populations [20–24].

Other authors have argued that these increased risk estimates for intrauterine fetal demise and neonatal death may be artificially inflated due to the large proportion of preterm fetuses identified as growth-restricted using customized growth curves. These authors argue that the differences in risk stem from the manner in which the two types of growth curves are developed. Whereas population-based growth curves are constructed using actual birth weight (BW), customized growth curves are constructed using intrauterine fetal weight. Given that intrauterine fetal weight traditionally has been an underestimate of observed birth weight in preterm infants, more preterm infants will be classified as SGA using the customized growth curve. This could potentially explain the higher incidence of stillbirth and neonatal mortality that is observed in these SGA infants. Zhang et al. demonstrated that there was only a modest difference in perinatal death after adjusting for gestational age when comparing the two curves [25]. Furthermore, Hutcheon et al. demonstrated that the addition of maternal characteristics to gestational age and gender contributed little explanation for the variance observed in birth weight using the customized growth curve [26, 27].

While the use of customized growth curves is gaining popularity in European countries, this approach has yet to be widely accepted in the United States. Further trials to evaluate the antenatal detection rate of true pathologic FGR using both population-based and customized growth curves are necessary. Additionally, the practical aspects of introducing customized growth curves into daily obstetric practice warrants further investigation.

Quality of Evidence: Level B, Class II

2. Does antepartum surveillance with non-stress tests (NSTs) or biophysical profiles (BPPs) affect perinatal outcome in growth-restricted fetuses?

The well-established association between FGR and stillbirth has lead physicians to adopt a strategy of increased antenatal surveillance in such patients. The BPP and NST are the two most commonly employed strategies of assessing fetal well-being in women at high risk for stillbirth. The goal of these tests is to detect fetuses at risk for developing acidosis or hypoxemia in order for physicians to intervene prior to further deterioration in fetal status. Despite their widespread adoption into clinical medicine, RCTs demonstrating their efficacy in decreasing stillbirth are lacking.

The NST incorporates baseline fetal heart rate as well as measures of fetal heart rate variability. A reactive NST after 32 weeks' gestation is defined by the presence of at least two fetal heart rate accelerations of at least 15 beats per minute lasting for greater than 15 seconds over a 20-minutes period [28]. A reactive NST reflects adequate oxygenation of the fetus and is representative of an intact fetal central nervous system. Advantages of the NST include its ease of administration as well as its high negative predictive value of >99.8%; however, limitations include its high false positive rate of >50%, especially at early gestational ages, as well as its relatively high interobserver and intraobserver variability [28–30]. While NSTs have traditionally been performed twice weekly, there remains a lack of evidence to support this practice. In 2000, a RCT was performed comparing a regimen of twice weekly NSTs to fortnightly NSTs in a population of women with SGA fetuses with normal UA Doppler studies. There was no difference in neonatal outcomes between the two groups; however, there was an increased incidence of induction of labor in the twice weekly NST group [31].

The BPP is another method of antenatal surveillance which incorporates evaluation of AFI, fetal movement, fetal tone, and fetal breathing with or without a NST. When normal, each parameter receives two points, for a maximum of 10 points. The NST portion of the exam may be omitted, leaving a score of 8/8 as a maximum [28, 32, 33]. As fetal status deteriorates, there is progressive loss in fetal breathing and AFI followed by loss of fetal heart rate reactivity. Fetal movement and tone are typically the last parameters to become abnormal. Overall, abnormal BPP scores have been associated with worsening acid–base status at the time of delivery [34, 35]. Similar to the NST, the BPP also has been associated with a high false positive rate, and there is lack of high quality evidence from RCTs to support its use in the evaluation of high-risk pregnancies [36]. Kaur et al. evaluated the use of daily BPPs in preterm fetuses with severe FGR (<1000 g with abnormal UA Doppler indices). Results from this study demonstrated that the BPP was not reliable in the evaluation of preterm severe FGR given both its high false positive and false negative rates [37].

The BPP also gives important information regarding AFI. Amniotic fluid index has been shown to progressively decrease in cases of FGR [38, 39]. A normal AFI is typically associated with adequate placental perfusion; whereas, a low AFI may be a sign of worsening placental dysfunction. Low AFI may also be found in cases of membrane rupture or congenital fetal abnormalities. A 1999 meta-analysis demonstrated that oligohydramnios (AFI < 5 cm) was associated with an increased rate of Cesarean section for fetal distress as well as low 5-minutes Apgar scores; however, oligohydramnios was not associated with fetal acidosis [40]. Alternatively, in a retrospective study of preterm FGR cases only, Scrifres et al. identified oligohydramnios as an independent predictor of perinatal mortality [41]. Regardless, the finding of oligohydramnios on ultrasound always warrants further fetal evaluation in an attempt to establish an etiology.

Quality of Evidence: Level B, Class IIa

3. What is the predictive value of Doppler studies in identifying fetuses at risk for adverse pregnancy outcomes when performed on growth-restricted fetuses in the third trimester?

More recent data has suggested that changes in fetal parameters as reflected by NSTs or BPPs are rather late occurrences in the series of events leading to fetal demise [42]. In fact, fetal acidosis may already be present in a proportion of fetuses displaying abnormalities in these antenatal tests. This has led to the investigation of other parameters which can be used in the evaluation of the growth-restricted fetus. Doppler interrogation of fetal vessels has become a common strategy in the evaluation and surveillance of FGR. The most common vessels which are evaluated include the UA, middle cerebral artery (MCA), and ductus venosus (DV). In normal gestations, placental resistance declines with advancing gestation leading to an increased amount of forward diastolic flow in the UA. With progressive uteroplacental insufficiency, there is elevated placental resistance leading to decreased forward diastolic flow which can progress to absent or even reversed diastolic flow in the most severe cases. UA Doppler is reported as a systolic to diastolic ratio (S/D) or as a PI [systolic – diastolic flow/mean]. The fetal MCA is typically a high impedance vascular bed with low end-diastolic velocity. In cases of progressive FGR, there is thought to be preferential shunting of blood toward vital organs such as the brain and heart at the expense of visceral organs, resulting in a lower MCA S/D ratio or PI. This phenomenon is known as the "brain-sparing effect." Finally, evaluation of the fetal venous system is an indirect measure of fetal cardiac compliance. Doppler interrogation of the DV produces a tri-phasic waveform comprised of S, D, and a waves. The S and D waves occur with ventricular contraction and then passive diastolic filling, respectively. The a wave is a reflection of ventricular filling which occurs during atrial systole or "atrial kick." With worsening right ventricular dysfunction, the a wave will become decreased or even reversed. This reflects decreased or reversed forward flow during atrial systole [4]. Examples of normal waveforms for each of these vessels are shown in Figure 43.1.

Multiple studies have evaluated the association between abnormal UA Doppler parameters and adverse perinatal outcomes. Studies evaluating fetal blood samples from cordocentesis specimens have shown an increased incidence of both hypoxia and acidosis with worsening UA Doppler studies [43, 44]. Abnormal UA Doppler studies have also been associated with other adverse perinatal outcomes such as neonatal intensive care unit (NICU) admission, low Apgar scores, and fetal distress, with absent or reversed end diastolic flow being the most ominous finding and associated with the highest risk of perinatal mortality [45–47]. Recently, Vergani et al. evaluated predictors of adverse neonatal outcomes in both late preterm and term growth-restricted neonates. Results from this study demonstrated that gestational age was the most important predictor of adverse outcome in term infants; however, in preterm infants, UA PI was found to be an independent predictor of adverse outcome [48].

There have also been multiple RCTs evaluating the efficacy of UA Doppler surveillance in improving perinatal outcome. When including only those studies which were performed in high-risk populations, improved outcomes with the use of Doppler surveillance has been demonstrated in the majority of studies; however, there are limitations in sample size, methodology, and randomization. In order to surpass these issues, results from these trials have been synthesized in meta-analyses in order to determine a more accurate effect size. Table 43.1 shows a summary of these results in the current published literature [49–52]. Of note, each of these studies shows a decrease in perinatal mortality with the use of Doppler surveillance in high-risk pregnancies such as those with FGR. Additionally, these meta-analyses also showed a decreased risk of antenatal admission, inductions of labor, and Cesarean section in the groups monitored with UA Doppler.

Quality of Evidence: Level A, Class I

The use of MCA Doppler studies in the routine surveillance of FGR has not been as widely accepted in clinical practice. In an observational study, Mari et al. demonstrated a lower risk of adverse outcomes in growth-restricted fetuses with a normal MCA PI compared to those with an abnormal MCA PI [53]. Nanthakomon et al. showed that growth-restricted fetuses with a normal UA PI but abnormal MCA PI had

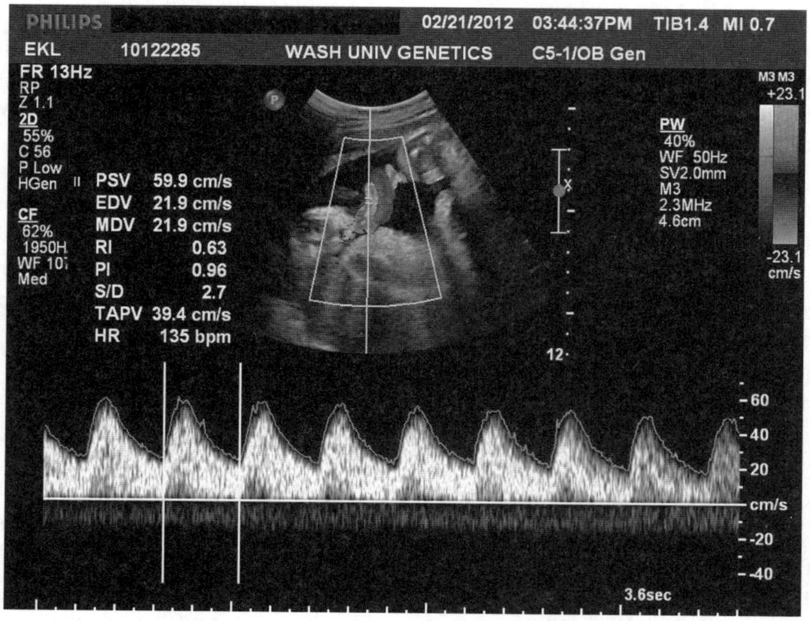

(a)

Figure 43.1 Normal Doppler Waveforms in (a) the umbilical artery, (b) the middle cerebral artery, and (c) the ductus venous.

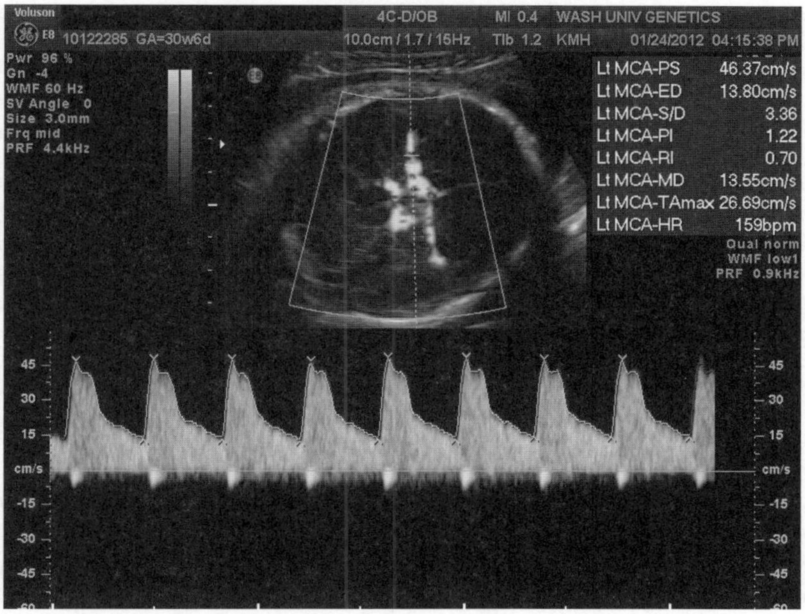

(b)

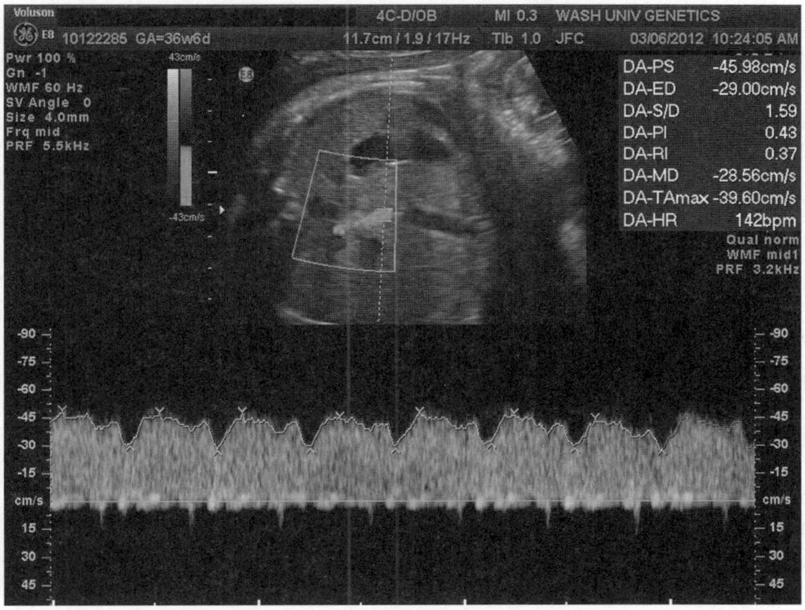

(c)

Figure 43.1 *(Continued)*

worse outcomes compared to those with normal UA and MCA PIs [54]. Furthermore, a longitudinal study by Hecher et al. has demonstrated progressive abnormality in the MCA PI as early-onset FGR worsens [39]. Unfortunately, this finding has not been consistently replicated in other studies [42, 55]. More recently, it has been suggested that the MCA peak systolic velocity (PSV) may also be an informative marker in evaluating FGR, and trends in both the MCA PI and MCA PSV may provide more useful clinical information than single measurements [56]. Additionally, the cerebroplacental ratio (CPR) has been shown to be predictive of adverse perinatal outcome [57, 58]. This parameter is calculated by dividing the MCA PI value by the UA PI value and, therefore, incorporates information regarding placental status and subsequent fetal response. Finally, it has also been suggested that MCA Doppler studies also may have utility when performed in the third trimester in pregnancies complicated by FGR; however, there remain no RCTs available to guide the use of MCA Doppler in the clinical management of FGR [59, 60].

Table 43.1 Summary results of currently published meta-analyses comparing routine umbilical artery Doppler evaluation versus no umbilical artery Doppler evaluation in high risk pregnancies

Authors	Year	Number of trials included	OR (95% CI)	Improvement in perinatal outcome
Alfirevic & Neilson	1995	12	0.62 (0.15–0.55)	Yes
Maulik et al.	1998	3	0.19 (0.06–0.63)	Yes
Westergaard et al.	2001	6	0.66 (0.36–1.22)	Yes[a]
Cochrane Review	2010	18	0.71 (0.53–0.98)	Yes

OR, odds ratio and CI, confidence interval.
[a]Finding not statistically significant.

Quality of Evidence: Level B, Class IIb

Interrogation of the fetal venous circulation provides indirect information regarding the status of the fetal cardiovascular system in response to FGR. Baschat et al. has shown that growth-restricted fetuses with abnormal venous flow have a higher rate of adverse perinatal outcomes compared to those with Doppler abnormalities in only the UA or MCA [61]. Turan et al. showed that an absent/reversed a wave in the DV lasting >seven days had 100% sensitivity and 80% specificity for detecting stillbirth; however, this finding was unrelated to neonatal morbidity and mortality [62]. A systematic review and meta-analyses demonstrated a modest predictive ability of abnormal DV Doppler for the prediction of perinatal mortality with a positive likelihood ratio of 4.21 (95% confidence interval (CI) 1.98–8.96) and a negative likelihood ratio of 0.43 (95% CI 0.30–0.61) [63].

The optimal strategy of incorporating Doppler studies and fetal well-being assessment with BPP and NST is still under investigation. Cosmi et al. evaluated a group of 145 growth-restricted fetuses with abnormal UA Doppler studies and divided them into two groups: Group 1: all indices (MCA, DV, and AFI) became abnormal preceding a non-reassuring BPP or NST; Group 2 : 1 or more indices were normal at the time of delivery. Although there was no statistically significant difference in perinatal morbidity and mortality between the two groups, UA reversed flow and DV absent/reversed flow were independently associated with adverse outcome [38]. In another study comparing NST, computerized fetal heart rate analysis, BPP, and arterial and venous Doppler, venous Doppler was found to be the most predictive of acidemia with a sensitivity of 73% and specificity of 90% [64]. Furthermore, Baschat et al. has shown that both multivessel Doppler assessment and BPP evaluation can effectively risk-stratify growth-restricted fetuses; however, their results do not consistently correlate with each other [65]. This finding would suggest that complementary use of these two modalities would be most effective. Prior studies have shown that multivessel Doppler may only identify fetuses at high risk for demise 24 hours earlier than BPP [42, 66]. A 2004 decision analysis evaluated four strategies of antepartum FGR assessment including Doppler + BPP, BPP only, Doppler only, and no testing. This analytic model actually demonstrated that BPP only was the best strategy to guide physicians on the timing of delivery in preterm growth-restricted fetuses [67]. Most recently, the Trial of Umbilical and Fetal Flow in Europe (TRUFFLE) was undertaken to evaluate the role of venous Doppler evaluation as a trigger for delivery in preterm FGR. This multicenter RCT randomized women with singleton gestations with preterm FGR (26–32 weeks) and elevated UA Doppler studies to one of three groups as a trigger for delivery: (i) reduced short-short term variation on cardiotocography monitoring; (ii) early DV changes of elevated PI; or (iii) late DV changes of absent or reversed a-wave. There was no significant difference in the primary outcome of survival without neurodevelopmental impairment at age two among the three groups. There was a significant increase in intact survival for infants randomized to delivery on the basis of late DV changes compared to cardiotocography monitoring; however, this was at the expense of an increased, but non-significant, risk of mortality [68]. Based on the available data, the role of multi-vessel fetal Doppler interrogation in the clinical management of the growth-restricted infant remains uncertain.

Quality of Evidence: Level B, Class IIb

4. What is the optimal timing of delivery in growth-restricted fetuses?

Based on the above data, the optimal surveillance strategy to prevent adverse perinatal outcome in growth-restricted fetuses remains uncertain [36]. This produces a clinical dilemma in determining optimal timing of delivery for these fetuses. In cases of maternal distress or imminent fetal compromise, the decision to deliver is straightforward; however, the majority of cases of FGR require the clinician to weigh the risk of stillbirth with the risks of prematurity and neonatal death in determining optimal delivery timing.

To date, the only RCT to evaluate timing of delivery for preterm FGR is the Growth Restriction Intervention Trial (GRIT) [69]. This was a multicenter RCT which compared immediate delivery vs. delayed delivery in pregnant women between 24 and 36 weeks' gestation in situations in which the obstetrician was uncertain as to whether to deliver based on current ultrasound and UA Doppler surveillance. On average, patients in the delayed delivery group remained pregnant for an additional four days. Overall, there were more intrauterine fetal deaths in the delayed group but fewer neonatal deaths. There was no significant difference in infant survival to the time of hospital discharge between the two groups. At two-year follow-up, there also was no difference in mortality or severe disability between the two groups. The severe disability that was observed in this study was limited to the group of patients who were delivered <31 weeks, likely secondary to prematurity-associated complications [70]. Most recently, long-term outcomes for a subset of patients from GRIT were published. These results demonstrated no clinically significant differences between the immediate and delayed delivery group at 9–13 years [71]. Based on these findings, the authors suggest that brain development cannot be improved by immediate delivery in cases of uncertainty, owing to the fact that the fetal neurologic insult has likely already occurred by the time signs of fetal compromise are evident on antenatal surveillance.

Quality of Evidence: Level B, Class IIb

While it is common practice to deliver the growth-restricted fetus at term, there is limited evidence to support or oppose this practice. Concerns over increased obstetric intervention and failed attempts at vaginal delivery with induction of labor may influence providers to proceed with expectant management and close antenatal surveillance. The Disproportionate Intrauterine Growth Intervention Trial at Term (DIGITAT) is the only RCT which specifically addresses this topic [72]. In this trial, patients beyond 36 weeks' gestation were randomized to induction of labor versus expectant management. There was no significant difference in their primary composite outcome of adverse neonatal outcome or in the rate operative vaginal delivery or Cesarean section. There were no fetal or neonatal deaths in either of the study arms, although this study was not powered to evaluate the rare outcome of stillbirth, which is generally considered to be unacceptable in an expectantly managed fetus at term. There was no difference in developmental or behavioral outcomes between the two groups at two-year follow up [73].

Quality of Evidence: Level B, Class IIb

5. Should supplementation with vitamins and antioxidants play a role in the prevention or treatment of FGR?

Multiple interventions have been evaluated for the prevention and treatment of FGR; however, studies of these interventions have demonstrated little impact on the clinical course and sequelae of FGR. Neither plasma volume expansion, administration of glucose/amino acids nor fish oil supplementation has proven to be effective prevention or treatment strategies for FGR [74–76]. In 1987, Nicolaides et al. demonstrated that continuously-administered humidified maternal oxygen increased fetal pO2 to within or near the normal range in cases of severe FGR when assessed by cordocentesis [77]. Additional studies have confirmed this finding, while also suggesting a significant improvement in perinatal mortality in the oxygen-treated groups [78, 79]. Methodologic concerns regarding blinding, selection bias, and use of placebo limit the clinical application of these results. To date, the only double-blind RCT on this subject demonstrated no benefit of chronic oxygen therapy on perinatal mortality in fetuses with absent end-diastolic flow (AEDF); however, this study was underpowered for the primary outcome [80]. Based on the results of this study as well as concern regarding maternal toxicity from hyperoxygenation, this therapy currently cannot be recommended for the treatment of FGR.

Quality of Evidence: Level B, Class III

The anti-oxidant effects of both Vitamins C and E also have been evaluated as potential targets for FGR prevention. Initial small RCTs demonstrated no benefit of Vitamin C and E supplementation on the prevention of FGR [81, 82]. These results have been confirmed in more recent multicenter RCTs [83, 84]. Data from the Australian Collaborative Trial of Supplements (ACTS) demonstrated a non-significant risk reduction (Risk Ratio (RR) 0.87, 0.66–1.16) in infant birth weight < 10th percentile in those in the supplement group [84]. Of note, this study included FGR as one of its primary outcomes, as opposed to the prior large trials which have been designed specifically to evaluate the primary outcome of pre-eclampsia. The majority of these RCTs focus on supra-physiologic doses of 1000 mg Vitamin C and 400 IU Vitamin E. At these doses, there has even been some suggestion of fetal harm. Poston et al. observed an increased risk of low birth weight infants (<2500 g) in patients treated with Vitamin C and E; however, there was no statistically significant difference in the proportion of babies weighing <5th percentile [85]. Subsequently, Xu et al. observed an increased risk of preterm premature rupture of membranes and fetal loss/perinatal death in those supplemented with Vitamin C and E [86]. Most recently, a systematic review and meta-analysis demonstrated no significant benefit to Vitamin C and E supplementation in the prevention of FGR (RR 0.99, 0.91–1.06) as well as no increased risk of any adverse fetal or perinatal outcome [87].

Quality of Evidence: Level A, Class III

Perhaps the most promising intervention for the prevention of FGR is low dose aspirin. Low-dose aspirin has been studied for the prevention of pre-eclampsia for many years, with conflicting results. Low-dose aspirin is hypothesized to act by inhibiting thromboxane-mediated vasoconstriction and pathologic coagulation in the placenta. While multiple RCTs have shown no improvement in infant birth weight when evaluated as a secondary outcome, a recent meta-analysis shows a greater than 50% risk reduction in FGR (RR 0.44, 0.30–0.65) when low dose aspirin is initiated prior to 16 weeks' gestation [88–92]. Additional RCTs to confirm this finding are necessary.

Quality of Evidence: Level A, Class IIa

6. What is the association between FGR and both short-term and long-term neonatal health consequences?

Growth-restricted fetuses are at increased risk for hypothermia, hypoglycemia, polycythemia, hyperbilirubinemia and apnea in the neonatal period. A higher proportion of growth-restricted fetuses also have UA pH values <7.0 and Apgar scores <7 [93]. Although earlier studies initially suggested that FGR was associated with accelerated fetal lung maturity and increased survival, larger, population-based studies have refuted this notion and demonstrated that FGR is actually associated with increased perinatal morbidity and mortality [93–97]. After retrospectively reviewing a large database of NICU summaries, Garite et al. concluded that FGR was associated with an increased risk for need for respiratory support, retinopathy of prematurity, necrotizing enterocolitis, and perinatal mortality in neonates born between 25 and 32 weeks, even after adjusting for gestational age [98]. Literature has been inconclusive regarding the association of cerebral palsy and FGR. Most recently, the Surveillance of Cerebral Palsy in Europe (SCPE) Collaborative Group reported a 4–6 fold increased risk of cerebral palsy in infants delivered between 32 and 42 weeks with a birth weight <10th percentile [99]. For very preterm infants, the risk is less clear given the difficulty in separating contributions from FGR versus contributions from early prematurity alone. A more recent focus has been on the association of adverse neurodevelopmental outcome and FGR. Multiple prospective studies have demonstrated that growth-restricted infants have decreased cognitive function compared to gestationally-age matched controls [100–104]. In 2007, Leitner et al. followed 123 growth-restricted infants from birth to ages 9–10. Observations from this study included decreased cognition, neurodevelopmental performance, and school achievement at 9–10 years in growth-restricted infants compared to matched appropriate for gestational age (AGA) controls. Children in these studies who demonstrated evidence of "catch-up" in their somatic growth had more favorable outcomes compared to those children whose somatic growth continued to lag [105]. Most recently, Figueras et al. demonstrated a higher level of neurodevelopmental impairment among a subgroup of preterm growth-restricted newborns with abnormal MCA Doppler PI <5th percentile [106]. Despite these findings, results from these studies remain limited given the different definitions used to define FGR, varying instruments used to evaluate neurodevelopmental performance, and wide range of follow up periods. A summary of results from these studies is shown in Table 43.2 [100–108]. Finally, evolving research regarding the developmental origins of human disease suggest that FGR is associated with an increased risk for cardiovascular disease, type 2 diabetes, and hypertension in adulthood. This theory proposes that these chronic disease states are a result of fetal adaptive responses to intrauterine insults, such as undernutrition. Specifically, slow growth in utero may lead to accelerated weight gain in childhood, resulting in disturbances in the metabolic profile. Such adaptive responses likely lead to altered gene expression as well as changes in tissue and organ development which are manifested later in life [109, 110].

7. In the setting of fetal macrosomia, does prophylactic induction of labor decrease the risk of Cesarean section?

Vaginal delivery of a macrosomic fetus can be associated with both maternal and neonatal morbidity and mortality. Maternal complications include increased risk for postpartum hemorrhage and third and fourth degree perineal lacerations [111, 112]. Macrosomic infants are also at increased risk for shoulder dystocia and brachial plexus injury, both of which occur more commonly in diabetic patients [113, 114]. Finally, macrosomic infants also have a higher incidence of meconium aspiration syndrome and a higher risk of requiring assisted ventilation at delivery [111].

In order to reduce these risks, many obstetricians have proposed elective induction of labor for fetuses which appear to be macrosomic or LGA by sonographic EFW. It has been thought that this policy would decrease the rate of Cesarean delivery for cephalopelvic disproportion as well as decrease the risk of infant and maternal trauma from difficult vaginal deliveries. Results from multiple observational studies comparing expectant management to labor induction for macrosomia actually demonstrated the opposite effect. The majority of these studies show a decreased risk of Cesarean delivery in patients who were managed expectantly and no difference in the risk of operative vaginal delivery or shoulder dystocia [115–120]. Additionally, a cost-effectiveness analysis suggested that expectant management is the most cost-effective approach to fetal macrosomia [121].

Few RCTs on this topic are available to guide clinical decision-making. Gonen et al. randomized 273 women to expectant management versus labor induction after 38 completed weeks' gestation and observed no statistically significant difference in the incidence of Cesarean delivery, operative vaginal delivery, and shoulder dystocia between the two groups. These findings persisted even when nulliparous and multiparous women were analyzed separately [122]. Combining results from this RCT and two other unpublished trials, a Cochrane review found no statistically significant difference in the incidence of Cesarean section (RR 0.96, 0.67–1.38), operative vaginal delivery (RR 1.02, 0.60–1.74) or shoulder dystocia (RR 1.06, 0.44–2.56) between patients who were induced versus those who were managed expectantly. Notably, there were two cases of brachial plexus injury and four clavicular fractures in the expectantly managed group while none were observed in the induction group [123]. Criticisms of the included trials include lack of power to determine a difference in rare

Table 43.2 Summary of results from recently-published studies evaluating neurodevelopmental outcomes associated with FGR

Authors	Year	Study design	Inclusion criteria	SGA/FGR definition	Findings
Wienerroither et al.	2001	Prospective cohort	23 FGR patients compared to gestational-age matched AGA controls	Abdominal circumference < 10th%ile and UA absent/reverse flow	Lower intellectual development in FGR patients; no difference in social development
Paz et al.	2001	Retrospective cohort	Cohort of 13 454 term infants	Birth weight < 10th%ile	Decreased intelligence scores at age 17 in FGR patients
Geva et al.	2006	Prospective cohort	123 patients compared to 63 matched controls	Birth weight < 10th%ile	Lower intelligence scores at age nine in FGR patients; more frequent neuropsychologic difficulties in FGR patients
Leitner et al.	2007	Prospective cohort	123 SGA infants compared to 63 matched AGA controls	Birth weight < 10th%ile	Lagging somatic growth, neurodevelopmental performance, cognition, and school achievement at age 9–10 in FGR patients; somatic catch-up at ages two and nine correlated with more favorable outcomes at age 9–10
Procianoy et al.	2009	Prospective cohort	55 SGA preterm infants compared to 41 AGA preterm infants; all enrolled infants had a BW < 1500 g	Birth weight < 10th%ile	Similar Bayley scores up to 24 months
Baschat et al.	2009	Prospective cohort	113 patients with FGR	Abdominal circumference < 5th%ile with abnormal UA Dopplers	UA-REDV is associated with increased likelihood for global delay at two years of age
Morsing et al.	2011	Prospective cohort	34 preterm infants with FGR, 34 matched preterm AGA infants, 34 term AGA	Birth weight less than 2 standard deviations of the mean with UA absent/reversed end diastolic flow	Lower cognitive outcomes at five to eight years of age in preterm FGR compared to both control groups. Results limited to male infants only.
Guellec et al.	2011	Prospective cohort	2357 preterm SGA (<33 weeks) infants. SGA compared to mild SGA (10–20th%ile) compared to AGA	Birth weight < 10th%ile	Increase in adverse neurodevelopmental outcomes in SGA only in the 29–32 week group. Mild SGA was associated with increased cognitive deficiency and behavioral problems
Figueras et al.	2011	Prospective cohort	126 preterm FGR (<34 weeks) infants compared to matched AGA controls. Subgroup analysis of FGR infants with MCA PI <5th%ile	Birth weight < 10th%ile with abnormal UA Doppler	Lower neurobehavioral scores in the areas of habituation, motor system, social interaction and attention in the FGR infants with abnormal MCA Doppler studies

FGR, fetal growth restriction; AGA, appropriate for gestational age; SGA, small for gestational age; UA, umbilical artery; MCA, middle cerebral artery; PI, pulsatility index; REDV, reversed end diastolic flow.

outcomes even after combining them in a meta-analysis, varying definitions of macrosomia, and late gestational age at the time of induction, possibly mitigating any associated benefit. Additionally, the RCT by Gonen et al. excluded patients with diabetes. Despite these criticisms, the current available data suggests that there is no benefit to prophylactic induction of labor for fetuses with suspected LGA or macrosomia.

Quality of Evidence: Level B, Class IIb

8. At which threshold of EFW should Cesarean delivery be offered in order to prevent shoulder dystocia?

Although fetal macrosomia is a risk factor for shoulder dystocia, a large proportion of cases occur in AGA fetuses. Although Cesarean delivery will prevent shoulder dystocia, the appropriate threshold of fetal weight at which to offer this intervention is inconsistent in the literature. Furthermore, brachial plexus injuries have been reported following Cesarean delivery. Determining an EFW threshold at which to offer Cesarean delivery that will minimize brachial plexus injury but not substantially contribute to the increasing Cesarean delivery rate has been a subject of debate.

Routine Cesarean delivery has not been found to substantially decrease the number of shoulder dystocia cases when employed at an EFW of 4000 g in the non-diabetic population [113, 124, 125]. Ecker et al. found that in order to prevent a single case of brachial plexus injury, 192 cesareans would need to be performed at a threshold of 4000 g, 51 at a threshold of 4500 g, and 19 at a threshold of 5000 g. However, given that only ~10% of brachial plexus injuries are permanent, the number of Cesareans needed to prevent one *permanent* brachial plexus injury would be substantially higher [114]. Bryant et al. also established that between 155 and 588 Cesareans would need to be performed to prevent one permanent brachial plexus injury if using a threshold of 4500 g [126]. In a retrospective analysis, Gonen et al. demonstrated that only one case of brachial plexus injury was prevented after implementing a policy of elective Cesarean delivery for suspected macrosomia >4500 g over a four year period [115].

The sonographic prediction of macrosomia has shown to be imperfect in multiple studies. With the commonly used Hadlock formula for estimating fetal weight, there is still 16–20% variability around the estimate [3]. Taking into account these sonographic imperfections, Rouse et al. performed a decision and cost-effectiveness analysis comparing three strategies: (i) management without ultrasound; (ii) ultrasound and Cesarean delivery for EFW >4000 g; and (iii) ultrasound and Cesarean delivery for EFW > 4500 g. Using a threshold of 4500 g, 3695 cesarean deliveries would need to be performed to prevent one permanent brachial plexus injury at a cost of $8.7 million for each injury prevented [127].

Given that shoulder dystocia occurs more commonly at any given birth weight in the diabetic population, this population has been analyzed separately in many studies. Thresholds ranging from 4000 to 5000 g have been proposed [113, 114, 126]. In the decision analysis by Rouse et al., 489 Cesarean deliveries were needed to prevent one permanent injury using the 4000 g threshold and 443 using the 4500 g threshold [127]. (Table 43.3) Taking into account the above data, the American College of Obstetricians and Gynecologists currently recommends offering prophylactic Cesarean delivery in the setting of an EFW >4500 g in diabetic patients and >5000 g in non-diabetic patients [128].

Quality of Evidence: Level C, Class IIb

Conclusions

Regarding the patient in the first clinical scenario, you continue to follow fetal growth with serial ultrasounds and UA Doppler studies. You counsel the patient that her baby is at increased risk for perinatal morbidity and mortality; however, you monitor her with twice weekly NSTs for the

Table 43.3 Number of cesarean deliveries necessary to prevent shoulder dystocia at varying estimated fetal weight thresholds

Author	Year	Estimated fetal weight threshold (g)	Number of cesareans needed to prevent one brachial plexus injury	Type of brachial plexus injury
Ecker et al.	1997	4000	192	All
Ecker et al.	1997	4500	51	All
Ecker et al.	1997	5000	19	All
Bryan et al.	1998	4500	155–588	Permanent only
Rouse et al.	1996	4500	3695	Permanent only
Diabetic patients only				
Rouse et al.	1996	4000	489	Permanent only
Rouse et al.	1996	4500	443	Permanent only

remainder of her pregnancy in an attempt to decrease that risk. You also counsel her that currently there is no effective strategy to treat FGR in pregnancy. When the patient reaches term, you induce labor and she has a successful vaginal delivery of a healthy male infant. Regarding the patient in the second clinical scenario, you continue to expectantly manage her pregnancy despite her LGA growth pattern. Three weeks later, she has a repeat ultrasound for fetal growth which demonstrates an EFW of 4020 g. Based on the current evidence, you continue to expectantly manage her, and she presents in spontaneous labor at 40 weeks. She has an uncomplicated normal spontaneous vaginal delivery.

Fetal growth disorders, such as those outlined in the above clinical scenarios, are commonly encountered in routine obstetric practice. While there is evidence to guide many management decisions, there still remain multiple clinical questions that warrant further investigation. Until data from large RCTs are available, clinicians must individualize patient care by assimilating the current available evidence outlined in this chapter.

References

1 Hadlock, F.P., Harrist, R.B., Sharman, R.S. et al. (1985). Estimation of fetal weight with the use of head, body, and femur measurements – a Prospective Study. *Am. J. Obstet. Gynecol.* **151**: 333–337.

2 Shepard, M.J., Richards, V.A., Berkowitz, R.L. et al. (1982). An evaluation of two equations for predicting fetal weight by ultrasound. *Am. J. Obstet. Gynecol.* **142**: 47–54.

3 Hadlock, F.P., Deter, R.L., Harrist, R.B., and Park, S.K. (1984). Estimating fetal age: computer-assisted analysis of multiple fetal growth parameters. *Radiology* **152**: 497–501.

4 Galan, H.L., Pandipati, S., and Filly, R.A. (2008). Ultrasound evaluation of fetal biometry and normal and abnormal fetal growth. In: *Ultrasonography in Obstetrics and Gynecology*, 5e (ed. P.W. Callen), 225–265. Philadelphia: Saunders Elsevier.

5 Naeye, R.L. (1967). Prenatal organ and cellular growth with various chromosomal disorders. *Biol. Neonat.* **11**: 248–260.

6 Khoury, M.J., Erickson, J.D., Cordero, J.F., and McCarthy, B.J. (1998). Congenital malformations and intrauterine growth retardation: a population study. *Pediatrics* **82**: 83–90.

7 Fowler, K.B., Stagno, S., Pass, R.F. et al. (1992). The outcome of congenital cytomegalovirus infection in relation to maternal antibody status. *N. Engl. J. Med.* **326**: 663–667.

8 Cunningham, F.G., Cox, C.M., Harstad, T.W. et al. (1990). Chronic renal disease and pregnancy outcome. *Am. J. Obstet. Gynecol.* **163**: 453–459.

9 Kupferminc, M.J., Peri, H., Zwang, E. et al. (2000). High prevalence of the prothrombin gene mutation in women with intrauterine growth retardation, abruptio placentae and second trimester loss. *Acta Obstet. Gynecol. Scand.* **79**: 963–967.

10 Ounsted, M., Moar, V.A., and Scott, A. (1985). Risk factors associated with small-for-dates and large-for-dates infants. *BJOG* **92**: 226–232.

11 American College of Obstetricians and Gynecologists (2000). *Fetal Macrosomia. ACOG Practice Bulletin No. 22*. Washington DC: American College of Obstetricians and Gynecologists.

12 Okun, N., Verma, A., Mitchell, B.F., and Flowerdew, G. (1997). Relative importance of maternal constitutional factors and glucose intolerance of pregnancy in the development of newborn macrosomia. *J. Matern. Fetal Med.* **6**: 285–290.

13 Benacerraf, B.R., Gelman, R., and Frigoletto, F.D. Jr. (1998). Sonographically estimated fetal weights: accuracy and limitation. *Am. J. Obstet. Gynecol.* **159**: 1118–1121.

14 Pollack, R.N., Hauer-Pollack, G., and Divon, M.Y. (1992). Macrosomia in postdates pregnancies: the accuracy of routine ultrasonographic screening. *Am. J. Obstet. Gynecol.* **167**: 7–11.

15 Sandmire, H.F. (1993). Whither ultrasonic prediction of fetal macrosomia? *Obstet. Gynecol.* **82**: 860–862.

16 Gardosi, J., Mongelli, M., Wilcox, M., and Chang, A. (1995). An adjustable fetal weight standard. *Ultrasound Obstet. Gynecol.* **6**: 168–174.

17 Gardosi, J. and Francis, A. (2009). A customized standard to assess fetal growth in a US population. *Am. J. Obstet. Gynecol.* **201**: 25e1–25e7.

18 Gardosi, J. and Francis, A. (2009). Adverse pregnancy outcome and association with small for gestational age birthweight by customized and population-based percentiles. *Am. J. Obstet. Gynecol.* **201**: 28.e1–28.e8.

19 Odibo, A.O., Francis, A., Cahill, A.G. et al. (2011). Association between pregnancy complications and small-for-gestational-age birth weight defined by customized fetal growth standard versus a population-based standard. *J. Matern. Fetal Med.* **24**: 411–417.

20 de Jong, C.L.D., Gardosi, J., Dekker, G.A. et al. (1998). Application of a customized birthweight standard in the assessment of perinatal outcome in a high risk population. *BJOG* **105**: 531–535.

21 Clausson, B., Gardosi, J., Francis, A., and Cnattingius, S. (2001). Perinatal outcome in SGA births defined by customized versus population-based birthweight standards. *BJOG* **108**: 830–834.

22 Ego, A., Subtil, D., Grange, G. et al. (2006). Customized versus population-based birth weight standards for identifying growth restricted infants: a French multicenter study. *Am. J. Obstet. Gynecol.* **194**: 1042–1049.

23 Figueras, F., Figueras, J., Meler, E. et al. (2007). Customised birthweight standards accurately predict perinatal morbidity. *Arch. Dis. Child. Fetal Neonatal Ed.* **92**: F277–F280.

24 Bukowski, R., Uchida, T., Smith, G.C.S. et al. (2008). Individualized norms of optimal fetal growth. *Obstet. Gynecol.* **111**: 1065–1076.

25 Zhang, X., Platt, R.W., Cnattingius, S. et al. (2007). The use of customized versus population-based birthweight standards in predicting perinatal mortality. *BJOG* **114**: 474–477.

26 Hutcheon, J.A., Zhang, X., Cnattingius, S. et al. (2008). Customised birthweight percentiles: does adjusting for maternal characteristics matter? *BJOG* **115**: 1397–1404.

27 Hutcheon, J.A., Walker, M., and Platt, R.W. (2001). Assessing the value of customized birth weight percentiles. *Am. J. Epidemiol.* **173**: 459–467.

28 American College of Obstetricians and Gynecologists (2014). *Antepartum Fetal Surveillance. ACOG Practice Bulletin No.145.* Washington DC: American College of Obstetricians and Gynecologists.

29 Cheng, L.C., Gibb, D.M., Ajayi, R.A., and Soothill, P.W. (1992). A comparison between computerized (mean range) and clinical visual cardiotocographic assessment. *BJOG* **99**: 817–820.

30 Evertson, L.R., Gauthier, R.J., Schifrin, B.S., and Paul, R.H. (1979). Antepartum fetal heart rate testing I. Evolution of the non-stress test. *Am. J. Obstet. Gynecol.* **133**: 29–33.

31 McCowan, L.M., Harding, J.E., Roberts, A.B. et al. (2000). A pilot randomized controlled trial of two regimens of fetal surveillance for small-for-gestational-age fetuses with normal results of umbilical artery Doppler velocimetry. *Am. J. Obstet. Gynecol.* **182** (Part 1): 81–86.

32 Manning, F.A., Platt, P.D., and Sipos, L. (1980). Antepartum fetal evaluation: development of a fetal biophysical profile. *Am. J. Obstet. Gynecol.* **136**: 787–795.

33 Manning Fa, M.I., Lange, I.R., Harman, C.R., and Chamberlain, P.F. (1987). Fetal biophysical profile scoring: selective use of the nonstress test. *Am. J. Obstet. Gynecol.* **156**: 709–712.

34 Vintzileos, A.M., Fleming, A.D., Scorza, W.E. et al. (1991). Relationship between fetal biophysical activities and umbilical cord gas values. *Am. J. Obstet. Gynecol.* **165**: 707–713.

35 Manning, F.A., Snijders, R., Harman, C.R. et al. (1993). Fetal biophysical profile score VI. Correlation with antepartum umbilical venous fetal pH. *Am. J. Obstet. Gynecol.* **169**: 755–763.

36 Grivell, R.M., Wong, L., and Bhatia, V. (2009). Regimens of fetal surveillance for impaired fetal growth. *Cochrane Database Syst. Rev.* (**21**): CD007113. doi: 10.1002/14651858.

37 Kaur, S., Picconi, J.L., Chadha, R. et al. (2008). Biophysical profile in the treatment of intrauterine growth-restricted fetuses who weigh <1000 g. *Am. J. Obstet. Gynecol.* **199**: 264.e1–264.e4.

38 Cosmi, E., Ambrosini, G., D'Antona, D. et al. (2005). Doppler, cardiotocography, and biophysical profile changes in growth-restricted fetuses. *Obstet. Gynecol.* **106**: 1240–1245.

39 Hecher, K., Bilardo, C.M., Stigter, R.H. et al. (2001). Monitoring of fetuses with intrauterine growth restriction: a longitudinal study. *Ultrasound Obstet. Gynecol.* **18**: 571–577.

40 Chauhan, S.P., Sanderson, M., Hendrix, N.W. et al. (1999). Perinatal outcome and amniotic fluid index in the antepartum and intrapartum periods: a meta-analysis. *Am. J. Obstet. Gynecol.* **181**: 1473–1478.

41 Scrifres, C.M., Stamilio, D., Macones, G.A., and Odibo, A.O. (2009). Predicting perinatal mortality in preterm intrauterine growth restriction. *Am. J. Perinatol.* **26**: 723–728.

42 Baschat, A.A., Gembruch, U., and Harman, C.R. (2001). The sequence of changes in Doppler and biophysical parameters as severe fetal growth restriction worsens. *Ultrasound Obstet. Gynecol.* **18**: 571–577.

43 Nicolaides, K.H., Bilardo, C.M., Soothill, P.W. et al. (1988). Absence of end diastolic frequencies in umbilical artery: a sign of fetal hypoxia and acidosis. *BMJ* **297**: 1026–1027.

44 Weiner, C.P. (1990). The relationship the umbilical artery systolic/diastolic ratio and umbilical blood gas measurements in specimens obtained by cordocentesis. *Am. J. Obstet. Gynecol.* **162**: 1198–1202.

45 Karsdorp, V.H., van Vugt, J.M., van Geijn, H.P. et al. (1994). Clinical significance of absent or reversed end diastolic velocity waveforms in umbilical artery. *Lancet* **344**: 1664–1668.

46 Hartung, J., Kalache, K.D., Heyna, C. et al. (2005). Outcome of 60 neonates who had ARED flow prenatally compared with a matched control group of appropriate-for-gestational-age preterm neonates. *Ultrasound Obstet. Gynecol.* **25**: 566–572.

47 Maulik, D., Mundy, D., Heitmann, E., and Maulik, D. (2011). Umbilical artery Doppler in the assessment of fetal growth restriction. *Clin. Perinatol.* **38**: 65–82.

48 Vergani, P., Roncaglia, N., Ghidini, A. et al. (2010). Can adverse neonatal outcome be predicted in late preterm or near term fetal growth restriction? *Ultrasound Obstet. Gynecol.* **36**: 166–170.

49 Alfirevic, Z. and Neilson, J.P. (1995). Doppler ultrasonography in high-risk pregnancies: systematic review with meta-analysis. *Am. J. Obstet. Gynecol.* **2**: 1379–1387.

50 Maulik, D., Figueroa, R., Sicuranza, G. et al. (1998). Doppler fetal surveillance in clinical practice: evidence based guidelines. *J. Fertil Reprod.* **2**: 5–6.

51 Westergaard, H.B., Langhoff-Roos, J., Lingman, G. et al. (2001). A critical appraisal of the use of umbilical artery Doppler ultrasound in high risk pregnancies: use of meta-analyses in evidence-based obstetrics. *Ultrasound Obstet. Gynecol.* **17**: 466–476.

52 Alfirevic, Z., Stampalija, T., and Gyte, G.M. (2010). Fetal and umbilical Doppler ultrasound in high-risk pregnancies. *Cochrane Database Syst. Rev.* (**20**): CD007529. doi: 10.1002/14651858.

53 Mari, G. and Deter, R.L. (1992). Middle cerebral artery flow velocity waveforms in normal and small-for-gestational-age fetuses. *Am. J. Obstet. Gynecol.* **166**: 1262–1270.

54 Nanthakomon, T. and Uerpairojkit, B. (2010). Outcome of small-for-gestational-age fetuses according to umbilical artery Doppler: is there any yield from additional middle cerebral artery Doppler? *J. Matern. Fetal Neonatal Med.* **23**: 900–905.

55 Ferrazzi, E., Bozzo, M., Rigano, S. et al. (2002). Temporal sequence of abnormal Doppler changes in the peripheral and central circulatory systems of the severely growth-restricted fetus. *Ultrasound Obstet. Gynecol.* **19**: 140–146.

56 Mari, G., Hanif, F., Kruger, M. et al. (2007). Middle cerebral artery peak systolic velocity: a new Doppler parameter in the assessment of growth-restricted fetuses. *Ultrasound Obstet. Gynecol.* **29**: 310–316.

57 Bahado-Singh, R.O., Kovanci, E., Jeffres, A. et al. (1999). The Doppler cerebroplacental ratio and perinatal outcome in intrauterine growth restriction. *Am. J. Obset. Gynecol.* **180**: 750–756.

58 Odibo, A.O., Riddick, C., Pare, E. et al. (2005). Cerebroplacental Doppler ratio and adverse perinatal outcomes in intrauterine growth restriction: evaluating the impact of using gestational age-specific reference values. *J. Ultrasound Med.* **24**: 1223–1228.

59 Severi, F.M., Bocchi, C., Visentin, A. et al. (2002). Uterine and fetal cerebral Doppler predict the outcome of third-trimester small-for-gestational age infants born at term gestation. *Am. J. Obstet. Gynecol.* **19**: 225–228.

60 Hershokovitz, R., Kingdom, J.C., Geary, M., and Rodeck, C.H. (2000). Fetal cerebral blood flow redistribution in late gestation: identification of compromise in small fetuses with normal umbilical artery Doppler. *Ultrasound Obstet. Gynecol.* **15**: 209–212.

61 Baschat, A.A., Gembruch, U., Reiss, I. et al. (2000). Relationship between arterial and venous Doppler and perinatal outcome in fetal growth restriction. *Ultrasound Obstet. Gynecol.* **16**: 407–413.

62 Turan, O.M., Turan, S., Berg, C. et al. (2011). Duration of persistent abnormal ductus venosus flow and its impact on perinatal outcome in fetal growth restriction. *Ultrasound Obstet. Gynecol.* **38**: 295–302.

63 Morris, R.K., Selman, T.J., Verma, M. et al. (2010). Systematic review and meta-analysis of the test accuracy of ductus venosus Doppler to predict compromise of fetal/neonatal wellbeing in high risk pregnancies with placental insufficiency. *Eur. J. Obstet. Gynecol. Reprod. Biol.* **152**: 3–12.

64 Turan, S., Turan, O.M., Berg, C. et al. (2007). Computerized fetal heart rate analysis, Doppler ultrasound and biophysical profile score in the prediction of acid-base status of growth-restricted fetuses. *Ultrasound Obstet. Gynecol.* **30**: 750–756.

65 Baschat, A.A., Galan, H.L., Bhide, A. et al. (2006). Doppler and biophysical assessment in growth restricted fetuses: distribution of test results. *Ultrasound Obstet. Gynecol.* **27**: 41–47.

66 Romero, R., Kalache, K.D., and Kadar, N. (2002). Timing of delivery of the preterm severely growth-restricted fetus: venous Doppler, cardiotocography or the biophysical profile? *Ultrasound Obstet. Gynecol.* **19**: 118–121.

67 Odibo, A.O., Quinones, J.N., Lawrence-Cleary, K. et al. (2004). What antepartum fetal test should guide the timing of delivery of the preterm growth-restricted fetus? A decision-analysis. *Am. J. Obstet. Gynecol.* **191**: 1477–1482.

68 Lees, C.C., Marlow, N., van Wassenaer-Leemhuis, A. et al. (2015). 2 year neurodevelopmental and intermediate perinatal outcomes in infants with very preterm fetal growth restriction (TRUFFLE): a randomized trial. *Lancet* **385**: 2162–2172.

69 Growth Restriction Intervention Trial study group (2003). A randomized trial of timed delivery for the compromised preterm fetus: short term outcomes and Bayesian interpretation. *BJOG* **110**: 27–32.

70 Thornton, J.G., Hornbuckle, J., Vail, A. et al., GRIT study group(2004). Infant wellbeing at 2 years of age in the growth restriction intervention trial (GRIT): multicentred randomized controlled trial. *Lancet* **364**: 513–520.

71 Walker, D.M., Marlow, N., Upstone, L. et al. (2010). The growth restriction intervention trial: long-term outcomes in a randomized trial of timing of delivery in fetal growth restriction. *Am. J. Obstet. Gynecol.* **204**: 34.e1–34.e9.

72 Boers, K.E., Vijgen, S.M.C., Bijlenga, D. et al. (2010). Induction versus expectant monitoring for intrauterine growth restriction at term: randomized equivalence trial (DIGITAT). *BMJ* **341**: c7087.

73 van Wyk, L., Boers, K.E., van der Post, J. et al. (2012). Effects on (neuro)developmental and behavioral outcome at 2 years of age of induced labor compared with expectant management in intrauterine growth-restricted infants: long-term outcomes of the DIGITAT trial. *Am. J. Obstet. Gynecol.*, 206(5): 406.e1–7.

74 Olsen, S.F., Secher, N.J., Tabor, A. et al. (2000). Randomised clinical trials of fish oil supplementation in high risk pregnancies. *BJOG* **107**: 382–395.

75 Gulmezoglu, M., de Onis, M., and Villar, J. (1997). Effectiveness of interventions to prevent or treat impaired fetal growth. *Obstet. Gynecol. Surv.* **52**: 139–149.

76 Nicolini, U., Hubinont, C., Santolaya, J. et al. (1990). Effects of fetal intravenous glucose challenge in normal and growth retarded fetuses. *Horm. Metab. Res.* **22**: 426–430.

77 Nicolaides, K.H., Campbell, S., Bradley, R.J. et al. (1987). Maternal oxygen therapy for intrauterine growth retardation. *Lancet* **1**: 942–945.

78 Battaglia, C., Artini, P.G., D'Ambrogio, G. et al. (1992). Maternal hyperoxygenation in the treatment of intrauterine growth restriction. *Am. J. Obstet. Gynecol.* **167**: 430–435.

79 Johanson, R., Lindow, S.W., van der Elst, C. et al. (1995). A prospective randomized comparison of the effect of continuous oxygen therapy and bedrest on fetuses with absent end diastolic flow on umbilical artery Doppler waveform analysis. *BJOG* **102**: 662–665.

80 Lindow, S.W., Mantel, G.D., Anthony, J., and Coetzee, E.J. (2002). A double-blind randomized controlled trial of continuous oxygen therapy for compromised fetuses. *BJOG* **109**: 509–513.

81 Beazley, D., Livingston, J., Kao, L., and Sibai, B. (2002). Vitamin C and E supplementation in women at high risk for preeclampsia: a double-blind placebo controlled trial. *Am. J. Obstet. Gynecol.* **187**: S216.

82 Chappell, L.C., Seed, P.T., Briley, A.L. et al. (1999). Effect of antioxidants on the occurrence of pre-eclampsia in women at increased risk: a randomized trial. *Lancet* **354**: 810–816.

83 Roberts, J.M., Myatt, L., Cy, S. et al. (2010). Vitamins C and E to prevent complications of pregnancy-associated hypertension. *N. Engl. J. Med.* **362**: 1282–1291.

84 Rumbold, A.R., Crowther, C.A., Haslam, R.R., and Dekker, G.A. (2006). Robinson JS for the ACTS study group. Vitamins C and E and the risks of pre-eclampsia and perinatal complications. *N. Engl. J. Med.* **354**: 1796–1806.

85 Poston, L., Briley, A.L., Seed, P.T. et al. (2006). Vitamins in pre-Eclampsia (VIP) trial consortium. Vitamin C and vitamin E in pregnant women at risk for pre-eclampsia (VIP trial): randomized placebo-controlled trial. *Lancet* **367**: 1145–1154.

86 Xu, H., Perez-Cuevas, R., Xiong, X. et al. (2010). An international trial of anti-oxidants in the prevention of preeclampsia (INTAPP). *Am. J. Obstet. Gynecol.* **202**: 239e1–239e10.

87 Conde-Agudelo, A., Romero, R., Kusanovic, J.P., and Hassan, S.S. (2011). Supplementation with vitamins C and E during pregnancy for the prevention of preeclampsia and other adverse maternal and perinatal outcomes: a systematic review and metaanalysis. *Am. J. Obstet. Gynecol.* **204**: 503e1–503e12.

88 Golding, J. (1998). The Jamiaca Low Dose Aspirin Study Group. A randomized trial of low dose aspirin for primiparae in pregnancy. *BJOG* **105**: 293–299.

89 Subtil, D., Goeusse, P., Puech, F. et al. (2003). Aspirin (100mg) used for prevention of pre-eclampsia in nulliparous women: the Essai regional Aspirine mere-enfant study (part 1). *BJOG* **110**: 475–484.

90 Sibai, B.M., Caritis, S.N., Thom, E. et al. (1993). Prevention of preeclampsia with low-dose aspirin in healthy, nulliparous pregnant women. *N. Engl. J. Med.* **329**: 1213–1218.

91 Caritis, S., Sibai, B., Hauth, J. et al. (1998). Low-dose aspirin to prevent preeclampsia in women at high risk. *N. Engl. J. Med.* **338**: 701–705.

92 Bujold, E., Roberge, S., Lacasse, Y. et al. (2010). Prevention of preeclampsia and intrauterine growth restriction with aspirin started in early pregnancy. *Obstet. Gynecol.* **116**: 402–414.

93 McIntire, D.D., Bloom, S.L., Casey, B.M., and Leveno, K.J. (1999). Birth weight in relation to morbidity and mortality among newborn infants. *N. Engl. J. Med.* **340**: 1244–1248.

94 Gluck, L. and Kulovich, M.V. (1973). Lecithin/sphingomyelin ratios in amniotic fluid in normal and abnormal pregnancy. *Am. J. Obstet. Gynecol.* **115**: 539–546.

95 Procianoy, R.S., Garcia-Prats, J.A., Adams, J.M. et al. (1980). Hyaline membrane disease and intraventricular haemorrhage in small for gestational age infants. *Arch. Dis. Child.* **55**: 502–505.

96 Bernstein, I., Horbar, J., Badger, G. et al. (2000). Morbidity and mortality among very-low-birth-weight neonates with intrauterine growth restriction. *Am. J. Obstet. Gynecol.* **182**: 198–206.

97 Lackman, F., Capewell, V., Richardson, B. et al. (2001). The risks of spontaneous preterm delivery and perinatal mortality in relation to size at birth according to fetal versus neonatal growth standards. *Am. J. Obstet. Gynecol.* **184**: 946–953.

98 Garite, T.J., Clark, R., and Thorp, J.A. (2004). Intrauterine growth restriction increases morbidity and mortality among premature neonates. *Am. J. Obstet. Gynecol.* **191**: 481–487.

99 Surveillance of cerebral palsy in Europe (2000). A collaboration of cerebral palsy surveys and registers. Surveillance of cerebral palsy in Europe (SCPE). *Dev. Med. Child Neurol.* **42**: 816–824.

100 Weinerroither, H., Steiner, H., Tomaselli, J. et al. (2001). Intrauterine blood flow and long-term intellectual, neurologic, and social development. *Obstet. Gynecol.* **97**: 449–453.

101 Geva, R., Eshel, R., Leitner, Y. et al. (2006). Neuropsychological outcome of children with intrauterine growth restriction: a 9-year prospective study. *Pediatrics* **118**: 91–100.

102 Baschat, A.A., Viscardi, R.M., Hussey-Gardner, B. et al. (2009). Infant neurodevelopment following fetal growth restriction: relationship with antepartum surveillance patterns. *Ultrasound Obstet. Gynecol.* **33**: 44–50.

103 Guellec, I., Lapillonne, A., Renolleau, S. et al. (2011). Neurologic outcomes at school age in very preterm infants born with severe or mild growth restriction. *Pediatrics* **127**: e883–e891.

104 Morsing, E., Asard, M., Ley, D. et al. (2011). Cognitive function after intrauterine growth restriction and very preterm birth. *Pediatrics* **127**: e874–e882.

105 Leitner, Y., Fattal-Valevski, A., Geva, R. et al. (2007). Neurodevelopmental outcome of children with intrauterine growth retardation: a longitudinal, 10-year prospective study. *J. Child Neurol.* **22**: 580–587.

106 Figueras, F., Cruz-Martinez, R., Sanz-Cortes, M. et al. (2011). Neurobehavioral outcomes in preterm, growth-restricted infants with and without prenatal advanced signs of brain-sparing. *Ultrasound Obstet. Gynecol.* **38**: 288–294.

107 Procianoy, R., Koch, M.S., and Silveira, R. (2009). Neurodevelopmental outcome of appropriate and small for gestational age very low birth weight infants. *J. Child Neurol.* **24**: 788–794.

108 Paz, I., Laor, A., Gale, R. et al. (2001). Term infants with fetal growth restriction are not at increased risk for low intelligence scores at age 17. *J. Pediatr.* **138**: 87–91.

109 Gluckman, P.D., Hanson, M.A., Cooper, C., and Thornburg, K.L. (2008). Effect of in utero and early-life conditions on adult health and disease. *N. Engl. J. Med.* **359**: 61–73.

110 Barker, D.J.P. (2006). Adult consequences of fetal growth restriction. *Clin. Obset. Gynecol.* **49**: 270–283.

111 Gregory, K.D., Henry, O.A., Ramicone, E. et al. (1998). Maternal and infant complications in high and normal weight infants by method of delivery. *Obstet. Gynecol.* **92**: 507–513.

112 Handa, V.L., Danielsen, B.H., and Gilbert, W.M. (2001). Obsetric anal sphincter lacerations. *Obstet. Gynecol.* **98**: 225–230.

113 Langer, O., Berkus, M.D., Huff, R.W., and Samueloff, A. (1991). Shoulder dystocia: should the fetus weighing greater than or equal to 4000 grams be delivered by cesarean section? *Am. J. Obstet. Gynecol.* **165**: 831–837.

114 Ecker, J.L., Greenberg, J.A., Norwitz, E.R. et al. (1997). Birth weight as a predictor of brachia plexus injury. *Obstet. Gynecol.* **89**: 643–647.

115 Gonen, R., Bader, D., and Ajami, M. (2000). Effects of a policy of elective cesarean delivery in cases of suspected fetal macrosomia on the incidence of brachial plexus injury and the rate of cesarean delivery. *Am. J. Obstet. Gynecol.* **183**: 1296–1300.

116 Nesbitt, T.S., Gilbert, W.M., and Herrchen, B. (1998). Shoulder dystocia and associated risk factors with macrosomic infants born in California. *Am. J. Obstet. Gynecol.* **179**: 476–480.

117 Boulet, S.L., Alexander, G.R., Salihu, H.M., and Pass, M. (2003). Macrosomic births in the United States: determinants, outcomes, and proposed grades of risk. *Am. J. Obstet. Gynecol.* **188**: 1372–1378.

118 Friesen, C.D., Miller, A.N., and Rayburn, W.F. (1995). Influence of spontaneous or induced labor on delivering the macrosomic fetus. *Am. J. Perinatol.* **12**: 63–66.

119 Leaphart, W.L., Meyer, M.C., and Capeless, E.L. (1997). Labor induction with a prenatal diagnosis of fetal macrosomia. *J. Matern. Fetal Med.* **6**: 99–102.

120 Combs, C.A., Singh, N.B., and Khoury, J.C. (1993). Elective induction versus spontaneous labor after sonographic diagnosis of fetal macrosmia. *Obstet. Gynecol.* **81**: 492–496.

121 Herbst, M.A. (2005). Treatment of suspected fetal macrosomia: a cost-effectiveness analysis. *Am. J. Obstet. Gynecol.* **193**: 1035–1039.

122 Gonen, O., Rosen, D.J.D., Dolfin, Z. et al. (1997). Induction of labor versus expectant management in macrosmia: a randomized study. *Am. J. Obstet. Gynecol.* **89**: 913–917.

123 Irion, O. and Boulvain, M. (2000). Induction of labour for suspected fetal macrosomia. *Cochrane Database Syst. Rev.* (**2**): CD000938. doi: 10.1002/14651858.CD000938.

124 Delpapa, E.H. and Mueller-Heubach, E. (1991). Pregnancy outcome following ultrasound diagnosis of macrosomia. *Obstet. Gynecol.* **78**: 340–343.

125 Gross, S.J., Shime, J., and Farine, D. (1987). Shoulder dystocia: predictors and outcome. A five-year review. *Am. J. Obstet. Gynecol.* **156**: 334–336.

126 Bryant, D.R., Leonardi, F.R., Landwehr, J.B., and Bottoms, S.F. (1998). Limited usefulness of fetal weight in predicting neonatal brachial plexus injury. *Am. J. Obstet. Gynecol.* **179**: 686–689.

127 Rouse, D.J., Owen, J., Goldenberg, R.L., and Cliver, S.P. (1996). The effectiveness and costs of elective cesarean delivery for fetal macrosomia diagnosed by ultrasound. *JAMA* **276**: 1480–1486.

128 American College of Obstetricians and Gynecologists (2002). *Shoulder Dystocia. ACOG Practice Bulletin No. 40.* Washington DC: American College of Obstetricians and Gynecologists.

44

CHAPTER 44
Multiple pregnancies and births

Isaac Blickstein and Oren Barak

Obstetrics and Gynecology, Kaplan Medical Center, Rehovot, The Hadassah-Hebrew University School of Medicine, Jerusalem, Israel

The natural pattern of plurality exhibits the relative rare birth of twins (about 1 per 80–100 births) and the extremely rare occurrence of high-order multiple pregnancies. The rarity of high-order multiple pregnancies can be appreciated by the quasi-mathematical Hellin–Zellany rule for twins, triplets, and quadruplets [1]. According to this law, if the frequency of twins in a population is 1/N, then the frequency of triplets will be $1/N^2$ and that of quadruplets $1/N^3$.

The Hellin–Zellany appears to be quite accurate as long as a population remains homogenous and enjoys natural conceptions. Otherwise, it became clear that deviations from the rule often exist because of racial differences in the frequency of dizygotic (DZ) twinning. The next significant deviation appeared after the emergence of effective infertility treatment when physician-made (iatrogenic) multiple pregnancies are now seen in almost all countries, with frequencies approaching 50% of twins and more than 75% of high-order multiple pregnancies. The contribution of infertility treatment to perinatal medicine can be appreciated from data of the Israel Neonatal Network. The data indicate that among infants weighing less than 1500 g, 10% of singletons were conceived by assisted reproduction compared with 60% of twins and 90% of triplets [2]. More recently, Tul et al. [3] found that the incidence of twins after assisted reproduction (Assisted Reproductive Technologies (ARTs)) born at <32 weeks increased 27-fold from 1987 to 2010 and has not reduced from its peak incidence over the last decade.

Biology

Most spontaneous human conceptions (>99.2%) emerge from a single zygote (i.e. monozygotic, (MZ)), whereas in the remaining cases, more than one ovum is ovulated and fertilized, resulting in polyzygotic conceptions (dizygotic (DZ), trizygotic, etc.). This phenomenon appears to occur more often in taller, older, parous, heavier, and black women. Although direct and indirect evidence point to a genetic predisposition of DZ twining, the exact mechanism whereby the ovary is naturally hyperstimulated is basically unknown. In contrast, all infertility treatments are associated with ovarian stimulation and polyovulation.

The vast majority of MZ conceptions result in singleton birth. In only a small fraction of the cases (0.4% of all natural conceptions) the zygote splits to form an MZ twin gestation. The only factor known to increase the frequency of MZ twins is assisted reproduction [4]; however, the true incidence of zygotic splitting following ART is unknown. In a large study of single-embryo transfers, a sixfold increase in zygotic splitting was found, and this incidence was not influenced by using fresh versus frozen-thawed embryos or by performing embryo transfers during a spontaneous versus an induced cycle [4]. Regardless, the mechanism of spontaneous zygotic splitting is unclear. A recent hypothesis suggests that the potential to undergo splitting might be an inherent characteristic of the oocyte [5].

From a clinical point of view, the placental arrangement (i.e. chorionicity and amnionicity) are more important than zygosity. DZ twins have two placentas (separate or fused), each with its chorion and amnion, forming the so-called dichorionic (DC) placenta. Placentation of the MZs, are assumed to depend on the stage of embryonic development at which the split occurs. Early splits (about one third) result in DC placentas, whereas later splits result in monochorionic (MC) placentas. Moreover, if the amnion has not yet differentiated, the MC placenta includes two amniotic sacs: the monochorionic–diamniotic (MCDA) placenta (about two-thirds of the cases). If the split occurs later than eight days after fertilization, a monochorionic–monoamniotic (MCMA) placenta develops. Finally, even later splits result in all varieties of conjoined twins. This construct of events appearing in every textbook, is unproven, as evidenced by the recent controversy regarding the quasi-accepted relationship between the timing of zygotic splitting and placentation [6, 7].

Evidence-Based Obstetrics and Gynecology, First Edition. Edited by Errol R. Norwitz, Carolyn M. Zelop, David A. Miller, and David L. Keefe.

In any case, because MZs with a DC placenta cannot be differentiated clinically from same-sex DZ twins (half of the DZs) who also have a DC placenta, zygosity can be determined with certainty only in the DC-unlike-sex twins (all must be DZs) and in twins with an MC placenta (all must be MZs). Simple calculation reveals that we are blind to zygosity in about 45% of the cases, and zygosity determination, if required, must be performed by DNA testing. Importantly, nothing should be said about zygosity to parents of same-sex twins with a DC placenta.

Maternal consequences

The significant changes in women's role in western societies witnessed after World War II, facilitated by effective contraception, allowed ample time to achieve education and a career, but resulted in increased maternal age at first delivery. Because age and fecundity are inversely related, infertility treatment to achieve a pregnancy often becomes inevitable. Because all infertility treatments carry an increased risk of multiple gestations, the end result of these socio-medical trends is an increased age of the cohort of mothers of multiples. US data clearly illustrate that the increase in maternal age is more prominent in high-order multiple pregnancies than in twins and in twins than in singletons, with a net result of multiples being more often delivered to older mothers in whom chronic disease conditions have already accumulated [8, 9].

Older maternal age frequently combines with the inevitable overwhelmed maternal homeostasis. Consider the fact that the average singleton, twin, and triplet has a similar birthweight until 28 weeks (around 1000 g). Thus, by 28 weeks, the mother of twins and the mother of triplets has accumulated twice and three times the fetal mass of singletons, respectively. This excess of fetal mass must come from either existing maternal resources or from supplemental energy. It is thus clear that during the third trimester all maternal systems in a multiple pregnancy are overwhelmed and some may be only a step away from clinical insufficiency.

Two examples vividly demonstrate the situation. The first is the increased frequency of clinically significant anemia during twin gestation as a result of either depleted maternal iron stores or from inadequate iron supplementation [10]. A second example relates to the increased cardiac output [11, 12]. Kuleva et al. [12] demonstrated a significantly higher increasing cardiac output throughout pregnancy in multiple as compared to a singleton gestation. It has been estimated that in the worst-case scenario (e.g. preterm labor due to infection in a multiple pregnancy) the cardiac output may exceed $10\,l\,min^{-1}$ (two to three times the normal value). It is therefore understandable why cardiac function so easily turns into dysfunction. Ghi et al. [13] showed that in uncomplicated twin gestations, significant changes in maternal systolic and diastolic function occur from the first to the third trimester. However, whereas diastolic parameters normalize after pregnancy, a relative systolic dysfunction persists after delivery.

Regardless of the altered maternal physiology in a multiple pregnancy, some maternal disease conditions are more frequent in these gestations. Foremost are hypertensive disorders which are two to three times more frequent [14] and their most dangerous complication – eclampsia – is six times more frequent among mothers of multiple gestations [15]. Moreover, pre-eclamptic toxemia (PET) occurs earlier in multiples than in singletons and often occurs in a more severe form [16]. Because triplets and other high-order multiples were rare in the past, scant data exist on hypertensive disorders in high-order multiple pregnancies. Along with the current epidemic dimensions of multiple gestations it has been shown that the risk of hypertensive disorders is plurality dependent, whereby the risk in triplets is higher than that in twins, and the risk in twins is higher than that in singletons [17]. This may suggest that hyperplacentation is an important reason for the higher incidence of pre-eclampsia in multiples. It is unknown why PET is more frequent in multiples. One potential explanation comes from a recent population-based study [18] that reiterated the exceptionally important association between the high pre-gravid body mass index (BMI) (rather than weight gain) and pre-eclampsia. Another theory suggested a higher incidence of hypertensive disorders in DZ twins (more "immunogenic" difference) than in MZ twins. A recent study, confirmed previous smaller studies that appear to disprove this theory [19].

In contrast to the clear association to pre-eclampsia, data are still conflicting about the relationship of multiple pregnancy and gestational diabetes. It appears that most tests to detect glucose intolerance showed a diabetogenic effect of multiple gestations, without a significantly increased rates of gestational diabetes. However, as with pre-eclampsia [17], it was shown that the risk of gestational diabetes is plurality dependent [20] pointing, at least in a teleological way, to hyperplacentosis as a potential common denominator for both gestational diabetes and hypertension. Yet, another common denominator – pregravid obesity – seems to equally important [18].

Whereas it is clear how hypertensive disorders influence a multiple pregnancy, the effect of gestational diabetes is less robust. Fox et al. [21] suggested that it is not clear that glycemic control in twin pregnancy is improving outcome and was in fact associated with an increased risk of small for gestational age (SGA) infants. A study by Simões et al. [22] found also that pre-gravid obesity appears to predispose women to gestational diabetes. They showed that twins from the gestational diabetes group had more respiratory distress syndrome and had a threefold, but not significantly, increased perinatal mortality rate. Birth weight characteristics were similar in both groups.

Mothers of multiples are at considerably greater risk of preterm labor and delivery. Many prophylactic measures, including progestatives, cervical sutures (cerclage), beta-sympathominetics, bed rest, and hospitalization, failed to significantly reduce this complication. Nevertheless, expecting mothers of multiples are frequently asked to leave work and to conduct a more sedentary lifestyle.

Table 44.1 lists the most common maternal complications during multiple gestations.

Fetal–neonatal consequences

In all mammals, an inverse relationship exists between litter size and both gestational age and birthweight. In the human, the average gestational age at birth is around 40 weeks for singletons, 35.3 weeks for twins, 31.9 weeks for triplets, and 29.5 weeks for quadruplets [23]. Although multiple pregnancies display many specific complications, the consequences of preterm birth are by far the most common and most important in terms of morbidity and mortality.

Malformations

Multiples are notorious for an increased risk of malformations. However, the increased risk is mainly related to MZ twinning whereas the malformation rates of each of the DZ twins is similar to that of singletons [24]. Nonetheless, the mother of DZ twins has an increased risk that one of the twins will be affected. In contrast, the higher malformation rate among MZs is explained by the hypothesis of a common teratogen: the one that causes the split of the zygote might be also responsible for the malformation.

Table 44.1 Maternal complications more frequently seen in multiple pregnancies

Hypertensive diseases
- Pre-eclamptic toxemia
- Hemolysis, elevated liver enzymes, low platelets (HELLPs) syndrome
- Acute fatty liver
- Pregnancy-induced hypertension
- Chronic hypertension
- Eclampsia

Anemia

Gestational diabetes mellitus (?)

Premature contractions and labor
- Complications associated with tocolysis

Delivery-associated complications
- Cesarean section
- Operative delivery
- Premature rupture of membranes
- Postpartum endometritis
- Placental abruption

Table 44.2 Categories of structural defects in twins

Category	Defect
Malformations more common in twins than in singletons	Neural tube defects Hydrocephaly Congenital heart disease Esophageal and anorectal atresias Intersex Genitourinary tract anomalies Amniotic band syndrome
Malformations unique to monozygotic twins	TRAP sequence Conjoined twins Twin embolization syndrome
Placental malformations	Single umbilical artery Twin–twin transfusion syndrome Velamentous cord insertion Selective growth restriction Twin anemia–polycythemia sequence
Deformations due to intrauterine crowding	Skeletal (postural) abnormalities; i.e. clubfoot, dolichocephalus

Malformations among multiples are grouped into four types (Table 44.2) [24]. The first type includes malformations that are more frequent among multiples, especially those of the central nervous and the cardiovascular systems. The second type involves malformations specific to MZ twinning such as twin reverse arterial perfusion (TRAP) sequence and the various forms of conjoined twins. The third type relates to consequences of placental malformations, in particular the MC placenta, resulting in the twin–twin transfusion syndrome (TTTS), selective intrauterine growth restriction (sIUGR), and twin anemia–polycythemia sequence (TAPS). Finally, the fourth type involves skeletal abnormalities such as clubfoot that are caused by intrauterine fetal crowding.

Some malformations can have a major impact on the normal twin. For instance, in the TRAP sequence, the circulation of the severely anomalous twin is entirely supported by the normal (pump) twin. Sooner or later, this cardiac overload will lead to cardiac insufficiency in the normal twin. Another example is the case in TTTS whereby both twins are usually completely normal, but the anomalous transplacental shunt of blood can cause serious morbidity in both twins. The most striking example is the case of single fetal demise in MC twins, whereby the surviving fetus dies in utero soon after the death of the first twin. Alternatively, the surviving twin can be seriously damaged (see later). A final example is the presence of an anencephalic twin which may be surrounded by severe polyhydramnios, increasing the risk of preterm birth. In such discordant lethal malformations, the risk of reducing the anencephalic twin should be weighed against the risk of endangering the normal fetus by the procedure-related preterm birth.

In contrast to structural malformations, chromosomal anomalies are not more frequent among multiples. For example, each member of the multiple gestation has the same maternal-age-dependent risk for trisomy 21. However, as with the probability calculations for structural anomalies, the risk for a mother that one of her twins will have trisomy 21 is greater than that of a mother of a singleton. Roughly, the risk for the mother that one of her twins will have trisomy 21 is 5/3 the risk of a mother of a singleton of the same age [25].

Because multiples are commonly seen in older mothers and invasive cytogenetic procedures (amniocentesis or chorionic villus sampling) carry a higher risk of pregnancy loss when performed in multiples, there is a genuine need for non-invasive maternal screening of aneuploidy to minimize the need for invasive procedures in these premium pregnancies. Regrettably, screening tests like the PAPP-A and inhibin and the triple test (second trimester maternal serum human chorionic gonadotropin (hCG) or free beta-hCG, alpha-fetoprotein, and unconjugated estriol) have a significantly lower prediction for trisomy 21 in multiples compared with singletons. An advance in this area is the implementation of nuchal translucency thickness measurement with or without biochemical markers in screening for aneuploidy [26]. Sarno et al. [27] examined the role of cell-free DNA testing in twin pregnancies and showed that the fetal fraction is lower (except for MZ twins where it is rather higher) and the failure rate is higher compared to singletons. The authors maintained that, at present, the data were too small for a fair assessment of performance of screening for trisomy 21, but it may be similar to that in singleton pregnancies.

Most structural anomalies can be detected by comprehensive sonographic and echocardiographic scans as well as Doppler velocimetry are able to detect many structural and functional cardiovascular anomalies. When a malformed twin is found the question of selective reduction of the anomalous twin might be discussed with the parents. In multichorionic multiples, reduction is accomplished by ultrasound-guided intracardiac injection of potassium chloride. However, because of the risk to the survivor in MC sets, highly invasive procedures are used to interrupt the umbilical circulation of the anomalous twin. In some instances, for example in the TRAP sequence, intrafetal radiofrequency might be employed to reduce the malformed twin.

All invasive procedures (amniocentesis, chorionic villus sampling, and the reduction methods) are associated with the risk of 5–10% of membrane rupture and loss of the entire pregnancy. When an invasive procedure is considered during the second trimester, the risk of extremely preterm birth of the normal twin is apparent. In some countries without an upper limit of gestational age for fetal reduction, invasive diagnostic methods might be deferred until 32 weeks, thus minimizing the risk of procedure-related preterm birth.

Embryonic and fetal demise

With the advent of sonography, it was clear that more twin pregnancies are generated than born. The early loss of one twin was eventually called vanishing twin syndrome (VTS) to denote the disappearance of an embryonic structure during the first trimester [28]. This spontaneous reduction appears to be the natural equivalent of intentional multifetal pregnancy (numerical) reduction.

Logically, the true frequency of VTS is unless sonography is performed at an early stage. One estimate of VTS frequency comes from iatrogenic conceptions: Spontaneous reduction of one or more gestational sacs or embryos occurred before the 12th week of gestation in 36% of twin, 53% of triplet, and 65% of quadruplet pregnancies [29]. Similarly, Pinborg et al. [30] found that 1 in 10 in vitro fertilization (IVF) singletons originates from a twin gestation.

Single fetal death occurring beyond the first trimester is also more common in multiples. In DC twins, it is believed that the risk to the surviving twin is extremely low and present only if there is an external insult such as maternal disease. In contrast, single fetal death in MC twins has an entirely different implication [31].

The chance of serious damage in the survivor is significant and estimated to be between 20% and 30%. The most recent meta-analysis [32] suggests that after single fetal demise, the death of the co-twin follows in about 15% (compared to 3% in DC twins), there is a higher rates for preterm delivery (68% vs. 54%), higher abnormal postnatal cranial imaging (34% vs. 16%) and neurodevelopmental impairment (26% versus 2%).

Although the consequences of single fetal death in MC twins is termed "twin embolization syndrome", this pathogenesis was discarded in the early 1990s, and replaced by the ischemic theory, which postulates that blood is acutely shunted from the live twin to the low-resistance circulation of the deceased fetus, causing acute hypovolemia, ischemia, and end organ damage in the survivor.

Usually, the diagnosis of single fetal death is delayed. The question then arises whether prompt delivery is indicated. Data suggest that acute blood loss occurs just before the time of death of the surviving twin, and therefore it is unlikely that prompt delivery of the survivor twin could decrease the associated high mortality and morbidity rates [33]. Thus, a conservative management is advocated in such cases, especially remote from term, and to use ultrasound and magnetic resonance imaging (MRI) to exclude brain lesions at 31–32 weeks' gestation.

Twin–twin transfusion syndrome

TTTS is seen mainly (or only) in the MC-diamniotic variety [34]. The plethora of studies on TTTS may lead to the wrong impression about its frequency. In fact, TTTS occurs in about 10% of MC twins, and about half are of mild severity [35]. Nonetheless, early onset (before 20 weeks' gestation) severe TTTS, unless intensively treated, is associated with 100% mortality of both twins.

The pathogenesis of TTTS is shunting of blood from one twin (the donor) to the other (the recipient) via transplacental arteriovenous anastomoses, with a paucity of compensating veno-venous and arterio-arterial connections. Nikkels et al. [36] evaluated the angioarchitecture of MC placentas and found that mortality was highest in the absence of an arterio-arterial anastomosis and lowest in the presence of an arterio-arterial anastomosis.

Once the cardiac overload of the recipient is significant enough (seen as tricuspid regurgitation in early echocardiography) polyhydramnios ensues and together with atrial natriuretic peptide that will cause poor micturition in the hypovolemic donor (absent bladder and oligohydramnios – the so-called "stuck twin sign" on sonography). Indeed, there is no TTTS without the so-called twin oligo-polyhydramnios sequence (TOPS) [37]. Subsequently, no bladder will be seen in the donor, followed by pathological Doppler flows in the umbilical artery, fetal hydrops, and death. The most useful classification of TTTS is termed Quintero's staging [38] which includes five stages:

(1) *Stage 1.* polyhydramnios (maximal vertical pocket (MVP), of 8 cm or more) in the recipient and oligohydramnios (MVP of 2 cm or less) in the donor twin (Figure 44.1);
(2) *Stage 2.* Absent visualization of the bladder in the donor twin;
(3) *Stage 3.* Critically abnormal Doppler studies (CADs) defined by at least one of the following: (i) absent end diastolic velocity (AEDV) or reverse end-diastolic velocity in the umbilical artery (REDV), (ii) reverse flow in the ductus venosus (RFDV), or (iii) pulsatile umbilical venous flow (PUVF);
(4) *Stage 4.* Presence of hydrops in either twin;
(5) *Stage 5.* Intrauterine fetal death of either twin.

Of several treatment modalities proposed in the past for TTTS, laser photocoagulation emerged as the treatment of choice [39]. Laser photocoagulation is usually performed in stages 2–4 TTTS between 16 and 28 weeks' gestation. It is debatable if such an intervention should be done for stage 1, before/after these gestational weeks, or in cases with a short cervix. In a meta-analysis of 10 articles [40], a higher overall survival (OR 2.04), a lower neonatal death and neurological morbidity (OR 0.24; OR 0.2, respectively) were found in the group treated with laser photocoagulation. Alternatively, one may use amnioreduction (sometimes repeated procedures) when laser treatment is not available. In some instances intervention is used to buy time (i.e. increasing gestational age to the point of viability) rather than for solving the problem of the intertwin shunt.

In the classic neonatal presentation of TTTS, albeit no longer used antepartum, the twins are discordant in size (at least 20–25%) and in hemoglobin levels (at least 5 g dl^{-1}). The donor is usually pale and anemic, whereas the recipient is polycythemic [34]. At present, it is known that discordant growth is not directly related (but may occur in addition) to TTTS but to unequal sharing of the placenta. If the smaller twin is growth restricted the situation is termed selective

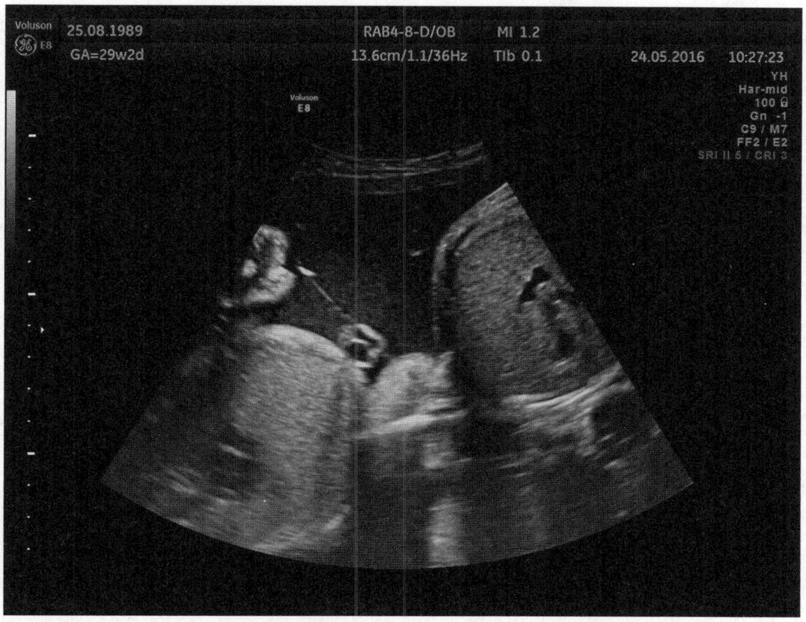

Figure 44.1 Twin oligopolyhydramnios sequence in a monochorionic pair. This is the first sign of twin–twin transfusion. Source: Figure courtesy of Dr. Y. Hazan, Kaplan Medical Center. Reproduced with permission.

IUGR (sIUGR, see below). It also became apparent that a significant difference in hemoglobin levels without TTTS are seldom seen (5% of the cases), but encountered mainly following failure to photocoagulate all arterio-venous (AV) anastomoses. This TAPS is a relatively new diagnosis and can be easily reached with Doppler measurements of the peak systolic velocity in the middle cerebral artery [41]. At present, the clinical significance of TAPS and its proper management are not established.

Fetal growth

Multiples grow in utero to the same extent as singletons until about 28 weeks, thereafter, growth curves show a clear decelerating trend compared with that of singletons. The higher risk of delivering low birthweight (LBW) infants in a multiple birth is well known, as is the advantage for the multiparous patient. Analysis of population-based data found that overall, the risk of having at least one very low birthweight (VLBW, <1500 g) infant was 1:5 among nulliparous women and 1:12 among multiparous women [42, 43]. The risk of having two VLBW twins among nulliparas (1:11) was double that of multiparas (1:22) [43]. A similar trend and similar frequencies, but for extremely LBW (<1000 g) babies, were found in the analysis of triplets [44].

The most common growth aberration in multiples is birth weight discordance (relative growth restriction) [45]. Birth weight discordance occurs whenever a significant difference exists in birth weights between the larger and the smaller fetus/infant of a multiple pregnancy set. In fact, one rarely finds that all members of the set have the same birth weight as some variation is expected between siblings and therefore the magnitude of the difference – the degree of discordance – must be incorporated in the definition. At present, the percent definition is usually employed, whereby the birth weight disparity is calculated as a percentage of the larger infant. Because the definition does not refer to the actual size of the twins, the same degree of discordance (e.g. 20%) may be assigned to a twin pair weighing 1500 and 1200 g and to a pair weighing 3000 and 2400 g. The analysis shows that about 75% of twins exhibit less than 15% discordance, about 20% are 15–25% discordant, and about 5% are more than 25% discordant [45].

The definition of birthweight discordance is even more complex in triplets. Using the same percent definition as used for twins will ignore the middle-sized triplet. Therefore, the true estimation of intertriplet relationship requires a different approach, in which the middle sized triplet is defined in relation to the difference between the larger and the smaller triplets [46].

It has also been determined that at lower levels of discordance either twin can be the smaller but the likelihood of the second-born twin being the smaller increases with increasing discordance levels [45]. At levels greater than 25%, the smaller twin was three to six times more often the second born.

The clinical approach to the level of discordance is generally accepted: observation for the lowest and intervention for and highest degrees of discordance. It has been suggested that at lower levels (i.e. <25%) discordance might even be an adaptive measure to promote maturity (i.e. delivery at a more advanced gestational age) by reducing the inevitable uterine overdistention [47]. It has been repeatedly shown that the larger the discordance the greater is the risk that the smaller twin will be also growth restricted, associated with anomalies and increased risk perinatal morbidity and mortality [48, 49]. As with singletons, growth restriction indicates special attention. The main problem with the accurate prediction of birth weight discordance is the plus/minus construct that exists in estimated fetal weights (EFWs). For example, 0% birth weight discordance can be estimated to be 18.1% discordance when one is +10% overestimated and the other is −10% underestimated. With this caveat in mind, other methods to circumvent this inherent problem of sonographic estimation of birth weight discordance were tested, but none is perfect.

Analysis of a large data set revealed that mortality rate of the smaller twin in a discordant pair (>25%) was apparent mainly if the smaller twins was also SGA [50]. In fact, even in severely discordant twin pairs, about 40% do not comprise a growth-restricted fetus. Thus, Identification of this group (severely discordant but appropriate for gestational age) is an imperative step in the management of birth weight discordance in twin gestations and in avoiding unnecessary interventions that may lead to iatrogenic prematurity.

Selective IUGR in MC pairs poses additional problems. Firstly, the etiology is probably a result of unequal placental sharing [51]. Secondly, at times, sIUGR in MC twins is commonly associated with both genuine or relative growth restriction. Finally, when growth restriction is severe enough, fetal death may result. In contrast to DC twins, single fetal death in a MC pair endangers the survivor. Clinical dilemmas may arise, especially remote from term, when a decision to save the ailing fetus may endanger the healthy fetus with potential risks of extreme preterm birth. At present, sIUGR in MC twins is categorized according to the umbilical artery Doppler values, but it is unclear at which stage intervention (in the form of early delivery or conversely – by preventive fetocide) might be indicated [52].

Fetal assessment

Fetal assessment in multiples is similar to that in singletons, although it is more complicated and more frequent [53, 54]. For instance, with the availability of modern equipment, fetal heart rate is currently traced for both twins at the same time. Intrapartum dual tracing is as important as during pregnancy, and once the membranes are ruptured, the presenting twin might be traced with a scalp electrode while the nonpresenting twin is followed with an external Doppler electrode.

Ultrasound is indispensable in the assessment of twins. This begins with chorionicity and amnionicity determination (preferably during the first trimester) (Figures 44.2 and 44.3), nuchal translucency measurement, anatomical scan, echocardiography, and growth estimation. The fetal biophysical profile is similarly assessed individually. Doppler velocimetry is frequently employed to assess various fetal vessels.

Delivery considerations

Timing

Almost 80–90% of twins and practically all high-order multiple pregnancies initiate spontaneous labor at less than

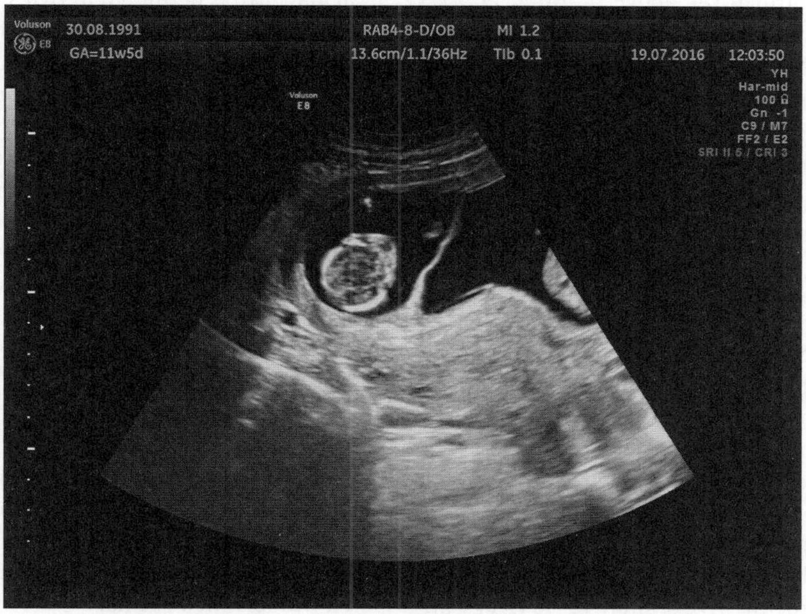

Figure 44.2 The so-called lambda ("twin pick") sign seen by transabdominal ultrasound at 11 weeks. The presence of decidual tissue between the two double layers of each gestational sac is evidence of dichorionicity. Source: Figure courtesy Dr. Y. Hazan, Kaplan Medical Center. Reproduced with permission.

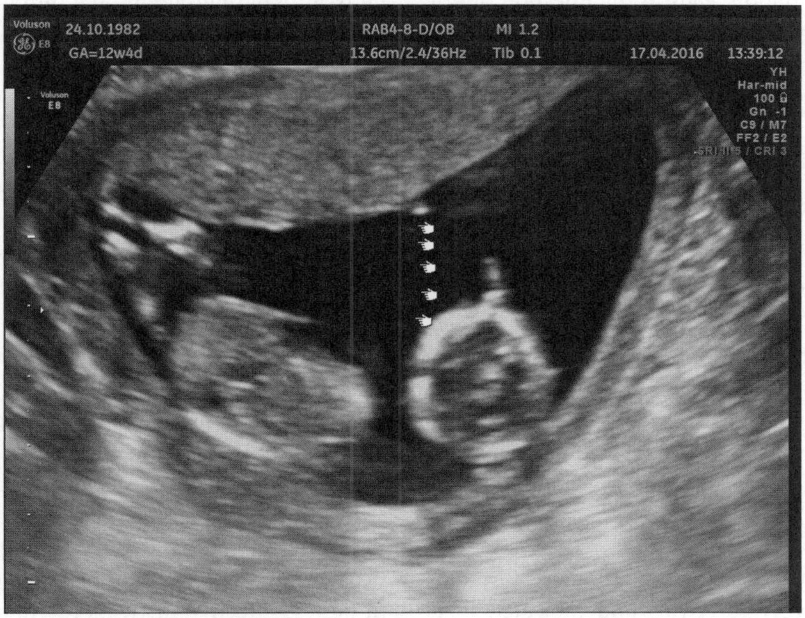

Figure 44.3 The absence of the lambda sign is suggestive of monochorionicity. The very thin membrane may sometimes be elusive and might be depicted toward the end of the first trimester. Source: Figure courtesy Dr. Y. Hazan, Kaplan Medical Center. Reproduced with permission.

38 weeks' gestation. In recent years, data have suggested that at least for twins, "term" by singleton standards (i.e. 40 weeks) might be inappropriate and could carry a similar risk to post-term singletons. This concept emerged from data suggesting that neonatal mortality [55] and morbidity [56] are increased after 37 completed weeks compared with singletons, and the concept that twins should be delivered by 37 or 38 weeks comes from evidence that the fetal systems of the multiple pregnancy might mature by this date [55].

More recent data confirmed the above. Kahn et al. [57] showed that at 36–37 weeks gestation the prospective risk for fetal death for twins equals that of post-term singletons. The same prospective risk for triplets is seen even earlier at about 28–30 weeks [58]. A recent Cochrane review [59] reviewed two randomized trials addressing the timing of delivery. This review did not find any significant difference between early birth at 37 weeks and expectant management. They concluded that early birth at 37 weeks' gestation compared with ongoing expectant management for women with an uncomplicated twin pregnancy does not appear to be associated with an increased risk of harms [59]. Another meta-analysis including the same data found a lower rate of serious adverse outcomes with a planned early (37 weeks) delivery group [60].

Great controversy exists regarding elective preterm (at 34–35 weeks) delivery of MC twins. This initiative started from the finding of increase prospective risk of intrauterine death in uncomplicated MC twins [61, 62]. As the reported deaths in uncomplicated MC twins after 32–33 weeks are in essence "unexpected", it is possible to reduce this risk by either elective preterm birth (presumably by cesarean section) after 33 weeks' gestation or by intensive fetal surveillance. This latter option leads to the question of how intensive is intensive enough. It should be stressed that the initially reported high risk was not universally confirmed [63] and was never tested prospectively.

Data related to timing of delivery of monoamniotic twins – a "ticking bomb" situation for cord entanglement and fetal demise – are even less robust [64]. A recent retrospective study found that with close surveillance, whether inpatients or outpatients, the risk of intrauterine fetal death before 33 weeks of gestation was nil and the risk of neonatal death resulting from prematurity was less than 2% – findings that led to the recommendation of close in/outpatients surveillance starting at 26–28 weeks and consideration of elective preterm delivery at 33 weeks gestation [65]. This logical approach for such was adopted by most guidelines, without any clear evidence.

Mode of delivery

Many reasons exist why cesarean section is the most common mode of delivery for twins and indicated in all high-order multiple pregnancies [66]. Because twin gestations often involve maternal and fetal complications and are quite often considered "premium" pregnancies, many clinicians follow the principle "no high-risk pregnancy should end with a high-risk delivery", and deliver twins by cesarean section for many subtle reasons other than clear-cut, evidence-based indications. Thus, the decision for an abdominal birth in twins, intentionally or not, is based on qualitative variables that were not quantified by randomized trials and on quantitative variables that suggest no advantage for a cesarean delivery in the majority of cases [66].

Vaginal birth is permitted in twins whenever the first twin is in vertex presentation. Breech delivery of the second twin or internal podalic version of a transverse-lying second twin are also permitted. These recommendations for delivery of vertex/nonvertex sets are currently based on the large Canadian randomized trial [67]. This study (and its secondary analysis on neurodevelopment) is, at present, the best that we have. After a very long recruitment period, the Twin Birth Study showed that, between 32 + 0 and 38 + 6 weeks gestation, the rate of cesarean delivery was 90.7% in the planned-cesarean-delivery group (i.e. some 10% delivered vaginally before the planned cesarean delivery) and was 43.8% in the planned-vaginal-delivery group (i.e. only 56% of planned vaginal births ended vaginally). Moreover, planned abdominal birth did not significantly change the risk of fetal/neonatal death, serious neonatal morbidity, and long-term neurological outcome as compared with planned vaginal delivery. However, planned cesarean birth did not significantly increase the risk of maternal morbidity, as compared with planned vaginal delivery. Thus the conclusions of this study appear to satisfy both proponents and opponent of vaginal births of vertex–nonvertex twins [68].

When a multiple birth is anticipated, the immediate neonatal treatment of an infant of a multiple pregnancy is not different from treating a singleton, except that twins come in pairs, and triplets come in sets. This means more staff available in the delivery suite, more cribs available in the nursery, and more stations are ready in the neonatal intensive care unit (NICU). If the availability of NICU cribs lags behind the increased production of multiples, a serious public health situation might be created.

Outcome

The overall outcome for multiples is worse compared with that for singletons. For instance, the increased risk of cerebral palsy among multiples is clear: roughly 20-fold for triplets and eightfold for twins as compared to singletons [69]. This increase in cerebral palsy rate with the number of fetuses seems to be exponential.

Another example is that the usual prophylactic dose of corticosteroids given to preterm singleton pregnancies appears to be less effective in twins to enhance lung maturity and reduce the risk of neonatal respiratory distress.as it is for singletons [70, 71]. This diminished effect is also seen, but to a lesser extent, for the effect of corticosteroids on the incidence of intraventricular hemorrhage (IVH) [72].

Regardless of these and other specificities related to the multiples, by far the most important issues influencing outcome of multiples are gestational age and birth weight. Indeed, the latest USA figures suggest that the incidence rate of very preterm births (<32 weeks) for singletons was 1.23%, as compared to 10.58% for twins and 39.27% for triples. These figures translate into the incidence rate of 1.07% low birth rate (<1500 g) singletons, as compared to 9.56% for twins and 36.96% for triplets [23].

Summary: Prevention vs. cure

It is evident that multiple pregnancies and births are a true challenge for all medical disciplines involved in caring for the mother, fetuses, and infants. At the same time, the increase in iatrogenic multiple births may have an anti-evolution effect with as yet unknown consequences.

The epidemic dimensions of multiple births, and especially of high-order multiple pregnancies, became clear toward the end of the 1980s as an aftershock resulting from effective infertility treatment. To amend this untoward consequence of infertility treatment, clinicians proposed to reduce the number of embryos during pregnancy [73]. Multifetal pregnancy reduction, soon became a popular "cure" of the side effects of infertility treatment. This procedure, performed during the early second trimester via the transvaginal or transabdominal route, carries a risk of about 5% total loss, as well as a risk for significant maternal psychological morbidity. However, multifetal pregnancy reduction is certainly associated with better outcomes because fewer fetuses will expectedly do better than more fetuses.

In every aspect of medicine, prevention is better than cure. In terms of infertility treatment, this means transferring fewer embryos in IVF programs and canceling ovulation induction cycles when more than one ripe follicle is visualized [74]. Obviously, such preventive measures will reduce the overall success rates, although it is debatable if birth of several severely premature infants constitutes any measure of success.

The change in attitude, mainly by infertility experts lead to the praiseworthy decline of triplets rate [75], however, this was probably achieved in expense of further increased incidence of twins after ART [3].

References

1 Blickstein, I. and Keith, L.G. (2002). Latrogenic multiple pregnancy. *Semin. Neonatol.* **7**: 169–176.

2 Shinwell, E.S., Shinwell, E.S., Blickstein, I. et al. (2003). Excess risk of mortality in very low birthweight triplets: a National, Population Based Study. *Arch. Dis. Child. Fetal Neonatal Ed.* **88**: F36–F40.

3 Tul, N., Lucovnik, M., Verdenik, I. et al. (2013). The contribution of twins conceived by assisted reproduction technology to the very preterm birth rate: a Population-Based Study. *Eur. J. Obstet. Gynecol. Reprod. Biol.* **171**: 311–313.

4 Blickstein, I., Jones, C., and Keith, L.G. (2003). Zygotic-splitting rates after single-embryo transfers in in vitro fertilization. *N. Engl. J. Med.* **348**: 2366–2367.

5 Blickstein, I. and Keith, L.G. (2007). On the possible cause of monozygotic twinning: lessons from the 9-banded armadillo and from assisted reproduction. *Twin Res. Hum. Genet.* **10**: 394–399.

6 Herranz, G. (2015). The timing of monozygotic twinning: a criticism of the common model. *Zygote* **23**: 27–40.

7 Gardner, R.L. (2014). The timing of monozygotic twinning: a pro-life challenge to conventional scientific wisdom. *Reprod. Biomed. Online* **28**: 276–278.

8 Blickstein, I. (2003). Motherhood at or beyond the edge of reproductive age. *Int. J. Fertil Womens Med.* **48**: 17–24.

9 Prapas, N., Kalogiannidis, I., Prapas, I. et al. (2006). Twin gestation in older women: antepartum, intrapartum complications, and perinatal outcomes. *Arch. Gynecol. Obstet.* **273**: 293–297.

10 Blickstein, I., Goldschmit, R., and Lurie, S. (1995). Hemoglobin levels during twin vs. singleton pregnancies. Parity makes the difference. *J. Reprod. Med.* **40**: 47–50.

11 Kametas, N.A., McAuliffe, F., Krampl, E. et al. (2003). Maternal cardiac function in twin pregnancy. *Obstet. Gynecol.* **102**: 806–815.

12 Kuleva, M., Youssef, A., Maroni, E. et al. (2011). Maternal cardiac function in normal twin pregnancy: a longitudinal study. *Ultrasound Obstet. Gynecol.* **38**: 575–580.

13 Ghi, T. et al. (2015). Maternal cardiac evaluation during uncomplicated twin pregnancy with emphasis on the diastolic function. *Am. J. Obstet. Gynecol.* **213** (**3**): 376.e1–376.e8.

14 Sibai, B.M., Hauth, J., Caritis, S. et al. (2000). Hypertensive disorders in twin versus singleton gestations. National Institute of Child Health and Human Development Network of Maternal-Fetal Medicine Units. *Am. J. Obstet. Gynecol.* **182**: 938–942.

15 Douglas, K.A. and Redman, C.W. (1994). Eclampsia in the United Kingdom. *BMJ* **309**: 1395–1400.

16 Blickstein, I., Ben-Hur, H., and Borenstein, R. (1992). Perinatal outcome of twin pregnancies complicated with pre-eclampsia. *Am. J. Perinatol.* **9**: 258–260.

17 Skupski, D.W., Nelson, S., Kowalik, A. et al. (1996). Multiple gestations from in vitro fertilization: successful implantation alone is not associated with subsequent pre-eclampsia. *Am. J. Obstet. Gynecol.* **175**: 1029–1032.

18 Lucovnik, M., Blickstein, I., Verdenik, I. et al. (2014). Impact of pre-gravid body mass index and body mass index change on pre-eclampsia and gestational diabetes in singleton and twin pregnancies. *J. Matern. Fetal Neonatal Med.* **27**: 1901–1904.

19 Lučovnik, M., Blickstein, I., Lasič, M. et al. (2016). Hypertensive disorders during monozygotic and dizygotic twin gestations: a population-based study. *Hypertens Pregnancy* **15**: 1–6.

20 Sivan, E., Maman, E., Homko, C.J. et al. (2002). Impact of fetal reduction on the incidence of gestational diabetes. *Obstet. Gynecol.* **99**: 91–94.

21 Fox, N.S., Gerber, R.S., Saltzman, D.H. et al. (2016). Glycemic control in twin pregnancies with gestational diabetes: are we improving or worsening outcomes? *J. Matern. Fetal Neonatal Med.* **29**: 1041–1045.

22 Simões, T., Queirós, A., Correia, L. et al. (2011). Gestational diabetes mellitus complicating twin pregnancies. *J. Perinat. Med.* **39**: 437–440.

23 Hamilton, B.E., Martin, J.A., Osterman, M.J. et al. (2015). Births: final data for 2014. *Natl. Vital. Stat. Rep.* **64**: 1–64.

24 Blickstein, I. and Smith-Levitin, M. (1998). Multifetal pregnancy. In: *Fetal Disorders: Diagnosis and Management* (ed. B.M. Petrikovsky), 223. New York, NY: Wiley.

25 Meyers, C., Adam, R., Dungan, J., and Prenger, V. (1997). Aneuploidy in twin gestations: when is maternal age advanced? *Obstet. Gynecol.* **89**: 248–251.

26 Prats, P., Rodríguez, I., Comas, C., and Puerto, B. (2014). Systematic review of screening for trisomy 21 in twin pregnancies in first trimester combining nuchal translucency and biochemical markers: a meta-analysis. *Prenat. Diagn.* **34**: 1077–1083.

27 Sarno, L., Revello, R., Hanson, E. et al. (2016). Prospective first-trimester screening for trisomies by cell-free DNA testing of maternal blood in twin pregnancy. *Ultrasound Obstet. Gynecol.* **47**: 705–711.

28 Landy, H.J. and Keith, L.G. (1998). The vanishing twin: a review. *Hum. Reprod Update* **4**: 177–183.

29 Dickey, R.P. (2005). Embryonic loss in iatrogenic multiples. *Obstet. Gynecol. Clin. North Am* **32**: 17–27.

30 Pinborg, A., Lidegaard, O., la Cour Freiesleben, N., and Andersen, A.N. (2005). Consequences of vanishing twins in IVF/ICSI pregnancies. *Hum. Reprod.* **20**: 2821–2829.

31 Blickstein, I. and Perlman, S. (2013). Single fetal death in twin gestations. *J. Perinat. Med.* **41**: 65–69.

32 Hillman, S.C., Morris, R.K., and Kilby, M.D. (2011). Co-twin prognosis after single fetal death: a systematic review and meta-analysis. *Obstet. Gynecol.* **118** (**4**): 928–940.

33 Nicolini, U. and Poblete, A. (1998). Fetal blood sampling immediately before and within 24 hours of death in monochorionic twin pregnancies complicated by single intrauterine death. *Am. J. Obstet. Gynecol.* **179**: 800–803.

34 Blickstein, I. (1990). The twin–twin transfusion syndrome. *Obstet. Gynecol.* **76**: 714–722.

35 Lewi, L., Jani, J., Blickstein, I. et al. (2008). The outcome of monochorionic diamniotic twin gestations in the era of invasive fetal therapy: a prospective cohort study. *Am. J. Obstet. Gynecol.* **199**: 514.e1–514.e8.

36 Nikkels, P.G., Hack, K.E., and van Gemert, M.J. (2008). Pathology of twin placentas with special attention to monochorionic twin placentas. *J. Clin. Pathol.* **61**: 1247–1253.

37 Wee, L. and Fisk, N.M. (2002). The twin–twin transfusion syndrome. *Semin. Neonatol.* **7**: 187–202.

38 Quintero, R.A., Morales, W.J., Allen, M.H. et al. (1999). Staging of twin–twin transfusion syndrome. *J. Perinatol.* **19**: 550–555.

39 Senat, M.V., Deprest, J., Boulvain, M. et al. (2004). Endoscopic laser surgery versus serial amnioreduction for severe twin-to-twin transfusion syndrome. *N. Engl. J. Med.* **351**: 136–144.

40 Rossi, A.C. and D'Addario, V. (2008). Laser therapy and serial amnioreduction as treatment for twin–twin transfusion syndrome: a metaanalysis and review of literature. *Am. J. Obstet. Gynecol.* **198**: 147–152.

41 Slaghekke, F., Kist, W.J., Oepkes, D. et al. (2010). Twin anemia-polycythemia sequence: diagnostic criteria, classification, perinatal management and outcome. *Fetal Diagn. Ther.* **27**: 181–190.

42 Blickstein, I. (2002). Normal and abnormal growth of multiples. *Semin. Neonatol.* **7**: 177–185.

43 Blickstein, I., Goldman, R.D., and Mazkereth, R. (2000). Risk for one or two very low birth weight twins: a population study. *Obstet. Gynecol.* **96**: 400–402.

44 Blickstein, I., Jacques, D.L., and Keith, L.G. (2002). The odds of delivering one, two or three extremely low birth weight (<1000 g) triplet infants: a study of 3288 sets. *J. Perinat. Med.* **30**: 359–363.

45 Blickstein, I. and Kalish, R.B. (2003). Birthweight discordance in multiple pregnancy. *Twin Res.* **6**: 526–531.

46 Blickstein, I., Jacques, D.L., and Keith, L.G. (2003). A novel approach to intertriplet birth weight discordance. *Am. J. Obstet. Gynecol.* **188**: 1026–1030.

47 Blickstein, I., Goldman, R.D., and Mazkereth, R. (2000). Adaptive growth restriction as a pattern of birth weight discordance in twin gestations. *Obstet. Gynecol.* **96**: 986–990.

48 Branum, A.M. and Schoendorf, K.C. (2003). The effect of birth weight discordance on twin neonatal mortality. *Obstet. Gynecol.* **101**: 570–574.

49 Wen, S.W., Fung, K.F., Huang, L. et al., Fetal and Infant Health Group of the Canadian Perinatal Surveillance System(2005). Fetal and neonatal mortality among twin gestations in a Canadian population: the effect of intrapair birthweight discordance. *Am. J. Perinatol.* **22**: 279–286.

50 Blickstein, I. and Keith, L.G. (2004). Neonatal mortality rates among growth-discordant twins, classified according to the birth weight of the smaller twin. *Am. J. Obstet. Gynecol.* **190**: 170–174.

51 Lewi, L., Cannie, M., Blickstein, I. et al. (2007). Placental sharing, birthweight discordance, and vascular anastomoses in monochorionic diamniotic twin placentas. *Am. J. Obstet. Gynecol.* **197**: 587.e1–587.e8.

52 Valsky, D.V., Eixarch, E., Martinez, J.M. et al. (2010). Selective intrauterine growth restriction in monochorionic twins: pathophysiology, diagnostic approach and management dilemmas. *Semin. Fetal. Neonatal. Med.* **15**: 342–348.

53 Blickstein, I., Arabin, B., Chervenak, F.A. et al. (2007). The Istanbul international consensus statement on the perinatal care of multiple pregnancy. *J. Perinat. Med.* **35**: 465–467.

54 Blickstein, I., Arabin, B., Lewi, L. et al. (2010). A template for defining the perinatal care of monochorionic twins: the Istanbul international ad hoc committee. *J. Perinat. Med.* **38**: 107–110.

55 Minakami, H. and Sato, I. (1996). Reestimating date of delivery in multifetal pregnancies. *JAMA* **275**: 1432–1434.

56 Luke, B., Bigger, H.R., Leurgans, S., and Sietsema, D. (1996). The cost of prematurity: a case-control study of twins vs singletons. *Am. J. Public Health* **86**: 809–814.

57 Kahn, B., Lumey, L.H., Zybert, P.A. et al. (2003). Prospective risk of fetal death in singleton, twin, and triplet gestations: implications for practice. *Obstet. Gynecol.* **102**: 685–692.

58 Sairam, S., Costeloe, K., and Thilaganathan, B. (2002). Prospective risk of stillbirth in multiple-gestation pregnancies: a population-based analysis. *Obstet. Gynecol.* **100**: 638–641.

59 Dodd, J.M., Deussen, A.R., Grivell, R.M., and Crowther, C.A. (2014). Elective birth at 37 weeks' gestation for women with an uncomplicated twin pregnancy. *Cochrane Database Syst. Rev.* (**2**): CD003582. doi: 10.1002/14651858.

60 Saccone, G. and Berghella, V. (2016). Planned delivery at 37 weeks in twins: a systematic review and meta-analysis of randomized controlled trials. *J. Matern. Fetal Neonatal Med.* **29**: 685–689.

61 Barigye, O., Pasquini, L., Galea, P. et al. (2005). High risk of unexpected late fetal death in monochorionic twins despite intensive ultrasound surveillance: a cohort study. *PLoS Med.* **2**: e172.

62 Breathnach, F.M., FM, M.A., Geary, M. et al., for the Perinatal Ireland Research Consortium(2012). Optimum timing for planned delivery of uncomplicated monochorionic and dichorionic twin pregnancies. *Obstet. Gynecol.* **119**: 50–59.

63 Simões, T., Queirós, A., Marujo, A.T. et al. (2016). Prospective risk of intrauterine death of monochorionic twins: update. *J. Perinat. Med.* **44** (**8**): 871–874. pii: /j/jpme.ahead-of-print/jpm-2015-0319.

64 Shub, A. and Walker, S.P. (2015). Planned early delivery versus expectant management for monoamniotic twins. *Cochrane Database Syst. Rev.* (**4**): CD008820. doi: 10.1002/1465185.

65 Van Mieghem, T., De Heus, R., Lewi, L. et al. (2014). Prenatal management of monoamniotic twin pregnancies. *Obstet. Gynecol.* **124**: 498–506.

66 Blickstein, I. (2000). Cesarean section for all twins? *J. Perinat. Med.* **28**: 169–174.

67 Barrett, J.F., Hannah, M.E., Hutton, E.K. et al., Twin Birth Study Collaborative Group(2013). A randomized trial of planned cesarean or vaginal delivery for twin pregnancy. *N. Engl. J. Med.* **369**: 1295–1305.

68 Blickstein, I. (2016). Delivery of vertex/nonvertex twins: did the horses already leave the barn? *Am. J. Obstet. Gynecol.* **214**: 308–310.

69 Blickstein, I. (2002). Cerebral palsy in multifoetal pregnancies. *Dev. Med. Child Neurol.* **44**: 352–355.

70 Blickstein, I., Shinwell, E., and Reichman, B. (2005). Plurality-dependent risk of respiratory distress syndrome among very low birth infants who had complete, partial, or no antepartum corticosteroid treatment. *Am. J. Obstet. Gynecol.* **192**: 360–364.

71 Choi, S.J., Song, S.E., Seo, E.S. et al. (2009). The effect of single or multiple courses of antenatal corticosteroid therapy on neonatal respiratory distress syndrome in singleton versus twin pregnancies. *Aust. N. Z. J. Obstet. Gynaecol.* **49**: 173–179.

72 Blickstein, I., Shinwell, E., Lusky, A., and Reichman, B. (2006). Plurality-dependent risk of severe intraventricular hemorrhage among very low birth weight infants and antepartum corticosteroid treatment. *Am. J. Obstet. Gynecol.* **194**: 1329–1333.

73 Evans, M.I., Andriole, S., and Britt, D.W. (2014). Fetal reduction: 25 years' experience. *Fetal Diagn. The.r* **35**: 69–82.

74 Adashi, E.Y. (2016). Seeing double: a nation of twins from sea to shining sea. *Am. J. Obstet. Gynecol.* **214**: 311–313.

75 Martin, J.A., Osterman, M.J., and Declines in Triplet, T.M.E. (2016). Higher-order multiple births in the United States, 1998–2014. *NCHS Data Brief* **243**: 1–8.

45 CHAPTER 45

Intrauterine fetal demise

Rana Snipe Berry

Department of Obstetrics and Gynecology, Indiana University School of Medicine, Indianapolis, IN, USA

Introduction

There is no universally accepted definition of when a fetal death is called a stillbirth, and the meaning of this term varies internationally [1]. The definition of a stillborn recommended by WHO for international comparison is a baby born with no signs of life at or after 28 weeks' gestation, fetal weight ≥1000 g, or ≥35 cm by crown-heel length [2]. A more common definition of stillbirth is fetal death that occurs at greater than 20 weeks gestation or with a fetal weight of >500 g when gestational age is uncertain, all with no evidence of life at birth [3].

More than 8000 babies are stillborn daily, which represents 2% of deliveries world-wide. There are geographical and socio-economic disparities in stillbirths, with 98% of stillbirth occurring in low- and middle-income countries [4]. Sub-Saharan Africa, South Asia, and eastern Mediterranean locales have the highest rates. There are complex contributing factors including poverty and lack access to quality maternal care that affect these numbers.

In the United States, stillbirth occurs in 1 of 160 pregnancies, accounting for about 26 000 stillbirths annually. The US stillbirth rate in 2013 was 5.96/1000 births, which is similar to the 2012 rate [5]. As world data exhibit disparities, so do national data. The fetal mortality rate for non-Hispanic black women has remained more than twice the rate for non-Hispanic white or Asian or Pacific Islander women. The rate for American Indian, Alaskan Native, and Hispanic women are also higher than the rate for non-Hispanic white women [5].

Stillbirth creates a complex socio-emotional and critical care environment for providers and families affected by it. Both providers and patients experience feelings unlike those exhibited in any other medical encounter. Obstetric providers are particularly disadvantaged as they are usually in situations of shepherding life into the world. This experience of stillbirth is the opposite, therefore providers may feel like the management of the death of a baby is out of their scope of comfort [6].

Guidance is needed to understand the nuances of the provision of care when: (i) a stillbirth presents; (ii) caring for a family who has previously experienced a stillbirth; and (iii) pregnancy is complicated by a medical condition, such as intrahepatic cholestasis of pregnancy (ICP), for which management hinges around the prevention of stillbirth.

CLINICAL VIGNETTE 1: STILLBIRTH ON CALL

The intern calls about a patient in triage. Ms. Tonya Aronson is a 25-year-old African-American g2p1001 at 37 + 4 weeks gestational age, dated by a six weeks ultrasound who presents to triage complaining of decreased fetal movement since the day prior. Fetal heart tones cannot be heard in triage. An ultrasound performed at bedside confirms no cardiac activity. Her past medical history includes obesity. Her prior pregnancy was a term uncomplicated vaginal delivery. She wants to discuss the delivery and to know the best way to determine what happened to cause the death. She was told that the "cord is around the neck" and wants more information about this as a cause.

When a stillbirth is diagnosed, a complex conversation must occur between providers and the family who has experienced the loss. Providers are often uncomfortable with the conversation and unsure of how to effectively and simultaneously provide evidence-based compassionate care, counsel on choices for care and delivery, and make recommendations for an accurate assessment. Care providers must also navigate a high level of sadness and possible feelings of blame [7]. In this environment, the three actions that are most pressing are comfort of the patient and family, care of

Evidence-Based Obstetrics and Gynecology, First Edition. Edited by Errol R. Norwitz, Carolyn M. Zelop, David A. Miller, and David L. Keefe.

the pregnancy and delivery, and planning for an assessment of etiology.

Compassionate care

Patients have a multitude of unique needs at the time of a stillbirth. The obstetric care team is accustomed to joyous celebrations of life and in the setting of stillbirth, life, and death intersect in a painful way unique to this tragedy. It may be difficult to match the skills and training of obstetric nurses and physicians to the needs of a grieving family. The care of a grieving family at this intersection has great implications for the rest of their lives [8]. Parents may recall the words used by the physician, and his or her ability to interact with them for many years following the death of their child [7]. In addition, the attitudes and skills of the physician may affect the parents' comfort level with ongoing management and their ability to trust in the care they are given [7]. "While it is clear that stillbirth places women at risk for complicated mourning, many mothers may not experience hospital-based interventions specifically targeted at their needs; moreover, it is unknown whether or not these interventions, even when experienced, are helpful" [8].

The experiences that parents and families have in the setting of stillbirth care delivery – including at the time of diagnosis, during and after delivery, and in follow-up care – will be the most cognizant memories of their still babies, so it is of paramount importance that providers are giving appropriate care during this human tragedy. Parents of stillborns wish to have the depth and duration of their grief acknowledged by providers [9]. A 2016 review has confirmed that "providing parents with understandable information, discussing options with them and tailoring care to their individual needs" were common themes [6]. This review has led to clinical and training recommendations that may improve care for bereaved parents.

This type of emerging evidence illustrates that compassionate care, specifically designed for care of families experiencing stillbirth, has unique components and that it can be done satisfactorily. In Gold's comprehensive review of over 6000 perinatal losses, she determined the best and worst practices for providers in this setting based on qualitative evidence. Constant themes emerge in studies of best practice care for stillbirth and neonatal loss to produce the optimal parental experience [7–9]. Best practices include themes related to respect, the provision of easy to understand information and time for processing, attention to the setting of care, creation of memories, appropriate aftercare instructions, and timely referral and follow-up care [10]. Despite a paucity of evidence of effectiveness, literature suggests that meaningful and appropriate interventions should be employed to improve the psychological well-being of bereaved parents [11].

There is also emerging evidence describing how providers are affected by stillbirth. There is an understanding that providers experience overlapping responses: the humane feeling of sadness for someone who has experienced a tragedy and, concurrently, the feeling of bearing the weight of professional responsibility for the event [12]. Trinidad and Kelley also give unique insights into the thoughts of providers during this time. Their study highlighted feelings of lack of preparation, inadequacy, and fear of blame. In their qualitative analysis, providers tended to want to find answers, reassure patients of the competence of the team, and generally felt ill-prepared to move from the role of physician to counselor [9].

Choices for care and delivery

One of the most pertinent and important decisions to be made with the family is a plan for delivery. The delivery choice should be individualized based upon gestational age, maternal diagnosis and condition, obstetric surgeries, and parental desires [13, 14].

A comprehensive review was undertaken in 2015 which addressed the available date to support choices based on gestational age and prior uterine surgery [15]. This paper summarized several protocols for delivery including both dilation and evacuation (D + E) or induction of labor in the second trimester and induction of labor or repeat c-section in the third trimester. In the second trimester, important parameters such as complications, cost, and grief resolution were examined. Dilation and evacuation is associated with less complication with experienced providers and lower cost, while time to grief resolution was similar with the two methods [15]. Regarding delivery guidelines in the third trimester the authors state, "The ideal management for stillbirths that occur after 28 weeks' gestation has not been determined; however, cesarean delivery should be avoided unless medically necessary for maternal indications" [15]. American College of Obstetricians and Gynecologists (ACOG) recommends that induction of labor be managed according to usual obstetrical protocols in these cases [14]. Treatment must be tailored individually to women with a prior uterine scar. Both D + E and induction of labor may be acceptable alternatives in the second trimester in these women. In the third trimester, a prior classical incision necessitates a repeat c-section, but a prior low transverse incision may be managed with induction of labor with a cervical ripening balloon and/or standard Pitocin protocols. Best evidence suggests that thorough counseling regarding risks and benefits of each option is necessary in every case.

Assessment

The evaluation of stillbirth provides important information for grieving families to help with maternal care as well as guide the management of future pregnancies [13, 14]. The purpose of the evaluation is to identify a cause of the fetal death as well as any potential contributing factors.

It is understood that currently, the optimal laboratory evaluation of stillbirth is controversial, neither has the most cost-effective approach been determined [16]. Any useful workup must consider cost as well as potential yield. This is especially valuable in low-resource settings. A systematic assessment, using the clinical setting as context, is generally understood to be the best approach for determining the cause of death in stillbirth.

There are multiple approaches to the evaluation process of a stillborn. One approach is based in the theory that the most and best information is obtained through a comprehensive evaluation for every still born baby [17]. The institution that utilizes this philosophy and therefore, employs the most systematic and thorough assessments, reports that they find cause in >75% cases [17]. It has been shown that a comprehensive protocol for post-mortem investigations for stillbirth can reduce the lack of explanation to less than one in seven [18–20].

Despite a sometimes thorough "workup," defined by Gordijn et al. as "a systematic approach to diagnostic investigation," many stillbirths are still considered "unexplained" [21]. The specific causes identified and the proportion of "unexplained" stillbirths are directly related to the system used to classify them [22]. The proportion of stillbirths who remain "unexplained" varies in different series from 15% to 75% [22]. It is known that thorough evaluation offers the best outcomes for patients and may aid in prevention of recurrence.

Just as causes of stillbirth differ in the developed vs. developing world, so do the recommendations for basic workup protocols. A workup in the developing world will include: a thorough history, narrative of events leading to delivery, possible identification of maternal comorbid conditions, and time of demise.

In the developed world, the basic workup will be a bit more robust. One example, as published by the American College of Obstetrics and Gynecology, includes: a detailed maternal and family history, fetal physical exam, fetal autopsy, placental pathology, fetal karyotype, and maternal laboratory evaluation. The maternal laboratory evaluation consists of routine prenatal labs, a complete blood count, Kleihauer Betke, human parvovirus B-19 IgG and IgM, syphilis, lupus anticoagulant, anticardiolipin antibodies, thyroid-stimulating hormone, and antibody, glucose, and toxicology screening [14]. In special cases, a thrombophilia workup may be considered [14, 16, 23–25].

Studies show that the tests of most yield are autopsy, pathologic examination of placenta, membranes, and cord, and karyotype [24]. If autopsy is declined, parents should be offered alternatives such as a full external exam by a perinatal pathologist with or without selected biopsies, full external exam with organ-sparing autopsy, head-sparing autopsy, magnetic resonance imaging (MRI), or ultrasound [14]. Most pathologic exams will also generally include photographs, x-rays, and measurements.

Genetic abnormalities account approximately 6–12% of stillbirths [25]. While the recommendation for karyotype still exists from major organizations, it is increasingly being replaced with a recommendation for more sensitive microarray analysis. It has been shown that microarray analysis detects abnormalities in stillbirth samples more often than karyotype analysis. Given this, microarray analysis is more likely than karyotype analysis to provide a genetic diagnosis [26]. Another major advantage of microarray is that samples may be harvested from nonviable tissue. This feature has been proven to be especially valuable in analyses of stillbirths with congenital anomalies or in cases in which karyotype results cannot be obtained [26]. When karyotype is employed, however, the most high yield specimens come from amniotic fluid. It is recommended that amniocentesis to obtain this fluid be undertaken prior to delivery [14].

The optimal evaluation of stillbirth remains controversial. Investigations are still ongoing to determine which combinations of studies and which approaches give the most yield from the perimortem investigation.

The autopsy

Although not all post-mortem investigations can adequately explain the cause of a stillbirth, in a significant proportion of cases, perinatal autopsies add additional information, rule out possible causes, and can even lead to changes of diagnosis [27].

Autopsy is known to be the single most important test in the determination of cause of a fetal death [23]. It helps to identify gross defects and morphological abnormalities as well as subtle findings that would be missed without it. The information gathered during autopsy helps with counseling for subsequent pregnancies. This single component of the evaluation for stillbirth and has been reported to provide additional important information to in 26–51% of cases [13].

Despite the known importance of autopsy, it is difficult to get parents to agree to one. It is also difficult to consent for it. The best evidence for communication surrounding autopsy suggests that the clinician discussing autopsy will ideally have [10]:

1. An established rapport with the parents
2. Detailed knowledge of autopsy procedures
3. Good communication skills
4. Significant clinical experience

And will:

5. Consider cultural or religious beliefs relating to autopsy
6. Provide written information about autopsy

7. Discuss with the parents:
   - The value of an autopsy
   - Options for full, limited, or stepwise autopsy
   - Issues related to retained fetal tissues
   - The possibility that a cause may not be found
   - Requirement for and cost (if any) related to transfer of the baby to another facility
   - Cost (if any) to the parents of the autopsy
   - Appearance of the baby following autopsy
   - The likely timeframe for results to become available
   - Arrangements for communicating results (e.g. appointment following results availability).

Communication around autopsy

As helpful as workup may be, communication surrounding workup is difficult, specifically discussions regarding autopsy [28]. A 2013 Cochrane Review by Horey et al. speaks to the inconsistencies often apparent in these situations, "support for parents making decisions about autopsy or other post-mortem examinations after stillbirth must rely on the ad hoc knowledge and experience of those involved at the time" [29].

The same 2013 review speaks to the lack of data we have regarding communication in this realm. They cite "insufficient evidence from randomized controlled trials that interventions which aim to provide counseling or psychological support to mothers, fathers, or families who have experienced perinatal death" are of any benefit [28]. Similarly, a Cochrane 2008 review could not make any evidence-based recommendations concerning the effectiveness of interventions for provision of support to families grieving perinatal death [30].

The ACOG Practice Bulletin on Management of Stillbirth states that support should include emotional support and communication of results. The practice bulletin advises consideration of referrals to support personnel such as counselors, clergy, peer support, bereavement counseling, or mental health networks [14]. The 2016 review by Ellis et al. concludes that parents want improved training so that staff can provide tailored discussions and written information to help them make informed decisions about post-mortem and funeral arrangements [6]. They also conclude that staff should be trained to discuss information regarding post-mortem and funeral arrangement options with parents in a clear and empathic manner [6].

The umbilical cord

The umbilical cord is a source often "blamed" for a stillbirth, particularly with an otherwise unknown cause. It is known that up to 30% of pregnancies that end in live births are complicated by nuchal cords and true knots [31]. To attribute the cause to cord accident alone, other recognized causes of stillbirth should be excluded through a careful and systematic evaluation. There "should be evidence of cord occlusion and hypoxia on perinatal postmortem examination and histologic examination of the placental and umbilical cord" [32]. ACOG gives further guidelines, requiring "evidence of obstruction or circulatory compromise on umbilical cord examination. In addition, other causes should be excluded" [14].

Many authors suggest very specific criteria that must be met in order to diagnose stillbirth secondary to hypoxia and asphyxia by acute cord compression [33–35]. Parast and co-workers propose vascular ectasia and thrombosis within the umbilical cord, chorionic plate, or stem villi as minimal histologic criteria suggestive of cord accident [33] For a probable diagnosis, they require the previous findings as well as regional distribution of avascular villi or villi showing stromal karyorrhexis [33]. This study suggested that cord accidents may be implicated wrongly in many cases, but may however be a true cause in a large percentage of stillbirth cases with an "unknown cause." Given these discrepancies, most investigators believe that cord accident is a potentially preventable cause of stillbirth which deserves more comprehensive investigation [25].

CLINICAL VIGNETTE 2: INTRAHEPATIC CHOLESTASIS OF PREGNANCY AND STILLBIRTH

Ms. Arely Hernandez, a Chilean 34-year-old g4p2012, presents to clinic at 34 weeks, dated by an eight weeks US. Her pregnancy has been uncomplicated to date. She presented to triage a few days ago, with complaints of itching all over, worsening over the last week and a half, and now with itching of the palms of her hands and soles of her feet, all worse at night. She presented to the office, where her labs were reviewed. She was found to have elevated bile acids (40 μmol) and placed on ursodiol. You tell her that you will watch her closely and then plan for induction of labor to prevent the possibility of stillbirth. She is afraid and wants to know the evidence surrounding the relationship between stillbirth and ICP, particularly for delivery timing and prevention.

ICP is the most common pregnancy-associated liver disorder. The incidence is reported to be between 0.2% and 2%, but is known to vary with geography and ethnicity. ICP is most common in South America and Northern Europe [36]. The clinical definition of ICP is pruritus in the absence of a rash with onset in the third trimester of pregnancy, which is associated with abnormal liver function in the absence of other liver disease and which resolves following delivery [37]. The major sequelae of ICP are premature birth, fetal distress, and intrauterine fetal demise (IUFD). The etiology of ICP is multifactorial and has been shown to involve genetic, hormonal, and environmental factors.

ICP has been commonly associated with stillbirth, but there is controversy surrounding the relationship. A 2014 study by Geenes et al., the largest prospective study of perinatal outcomes in women with severe ICP, showed significant positive correlations between maternal serum bile acid levels and adverse fetal outcomes which included preterm delivery, spontaneous preterm delivery, meconium staining of the amniotic fluid, and stillbirth [36] In this study, the rate of stillbirth was three times higher than baseline in women with bile acids >40 μmol l^{-1} or severe ICP [36]. Some have postulated that 100 μmol l^{-1} is the threshold at which to hold concern for fetal demise [38].

Conversely, an earlier 2014 review of unexplained stillbirth did not find any association between stillbirth and ICP [39]. A study by the Stillbirth Collaboration Network found that the proportion of women with elevated levels of bile acids was similar in women with stillbirth and live births using either ≥10 or ≥40 μmol l^{-1} as a threshold [40]. Furthermore, in other studies, an increased risk of stillbirth has not been definitively linked to either symptom or lab severity. In summary, it is uncertain whether there is a critical bile acid threshold below which adverse pregnancy outcome can be avoided.

There are many hypotheses surrounding the mechanism of stillbirth with ICP, but none proven. This makes management of the disease and careful planning regarding risks and benefits of continuing a pregnancy all the more difficult.

Although controversy exists, the therapeutic goals are to reduce maternal symptoms and to avoid fetal distress and death. To this end, active management of pregnancy with ICP has been a standard international practice with the goal of delivery at <39 weeks. Active management has been defined in various ways, but in most cases means closer fetal surveillance and induction of labor at 37 weeks gestation. Some practitioners advocate for amniocentesis at 36 weeks, to detect meconium = -stained amniotic fluid, which is thought to be a strong predictor of risk. It is, however, unknown if the meconium is the cause of the death, or simply a marker of a distressed fetus.

At least one major practice authority, the Royal College of Obstetricians and Gynecologists (RCOG), has moved from recommending active management in all cases, to a recommendation of individual management based on risk benefit discussions with patients [41].

Based on the available evidence, RCOG recommends that a discussion should be had regarding induction of labor after 37 weeks. Per this guideline, the discussion should detail the increased risk of perinatal and maternal morbidity, that the case for intervention may be stronger in those with more severe lab abnormalities, but not necessarily beneficial for others, and lastly, that stillbirth is not able to be predicted if the pregnancy continues [41]. In the United States, antepartum fetal surveillance is recommended by The Society for Maternal-Fetal Medicine, but the ideal type, duration, and frequency of monitoring has not been identified [42]. There are currently no available evidence based recommendations for fetal monitoring.

A Cochrane review in 2013 found "insufficient evidence to recommend early term delivery in obstetric cholestasis." The review determined that, while ursodiol improves maternal pruritus to a small degree, there is insufficient evidence to recommend it to improve fetal outcomes. The current recommendation, by the European Association for the Study of the Liver, is ursodiol at 10–20 mg kg^{-1} per day, divided into two doses, as the first-line treatment for ICP [43].

It is thought that a decrease in serum bile acids and transaminases may contribute to better fetal outcomes. Most management strategies do still employ the recommendation of delivery between 37 and 38 weeks or sooner with documented lung maturity. A recent view by Diken et al. provides an algorithm for practitioners to follow when caring for patients with ICP [44].

CLINICAL VIGNETTE 3: PREGNANCY WITH PRIOR STILLBIRTH

Ms. Jocelyn Manning is a 27-year-old g2p0100 who presents for new obstetrics (OB) care at 11 weeks gestation. A healthy young woman, with obstetric history significant for a prior stillbirth at 28 weeks. Her stillborn baby, "Saraya" was delivered at another hospital and there are no records available, but she knows that the baby was "IUGR." At that time, she was diagnosed in the office with IUFD and was induced and delivered vaginally. She wants the best care possible for this pregnancy, and asks you to address what her care will consist of, and to address how it will be different from a routine pregnancy.

Care of a pregnancy following a stillbirth can be difficult. Loss of a pregnancy is a significant event that may sometimes amount to a crisis in a woman's life [45]. Evidence-based consensus for the optimal management of subsequent pregnancy following a fetal loss, especially an unexplained fetal death, is lacking [46]. Caring for a pregnancy following this crisis-level event is a complex situation for provider and patient with increased psychosocial needs for the family and extra care and planning on the part of the provider.

In an extensive review by Lamb, four recurring issues surrounding perinatal loss and subsequent pregnancy were identified: the effect of the grief process on the subsequent pregnancy; parental coping mechanisms during the subsequent pregnancy; replacement or vulnerable child syndrome; and parenting issues with the subsequent live-born child [45]. The first three are important to recognize as key components in planning for care during the follow-up pregnancy, the fourth is important in neonatal care.

It has been shown that women experience specific anxieties and grief before and during a pregnancy preceded by a loss. The type and levels of grief vary by study, but at least one suggests that grief may be impacted positively by knowing the exact cause of the preceding loss (chromosomal abnormality implicated in a miscarriage, for example) [47]. Multiple investigators have studied the coping mechanisms that women employ with a pregnancy after a loss. Anxiety and depression are commonly experienced by women in a pregnancy marked by a prior loss [45]. Intensified anxiety surrounding routine prenatal tests and the anniversary of the previous loss are also well documented in the literature [48]. Replacement or vulnerable child syndrome has been described in the literature and is characterized by parents using another pregnancy and subsequent child as a substitution for the child that they previously lost [49]. All of the above need to be acknowledged as possible reactions and providers should be readily armed to provide holistic and multidisciplinary care for these women and families.

The best guidance for care for a pregnancy following stillbirth comes from qualitative data. One of the key components of care is "in-depth exploration of what the loss meant to the parents and how it may affect their current pregnancy" [45]. This early step is vital to creating an environment of trust and acknowledgement that the prior pregnancy was real and important. Many studies also document the importance of verbally documenting milestones or critical points in the pregnancy and providing "longer scheduled appointments" to allow for open discussion of emotions and concerns [48, 49].

The Lamb review, supported by others, suggests specific interventions including "... an increase in frequency of prenatal visits, validation of the patient's concerns regarding the previous loss, ... specific prenatal care group visits with other families with a previous pregnancy loss, and the incorporation of other formal counseling as needed" [45].

In the study by O'Leary et al., the most important idea regarding subsequent pregnancies was an "intergenerational acknowledgment of the ongoing relationship to the deceased child as an important, though absent family member, especially during the pregnancy that followed" [50]. Although this study specifically examined the parent/grandparent relationship, it is likely that this sentiment is a general one. It is well known that parents want their babies lives to be acknowledged and providers must incorporate acknowledgment of the "absent family member" while providing care.

Summary

In summary, stillbirth is a difficult and tragic event for which obstetric providers must learn to care. There are many areas of ongoing investigation where there is newly emerging evidence for best practices in care delivery. A few situations which warrant special consideration are: care for a family presenting with a current stillbirth, management of pregnancies complicated by a condition, such as ICP, that portends risk of stillbirth, and the provision of care for families with a history of stillbirth.

In the care of families presenting with stillbirth, we have highlighted recent literature regarding compassionate care and communication, specifically addressing communication around autopsy. We have discussed the current best assessment practices including autopsy and genetic analysis and the possible role of the umbilical cord in some stillbirths.

ICP is thought to increase risk of stillbirth. Management of pregnancies affected by it must weigh the risks of early delivery with the risk of fetal demise with ongoing pregnancy. We have discussed current recommendations and rationale behind them.

Finally, we reviewed recent recommendations regarding the provision of increased levels of care for a pregnancy with history of a prior stillbirth. We discussed the complex psychosocial environment in which this care must be given and some provider-led actions that acknowledge the prior pregnancy and provide the necessary holistic care for the current pregnancy.

References

1 The Partnership for Maternal, Newborn and Children's Health (2011). Make stillbirths count. In: *Knowledge Summary #13: Women's and Children's Health*. Rome: WHO.

2 World Health Organization (WHO) (2015). Stillbirths. In: *Maternal, Newborn, Child, and Adolescent Health Topics*. Rome: WHO.

3 Kowaleski, J. (1997). *State Definitions and Reporting Requirements for Live Births, Fetal Deaths, and Induced Terminations of Pregnancy*. Hyattsville, MD: National Center for Health (NCFH) Statistics.

4 Lawn, J.E. et al. Stillbirths: rates, risk factors, and acceleration towards 2030. *Lancet* **387** (**10018**): 587–603.

5 MacDorman, M.F. and Gregory, E.C. (2015). Fetal and perinatal mortality: United States, 2013. *Natl. Vital. Stat. Rep.* **64** (**8**): 1–24.

6 Ellis, A. et al. (2016). Systematic review to understand and improve care after stillbirth: a review of parents' and healthcare professionals' experiences. *BMC Pregnancy Childbirth* **16** (**1**): 1–19.

7 Gold, K.J. (2007). Navigating care after a baby dies: a systematic review of parent experiences with health providers. *J. Perinatol.* **27** (**4**): 230–237.

8 Cacciatore, J. and Bushfield, S. (2007). Stillbirth: the mother's experience and implications for improving care. *J. Soc. Work End Life Palliat. Care* **3** (**3**): 59–79.

9 Kelley, M.C. and Trinidad, S.B. (2012). Silent loss and the clinical encounter: parents' and physicians' experiences of stillbirth-a qualitative analysis. *BMC Pregnancy Childbirth* **12**: 137.

10 Queensland Clinical Guidelines Stillbirth care. Guideline No. MN11.24-V4-R16. Queensland Health. 2018. Most updated version available from: http://www.health.qld.gov.au/qcg

11 Fenwick, J. et al. (2007). Providing perinatal loss care: satisfying and dissatisfying aspects for midwives. *Women Birth* **20**.

12 Nuzum, D., Meaney, S., and O'Donoghue, K. (2014). The impact of stillbirth on consultant obstetrician gynaecologists: a qualitative study. *BJOG* **121** (**8**): 1020–1028.

13 Silver, R.M. and Heuser, C.C. (2010). Stillbirth workup and delivery management. *Clin. Obstet. Gynecol.* **53** (**3**): 681–690.

14 American College of Obstetrics and Gynecology (2009). Management of Stillbirth. In: *Practice Bulletin 102*. Washington, DC: ACOG.

15 Chakhtoura, N.A. and Reddy, U.M. (2015). Management of stillbirth delivery. *Semin. Perinatol.* **39** (**6**): 501–504.

16 Silver, R.M. et al. (2007). Work-up of stillbirth: a review of the evidence. *Am. J. Obstet. Gynecol.* **196** (**5**): 433–444.

17 Pauli, R.M. and Reiser, C.A. (1994). Wisconsin Stillbirth Service Program: II. Analysis of diagnoses and diagnostic categories in the first 1,000 referrals. *Am. J. Med. Genet.* **50** (**2**): 135–153.

18 Dickinson, J.E. (2011). The continuing dilemma of stillbirth. *Aust. N. Z. J. Obstet. Gynaecol.* **51** (**1**): 1–2.

19 Flenady, V. et al. Stillbirths: the way forward in high-income countries. *Lancet* **377** (**9778**): 1703–1717.

20 Gordijn, S.J., Erwich, J.J., and Khong, T.Y. (2002). Value of the perinatal autopsy: critique. *Pediatr. Dev. Pathol.* **5** (**5**): 480–488.

21 Facchinetti, G.A., Dekker, D.B., and Saade, G. (2010). *Stillbirthding and Management*, 136. London: Informa Healthcare.

22 VanderWielen, B. et al. (2011). Wisconsin stillbirth services program: a multifocal approach to stillbirth analysis. *Am. J. Med. Genet. A* **155** (**5**): 1073–1080.

23 Silver, R.M. et al. (2011). Stillbirth Collaborative Research Network Writing Group. Association between stillbirth and risk factors known at pregnancy confirmation. *JAMA* **306** (**22**): 2469.

24 Silver, R.M. (2012). Optimal "work-up" of stillbirth: evidence! *Am. J. Obstet. Gynecol.* **206** (**1**): 1–2.

25 Stillbirth Collaborative Research Network Writing Group (2011). Causes of death among stillbirths. *JAMA* **306** (**22**): 2459–2468.

26 Reddy, U.M. et al. (2012). Karyotype versus microarray testing for genetic abnormalities after stillbirth. *N. Engl. J. Med.* **367** (**23**): 2185–2193.

27 Wagner, C.L., Goldstein, M., and Conradi, S.E. (2005). Changing a diagnosis: the importance of neonatal autopsy. *J. Perinatol.* **25** (**1**): 69–71.

28 Koopmans, L., Wilson, T., Cacciatore, J., and Flenady, V. (2013). Support for mothers, fathers and famillies after perinatal death. *Cochrane Database Syst. Rev.* doi: 10.1002/14651858.CD000452.pub3.

29 Horey, D. et al. (2013). Interventions for supporting parents' decisions about autopsy after stillbirth. *Cochrane Database Syst. Rev.* (**2**): Cd009932. doi: 10.1002/14651858.CD009932.pub2.

30 Flenady, V. and Wilson, T. (2008). Support for mothers, fathers and families after perinatal death. *Cochr Data Syst Rev* (**1**): doi: 10.1002/14651858.CD000452.pub3.

31 Clapp, J.F. 3rd et al. (2003). The natural history of antenatal nuchal cords. *Am. J. Obstet. Gynecol.* **189** (**2**): 488–493.

32 Reddy, U.M. et al. (2009). Stillbirth classification—developing an international consensus for research: executive summary of a National Institute of Child Health and Human Development Workshop. *Obstet. Gynecol.* **114** (**4**): 901–914.

33 Ryan, W.D. et al. (2012). Placental histologic criteria for diagnosis of cord accident: sensitivity and specificity. *Pediatr. Dev. Pathol.* **15** (**4**): 275–280.

34 Pinar, H. and Carpenter, M. (2010). Placenta and umbilical cord abnormalities seen with stillbirth. *Clin. Obstet. Gynecol.* **53** (**3**): 656–672.

35 Ptacek, I. et al. (2014). Systematic review of placental pathology reported in association with stillbirth. *Placenta* **35** (**8**): 552–562.

36 Geenes, V. et al. (2014). Association of severe intrahepatic cholestasis of pregnancy with adverse pregnancy outcomes: a prospective population-based case-control study. *Hepatology* **59** (**4**): 1482–1491.

37 Geenes, V. (2009). Intrahepatic cholestasis of pregnancy. *World J. Gastroenterol.* **15** (**17**): 2049.

38 Glantz, A., Marschall, H.U., and Mattsson, L.A. (2004). Intrahepatic cholestasis of pregnancy: relationships between bile acid levels and fetal complication rates. *Hepatology* **40** (**2**): 467–474.

39 Henderson, C.E. et al. (2014). Primum non nocere: how active management became modus operandi for intrahepatic cholestasis of pregnancy. *Am. J. Obstet. Gynecol.* **211** (**3**): 189–196.

40 Silver, R.M. et al. (2014). Bile acids in a multicenter, population-based case-control study of stillbirth. *Am. J. Obstet. Gynecol.* **210** (**5**): 460.e1–460.e9.

41 Royal College of Obstetricians and Gynaecologists (RCOG) (2011). *Obstetric Cholestasis*. RCOG Green-Top Guideline Number 43, 1–14. London: RCOG.

42 Modern Medicine Network (2011). Understanding Intrahepatic Cholestasis of Pregnancy. *Contemporary OB/GYN* 22–26.

43 European Association for the Study of the Liver (2009). EASL Clinical Practice Guidelines: Management of cholestatic liver diseases. *J. Hepatol.* **51** (**2**): 237–267.

44 Diken, Z., Usta, I.M., and Nassar, A.H. (2014). A clinical approach to intrahepatic cholestasis of pregnancy. *Am. J. Perinatol.* **31** (**1**): 1–8.

45 Lamb, E.H. (2002). The impact of previous perinatal loss on subsequent pregnancy and parenting. *J. Perinat. Educ.* **11** (**2**): 33–40.

46 Rowland, A. and Goodnight, W.H. (2009). Fetal loss: addressing the evaluation and supporting the emotional needs of parents. *J. Midwifery Womens Health* **54** (**3**): 241–248.

47 Nikcevic, A.V. et al. (1999). Investigation of the cause of miscarriage and its influence on women's psychological distress. *Br. J. Obstet. Gynaecol.* **106** (**8**): 808–813.

48 Armstrong, D. and Hutti, M. (1998). Pregnancy after perinatal loss: the relationship between anxiety and prenatal attachment. *J. Obstet. Gynecol. Neonatal. Nurs.* **27** (**2**): 183–189.

49 Robertson, P.A. and Kavanaugh, K. (1998). Supporting parents during and after a pregnancy subsequent to a perinatal loss. *J. Perinat. Neonatal Nurs.* **12** (**2**).

50 O'Leary, J., Warland, J., and Parker, L. (2011). Bereaved parents' perception of the grandparents' reactions to perinatal loss and the pregnancy that follows. *J. Fam. Nurs.* **17** (**3**): 330–356.

46

CHAPTER 46
Fetal anomalies

Ashley T. Peterson and Sabrina D. Craigo

Division of Maternal-Fetal Medicine, Department of Obstetrics and Gynecology, Tufts Medical Center, Boston, MA, USA

CLINICAL VIGNETTE

A 28-year-old nulliparous patient at 17 weeks gestational age presents for a scheduled prenatal visit. The patient has an unremarkable medical, obstetric, and family history. She relates that a friend recently had a child diagnosed with a major congenital anomaly at the time of birth. She would like to know her chances for prenatal detection of major fetal anomalies as well as options for treatment and any potential risks to her or the fetus if a major anomaly is diagnosed.

Introduction and background

The presence of fetal anomalies complicate between 2% and 3% of all pregnancies [1]. The World Health Organization estimates that more than a quarter-million neonatal deaths are associated with congenital anomalies annually worldwide. Major anomalies are an important contributor to chronic illness and disability and can have significant impact on the patient, family, and healthcare system. The most common major anomalies are cardiovascular and neural tube defects. The most common chromosome abnormality associated with anomaly is Trisomy 21, or Down syndrome. Causes can be genetic, infectious, drug-related or environmental. Some anomalies may be prevented via the avoidance of known or suspected teratogens (alcohol), supplementation of nutrition (folate), administration of vaccines (rubella), or control of chronic maternal illnesses (diabetes). In addition, screening programs exist to improve rates of prenatal detection and aid in parental counseling and guide individual pregnancy management.

Genetics

Patients with structural ultrasound anomalies, especially more than one major anomaly, should be offered diagnostic testing. In the literature, the risk of chromosome abnormalities in a fetus with major anomalies varies (rates of 2–35% have been reported) and depends on the number and the type of fetal systems involved. A retrospective study at a single institution that included 2806 fetuses with malformations detected on ultrasound found multisystem malformations were associated with a higher rate of abnormal karyotype (29%) than isolated malformations (2%) [2]. Similarly, Rizzo et al. included 425 fetuses with abnormal karyotypes and reported multiple anomalies were more likely to be associated with an abnormal karyotype than an isolated anomaly (35.0% versus 8.9%) [3]. A 2005 retrospective review of a low-risk population in Belgium reported a statistically significant difference in abnormal chromosomes for fetuses with multiple malformations (18.8%) compared with isolated malformations (9.3%) [4]. Furthermore, isolated malformations of cystic hygroma or hydrops were statistically more likely to be associated with abnormal karyotype compared to all other organ systems ($p < 0.001$). Conversely, isolated malformations of the urinary tract were significantly less likely to be associated with abnormal karyotype than anomalies of other systems.

Chromosomal microarray analysis has also been studied and reported to improve diagnosis of cytogenetic aberrations in fetuses with structural anomalies over traditional karyotyping. In a prospective multi-center study, microarray detected clinically relevant deletions or duplications in 6.0% of subjects with anomaly on ultrasound ($N = 1109$) when the fetal karyotype was normal [5]. This confirms an earlier systematic review that reports microarray detects clinically significant genomic alterations in 5.2% of patients with an ultrasound anomaly and a normal karyotype [6]. Microarray will detect deletions and duplications that will be missed on traditional karyotype, however it will miss inversions and balanced translocations, which are associated with 6.7% (95% confidence limits, 3.1–10.3%) of structural anomalies [7]. Thus, for patients with at least one major structural anomaly on ultrasound, microarray is recommended and

Evidence-Based Obstetrics and Gynecology, First Edition. Edited by Errol R. Norwitz, Carolyn M. Zelop, David A. Miller, and David L. Keefe.

can replace fetal karyotype; for patients with normal ultrasound findings, traditional karyotype for prenatal diagnosis is preferred [8].

Associated findings

A retrospective study from a single institution of 250 pregnancies noted to have severe oligohydramnios (anhydramnios) reported fetal anomalies in 50.7% of second-trimester cases and 22.1% of third-trimester cases [9]. Severe oligohydramnios was associated with renal anomalies most often (65.2%). Similarly, a 2011 single-institution retrospective study of 28 555 third-trimester ultrasounds reported major fetal malformations were more common in pregnancies with oligohydramnios (25%) and borderline amniotic fluid index (AFI) (10%) than normal AFI (2%), $p < 0.001$ [10].

The presence of a single umbilical artery has been known to be associated with congenital anomalies, but the degree of association varies depending on the study design. A meta-analysis that included studies spanning four decades found a 27% incidence of congenital malformation associated with a single umbilical artery among live-born singleton pregnancies, 7% of which were major renal anomalies [11]. Additionally, when the analysis expanded the sample from live-born pregnancies to include fetal autopsies, abortions and demised fetuses, single-umbilical cord arteries were associated with congenital anomalies in two-thirds of cases. A large Canadian population-based study found single umbilical artery occurred in 0.44% of singleton pregnancies and was associated with an almost sevenfold increased risk of co-occurring fetal anomalies, with genitourinary anomalies being most common [12]. A smaller, single-institution retrospective cohort study of singleton pregnancies undergoing routine anatomic survey found fetuses with a single umbilical artery were associated with significantly increased risk of renal and cardiac malformations, with adjusted odds ratios of 3.0 and 21.0 respectively [13].

Twinning is associated with an increased risk of congenital anomalies. Data from the 1980 Metropolitan Atlanta Congenital Defects Program reported that twins have almost a 50% higher likelihood of anomalies, and even more so with same-sex (likely monozygous) twinning [14]. An analysis of nine international registries reported an overall congenital malformation relative risk of 1.25 (95% CI, 1.21–1.28) in twins compared with singletons [15]. Additionally, this study reported anomalies were more likely to occur in twin pregnancies across all systems. Rates of cardiac anomalies in particular have been reported as occurring more frequently in twin gestations. One population-based study in Northern Ireland reported increased rates of fetal cardiovascular system anomalies in same-sex twins (91.0/10 000) versus singletons (66.4/10 000) [16]. A smaller study of twins from Spain reported similar overall rates of fetal anomalies in twins and singletons, but significantly higher relative risk of central nervous system (CNS), cardiovascular system, and genitourinary system anomalies in same-sex twins than singletons [17].

Imaging

Ultrasound screening is used to detect anomalies before birth. Three large trials (the Eurofetus study, the RADIUS study, and the Helsinki Ultrasound Trial) have been published that report varying sensitivities for ultrasound detection of fetal anomalies ranging from 35% to 56% [18–20]. The Eurofetus study, a large multi-center prospective trial of 3685 fetuses with structural malformations, deformations and dysplasias, reported a sensitivity of 61.4% (CI 95%, 59.8–63.0%) for routine ultrasound examination. Limited to major fetal anomalies, the sensitivity increased to 73.7% with higher rates for CNS (88.3%) and urinary tract (84.8%) abnormalities. The Helsinki Study group noted prenatal detection incurred a lower perinatal mortality rate, while the RADIUS study group's findings did not. The difference in perinatal mortality rate between the two studies may be a reflection of their respective study designs (the RADIUS study group examined a low-risk population and the Helsinki trial was population-based), or the rate of termination between the two countries.

Prenatal ultrasound imaging has been thought to be suboptimal in the detection of fetal anomalies in the presence of oligohydramnios or maternal obesity. Few studies have specifically looked at the effect of low amniotic fluid volume on the detection of fetal anomalies. A study of 345 pregnancies ranging from 16 to 38 weeks affected by premature rupture of membranes (175 with oligohydramnios, 170 without oligohydramnios) showed no difference in detection of major fetal anomalies with rates of 7.4% and 10%, respectively [21]. With respect to maternal obesity, one retrospective cohort study of 11 135 singleton pregnancies at a single institution reported lower detection rates of congenital anomalies on both standard and targeted ultrasounds as maternal body mass index (BMI) increased. Detection rates for normal BMI, overweight, Class I, II, and III obesity were reported as 66%, 49%, 48%, 42%, and 25%, respectively [22].

The role of additional imaging modalities for detection of fetal anomalies, such as 3D ultrasound imaging and magnetic resonance imaging (MRI) remains adjunctive. For specific situations or anomalies, there may be a role in using additional modalities for prenatal counseling and postnatal therapy. Fetal MRI has been in use since 1983 and gained more traction in the 1990s after technical advancements improved accuracy with ultrafast T2-weighted sequences. A systematic review of the literature in 2014 analyzed the additional value added by fetal MRI to CNS abnormalities detected by ultrasound. The review found that fetal MRI results confirmed ultrasound-detected CNS abnormalities in 65.4% of fetuses and reported pooled sensitivity and specificity of MRI was 97% (95% CI, 95–98%) and 70% (95% CI, 58–81%) [23]. Strikingly, this review found that fetal MRI results differed from ultrasound in 30.2% and thereby significantly altered counseling and pregnancy management. To date, there has been one prospective blinded case–control study comparing the sensitivity and specificity of 2D ultrasound, 3D ultrasound and MRI in detection of fetal anomalies. Goncalves et al. reported fetal MRI, 2D ultrasound, and 3D ultrasound had similar sensitivities (80%, 78%, and 76% respectively) for overall detection of congenital anomalies [24]. For detection of CNS anomalies, fetal MRI was found to be statistically significantly more sensitive than 3D ultrasound but similar to 2D ultrasound. In 22.2% of cases, fetal MRI was found to provide additional information over ultrasound that affected prognosis, counseling, and or management.

Fetal echocardiography is widely used to aid in the prenatal detection of cardiac anomalies. To date, there are no evidence based appropriate use criteria that have been developed for referral of women for fetal echocardiography. A single center retrospective study in 2014 revealed that reported that suspicion of congenital heart disease on screening ultrasound was most predictive of positive echocardiogram findings (59.9% prevalence, 85% CI, 56.7–63.1%) [25]. A high prevalence of congenital heart disease was also seen in fetuses with a known chromosome abnormality (42.4% prevalence, 95% CI, 25.6–59.3%), incomplete screening exam (33.3% prevalence, 95% CI, 14.5–52.2%), known twin-to-twin transfusion syndrome (28.6% prevalence, 95% CI, 4.9–52.2%), and extracardiac anomalies on screening ultrasound (21.2% prevalence, 95% CI, 15.6–26.9%). The prevalence of congenital heart disease was also found to be increased if the patient was referred for more than one indication, ranging from 26% for one indication to 53% for three indications.

Fetal surgery

Prenatal intervention with fetal surgery has been a possibility in select cases of major anomalies for over two decades at highly specialized centers with the goal of improving outcomes. Fetal surgery can be performed via open hysterotomy or minimally invasive techniques (fetoscopy) for a narrow set of indications involving anomalies such as neural tube defects, fetal lung lesions, congenital diaphragmatic hernia, skeletal dysplasias, sacrococcygeal teratomas, and obstructive uropathy. The literature has been largely limited to case series and cohort studies. One randomized controlled trial (Management of Myelomeningocele Study, also known as MOMS) compared prenatal and postnatal repair of myelomeningocele with hindbrain herniation and showed a clear survival benefit for fetal surgery before 26 weeks compared with postnatal repair for eligible cases and the trial was stopped for efficacy [26]. Prenatal surgery in this trial was shown to improve rates of fetal death, neonatal death and need for placement of cerebrospinal fluid shunt in first 12 months of life (68% versus 98%, relative risk, 0.70; 97.7% confidence interval [CI], 0.58–0.84; $P < 0.001$). Fetal lung lesions, such as congenital cystic adenomatoid malformation or bronchopulmonary sequestration) have been managed both prenatally and postnatally based on the presence of hydrops and gestational age at discovery. Two case series have noted that for those fetuses with hydrops and polyhydramnios less than 32 weeks gestation, fetal surgery, and thoracoamniotic shunting appears to improve survival [27, 28]. Management of fetal sacrococcygeal teratoma with prenatal surgery has also been reported in case series and found to be successful in the presence of co-occurring hydrops, with reported survival rates of 30% and 55% for minimally invasive and open techniques [29, 30].

Delivery mode and timing

In the majority of cases, mode of delivery is not affected by the presence of a congenital anomaly and most affected pregnancies will, similarly, not require a preterm or early term delivery. However, it is reasonable to assume that cesarean delivery should be considered if the anomaly results in cephalopelvic disproportion, causes fetal soft tissue trauma during vaginal delivery, or the malformation affects the ability to assess fetal wellbeing in labor [31]. Four retrospective studies have been conducted that compare mode of delivery for meningomyelocele and no significant differences were found in short-term neonatal outcomes in those delivered via vaginal or abdominal routes [32–35]. There is no evidence that cesarean delivery is beneficial for fetuses with ventral wall defects, such as omphalocele. The data has been mixed with respect to outcomes for fetuses affected by gastroschisis; however, there is a large amount of confounding bias given studies that have been conducted are largely retrospective. In the last decade, six retrospective studies have been published that show no added benefit of cesarean delivery over vaginal delivery for fetal gastroschisis [36–40]. In cases of cystic hygroma, cesarean delivery may be optimal for management of large anterior lymphangiomas obstructing the airway, though there are no data to support this recommendation. In the event that an EXIT (ex utero intrapartum therapy) procedure is indicated for successful delivery and intubation of a neonate with a lung mass causing airway compromise, cesarean delivery is necessary and is often a planned preterm delivery [41, 42]. Delivery for sacrococcygeal teratoma is often via cesarean, most commonly for either tumor size (more than 5 cm) or for obstetric indications, though this has not been well studied and published literature is limited to a case series and a survey of providers' experience [43, 44].

Some anomalies may benefit from late preterm or early term delivery, however in the case of most individual anomalies this is not well studied and is often based on clinical experience and expert recommendations [45]. In the case of fetal gastroschisis, the management has been controversial and the reported data has been conflicting. One randomized controlled trial compared elective delivery at 36 weeks versus spontaneous labor for fetal gastroschisis and no benefit was found for elective preterm delivery [46]. Though a number of retrospective studies support this finding, other retrospective studies have shown that elective preterm or elective cesarean delivery for gastroschisis before 36 weeks may be associated with earlier enteral feeding of neonates and fewer neonatal complications [39, 47, 48].

Fetal risks

Congenital anomalies and malformation syndromes are a risk factor for stillbirth [49, 50]. A retrospective cohort study spanning two decades at a single institution compared stillbirth rates between anomalous and nonanomalous pregnancies and noted stillbirth to be significantly higher for fetuses with anomalies, (adjusted odds ratio [OR] 15.17, 95% confidence interval [CI] 11.03–20.86) [51]. Notably, the stillbirth rate more than doubled when the fetus was growth restricted. A nested case-control study by the Italian Stillbirth Study Group similarly reported fetal malformations were significantly related to risk of stillbirth (OR 7.96, 95% CI 2.69–23.55) [52].

Pregnancies complicated by fetal anomaly are at increased risk of preterm birth. A secondary analysis of a large, prospective multi-center study (the first and second trimester evaluation of risk (FASTER) Trial) included 33 020 liveborn singletons and found that birth defects were associated with preterm delivery and low birth weight [53]. Birth defects were defined as either chromosome or structural anomalies. Infants with birth defects were 2.7, 7.0, and 11.5 times more likely to deliver before 37, 34, and 32 weeks, respectively, than unaffected infants. A strength of the FASTER Trial was the use of propensity scoring to attempt to control for confounders such as sociodemographic risk factors, environmental exposures, obstetric history, and pregnancy complications.

For twin pregnancies, two retrospective studies reported lower gestational age at delivery and lower birth weight when complicated by an anomalous twin [54, 55]. In a more recent retrospective analysis of expectantly managed twins where one twin had a lethal anomaly, there was no difference in gestational age at delivery for twins with an anomalous fetus (254 days gestational age at delivery) versus twins without structural anomalies (254 days) [56].

Termination

After a fetal anomaly is diagnosed, upwards of 41% of pregnancies are electively terminated. While the RADIUS trial showed no increase in the rate of terminations for fetal abnormalities with routine ultrasound screening, both the Helsinki Trial and the Eurofetus Study reported an increase in termination of pregnancy. Rates of termination vary based on type of anomaly and severity. In a study of population registries encompassing 11 European nations, 44% of pregnancies with prenatal detection of severe fetal anomalies were electively terminated [57]. The highest rates for termination were reported for CNS abnormalities and severe genitourinary system anomalies. Termination rates were reported as 85%, 66%, 61%, and 52% for anencephaly, encephalocele, spina bifida, and bilateral renal agenesis, respectively. In the Eurofetus study, 41% of pregnancies complicated by severe fetal anomaly ended in elective termination with 27% of pregnancies with any major anomaly ending in elective termination. In a prospective, single institution US study of 53 000 pregnancies, elective termination for severe CNS anomalies occurred at a rate of 72.5% versus 37.1% for severe non-CNS anomalies [58]. Additionally, termination rates were inversely correlated with maternal age and level of education.

Following termination of pregnancy, autopsy may be performed to confirm prenatal diagnosis and enhance preconception counseling for future pregnancies. Most studies conducted have been retrospective and several cite a high rate of concordance of major anomalies found on prenatal ultrasound and postmortem examination. Of the number of retrospective studies, two were cohort studies that specifically looked at fetuses aborted for structural malformations. A German cohort of 183 pregnancies terminated prior to the 24th week reported 78% concordance of autopsy and prenatal ultrasound, with 20% additional anomalies detected on autopsy [59]. A Norwegian retrospective cohort of 288 second trimester terminations for fetal malformations reported 58.4% complete agreement between prenatal ultrasound and fetal autopsy. One prospective cohort study at a single tertiary care center found 100% concordance in detection of major anomalies and 77% concordance for minor anomalies [60]. An additional 20% of minor anomalies were detected on autopsy alone. A minority (3%) of the anomalies detected by ultrasound were not concordant with autopsy results.

Maternal risks

Most fetal anomalies carry no maternal risks other than psychological distress, such as anxiety or depression [61]. A prospective observational study of women's acute perceptions after ultrasound diagnosis of anomaly found higher rates of depression, suicidal ideation, and social dysfunction compared to those with normal ultrasound findings [62]. A limitation of this study was that the cohort had significantly lower education level than the comparison group. In a qualitative study, patients reported wanting realistic information specific to their situation and experiencing increased anxiety if receiving conflicting information [63].

For those who undergo invasive fetal surgeries, there are maternal risks including surgical morbidity and future uterine rupture. Risk for uterine rupture after open fetal surgery at one experienced center is 6–14%, significantly higher than after a primary low transverse cesarean and closer to the risk of a classical hysterotomy scar [64, 65]. Endoscopic fetal procedures have less morbidity than open hysterotomy procedures. A single-institution retrospective analysis showed endoscopic procedures have significantly less morbidity compared with the open hysterotomy group regarding delivery mode, intensive care unit stay, length of hospital stay, and need for blood transfusions [66].

The development of mirror syndrome is rare, but is a potentially significant risk to the patient whose pregnancy is complicated by hydrops fetalis. A 2010 systematic review of the literature included 56 cases of mirror syndrome, of which 23.2% were associated with fetal malformations [67]. Structural anomalies associated with mirror syndrome include Ebstein's anomaly, sacrococcygeal teratoma, aortic stenosis and aneurysm of the vein of Galen. Maternal symptoms in all cases appeared preterm, and only a few pregnancies continued to term. Though the exact pathophysiology of mirror syndrome is unclear, the cases demonstrate how fetal symptoms of hydrops can be mirrored in maternal symptoms. The most common symptoms reported are maternal weight gain and edema (89.3%), hypertension (60.7%) mild anemia, and hemodilution (46.4%). More than one fifth of pregnancies complicated by mirror syndrome resulted in pulmonary edema. Severe maternal complications were reported in more than one-fifth of mirror syndrome cases. In this review, maternal symptoms associated with mirror syndrome resolved within a mean of 8.9 days after either successful treatment of fetal symptoms or the delivery/termination of the pregnancy.

Fetal tumors are a rare event that can also lead to maternal symptoms. Cases of fetal neuroblastoma inducing maternal symptoms consistent with catecholamine excess have been reported in the literature [68]. In a case series of six pregnancies, fetal adrenal tumors caused maternal symptoms of sweating, tingling of the extremities, palpitations, and hypertension that resolved following delivery of the infant [69]. Maternal urine catecholamines were negative postpartum in the cases described, though there is evidence that if collected antepartum they would likely be elevated.

Conclusions

The screening and detection of fetal anomalies can improve the management and counseling for patients with affected pregnancies. Options for management include diagnostic testing, fetal surgery, delivery planning, and offering termination. A review of the literature reveals a paucity of randomized controlled trials regarding obstetric management of fetal anomalies; however systematic reviews, population studies, retrospective studies, and case series have been published that can aid in directing care for affected pregnancies.

Genetics

Level B evidence

- Fetal anomalies of multiple systems are more likely to be associated with abnormal karyotypes than isolated anomalies.
- Microarray analysis increases detection of clinically significant genetic abnormalities over fetal karyotype when fetal anomaly is detected on ultrasound.

Associated findings

Level B evidence

- Oligohydramnios as an ultrasound finding is associated with the presence of fetal anomalies, and is more often associated with genitourinary anomalies.
- Single umbilical artery as an ultrasound finding is associated with increased rates of fetal anomalies.
- Twinning is associated with higher rates of fetal anomaly.

Imaging

Level B evidence

- Low amniotic fluid volume has not been shown to compromise the detection of fetal anomaly by ultrasound.
- Maternal obesity is associated with lower prenatal ultrasound detection rates of fetal anomalies.
- Fetal MRI can be reliably used as adjunctive imaging to confirm ultrasound-detected CNS anomalies.
- Suspicion of fetal cardiac anomaly or more than one indication for ordering additional testing is predictive of a positive fetal echocardiography.

Fetal surgery

Level B evidence

- Fetal surgery for myelomeningocele with hindbrain herniation, compared with postnatal repair, improves outcomes.

Level C evidence

- For a narrow set of indications, fetal surgery is possible to improve outcomes.

Delivery mode and timing

Level B evidence

- Cesarean delivery is necessary when an EXIT procedure is planned for fetal anomalies.
- The optimal timing of delivery for pregnancies complicated by gastroschisis remains uncertain.

Level C evidence

- If cephalopelvic disproportion is suspected given a particular fetal anomaly, cesarean section may be indicated.

Fetal risks
Level B evidence
• The presence of fetal anomalies is associated with higher rates of stillbirth.
• Pregnancies complicated by fetal anomaly are associated with higher rates of preterm birth.
• Twin pregnancies complicated by an anomalous fetus are at risk for lower birth weight and lower gestational age at delivery for non-anomalous twin.

Termination
Level B evidence
• Fetal autopsy performed after a termination procedure for a prenatal diagnosis of a major anomaly can detect additional anomalies.

Maternal risks
Level B evidence
• Diagnosis of fetal anomalies is associated with adverse psychological effects, such as anxiety, in the short-term.
• Fetal surgery can result in increased maternal morbidity, specifically future risk of uterine rupture.

Level C evidence
• Mirror syndrome is a rare occurrence in pregnancies complicated by hydrops fetalis which can be associated with fetal anomalies.
• Fetal tumors, such as neuroblastoma, have been reported to cause maternal symptoms and associated morbidity.

References

1 EUROCAT Working Group (2002). *Appendix 7 and Appendix 8 in Report 8: Surveillance of Congenital Anomalies in Europe 1980–99.* University of Ulster.

2 Nicolaides, K.H., Snijders, R.J.M., Gosden, C.M. et al. (1992). Ultrasonographically detectable markers of fetal chromosomal abnormalities. *Lancet* **340** (**8821**): 704–707.

3 Rizzo, N., Pittalis, M.C., Pilu, G. et al. (1996). Distribution of abnormal karyotypes among malformed fetuses detected by ultrasound throughout gestation. *Prenat. Diagn.* **16** (**2**): 159–163.

4 Staebler, M., Donner, C., Van Regemorter, N. et al. (2005). Should determination of the karyotype be systematic for all malformations detected by obstetrical ultrasound? *Prenat. Diagn.* **25** (**7**): 567–573.

5 Wapner, R.J., Martin, C.L., Levy, B. et al. (2012). Chromosomal microarray versus karyotyping for prenatal diagnosis. *N. Engl. J. Med.* **367** (**23**): 2175–2184.

6 Hillman, S.C., Pretlove, S., Coomarasamy, A. et al. (2011). Additional information from array comparative genomic hybridization technology over conventional karyotyping in prenatal diagnosis: a systematic review and meta-analysis. *Ultrasound Obstet. Gynecol.* **37** (**1**): 6–14.

7 Warburton, D. (1991). De novo balanced chromosome rearrangements and extra marker chromosomes identified at prenatal diagnosis: clinical significance and distribution of breakpoints. *Am. J. Hum. Genet.* **49** (**5**): 995–1013.

8 The use of chromosomal microarray analysis in prenatal diagnosis (2013). Committee opinion no. 581. American College of Obstetricians and Gynecologists. *Obstet. Gynecol.* **122**: 1374–1377.

9 Shipp, T.D., Bromley, B., Pauker, S. et al. (1996). Outcome of singleton pregnancies with severe oliogohydramnios in the second and third trimesters. *Ultrasound Obstet. Gynecol.* **7** (**2**): 108–113.

10 Petrozella, L.N., Dashe, J.S., McIntire, D.D., and Leveno, K.J. (2011). Clinical significance of borderline amniotic fluid index and ahydramnios in preterm pregnancy. *Obstet. Gynecol.* **117** (**2 Pt 1**): 338–342.

11 Thummala, M.R., Raju, T.N., and Langenberg, P. (1998). Isolated single umbilical artery anomaly and the risk for congenital malformations: a meta-analysis. *J. Pediatr. Surg.* **33** (**4**): 580–585.

12 Murphy-Kaulbeck, L., Dodds, L., Joseph, K.S., and Van den Hof, M. (2010). Single umbilical artery risk factors and pregnancy outcomes. *Obstet. Gynecol.* **116** (**4**): 843–850.

13 Hua, M., Odibo, A.O., Macones, G.A. et al. (2010). Single umbilical artery and its associated findings. *Obstet. Gynecol.* **115** (**5**): 930–934.

14 Layde, P.M., Erickson, J.D., Falek, A., and McCarthy, B.J. (1980). Congenital malformation in twins. *Am. J. Hum. Genet.* **32** (**1**): 69–78.

15 Mastroiacovo, P., Castilla, E.E., Arpino, C. et al. (1999). Congenital malformations in twins: an international study. *Am. J. Med. Genet.* **83** (**2**): 117–124.

16 Little, J. and Nevin, N.C. (1989). Congenital anomalies in twins in Northern Ireland. III: anomalies of the cardiovascular. System 1974-1979. *Acta Geneti. Med. Gemellol. (Roma)* **38** (**1–2**): 27–35.

17 Ramos-Arroyo, M.A. (1991). Birth defects in twins: study in a Spanish population. *Acta Genet. Med. Gemellol. (Roma)* **40** (**3–4**): 337–344.

18 Grandjean, H., Larroque, D., and Levi, S. (1998). Sensitivity of routine ultrasound screening of pregnancies in the Eurofetus database. The Eurofetus team. *Ann. N. Y. Acad. Sci.* **847**: 118–124.

19 Crane, J.P., LeFevre, M.L., Winborn, R.C. et al. (1994). A randomized trial of prenatal ultrasonographic screening: impact on the detection, management and outcome of anomalous fetuses. The RADIUS study group. *Am. J. Obstet. Gynecol.* **171** (**2**): 392–399.

20 Saari-Kemppainen, A., Karjalainen, O., Ylöstalo, P., and Heinonen, O.P. (1994). Fetal anomalies in a controlled one-stage ultrasound screening trial. A report from the Helsinki ultrasound trial. *J. Perinat. Med.* **22** (**4**): 279–289.

21 Levine, D., Goldstein, R.B., Callen, P.W. et al. (1997). The effect of oligohydramnios on detection of fetal anomalies with sonography. *AJR Am. J. Roentgenol.* **168** (**6**): 1609–1611.

22 Dashe, J.S., McIntire, D.D., and Twickler, D.M. (2009). Effect of maternal obesity on the ultrasound detection of anomalous fetuses. *Obstet. Gynecol.* **113** (**5**): 1001–1007.

23 Rossi, A.C. and Prefumo, F. (2014). Additional value of fetal magnetic resonance imaging in the prenatal diagnosis of central

nervous system anomalies: a systematic review of the literature. *Ultrasound Obstet. Gynecol.* **44** (**4**): 388–393.

24 Goncalves, L.F., Lee, W., Mody, S. et al. (2016). Diagnostic accuracy of ultrasonography and magnetic resonance imaging for the detection of fetal anomalies – a blinded case-control study. *Ultrasound Obstet. Gynecol.* **48** (**2**): 185–192.

25 Wright, L., Stauffer, N., Samai, C., and Oster, M. (2014). Who should be referred? An evaluation of referral indications for fetal echocardiography in the detection of structural congenital heart disease. *Pediatric Cardiol.* **35** (**6**): 928–933.

26 Adzick, N.S., Thom, E.A., Spong, C.Y. et al. (2011). A randomized trial of prenatal versus postnatal repair of myelomeningocele. *N. Engl. J. Med.* **364** (**11**): 993–1004.

27 Dommergues, M., Louis-Sylvestre, C., Mandelbrot, L. et al. (1997). Congenital adenomatoid malformation of the lung: when is active fetal therapy indicated? *Am. J. Obstet. Gynecol.* **177** (**4**): 953–958.

28 Adzick, N.S., Harrison, M.R., Crombleholme, T.M. et al. (1998). Fetal lung lesions: management and outcome. *Am. J. Obstet. Gynecol.* **179** (**4**): 884–889.

29 T, V.M., Al-Ibrahim, A., Deprest, J. et al. (2014). Minimally invasive therapy for fetal sacrococcygeal teratoma: case series and systematic review of the literature. *Ultrasound. Obstet. Gynecol.* **43** (**6**): 611–619.

30 Wilson, R.D., Hedrick, H.L., Flake, A.W. et al. (2009). Sacrococcygeal teratomas: prenatal surveillance, growth, and pregnancy outcome. *Fetal. Diagn. Ther.* **25** (**1**): 15–20.

31 Wilkins-Haug, L. (1999). Considerations for delivery of infants with congenital abnormalities. *Obstet. Gynecol. Clin. North Am.* **26** (**2**): 399–412.

32 Bensen, T., Dillard, R.G., and Burton, B.K. (1988). Open spina bifida: does cesarean section delivery improve prognosis? *Obstet. Gynecol.* **71** (**4**): 532–534.

33 Luthy, D.A., Wardinsky, T., Shurtleff, D.B. et al. (1991). Cesarean section before the onset of labor and subsequent motor function in infants with meninigomyelocele diagnosed antenatally. *N. Engl. J. Med.* **324** (**10**): 662–666.

34 Sakala, E.P. and Andree, I. (1990). Optimal route of delivery for meningomyelocele. *Obstet. Gynecol. Surv.* **45** (**4**): 209–212.

35 Hill, A.E. and Beattie, F. (1994). Does cesarean section delivery improve neurological outcome in open spina bifida? *Eur. J. Pediatr. Surg.* **4** (**Suppl 1**): 32–34.

36 Abdel-Latif, M.E., Bolisetty, S., Abeywardana, S., and Lui, K. (2008). Australian and New Zealand neonatal network. Mode of delivery and neonatal survival of infants with gastroschisis in Australia and New Zealand. *J. Pediatr. Surg.* **43** (**9**): 1685–1690.

37 Baud, D., Lausman, A., Alfaraj, M.A. et al. (2013). Expectant management compared with elective delivery at 37 weeks for gastroschisis. *Obstet. Gynecol.* **121** (**5**): 990–998.

38 Boutros, J., Regier, M., Skarsgard, E.D., and Network, C.P.S. (2009). Is timing everything? The influence of gestational age, birth weight, route, and intent of delivery on outcome in gastroschisis. *J. Pediatr. Surg.* **44** (**5**): 912–917.

39 Hadidi, A., Subotic, U., Goeppl, M., and Waag, K.L. (2008). Early elective cesarean delivery before 36 weeks vs late spontaneous delivery in infants with gastroschisis. *J. Pediatr. Surg.* **43** (**7**): 1342–1346.

40 Snyder, C.L. and St Peter, S.D. (2005). Trends in mode of delivery for gastroschisis infants. *Am. J. Perinatol.* **22** (**7**): 391–396.

41 Bouchard, S., Johnson, M.P., Flake, A.W. et al. (2002). The EXIT procedure: experience and outcome in 31 cases. *J. Pediatr. Surg.* **37** (**3**): 418–426.

42 Hedrick, H.L., Flake, A.W., Crombleholme, T.M. et al. (2005). The ex utero intrapartum therapy procedure for high-risk fetal lung lesions. *J. Pediatr. Surg.* **40** (**6**): 1038–1043.

43 Gross, J., Renzie, R.J., Sermer, M. et al. (1987). Sacrococcygeal teratoma: prenatal diagnosis and management. *Am. J. Obstet. Gynecol.* **156** (**2**): 393–396.

44 Bond, S.J., Harrison, M.R., Schmidt, K.G. et al. (1990). Death due to high output failure in fetal sacrococcygeal teratoma. *J. Pediatr. Surg.* **25** (**12**): 1287–1291.

45 Craigo, S.D. (2011). Indicated preterm birth for fetal anomalies. *Semin. Perinatol.* **35**: 270–276.

46 Logghe, H.L., Mason, G.C., Thornton, J.G., and Stringer, M.D. (2005). A randomized controlled trial of elective preterm delivery of fetuses with gastroschisis. *J. Pediatr. Surg.* **40** (**11**): 1726–1731.

47 How, H.Y., Harris, B.J., Pietrantoni, M. et al. (2000). Is vaginal delivery preferable to elective cesarean delivery in fetuses with a known ventral wall defect? *Am. J. Obstet. Gynecol.* **182** (**6**): 1527–1534.

48 Serra, A., Fitze, G., Kamin, G. et al. (2008). Preliminary report on elective preterm delivery at 34 weeks and primary abdominal closure for the management of gastroschisis. *Eur. J. Pediatr. Surg.* **18** (**1**): 32–37.

49 Pauli, R.M. and Reiser, C.A. (1994). Wisconsin stillbirth service program: II. Analysis of diagnoses and diagnostic categories in the first 1,000 referrals. *Am. J. Med. Genet.* **50** (**2**): 135–153.

50 Getahun, D., Ananth, C.V., and Kinzler, W.L. (2007). Risk factors for antepartum and intrapartum stillbirth: a population-based study. *Am. J. Obstet. Gynecol.* **196** (**6**): 499–507.

51 Frey, H.A., Odibo, A.O., Dicke, J.M. et al. (2014). Stillbirth risk among fetuses with ultrasound-detected isolated congenital anomalies. *Obstet. Gynecol.* **124** (**1**): 91–98.

52 Facchinetti, F., Alberico, S., Benedetto, C. et al. (2011). Italian stillbirth study group. A multicenter, case-control study on risk factors for antepartum stillbirth. *J. Matern. Fetal. Neonatal. Med.* **24** (**3**): 407–410.

53 Dolan, S.M., Gross, S.J., Merkatz, I.R. et al. (2007). For the FASTER trial research consortium. The contribution of birth defects to preterm birth and low birth weight. *Obstet. Gynecol.* **110** (**2 Pt 1**): 318–324.

54 Malone, F.D., Craigo, S.D., Chelmow, D., and D'Alton, M.E. (1996). Outcome of twin gestations complicated by a single anomalous fetus. *Obstet. Gynecol.* **88** (**1**): 1–5.

55 Gul, A., Cebeci, A., Aslan, H. et al. (2005). Perinatal outcomes of twin pregnancies discordant for major fetal anomalies. *Fetal. Diagn. Ther.* **20** (**4**): 244–248.

56 Linskens, I.H., van Elburg, R.M., Oepkes, D. et al. (2011). Expectant management in twin pregnancies with discordant structural fetal anomalies. *Twin Res. Hum. Genet.* **14** (**3**): 283–289.

57 Garne, E., Loane, M., Dolk, H. et al. (2005). Prenatal diagnosis of severe structural congenital malformations in Europe. *Ultrasound Obstet. Gynecol.* **25** (**1**): 6–11.

58 Schectman, K.B., Gray, D.L., Baty, J.D., and Rothman, S.M. (2002). Decision-making for termination of pregnancies with fetal anomalies: analysis of 53,000 pregnancies. *Obstet. Gynecol.* **99**: 2, 216–222.

59 Tennstedt, C., Chaoui, R., Bollmann, R. et al. (1998). Correlation of prenatal ultrasound diagnosis and morphological findings of fetal autopsy. *Pathol. Res. Pract.* **194** (**10**): 721–724.

60 Akgun, H., Basbug, M., Ozgun, M.T. et al. (2007). Correlation between prenatal ultrasound and fetal autopsy findings in fetal anomalies terminated in the second trimester. *Prenat. Diagn.* **27** (**5**): 457–462.

61 Kemp, J., Davenport, M., and Pernet, A. (1998). Antenatally diagnosed surgical anomalies: the psychological effect of parental antenatal counseling. *J. Pediat. Surg.* **33** (**9**): 1376–1379.

62 Kaasen, A., Helbig, A., Malt, U.F. et al. (2010). Acute maternal social dysfunction, health perception and psychological distress after ultrasonographic detection of a fetal structural anomaly. *BJOG* **117** (**9**): 1127–1138.

63 Miquel-Verges, F., Woods, S.L., Aucott, S.W. et al. (2009). Prenatal consultation with a neonatologist for congenital anomalies: parental perceptions. *Pediatrics* **124** (**4**): e573–e579.

64 Wilson, R.D., Johnson, M.P., Flake, A.W. et al. (2004). Reproductive outcomes after pregnancy complicated by maternal-fetal surgery. *Am. J. Obstet. Gynecol.* **191** (**4**): 1430–1436.

65 Wilson, R.D., Lemerand, K., Johnson, N.P. et al. (2010). Reproductive outcomes after pregnancy complicated by open maternal-fetal surgery (1996-2007). *Am. J. Obstet. Gynecol.* **203** (**3**): 209e1–209e6.

66 Golombeck, K., Ball, R.H., Lee, H. et al. (2006). Maternal morbidity after maternal-fetal surgery. *Am. J. Obstet. Gynecol.* **194** (**3**): 834–839.

67 Braun, T., Brauer, M., Fuchs, I. et al. (2010). Mirror syndrome: a systematic review of fetal associated conditions, maternal presentation and perinatal outcome. *Fetal. Diagn. Ther.* **27** (**4**): 191–203.

68 Newton, E.R., Louis, F., Dalton, M.E., and Feingold, M. (1985). Fetal neuroblastoma and catecholamine-induced maternal hypertension. *Obstet. Gynecol.* **65** (**3 Suppl**): 49S–52S.

69 Voute, P.A., Wadman, S.K., and Van Putten, W.J. (1970). Congenital neuroblastoma: symptoms in the mother during pregnancy. *Clin. Pediatr. (Phila)* **9** (**4**): 206–207.

47

CHAPTER 47

Antepartum/intrapartum fetal surveillance

David A. Miller
Division of Maternal-Fetal Medicine, Department of Obstetrics and Gynecology, Keck School of Medicine, University of Southern California, Los Angeles, CA, USA

Introduction

Electronic fetal heart rate monitoring (EFM) was introduced into clinical practice during an era in which intrapartum fetal hypoxia was thought to be the primary cause of cerebral palsy (CP). Based on this assumption, EFM offered the hope of detecting intrapartum fetal oxygen deprivation so that early intervention could prevent CP [1]. When EFM replaced the traditional practice of intermittent auscultation in the 1970s, a series of non-randomized studies reported significantly lower perinatal mortality rates in electronically monitored patients [2–12]. However, subsequent randomized trials failed to demonstrate consistent improvements in either perinatal morbidity or mortality when the new technology was compared to intermittent auscultation summarized in Table 47.1 [13–24].

Randomized trials of EFM versus intermittent auscultation

In 2006, a Cochrane review of these studies concluded that EFM was associated with an increased rate of cesarean delivery compared with intermittent fetal heart rate (FHR) auscultation during labor [25]. In the 1970s, four randomized trials compared EFM to intermittent auscultation during labor [13–16]. Together, these four trials included 2027 patients, and each of the four trials demonstrated a significantly higher rate of cesarean birth in the electronically-monitored groups. Subsequently seven randomized trials were published on the same topic, six of which included data regarding overall cesarean rates [17–22]. These six trials included a total of 20 640 patients. None of the trials published after 1980 demonstrated a higher rate of cesarean delivery in women managed with EFM compared with those managed with intermittent auscultation.

To date, no randomized, controlled trial has confirmed the original assumption that EFM can prevent CP. Retrospective studies have demonstrated that more than 90% of CP cases may have no identifiable link to intrapartum hypoxia. Such cases cannot reasonably be expected to be detectable or preventable by refinements in the management of labor, including interpretation and management of intrapartum EFM [26, 27]. The false-positive rate of EFM for predicting CP has been reported to exceed 99%, yielding a positive predictive value of less than 1% [28, 29]. Potential explanations for this imprecision include the relative rarity of intrapartum hypoxic neurologic injury, the mitigating interventions that frequently are triggered by FHR "abnormalities", the amount of time that separates EFM from the later diagnosis of CP, and finally, the fact that EFM is a screening test rather than a diagnostic test. Despite these limitations, some form of intrapartum fetal monitoring is necessary, even in low-risk pregnancies. The only form of intrapartum fetal monitoring that has been demonstrated in randomized trials to be equivalent to EFM in safety and efficacy is intermittent auscultation conducted under research protocols employing one-on-one nursing care. No study has demonstrated that such an approach is as cost-effective as EFM, much less more cost effective. Therefore, principles of patient safety dictate that future efforts should focus on standardization and simplification of EFM as it is used in contemporary clinical practice. These efforts should include promulgation of standardized definitions, simplification of interpretation and development of practical, evidence-based approaches to management.

The evolution of standardized FHR definitions

Electronic FHR monitoring was introduced into clinical practice before consensus was achieved regarding standardized

Evidence-Based Obstetrics and Gynecology, First Edition. Edited by Errol R. Norwitz, Carolyn M. Zelop, David A. Miller, and David L. Keefe.

Table 47.1 Randomized trials of EFM versus Intermittent auscultation

Author [Reference]	Number of patients	EFM impact on					
		Cesarean rate	Perinatal mortality	Apgar scores	Umbilical cord blood pH	NICU admissions	Neonatal neurologic abnormalities
Haverkamp et al. [13]	483	Increase	No difference	No difference	No difference	No difference	No difference
Renou et al. [14]	350	Increase	No difference	No difference	Higher cord pH In EFM group	Fewer NICU admissions in EFM group	Fewer neonatal neurologic abnormalities in EFM group
Kelso et al. [15]	504	Increase	No difference	No difference	No difference	No difference	No difference
Haverkamp et al. [16]	690	Increase	No difference	No difference	No difference	No difference	No difference
Wood et al. [17]	989	No difference	No difference	No difference	No difference	No difference	No difference
MacDonald et al. [18]	12 964	No difference	No difference	No difference	No difference	No difference	Fewer neonatal seizures in EFM group
Neldam et al. [19]	969	No difference	No difference	No difference	No difference	No difference	No difference
Luthy [23]	246	No difference	No difference	No difference	No difference	No difference	No difference
Vintzileos [20]	1 428	No difference	Fewer perinatal deaths in EFM group	No difference	No difference	No difference	No difference
Herbst & Ingemarrson [21]	4 044	No difference	No difference	No difference	No difference	No difference	No difference

definitions of FHR patterns. This resulted in wide variations in the description and interpretation of common FHR observations. In 1995 and 1996, the National Institute of Child Health and Human Development (NICHD) convened a workshop to develop "standardized and unambiguous definitions for fetal heart rate tracings" [30]. In 2005 and 2006, the NICHD definitions were endorsed by the American College of Obstetricians and Gynecologists (ACOG), The Association of Women's Health, Obstetric and Neonatal Nurses (AWHONN) and the American College of Nurse Midwives (ACNM) [31–33]. In 2008, a second NICHD consensus panel was convened to review and update the standardized definitions published in 1997 and to reach consensus regarding basic principles of FHR interpretation [34]. The standardized NICHD FHR definitions published in 2008 are summarized in Table 47.2.

The 2008 NICHD consensus report

In addition to clarifying and reaffirming the standardized FHR definitions proposed in the 1997 NICHD consensus report, the 2008 report recommended a simplified system for classifying FHR tracings using baseline rate, variability and decelerations to group FHR tracings into three categories as summarized in Table 47.3.

The proposed FHR categories represent a shorthand method of defining FHR tracings. Category II, in particular, includes a very wide range of FHR tracings with variable clinical significance. Consequently, categories alone do not provide sufficient information for accurate communication of FHR patterns. Categories specifically do not replace a full description of baseline rate, variability, accelerations, decelerations, sinusoidal pattern, and changes or trends over time. The 2008 NICHD consensus report also made recommendations regarding uterine activity. Normal uterine contraction frequency was defined as five or fewer contractions in a 10-minute window averaged over 30 minutes. Contraction frequency of more than 5 in 10 minutes averaged over 30 minutes was defined as tachysystole. The terms hyperstimulation and hypercontractility have been defined inconsistently in the literature, therefore the consensus report recommended that they be abandoned [34]. Contraction frequency alone is a partial assessment of uterine activity. Other factors such as duration, intensity, relaxation time between contractions and resting uterine tone between contractions are equally important in clinical practice. Recommendations of the 2008 NICHD report are summarized in ACOG Practice Bulletins 106 and 116 [29, 36].

NICHD definitions – general considerations

The standardized definitions proposed by the NICHD in 1997 and reaffirmed in 2008 apply to the interpretation of FHR patterns produced by a direct fetal electrode detecting the fetal electrocardiogram (ECG), or by an external Doppler device detecting fetal cardiac motion using the autocorrelation technique. Autocorrelation, used in modern FHR monitors, is a computerized method of minimizing the artifact associated with Doppler ultrasound calculation of the FHR. Patterns are categorized as baseline, periodic, or episodic.

- Baseline patterns include baseline rate and variability.
- Periodic and episodic patterns include FHR accelerations and decelerations.
- Periodic patterns are those associated with uterine contractions.
- Episodic patterns are those not associated with uterine contractions.
- A number of FHR characteristics are dependent upon gestational age, so gestational age must be considered in the full evaluation of the pattern.
- In addition, the FHR tracing should be evaluated in the context of maternal medical condition, prior results of fetal assessment, medications, and other factors.
- FHR patterns do not occur alone and generally evolve over time.
- A full description of a FHR tracing requires assessment of uterine activity as well as a qualitative and quantitative description of all components, including baseline rate, variability, accelerations, decelerations and changes or trends over time.

Baseline

Baseline FHR is defined as the approximate mean FHR rounded to increments of 5 bpm during a 10-minute segment, excluding accelerations, decelerations, and periods of marked variability. Baseline rate is defined as a single number (for example 145 bpm), not as a range (for example "140–150 bpm" or "140s"). In any 10-minute window the minimum baseline duration must be at least two minutes (not necessarily contiguous) or the baseline for that period is deemed indeterminate. If the baseline during any 10 minute segment is deemed indeterminate, it may be necessary to refer to previous 10-minute segment(s) for determination of the baseline.

Fetal heart rate variability

Variability is defined as fluctuations in the baseline FHR that are irregular in amplitude and frequency. Variability is quantitated in beats per minute and is measured from the peak to the trough in beats per minute. No distinction is made between "short-term" ("beat-to-beat") variability and "long-term" variability because in actual practice they are visually determined as a unit. Standardized NICHD nomenclature classifies variability as absent, minimal, moderate or marked. Variability is defined as absent when the amplitude range of the FHR fluctuations is undetectable to the unaided eye. Variability is defined as minimal when the amplitude range is detectable but less than or equal to five beats per

Table 47.2 Standard fetal heart rate definitions

Pattern	Definition
Baseline	The mean FHR rounded to increments of 5 beats per min during a 10 min segment, excluding accelerations, decelerations and periods of marked FHR variability The baseline must be for a minimum of 2 min (not necessarily contiguous) in any 10-min segment, or the baseline for that segment is defined as "indeterminate"
Tachycardia	Baseline FHR greater than 160 beats per min
Bradycardia	Baseline FHR less than 110 beats per min
Baseline variability	Fluctuations in the FHR baseline that are irregular in amplitude and frequency. Variability is measured from the peak to the trough of the FHR fluctuations and is quantified in beats per min. Variability is classified as follows Absent – amplitude range undetectable Minimal– amplitude range detectable but ≤5 beats per min Moderate – amplitude range 6–25 beats per min Marked – amplitude range > 25 beats, per min No distinction is made between: short term variability (or beat-to-beat variability or R-R wave period differences in the electrocardiogram) and long-term variability because in actual practice they are visually determined as a unit
Acceleration	A visually apparent abrupt increase (onset to peak <30 s) in the FHR from the baseline At 32 weeks of gestation and beyond, an acceleration has a peak at least 15 heats per min above baseline sod a duration of at least 15 s but less than 2 min Before 32 weeks of gestation, an acceleration has peak at least 10 beats per min above baseline and a duration of at least 10 s but less than 2 min Prolonged acceleration lasts ≥2 min but <10 min If an acceleration lasts ≥10 min, if is a baseline change
Early deceleration	In association with a uterine contraction, a visually apparent, gradual (onset to nadir ≥30 s) decrease in FHR with return to baseline In general, the nadir of the deceleration occurs at the same time as the peat of the contraction
Late deceleration	In association with a uterine contraction, a visually apparent, gradual (onset to nadir ≥30 s) decrease in FHR with return to baseline In general, the onset, nadir, and recovery of the deceleration occur after the beginning, peak, and end of the contraction, respectively
Variable deceleration	An abrupt (onset to nadir <30 s), visually apparent decrease in the FHR below the baseline The decrease in FHR is at least 15 beats per min and lasts at least 15 s but less than 2 min
Prolonged deceleration	Visually apparent decrease in the FHR at least 15 beats per min below the baseline lasting at least 2 min but less than 10 min from onset to return to baseline
Periodic deceleration	Accompanies a uterine contraction
Episodic deceleration	Does not accompany a uterine contraction
Sinusoidal pal tern	Visually apparent, smooth, sine wave-like undulating pattern in FHR baseline with a cycle frequency of 3–5 per min which persists for ≥20 min.

Source: Adapted from: Macones GA, Hankins GD, Spong CY, Hauth J/Moore T. The 2008 National Institute of Child Health and Human Development workshop report on electronic fetal monitoring: update on definitions, interpretation, and research guidelines. Obstet Gynecol. 2008 Sep;112(3):661–666 [35].

Table 47.3 Fetal heart rate categories

Category I requires all of the following
Baseline rate: 110–160 bpm
Variability: Moderate
Accelerations: Present or absent
Decelerations: No late, variable or prolonged decelerations
Category II
Any FHR tracing that does not meet criteria for classification in Category I or Category III
Category III requires at least one of the following
Absent variability with recurrent late decelerations
Absent variability with recurrent variable decelerations
Absent variability with bradycardia for at least 10 min
Sinusoidal pattern for at least 20 min

minute. When the amplitude range of the fluctuations is 6–25 beats per minute, variability is defined as moderate (Figure 47.1). Finally, variability is defined as marked when the amplitude range is greater than 25 beats per minute.

Acceleration

Acceleration is defined as an abrupt (onset to peak <30 seconds) increase in FHR above the baseline. The peak is at least 15 bpm above the baseline and the acceleration lasts at least 15 seconds from the onset to return to baseline. Before 32 weeks of gestation, an acceleration is defined as having a peak at least 10 bpm above the baseline and a duration of at least 10 seconds. An acceleration lasting at least 2 minutes but less than 10 minutes is defined as a prolonged acceleration. An acceleration lasting 10 minutes or longer is defined as a baseline change. Accelerations that are provoked by fetal stimulation have the same clinical significance as spontaneous accelerations [34].

Decelerations

Decelerations in the FHR are categorized as early, late, variable or prolonged and are quantitated by depth in bpm below the baseline and duration in minutes and seconds. An abrupt deceleration reaches its nadir in less than 30 seconds. A gradual deceleration reaches its nadir in ≥30 seconds. Decelerations that occur with at least 50% of uterine contractions in 20 minute period are defined as recurrent. Decelerations occurring with fewer than 50% of contractions in a 20-minute period are defined as intermittent. Decelerations may be accompanied by other characteristics such as slow return of the FHR after the end of the contraction, biphasic decelerations, tachycardia following variable deceleration(s), accelerations preceding and/or following decelerations (sometimes called shoulders or overshoots), and fluctuations in the FHR in the trough of the deceleration. The clinical significance of these characteristics requires further research investigation; therefore, they are not included in standard NICHD terminology. Classification of decelerations as "mild", "moderate", or "severe" has not been shown to correlate with metabolic acidemia or newborn outcome independent of known confounding factors such as baseline rate, moderate variability, accelerations, and frequency of decelerations. Therefore, such classification is not included in standardized NICHD terminology [34].

Early deceleration

Early deceleration is defined as a gradual (onset to nadir <30 seconds) decrease in FHR from the baseline and subsequent return to baseline associated with a uterine

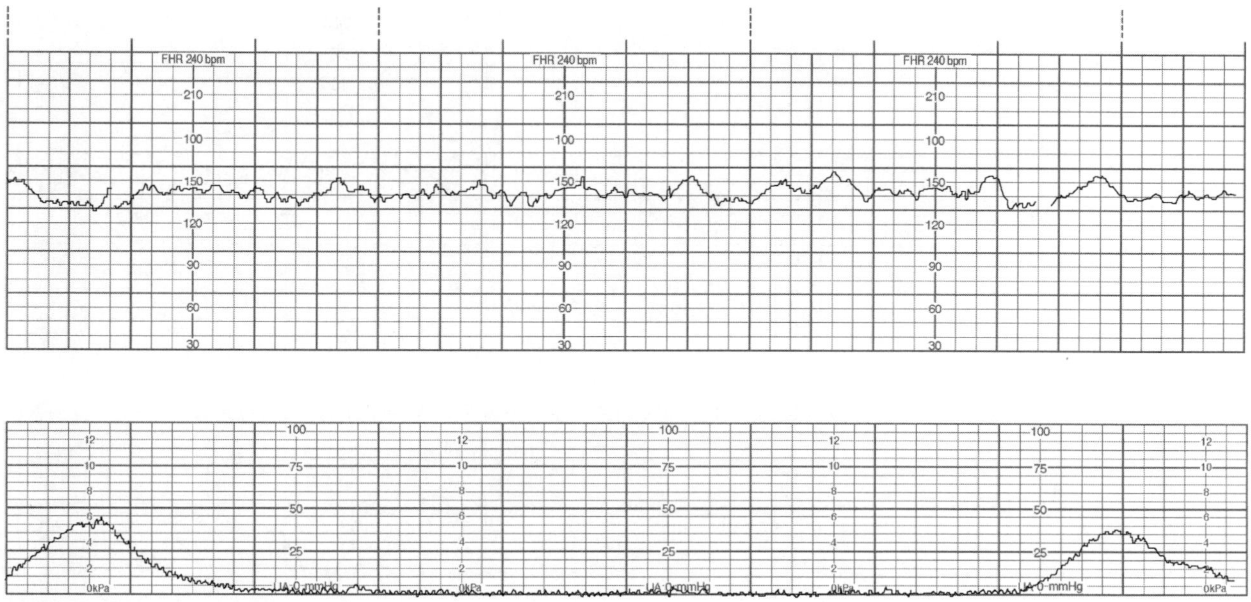

Figure 47.1 Fetal heart rate.

contraction (Figure 47.2). The onset, nadir, and recovery of the deceleration occur at the same time as the beginning, peak, and end of the contraction, respectively.

Late deceleration

Late deceleration of the FHR is defined as a gradual (onset to nadir ≥30 seconds) decrease of the FHR from the baseline and subsequent return to the baseline associated with a uterine contraction (Figure 47.3). In most cases the onset, nadir, and recovery of the deceleration occur after the beginning, peak, and ending of the contraction, respectively.

Variable deceleration

Variable deceleration of the FHR is defined as an abrupt (onset to nadir <30 seconds) decrease in FHR below the baseline (Figure 47.4). The decrease is at least 15 bpm below the baseline and the deceleration lasts at least 15 seconds and <2 minutes from onset to return to baseline. Variable decelerations can occur with or without uterine contractions.

Prolonged deceleration

Prolonged deceleration of the FHR is defined as a decrease (either gradual or abrupt) in FHR at least 15 bpm below the baseline lasting at least 2 minutes from onset to return to baseline. According to NICHD terminology, a prolonged deceleration lasting 10 minutes or longer is defined as a baseline change.

Sinusoidal pattern

The sinusoidal pattern is a smooth, sine wave-like undulating pattern in FHR baseline with a cycle frequency of three to five per minute that persists for at least 20 minutes (Figure 47.5). It is specifically excluded from the definition of variability. The sinusoidal pattern can be distinguished from variability

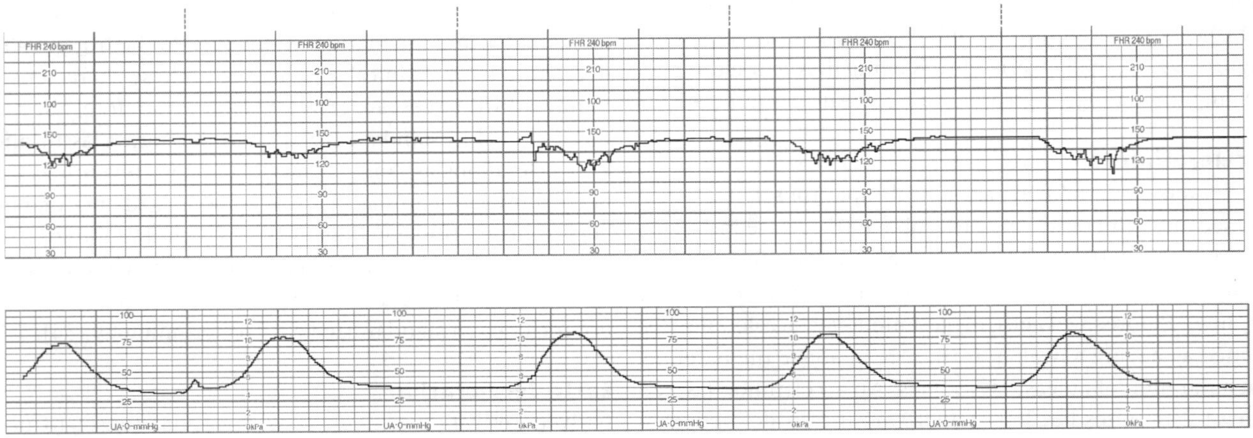

Figure 47.2 Early decelerations.

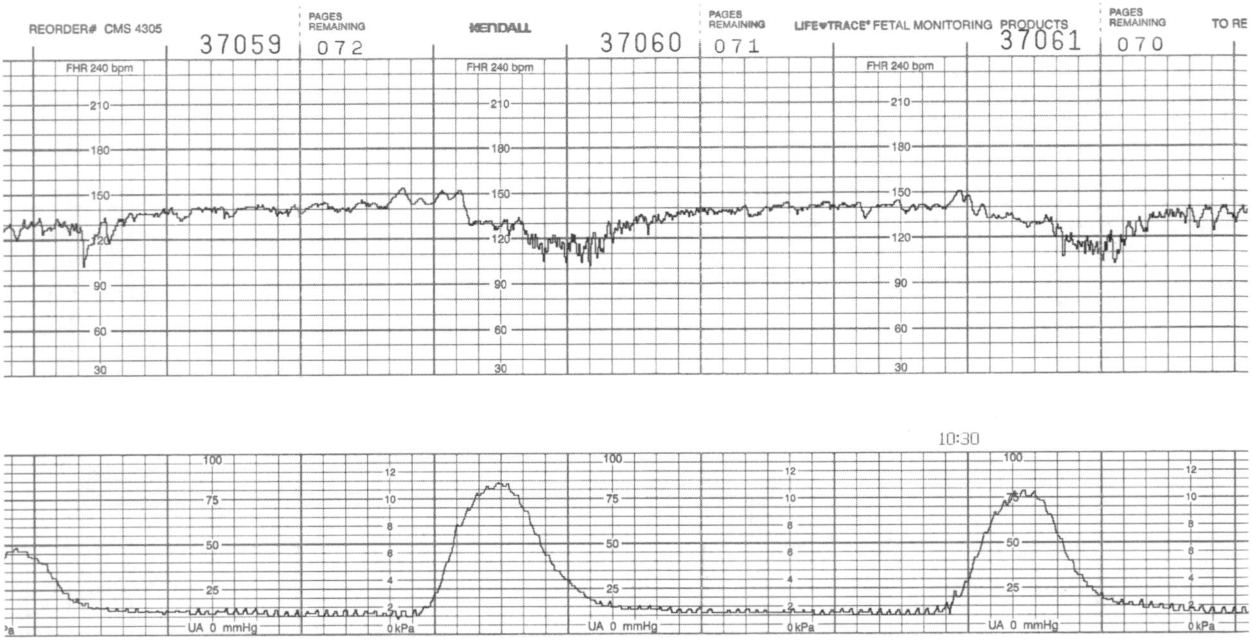

Figure 47.3 Late decelerations.

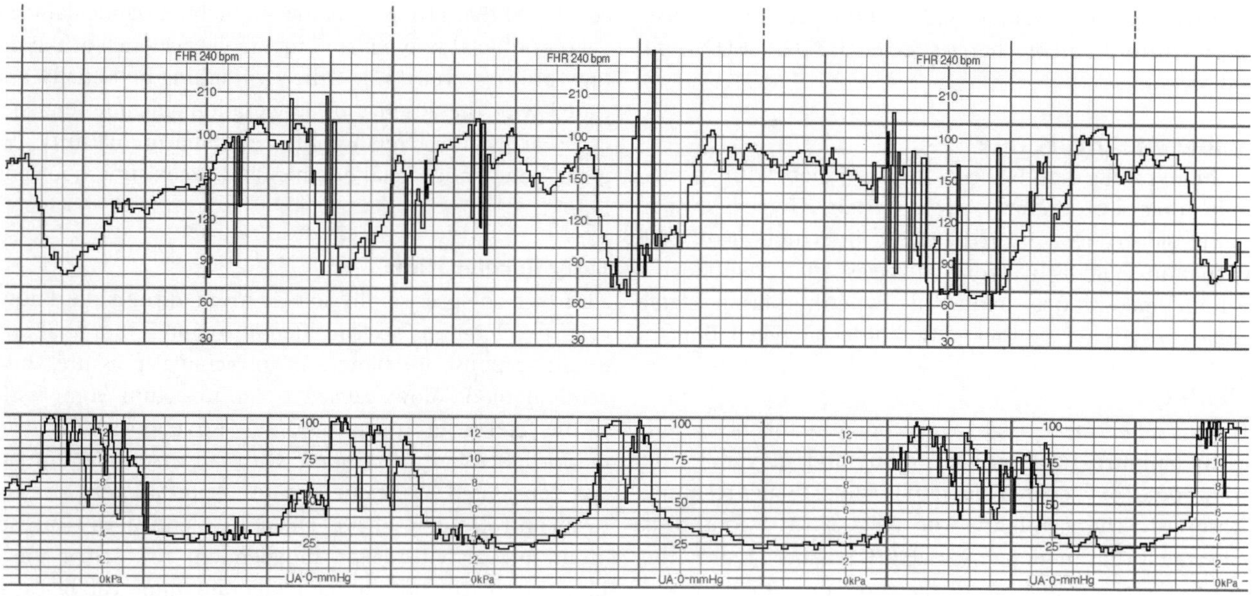

Figure 47.4 Variable decelerations.

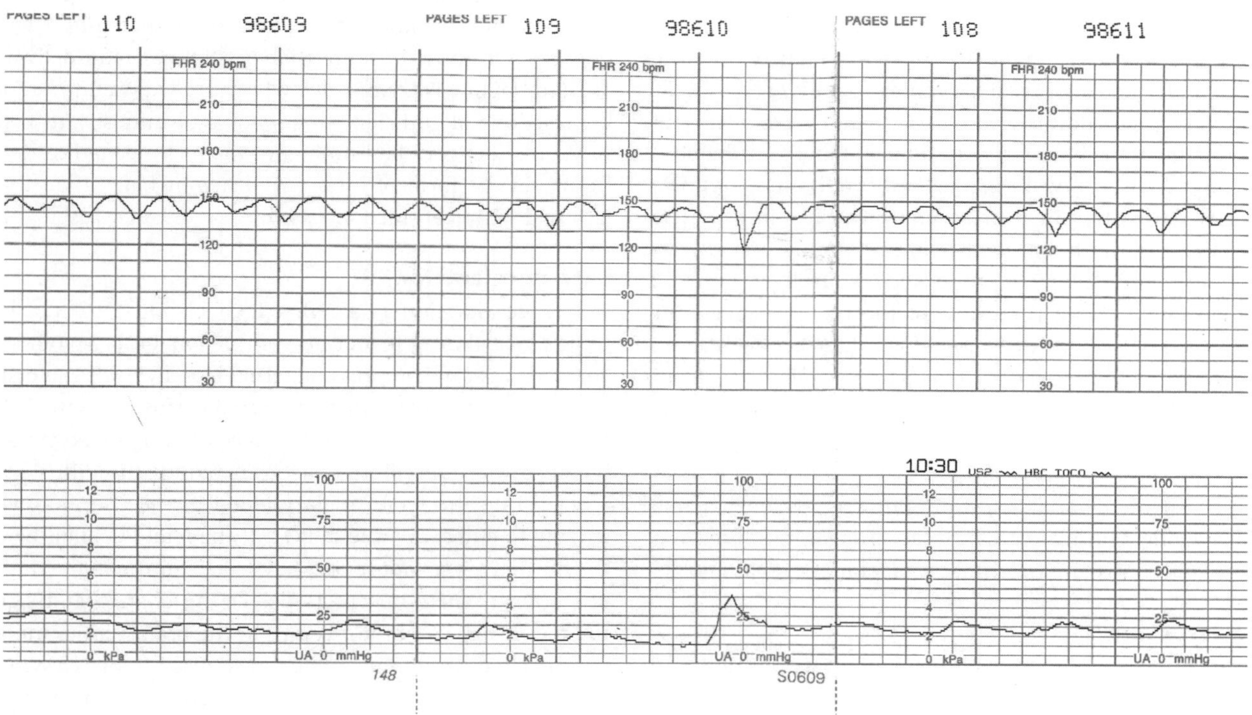

Figure 47.5 Sinusoidal pattern.

because it is characterized by fluctuations in the baseline that are regular in amplitude in frequency.

Physiology of fetal heart rate patterns

Many factors interact to regulate the FHR, including cardiac pacemakers, the cardiac conduction system, autonomic innervation (sympathetic, parasympathetic), humoral factors (catecholamines), extrinsic factors (medications), and local factors (calcium, potassium). Fluctuations in PO2, PCO2, and blood pressure are detected by chemoreceptors and baroreceptors located in the aortic arch and carotid arteries. Signals from these receptors are processed in the medullary vasomotor center, possibly with regulatory input from higher centers in the hypothalamus and cerebral cortex. Sympathetic and parasympathetic signals from the medullary vasomotor center modulate the FHR in response to moment-to-moment changes in fetal PO2, PCO2, and blood pressure.

Baseline fetal heart rate

Fetal bradycardia may be seen in association with maternal beta-blocker therapy, hypothermia, hypoglycemia, hypothyroidism, fetal heart block, or interruption of fetal oxygenation. Fetal tachycardia may be associated with fever, infection, medications, maternal hyperthyroidism, fetal anemia, arrhythmia, or interruption of fetal oxygenation.

Variability

With every heartbeat, slight corrections in the heart rate help to optimize fetal cardiac output and maximize the distribution of oxygenated blood to the fetal tissues resulting in observed FHR variability. The 2008 NICHD consensus report stated that moderate variability reliably predicts the absence of fetal metabolic acidemia at the time it is observed [34]. However, the converse is not true. Minimal or absent variability alone do not confirm the presence of fetal metabolic acidemia [34]. In 2014, Neonatal Encephalopathy Task Force of ACOG and the American Academy of Pediatrics (AAP) published a consensus report identifying moderate variability as a FHR observation that reliably excludes damaging degrees of fetal hypoxia and metabolic acidemia at the time it is observed [37]. Other conditions potentially associated with minimal or absent variability include fetal sleep cycle, arrhythmia, medications, extreme prematurity, congenital anomalies, or pre-existing neurologic injury. It is important to note that most of the literature regarding "decreased" variability does not differentiate between absent variability (amplitude range undetectable) and minimal variability (amplitude range detectable but ≤5 bpm). Therefore, it is not possible to draw valid conclusions regarding the relative clinical significance of these two categories. The significance of marked variability is not known. Possible explanations include a normal variant or an exaggerated autonomic response to transient interruption of fetal oxygenation.

Accelerations

Accelerations in FHR frequently occur in association with fetal movement, possibly as a result of stimulation of peripheral proprioceptors, increased catecholamine release and autonomic stimulation of the heart. Another suspected mechanism of FHR acceleration is transient compression of the umbilical vein, resulting in decreased fetal venous return and a reflex rise in heart rate. The 2008 NICHD consensus report stated that FHR accelerations variability reliably predict the absence of fetal metabolic acidemia at the time they are observed [34]. However, the converse is not true. The absence of accelerations does not confirm the presence of fetal metabolic acidemia or ongoing hypoxic injury [34]. In 2014, the ACOG-AAP Neonatal Encephalopathy Taskforce concluded that FHR accelerations reliably exclude damaging degrees of fetal hypoxia and metabolic acidemia at the time they are observed [37]. Other conditions potentially associated with the absence of accelerations include fetal sleep cycle, arrhythmia, medications, extreme prematurity, congenital anomalies, fetal anemia, and preexisting neurologic injury.

Early deceleration

Although the precise physiologic mechanism is not known, early decelerations are considered to represent a fetal autonomic response to changes in intracranial pressure and/or cerebral blood flow caused by intrapartum compression of the fetal head during uterine contractions. Early decelerations are not correlated with adverse outcome and are considered clinically benign. Appropriately designed case-control studies have failed to identify any measure of uterine activity as an independent risk factor for CP [26, 38–40]. The notion that fetal brain injury can be caused by mechanical forces of labor is further challenged by level II evidence from a large cohort study comparing neonatal outcomes of more than 380 000 spontaneous vaginal deliveries to those of more than 33 000 cesarean deliveries without labor [41]. Neonates who were exposed to uterine contractions of sufficient frequency and intensity to result in vaginal delivery had no higher rates of mechanical brain injury, in the form of intracranial hemorrhage, than those exposed to no contractions at all.

Late deceleration

A late deceleration is a reflex fetal response to transient hypoxemia during a uterine contraction [42]. Myometrial contractions can compress maternal blood vessels traversing the uterine wall and reduce maternal perfusion of the intervillous space of the placenta. Reduced delivery of oxygenated blood to the intervillous space can reduce the diffusion of oxygen into the fetal capillary blood in the chorionic villi, leading to a decline in fetal PO2. If the fetal PO2 falls below the normal range (approximately 15–25 mmHg in the umbilical artery), chemoreceptors detect the change and signal the medullary vasomotor center in the brainstem to initiate a protective autonomic reflex response. Initially, sympathetic outflow causes peripheral vasoconstriction, shunting oxygenated blood flow away from non-vital vascular beds and toward vital organs such as the brain, heart and adrenal glands. The resulting increase in fetal blood pressure is detected by baroreceptors, which trigger a parasympathetic reflex slowing of the heart rate to reduce cardiac output and return the blood pressure to normal. After the contraction, fetal oxygenation is restored, autonomic reflexes subside and the FHR gradually returns to baseline. This combined sympathetic-parasympathetic reflex response to transient interruption of fetal oxygenation, summarized in Figure 47.6, has been confirmed in animal studies [42–51].

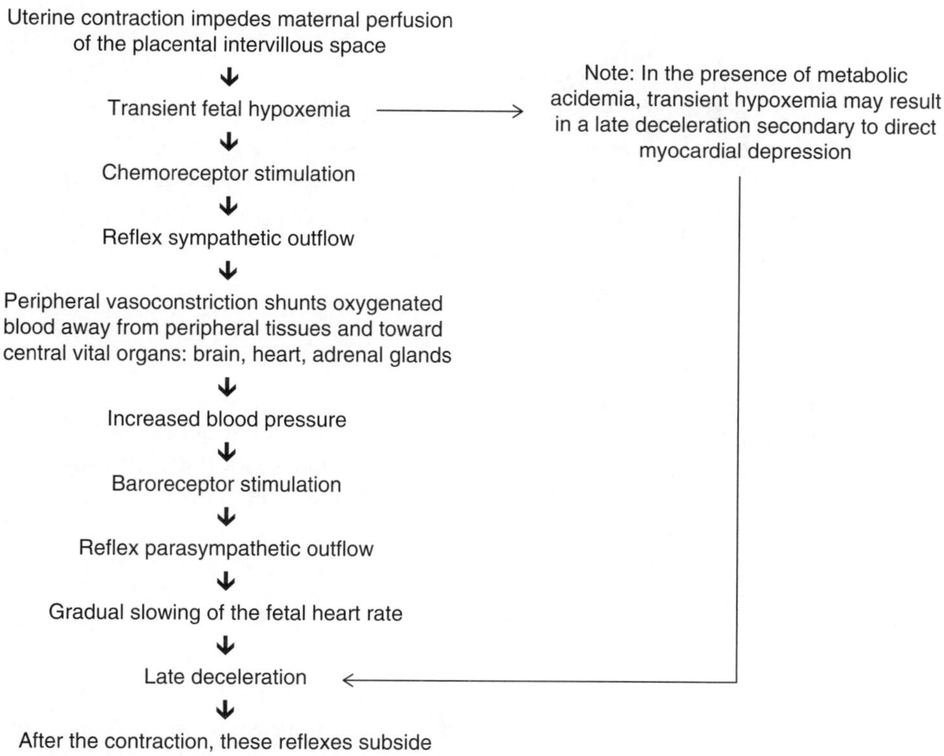

Figure 47.6 Mechanisms of late deceleration.

Occasionally, fetal oxygenation can be interrupted sufficiently to cause metabolic acidemia. In that event, a late deceleration may result from direct hypoxic myocardial depression [42]. Since this mechanism requires metabolic acidemia, it can be excluded by the observation of moderate variability or accelerations [34].

Variable deceleration

A variable deceleration represents a fetal autonomic reflex response to transient mechanical compression of the umbilical cord [47, 52–60]. Initially, compression of the umbilical cord occludes the thin-walled, compliant umbilical vein, decreasing fetal venous return and triggering a baroreceptor-mediated reflex rise in FHR (previously described as a "shoulder"). Further compression occludes the umbilical arteries, causing an abrupt increase in fetal peripheral resistance and blood pressure. Baroreceptors detect the abrupt rise in blood pressure and signal the medullary vasomotor center in the brainstem which, in turn, triggers an increase in parasympathetic outflow and an abrupt decrease in heart rate. As the cord is decompressed, this sequence of events occurs in reverse.

Prolonged deceleration

If the physiologic mechanisms responsible for late or variable decelerations persist, a deceleration can last two minutes or longer. A deceleration lasting 2 minutes but less than 10 minutes is defined as a prolonged deceleration. A deceleration lasting 10 minutes or longer is defined as a baseline change.

Sinusoidal pattern

Although the pathophysiologic mechanism is not known, this pattern classically is associated with severe fetal anemia. Variations of the pattern have also been described in association with administration of narcotic analgesics and chorioamnionitis.

Interpretation

Intrapartum FHR monitoring is intended to assess the adequacy of fetal oxygenation during labor. Fetal oxygenation involves the transfer of oxygen from the environment to the fetus along a pathway that includes the maternal lungs, heart, vasculature, uterus, placenta, and umbilical cord. Fetal oxygenation also involves the fetal physiologic response to interruption of the oxygen pathway, including the sequential progression from fetal hypoxemia, to fetal hypoxia, metabolic acidosis, and finally, metabolic acidemia.

Interruption of oxygen transfer from the environment to the fetus

Oxygen is carried from the environment to the fetus by maternal and fetal blood along a pathway that includes the

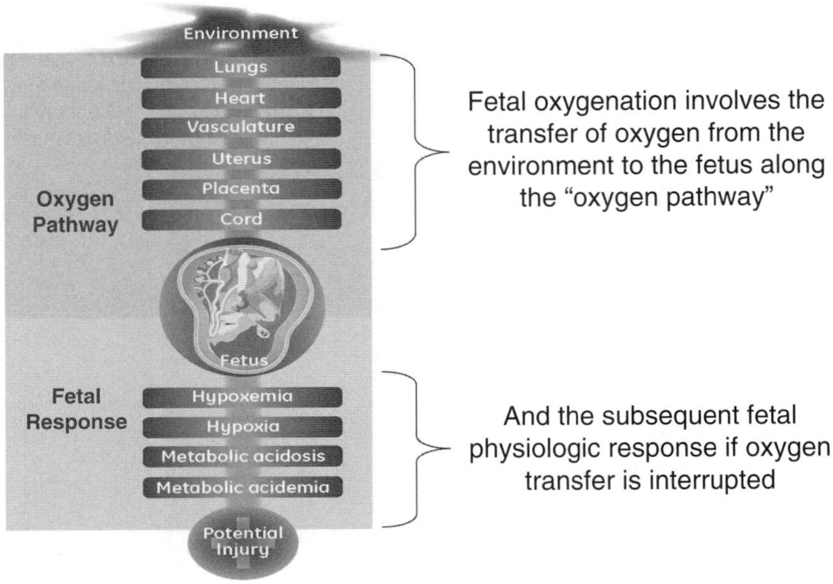

Figure 47.7 Components of fetal oxygenation.

maternal lungs, heart, vasculature, uterus, placenta, and umbilical cord (Figure 47.7).

Interruption of the oxygen pathway at one or more points can result in a FHR deceleration. For example, interruption of the oxygen pathway by compression of the umbilical cord can result in a variable deceleration [29, 52]. A late deceleration can result from reduced placental perfusion during a uterine contraction [42]. Interruption at any point along the pathway can result in a prolonged deceleration. Examples at each point are illustrated in Table 47.4.

Variable, late, and prolonged decelerations all share a common initiating event: interruption of the oxygen pathway at one or more points. *The first principle of standardized intrapartum FHR interpretation is that all FHR decelerations that have potential clinical significance (variable, late, or prolonged) reflect interruption of the pathway of oxygen transfer from the environment to the fetus at one or more points.*

Interruption of fetal oxygenation has the potential to result in hypoxic neurologic injury. The pathway from normal fetal oxygenation to potential hypoxic injury includes a series of sequential physiologic steps. The first step, hypoxemia, is defined as decreased oxygen content in the blood. Hypoxemia can lead to reduced oxygen content in the tissues, termed hypoxia. Tissue hypoxia can trigger anaerobic metabolism, lactic acid production, and metabolic acidosis in the tissues. Eventually, the blood pH can fall, causing metabolic acidemia. The 2008 NICHD Research Planning Workshop, and the 2014 ACOG-AAP Neonatal Encephalopathy Task Force identified moderate variability and accelerations as the two FHR characteristics that reliably exclude damaging degrees of fetal hypoxia or metabolic acidemia [34, 37]. *The second principle of intrapartum FHR interpretation is that moderate variability or accelerations reliably exclude damaging degrees of fetal hypoxia or fetal metabolic acidemia at the time they are observed.*

Criteria for hypoxic neurologic injury

In 1999 and 2003, the International Cerebral Palsy Task Force, ACOG, and AAP published consensus statements identifying significant fetal metabolic acidemia (umbilical artery pH < 7.0 and base deficit $\geq 12\ \text{mmol}\,l^{-1}$) as an essential precondition to acute intrapartum hypoxic neurologic injury in the form of CP [35, 61]. Other criteria are summarized in Tables 47.5 and 47.6.

Table 47.4 Potential causes of prolonged deceleration

Oxygen pathway	Examples of potential causes of interruption
Maternal lungs	Maternal apnea during a convulsion
Heart	Acute reduction in cardiac output during arrhythmia
Vasculature	Acute hypotension due to regional anesthesia or supine position
Uterus	Uterine rupture or excessive uterine activity
Placenta	Placental abruption
Umbilical cord	Compression or prolapse

Table 47.5 Essential criteria that define an acute intrapartum event sufficient to cause cerebral palsy (must meet all four)

1. Umbilical cord arterial blood pH <7 and base deficit ≥12 mmol l^{-1}
2. Early onset of severe or moderate neonatal encephalopathy in infants born at 34 or more weeks of gestation
3. Cerebral palsy of the spastic quadriplegic or dyskinetic type
4. Exclusion of other identifiable etiologies such as trauma, coagulation disorders, infectious conditions or genetic disorders

Table 47.6 Criteria that collectively suggest the event occurred within 48 hours of birth

1. A sentinel hypoxic event immediately before or during labor
2. A sudden and sustained fetal bradycardia or the absence of FHR variability in the presence of persistent late or variable decelerations, usually after a hypoxic sentinel event when the pattern was previously normal
3. Apgar scores of 0–3 beyond 5 min
4. Onset of multisystem involvement within 72 hr of birth
5. Early imaging study showing evidence of acute non-focal cerebral abnormality

The 2014 ACOG-AAP Task Force report reaffirmed that "in a fetus exhibiting either moderate variability or accelerations of the FHR, damaging degrees of hypoxia-induced metabolic acidemia can reliably be excluded" [37]. Unlike its predecessor, the 2014 Task Force report did not identify metabolic acidemia as an absolute requirement to diagnose intrapartum hypoxic neurologic injury. Intrapartum FHR monitoring interpretation can be summarized in two central principles that are illustrated in Figure 47.8.

A simplified, standardized approach to management

The ability to distill intrapartum FHR monitoring into two evidence-based principles of interpretation permits the development of a simplified, standardized approach to management [62]. The management algorithm described below incorporates standard FHR definitions and simplified principles of interpretation. It does not include adjunctive tests of fetal status that are not commonly used in the United States, such as fetal scalp blood sampling, fetal pulse oximetry or fetal ST-segment analysis. The management recommendations are consistent with those proposed by ACOG [36].

Confirm fetal heart rate and uterine activity

The objective of standardized EFM management is to identify and minimize potential sources of preventable error. The first step is to confirm that the monitor is recording the FHR and uterine activity adequately to permit informed management decisions (Figure 47.9). If external monitoring does not provide adequate information, placement of a fetal scalp electrode and/or intrauterine pressure catheter should be considered.

Evaluate FHR components

Thorough evaluation of a fetal monitor tracing includes assessment of uterine contractions along with all FHR components: baseline rate, variability, accelerations, decelerations, sinusoidal pattern, and changes or trends over time. If a tracing meets criteria for inclusion in Category I, it is considered normal. In low-risk patients, the FHR tracing should be reviewed at least every 30 minutes during the active phase of the first stage of labor and at least every

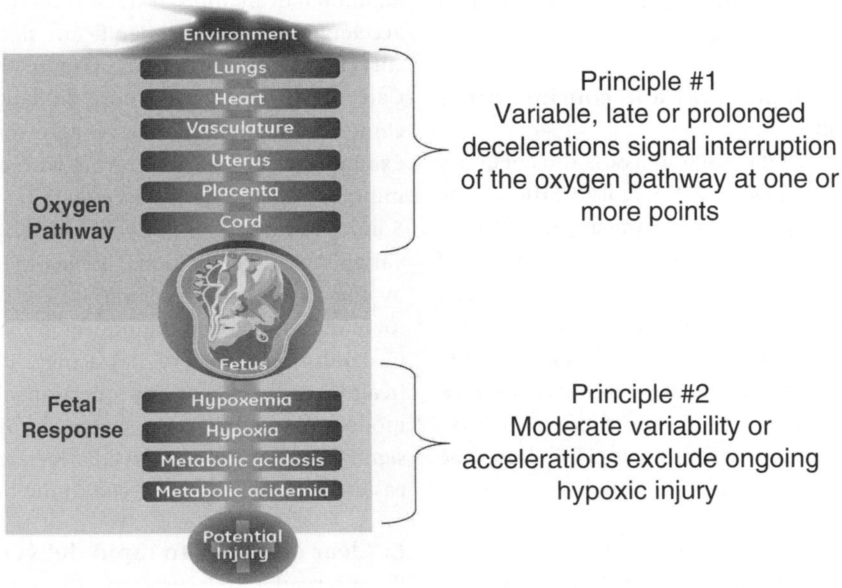

Figure 47.8 Two central principles of electronic intrapartum fetal heart rate monitoring.

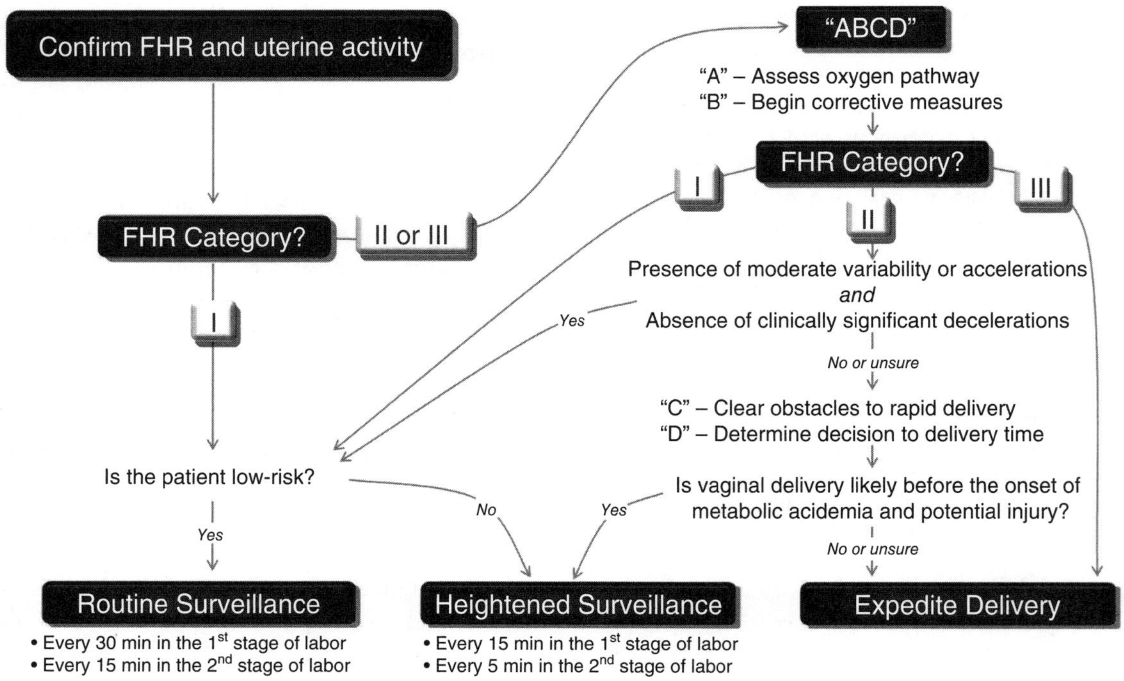

Figure 47.9 Intrapartum FHR monitoring management decision algorithm.

15 minutes during the second stage [29, 63, 64]. In high-risk patients, the corresponding frequency of review is at least every 15 minutes during the active phase of the first stage and at least every 5 minutes during the second stage. As recommended by ACOG and the AWHONN, documentation should be performed periodically [29, 64, 65]. The content and frequency of documentation should be determined by the clinical scenario and applicable institutional policies.

If a FHR tracing does not meet criteria for classification in Category I, a systematic "ABCD" approach can help ensure that important considerations are not overlooked and that decisions are made in a timely fashion (Table 47.7).

A: ***Assess the oxygen pathway and consider other causes of FHR changes

Intrapartum FHR monitoring is used to assess the adequacy of fetal oxygenation during labor. A Category I FHR tracing indicates normal fetal oxygenation. A tracing that moves beyond Category I raises the possibility of interruption of fetal oxygenation at one or more points along the oxygen pathway. Therefore, when a tracing moves beyond Category I, the oxygen pathway should be assessed systematically (Table 47.7). In addition, several factors can affect the FHR tracing by mechanisms other than interruption of oxygenation. The factors summarized in Table 47.8 should be identified and addressed as clinically indicated.

B: Begin corrective measures as indicated

Interruption of the oxygen pathway should be addressed with appropriate conservative corrective measures [36, 62–65]. Table 47.7 summarizes common measures to consider at each level.

Re-evaluate the FHR tracing

After beginning conservative corrective measures, the FHR tracing should be reevaluated within a reasonable time frame. If the tracing returns to Category I, surveillance can be resumed. If the tracing progresses to Category III despite corrective measures, expedited delivery should be considered. Tracings that remain in Category II require additional evaluation. If there is moderate variability and/or accelerations without significant decelerations, continued surveillance is appropriate (Figure 47.9). However, some Category II tracings are more difficult to interpret, and the clinical team might not always agree on the level of risk. One example is a Category II tracing with a normal baseline rate, minimal variability, no accelerations but no decelerations. Some clinicians might be concerned by the lack of moderate variability or accelerations, while others might be comforted by the absence of decelerations. A standardized approach to management can minimize the controversy generated by confusing Category II tracings. If any member of the healthcare team has any question about the presence of moderate variability, the presence of accelerations or the significance of any observed decelerations, the safest and easiest approach is to proceed to the next step.

C: Clear obstacles to rapid delivery

If conservative measures do not correct the FHR tracing to the satisfaction of the clinicians involved, it is prudent to

Table 47.7 A standardized "ABCD" approach to intrapartum EFM management

	"A" **Assess oxygen pathway**	"B" **Begin corrective measures if indicated**		"C" **Clear obstacles to rapid delivery**	"D" **Determine decision to delivery time**
Lungs	An way mid breathing	Supplemental oxygen	Facility	OR availability Equipment	facility response time
Heart	Heart rate and rhythm	Position change Haid bolus Correct hypotension	Staff	Consider notifying: Obstetrician Surgical assistant Anesthesiologist Neonatologist Pediatrician Nursing staff	Consider staff: Avail ability Training Experience
Vasculature	Blood pressure Volume status		Mother	Consider: informed consent Anesthesia options Laboratory tests Blood products intravenous access Urinary catheter Abdominal prep Transfer to OR	Surgical considerations (prior abdominal or uterine surgery) Medical considerations (obesity, hypertension, diabetes, lupus erythematosus (SLE) Obstetric considerations (parity, pelvimetry, placental location)
Uterus	Contraction strength Contraction frequency Baseline uterine tone Exclude uterine rupture	Stop or reduce stimulant Consider uterine relaxant	Fetus	Consider Fetal number Estimated fetal weight Gestational age Presentation Position	Consider factors-such as: Estimated fetal weight Gestational age Presentation Position
Placenta	Placental separation				
Cord	Vaginal exam Exclude cord prolapse	Consider amnioinfusion	Labor	Consider IUPC	Consider factors such as: Arrest disorder Protracted labor Poor expulsive efforts

Table 47.8 Several maternal and fetal factors can influence tie appearance of the FHR tracing but are not specifically related to fetal oxygenation

Factor	Reported FHR associations
Fever/infection	Increased baseline rate, decreased variability
Medications	Effects depend upon specific medication and may include changes in baseline rate, frequency and amplitude of accelerations, variability and sinusoidal pattern
Hyperthyroidism	Tachycardia, decreased variability
Prematurity	Increased baseline rate, decreased variability, reduced frequency and amplitude of accelerations
Fetal anemia	Sinusoidal pattern, tachycardia
Fetal heart block	Bradycardia, decreased variability
Fetal tachyarrhythmia	Variable degrees of tachycardia, decreased variability
Congenital anomaly	Decreased variability, decelerations
Preexisting neurologic abnormality	Decreased variability, absent accelerations
Sleep cycle	Decreased variability, reduced frequency and amplitude of accelerations

plan ahead for the possible rapid delivery. This does not constitute a commitment to a particular time or method of delivery. It simply serves as a reminder of common sources of unnecessary delay so that they can be addressed in a timely manner. Because many of the considerations summarized in Table 47.7 are viewed by clinicians as "common sense", they may be overlooked, potentially jeopardizing patient safety and inviting criticism. One way to address this problem is to use a simple checklist that organizes potential sources of unnecessary delay into major categories and arranges them in non-random order. (See Table 47.7).

D: Decision-to-delivery time

After appropriate conservative measures have been implemented, it is sensible to take a moment to estimate the time needed to accomplish delivery in the event of a sudden emergency. This step should be addressed by the clinician ultimately responsible for performing operative delivery should it become necessary. The time between decision and delivery can be estimated systematically by considering individual characteristics of the facility, staff, mother, fetus, and labor. (Table 47.7)

Delivery

Management steps A, B, C, and D are amenable to standardization and represent the majority of decisions that must be made during labor. However, once they are exhausted, further management decisions require the individual judgment of the clinician who ultimately will assume responsibility for the safety of the mother and the fetus in the event that operative delivery becomes necessary.

Expectant management versus delivery

If conservative measures do not correct a persistent Category II FHR tracing, the clinician must decide whether to continue to await spontaneous vaginal delivery or to proceed with operative delivery. The decision balances the likelihood of safe vaginal delivery against the potential for fetal hypoxic injury. In 2013, Clark and colleagues proposed a standardized approach to the management of persistent Category II FHR tracings [66]. In the setting of moderate variability or accelerations and normal progress in the active phase or second stage of labor, the algorithm permits continued expectant management with close observation in most cases, regardless of the presence of decelerations. One exception is the scenario in which conservative measures fail to correct recurrent significant decelerations remote from delivery. Another is the setting in which vaginal bleeding and/or previous cesarean section(s) introduce the risks of placental abruption or uterine rupture. In such situations, further evaluation may be necessary and adherence to the algorithm should be individualized. Recommended management of prolonged decelerations includes discontinuation of the algorithm and initiation of appropriate corrective measures. If moderate variability and accelerations are absent, and recurrent significant decelerations fail to respond to corrective measures after approximately 30 minutes, delivery should be considered regardless of the stage of labor. If moderate variability and accelerations are absent *without* recurrent decelerations, the algorithm recommends observation for an hour, beyond which time persistence of the pattern warrants consideration of delivery. This algorithm reflects the consensus of 18 authors regarding one reasonable approach to persistent Category II FHR patterns. No single approach to such patterns has been demonstrated to be superior to all others. However, there is a growing body of evidence supporting the concept that the adoption of one appropriate management plan, by virtue of standardization alone, will yield results superior to those achieved by random application of several individually-equivalent approaches [66]. One of the most common preventable errors at this point is to postpone a clinically-necessary but difficult decision in the hope of spontaneous resolution. It is important to recognize that "deciding to wait" is distinctly different from "waiting to decide". The former reflects clinical judgment, while the latter suggests procrastination.

Adjunct methods of intrapartum fetal monitoring

Fetal pulse oximetry

Intrapartum reflectance fetal pulse oximetry is a modification of transmission pulse oximetry that indirectly measures the oxygen saturation of hemoglobin in fetal blood [67]. An intrauterine sensor placed in contact with fetal skin uses the differential absorbtion of red and infrared light by oxygenated and deoxygenated fetal hemoglobin to provide continuous estimation of fetal oxygen saturation. Sensors have been reported to obtain reliable signals 45–60% of the time [68]. In fetal sheep, normal aerobic metabolism is maintained at oxygen saturations above 30% [69, 70]. Below that level, metabolic acidosis, and eventually metabolic acidemia, may develop.

The inconclusive and inconsistent results of a number of randomized trials (References from above) led the manufacturer of the fetal pulse oximeter to announce that it would no longer distribute the sensors needed for the monitors, effectively withdrawing it from the market.

ST segment analysis

Study of the fetal ECG has produced some promising results. The S-T segment of the fetal ECG represents myocardial repolarization. Myocardial hypoxia can lead to elevation of the S-T segment and T wave secondary to catecholamine release, β-adrenoceptor activation, glycogenolysis, and tissue metabolic acidosis [71–73]. These observations led to the development of technology to analyze the fetal ECG plus the S-T waveform analysis (STAN) [74, 75].

A meta-analysis of four studies, including 9829 women, concluded that adjunctive S-T segment analysis was associated with significantly fewer cases of severe metabolic acidemia at birth, fewer cases of neonatal encephalopathy, and fewer operative vaginal deliveries [76]. However, there were no significant differences in cesarean delivery rates, low five-minute Apgar scores or neonatal intensive care unit (NICU) admissions. A recent multi-center randomized trial in the US, including over 11 000 women, showed no significant benefit of STAN in perinatal outcome or operative delivery rates [77].

Summary

The greatest strength of intrapartum EFM is its ability to predict the absence of metabolic acidemia and hypoxic neurologic injury with an extremely high degree of reliability. Its greatest weakness is its inability to predict the presence of these conditions with any clinically relevant accuracy. The false-positive rate of EFM for predicting CP has been reported to exceed 99%, yielding a positive predictive value of less than 1% [28, 29]. Reasonable management decisions cannot be based on the results of a test that it is virtually always wrong. On the other hand, the negative predictive value of EFM is near 100%. A test that is virtually always right is the ideal foundation for rational decision-making. The interpretation and management method described in this chapter uses the exceptional negative predictive value of EFM to formulate a structured, systematic, non-random approach to intrapartum care. Standardization of FHR definitions and simplification of interpretation and management promote safety by reducing unnecessary complexity and minimizing reliance on random recall, consistent with basic principles of patient safety. Standardization and checklists can improve outcomes and reduce liability by providing a framework for clinicians of all educational backgrounds to apply and articulate a plan of management that is evidence-based, factually accurate and reasonable [78, 79].

References

1 Quilligan, E.J. and Paul, R.H. (1975). Fetal monitoring: is it worth it? *Obstet. Gynecol.* **45** (**1**): 96–100.

2 Chan, W.H., Paul, R.H., and Toews, J. (1973). Intrapartum fetal monitoring: maternal and fetal morbidity and perinatal mortality. *Obstet. Gynecol.* **41** (**1**): 7–13.

3 Kelly, V.C. and Kulkarni, D. (1973). Experiences with fetal monitoring in a community hospital. *Obstet. Gynecol.* **41** (**6**): 818–824.

4 Tutera, G. and Newman, R.L. (1975). Fetal monitoring: its effect on the perinatal mortality and caesarean section rates and its complications. *Am. J. Obstet. Gynecol.* **122** (**6**): 750–754.

5 Sibanda, J. and Beard, R.W. (1975). Influence on clinical practice of routine intra-partum fetal monitoring. *Br. Med. J.* **3** (**5979**): 341–343.

6 Shenker, L., Post, R.C., and Seiler, J.S. (1975). Routine electronic monitoring of fetal heart rate and uterine activity during labor. *Obstet. Gynecol.* **46** (**2**): 185–189.

7 Koh, K.S., Greves, D., Yung, S., and Peddle, L.J. (1975). Experience with fetal monitoring in a university teaching hospital. *Can. Med. Assoc. J.* **112** (**4**): 455–456, 459–460.

8 Lee, W.K. and Baggish, M.S. (1976). The effect of unselected intrapartum fetal monitoring. *Obstet. Gynecol.* **47** (**5**): 516–520.

9 Paul, R.H., Huey, J.R. Jr., and Yaeger, C.F. (1977). Clinical fetal monitoring: its effect on cesarean section rate and perinatal mortality: five-year trends. *Postgrad. Med.* **61** (**4**): 160–166.

10 Amato, J.C. (1977). Fetal monitoring in a community hospital. A statistical analysis. *Obstet. Gynecol.* **50** (**3**): 269–274.

11 Johnstone, F.D., Campbell, D.M., and Hughes, G.J. (1978). Has continuous intrapartum monitoring made any impact on fetal outcome? *Lancet* **1** (**8077**): 1298–1300.

12 Hamilton, L.A. Jr., Gottschalk, W., Vidyasagar, D. et al. (1978). Effects of monitoring high-risk pregnancies and intrapartum FHR monitoring on perinates. *Int. J. Gynaecol. Obstet.* **15** (**6**): 483–490.

13 Haverkamp, A.D., Thompson, H.E., McFee, J.G., and Cetrullo, C. (1976). The evaluation of continuous fetal heart rate monitoring in high-risk pregnancy. *Am. J. Obstet. Gynecol.* **125** (**3**): 310–320.

14 Renou, P., Chang, A., Anderson, I., and Wood, C. (1976). Controlled trial of fetal intensive care. *Am. J. Obstet. Gynecol.* **126** (**4**): 470–476.

15 Kelso, I.M., Parsons, R.J., Lawrence, G.F. et al. (1978). An assessment of continuous fetal heart rate monitoring in labor. A randomized trial. *Am. J. Obstet. Gynecol.* **131** (**5**): 526–532.

16 Haverkamp, A.D., Orleans, M., Langendoerfer, S. et al. (1979). A controlled trial of the differential effects of intrapartum fetal monitoring. *Am. J. Obstet. Gynecol.* **134** (**4**): 399–412.

17 Wood, C., Renou, P., Oats, J. et al. (1981). A controlled trial of fetal heart rate monitoring in a low-risk obstetric population. *Am. J. Obstet. Gynecol.* **141** (**5**): 527–534.

18 MacDonald, D., Grant, A., Sheridan-Pereira, M. et al. (1985). The Dublin randomized controlled trial of intrapartum fetal heart rate monitoring. *Am. J. Obstet. Gynecol.* **152** (**5**): 524–539.

19 Neldam, S., Osler, M., Hansen, P.K. et al. (1986). Intrapartum fetal heart rate monitoring in a combined low- and high-risk population: a controlled clinical trial. *Eur. J. Obstet. Gynecol. Reprod. Biol.* **23** (**1–2**): 1–11.

20 Vintzileos, A.M., Antsaklis, A., Varvarigos, I. et al. (1993). A randomized trial of intrapartum electronic fetal heart rate monitoring versus intermittent auscultation. *Obstet. Gynecol.* **81** (**6**): 899–907.

21 Herbst, A. and Ingemarsson, I. (1994). Intermittent versus continuous electronic fetal monitoring in labour: a randomised study. *Br. J. Obstet. Gynaecol.* **101** (**8**): 663–668.

22 Leveno, K.J., Cunningham, F.G., Nelson, S. et al. (1986). A prospective comparison of selective and universal electronic fetal monitoring in 34,995 pregnancies. *N. Engl. J. Med.* **315** (**10**): 615–619.

23 Luthy, D.A., Shy, K.K., van Belle, G. et al. (1987). A randomized trial of electronic fetal monitoring in preterm labor. *Obstet. Gynecol.* **69** (**5**): 687–695.

24 Grant, A., O'Brien, N., Joy, M.Y. et al. (1989 Nov 25). Cerebral palsy among children born during the Dublin randomized trial of intrapartum monitoring. *Lancet* **2** (**8674**): 1233–1236.

25 Alfirevic, Z., Devane, D., and Gyte, G.M. (2006). Continuous cardiotocography (CTG) as a form of electronic fetal monitoring

(EFM) for fetal assessment during labour. *Cochrane Database Syst. Rev.* (**3**): CD006066. doi: 10.1002/14651858.CD006066.

26 Nelson, K.B. and Ellenberg, J.H. (1986). Antecedents of cerebral palsy: multivariate analysis of risk. *N. Engl. J. Med* **315**: 81–86.

27 Blair, E. and Stanley, F.J. (1988). Intrapartum asphyxia: a rare cause of cerebral palsy. *J. Pediatr.* **112**: 515–519.

28 Nelson, K.B., Dambrosia, J.M., Ting, T.Y., and Grether, J.K. (1996). Uncertain value of electronic fetal monitoring in predicting cerebral palsy. *N. Engl. J. Med.* **334** (**10**, **7**): 613–618.

29 American College of Obstetricians and Gynecologists (2009). ACOG practice bulletin number 106: intrapartum fetal heart rate monitoring: nomenclature, interpretation, and general management principles. *Obstet. Gynecol.* **114**: 192–202.

30 (1997). Electronic fetal heart rate monitoring: research guidelines for interpretation. National Institute of Child Health and Human Development research planning workshop. *Am. J. Obstet. Gynecol.* **177** (**6**): 1385–1390.

31 American College of Obstetricians and Gynecologists (2005). ACOG practice bulletin. Clinical management guidelines for obstetricians-gynecologists, number 70 December 2005 (replaces practice bulletin number 62 may 2005). Intrapartum fetal heart rate monitoring. *Obstet. Gynecol.* **106**: 1453–1461.

32 Association of Women's Health, Obstetric and Neonatal Nurses (2005). *Fetal Heart Monitoring: Principles and Practices*, 3rde. Washington, DC: Association of Women's Health, Obstetric and Neonatal Nurses.

33 American College of Nurse-Midwives (2006). *Position Statement: Standardized Nomenclature for Electronic Fetal Monitoring*. Silver Spring, MD: American College of Nurse-Midwives.

34 Macones, G.A., Hankins, G.D., Spong, C.Y. et al. (2008). The 2008 National Institute of Child Health and Human Development workshop report on electronic fetal monitoring: update on definitions, interpretation, and research guidelines. *Obstet. Gynecol.* **112** (**3**): 661–666.

35 American College of Obstetricians and Gynecologists Task Force on Neonatal Encephalopathy and Cerebral Palsy, American College of Obstetricians and Gynecologists, American Academy of Pediatrics (2003). *Neonatal Encephalopathy and Cerebral Palsy: Defining the Pathogenesis and Pathophysiology ACOG*. Washington, DC: AAP.

36 American College of Obstetricians and Gynecologists (2010). Practice bulletin no. management of intrapartum fetal heart rate tracings. *Obstet. Gynecol.* **116**: 1232–1240.

37 American Academy of Pediatrics (2014). *Neonatal Encephalopathy and Neurologic Outcome*, 2nde. American College of Obstetricians and Gynecologists.

38 Nelson, K.B. and Ellenberg, J.H. (1985). Antecedents of cerebral palsy. Univariate analysis of risks. *Am. J. Dis. Child.* **139** (**10**): 1031–1038.

39 Badawi, N., Kurinczuk, J.J., Keogh, J.M. et al. (1998). Intrapartum risk factors for newborn encephalopathy: the western Australian case-control study. *BMJ* **317**: 1554–1558.

40 Suvanand, S., Kapoor, S.K., Reddaiah, V.P. et al. (1997). Risk factors for cerebral palsy. *Indian J. Pediatr.* **64**: 677.

41 Towner, D., Castro, M.A., Eby-Wilkens, E., and Gilbert, W.M. (1999). Effect of mode of delivery in nulliparous women on neonatal intracranial injury. *N. Engl. J. Med.* **341** (**23**): 1709–1714.

42 Martin, C.B. Jr., de Haan, J., van der Wildt, B. et al. (1979). Mechanisms of late decelerations in the fetal heart rate. A study with autonomic blocking agents in fetal lambs. *Eur. J. Obstet. Gynecol. Reprod. Biol.* **9** (**6**): 361–373.

43 Ball, R.H., Espinoza, M.I., and Parer, J.T. (1994). Regional blood flow in asphyxiated fetuses with seizures. *Am. J. Obstet. Gynecol.* **170**: 156–161.

44 Ball, R.H., Parer, J.T., Caldwell, L.E., and Johnson, J. (1994). Regional blood flow and metabolism ovine fetuses during severe cord occlusion. *Am. J. Obstet. Gynecol.* **171**: 1549–1555.

45 Cohn, H.E., Sacks, E.J., Heymann, M.A., and Rudolph, A.M. (1974). Cardiovascular response to hypoxemia and acidemia in fetal lambs. *Am. J. Obstet. Gynecol.* **120**: 817–824.

46 Field, D.R., Parer, J.T., Auslander, R.A. et al. (1990). Cerebral oxygen consumption during asphyxia in fetal sheep. *J. Dev. Physiol.* **14**: 131–137.

47 Itskovitz, J., LaGamma, E.F., and Rudolph, A.M. (1983). The effect of reducing umbilical blood flow on fetal oxygenation. *Am. J. Obstet. Gynecol.* **145**: 813–818.

48 Jensen, A., Roman, C., and Rudolph, A.M. (1991). Effects of reducing uterine blood flow on fetal blood flow distribution and oxygen delivery. *J. Dev. Physiol.* **15**: 309–323.

49 Peeters, L.L., Sheldon, R.D., Jones, M.D. et al. (1979). Blood flow to fetal organs as a function of arterial oxygen content. *Am. J. Obstet. Gynecol.* **135**: 637–646.

50 Reid, D.L., Parer, J.T., Williams, K. et al. (1991). Effects of severe reduction in maternal placental blood flow on blood flow distribution in the sheep fetus. *J. Dev. Physiol.* **15**: 183–188.

51 Richardson, B.S., Rurak, D., Patrick, J.E. et al. (1989). Cerebral oxidative metabolism during prolonged hypoxemia. *J. Dev. Physiol.* **11**: 37–43.

52 Itskovitz, J., LaGamma, E.F., and Rudolph, A.M. (1983). Heart rate and blood pressure responses to umbilical cord compression in fetal lambs with special reference to the mechanism of variable deceleration. *Am. J. Obstet. Gynecol.* **147**: 451–457.

53 Itskovitz, J., LaGamma, E.F., and Rudolph, A.M. (1987). Effect of cord compression on fetal blood flow distribution and O2 delivery. *Am. J. Physiol.* **252**: H100–H109.

54 James, L.S., Yeh, M.N., Morishima, H.O. et al. (1976). Umbilical vein occlusion and transient acceleration of the fetal heart rate. Experimental observations in subhuman primates. *Am. J. Obstet. Gynecol.* **126**: 276–283.

55 Lee, C.Y., Loreto, D., P.C., and O'Lane, J.M. (1975). A study of fetal heart rate acceleration patterns. *Obstet. Gynecol.* **45**: 142–146.

56 Lee, S.T. and Hon, E.H. (1963). Fetal hemodynamic response to umbilical cord compression. *Obstet. Gynecol.* **22**: 553–562.

57 Mueller-Heubach, E. and Battelli, A.F. (1982). Variable heart rate decelerations and transcutaneous PO_2 during umbilical

cord occlusion in fetal monkeys. *Am. J. Obstet. Gynecol.* **144**: 796–802.

58 Siassi, B., Wu, P.Y., Blanco, C., and Martin, C.B. (1979). Baroreceptor and chemorecephtor responses to umbilical cord occlusion in fetal lambs. *Biol. Neonate.* **35**: 66–73.

59 Towell, M.D. and Salvador, H.S. (1971). Compressionof the umbilical cord. In: *An Experimental Model in the Fetal Goat, Fetal Evaluation during Pregnancy and Labor* (ed. P. Crasignoni and G. Pardi), 143–156. New York, NY: Academia Press.

60 Yeh, M.N., Morishima, H.O., Niemann, W.E., and James, L.S. (1975). Myocardial conduction defects in association with compression of the umbilical cord. Experimental observations on fetal baboons. *Am. J. Obstet. Gynecol.* **121**: 951–957.

61 MacLennan, A. (1999). A template for defining a causal relation between acute intrapartum events and cerebral palsy: international consensus statement. *BMJ* **319** (**7216**): 1054–1059.

62 Miller, D.A. and Miller, L.A. (2012). Electronic fetal heart rate monitoring: applying principles of patient safety. *Am. J. Obstet. Gynecol.* **206** (**4**): 278–283.

63 American Academy of Pediatrics (2007). *American College of Obstetricians and Gynecologists: Guidelines for Perinatal Care*, 6the. Washington, DC: American Academy of Pediatrics.

64 ACOG and Association of Women's Health, Obstetric and Neonatal Nurses (2008). *Fetal Heart Monitoring (Position Statement)*. Washington, DC: ACOG.

65 Simpson, K.R. and James, D.C. (2005). Efficacy of intrauterine resuscitation techniques in improving fetal oxygen status during labor. *Obstet. Gynecol.* **105**: 1362–1368.

66 Parer, J.T., King, T., Flanders, S. et al. (2006). Fetal acidemia and electronic fetal heart rate patterns. Is there evidence of an association? *J. Matern. Fetal Neonatal Med.* **19** (**5**): 289–294.

67 Dildy, G.A., Clark, S.L., and Loucks, C.A. (1996a). Intrapartum fetal pulse oximetry: past, present, and future. *Am. J. Obstet. Gynecol.* **175** (**1**): 1–9.

68 Dildy, G.A., Clark, S.L., and Loucks, C.A. (1993). Preliminary experience with intrapartum fetal pulse oximetry in humans. *Obstet. Gynecol.* **81**: 630–635.

69 Oeseburg, B., Ringnalda, B.E.M., Crevels, J. et al. (1992). Fetal oxygenation in chronic maternal hypoxia: what's critical? *Adv. Exp. Med. Biol.* **317**: 499–502.

70 Nijland, R., Jongsma, H.W., Nijhuis, J.G. et al. (1995). Arterial oxygen saturation in relation to metabolic acidosis in fetal lambs. *Am. J. Obstet. Gynecol.* **172**: 810–819.

71 Widmark, C., Jansson, T., Lindecrantz, K., and Rose'n, K.G. (1991). ECG waveform, short term heart rate variability and plasma catecholamine concentrations in response to hypoxia in intrauterine growth retarded Guinea pig fetuses. *Dev. Physiol.* **15**: 161–168.

72 Rosén, K.G., Dagbjartsson, A., Henriksson, B.A. et al. (1984). The relationship between circulating catecholamine and ST waveform in the fetal lamb electrocardiogram during hypoxia. *Am. J. Obstet. Gynecol.* **149**: 190–195.

73 Hökegård, K.H., Eriksson, B.O., Kjellemer, I. et al. (1981). Myocardial metabolism in relation to electrocardiographic changes and cardiac function during graded hypoxia in the fetal lamb. *Acta Physiol. Scand.* **113**: 1–7.

74 Lilja, H., Karlsson, K., Lindecrantz, K., and Rosén, K.G. (1989). Microprocessor based vaveform analysis of the fetal electrocardiogram during labor. *Int. J. Gynecol. Obstet.* **30**: 109–116.

75 Arulkumaran, S., Lilja, H., Lindecrantz, K. et al. (1990). Fetal ECG waveform analysis should improve fetal surveillance in labour. *J. perinatal. Med.* **18**: 13–22.

76 Neilson, J.P. (2006). Fetal electrocardiogram (ECG) for fetal monitoring during labour. *Cochrane Database of Syst. Rev.* (**3**): CD000116. doi: 10.1002/14651858.CD000116.pub2.

77 Belfort, M.A., Saade, G.R., Thom, E. et al. (2015). A randomized rial of intrapartum fetal ECG ST-segment analysis. *N. Engl. J. Med.* **373**: 632–641.

78 Clark, S.L., Belfort, M.A., Byum, S.L. et al. (2008). Improved outcomes, fewer cesarean deliveries, and reduced litigation: results of a new paradigm in patient safety. *Am. J. Obstet. Gynecol.* **199** (**2**): 105e1–105e7.

79 Pettker, C.M., Thung, S.F., Norwitz, E.R. et al. (2009). Impact of a comprehensive patient safety strategy on obstetric adverse events. *Am. J. Obstet. Gynecol.* **200** (**5**): 492.e1–e8.

48

CHAPTER 48
Hydrops fetalis

Joong Shin Park
Department of Obstetrics and Gynecology, Seoul National University College of Medicine, Seoul National University Hospital, Seoul, Korea

CLINICAL SCENARIO

A nulliparous 36-year-old woman in 21 weeks gestation was referred for a cystic chest mass found in the midtrimester screening ultrasonography (USG). Her obstetric history was unremarkable, including serum screening test for Down syndrome.

USG in our center showed multiple cystic and echolucent pulmonary mass filling the left chest of the fetus, with the measured size of $5.14 \times 3.96 \times 3.57\,cm^3$. The mass was displacing the diaphragm toward the abdominal cavity and shifting the mediastinal structure to the right side, resulting in the displacement of the heart but with an intact morphology (Figure 48.1). Congenital pulmonary airway malformation (CPAM) was diagnosed after defining arterial supply from pulmonary artery. There were also findings of accompanying hydrops, including scalp edema and ascites. During the follow-up in outpatient clinic, the size of the cystic mass was increased up to 7.68 cm, with aggravation of hydrops at 24^{+5} weeks of gestation (Figures 48.2 and 48.3).

After counseling, we decided to perform a thoracoamniotic shunt. After injection of vecuronium into the umbilical cord for fetal sedation, thoracoamniotic shunt was placed under ultrasound guidance (Figure 48.4). After the procedure, the size of CPAM remained small and neither increase in the cystic size nor newly developed ascites was noted. In her 32 weeks of gestation, a 1.7 kg male baby was delivered because of premature rupture of membrane and preterm labor. The Apgar scores were 3 and 5 at one and five minutes respectively. After birth, the baby was admitted to neonatal intensive care unit (NICU) and was diagnosed as CPAM. The thoracoamniotic shunt was removed at bed side, and Lt. lobectomy operation was done 10 days later after birth.

Background

Hydrops fetalis is usually defined as the accumulation of excessive fluid in at least two fetal extravascular compartments and body cavities including scalp edema, body wall edema, pericardial effusion, pleural effusions, and ascites. Classically, it has been divided into two main entities based on etiology: immune (related to maternal alloimmunization to red cell antigens) and non-immune (related to a diversity of other causes). With the widespread use of Rhesus immune globulin for the prevention of RhD alloimmunization, most cases of hydrops were nonimmune [1]. Non-immune hydrops may be caused by a variety of conditions such as cardiovascular disorders, chromosomal abnormalities, infectious diseases, twin-to-twin transfusion syndrome, metabolic disorders, hematologic disorders, lymphatic dysplasia, structural anomalies(just like this scenario for CPAM), or tumors. However, in one third of the cases, the etiology is unknown.

Development of fetal hydrops associated with CPAM is caused by an impaired venous return because of compression of the vena cava or heart [2]. Polyhydramnios can be developed by decreased fetal swallowing amniotic fluid or by increased secretion of amniotic fluid by the CPAM. In about 10% of the cases, additional extra-pulmonary abnormalities may be found, such as cardiac failure, renal dysfunction, central nervous abnormalities, and gastrointestinal defects [3].

CPAM is a pulmonary mass derived from proliferation of bronchial structures, with an incidence of between 1 : 250 000 and 1 : 35 000 in livebirths [4–6]. The prognosis is highly variable, depending on the presence of fetal hydrops or the size of the mass [7]. The large mass size and secondary sequelae, including mediastinal shift, pulmonary hypoplasia, polyhydramnios, and hydrops are associated with adverse outcomes [8]. In the presence of large dominant cyst and hydrops, percutaneous aspiration or thoracoamniotic shunting can be considered [9].

Evidence-Based Obstetrics and Gynecology, First Edition. Edited by Errol R. Norwitz, Carolyn M. Zelop, David A. Miller, and David L. Keefe.

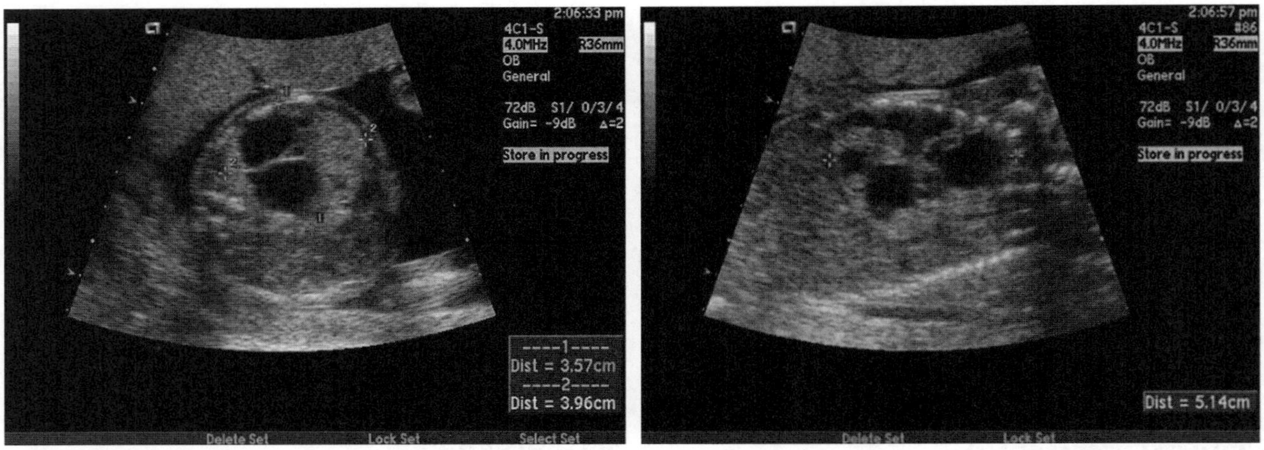

Figure 48.1 Congenital pulmonary airway malformation at presentation.

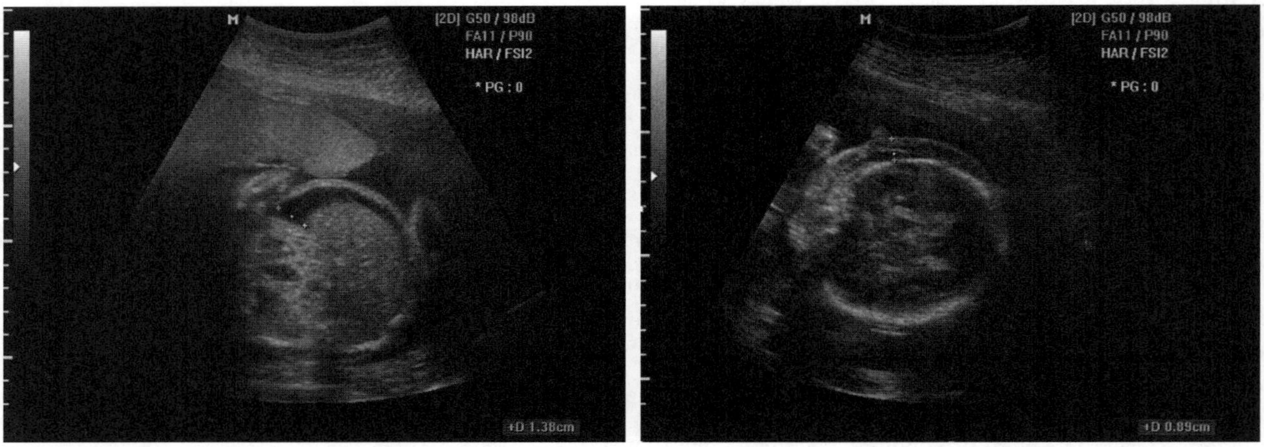

Figure 48.2 Associated findings of fetal hydrops (left: ascites, right: anasarca).

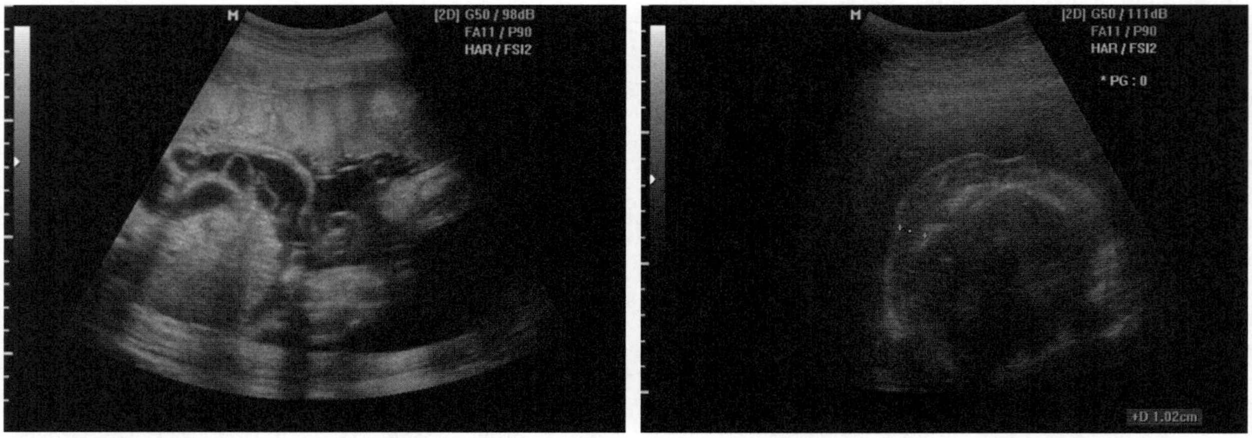

Figure 48.3 Aggravation of fetal hydrops at 24^{+5} weeks of gestation.

Although still controversial, treatment of choice after birth is complete resection of the CPAM even in asymptomatic neonates, because of the risks of infection and occult malignant transformation [10]. And the long term outcome of infants with CPAM following resection is usually excellent.

Clinical questions

In order to address the issues of most relevance to your patient and to help in searching the literature for the evidence regarding these issues, you should structure your clinical questions as recommended in Chapter 1.

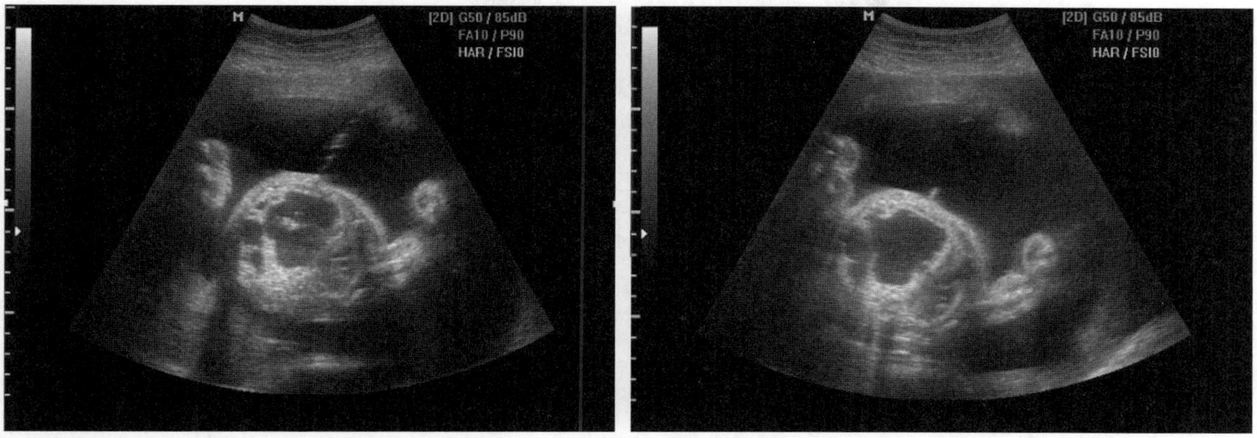

Figure 48.4 In utero treatments of thoracoamniotic shunting.

1. In cases with nonimmune hydrops fetalis, what is the distribution of the etiologies and rate of the occurrence?
2. How can we approach the diagnostic steps for underlying cause in cases with hydrops fetalis?
3. What is the chance of survival in cases with nonimmune hydrops fetalis?
4. How can we make the diagnosis of fetal CPAM and predict prognosis?
5. What's the in-utero treatment in CPAM?

Critical appraisal of the literature

1. In cases with non-immune hydrops fetalis, what is the distribution of the etiologies and rate of the occurrence?

Hydrops fetalis is nonspecific condition, as the final stage of a wide variety of disorders. With the widespread use of Rhesus immune globulin for the prevention of RhD alloimmunization, most remaining cases of hydrops fetalis are nonimmune. Nonimmune hydrops fetalis has a multifactorial cause as follows; cardiovascular, hematologic, chromosomal, syndromic, lymphatic dysplasia, inborn errors of metabolism, infectious, thoracic, urinary tract malformations, extra thoracic tumors, placental (twin to twin transfusion syndrome), gastrointestinal, and idiopathic. Understanding of the underlying disorder in cases with hydrops fetalis is very important for adequate management. However, the direct mechanisms responsible for generating hydrops fetalis are still unclear. The generalized edema of hydrops fetalis may particularly result from high interstitial fluid accumulation by low plasma oncotic pressure, high central venous pressure and reduced lymphatic flow owing to multi-organ failure in various pathologic conditions [11]. A large number of studies have investigated the etiologic classification in cases with nonimmune hydrops fetalis. Several systemic reviews and observational studies have addressed various causative disorders of the nonimmune hydrops fetalis and their percentage among the causes (Table 48.1). Although cardiovascular disorders including cardiac structural anomalies and rhythmic disorders are the most common cause of nonimmune hydrops fetalis, there are considerable hydropic cases with unknown etiology (idiopathic). After exclusion of the main causes of hydrops fetalis, hereditary disorder should be considered in unexplained cases. Metabolic disease, including lysosomal storage disease, is found in 1–2% of all nonimmune hydrops fetalis cases [26, 27]. The diagnosis of metabolic disease can be performed using cultured amniotic fluid cells for specific metabolites. In the South-East Asian population, alpha-thalassemia is common etiology of nonimmune hydrops fetalis [15, 16].

2. How can we approach the diagnostic steps for underlying cause in cases with hydrops fetalis?

Following the sonographic diagnosis of hydrops fetalis, the first step is to differentiate between immune and non-immune causes. This can be carried out by the maternal ABO/Rh blood typing and indirect Coombs test to screen for antibodies associated with blood group incompatibility. After the exclusion of immune causes, each potential condition of non-immune hydrops should be considered sequentially to find out the underlying disorder.

Careful sonographic scanning is one of the most important steps for identification of fetal structural anomalies or fetal tumors. And then, a comprehensive fetal echocardiography should be performed to examine cardiac structural or rhythmic abnormalities. A decrease of cardiac output with right atrial overload can be the primary cause in most cases of early hydrops fetalis. Inadequate cardiac output results from major cardiac anomalies such as atrioventricular septal defect, fast ventricular rate with suboptimal filling of the ventricles, or cardiomyopathy [28]. Doppler examination of middle cerebral artery (MCA) should also be performed to rule out fetal anemia as the cause of hydrops fetalis. An elevated peak systolic velocity of the MCA has been associated with fetal anemia even in cases of non-immune hydrops fetalis [29]. If the pregnant woman has a previous obstetric history of stillbirth or a hydrops fetus, lysosomal

Table 48.1 Distribution of cases with nonimmune hydrops fetalis in relation to etiologic classification

Study	No. of cases	Cardiovascular	Hematologic	Chromosomal	Syndromic	Lymphatic	Metabolic	Infectious	Thoracic	Urinary	Placental	Miscellaneous	Idiopathic
Hansmann et al. [12]	402	71	39	47	18	89		11	23	9		31	64
	100%	17.7%	9.7%	11.7%	4.5%	22.1%	0.0%	2.7%	5.7%	2.2%	0.0%	7.7%	15.9%
Machin [13]	1345	370	163	172		17	19	61	132	53	86	93	179
	100%	28%	12%	13%	0%	1%	1%	5%	10%	4%	6%	7%	13%
McCoy et al. [14]	82	19	4	13	9			3	11		5		18
	100%	23%	5%	16%	11%	0%	0%	4%	13%	0%	6%	0%	22%
Anandakumar et al. [15]	100	23	23	10	9			2	5		4		24
	100%	23%	23%	10%	9%	0%	0%	2%	5%	0%	4%	0%	24%
Yang et al. [16]	78	15	25	5		2		2	2			7	20
	100%	19%	32%	6%	0%	3%	0%	3%	3%	0%	0%	9%	26%
Lallemand et al. [17]	94	13		31	4	1		15	3	3	8	7	9
	100%	14%	0%	33%	4%	1%	0%	16%	3%	3%	9%	7%	10%
Swain et al. [18]	40	6	1	3	4			7	1	1	3		14
	100%	15%	3%	8%	10%	0%	0%	18%	3%	3%	8%	0%	35%
Heinonen et al. [19]	58	3		26	16			4	3			3	3
	100%	5%	0%	45%	28%	0%	0%	7%	5%	0%	0%	5%	5%
Ismail et al. [20]	55	5		14		6		8	6		3	2	11
	100%	9%	0%	25%	0%	11%	0%	15%	11%	0%	5%	4%	20%
Sohan et al. [1]	83	11	1	23	5	11		13	1		7	2	9
	100%	13%	1%	28%	6%	13%	0%	16%	1%	0%	8%	2%	11%
Hofstaetter et al. [21]	95	28		11		15		14	5		5	6	11
	100%	29%	0%	12%	0%	16%	0%	15%	5%	0%	5%	6%	12%
Simpson et al. [22]	30	6	3			3		1			6	1	10
	100%	20%	10%	0%	0%	10%	0%	3%	0%	0%	20%	3%	33%
Abrams et al. [23]	571	144	30	45	21	10	5	40	21		54	44	157
	100%	25%	5%	8%	4%	2%	1%	7%	4%	0%	9%	8%	27%
Czernik et al. [24]	68	12	8	4		17		2			4	6	15
	100%	18%	12%	6%	0%	25%	0%	3%	0%	0%	6%	9%	22%
Santo et al. [25]	71	6	1	2	2			12	13			4	31
	100%	8%	1%	3%	3%	0%	0%	17%	18%	0%	0%	6%	44%
Total (%)	3172	23.10%	9.40%	12.80%	2.80%	5.40%	0.80%	6.20%	7.10%	2.10%	5.80%	6.50%	17.80%

storage diseases should be considered. The precise maternal history should be also gathered regarding exposure to patients with *fifth disease* due to parvovirus B19. Parvovirus B19 is a potent inhibitor of hematopoiesis because it infects erythroid precursor cells. Infection with parvovirus B19 usually occurs through respiratory droplets, but it can be transmitted by blood and blood-derived products, and may also be transmitted vertically from mother to fetus. Maternal symptoms appear approximately 10–14 days after infection in about half of infected women, and the symptoms of infection include fever, arthralgia, and an exanthema on the upper body [30]. Parvovirus B19 IgM antibodies become detectable in maternal serum within 7–10 days after infection, peak at 10–14 days, and then decrease within two to three months. IgG antibodies rise more slowly and reach a plateau at four weeks after infection. The next step in diagnostic approach is usually maternal venipuncture. Maternal blood is used for serologic examinations such as syphilis, toxoplasmosis, rubella, cytomegalovirus, herpes simplex virus, and parvovirus. Amniocentesis or cordocentesis is performed for evaluation of chromosomal abnormalities, lysosomal disease, or viral infections. Fluorescent in situ hybridization (FISH) for major chromosomal abnormalities and polymerase chain reaction (PCR) for viral infections have shortened the time required to get the results of amniocentesis (Figure 48.5).

3. What is the chance of survival in cases with non-immune hydrops fetalis?

Although perinatal survival for non-immune hydrops fetalis has improved with advances in perinatal/neonatal medicine, the prognosis of non-immune hydrops fetalis is still problematic. The survival rate varied over a wide range depending on the underlying causes of hydrops fetalis [20, 23, 31]. Intrauterine interventions such as fetal transfusion for fetal anemia or laser coagulation for twin-to-twin transfusion syndrome are expected to improve the prognosis of hydrops fetalis, but the mortality rates reported by Simpson et al. were similar between the time periods 1990–1999 and 2000–2004 [22]. In a literature review, the survival rate of non-immune hydrops fetalis was 27% and 52% in prenatal and postnatal studies, respectively [25]. In the series of postnatal studies the survival rate with a wide range may result from diverse preterm delivery rates and neonatal care unit facilities. Postnatal studies also have the selection bias of only newborns that survive to birth excluding intrauterine fetal deaths and cases with termination of pregnancy. A study reviewed 30 cases with non-immune hydrops fetalis diagnosed in the first trimester reported that all cases resulted in abortion, intrauterine fetal death, or termination of pregnancy [32]. Therefore, the actual mortality rate among the cases with hydrops fetalis might be higher than that reported in the postnatal studies. The rate of survival beyond 28 days was between 8.6% and 47.9% in prenatal studies of non-immune hydrops fetalis (Table 48.2). The mortality rate was between 43% and 67% in live births with non-immune hydrops fetalis (Table 48.3).

4. How can we make the diagnosis of fetal CPAM and predict prognosis?

The CPAM can be diagnosed by antenatal ultrasound with a sonographic appearance of a cystic mass or solid echodense mass occupying a part or all of fetal thorax, with an absence of systemic blood supply. In color Doppler, arterial blood

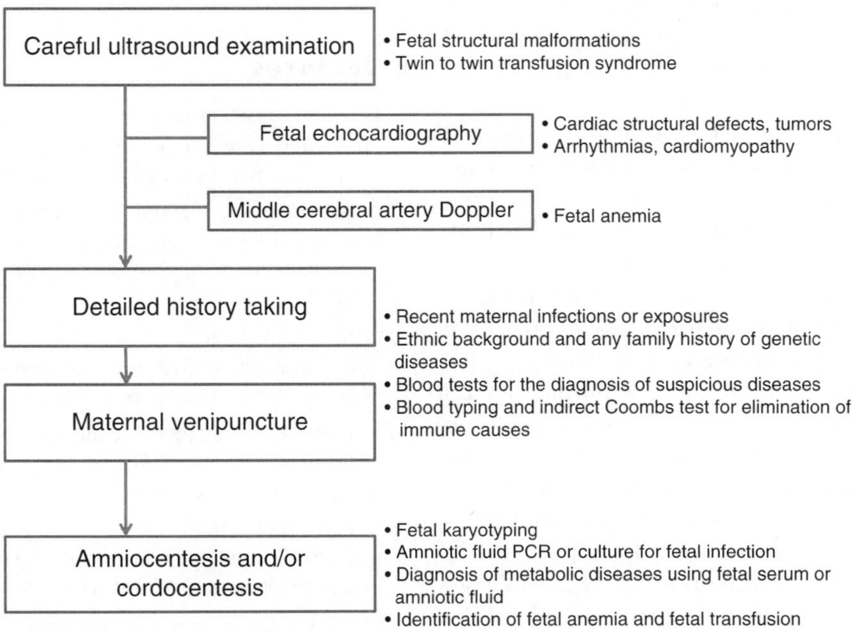

Figure 48.5 Flowchart for diagnostic approach of non-immune hydrops fetalis.

Table 48.2 Pregnancy outcome in prenatal studies of nonimmune hydrops fetalis

Study	Case number	Live birth	Termination pregnancy	Intrauterine death	Survival > 28 days (%)
McCoy et al. [14]	82	40		42	11 (13.4)
Swain et al. [18]	40	12	4	24	5 (12.5)
Heinonen et al. [19]	58	7	42	9	5 (8.6)
Ismail et al. [20]	55	24	21	10	15 (27.3)
Sohan et al. [1]	83	36	31	16	25 (30.1)
Santo et al. [25]	71	44	15	12	34 (47.9)
Total (%)	389	41.9	29.0	29.0	24.4

Table 48.3 Survival rate among live births with nonimmune hydrops fetalis

Study	Case number	Survivors (%)
Nakayama et al. [33]	51	21 (41.2)
Haverkamp et al. [34]	107	61 (57.0)
Simpson et al. [22]	30	10 (33.3)
Abrams et al. [23]	409	223 (54.5)
Czernik et al. [24]	68	28 (41.2)
Total	665	343 (51.5)

flow from pulmonary artery can be determined, and this can be used in the differential diagnosis from bronchopulmonary sequestration, which derives their blood supply from the systemic feeding vessel [35]. Other differential diagnoses of fetal thoracic masses include congenital diaphragmatic hernia, bronchogenic cyst, mediastinal cystic hygroma, bronchial atresia, or stenosis.

CPAM is subdivided into three types (type I, II, and III) based on their pathologic criteria proposed by Stocker et al. [36] and into two types (macrocystic and microcystic) based on their sonographic appearances in the classification proposed by Adzick et al. [37].

Known prenatal prognostic factors include the size and type of the mass, progression or regression of the mass size, cardiac axis deviation/mediastinum shift, development of hydrops and the presence of other anomalies [38]. Large cystic mass and microcystic type might have poor prognosis. There can be a mediastinal shifting because of compression effect of the mass and up to 15% of cases have bilateral involvement. And arising of fetal hydrops is the poorest prognostic feature. Unfortunately, no biochemical or sonographic markers have been available for prediction of regression or progress to hydrops. Recently, CVR (the CPAM volume ratio; obtained by dividing the CPAM volume by the head circumference) is known to be a useful sonographic indicator. The risk of developing hydrops is 80% in cases with CVR > 1.6, whereas the risk is only 2% in cases with CVR < 1.6 [39]. Fetal echocardiography also should be performed in all cases because there can be impaired cardiac function in large CPAMs and an increased risk of associated congenital cardiac anomalies.

5. What's the in-utero treatment in CPAM?

During antenatal period, the prognosis is generally good and fetal intervention for CPAM is not usually indicated. But in specific situations, in utero therapy may be required for fetal survival [8]. The decision for in utero therapy is made by some factors such as the development of fetal hydrops, presence of other associated anomalies, and gestational age. In cases considering fetal therapy, karyotyping may be performed.

In fetus with hydrops at 32 weeks or later, delivery and postnatal treatment for CPAM is usually planned. EXIT (ex-utero intrapartum treatment)-to-resection may be indicated in severe cases with mediastinal shift making ventilation difficult. In the fetus with a macrocystic CPAM and hydrops at 32 weeks or earlier, then fetal intervention like thoracoamniotic shunting can be considered. If the fetus is less than 32 weeks and there is no large cyst, an open maternal-fetal surgery such as fetal thoracotomy/lobectomy might be considered, but the evidence on the usefulness of fetal surgery is limited until now [9, 40].

References

1 Sohan, K. et al. (2001). Analysis of outcome in hydrops fetalis in relation to gestational age at diagnosis, cause and treatment. *Acta Obstetricia et Gynecologica Scandinavica* **80** (**8**): 726–730.

2 Wilson, R.D. et al. (2006). Cystic adenomatoid malformation of the lung: review of genetics, prenatal diagnosis, and in utero treatment. *American Journal of Medical Genetics. Part A* **140** (**2**): 151–155.

3 Schott, S. et al. (2009). Cystic adenomatoid malformation of the lung causing hydrops fetalis: case report and review of the literature. *Archives of Gynecology and Obstetrics* **280** (**2**): 293–296.

4 Laberge, J.M. et al. (2001). Outcome of the prenatally diagnosed congenital cystic adenomatoid lung malformation: a Canadian experience. *Fetal Diagnosis and Therapy* **16** (**3**): 178–186.

5 Laberge, J.M., Bratu, I., and Flageole, H. (2004). The management of asymptomatic congenital lung malformations. *Paediatric Respiratory Reviews* **5** (**Suppl A**): S305–S312.

6 Calvert, J.K. et al. (2006). Outcome of antenatally suspected congenital cystic adenomatoid malformation of the lung: 10 years' experience 1991-2001. *Archives of Disease in Childhood. Fetal and neonatal edition* **91** (**1**): F26–F28.

7 Gornall, A.S. et al. (2003). Congenital cystic adenomatoid malformation: accuracy of prenatal diagnosis, prevalence and outcome in a general population. *Prenatal Diagnosis* **23** (**12**): 997–1002.

8 Grethel, E.J. et al. (2007). Fetal intervention for mass lesions and hydrops improves outcome: a 15-year experience. *Journal of Pediatric Surgery* **42** (**1**): 117–123.

9 Adzick, N.S. et al. (1998). Fetal lung lesions: management and outcome. *American Journal of Obstetrics and Gynecology* **179** (**4**): 884–889.

10 Tsai, A.Y. et al. (2008). Outcomes after postnatal resection of prenatally diagnosed asymptomatic cystic lung lesions. *Journal of Pediatric Surgery* **43** (**3**): 513–517.

11 Bellini, C. et al. (2009). Etiology of nonimmune hydrops fetalis: a systematic review. *American Journal of Medical Genetics Part A* **149A** (**5**): 844–851.

12 Hansmann, M., Gembruch, U., and Bald, R. (1989). New therapeutic aspects in nonimmune hydrops fetalis based on four hundred and two prenatally diagnosed cases. *Fetal Therapy* **4** (**1**): 29–36.

13 Machin, G.A. (1989). Hydrops revisited: literature review of 1,414 cases published in the 1980s. *American Journal of Medical Genetics* **34** (**3**): 366–390.

14 McCoy, M.C. et al. (1995). Non-immune hydrops after 20 weeks' gestation: review of 10 years' experience with suggestions for management. *Obstetrics and Gynecology* **85** (**4**): 578–582.

15 Anandakumar, C. et al. (1996). Management of non-immune hydrops: 8 years' experience. *Ultrasound in Obstetrics & Gynecology* **8** (**3**): 196–200.

16 Yang, Y.H. et al. (1998). Etiology and outcome of hydrops fetalis. *Journal of the Formosan Medical Association* **97** (**1**): 16–20.

17 Lallemand, A.V., Doco-Fenzy, M., and Gaillard, D.A. (1999). Investigation of nonimmune hydrops fetalis: multidisciplinary studies are necessary for diagnosis – review of 94 cases. *Pediatric and Developmental Pathology* **2** (**5**): 432–439.

18 Swain, S. et al. (1999). Prenatal diagnosis and management of nonimmune hydrops fetalis. *The Australian & New Zealand Journal of Obstetrics & Gynaecology* **39** (**3**): 285–290.

19 Heinonen, S., Ryynanen, M., and Kirkinen, P. (2000). Etiology and outcome of second trimester non-immunologic fetal hydrops. *Acta Obstetricia et Gynecologica Scandinavica* **79** (**1**): 15–18.

20 Ismail, K.M. et al. (2001). Etiology and outcome of hydrops fetalis. *The Journal of Maternal-Fetal Medicine* **10** (**3**): 175–181.

21 Hofstaetter, C. et al. (2006). A cardiovascular profile score in the surveillance of fetal hydrops. *The Journal of Maternal-Fetal & Neonatal Medicine* **19** (**7**): 407–413.

22 Simpson, J.H. et al. (2006). Severity of non-immune hydrops fetalis at birth continues to predict survival despite advances in perinatal care. *Fetal Diagnosis and Therapy* **21** (**4**): 380–382.

23 Abrams, M.E. et al. (2007). Hydrops fetalis: a retrospective review of cases reported to a large national database and identification of risk factors associated with death. *Pediatrics* **120** (**1**): 84–89.

24 Czernik, C. et al. (2011). Hydrops fetalis – has there been a change in diagnostic spectrum and mortality? *The Journal of Maternal-Fetal & Neonatal Medicine* **24** (**2**): 258–263.

25 Santo, S. et al. (2011). Prenatal diagnosis of non-immune hydrops fetalis: what do we tell the parents? *Prenatal Diagnosis* **31** (**2**): 186–195.

26 Jauniaux, E. et al. (1990). Nonimmune hydrops fetalis associated with genetic abnormalities. *Obstetrics and Gynecology* **75** (**3**): 568–572.

27 Burin, M.G. et al. (2004). Investigation of lysosomal storage diseases in nonimmune hydrops fetalis. *Prenatal Diagnosis* **24** (**8**): 653–657.

28 Jauniaux, E. (1997). Diagnosis and management of early non-immune hydrops fetalis. *Prenatal Diagnosis* **17** (**13**): 1261–1268.

29 Hernandez-Andrade, E. et al. (2004). Fetal middle cerebral artery peak systolic velocity in the investigation of non-immune hydrops. *Ultrasound in Obstetrics & Gynecology* **23** (**5**): 442–445.

30 de Jong, E.P. et al. (2006). Parvovirus B19 infection in pregnancy. *Journal of Clinical Virology* **36** (**1**): 1–7.

31 Huang, H.R. et al. (2007). Prognostic factors and clinical features in liveborn neonates with hydrops fetalis. *American Journal of Perinatology* **24** (**1**): 33–38.

32 Has, R. (2001). Non-immune hydrops fetalis in the first trimester: a review of 30 cases. *Clinical and Experimental Obstetrics & Gynecology* **28** (**3**): 187–190.

33 Nakayama, H. et al. (1999). Long-term outcome of 51 liveborn neonates with non-immune hydrops fetalis. *Acta Paediatrica* **88** (**1**): 24–28.

34 Haverkamp, F. et al. (2000). Good prognosis for psychomotor development in survivors with nonimmune hydrops fetalis. *BJOG* **107** (**2**): 282–284.

35 Duncombe, G., Dickinson, J.E., and Kikiros, C.S. (2002). Prenatal diagnosis and management of congenital cystic adenomatoid malformation of the lung. *American Journal of Obstetrics and Gynecology* **187** (**4**): 950–954.

36 Stocker, J.T., Madewell, J.E., and Drake, R.M. (1977). Congenital cystic adenomatoid malformation of the lung. Classification and morphologic spectrum. *Human Pathology* **8** (**2**): 155–171.

37 Adzick, N.S. et al. (1985). Fetal cystic adenomatoid malformation: prenatal diagnosis and natural history. *Journal of Pediatric Surgery* **20** (**5**): 483–488.

38 Bunduki, V. et al. (2000). Prognostic factors associated with congenital cystic adenomatoid malformation of the lung. *Prenatal Diagnosis* **20** (**6**): 459–464.

39 Crombleholme, T.M. et al. (2002). Cystic adenomatoid malformation in prenatally diagnosed cystic volume ratio predicts outcome adenomatoid malformation of the lung. *Journal of Pediatric Surgery* **37** (**3**): 331–337.

40 Hedrick, H.L. et al. (2005). The ex utero intrapartum therapy procedure for high-risk fetal lung lesions. *Journal of Pediatric Surgery* **40** (**6**): 1038–1044.

CHAPTER 49
Malpresentation

Joseph G. Ouzounian and Shivani R. Patel
Division of Maternal-Fetal Medicine, Department of Obstetrics and Gynecology, University of Southern California, Keck School of Medicine, Los Angeles, CA, USA

Background

In early pregnancy fetuses have a variable lie within the uterus. As the pregnancy approaches the latter part of the third trimester, the majority of singleton pregnancies have a longitudinal lie and the fetus enters the pelvis with a cephalic presentation. In 3–4% of singleton pregnancies, the fetus is in a breech presentation at term, with the fetal buttocks entering the pelvis before the head [1]. Transverse lie, compound presentation, face presentation, and brow presentation together account for less than 1% of fetal positions at term. Such noncephalic presentations are referred to as malpresentation. In the past, many patients with breech presentation were delivered vaginally with the use of forceps. In recent years, however, the morbidity and mortality associated with this method and a lack of experienced clinicians has led practicing obstetricians to avoid this method of vaginal delivery. External cephalic version (ECV) can be considered in an effort to turn a fetus into a cephalic presentation and attempt vaginal delivery; otherwise, cesarean deliveries are performed.

Clinical questions

Critical appraisal of the literature

1. In patients with late third trimester malpresentation (population) what percentage (diagnostic test characteristics) are associated with known risk factors of breech presentation (outcome)?

There are numerous etiologies that are thought to cause late third trimester malpresentation. Maternal causes include uterine anomalies, uterine fibroids, uterine relaxation from increased parity, and a history of a breech delivery. Pregnancy related factors include polyhydramnios, oligohydramnios, fetal anomalies such as anencephaly, and site of placental implantation have all been linked to breech presentations in the third trimester.

Rayl et al. studied the characteristics associated with breech presentation, and reported that as birthweight decreased there was a continuous increase in the risk of malpresentation with every 500 g decrease in weight resulting in a 1.3-fold (95% CI 1.26–1.38) increase in the risk of breech presentation [2]. Their study also showed that with every five-year increase in maternal age the risk of breech presentation increased by 1.28-fold (95% CI 1.22–1.33). Furthermore, nulliparous women appeared to be at increased risk, and that with every week advancing gestational age the odds ratio for breech presentation decreased by 9% (OR 0.91, 95% CI 0.80–0.93) [2]. Other risk factors identified were fetal congenital anomalies (OR 2.1, 95% CI 1.7–2.7), maternal diabetes (OR 2.8, 95% CI 1.4–5.4), and smoking during pregnancy (1.3, 95% CI 1.2–1.4) [2].

Malpresentation can recur in subsequent pregnancies. Ford et al. evaluated the recurrence risk for breech presentation and showed that the relative risk for breech presentation in a second pregnancy was 3.2 (95% CI 2.8–3.6) and in a third pregnancy 13.9 (95% CI 8.8–22.1) [3]. Luterkort et al. also showed that fetuses in breech presentation had a smaller birth weight (3190 g vs. 3595 g) compared to those in vertex presentation [4]. It has been shown that in cases of breech presentation, 72.6% of the time the placenta is implanted in the cornual/fundal region while in cases of cephalic presentation this occurs in 4.8% of cases [5]. Finally, Dunn et al. evaluated pregnancies complicated by breech presentation at term and found that 22% of multiparous patients had a history of a breech delivery, further reinforcing this as a risk factor for malpresentation in subsequent pregnancies [6].

2. In patients with third trimester malpresentation (population) what is the effectiveness of cesarean delivery (intervention) in improving maternal and fetal outcomes (outcomes) compared to planned breech vaginal delivery (control)?

In current obstetric practice, most fetuses with malpresentation at term are delivered via cesarean section. Vaginal

Evidence-Based Obstetrics and Gynecology, First Edition. Edited by Errol R. Norwitz, Carolyn M. Zelop, David A. Miller, and David L. Keefe.

breech deliveries used to be common practice amongst obstetricians, but that has changed with a lack of experienced operators and the continued debate regarding the safety of breech vaginal delivery.

Cheng et al. published a review demonstrating that perinatal mortality was higher in breech infants delivered vaginally compared to those delivered via cesarean section (OR3.86, 95% CI 2.22–6.69) [7]. They also showed that maternal morbidity and mortality was lower in the planned vaginal delivery group than cesarean section group (OR 0.61, 95% CI 0.47–0.80) [7]. Golfier et al. looked at the difference in outcomes between planned vaginal breech delivery and cesarean section and found increased risks of a five minute APGAR <7 (relative risk (RR) 3.05, 95% CI 1.03–9.05), minor neurologic damage 1.7% vs. 0%, $p < 0.001$), fetal obstetrical trauma (RR 4.24, 95% CI 1.66–10.8), and infant transfer to the intensive care unit (RR 3.23, 95%CI 1.57–6.64) [8]. Overall maternal morbidity between the two groups showed no difference in this study (RR 0.65, 95%CI 0.44–0.94) [8]. Conversely, Irion et al. found that the rate of neonatal mortality (1.0% vs. 0.3%, $p = 0.38$) and neonatal morbidity (4.5% vs. 2.6%, $p = 0.22$) did not differ between the two groups, but that maternal morbidity was lower in the vaginal breech delivery group (17.7% vs. 28.1%, $p = 0.001$) [9]. Most recently the Term Breech Trial was published as the largest study looking at maternal and fetal outcomes from vaginal breech deliveries compared to breech cesarean deliveries [10]. In that study, perinatal/neonatal mortality or serious neonatal morbidity was lower in the planned cesarean section group when compared to the planned vaginal birth group (11.6% vs. 5.0%, $p < 0.0001$) [10]. There was no difference, however, in maternal mortality or serious morbidity between the two groups (3.9% vs. 3.2%, $p = 0.35$) [10].

Studies assessing long term outcome of breech infants in relation to route of delivery are limited. Danielian et al. showed that long-term handicap was no different in the two groups (20.7% in the elective cesarean group and 18.7% in the planned vaginal birth group) [11]. A follow-up to the Term Breech Trial was done which showed that there was no difference in risk of death or neurodevelopmental delay at age 2 between children born via vaginal breech delivery or breech cesarean section (2.8% vs. 3.1%, $p = 0.85$) [12].

In summary, current evidence appears to show that breech cesarean section may be safer for the infant in the perinatal period (Level I-A), but information regarding long-term outcome is less clear (Level II-B). Conversely, maternal morbidity appears to be decreased with vaginal breech delivery when compared to elective cesarean section (Level I-A).

3. In patients with third trimester malpresentation (population) what are the risks of undergoing external cephalic version (intervention and outcome) compared to not undergoing ECV (control)?

ECV is one option to potentially avoid cesarean delivery or a breech vaginal delivery with a case of malpresentation. However, ECV itself entails risk Pregnancy complications from ECV include rupture of membranes, labor, placental abruption, fetal heart rate abnormalities, and procedure failure. Maternal complications include pain and discomfort, bleeding, uterine rupture, and contractions.

Many of the studies done looking at the risks of ECV are small and many times without adequate power to reach significance. Thus, four review articles have been published pooling the data from smaller studies to provide information regarding the risk of ECV. In a study done by Nassar et al. 399 women identified to have breech presentation at 37 weeks underwent ECV. They found that 0.6% had an antepartum hemorrhage, 0.3% had a cord prolapse, 0.3% had premature rupture of membranes, 0.6% experienced a cord presentation, 1.5% had transient fetal bradycardia or tachycardia, 14.6% of infants had a one-minute APGAR <7, and 1.7% had a five-minute APGAR <7 [13]. In comparison to controls who did not undergo ECV, they found that the likelihood of cord prolapse and a one-minute APGAR <7 was lower in patients who did undergo ECV [13]. A systematic review of 11 studies reported that 35% of women reported mild to moderate pain and 4% complained of cardiac palpitations, and 1.5% were found to have fetomaternal hemorrhage with increased fetal cells in the maternal circulation [14]. Fetal heart rate tracing complications in this review included transient fetal bradycardia in up to 47% of cases, but decelerations necessitating delivery in only 1.1% of cases [14]. Only one study in this review looked at the risk of cord prolapse, placental abruption, premature rupture of membranes, and uterine rupture, and none were reported [14]. A third review of studies published over a 12 years span showed similar results to the previous two reviews. They found that transient fetal heart rate bradycardia occurred in 5.7% of cases, significant fetomaternal transfusion was found in 3.7%, and vaginal bleeding occurred in 0.47% (with approximately 50% of those undergoing an emergency cesarean section) [15]. The mean incidence of placental abruption was found to be 0.12% [15]. Lastly, Grootscholten et al. reviewed the data of 12 955 attempted cases of ECV [16]. They found an overall complication rate of 6.5% (95% CI 4.7–7.8). Specifically, the OR of placental abruption was 1.1 (95% CI 0.32–3.5), cord prolapse 1.1 (95% CI 0.19–6.2), vaginal bleeding 0.33 (95% CI 0.14–0.82), abnormal fetal heart rate tracing 1.3 (95% CI

0.94–1.9), fetomaternal hemorrhage 1.2 (95% CI 0.18–7.4), and rupture membranes 0.33 (95% CI 0.07–1.6) [16].

The most consistently reported complications associated with ECV include fetal heart rate abnormalities, vaginal bleeding, fetomaternal hemorrhage, ruptured membranes, and cord prolapse. Overall, though, rates for these complications are low, and the evidence supports ECV as a reasonably safe procedure that can help mitigate the need for cesarean section (Level I-A).

4. In patients with third trimester malpresentation (population) what maternal and fetal characteristics (tests) predict a successful external cephalic version (outcome)?

Many patients with breech presentation near term undergo ECV in an effort to turn the fetus to cephalic presentation and thus attempt a vaginal birth. Multiple factors, maternal, fetal, and pregnancy related, can affect the chances of a successful ECV. Overall success rates for ECV range from 35% to 86% (mean 58%) [17].

Ferguson et al. looked at maternal factors that lead to successful version and found that multiparous women (94.5% vs. 63.4%, $p = 0.0001$) were more likely to have successful ECV [18]. Aisenbrey et al. also looked at the importance of different maternal variables in predicting successful ECV [19], and showed that low uterine tone was the most important predictor of successful ECV (100% vs. 28%, $p < 0.001$) and maternal weight (< 68 kg or ≥68 kg) did not impact success (67% vs. 54%, $p = 0.15$). Additionally, they confirmed the findings of Ferguson et al. and showed that multiparous women (75% vs. 55%, $p < 0.05$) also had a higher chance of successfully flipping the baby to the cephalic position [19]. A meta-analysis looked at 53 publications regarding factors that lead to a successful ECV [20]. They found that a relaxed uterine tone after administration of a tocolysis yielded a higher chance of successful ECV (OR 18, 95% CI 12–29) and that maternal weight < 65 kg improved the chances of the procedure (OR 1.8, 95% CI 1.2–2.6) [20]. In many cases of attempted version a tocolytic agent is used to relax the uterus in an effort to increase the chances of a successful ECV. Marquette et al. studied the effect of ritodrine tocolysis on ECV and found that the rate of switching the fetus to cephalic presentation was greater in the tocolytic group than the placebo group (52% vs. 42%, $p = 0.028$) [21]. Collaris et al. compared nifedipine to terbutaline and found that ECV success rate did not differ between the two groups (34.1% vs. 52.2%, $p = 0.094$) [22]. Similarly Kok et al. found no difference with nifedipine in the outcome of ECV when compared to placebo (41.6% vs. 37.2%, RR 1.2, 95% CI 0.85–1.47) [23].

Additional fetal and pregnancy related factors have also been studied to assess the probability of switching the fetus to cephalic presentation. Ferguson et al. showed that women with a normal or increased amniotic fluid volume (79.7% vs. 33.3%, $p = 0.005$) were more likely to have a successful version [18]. Similarly Boucher et al. showed that success of ECV was directly related to amniotic fluid index (AFI). They found that the success rate with AFI < 10 cm was 41.9%, 10–15 cm was 51.9%, and AFI >15 cm was 64.5%, $p < 0.001$ [24]. In the study by Aisenbrey described above, they also found that a nonengaged fetus was more likely to undergo ECV(68% vs. 0%, $p < 0.001$) and that estimated fetal weight <3000 g or ≥3000 g did not impact their chances (62% vs. 62%, $p = 0.86$) [19]. Furthermore, they showed that a nonengaged fetal head (OR 9.4, 95% CI 6.3–14) and a palpable fetal head (OR 6.3, 95% CI 4.3–9.2) increase the chances of a successful ECV [20].

ECV appears to be a reasonable option in appropriately selected patients (Level I-A). Maternal characteristics that favor a successful version include a thin multiparous patient with relaxed uterine tone. Even though the evidence regarding tocolytic use is less clear, it does appear that uterine relaxation increases the success rate for ECV (Level I-B). Fetal and pregnancy-related factors that seem to be important in accomplishing a successful ECV include a nonengaged fetal head and normal amniotic fluid volume. A prior uterine incision is a relative contraindication to ECV, and decisions regarding the procedure in such women should be individualized (Level I-B).

References

1 Cunningham, F.G., Leveno, K.J., Bloom, S.L. et al. (2005). *Breech Presentation and Delivery. Williams Obstetrics*, 22e. New York: McGraw-Hill.

2 Rayl, J., Gibson, P.J., and Hickok, D.E. (1996). A population-based case-control study of risk factors for breech presentation. *Am. J. Obstet. Gynecol.* **174**: 28–32.

3 Ford, J.B., Roberts, C.L., Nassar, N. et al. (2010). Recurrence of breech presentation in consecutive pregnancies. *BJOG* **117**: 830–836.

4 Luterkort, M., Persson, P., and Weldner, B. (1984). Maternal and fetal factors in breech presentation. *Obstet. Gynecol.* **64** (**1**): 55–59.

5 Fianu, S. and Václavínková, V. (1978). The site of placental attachment as a factor in the aetiology of breech presentation. *Acta Obstet. Gynecol. Scand.* **57** (**4**): 371–372.

6 Dunn, L.J., Vanvoorhis, L., and Naper, J. (1965). Term breech presentation: a report of 499 consecutive cases. *Obstet. Gynecol.* **25**: 170–176.

7 Cheng, M. and Hannah, M. (1993). Breech delivery at term: a critical review of the literature. *Obstet. Gynecol.* **82** (**4 Pt 1**): 605–618.

8 Golfier, F., Vaudoyer, F., Ecochard, R. et al. (2001). Planned vaginal delivery versus elective caesarean section in singleton term breech presentation: a study of 1116 cases. *Eur. J. Obstet. Gynecol. Reprod. Biol.* **98** (**2**): 186–192.

9 Irion, O., Hirsbrunner Almagbaly, P., and Morabia, A. (1998). Planned vaginal delivery versus elective caesarean section: a study of 705 singleton term breech presentations. *Br. J. Obstet. Gynaecol.* **105** (**7**): 710–717.

10 Hannah, M.E., Hannah, W.J., Hewson, S.A. et al. (2000). Planned caesarean section versus planned vaginal birth for breech presentation at term: a randomised multicentre trial. *Lancet* **356** (**9239**): 1375–1383.

11 Danielian, P.J., Wang, J., and Hall, M.H. (1996). Long-term outcome by method of delivery of fetuses in breech presentation at term: population based follow up. *BMJ* **312**: 1451.

12 Whyte, H., Hannah, M.E., Saigal, S. et al. (2004). Outcomes of children at 2 years after planned cesarean birth versus planned vaginal birth for breech presentation at term: the international randomized term breech trial. *Am. J. Obstet. Gynecol.* **191** (**3**): 864–871.

13 Nassar, H., Roberts, C., Cameron, C., and Peat, B. (2006). Outcomes of external cephalic version and breech presentation at term, an audit of deliveries at a Sydney tertiary obstetric hospital, 1997-2004. *Acta Obstet. Gynecol. Scand.* **85** (**10**): 1231–1238.

14 Nassar, N., Roberts, C.L., Barratt, A. et al. (2006). Systematic review of adverse outcomes of external cephalic version and persisting breech presentation at term. *Paediatr. Perinat. Epidemiol.* **20** (**2**): 163–171.

15 Collaris, R. and Oei, S.G. (2004). External cephalic version: a safe procedure? A systematic review of version-related risks. *Acta Obstet. Gynecol. Scand.* **83**: 511–518.

16 Grootscholten, K., Kok, M., Oei, S.G. et al. (2008). External cephalic version-related risks: a meta-analysis. *Obstet. Gynecol.* **112** (**5**): 1143–1151.

17 American College of Obstetricians and Gynecologists (2000). *Task Force on Cesarean Delivery Rates: Evaluation of Cesarean Delivery*. Washington, DC: ACOG.

18 Ferguson, J.E., Armstrong, M., and Dyson, D.C. (1987). Maternal and fetal factors affecting success of antepartum external cephalic version. *Obstet. Gynecol.* **70** (**5**): 722–725.

19 Aisenbrey, G.A., Catanzarite, V.A., and Nelson, C. (1999). External cephalic version: predictors of success. *Obstet. Gynecol.* **94**: 783–786.

20 Kok, M., Cnossen, J., Gravendeel, L. et al. (2008). Clinical factors to predict outcome of external cephalic version: a metaanalysis. *Am. J. Obstet. Gynecol.* **199**: 630.e1–630.e7.

21 Marquette, G., Boucher, M., Theriault, D., and Rinfret, D. (1996). Does the use of tocolytic agent affect the success rate of external cephalic version? *Am. J. Obstet. Gynecol.* **175** (**4 Pt 1**): 859–861.

22 Collaris, R. and Tan, P.C. (2009). Oral nifepidine versus subcutaneous terbutaline tocolysis for external cephalic version: a double-blind randomised trial. *BJOG* **116**: 74–81.

23 Kok, M., Bais, J.M., van Lith, J.M. et al. (2008). Nifedipine as a uterine relaxant for external cephalic version: a randomized controlled trial. *Obstet. Gynecol.* **112** (**2 Pt 1**): 271–276.

24 Boucher, M., Bujold, E., Marquette, G.P., and Vezina, Y. (2003). The relationship between amniotic fluid index and successful external cephalic version: a 14-year experience. *Am. J. Obstet. Gynecol.* **189** (**3**): 751–754.

Peripartum complications

50

CHAPTER 50
Induction/augmentation of labor

Christine Farinelli[1], Lili Sheibani[2], and Deborah Wing[2]
[1] *Obstetrix Medical Group, Tucson Medical Center, Tucson, AZ, USA*
[2] *Maternal-Fetal Medicine, Department of Obstetrics and Gynecology, University of California, Irvine, Orange, CA, USA*

CLINICAL SCENARIO: INDUCTION OF LABOR

A 26-year-old gravida 1 para 0 presents to your office for her routine prenatal visit at 40 5/7 weeks gestation. She reports that she is feeling well, but has been experiencing irregular contractions for the past two days. She acknowledges that while she has felt fetal movements, they seem diminished in frequency as well as intensity.

On examination, she appears in no acute distress, with a fundal height appropriate to her gestational age. Her blood pressure is 120/70, pulse 76, and her urine dipstick is negative for protein, blood, or nitrites. Fetal heart tones by Doppler are 150 bpm. Her exam is notable for a 1 cm dilated, long, soft cervix.

The patient reports that her mother has recently arrived from outside of the country and departs again in two weeks. The patient enquires about scheduling an induction of labor to accommodate her mother's desire to be present for the birth of her grandchild.

Background

One of the most commonly performed obstetrical procedures in the United States, induction of labor, refers to the iatrogenic stimulation of uterine contractions in order to accomplish a vaginal delivery prior to the onset of spontaneous labor. The overall frequency of labor induction more than doubled in the United States between 1990 and 2012, rising from 9.5% to 23.3% [1]. Factors contributing to this rise include improved cervical ripening methods, patient and clinician desires to arrange convenient delivery times, relaxed attitudes toward marginal indications for inductions, and patient or provider concerns regarding the risks of fetal demise with expectant management near or after term [2].

Clinical questions: induction of labor

1. In pregnant term patients (population), does elective induction (intervention) lead to improved fetal or maternal outcomes?
2. In pregnant patients undergoing induction of labor (population), does transvaginal ultrasound or biochemical examinations (tests) predict labor induction success (outcome) better than cervical examination (comparison)?
3. In a pregnant patient with an unfavorable cervix (population), how do pharmacologic ripening methods (intervention) compare to mechanical methods (comparison) in terms of achieving successful vaginal deliveries (outcome)?
4. In a pregnant patient undergoing labor induction with oxytocin (population), do low dose protocols (intervention) lead to more cesareans (outcome) than high dose protocols (comparison)?
5. In pregnant patients undergoing induction of labor (population), what constitutes a failed induction (outcome)?

Critical appraisal of the literature

1. In pregnant term patients (population), does elective induction (intervention) lead to improved fetal or maternal outcomes?

Labor may be induced for either maternal or fetal indications. Induction of labor is undertaken when both of the following criteria are met [3]:

- Continuing the pregnancy is believed to be associated with greater maternal or fetal risk than intervention to deliver the pregnancy, and
- There is no contraindication to vaginal birth, including prior classical uterine incision, prior transmural uterine incision entering the uterine cavity, active genital herpes infection, placenta or vasa previa, umbilical cord prolapse, transverse fetal lie.

The magnitude of risk is influenced by factors such as gestational age, fetal lung maturity status, severity of the

Evidence-Based Obstetrics and Gynecology, First Edition. Edited by Errol R. Norwitz, Carolyn M. Zelop, David A. Miller, and David L. Keefe.

Table 50.1 Indications for labor induction

Accepted absolute indications	Relative indications
Hypertensive disorders • Pre-eclampsia/eclampsia *Maternal medical conditions* • Diabetes mellitus • Renal disease • Chronic pulmonary disease	*Hypertensive disorders* • Chronic hypertension *Maternal medical conditions* • Systemic lupus erythematosus • Gestational diabetes • Hypercoagulable disorders • Cholestasis of pregnancy
Prelabor rupture of membranes	*Polyhydramnios*
Chorioamnionitis	*Fetal anomalies requiring specialized neonatal care*
Fetal compromise • Fetal growth restriction • Isoimmunization • Nonreassuring antepartum fetal testing • Oligohydramnios	*Logistic factors* • Risk of rapid labor • Distance from hospital • Psychosocial indications • Advanced cervical dilation
Fetal demise	*Previous stillbirth*
Post-term pregnancy (≥42 wk)	*Late term pregnancy (≥41 wk)*

clinical condition, and cervical status. Appropriately timed induction of women with pregnancy complications can improve maternal-fetal outcomes (Table 50.1) [4]. This appears particularly true in women with some of the hypertensive complications of pregnancy. In the monitoring for hypertensive disorders of pregnancy between 34 and 37 weeks of gestation (HYPITAT) trial, a small (n = 756) but nonetheless well-designed study, singleton pregnancies at 36–41 weeks gestation complicated by gestational hypertension or mild pre-eclampsia were randomized to induction (n = 377) vs. expectant management (n = 379). Of women randomized, 177 (31%) allocated to induction of labor developed poor maternal outcome (maternal mortality or morbidity including eclampsia, hemolysis, elevated liver enzymes and low platelet (HELLP) syndrome, pulmonary edema, thromboembolic disease, or placental abruption), whereas 166 (44%) of women who underwent expectant management suffered from poor outcomes (RR 0.71, [95% CI 0.59–0.86], p = 0.0001). There were no cases of maternal or neonatal death or eclampsia [5]. Based on these findings, induction of labor for gestational hypertension or pre-eclampsia without severe features is advised at 37 weeks' gestation (Level of evidence A).

Overall, there is only limited high quality evidence establishing any benefits for specific medical and obstetrical indications for induction [6]. The risks of iatrogenic late preterm birth appear to outweigh any theoretical benefits when the indication for delivery is "soft," such as suspected macrosomia without maternal diabetes, uncomplicated chronic hypertension, or history of fetal, maternal, or obstetric complication in a previous pregnancy [7, 8].

In comparison to indicated induction where the maternal or fetal health is considered to be in jeopardy, elective induction refers to the iatrogenic stimulation of labor in the absence of maternal or obstetrical indications. The major concerns associated with elective induction of labor at term are the potential for increased rates of cesarean delivery, iatrogenic prematurity, and cost. Another concern is that maternal-fetal medical benefits, such as reduction in stillbirth, have not been proven. Nevertheless, there are potential advantages to scheduled induction of labor, such as avoiding the risk of delivery en route to the hospital if labor is rapid or the patient lives far away, and avoiding sudden disruption of the patient's (and provider's) work and non-work related responsibilities. There are insufficient data to support a policy of routine elective induction of labor at term. Large, randomized trials with emphasis on maternal and neonatal safety, determination of neonatal benefit as a reflection of reduced unexplained fetal death, and cost-benefit analyses are needed.

In a 2014 study, Baitlit et al. compared maternal and neonatal outcomes in nulliparous women with non-medically indicated induction at term vs. expectant management. They concluded that at 39 weeks of gestation, nonmedically indicated induction is associated with lower maternal and neonatal morbidity than expectant management. When induced women were compared with expectantly managed women at the same gestational age, they did not find a substantial increase in the cesarean delivery rate in the induced group [9] (Level of evidence B).

Preventive or risk-based induction has also been termed Active Management of Risk in Pregnancy at Term (AMOR-IPAT), or non-indicated but risk-based induction. Nicholson et al. performed a meta-analysis of the associations between the regular use of modeled risk based non-indicated term labor induction and rate of adverse outcomes. The use of preventive induction, as compared with the standard approach, was associated with a more favorable pattern of birth outcomes. Certain types of non-indicated induction may be beneficial for maternal-fetal outcome; however, evidence of the benefits of preventive induction for specific indications is limited [10]. (Level of evidence B).

Currently, there is expert consensus that elective induction should not be performed before 39 weeks gestation; however there is insufficient evidence to recommend for or against induction of labor at ≥39 weeks of gestation [11]. Adequately powered randomized clinical trials are needed to study the risks of non-indicated term labor induction (Level of evidence C).

The risk of cesarean delivery with elective induction has remained controversial, secondary to differing control groups (either patients undergoing spontaneous labor or expectant management) in the currently published literature. When comparing elective induction outcomes to spontaneous labor, an increased risk of cesarean delivery is noted, as in one of the largest observational studies of elective induction in low risk women, which included 1847 women undergoing elective induction and 35 597 spontaneously laboring women [12]. In this study, the World Health Organization's Global Survey on Maternal and Perinatal Health in Latin America Study Group observed cesarean rates of 11.7% with elective induction and 8.6% after spontaneous labor (crude RR 1.36, 95% CI 1.19–1.55). The increased risk of operative delivery appears particularly noteworthy in nulliparous women. This is best illustrated by a matched cohort study that compared the fetomaternal outcomes of 7683 women who underwent electively induced labor to 7683 women who experienced spontaneous labor [13]. All of the women were nulliparous with singleton pregnancies in cephalic presentation, gestational age 266–287 days, and birth weight 3000–4000 g. Information on cervical status and use of cervical ripening agents was not available. Elective induction led to statistically significant higher rates of cesarean delivery (10% vs. 7%), instrumental delivery (32% vs. 29%), and use of epidural anesthesia (80% vs. 58%). The higher cesarean rate was attributed to an increased frequency of intervention for failure to progress in the first stage of labor. Similar findings have been reported in multiple cohort studies of nulliparous women with vertex, singleton term pregnancies delivering in the United States [14–20]. These studies consistently showed that the rate of cesarean delivery was increased approximately twofold in women who underwent elective or medical induction of labor compared to those who experienced spontaneous labor.

However, if patients undergoing elective induction are compared to those receiving expectant management rather than those undergoing spontaneous labor, the risk of cesarean delivery appears to be decreased. Women in spontaneous labor, such as in those studies noted above, may not be an appropriate control group for studies evaluating elective induction outcomes. Using them as controls biases differences in cesarean rates to favor the control group because many patients managed expectantly would have gone on to have an indicated cesarean delivery rather than spontaneous labor. Also, in practical terms, a physician cannot decide between spontaneous labor and induction on a given day, but between expectant management and induction. When cesarean delivery rates have been compared for induced labors vs. expectant management at the same gestational age, the differences in cesarean delivery rates were small and favored the induction groups [21, 22]. In a 2012 Cochrane Review of randomized trials in which a policy of induction "at or beyond term" was compared with expectant management, cesarean delivery rate was 11% lower in the induction group (relative risk [RR] 0.89, 95% CI 0.81–0.97). Of note 17 of the 21 trials included in this analysis involved women >41 weeks of gestation [23]. In another systematic review of randomized trials in which induction at "term" was compared with expectant management, the cesarean delivery rate was 13% lower in the induction group (RR 0.87, 95% CI 0.82–0.92). The findings in the latter study were for pregnancies at 37 to <42 weeks gestation [24] (Level of evidence A).

Another issue when evaluating the risk of cesarean delivery is parity. In comparison to nulliparas, most studies in multiparous women have not shown an increased risk of cesarean delivery with induction of labor [25]. Almost all of these reports were retrospective, but one small randomized trial confirmed these findings [26]. One of the largest series was a population-based cohort study that compared the risk of cesarean delivery in 1775 healthy, low risk multiparous women at term who underwent induction without an identifiable indication to 5785 similar women who entered labor spontaneously [27]. Cervical ripening agents were used in women with unfavorable cervices. The overall cesarean delivery rate was similar for induced and spontaneous labors, 3.8% and 3.6%, respectively (RR 1.07, 95% CI 0.91–1.39). Although the cesarean delivery rate was higher in women with a previous cesarean delivery, the rate did not differ significantly for induced and spontaneous labors (30.5% and 30.7%, respectively).

Even when inductions for medical indications are included, multiparas have a relatively low rate of cesarean delivery. In one retrospective cohort study, the rates of cesarean delivery in multiparas in spontaneous labor (n = 7208), induced with oxytocin (n = 2190), and induced with cervical ripening agents (n = 239) were 4.2%, 6.3%, and 14.2%, respectively [28]. Oxytocin-induced multiparas were 37% more likely to require cesarean than those with spontaneous labor (OR, 1.37; 95% CI, 1.10–1.71) and nearly three times more likely to undergo cesarean when cervical ripening agents were used (OR, 2.82; 95% CI, 1.84–4.53) (Level of evidence B).

If successful elective induction is defined as achieving a vaginal birth while avoiding excessive costs and admission to a special care nursery, then the best candidates are women (nulliparous or multiparous) with well-dated pregnancies of at least 39 weeks of gestation and favorable cervices. The excess neonatal morbidity of earlier intervention was illustrated in a prospective observational study that compared the outcome of 790 planned elective inductions at 37–38 weeks of gestation with the outcome of 2004 planned elective inductions at ≥39 weeks of gestation [29]. Earlier induction was associated with a significantly higher risk of neonatal intensive care unit (NICU) admission (7.7% vs. 3.0%) (Level of evidence B).

The major pediatric concerns with regards to elective delivery include neonatal respiratory problems. Respiratory problems can result from inadvertent delivery of a premature infant or transient tachypnea related to cesarean delivery after failed induction. However, several, primarily retrospective, studies have not shown a marked impairment in neonatal outcome when elective induction of labor was undertaken at term in well-dated pregnancies [30–34].

There may, in fact, be a slight benefit as fewer electively induced infants have meconium passage when compared to spontaneously labored infants. Macrosomia also may be reduced [35] (Level of evidence B).

The risk of respiratory morbidity was illustrated in a retrospective review of infants with respiratory distress or transient tachypnea of the newborn admitted to the NICU following elective delivery at term [36]. The data were stratified by gestational age and route of delivery with a baseline incidence of respiratory distress syndrome of 2.2/1000 deliveries (95% CI 1.7–2.7/1000) and transient tachypnea of 5.7/1000 (95% CI 4.9–6.5/1000) at term. The frequencies of respiratory morbidity following vaginal or cesarean delivery increased with decreasing gestational age, with the highest risk associated with cesarean after labor at 37–38 weeks gestation (57.7/1000 deliveries, 95% CI 26.7–107.1/1000). Delivery by cesarean without preceding labor increased the frequencies of respiratory morbidities even higher across all gestational ages. These data provide support for delaying elective delivery until 39 weeks of gestation (Level of evidence B).

A study using decision analysis analyzed the economic consequences of elective induction of labor at term in a cohort of 100 000 women for whom an initial decision was made to either induce labor at 39 weeks of gestation or follow expectantly through the remainder of pregnancy [37]. All patients in this model underwent elective induction at 42 weeks. Using baseline estimates, the investigators concluded that elective induction would result in more than 12 000 excess cesareans, imposing an annual cost to the medical system of nearly $100 million. A policy of induction at any gestational age, regardless of parity or cervical ripeness, required economic expenditures by the medical system. Although never cost saving, inductions were less expensive at later gestational ages, for multiparous patients, and for those women with a favorable cervix. The inductions most costly to the healthcare system were those performed in nulliparas with unfavorable cervices at 39 weeks. When nulliparous women with favorable cervices undergo labor induction, the estimated cost is approximately halved compared to nulliparas with unfavorable cervices; however, it still resulted in overall added expenditures and additional cesarean deliveries (Level of evidence B).

2. In pregnant patients undergoing induction of labor (population), does transvaginal ultrasound or biochemical examinations (tests) predict labor induction success (outcome) better than cervical examination (comparison)?

Cervical status is one of the most important factors for predicting the likelihood of successfully inducing labor. For this reason, a cervical examination should be performed before initiating attempts at induction. There are several cervical scoring systems available for this purpose [38], although the modified Bishop score is the system most commonly used in clinical practice in the United States [39]. This system tabulates a score based upon the station of the presenting part and four characteristics of the cervix: dilatation, effacement, consistency, and position (Table 50.2). If the Bishop score is high (variously defined as ≥5 or ≥8), the likelihood of vaginal delivery is similar whether labor is spontaneous or induced [40]. In contrast, a low Bishop score is predictive that induction will fail and result in cesarean delivery. These relationships are particularly strong in nulliparous women who undergo induction [11, 41], although Bishop scoring was originally described in multiparous women. Of note, the relationship between a low Bishop score and failed induction, prolonged labor, and a high cesarean birth rate was first described prior to widespread use of cervical ripening agents [42].

Table 50.2 Modified Bishop score

Score	0	1	2	3
Parameter				
Dilatation (cm)	Closed	1–2	3–4	5 or more
Effacement (%)	0–30	40–50	60–70	80 or more
Length[a] (cm)	*>4*	*2–4*	*1–2*	*1–2*
Station	−3	−2	−1 or 0	+1 or +2
Consistency	Firm	Medium	Soft	
Cervical Position	Posterior	Midposition	Anterior	

[a]Modification by Calder AA, Brennand, J.E. Labor and normal delivery: Induction of labor. Curr Opin Obstet Gynecol 1991 3:764. This modification replaces percent effacement as one of the parameters of the Bishop score.

Source: Bishop EH: *Pelvic Scoring For Elective Induction.* Obstet Gynecol 24:266, 1964.

In observational studies, other characteristics associated with successful induction include multiparity, tall stature (over 5 ft 5 in.), increasing gestational age, non-obese maternal weight or body mass index, and infant birth weight less than 3.5 kg [43, 44]. However, these characteristics are predictive of success even in spontaneous labors, which suggests they are more predictive of the route of delivery than the likelihood that the patient will reach the active phase of labor.

Because of the risk of cesarean delivery and the rising costs of health care associated with labor induction, some researchers have tried to identify, with varying success, biochemical and biophysical assays to predict the probability of vaginal delivery following labor induction [45–48]. These measures include digital evaluation of the cervix, ultrasonographic cervical length measurements, and use of fetal fibronectin (fFN) before labor induction.

Cervical length is predictive of the likelihood of spontaneous onset of labor post-term [49]. Sonographic assessment of cervical length for predicting the outcome of labor induction has been evaluated in numerous studies. A systematic review of 20 prospective studies found that cervical length was predictive of successful induction (likelihood ratio of a positive test, 1.66; 95% CI 1.20–2.31) and failed induction (likelihood ratio of a negative test, 0.51; 95% CI, 0.39–0.67) [50]. However, sonographic cervical length performed poorly for predicting vaginal delivery within 24 hours (sensitivity 59%, specificity 65%), vaginal delivery (sensitivity 67%, specificity 58%), achieving active labor (sensitivity 57%, specificity 60%), and delivery within 24 hours (sensitivity 56%, specificity 47%), and did not perform significantly better than the Bishop score for predicting a successful induction. These data are limited by substantial heterogeneity among the studies. The role of ultrasound examination as a tool for selecting women likely to have a successful induction is uncertain at this time.

In a study from Verhoeven et al., they performed a systematic review and meta-analysis to assess the predictive capacity of transvaginal sonographic assessment of the cervix for outcome of induction. This study included 31 studies reporting on both cervical length and outcome of delivery. Sensitivity of cervical length in the prediction of cesarean delivery ranged from 0.14 to 0.92 and specificity ranged from 0.35 to 1.00. For cervical wedging in the prediction of failed induction of labor summary point estimates of sensitivity/specificity were 0.37/0.80. They concluded that cervical length measured sonographically at or near term have moderate capacity to predict the outcome of delivery after induction [51] (Level of evidence B). Overall, the role of ultrasound examination as a tool for selecting women likely to have a successful induction is uncertain at this time.

The presence of an elevated fFN concentration in cervicovaginal secretions has also been used to predict uterine readiness for induction. fFN is thought to represent a disruption or inflammation of the chorionic-decidual interface. In several studies, women with a positive fFN result had a significantly shorter interval until delivery than those with a negative fFN result [52] and there was reduction in the frequency of cesarean delivery [53]. Positive fFN results were predictive of a shorter interval to delivery, even in nulliparas with low (<5) Bishop scores [54]. However, there are other investigations which did not confirm these findings [48, 55].

The Bishop score appears to be the best available tool for predicting the likelihood that induction will result in vaginal delivery. This conclusion is based on systematic reviews of controlled studies that found the Bishop score was as, or more, predictive of the outcome of labor induction than fFN [45] or sonographic measurement of cervical length [45, 52, 56], and that dilatation was the most important element of the Bishop score [45] (Level of evidence B).

3. In a pregnant patient with an unfavorable cervix (population), how do pharmacologic ripening methods (intervention) compare to mechanical methods (comparison) in terms of achieving vaginal deliveries (outcome)?

Cervical ripening is a complex process that results in physical softening and distensibility of the cervix, ultimately leading to partial cervical effacement and dilatation [57]. The methodology falls into two main categories: (i) mechanical (physical), such as disruption of the fetal membranes or insertion of dilators or a balloon catheter, and (ii) application of cervical ripening agents, such as prostaglandin compounds or oxytocin (Table 50.3).

Table 50.3 Methods of cervical ripening

Pharmacologic methods	Mechanical methods
Oxytocin Prostaglandins • E_2 (dinoprostone, Prepidil™ gel, and Cervidil time-released vaginal insert) • E_1 (misoprostol, Cytotec™) Estrogen Relaxin Hyaluronic acid Progesterone receptor antagonists	Membrane stripping Amniotomy Mechanical dilators • Laminaria tents • Dilapan • Lamicel • Transcervical balloon catheters ◦ With extra-amniotic saline infusion ◦ With concomitant oxytocin administration

Mechanical methods are among the oldest approaches used to promote cervical ripening. Advantages of these techniques compared to pharmacologic methods include their low cost, low risk of tachysystole, few systemic side effects, and convenient storage requirements (no refrigeration or expiration) [58]. Comparing mechanical methods with placebo or no treatment [58], tachysystole with fetal heart rate changes was not reported. The risk of cesarean birth was similar between groups (34%; RR 1.00; 95% CI: 0.76–1.30, n = 416, 6 studies). There were no reported cases of severe neonatal and maternal morbidity among them. The risk of tachysystole was reduced when compared with all prostaglandins. Compared with oxytocin in women with unfavorable cervix, mechanical methods reduce the risk of cesarean delivery. Disadvantages of mechanical methods include a small increase in the risk of maternal and neonatal infection from introduction of a foreign body [59], the potential for disruption of a low-lying placenta, and some maternal discomfort upon manipulation of the cervix. The most common mechanical methods are stripping (or sweeping) of the fetal membranes, placement of hygroscopic dilators within the endocervical canal, and insertion of a balloon catheter above the internal cervical os (with or without infusion of extra-amniotic saline).

The efficacy of membrane sweeping was demonstrated in a meta-analysis of 22 trials in which 20 compared sweeping of membranes to no treatment, three compared sweeping to prostaglandin administration, and one compared sweeping to oxytocin administration before formal induction of labor [60]. Compared to no intervention, membrane sweeping was associated with reduced frequency of pregnancy continuing beyond 41 weeks (RR 0.59, 95% CI 0.46–0.74) and 42 weeks of gestation (RR 0.28, 95% CI 0.15–0.50), and reduced frequency of formal induction (RR 0.72, 95% CI 0.52–1.00).

The cesarean delivery rate was not altered; the change in Bishop score was not assessed. Overall, eight women would need to undergo membrane sweeping to avoid one formal induction of labor. There was no increased risk of maternal or neonatal infection, but minor maternal discomforts were common. Compared to no intervention, weekly membrane stripping at term shortens the interval of time to onset of spontaneous labor and reduces the need for formal induction. Current recommendations are to begin stripping membranes at more than 37 weeks gestation in patients who wish to hasten the onset of labor [6] (Level of evidence A).

Amniotomy appears to be an effective method of labor induction, but can only be performed in women with partially dilated and effaced cervices. A Cochrane review of randomized trials found the combination of amniotomy plus intravenous oxytocin administration was more effective than amniotomy alone for induction of labor [61] (Level of evidence A). With the combined regimen, fewer women were undelivered at 24 hours than with amniotomy alone (RR 0.13, 95% CI 0.04–0.41). To achieve the greatest impact on duration of labor, amniotomy should be performed as early as possible and oxytocin should be initiated immediately thereafter [62]. There are inadequate data for assessing the efficacy of the combination of amniotomy plus intravenous oxytocin administration compared to intravenous oxytocin alone [63]. There are limited data suggesting the efficacy of amniotomy plus oxytocin is similar to that of prostaglandins alone [61].

Hygroscopic dilators are safe and effective for dilating the cervix, although they are used primarily during pregnancy termination rather than for pre-induction cervical ripening of term pregnancies. A meta-analysis of randomized trials comparing hygroscopic dilators to placebo or no treatment found that pregnant women in both groups had similar rates of not achieving a vaginal delivery by 24 hours (RR 0.90; 95% CI 0.64–1.26), cesarean deliveries (RR 0.98; 95% CI 0.74–1.30), and infection [58]. These data suggest that although hygroscopic dilators can dilate the cervix, they are inadequate for improving the outcome of induction. However, no large trials have been performed and there are no high-quality comparative studies evaluating the optimal use of hygroscopic dilators with other modalities, such as amniotomy, to improve the rate of successful induction. A significant disadvantage of the use of laminaria for cervical ripening is patient discomfort both at the time of insertion and with progressive cervical dilatation. With other equally effective agents available, there is no obvious benefit to support their routine use for labor induction at term (Level of evidence A).

Transcervical balloon catheters appear to be as effective for preinduction cervical ripening as prostaglandin E2 (PGE2) gel and intravaginal misoprostol in most studies [64–70] (Level of evidence A). A meta-analysis on intravaginal misoprostol vs. transcervical Foley catheter (nine studies included, n = 1603) revealed no significant difference in mean time to delivery (mean difference 1.08 ± 2.19 hours shorter for misoprostol, p = 0.25), rate of cesarean delivery (RR 1.0; 95% CI 0.77–1.28), or rate of chorioamnionitis (RR 1.13; 95% CI 0.61–2.09) [70]. As anticipated, transcervical balloon catheters were associated with a lower incidence of tachysystole. The combination of a balloon catheter plus administration of a prostaglandin does not appear to be more effective than prostaglandins alone [69]. While the risk of infection may theoretically be associated with the insertion of a foreign object in the cervix, existing meta-analysis data did not show evidence of an increased risk of infectious morbidity. This technique is a superior method of preinduction cervical ripening when compared with intravenous oxytocin and has been associated with a lower rate of cesarean delivery in one investigation [58]. Some studies show more rapid cervical ripening, a shortened induction to delivery interval, and reduced frequency of patients undelivered in 24 hours when combining a transcervical balloon catheter with a pharmacologic method of cervical ripening such as a prostaglandin [66], whereas others do not [64]. Sciscione et al. [69], in a study examining 126 women, found no increased risk of preterm delivery in subsequent pregnancies following the placement of balloon catheters in the lower uterine segment (Level of evidence A).

The use of the Atad double-balloon device has also been described in a limited group of studies [70–72]. One investigation included 95 women with Bishop scores <4 and randomly assigned them to vaginally administered PGE2, Atad balloon dilator technique, or continuous oxytocin for labor induction. They found a significant mean change in Bishop score after 12 hours in the PGE2 group and Atad balloon dilator group of 5 compared with 2.5 in the oxytocin group. In addition they found a higher rate of failed induction in the oxytocin group (58%) compared with 20% in the PGE2 and 5.7% in the Atad balloon dilator groups. Vaginal delivery rates in the oxytocin group were 26.7% compared with 77% and 70% in the Atad balloon dilator and PGE2 groups, respectively. There are no comparative studies of single to double-balloon catheters.

In comparison to mechanical methods, randomized trials have established that prostaglandins (PG E2, F2-alpha, and E1) are also effective for both cervical ripening and labor induction [73–76]. The efficacy of locally applied prostaglandins (vaginal or intracervical) for cervical ripening and labor induction as compared with oxytocin (alone or in combination with amniotomy) has been demonstrated in a Cochrane review involving more than 10 000 women. Vaginal PGE2 compared with placebo reduced the likelihood of vaginal delivery not being achieved within 24 hours, the risk of the cervix remaining unfavorable or unchanged, and the need for oxytocin. There was no difference between cesarean delivery rates, although PGE2 use increased the risk of uterine tachysystole with fetal heart rate changes. The various administration vehicles (tablet, gel, and timed-release pessary) appear to be as efficacious as each other [76]. The optimal route, frequency, and dose of prostaglandins of all types and formulations for cervical ripening and labor induction have not been determined (Level of evidence A).

Although oxytocin is an effective means of labor induction in women with a favorable cervix, it is less effective as a cervical ripening agent. Many randomized controlled trials comparing oxytocin with various prostaglandin formulations and other methods of cervical ripening confirm this observation. Lyndrup et al. [77] compared the efficacy of labor induction with vaginal PGE2 with continuous oxytocin infusion in 91 women with an unfavorable cervix (Bishop score < 6). They found PGE2 more efficacious for labor induction in 12–24 hours, with fewer women undelivered at 24 hours. However, by allowing the inductions to proceed for 48 hours, they found no difference in vaginal delivery rates after 48 hours between the two groups. In a larger study involving 200 women with an unfavorable cervix undergoing labor induction, vaginally applied PGE2 was compared with continuous oxytocin infusion [78]. These investigators found a shorter time interval to active labor, a significantly greater change in Bishop score, fewer failed inductions, and fewer multiple-day inductions with PGE2 compared with oxytocin. No difference in the rate of cesarean delivery was found between the groups overall. In a Cochrane review of 110 trials including more than 11 000 women comparing oxytocin with any vaginal prostaglandin formulation for labor induction, oxytocin alone was associated with an increase in unsuccessful vaginal delivery within 24 hours (52% vs. 28%, RR 1.85, 95% CI 1.41–2.43). There was no difference in the rate of cesarean delivery between groups. When intracervical prostaglandins were compared with oxytocin alone for labor induction, oxytocin alone was associated with an increase in unsuccessful vaginal delivery within 24 hours (51% vs. 35%, RR 1.49, 95% CI 1.12–1.99) and an increase in cesarean delivery (19% vs. 13%, RR 1.42, 95% CI 1.11–1.82) [79] (Level of evidence A).

4. In a pregnant patient undergoing labor induction with oxytocin (population), do low dose protocols (intervention) lead to more cesareans (outcome) than high dose protocols (comparison)?

Oxytocin is a polypeptide hormone produced in the hypothalamus and secreted from the posterior lobe of the pituitary gland in a pulsatile fashion. It is identical to its synthetic analog (pitocin), which is among the most potent uterotonic agents known. Synthetic oxytocin is an effective means of labor induction [79]. Oxytocin is most often given intravenously because when given orally the polypeptide is degraded to small, inactive forms by gastrointestinal enzymes. The plasma half life is short, estimated at three to six minutes [80], and steady-state concentrations are reached within 30–40 minutes of initiation or dose change [81].

The optimal regimen for oxytocin administration is debatable, although success rates for varying protocols are similar. Protocols differ as to the initial dose (0.5–6 mU min^{-1}), incremental time period (10–60 minutes), and maximum dose (16–64 mU min^{-1}) [3]. Success rates for the varying protocols are strikingly similar. Several experts have suggested that implementation of a standardized protocol is desirable to minimize errors in oxytocin administration [82–84]. A literature review of randomized clinical trials of high vs. low dose oxytocin regimens for augmentation or induction of labor concluded high-dose oxytocin decreased the time from admission to vaginal delivery, but did not decrease the incidence of cesarean delivery compared with low-dose therapy [85]. Only one double-blinded randomized trial has been published, and had the same findings [86]. High dose regimens are associated with a higher rate of tachysystole then low dose regimens, and in some studies this has resulted in a higher rate of cesarean for fetal distress [87], but no significant differences in neonatal outcomes have been noted [88]. A large observational study produced by the Consortium on Safe Labor evaluated 7775 nulliparous and 7280 multiparous patients, with similar results to the randomized trials [89]: no differences in rate of cesarean delivery or other perinatal outcomes. The Safe Labor Project is a retrospective observational study conducted by the Eunice Kennedy Shriver National Institute of Child Health and Human Development, National Institutes of Health, in collaboration with several institutions across the United States. In this particular evaluation of oxytocin regimens, six hospitals provided data on 15 054 women who were grouped based on their starting oxytocin doses (1, 2, or 4 mU min^{-1}). Interestingly, the high dose regimen (starting dose of 4 mU min^{-1} with increases of 4 mU min^{-1}) was associated with reduced risks of meconium staining, chorioamnionitis, and newborn fever in multiparous patients.

The oxytocin dose is typically increased until there is normal progression of labor, or strong contractions occurring at two to three minutes intervals, or uterine activity reaches 150–350 Montevideo units (i.e. the peak strength of contractions in mmHg measured by an internal monitor multiplied by their frequency per 10 minutes). There is no benefit to increasing the dose after one of these endpoints has been achieved. In addition, two randomized trials found there was no significant benefit in continuing oxytocin infusion after the onset of active labor [90, 91].

Low-dose protocols attempt to mimic endogenous maternal physiology [3]. Oxytocin is initiated at 0.5–1 mU min^{-1} and increased by 1 mU min^{-1} at 40–60-minutes intervals. Slightly higher doses beginning at 1–2 mU min^{-1} increased by 1–2 mU min^{-1}, with shorter incremental time intervals of 15–30 minutes have also been recommended [92]. Pulsatile oxytocin administration at 8–10-minutes intervals is considered a variant of low-dose oxytocin administration and may better simulate normal labor. It has the advantage of reducing total oxytocin requirements by 20–50% compared to nonpulsatile regimens [93–95].

High-dose oxytocin regimens are often employed in active management of labor protocols. Examples of these protocols include an initial oxytocin dose of 6 mU min^{-1} increased by 6 mU min^{-1} at 20 minutes intervals [93] or an initial dose at 4 mU min^{-1} with 4 mU min^{-1} incremental increases [41]. It is important to note that active management of labor protocols do not consist merely of the dosing for oxytocin, but are actually multi-faceted strategies which include one to one nursing care and early amniotomy within an hour of active labor diagnosis [96] (Level of evidence B).

In a systematic review comparing high dose and low dose infusions for induction of labor, nine trials involving 2391 women and their babies were included in the review. Their findings did not provide evidence that high-dose oxytocin increases vaginal delivery within 24 hours or the cesarean delivery rate. Additionally, they did not find a decrease in induction to delivery time, although results may be confounded by poor quality trials [97] (Level of evidence B).

5. In pregnant patients undergoing induction of labor (population), what constitutes a failed induction (outcome)?

Vaginal delivery is the goal of the induction process; however, this occurs less often than when women labor spontaneously. It is important to allow adequate time for cervical ripening and development of an active labor pattern before determining that an induction has failed. One group proposed that failed induction be defined as the inability to achieve cervical dilatation of 4 cm and 80% effacement or 5 cm (regardless of effacement) after a minimum of 12–18 hours of both oxytocin administration and membrane rupture [98]. They also specified that uterine contractile activity should reach 5 contractions per 10 minutes or 250 Montevideo units, which is the minimum level achieved by most women whose labor is progressing normally. The goal is to minimize the number of cesarean deliveries performed for failed induction in patients who are progressing slowly because they are still in the latent phase of labor [41, 99, 100]. Once induced women enter active labor, progression should be comparable to progression in women with spontaneous active labor, or faster [101].

The utility of administering oxytocin for at least 10–12 hours after membrane rupture is illustrated by the following examples:

- An Australian researcher evaluated a group of 978 nulliparous women after either artificial or spontaneous rupture of membranes to determine factors that could predict failed induction [102]. There was a direct correlation between increasing duration of the latent phase and the probability of cesarean birth. After 10 hours of oxytocin administration, the 8% of women not in the active phase of labor had an approximately 75% chance of being delivered by cesarean for failed induction; after 12 hours of oxytocin administration, the chance of cesarean was almost 90%.
- Two large studies that required a minimum of 12 hours of oxytocin administration after membrane rupture before diagnosing failed labor induction reported that vaginal delivery occurred in 75% of all nulliparas and that failed labor induction was eliminated as an indication for cesarean [100]. Also, for nulliparous women with an unfavorable cervix, the overall rate of vaginal delivery was 63%, with most of the 95% of women who completed latent phase delivering vaginally and approximately 40% of the remaining 5% of women achieving vaginal deliveries as well [103].
- Membrane rupture and oxytocin administration should in most cases be a prerequisite before diagnosing a failed induction of labor. Additionally, experts have proposed waiting at least 24 hours in the setting of both oxytocin and ruptured membranes before making the diagnosis [104] (Level of evidence C).

CLINICAL SCENARIO: AUGMENTATION OF LABOR

A 26-year-old gravida 1 para 0 at 38 5/7 weeks gestation presents to labor and delivery complaining of painful uterine contractions occurring every three to five minutes. She reports good fetal movement and some vaginal spotting today noted on her underwear. Her pregnancy has been uncomplicated prior to this. Physical examination in triage reveals her vital signs to be stable and her cervix to be 4 cm dilated, 75% effaced, and the fetal vertex at −2 station. The fetal heart rate tracing is Category 1. The patient is admitted for labor. However, upon repeat vaginal exam in two hours, her cervix is unchanged.

Background

Most guidelines for normal human labor progress are derived from Friedman's clinical observations of women in labor [105]. He divided labor into three functional divisions: the preparatory division, dilatational division, and pelvic division. The preparatory division is better known as the latent phase, during which little cervical dilatation occurs but considerable changes are taking place in the connective tissue components of the cervix. The dilatation division or active phase is the time period when dilatation proceeds at its most rapid rate to complete cervical dilatation. These two phases together make up the first stage of labor. The pelvic division or second stage of labor refers to the time of full cervical dilatation to the delivery of the infant. The third stage of labor refers to the time from the delivery of the infant to expulsion of the placenta.

Subsequent observations challenge Friedman's original labor curves. Zhang and colleagues for the Consortium on

Safe Labor [106] determined that the active phase of labor as described by Friedman may not actually begin until 5 cm dilation in multiparas and even later in nulliparas. Nineteen hospitals provided data for this analysis, which included 62 415 parturients who had singleton, term, spontaneous labors, and vaginal deliveries. Importantly, prior to 6 cm of dilation, a two-hour threshold for diagnosing labor arrest may be too brief while a four-hours threshold may be too lengthy after 6 cm of dilation. While cervical dilation does accelerate as labor advances, a precipitous dilation as described by Friedman may not necessarily occur, especially in nulliparas.

Diagnoses of abnormal labor, such as protracted labor or an arrest disorder, require prompt evaluation of uterine activity, fetal heart rate status, fetal position, clinical pelvimetry, and a reevaluation of estimated fetal weight. Decisions then may be made regarding interventions, such as increasing or initiating oxytocin, amniotomy, or proceeding with operative vaginal or cesarean delivery. (Level of evidence C).

Clinical questions: augmentation of labor

6. In a pregnant patient experiencing a protracted latent phase of labor (population), how does therapeutic rest compare to active management (comparison)?

7. In a pregnant patient experiencing a protracted active phase of labor (population), does low dose or high dose oxytocin (comparison) improve vaginal delivery rates (outcome)?

8. Does a prolonged second stage of labor (population) affect maternal or neonatal morbidity (outcome)?

9. Compared to patients who do not receive conduction anesthesia (i.e. epidural or combined spinal epidural; comparison), do patients receiving conduction anesthesia (population) experience prolonged labor courses (outcome)?

Critical appraisal of the literature

6. In a pregnant patient experiencing a protracted latent phase of labor (population), how does therapeutic rest compare to active management (comparison)?

The onset of latent labor is considered to be the point at which regular uterine contractions are perceived. Friedman found the mean duration of latent labor was 6.4 hours for nulliparas and 4.8 for multiparas. The 95th percentiles for maximum length in latent labor was 20 hours for nulliparous women and 14 hours for multiparous women [107]. These were considered the upper limits for time spent in latent labor [105]. However, with the recent analyses of the Consortium on Safe Labor, many of the traditional understandings of labor are now being reconsidered. Duration of labor prior to 6 cm dilation actually appears similar in nulliparous and multiparous women, with the 95th percentiles indicating that a woman may require six hours to progress from 4 to 5 cm dilation, and three hours to progress from 5 to 6 cm (median duration 1.3 hours and 0.8 hours respectively). After 6 cm dilation, multiparous women exhibit faster labor, unlike nulliparous women for whom no traditional transition point to "active" labor is seen. Almost all women who achieved a spontaneous vaginal delivery had a 95th percentile of first stage of labor of less than two hours [108]. Duration of labor, based on dilation at admission to dilation of 10 cm, ranged from 3.8 to 8.4 hours (medians) and 12.7 to 20 (95th percentiles) in nulliparous women.

Latent phase arrest implies that labor has not truly begun. Prolonged latent phase refers to a latent phase lasting longer than the 95th percentiles per Friedman [105]. Because the duration of latent labor is highly variable, expectant management is most appropriate. Some women can spend days in latent labor; provided there is no indication for delivery, awaiting active labor is appropriate. If expeditious delivery is indicated, then augmentation of labor may be initiated with a pharmacologic agent such as oxytocin. Another option is to administer "therapeutic rest," especially if contractions are painful or the patient is exhausted, with an analgesic agent such as morphine. A recommended dosing regimen is a single administration of 15–20 mg of morphine subcutaneously or intramuscularly. Often this will help abate or alleviate painful contractions and allow the patient to rest comfortably until active labor begins. The onset of regular contractions is often unpredictable after amniotomy and, therefore, such therapy is not recommended in nulliparas with prolonged latent phase. Early amniotomy may increase the risk of prolonged membrane rupture and its associated infectious morbidity.

Few randomized clinical trials have been published regarding treatment of a prolonged latent phase. However, Nachum et al. in a small study of 213 women compared oxytocin augmentation, amniotomy, or a combination of both with the findings that the combination arm had a shorter time from augmentation to the beginning of active phase as well as a shorter first stage of labor [109]. Notably, only 80 of the women were primiparous, and inclusion criteria required the subjects to be dilated at least 2–4 cm prior to augmentation. (Level of evidence: B).

7. In a pregnant patient experiencing a protracted active phase of labor (population), does low dose or high dose oxytocin (comparison) improve vaginal delivery rates (outcome)?

According to traditional understandings of labor, arrest of labor is defined as cessation of previously normal active phase cervical dilatation for a period of two hours or more [105]. Evaluation of this disorder includes an assessment of uterine activity with an intrauterine pressure catheter (IUPC), performance of clinical pelvimetry, and evaluation of fetal presentation, position, station, and estimated fetal weight. Amniotomy and oxytocin therapy can be initiated if uterine activity is found to be inadequate. The majority of gravidas respond to this intervention, and resume progression of cervical dilatation and achieve vaginal delivery. While the definition reflects a two hours window prior to diagnosis of arrest, Rouse et al. [110] found that at least four hours may be permissible before making this diagnosis without incurring additional maternal or fetal compromise. With the new labor curves produced by the Consortium of Safe Labor, the definition of arrest of labor is now dependent on parity as well as admission dilation. However, these data appear to support Rouse's findings as well [108].

If uterine activity is found to be suboptimal, the most common remedy is oxytocin augmentation, because once labor is initiated, the uterus becomes more sensitive to oxytocin stimulation. Various oxytocin dosing regimens have been described in the obstetric literature. Local protocols for oxytocin administration should specify the dose of oxytocin being delivered (milliunits per minute) as opposed to the volume of fluid being infused (milliliters per minute), initial dose, incremental increases with periodicity, and maximum dose. While oxytocin currently is used in a majority of labors in the United States, it is important for clinicians to recognize that it is also the medication implicated in approximately half of all paid obstetric litigation claims and is the medication most commonly associated with preventable adverse events during childbirth [111].

Satin et al. [112] studied the differences in outcomes when oxytocin was used to augment, as opposed to induce, labor. These investigators prospectively studied 2788 consecutive women with singleton pregnancies. Indications for oxytocin stimulation were divided into augmentation ($n = 1676$) and induction ($n = 1112$). The low-dose regimen consisted of a starting dose of $1\,mU\,min^{-1}$ with incremental increases of $1\,mU\,min^{-1}$ at 20-minutes intervals until $8\,mU\,min^{-1}$, then $2\,mU\,min^{-1}$ increases up to a maximum of $20\text{-}mU\,min^{-1}$, and was used first for five months in 1251 pregnancies. The high-dose regimen consisted of a starting dose of $6\,mU\,min^{-1}$ with increases of $6\,mU\,min^{-1}$ at 20-minutes intervals up to a maximum dose of $42\,mU\,min^{-1}$, and was used for the subsequent five months in 1537 pregnancies. Labor augmentation was more than three hours shorter in the high-dose group compared with that of the low-dose group. High-dose augmentation resulted in fewer cesarean deliveries for labor dystocia and fewer failed inductions when compared with the low-dose regimen, although cesarean deliveries for fetal distress were performed more frequently.

Wei et al. evaluated high dose compared to low dose oxytocin protocols in a meta-analysis of oxytocin for labor augmentation, which included 10 trials and 5423 women [113]. A 15% reduction in the rate of cesarean delivery was noted in the high dose group, as well as a decrease in labor duration (mean difference – 1.54 hours, 95% CI −2.44 to −0.64). Tachysystole was increased in the high dose group (RR 1.91, 1.49–2.35) but no significant differences were noted in fetal heart rate abnormalities, fetal distress, five minutes Apgar <7, cord pH <7.10, or NICU admissions.

Varying dosing intervals have also been studied [114, 115] and, in contemporary practice, vary from 15 to 40 minutes. One comparison of the efficacy and outcomes with differing oxytocin dosing intervals [112] included 1801 consecutive pregnancies receiving high-dose oxytocin (starting dose of $6\,mU\,min^{-1}$ with incremental increases of $6\,mU\,min^{-1}$) at 20- and 40-minutes intervals. In this study, 949 women received oxytocin at 20-minutes intervals ($n = 603$ labor augmentations and $n = 346$ labor inductions) and 852 women received oxytocin at 40-minutes dosing intervals ($n = 564$ labor augmentations and $n = 288$ labor inductions). The rates of cesarean delivery for dystocia or fetal distress were not statistically different between groups; however, the 20-minutes regimen for augmentation was associated with a significant reduction in cesareans for dystocia (8% vs. 12%, $p = 0.05$). The incidence of uterine tachysystole was greater with the 20-minutes regimen compared to the 40-minutes regimen (40% vs. 31%; $p = 0.02$). Neonatal outcomes were unaffected by the dosing interval. The authors concluded that the 40-minutes dosing interval offered no clear advantage over the 20-minutes interval and that both were safe and efficacious.

Recently, attention has been turned to misoprostol solution as an alternative augmentation agent. Ho et al. [116] evaluated a solution of 200 mcg misoprostol dissolved in 200 ml tap water randomized against intravenous oxytocin in 231 women. The results of this admittedly small study revealed promising results with similar rates of vaginal delivery between the two groups and no difference noted in side effects of neonatal outcomes. Bleich et al. conducted a slightly larger investigation in 350 women who were randomized to either oral misoprostol or intravenous oxytocin. No difference in time interval from initiation of augmentation to delivery or any significant difference in maternal or neonatal outcomes was noted. While women in the misoprostol arm did experience more uterine tachysystole, there was no difference in cesarean deliveries for nonreassuring fetal heart rate patterns [117].

8. Does a prolonged second stage of labor (population) affect maternal or neonatal morbidity (outcome)?

The median duration of the second stage is 50–60 minutes for nulliparas and 20–30 minutes for multiparas, but this is highly variable [118, 119]. In classic obstetrical teaching, the upper limit for the duration of the second stage of labor was considered to be two hours. Factors influencing the length of the second stage include parity, maternal size, birth weight, occiput posterior position, fetal station at complete dilatation, and, potentially, conduction anesthesia [120]. Currently, the American College of Obstetricians and Gynecologists' guidelines [121] for the definition of prolonged second stage, provided the fetal heart rate tracing is normal and there is some degree of labor progress, are as follows: For nulliparous women, the diagnosis should be considered when the second stage exceeds three hours if regional anesthesia has been administered or two hours if no regional anesthesia is used and in multiparous women, the diagnosis can be made when the second stage exceeds two hours with regional anesthesia or one hour without. The Consortium on Safe Labor determined that in the second stage of labor, the 95th percentiles for nulliparous women with and without regional analgesia were 3.6 and 2.8 hours respectively [106]. Janakiraman et al. compared the second stage in 3139 induced women to that of 11 588 women in spontaneous labor [122]. No differences in the length of second stage or the risk of a prolonged second stage were noted between the groups, although the induced nulliparas appeared to be at increased risk of postpartum hemorrhage and cesarean delivery (4.2% vs. 2.0%, OR 1.62, 95% CI 1.02–2.58; 10.9% vs. 7.2%, OR 1.32, 95% CI 1.01–1.71 respectively).

Many authors have studied the perinatal and maternal effects of a prolonged second stage, although no meta-analysis or Cochrane review currently exists. Several studies found no increase in infant morbidity or mortality with a second stage lasting longer than two hours [123–125], although the rate of vaginal delivery precipitously decreases after three hours in the second stage. However, a recent population based cohort study by Allen et al. examined 63 404 nulliparous women and found increased risks of low five-minutes Apgar score, birth depression, and admission to the NICU with increasing duration of the second stage greater than three hours [125]. This study by Allen et al. is the largest thus far evaluating neonatal and maternal outcomes with prolonged second stage. In this study, as well as others, there is evidence that maternal morbidities including perineal trauma, chorioamnionitis, instrumental delivery, and postpartum hemorrhage increase with prolonged second stages greater than two hours (Level of evidence C).

9. Compared to patients who do not receive conduction anesthesia (i.e. epidural or combined spinal epidural; comparison), do patients receiving conduction anesthesia (population) experience prolonged labor courses (outcome)?

Conduction anesthesia's effect on the rate of cervical change remains controversial. In a recent meta-analysis [126], 15 randomized controlled trials including 4619 patients compared the effects of epidural anesthesia to parenteral opioid. The incidence of cesarean section was the same between the groups, although the incidence of operative vaginal delivery was increased in the conduction anesthesia group (OR 1.92; 95% CI 1.52–1.22). It has been difficult to establish whether this increase in operative vaginal delivery was due to a direct effect of the epidural analgesia on the rate of labor or an indirect effect, such as resident training. No difference in the duration of the first stage was noted; however, the second stage was prolonged by approximately 16 minutes (95% CI 10–23 minutes). This statistically significant finding lacks clinical relevance [126].

It has also been suggested that receiving epidural anesthesia during latent labor, as opposed to during the active phase, results in prolongation of the labor, such that many practitioners refrain from administering epidural analgesia until the patient reaches 4 cm or more dilation. An investigation including 12 693 nulliparas randomized subjects to receive early epidural analgesia (at first request if cervical dilation was at least 1 cm) compared with late epidural analgesia (parenteral meperidine until cervical dilation of 4 cm was achieved) [127]. The median cervical dilation at the time of epidural placement was 1.6 cm for the early group and 5.1 for the late group. These researchers found no difference in the incidence of cesarean birth, operative vaginal delivery, or length of first or second stages of labor (Level of evidence A).

CLINICAL SCENARIO: MID-TRIMESTER INDUCTION OF LABOR

A 37-year-old gravida 2 para 1 was diagnosed with a lethal fetal anomaly during her routine second trimester anatomy sonogram. After reviewing her options for pregnancy termination vs. continuation, the patient decides to continue the pregnancy, with plans for comfort care upon delivery. However, at 22 weeks gestation, a fetal demise is diagnosed. The patient wants to know what her options are regarding modes of delivery at this time.

Background

In particular circumstances, such as when a fetus has died in utero or in cases of termination of pregnancy where a fetus would not survive or would survive but with significant handicaps, a woman may need to give birth prior to spontaneous labor. Several delivery options are available for these women, and the decision as to which option is chosen depends upon physician expertise, gestational age, clinical circumstances, and the patient's preferences. Many women will desire immediate delivery secondary to the emotional difficulties of continuing to carry a nonviable fetus; however, some would prefer expectant management in order to avoid an induction of labor. In most cases, there is no medical urgency for immediate delivery. Expectant management raises concerns regarding consumptive coagulopathy and intrauterine infection, but these are rarely associated with prolonged expectant management. Some studies report that 80–90% of women will spontaneously labor within two weeks of a fetal demise, but the latency period may be longer [128].

Clinical question: mid-trimester induction of labor

Critical appraisal of the literature

10. In patients requiring a mid-trimester induction of labor secondary to a lethal anomaly or fetal demise (population), is maternal morbidity (outcome) increased with an induction of labor or with a dilation and evacuation procedure (intervention)?

Options of delivery include induction of labor and dilation and evacuation (D&E), among others (Table 50.4). The decision for which mode of delivery to choose must be individualized by practitioner experience, gestational age, and patient's desires. The emotional and psychological factors vary with each patient, with one advantage of induction being the delivery of an intact fetus whereas an advantage of D&E may be avoiding a prolonged induction.

Most of the research available regarding modes of delivery for mid trimester delivery are extrapolated from the investigations performed regarding second trimester elective abortions. One study evaluated patients undergoing surgical termination between 14 and 23 6/7 weeks of gestation and women undergoing labor induction, which revealed an overall lower rate of complications in those undergoing D&E (4% vs. 29%) [129]. The groups were similar, however, in their need for blood transfusion, infection, cervical laceration, maternal organ damage, and hospital readmission. A more recent study retrospectively analyzed 94 women undergoing D&E vs. 126 women undergoing induction. Midtrimester D&E was associated with more cervical injury, but the induction group had higher rates of retained placenta requiring curettage. Serious complications, including blood transfusion, need for major additional surgery, serious maternal morbidity or maternal death, was similar in the two groups (2%) [130]. Cochrane reviewers recently concluded that D&E is superior to intra-amniotic instillation of prostaglandin F2-alpha and may be favored over mifepristone and misoprostol, but larger randomized studies are necessary to confirm these latter findings [131]. At this time, both methods of delivery are considered reasonably safe.

Several methods of labor induction have been utilized, with no standard protocol currently accepted. In the 1940s, physicians attempted to "salt out" the fetus by injecting hypertonic agents into the amniotic cavity. Hypertonic saline thus became the mainstay of second trimester medical abortion through the 1970s. However, significant risks associated with this method included hypernatremia, coagulopathy, and massive hemorrhage requiring blood transfusions [132]. Instillation regimens utilizing hyperosmolar urea were associated with less coagulopathy and hypernatremia than saline. However, the urea regimens have not been compared to more recent induction protocols. Hyperosmolar regimens often require concomitant use of medical induction agents, such as oxytocin, to stimulate contractions and delivery.

Table 50.4 Second trimester termination methods

Surgical techniques	Medical techniques
Dilatation and evacuation	Intravenous oxytocin
	Intra-amniotic hyperosmotic fluid
Laparotomy	20% saline
Hysterotomy	30% urea
Hysterectomy	Prostaglandins E2, F2 alpha, E1, and analogues
	RU-486 (mifepristone)
	Various combinations of above

More recent protocols have implemented regimens with gemeprost or misoprostol, both PGE_1 analogues; however, a meta-analysis of randomized trials comparing the two medications reported that misoprostol suppositories were associated with a reduced need for narcotic analgesia and surgical evacuation of the uterus [133]. (Level of evidence: A). The application of gemeprost is limited secondary to its expense, instability at room temperature, and narrow routes of administration. It is also not currently available in the United States. At this time, the World Health Organization also recommends the use of mifepristone prior to PGE1 analogues for expeditious and safe second trimester abortions. Mifepristone, as an antiprogestin, increases uterine sensitivity to prostaglandins, permitting lower doses, and minimizing side effects [133]. However, current studies do not reveal any advantage of pretreatment with mifepristone for induction in second trimester fetal demise [134–136].

When planning an induction of labor, gestational age plays a significant role regarding the methods of induction. When the gestational age is less than 28 weeks, the uterus is less sensitive to oxytocin and, therefore, prostaglandins or mechanical devices may be required to commence labor. Current induction protocols vary by dose, route, and gestational age. While side effects (uterine tachysystole, nausea, vomiting, diarrhea) and safety remain important considerations for the patient in these circumstances, the fetal well-being is no longer an issue [137].

Women with a prior cesarean birth are candidates for induction of labor in these circumstances as well. A recent review by Berghella et al. reported an incidence of uterine rupture of 0.4%, hysterectomy 0%, and transfusion 0.2% for women undergoing second trimester misoprostol terminations [138]. Patients may elect for a repeat cesarean delivery but the risks and benefits should be carefully considered (Level of evidence B).

References

1 Martin, J.A., Hamilton, B.E., Osterman, M.J.K. et al. (2013). Births: final data for 2012. *Natl. Vital. Stat. Reports* **62** (**9**. Hyattsville, MD: National Center for Health Statistics).

2 Rayburn, W.F. and Zhang, J. (2002). Rising rates of labor induction: present concerns and future strategies. *Obstet. Gynecol.* **100**: 164.

3 ACOG Committee on Practice Bulletins (2009). ACOG practice bulletin no. 107: induction of labor. *Obstet. Gynecol.* **114**: 386.

4 Nicholson, J.M., Parry, S., Caughey, A.B. et al. (2008). The impact of the active management of risk in pregnancy at term on brith outcomes: a randomized clinical trial. *Am. J. Obstet. Gynecol.* **198**: 511.e1.

5 Koopmans, C.M., Bijlenga, D., Groen, H. et al. (2009). Induction of labour vs. expectant management for gestational hypertension or mild pre-eclampsia after 36 weeks' gestation (HYPITAT): a multicentre, open-label randomised controlled trial. *Lancet* **374**: 979.

6 Mozurkewich, E., Chilimigras, J., Koepke, E. et al. (2009). Indications for induction of labour: a best-evidence review. *BJOG* **116**: 626.

7 Laughon, S.K., Reddy, U.M., Sun, L., and Zhang, J. (2010). Precursors for late preterm birth in singleton gestations. *Obstet. Gynecol.* **116**: 1047.

8 Hibbard, J.U., Wilkins, I., Sun, L. et al. (2010). Respiratory morbidity in late preterm births. *JAMA* **304**: 419.

9 Bailit, J.L., Grobman, W., Zhao, Y. et al. (2015). Nonmedically indicated induction vs. expectant treatment in term nulliparous women. *Am. J. Obstet. Gynecol.* **212**: 103.e1.

10 Nicholson, J.M., Kellar, L.C., Henning, G.F. et al. (2015). The association between the regular use of preventive labour induction and improved term birth outcomes: findings of a systematic review and meta-analysis. *BJOG* **122**: 773.

11 American College of Obstetricians and Gynecologists. ACOG committee opinion no. 561 (2013). Nonmedically indicated early-term deliveries. *Obstet. Gynecol.* **121**: 911.

12 Guerra, G.V., Cecatti, J.G., Souza, J.P. et al. (2011). Elective induction vs. spontaneous labour in Latin America. *Bull. World Health Organ.* **89**: 657.

13 Cammu, H., Martens, G., Ruyssinck, G., and Amy, J.J. (2002). Outcome after elective labor induction in nulliparous women: a matched cohort study. *Am. J. Obstet. Gynecol.* **186**: 240.

14 Prysak, M. and Castronova, F.C. (1998). Elective induction vs. spontaneous labor: a case-control analysis of safety and efficacy. *Obstet. Gynecol.* **92**: 47.

15 Seyb, S.T., Berka, R.J., Socol, M.L., and Dooley, S.L. (1999). Risk of cesarean delivery with elective induction of labor at term in nulliparous women. *Obstet. Gynecol.* **94**.

16 Vrouenraets, F.P., Roumen, F.J., Dehing, C.J. et al. (2005). Bishop score and risk of cesarean delivery after induction of labor in nulliparous women. *Obstet. Gynecol.* **105**: 690.

17 Luthy, D.A., Malmgren, J.A., and Zingheim, R.W. (2004). Cesarean delivery after elective induction in nulliparous women: the physician effect. *Am. J. Obstet. Gynecol.* **191**: 1511.

18 Vahratian, A., Zhang, J., Troendle, J.F. et al. (2005). Labor progression and risk of cesarean delivery in electively induced nulliparas. *Obstet. Gynecol.* **105**: 698.

19 Yeast, J.D., Jones, A., and Poskin, M. (1999). Induction of labor and the relationship to cesarean delivery: a review of 7001 consecutive inductions. *Am. J. Obstet. Gynecol.* **180**: 628.

20 Ehrenthal, D.B., Jiang, X., and Strobino, D.M. (2010). Labor induction and the risk of a cesarean delivery among nulliparous women at term. *Obstet. Gynecol.* **116**: 35.

21 Caughey, A.B., Nicholson, J.M., Cheng, Y.W. et al. (2006). Induction of labor and cesarean delivery by gestational age. *Am. J. Obstet. Gynecol.* **195**.

22 Osmundson, S., Ou-Yang, R.J., and Grobman, W.A. (2011). Elective induction compared with expectant management in nulliparous women with an unfavorable cervix. *Obstet. Gynecol.* **117**: 583.

23 Gülmezoglu, A.M., Crowther, C.A., Middleton, P., and Heatley, E. (2012). Induction of labour for improving birth outcomes for women at or beyond term. *Cochrane Database Syst. Rev.* (**6**): CD004945. doi: 10.1002/14651858.CD004945.pub3.

24 Mishanina, E., Rogozinska, E., Thatthi, T. et al. (2014). Use of labour induction and risk of cesarean delivery: a systematic review and meta-analysis. *CMAJ* **186**: 665.

25 Moore, L.E. and Rayburn, W.F. (2006). Elective induction of labor. *Clin. Obstet. Gynecol.* **49**: 698.

26 Nielsen, P.E., Howard, B.C., Hill, C.C. et al. (2005). Comparison of elective induction of labor with favorable bishop scores vs. expectant management: a randomized clinical trial. *J. Matern. Fetal Neonatal Med.* **18**: 59.

27 Dublin, S., Lydon-Rochelle, M., Kaplan, R.C. et al. (2000). Maternal and neonatal outcomes after induction of labor without an identified indication. *Am. J. Obstet. Gynecol.* **183**: 986.

28 Battista, L., Chung, J.H., Lagrew, D.C., and Wing, D.A. (2007). Complications of labor induction among multiparous women in a community-based hospital system. *Am. J. Obstet. Gynecol.* **197**: 241.e1.

29 Clark, S.L., Miller, D.D., Belfort, M.A. et al. (2009). Neonatal and maternal outcomes associated with elective term delivery. *Am. J. Obstet. Gynecol.* **200**: 156.e1.

30 Smith, L.P., Nagourney, B.A., McLean, F.H., and Usher, R.H. (1984). Hazards and benefits of elective induction of labor. *Am. J. Obstet. Gynecol.* **148**: 579.

31 Vierhout, M.E., Out, J.J., and Wallenburg, H.C. (1985). Elective induction of labor: a prospective clinical study, 1: obstetric and neonatal effects. *J. Perinat. Med.* **13**: 155.

32 Macer, J.A., Macer, C.L., and Chan, L.S. (1992). Elective induction vs. spontaneous labor: a retrospective study of complications and outcomes. *Am. J. Obstet. Gynecol.* **166**: 1690.

33 Martin, D.H., Thompson, W., Pinkerton, J.H., and Watson, J.D. (1978). A randomized controlled trial of selective planned delivery. *BJOG* **85**: 109.

34 Tylleskär, J., Finnström, O., Leijon, I. et al. (1979). Spontaneous labor and elective induction – a prospective randomized study. 1: effects on mother and fetus. *Acta Obstet. Gynecol. Scand.* **58**: 513.

35 Zhang, X., Joseph, K.S., and Kramer, M.S. (2010). Decreased term and postterm birthweight in the US: impact of labor induction. *Am. J. Obstet. Gynecol.* **203**: 124.e1.

36 Morrison, J.J., Rennie, J.M., and Milton, P.J. (1995). Neonatal respiratory morbidity and mode of delivery at term: influence of timing of elective caesarean section. *BJOG* **102**: 101.

37 Kaufman, K.E., Bailit, J.L., and Grobman, W. (2002). Elective induction: an analysis of economic and health consequences. *Am. J. Obstet. Gynecol.* **187**: 858.

38 Cotzias, C.S., Paterson-Brown, S., and Fisk, N.M. (1999). Prospective risk of unexplained stillbirth in singleton pregnancies at term: population based analysis. *BMJ* **319**: 287.

39 Baacke, K.A. and Edwards, R.K. (2006). Preinduction cervical assessment. *Clin. Obstet. Gynecol.* **49**: 564.

40 Bishop, E.H. (1964). Pelvic scoring for elective induction. *Obstet. Gynecol.* **24**: 266.

41 Xenakis, E.M., Piper, J.M., Conway, D.L., and Langer, O. (1997). Induction of labor in the nineties: conquering the unfavorable cervix. *Obstet. Gynecol.* **90**: 235.

42 Johnson, D.P., Davis, N.R., and Brown, A.J. (2003). Risk of cesarean delivery after induction at term in nulliparous women with an unfavorable cervix. *Am. J. Obstet. Gynecol.* **188**: 1565.

43 Arulkumaran, S., Gibb, D.M., Tamby Raja, R.L. et al. (1985). Failed induction of labour. *Aust. N. Z. J. Obstet. Gynaecol.* **25**: 190.

44 Pevzner, L., Rayburn, W.F., Rumney, P.J., and Wing, D.A. (2009). Factors predicting successful labor induction with dinoprostone and misoprostol vaginal inserts. *Obstet. Gynecol.* **114**: 261.

45 Crane, J.M. (2006). Factors predicting labor induction success: a critical analysis. *Clin. Obstet. Gynecol.* **49**: 573.

46 Chandra, S., Crane, J.M., Hutchens, D., and Young, D.C. (2001). Transvaginal ultrasound and digital examination in predicting successful labor induction. *Obstet. Gynecol.* **98**: 2.

47 Kiss, H., Ahner, R., Hohlagschwandtner, M. et al. (2000). Fetal fibronectin as a predictor of term labor: a literature review. *Acta. Obstet. Gynecol. Scand.* **79**: 3.

48 Ojutiku, D., Jones, G., and Bewley, S. (2002). Quantitative fetal fibronectin as a predictor of successful induction of labour in post-date pregnancies. *Eur. J. Obstet. Gynecol. Reprod. Biol.* **101**: 143.

49 Pandis, G.K., Papageorghiou, A.T., Ramanathan, V.G. et al. (2001). Preinduction sonographic measurement of cervical length in the prediction of successful induction of labor. *Ultrasound Obstet. Gynecol.* **18**: 623.

50 Vankayalapati, P., Sethna, F., Roberts, N. et al. (2008). Ultrasound assessment of cervical length in prolonged pregnancy: prediction of spontaneous onset of labor and successful vaginal delivery. *Ultrasound Obstet. Gynecol.* **31**: 328.

51 Verhoeven, C.J., Opmeer, B.C., Oei, S.G. et al. (2013). Transvaginal sonographic assessment of cervical length and wedging for predicting outcome of labor induction at term: a systematic review and meta-analysis. *Ultrasound Obstet. Gynecol.* **42**: 500.

52 Hatfield, A.S., Sanchez-Ramos, L., and Kaunitz, A.M. (2007). Sonographic cervical assessment to predict the success of labor induction: a systematic review with meta-analysis. *Am. J. Obstet. Gynecol.* **197**: 186.

53 Sciscione, A., Hoffman, M.K., DeLuca, S. et al. (2005). Fetal fibronectin as a predictor of vaginal birth in nulliparas undergoing preinduction cervical ripening. *Obstet. Gynecol.* **106**: 980.

54 Garite, T.J., Casal, D., Garcia-Alonso, A. et al. (1996). Fetal fibronectin: a new tool for the prediction of successful induction of labor. *Am. J. Obstet. Gynecol.* **175**: 1516.

55 Reis, F.M., Gervasi, M.T., Florio, P. et al. (2003). Prediction of successful induction of labor at term: role of clinical history, digital examination, ultrasound assessment of the cervix, and fetal fibronectin assay. *Am. J. Obstet. Gynecol.* **189**: 1361.

56 Tanir, H.M., Sener, T., and Yildiz, Z. (2008). Digital and transvaginal ultrasound cervical assessment for prediction of successful labor induction. *Int. J. Gynaecol. Obstet.* **100**: 52.

57 Maul, H., Mackay, L., and Garfield, R.E. (2006). Cervical ripening: biochemical, molecular, and clinical considerations. *Clin. Obstet. Gynecol.* **49**: 551.

58 Boulvain, M., Kelly, A.J., and Lohse, C. (2001). Mechanical methods for induction of labor. *Cochrane Database Syst. Rev.* (**4**): CD001233. doi: 10.1002/14651858.CD001233.

59 Heinemann, J., Gillen, G., Sanchez-Ramos, L., and Kaunitz, A.M. (2008). Do mechanical methods of cervical ripening increase infectious morbidity? A systematic review. *Am. J. Obstet. Gynecol.* **199**.

60 Boulvain, M., Stan, C., and Irion, O. (2005). Membrane sweeping for induction of labour. *Cochrane Database Syst. Rev.* (**1**): CD000451. doi: 10.1002/14651858.CD000451.pub.

61 Howarth, G. and Botha, D.J. (2001). Amniotomy plus intravenous oxytocin for induction of labour. *Cochrane Database Syst. Rev.* (**3**): CD003250. doi: 10.1002/14651858.CD003250.

62 Selo-Ojeme, D.O., Pisal, P., Lawal, O. et al. (2009). A randomised controlled trial of amniotomy and immediate oxytocin infusion vs. amniotomy and delayed oxytocin infusion for induction of labour at term. *Arch. Gynecol. Obstet.* **279**: 813.

63 Bricker, L. and Luckas, M. (2000). Amniotomy alone for induction of labour. *Cochrane Database Syst. Rev.* (**4**): CD002862. doi: 10.1002/14651858.CD002862.

64 St Onge, R.D. and Connors, G.T. (1995). Preinduction cervical ripening: a comparison of intracervical prostaglandin E2 gel vs. the Foley catheter. *Am. J. Obstet. Gynecol.* **172**: 687.

65 Sciscione, A.C., Nguyen, L., Manley, J. et al. (2001). A randomized comparison of transcervical Foley catheter to intravaginal misoprostol for preinduction cervical ripening. *Obstet. Gynecol.* **97**: 603.

66 Chung, J.H., Huang, W.H., Rumney, P.J. et al. (2003). A prospective randomized controlled trial that compared misoprostol, Foley catheter, and combination misoprostol-Foley catheter for labor induction. *Am. J. Obstet. Gynecol.* **189**: 1031.

67 Fox, N.S., Saltzman, D.H., Roman, A.S. et al. (2011). Intravaginal misoprostol vs. Foley catheter for labour induction: a meta-analysis. *BJOG* **118**: 647.

68 Perry, K.G. Jr., Larmon, J.E., May, W.L. et al. (1998). Cervical ripening: a randomized comparison between intravaginal misoprostol and an intracervical balloon catheter combined with intravaginal dinoprostone. *Am. J. Obstet. Gynecol.* **178**: 1333.

69 Sciscione, A., Larkin, M., O'Shea, A. et al. (2004). Preinduction cervical ripening with the Foley catheter and the risk of subsequent preterm birth. *Am. J. Obstet. Gynecol.* **190**: 751.

70 Atad, J., Bornstein, K., Calderon, I. et al. (1991). Nonpharmaceutical ripening of the unfavorable cervix and induction of labor by a novel double balloon device. *Obstet. Gynecol.* **77**: 146.

71 Atad, J., Hallak, M., Auslender, R. et al. (1996). A randomized comparison of prostaglandin E2, oxytocin, and the double-balloon device in inducing labor. *Obstet. Gynecol.* **87**: 223.

72 Atad, J., Hallak, M., Ben-David, Y. et al. (1997). Ripening and dilatation of the unfavourable cervix for induction of labour by a double balloon device: experience with 250 cases. *BJOG* **104**: 29.

73 Alfirevic, Z. and Weeks, A. (2006). Oral misoprostol for induction of labour. *Cochrane Database Syst. Rev.* (**2**): CD001338. doi: 10.1002/14651858.CD001338.pub3.

74 Hofmeyr, G.J., Gulmezoglu, A.M., and Pileggi, C. (2010). Vaginal misoprostol for cervical ripening and induction of labour. *Cochrane Database Syst. Rev.* (**10**): CD000941. doi: 10.1002/14651858.CD000941.pub2.

75 Hughes, E.G., Kelly, A.J., and Kavanagh, J. (2001). Dinoprostone vaginal insert for cervical ripening and labor induction: a meta-analysis. *Obstet. Gynecol.* **97**: 847.

76 Kelly, A.J., Malik, S., Smith, L. et al. (2009). Vaginal prostaglandin (PGE2 and PGF2a) for induction of labour at term. *Cochrane Databae Syst. Rev.* (**4**): CD003101.

77 Lyndrup, J., Legarth, J., Dahl, C. et al. (1990). Induction of labour: the effect of vaginal prostaglandin or i. v. Oxytocin – a matter of time only? *Eur. J. Obstet. Gynecol. Reprod. Biol.* **37**: 111.

78 Pollnow, D.M. and Broekhuizen, F.F. (1996). Randomized, double-blind trial of prostaglandin E2 intravaginal gel vs. low-dose oxytocin for cervical ripening before induction of labor. *Am. J. Obstet. Gynecol.* **174**: 1910.

79 Kelly, A.J. and Tan, B. (2009). Intravenous oxytocin alone for cervical ripening and induction of labour. *Cochrane Database Syst. Rev.* (**4**): CD003246. doi: 10.1002/14651858.CD003246.

80 Ryden, G. and Sjoholm, I. (1971). The metabolism of oxytocin in pregnant and non-pregnant women. *Acta Obstet. Gynecol. Scand. Suppl.* **9**: 37.

81 Seitchik, J., Amico, J., Robinson, A.G., and Castillo, M. (1984). Oxytocin augmentation of dysfunctional labor. IV. Oxytocin pharmacokinetics. *Am. J. Obstet. Gynecol.* **150**: 225.

82 Freeman, R.K. and Nageotte, M.P. (2007). A protocol for use of oxytocin. *Am. J. Obstet. Gynecol.* **197**: 445.

83 Clark, S., Belfort, M., Saade, G. et al. (2007). Implementation of a conservative checklist-based protocol for oxytocin administration: maternal and neonatal outcomes. *Am. J. Obstet. Gynecol.* **197**: 480.e1.

84 Hayes, E.J. and Weinstein, L. (2008). Improving patient safety and uniformity of care by a standardized regimen for the use of oxytocin. *Am. J. Obstet. Gynecol.* **198**: 622.e1.

85 Patka, J.H., Lodolce, A.E., and Johnston, A.K. (2005). High- vs. low-dose oxytocin for augmentation or induction of labor. *Ann. Pharmacother.* **39**: 95.

86 Merrill, D.C. and Zlatnik, F.J. (1999). Randomized double-masked comparison of oxytocin for augmentation and induction of labor. *Obstet. Gynecol.* **94**: 455.

87 Satin, A.J., Leveno, K.J., Sherman, M.L., and McIntire, D. (1994). High-dose oxytocin: 20- vs. 40-minute dosage interval. *Obstet. Gynecol.* **83**: 234.

88 Smith, J.G. and Merrill, D.C. (2006). Oxytocin for induction of labor. *Clin. Obstet. Gynecol.* **49**: 594.

89 Zhang, J., Branch, D.W., Ramirez, M.M. et al. (2011). Oxytocin regimen for labor augmentation, labor progression, and perinatal outcomes. *Obstet. Gynecol.* **118**: 249.

90 Daniel-Spiegel, E., Weiner, Z., Ben-Shlomo, I., and Shalev, E. (2004). For how long should oxytocin be continued during induction of labour? *BJOG* **111**: 331.

91 Ustunyurt, E., Ugur, M., Ustunyurt, B.O. et al. (2007). Prospective randomized study of oxytocin discontinuation after the active stage of labor is established. *J. Obstet. Gynaecol. Res.* **33**: 799.

92 Blakemore, K.J., Qin, N.G., Petrie, R.H., and Paine, L.L. (1990). A prospective comparison of hourly and quarter-hourly oxytocin dose increase intervals for the induction of labor at term. *Obstet. Gynecol.* **75**: 757.

93 O'Driscoll, K., Foley, M., and Mac Donald, D. (1984). Active management of labor as an alternative to cesarean section for dystocia. *Obstet. Gynecol.* **63**: 485.

94 Willcourt, R.J., Pager, D., Wendel, J., and Hale, R.W. (1994). Induction of labor with pulsatile oxytocin by a computer-controlled pump. *Am. J. Obstet. Gynecol.* **170**: 603.

95 Odem, R.R., Work, B.A. Jr., and Bawood, M.Y. (1988). Pulsatile oxytocin for induction of labor: a randomized prospective controlled study. *J. Perinat. Med.* **16**: 31.

96 Frigoletto, F.D., Lieberman, E., Lang, J.M. et al. (1995). A clinical trial of active management of labor. *N. Eng. J. Med.* **333**: 745.

97 Budden, A., Chen, L.J., and Henry, A. (2014). High-dose vs. low-dose oxytocin infusion regimens for induction of labour at term. *Cochrane Database Syst. Rev.* (**10**): CD009701. doi: 10.1002/14651858.CD009701.pub2.

98 Lin, M.G. and Rouse, D.J. (2006). What is a failed labor induction? *Clin. Obstet. Gynecol.* **49**: 585.

99 Simon, C.E. and Grobman, W.A. (2005). When has an induction failed? *Obstet. Gynecol.* **105**: 705.

100 Rouse, D.J., Owen, J., and Hauth, J.C. (2000). Criteria for failed labor induction: prospective evaluation of a standardized protocol. *Obstet. Gynecol.* **96**: 671.

101 Hoffman, M.K., Vahratian, A., Sciscione, A.C. et al. (2006). Comparison of labor progression between induced and noninduced multiparous women. *Obstet. Gynecol.* **107**: 1029.

102 Beckman, M. (2007). Predicting a failed induction. *Aust. N. Z. J. Obstet. Gynaecol.* **47**: 394.

103 Rouse, D.J., Weiner, S.J., Bloom, S.L. et al. (2011). Failed labor induction: toward an objective diagnosis. *Obstet. Gynecol.* **117**: 267.

104 Spong, C.Y., Berghella, V., Wenstrom, K.C. et al. (2012). Prevention of the fist cesarean delivery: Eunice Kennedy Shriver National Institute of child health and development, Society for Maternal-Fetal Medicine, and American College of Obstetricians and Gynecologists workshop. *Obstet. Gynecol.* **120**: 1181–1193.

105 Friedman, E.A. (1972). An objective approach to the diagnosis and management of abnormal labor. *Bull. N. Y. Acad. Med.* **48**: 842.

106 Zhang, J., Troendle, J., Mikolajczyk, R. et al. (2010). The natural history of the normal first stage of labor. *Obstet. Gynecol.* **115**: 705.

107 Friedman, E.A. (1978). *Labor: Clinical Evaluation & Management*. New York, NY: Appleton-Century-Crofts.

108 Zhang, J., Landy, H.J., Branch, D.W. et al. (2010). Contemporary patterns of spontaneous labor with normal neonatal outcomes. *Obstet. Gynecol.* **116**: 1281.

109 Nachum, Z., Garmi, G., Kadan, Y. et al. (2010). Comparison between amniotomy, oxytocin or both for augmentation of labor in prolonged latent phase: a randomized controlled trial. *Reprod. Biol. Endocrinol.* **8**: 136.

110 Rouse, D.J., Owen, J., and Hauth, J.C. (1999). Active-phase labor arrest: oxytocin augmentation for at least 4 hours. *Obstet. Gynecol.* **93**: 323.

111 Clark, S.L., Simpson, K.R., Knox, G.E., and Garite, T.J. (2009). Oxytocin: new perspectives on an old drug. *Am. J. Obstet. Gynecol.* **200**: 35e.1.

112 Satin, A.J., Leveno, K.J., Sherman, M.L. et al. (1992). High- vs. low-dose oxytocin for labor stimulation. *Obstet. Gynecol.* **80**: 111.

113 Wei, S.Q., Luo, Z.C., Qi, H.P. et al. (2010). High-dose vs low-dose oxytocin for labor augmentation: a systematic review. *Am. J. Obstet. Gynecol.* **203**: 296.

114 Orhue, A.A. (1993). A randomised trial of 45 minutes and 15 minutes incremental oxytocin infusion regimes for the induction of labour in women of high parity. *BJOG* **100**: 126.

115 Orhue, A.A. (1993). A randomised trial of 30-min and 15-min oxytocin infusion regimen for induction of labor at term in women of low parity. *Int. J. Gynaecol. Obstet.* **40**: 219.

116 Ho, M., Cheng, S.Y., and Li, T.C. (2010). Titrated oral misoprostol solution compared with intravenous oxytocin for labor augmentation. *Obstet. Gynecol.* **116**: 612.

117 Bleich, A.T., Villano, K.S., Lo, J.Y. et al. (2011). Oral misoprostol for labor augmentation: a randomized controlled trial. *Obstet. Gynecol.* **118**: 1255.

118 Kilpatrick, S.J. and Laros, R.K. Jr. (1989). Characteristics of normal labor. *Obstet. Gynecol.* **74**: 85.

119 Allen, V.M., Baskett, T.F., O'Connell, C.M. et al. (2004). Maternal and perinatal outcomes with increasing duration of the second stage of labor. *Obstet. Gynecol.* **113**: 1248.

120 Piper, J.M., Bolling, D.R., and Newton, E.R. (1991). The second stage of labor: factors influencing duration. *Am. J. Obstet. Gynecol.* **165**: 976.

121 ACOG Committee on Practice Bulletins (2004). ACOG practice bulletin no. 49: dystocia and augmentation of labor. *Obstet. Gynecol.* 102.

122 Janakiraman, V., Ecker, J., and Kaimal, A.J. (2010). Comparing the second stage in induced and spontaneous labor. *Obstet. Gynecol.* **116**: 606.

123 Cohen, W.R. (1977). Influence of the duration of second stage labor on perinatal outcome and puerperal morbidity. *Obstet. Gynecol.* **49**: 266.

124 Menticoglou, S.M., Manning, F., Harman, C., and Morrison, I. (1995). Perinatal outcome in relation to second stage duration. *Am. J. Obstet. Gynecol.* **173**: 906.

125 Myles, T.D. and Santolaya, J. (2003). Maternal and neonatal outcomes in patients with a prolonged second stage of labor. *Obstet. Gynecol.* **102**: 52.

126 Halpern, S.H. and Abdallah, F.W. (2010). Effect of labor analgesia on labor outcome. *Curr. Opin. Anaesthesiol.* **23**: 317.

127 Wang, F., Shen, X., Guo, X. et al. (2009). Epidural analgesia in the latent phase of labor and the risk of cesarean delivery: a five year randomized controlled trial. *Anesthesiology* **111**: 871.

128 Silver, R.M. and Heuser, C.C. (2010). Stillbirth workup and delivery management. *Clin. Obstet. Gynecol.* **53**: 681.

129 Autry, A.M., Hayes, E.J., Jacobson, G.F., and Kirby, R.S. (2002). A comparison of medical induction and dilation and evacuation for second trimester abortion. *Am. J. Obstet. Gynecol.* **187**: 393.

130 Whitley, K.A., Trinchere, K., Prutsman, W. et al. (2011). Midtrimester dilation and evacuation vs. prostaglandin induction: a comparison of composite outcomes. *Am. J. Obstet. Gynecol.* **205**: 386.e1.

131 Lohr, P.A., Hayes, J.L., and Gemzell-Danielsson, K. (2008). Surgical vs. medical methods for second trimester induced abortion. *Cochrane Database Syst. Rev.* (**1**): CD006714. doi: 10.1002/14651858.CD006714.pub2.

132 Kafrissen, M.E., Barke, M.W., Workman, P. et al. (1983). Coagulopathy and induced abortion methods: rates and relative risks. *Am. J. Obstet. Gynecol.* **147**: 344.

133 Hammond, C. (2009). Recent advances in second-trimester abortion: an evidence based review. *Am. J. Obstet. Gynecol.* **200**: 347.

134 Wagaarachchi, P.T., Ashok, P.W., Narvekar, N.N. et al. (2002). Medical management of late intrauterine death using a combination of mifepristone and misoprostol. *BJOG* **109**: 443.

135 Fairley, T.E., Mackenzie, M., Owen, P., and Mackenzie, F. (2005). Management of late intrauterine death using a combination of mifepristone and misoprostol-experience of two regimens. *Eur. J. Obstet. Gynecol. Reprod. Biol.* **118**: 28.

136 Jannet, D., Aflak, N., Abankwa, A. et al. (1996). Termination of 2nd and 3rd trimester pregnancies with mifepristone and misoprostol. *Eur. J. Obstet. Gynecol. Reprod. Biol.* **70**: 159.

137 Dodd, J.M. and Crowther, C.A. (2010). Misoprostol for induction of labor to terminate pregnancy in the 2nd or 3rd trimester for women with a fetal anomaly or after intrauterine fetal death. *Cochrane Database Syst. Rev.* (**4**): CD004901. doi: 10.1002/14651858.CD004901.pub2.

138 Berghella, V., Airoldi, J., O'Neill, A.M. et al. (2009). Misoprostol for 2nd trimester pregnancy termination in women with prior cesarean: a systematic review. *BJOG* **116**: 1151.

51

CHAPTER 51

Postpartum hemorrhage

Alexandria J. Hill[1,2,3], Karin Fox[4,5], and Stephanie R. Martin[6]

[1] *High Risk Pregnancy Center, Las Vegas, NV, USA*
[2] *Texas A&M College of Medicine, College Station, TX, USA*
[3] *University of Arizona, Phoenix, AZ, USA*
[4] *Maternal-Fetal Medicine, Baylor College of Medicine, Houston, TX, USA*
[5] *Texas Children's Hospital, Pavilion for Women, Houston, TX, USA*
[6] *Clinical Concepts in Obstetrics, Scottsdale, AZ, USA*

Introduction

This chapter will focus specifically on the obstetrical patient experiencing a postpartum hemorrhage (PPH). The goal is to identify the emergency, explain the etiology, and understand general management tools to assist in decision-making during such emergencies. We introduce two clinical scenarios and lead you through management decisions for the event based on best available evidence.

Background

PPH remains a leading cause of maternal morbidity and mortality worldwide [1, 2], and the immediate postpartum period is the most common time for complications from hemorrhage [2]. The most frequent cause of PPH is uterine atony. Table 51.1 lists causes of PPH [1]. In industrialized nations, the prevalence of obesity, advancing maternal age, multiple gestations, rates of induction, cesarean delivery, and subsequent trials of labor after cesarean are on the rise, thereby increasing the overall potential for PPH. Definitions of PPH (also described as massive obstetrical hemorrhage, MOH) vary widely. In general, accepted definitions include estimated blood loss > 500 ml following a vaginal delivery or > 1000 ml following a cesarean delivery. It has been proposed that a drop in hematocrit by 10% or need for blood transfusion should also be criteria for the diagnosis of PPH [1, 3]. Other studies have defined PPH as a blood loss exceeding 1, 2.5 l, or need for at least 5 units of packed red blood cells (PRBCs) [4]. Management of acute PPH focuses initially on identifying and addressing underlying etiology (i.e. treatment of uterine atony or repair of a laceration). Maternal mortality in the United States declined dramatically over the last century, but reached a nadir in the late-1980s, but has had a small, but steady increase over the last 2 decades [5]. Although a majority of maternal deaths have been deemed unpreventable, hemorrhage is one of the identified preventable causes of maternal death, and thus the Joint Commission has recommended that protocols for rapid identification and response should be in place in the hospital setting [6]. *In this chapter, the focus will be on identifying causes of hemorrhage as well as treatments and outcomes of various interventions.*

Table 51.1 Acute causes of postpartum hemorrhage

Uterine atony
Lower genital tract lacerations (perineal, vaginal, cervical, periclitoral, labial, periurethral, rectal)
Upper genital tract lacerations (broad ligament)
Lower urinary tract lacerations (bladder, urethra)
Retained products of conception (placenta, membranes)
Invasive placentation (placenta accreta/increate/percreta)
Uterine rupture
Uterine inversion
Coagulopathy (hereditary, acquired)

CLINICAL SCENARIO 1

A 34-years-old G5P4004 at 39 weeks' gestation presents to the obstetrical triage unit with the chief complaint of contractions and leakage of fluid. On sterile vaginal examination, she is noted to be 8 cm/100% effaced/+2 station. You work with staff to get a peripheral IV placed, successfully, and soon after she precipitously delivers in the obstetrical triage unit. Uterine atony follows, accompanied by a large amount of bleeding from the vagina immediately after delivery of the placenta. You estimate a total blood loss of 1100 ml, including blood loss at the time of delivery.

Evidence-Based Obstetrics and Gynecology, First Edition. Edited by Errol R. Norwitz, Carolyn M. Zelop, David A. Miller, and David L. Keefe.

Clinical questions

1. In pregnant patients experiencing acute PPH (population) what are effective medical interventions (targeted test) that can be used to decrease further bleeding (outcome)?
2. In pregnant patients experiencing acute PPH (population) do invasive procedures (intervention) prevent further hemorrhage and decrease the need for hysterectomy (outcomes)?

General search strategy

Addressing the topic of PPH can be guided by first identifying the cause of the hemorrhage. One might begin with a broad search of PPH in common electronic databases such as MEDLINE and OVID, specifically searching for prospective studies, systematic reviews, and randomized trials regarding this subject. The Cochrane Library can assist in finding systematic reviews of treatment strategies in the various causes of PPH. These three search engines were used throughout this chapter for data retrieval.

Critical appraisal of the literature

1. In pregnant patients experiencing acute postpartum hemorrhage (population) what are effective medical interventions (targeted test) that can be used to decrease further bleeding (outcome)?

Search Strategy

- COCHRANE: postpartum hemorrhage.
- MEDLINE: postpartum hemorrhage AND interventions AND clinical trial AND (clinical trial OR case–control studies OR cohort studies OR meta-analysis).
- Hand-searching: references listed in the articles obtained.

Acute PPH is often defined as estimated blood loss of >500 ml after a vaginal delivery and > 1000 ml after a cesarean delivery. Quantification of PPH is often subjective and visual. Data indicate that blood loss in the obstetric patient is commonly underestimated by medical professionals including midwifes, nurses, and physicians [7–12]. Objective measures of blood loss including weighing of sponges, measurement of volume in premarked drapes and assessment of hemoglobin can assist in estimation of blood loss [13]. When a collection drape is used, studies have shown a reduction in maternal morbidity and mortality [13] yet no significant decrease in PPH severity [14].

Prevention of hemorrhage is an important component of the management of patients at the time of delivery. Active management of the third stage of labor (AMTSL) has proven to reduce the risk of PPH [15]. AMTSL includes: (i) use of prophylactic uterotonics; (ii) early cord clamping; and (iii) cord traction for delivery of the placenta. The uterotonic agent of choice has been oxytocin, which has proven more effective than prostaglandins [16]. Although AMTSL is easy to perform, many institutions worldwide perform only one or two of the necessary three components of AMTSL [17]. Continuing education and training for providers to consistently utilize AMTSL are necessary to reduce the incidence of highly morbid complications of PPH. The World Health Organization recommends inclusion of the three criteria for AMTSL to prevent PPH, yet recent findings indicate that the most protective measure of the three is immediate administration of oxytocin after delivery of the fetus (or the anterior shoulder) [18]. A recent double-blind, randomized controlled trial compared oxytocin alone to ergometrine (Syntometrine) plus oxytocin, finding that blood loss was less with the administration of both uterotonics, yet side effects of ergometrine were significant (nausea, vomiting, elevated blood pressures) [19]. Studies have been done on women with identifiable risk factors for PPH, such as a distended uterus (e.g.: polyhydramnios, multiple gestation, fetal macrosomia) or abnormal placentation (placenta previa, placenta accreta) and found that patients who received Hemabate and oxytocin (over either drug alone) prophylactically had significantly less bleeding than controls [20].

When PPH is identified, a general, stepwise approach is used. After vaginal delivery, the cervix and vagina should be well visualized and any bleeding lesions should be repaired. The uterus should also be examined for any retained products of conception and bimanually compressed to decrease immediate bleeding due to atony. If atony is felt to be the cause of hemorrhage, first line therapy is the administration of uterotonic medications and repletion of intravenous fluids and blood products as necessary. If hemorrhage persists, the decision is then made to either proceed with uterine packing or balloon tamponade, uterine artery embolization (UAE), or exploratory laparotomy to ligate vessels, place compression sutures, or a combination of these methods. Hysterectomy may be required should the other interventions fail, and if done in a timely manner, may be life-saving.

Commonly recommended uterotonics include: oxytocin (Pitocin®), methylergonovine (Methergine®), misoprostol (Cytotec®), and prostaglandin formulations such as $F_{2\alpha}$ (Hemabate®) and E_2 (Dinoprostone). Examples of uterotonic drugs, dosing, and route of administration can be found on Table 51.2 [1]. All uterotonics may cause nausea and/or vomiting. The physician must also be aware of the contraindications of specific uterotonic medications. For example, Methergine should be avoided in patients who are hypertensive or with a history of hypertension and Hemabate should be avoided in patients with active cardiac, pulmonary, renal, or hepatic disease [1]. Some uterotonic drugs have the advantage to be administered via more than one route, like misoprostol (Cytotec®), which can be given rectally, buccally or orally, and oxytocin, which may be given intravenously or intramuscularly. This is potentially advantageous for patients who do not have IV access or are unable to tolerate oral medications.

Misoprostol (Cytotec®) is a shelf-stable medication in tablet form that does not require refrigeration. This affords it

Table 51.2 Uterotonic medications

Agent	Dose	Route	Dosing frequency	Side effects	Contraindications
Oxytocin (Pitocin)	10–80 U in 1000 ml of crystalloid	*IV IM or IU	Continuous	N/V, emesis, water intoxication	None
Misoprostol (Cytotec)	600–1000 μg	*PR PO	Single dose	N/V, diarrhea, fever, chills	None
Methylergonovine (Methergine)	0.2 mg	*IM IU	Every 2–4 h	Hypertension, hypotension, N/V	Hypertension, preeclampsia
Prostaglandin $F_{2\alpha}$ (Hemabate)	0.25 mg	*IM IU	Every 15–90 min (8 dose max)	N/V, diarrhea, flushing, chills	Active cardiac, pulmonary, renal, or hepatic disease
Prostaglandin E_2 (Dinoprostone)	20 mg	PR	Every 2 h	N/V, diarrhea, fever, chills, headache	Hypotension

IV, intravenous; IM, intramuscular; IU, intrauterine; PR, per rectum; PO, per oral; *1st line; N/V, nausea and vomiting.

the potential benefit of use in remote, low-resource settings. A notable trend toward reduction in postpartum blood loss, drop in hemoglobin, and need for additional interventions was seen in patients that received misoprostol (600 mcg sublingually) versus placebo when they had an estimated blood loss >500 ml after a normal spontaneous vaginal delivery [21]. Misoprostol can also be administered rectally, up to 1000 mcg, and has been shown to decrease need for further intervention for PPH [22]. Although a randomized control trial comparing interventions for treatment of PPH showed insufficient evidence for misoprostol to be added to the current combination of oxytocin/ergometrine (Syntometrine), misoprostol showed a better clinical response when administered rectally than did IV Syntometrine. Misoprostol, however, is associated with a significant increase in maternal pyrexia and shivering [23].

Oxytocin, the most commonly used uterotonic, has a rapid onset of action and a short half-life. It can be administered intravenously or intramuscularly. When administered too rapidly, it can cause maternal hypotension [24]. Studies have shown that oxytocin administered in an immediate bolus (5 units over one minute) after cesarean delivery can be as effective in preventing PPH as a bolus plus an additional IV infusion (40 units in 500 ml saline over four hours). However, a decreased need for other uterotonics is seen when a continued IV infusion of oxytocin is administered after cesarean delivery [25]. Oxytocin agonists, such as Carbetocin, have been studied for their effectiveness in preventing PPH. A large Cochrane Database search revealed that Carbetocin reduced the need for other uterotonics (after cesarean delivery), need for uterine massage (after cesarean or vaginal delivery), and overall risk of PPH when compared to oxytocin [26]. Another medication that has been proposed to assist with management of PPH is estradiol. When compared to routine management of PPH (uterine massage and uterotonics), women experiencing acute PPH who received 4 mg estradiol benzoate intramuscularly had less blood loss and did not require hysterectomy as often [27], however this is not currently widely used.

Tranexamic acid acts as an antifibrinolytic agent, preventing breakdown of fibrin by plasmin [28], and has been used in trauma patients and gynecologic patients with significant menorrhagia to stop further bleeding. A recent randomized controlled trial confirmed data from prior studies [29–32] indicating that tranexamic acid administration can decrease intra- and post-operative blood loss in patients undergoing a cesarean delivery [28]. The WOMAN (World Maternal Antifibrinolytic) trial was designed to enroll patients with a PPH following the delivery of an infant via cesarean or vaginal delivery and randomized them to either tranexamic acid (1 g IV) or placebo (sodium chloride 0.9%), an analysis based on intent to treat. Enrollment is aimed at 15 000 women, with the aim to reduce mortality or need for hysterectomy in this patient population [2].

Recombinant factor VIIa (rFVIIa) has been administered in the setting of PPH, to improve coagulopathy, and may contribute to an improvement in predicted maternal mortality [33], however its use remains controversial. A notable decrease in prothrombin time (PT), to nearly a normal level, can be seen in patients who receive rFVIIa in the setting of massive hemorrhage and need for blood transfusion [34]. However, this medication may be ineffective in the setting of hypofibrinogenemia, due to the role of FVII in the coagulation cascade, such that factor VII cleaves fibrinogen to fibrin, which is then available for clot formation. Therefore, transfusion of cryoprecipitate must often precede administration of rFVIIa. Whether or not rFVIIa decreases the need for blood products is also questionable [33, 35]. Moreover, the dosing range of rFVIIa is very broad (16–128 mμg kg^{-1}) [36], and optimal dosing remains unknown. The disadvantages of rFVIIa are the possible complication of arterial thromboembolism due to activation of the clotting cascade and high cost per dose [37]. Its use has been limited in the obstetric context.

In the face of MOH, it is imperative to replete blood products appropriately and in a timely manner. Timely transfusion and resuscitation must be initiated during PPH and may be given concomitantly during both conservative and surgical methods to identify and stop hemorrhage. Continual assessment of bleeding activity, patient vital signs and symptoms is imperative, as obstetrical hemorrhage can rapidly deteriorate toward hypovolemic shock or disseminated intravascular coagulopathy. Blood products should be transfused as needed, and without unnecessary delay [38]. Trauma patients transfused at a ratio of 1 : 1 of fresh frozen plasma (FFP) to PRBC when compared to more traditional ratios of 1 : 4 or 1 : 5 showed increased survival [39].

Quantification of PPH is often subjective and visual. Data indicate that blood loss in the obstetric patient is commonly underestimated by medical professionals including midwifes, nurses, and physicians [7–12]. Objective measures of blood loss including weighing of sponges, measurement of volume in premarked drapes and assessment of hemoglobin can assist in estimation of blood loss [13]. When a collection drape is used, studies have shown a reduction in maternal morbidity and mortality [13] yet no significant decrease in PPH severity [14]. If collection tools are not utilized, training medical providers in assessment of blood loss has been shown to improve accuracy of blood loss estimation [40].

Although medical therapy can often slow hemorrhage due to uterine atony, surgical intervention, including hysterectomy, should be anticipated, particularly in patients with severe blood loss requiring blood transfusion. A three-year study of 117 major obstetrical hemorrhage patients in Dublin, Ireland found that in patients who received at least 5 units of PRBC (majority due to uterine atony) only 15% were managed successfully with medical therapy (oxytocin, misoprostol, Hemabate, ergometrine, or rarely, rFVIIa) alone [4].

Given that PPH is an unfortunately common morbidity in obstetrics, various protocols for management of PPH have been designed that decrease the need for blood products, prevent development of disseminated intravascular coagulation (DIC), and allow earlier resolution of maternal bleeding [41]. For example, investigators from the United Kingdom reviewed the use of the algorithm "HEMOSTASIS" (Help, Establish etiology, Massage the uterus, Oxytocin infusion and prostaglandins, Shift to operating room, Tamponade test, Apply compression sutures, Systemic pelvic devascularization, Interventional radiology, Subtotal/total abdominal hysterectomy) for women with >1500 ml blood loss. Use of this algorithm facilitated proper management as well as a decreased need for blood transfusions, hysterectomies, ICU admissions, and maternal mortality [42]. For institutions that do not routinely manage patients with uterotonics, protocols such as this are suggested to guide management of the PPH patient prior to moving toward operative techniques [43].

2. In pregnant patients experiencing acute postpartum hemorrhage (population) do invasive procedures (intervention) prevent further hemorrhage and decrease the need for hysterectomy (outcomes)?

Search Strategy

- COCHRANE: postpartum hemorrhage.
- MEDLINE: postpartum hemorrhage AND surgery AND hysterectomy AND (clinical trial OR case–control studies OR cohort studies OR meta-analysis).
- Hand-searching: references listed in the articles obtained.

A patient experiencing PPH, especially after a vaginal delivery, will often be managed first with uterotonic medications, manual compression of the uterus, and repair of any bleeding lacerations. Invasive procedures are often second-line therapy if the aforementioned methods are not successful. Invasive procedures reviewed will include uterine packing and tamponade, use of compression sutures, systemic devascularization (arterial ligation), and UAE. Current data will be reviewed regarding effectiveness of these methods in controlling bleeding and preventing the need for hysterectomy in an acute PPH patient.

Bimanual uterine compression and uterine tamponade

Bleeding from uterine atony can be controlled not only with uterotonic medications, but also with manual compression of the uterus. Classically, a single-handed Crede maneuver was described, whereby the uterine fundus is grasped through the abdominal wall between the provider's fingers and thumbs. While still a useful technique, it is difficult in overweight or obese patients and does not provide compression of the lower uterine segment. Bimanual compression can be performed by placing one hand placed intravaginally, just posterior to the cervix, and by placing other hand on the patient's abdomen, at the fundus, and "sandwiching" the uterus between the hands. This technique also allows the provider to pull the uterus slightly anteriorly, toward the symphysis pubis, providing further compression. This bimanual technique compresses the lower segment, places the uterine arteries on stretch, and applies pressure to the fundus.

While effective, manual compression is only a temporizing measure to treat immediate PPH. Intrauterine tamponade is another method to apply pressure to aid with hemostasis. Two main methods have been described in the literature, including uterine packing, using rolled gauze or balloon tamponade. Not only has intrauterine tamponade been used for atony, but also for bleeding due to uterine inversion, with the added benefit of providing structural support to prevent early recurrent uterine inversion [44, 45]. Use of gauze packing is a readily available, inexpensive and older technique that was endorsed in numerous textbooks in the 1930s and 1940s [46]. Gauze is placed manually or with long forceps at the fundus and layered within the uterine cavity until filled, and a "tail" of gauze is allowed to remain visible outside the introitus to monitor bleeding and allow for easy removal. Traditionally, laparotomy sponges tied together or rolled gauze has been used, to ensure that no packing material is retained. More recently, studies have evaluated the feasibility of use of specially saturated gauze, such as gauze saturated in chitosan to better achieve hemostasis, with promising results [47]. In this series of 19 cases of PPH, the need for hysterectomy was reduced by 75% compared to the rate prior to the introduction of chitosan-soaked gauze. Additionally, the authors concluded that as this gauze was easy to use, and inexpensive, it may prove useful in low-resource settings. Uterine packing has been shown via angiography not only to halt bleeding by placing pressure within the uterine cavity, but also to reduce the perfusion pressure and flow within the uterine arteries [48].

Balloon tamponade for uterine bleeding was introduced by Bakri et al. in 1992 [49]. In addition to the use of the Bakri® balloon, use of various types of easily accessible balloons has been described, including the use of a water or saline-filled condom tied to a straight catheter, a Sengstaken-Blakemore gastrointestinal balloon [50, 51], large Foley catheter, and Ebb® balloon [52]. In multiple retrospective and prospective studies, the use of uterine balloon tamponade was associated with a decrease in the need for invasive surgical interventions between 85% and 100%, and is also very useful for resource poor settings [53].

Systemic devascularization (arterial ligation)

Various vessels can be ligated in an attempt to stop PPH. In the face of PPH at time of cesarean delivery, the vessel most easily assessable, visualized, and palpable for ligation is the uterine artery. This vessel can be seen entering the inferior lateral borders of the lower uterine segment, adjacent to the internal cervical os. Ligation of the internal iliac artery, or hypogastric artery, may also be performed. The anterior division of this vessel feeds the uterus and vagina. This artery is retroperitoneal and thus dissection and ligation requires extensive experience and knowledge of this anatomical region, which can take time in the face of a rapid and life threatening obstetric hemorrhage. A long-term study reviewed cases of early PPH that required laparotomy in a 3-year time span in the 1980s and again in the 2000s. A significant decrease in need for hysterectomy has been described during this time frame (87.5% in the 1980s vs. 22.2% in the 2000s). The authors concluded that use of uterine or hypogastric artery ligation, is associated with successful control of PPH and the ability to avoid hysterectomy [54]. It should be noted that hypogastric artery ligation is a technically complex procedure, with which few obstetrical and gynecologic surgeons have extensive experience, and its utility may thereby be limited.

Approximately 40% of patients with attempt at internal iliac artery ligation ultimately required hysterectomy overall, but this varies by etiology of hemorrhage. Internal iliac artery ligation was successful in salvaging the uterus in 63.8% with uterine atony, 85.7% with placenta previa, and 21% of those who experienced uterine rupture [55]. Other studies have found that internal iliac artery ligation controlled PPH, thus preventing need for hysterectomy, in 75–82% of patients [56, 57]. A major limitation to performing this ligation is the technical expertise and experience operating in the retroperitoneal space, especially in the setting of hemorrhage. MRI has shown that the vast majority of patients show complete repermeation of the arteries even after bilateral internal iliac artery ligation [57].

Compression sutures

Another method to control hemorrhage in the postpartum patient is to use uterine compression sutures. The B-Lynch suture is the most well-known uterine compression suture. To perform this procedure, one should use a large absorbable suture and, in a running fashion, pass the suture through one corner of the hysterotomy, run the suture over the fundus, pass the suture transversely through the posterior lower uterine segment, back over the fundus to the anterior uterus, and then pass through the other corner of the hysterectomy allowing for the suture to then be tied in the anterior lower uterine segment region inferior to the hysterotomy. Proper step-by-step placement of this suture can be seen in Figure 51.1 [58]. Multiple studies looking at outcomes in patients who had compression sutures placed due to PPH found that 77–82% of women avoided hysterectomy [59–61]. Moreover, hysterectomy can be avoided in patients with B-Lynch sutures following unsuccessful vessel ligation; of 15 patients who underwent compression sutures for this purpose only 3 (20%) required hysterectomy [36].

A modification of the B-Lynch suture was proposed by Hayman in 2002, and is illustrated in Figure 51.2 [58]. The surgeon places two separate sutures through the lower uterine segment and each are tied separately at the fundus. This procedure does not require that a hysterotomy be made for evacuation of uterine contents and there is no need for excessive passes through the lower uterine segment. This technique was performed on 11 patients in an Italian study, who also received a protocol of uterotonics for PPH, and only one patient required hysterectomy [62]. There is little data to guide patient counseling regarding future childbearing or intrauterine scar formation after placement of compression sutures. Women have had imaging of the uterus or direct visualization of the uterus (hysterosalpingogram or hysteroscopy) after compression sutures with a uterine synechiae formation rate ranging from 26.7%

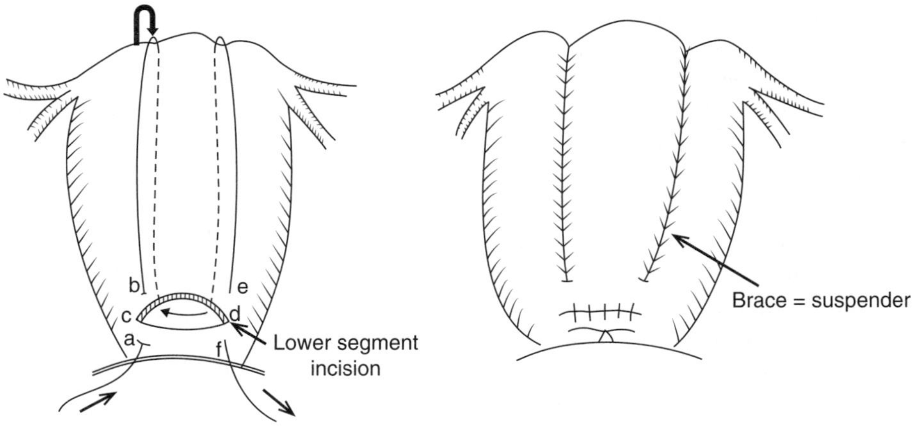

Figure 51.1 B-Lynch uterine compression suture.

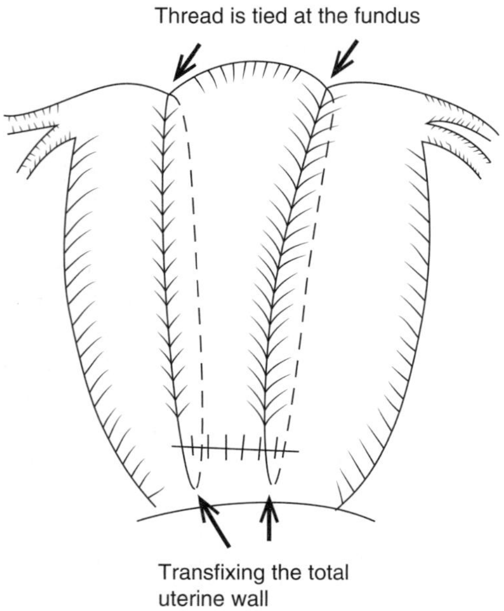

Figure 51.2 Hayman suture – Modified B-Lynch suture.

to 53.8% [63, 64]. Asherman syndrome has been noted in these patients at time of follow up, but successful subsequent pregnancies have also been reported [64].

Conservative surgical techniques have been reported to control excessive bleeding caused by uterine atony, cervical scar pregnancy, and uterine-cervical-vaginal tears, and in selected placenta previa and accreta cases at 12 institutions in Buenos Aires, Argentina [65]. In this series, hysterectomy was required in only 7.4% of women. The various surgical techniques evaluated were selective arterial ligation (bilateral uterine artery ligation, selective pelvic subperitoneal pedicle ligation) and compression procedures (B-Lynch, Hayman's, Pereira's, Cho's). Furthermore, patients were followed up with hysteroscopy and MRI, and of the 499 women who retained their uterus, 116 successful pregnancies were reported [65].

Uterine artery embolization (UAE)

UAE has been integrated in many institutions as an intervention to prevent further bleeding in the event of PPH. This procedure has the advantage of being minimally invasive, but requires the expertise of Interventional Radiology (IR). This can be a limitation for those institutions that do not have immediate access to an IR department, or when a patient must be moved long distances to a remote IR unit. UAE has been found to have a 90–95% [66–68] success rate overall with a 98% success rate with acute (or primary) PPH and a 94% success rate with PPH after cesarean deliveries [67]. Other studies have found an 82% success rate of UAE to prevent hysterectomy [69]. UAE also has proven successful in managing PPH patients when other methods such as uterine packing, compression sutures, balloon tamponade, or even hysterectomy have failed. It was found that 94% of patients who failed these methods were made hemostatic with UAE, and no immediate complications were associated with embolization [70]. Even in patients who experience PPH from placenta accreta, UAE has been successful. In 17 patients who underwent UAE to control hemorrhage from a placenta accreta, 14 (82.4%) ceased bleeding, whereas the remaining 3 required hysterectomy [71].

Complications following UAE are uncommon but include thrombus formation and ischemia. This includes emboli in the femoral artery (1 of 11 subjects), likely from particle migration [69] and lower extremity thrombus formation (1 of 26 subjects) [72]. For patients who failed arterial ligation and were treated with UAE (successful in 11 of 12 subjects), two complications were noted: lower extremity ischemia and nerve ischemia. Both resolved without residual complications [73]. An observational retrospective study reviewed deliveries that required blood transfusion for PPH that also underwent UAE or hysterectomy for treatment. Patients who underwent hysterectomy required double the amount of blood products than those who had an UAE. They also found that some patients treated with hysterectomy subsequently underwent UAE to reach hemostasis, where the reverse was true 1/10 of the time [74]. These data are not randomized and therefore may reflect selection bias. Questions also arise regarding fertility after UAE. A 10-year review at a single institution found that all women who underwent UAE for PPH had return of regular menses. Moreover, of the women who desired future childbearing, all were successful [75]. Resumption of menses after UAE ranges from 91% to 100% [68, 76].

The efficacy of invasive second-line treatment to stop PPH in women who failed first-line uterotonic or intrauterine tamponade were as follows (in descending order): UAE 86%, uterine compression sutures 75%, pelvic vessel ligation (internal iliac, uterine, or ovarian) 36% [77]. Some patients received more than one second-line treatment, and were more clinically complex. One fourth of the patients ultimately required hysterectomy [77]. Interestingly, in a 2007 study from the United Kingdom (UK), women often underwent surgical treatment for PPH without universally being treated with uterotonics, suggesting an opportunity for improved enforcement of a protocol of uterotonics prior to proceeding with operative techniques [43].

In conclusion, the treatment of PPH must be guided first by early recognition and treatment of the underlying etiology. Multiple medical and/or surgical treatment modalities may be required to attain sufficient control and to stabilize the patient. Hemorrhage with vessel ligation and salvaging of the uterus [55]. Compression sutures have been found to have a high success rate in preventing the need for hysterectomy [59–61], but the long-term effect they have on the uterine cavity is yet to be completely understood [63, 64]. Studies have shown that UAE is an effective adjunct that may not always negatively impact menstruation and fertility [68, 75, 76].

Conclusions

The patient in our scenario likely experienced an acute PPH from uterine atony. The patient can be managed medically with oxytocin IV as well as administration of uterotonics. Identification and repair of any vaginal or cervical lacerations is imperative. Since there is no direct visualization of the uterus after vaginal delivery, balloon tamponade or UAE may be considered. Early transfusion of blood and blood products to prevent hypovolemic shock and coagulopathy is essential. If compression techniques are ineffective, laparotomy should be considered. Compression sutures can be placed and uterine and/or ovarian vessels can be ligated. Finally, attempt at hypogastric artery ligation can be performed if the physician is able to visualize and adequately dissect the retroperitoneum. Finally, the physician can proceed with hysterectomy.

CLINICAL SCENARIO 2

A 34-year-old G6P5005 at 37 weeks' gestation presents to obstetrics (OB) triage with painful, regular contractions. She has a history of three prior, uncomplicated cesarean deliveries. She is visiting from out of town, and tells you that her OB told her no one should check her cervix as she has a previa. She denies any vaginal bleeding. You perform a quick bedside ultrasound and note an anterior placenta with multiple heterogeneous appearing areas within the placenta and a loss of the hyperechoic uterine-bladder interface.

Background

Placenta accreta is abnormal invasion of the placenta into the myometrium of the uterus, and is one of the most life threatening surgical encounters that the Obstetrician will face. The biggest risk factors for this invasive placentation are placenta previa and prior uterine surgery, most commonly cesarean delivery. The risk of an accreta increases with each prior cesarean delivery: 0.3% with 1, 0.6% with 2, 2.1% with 3, 2.3% with 4, and 6.7% with more than 4 [78]. When a previa is present, the risks are substantially higher: 3% with 1, 11% with 2, 40% with 3, 61% with 4, and 67% with more than 4 [78]. The region of involvement can be localized or extensive, and the depth and degree of invasion can be less than 50% of the myometrium (accreta), further into the myometrium (increta), or through the entire myometrium (percreta). Blood loss is extensive when an accreta is identified, and typically ranges from 3 to 5 l [79]. Complications at time of delivery include injury to surrounding organs such as bladder, bowel, or ureters, and massive hemorrhage leading to disseminated intravascular coagulopathy. Patients may ultimately require admission to the intensive care unit as they may experience complications associated with hemorrhagic shock and massive transfusion such as transfusion related acute lung injury, transfusion associated cardiopulmonary overload, electrolyte disturbances, or acute renal failure. Although the exact maternal mortality rate in women with placenta accreta is unknown, it has been reported to be as low as 1 in 1000 [72] to as high as 4–8% [80]. The incidence of placenta accreta is rising concomitantly with the increase in cesarean delivery rate, at an estimated 1 in every 533 pregnancies [81], to 1 in 1000 pregnancies [82], compared to 1 in every 4027 and 1 in every 2510 in the 1970s and 1980s respectively [83]. For these reasons, attempts to identify placental invasion antenatally and reduce morbidity have been areas of interest in clinical research.

Clinical questions

1. In pregnant patients with suspected abnormal placentation (population), can antenatal identification and preparatory measurements (intervention) decrease maternal comorbidities (outcomes)?
2. In pregnant patients with morbidly adherent placenta (placenta accreta, increta or percreta) (population), what are potential alternatives to hysterectomy (interventions) to assist with controlling/preventing hemorrhage (outcome)?

Critical appraisal of the literature

1. In pregnant patients with suspected abnormal placentation (population), can antenatal identification and preparatory measurements (intervention) decrease maternal comorbidities (outcomes)?
Search Strategy

- COCHRANE: placenta accrete.
- MEDLINE: placenta accreta AND postpartum hemorrhage AND interventions AND clinical trial AND (clinical trial OR case–control studies OR cohort studies OR meta-analysis).
- Hand-searching: references listed in the articles obtained.

A retrospective review of approximately 106 000 deliveries aimed to identify the most common reasons for peripartum, emergent (within 24 hours of delivery) hysterectomy [84]. Of the 39 emergent peripartum hysterectomies, placenta accreta was identified in 53.8% of the cases requiring emergent hysterectomy [84].

Various imaging modalities have been used to attempt to identify abnormal placentation prior to the time of delivery. As most all women undergo ultrasound during pregnancy, it is considered an ideal modality for initial screening for abnormal placentation and is relatively cost effective compared to MRI.

The following ultrasound findings have been associated with invasive placentation: inability to clearly identify the hypoechoic myometrial-retroplacental region; loss of the hyperechoic bladder-uterine serosa interface; myometrial thickness less than 1 mm; irregular lacunae in the placenta with turbulent flow; color Doppler showing increased vascularity near the bladder wall; and focal exophytic masses [85–87].

A meta-analysis in 2013 reviewed 23 studies, including 3707 pregnancies, to evaluate how well ultrasound identified invasive placentation [88]. They found that the sensitivity of ultrasound to detect invasive placentation was 90.72% with a specificity of 96.94%. Overall, the most accurate ultrasound identifier was color Doppler, with a sensitivity of 90.74%. Grayscale, however, has been shown to be comparable in other studies with a sensitivity of 77–87%, specificity of 96–98%, as well as a positive predictive value of 65–93% [89, 90]. Other studies have identified that the number of lacunae within the placenta, seen at approximately 15–20 weeks' gestation is the most predictive finding on ultrasound yielding a sensitivity of 79% and a positive predictive value of 92% [90].

A meta-analysis of 13 studies aimed to review the overall sensitivity and specificity of ultrasound and MRI at detecting invasive placentation [91]. Specificity and sensitivity of ultrasound was found to be 95% (CI 93–96%) and 83% (CI 77–88%) respectively, compared to 88% (CI 81–94%) and 82% (CI 72–90%) for MRI. In this review, the two modalities were not noted, after review with receiver operating characteristic analysis, to significantly differ.

Some experts have questioned if it is necessary to evaluate for placenta accreta in the antepartum period, and argue that the appearance of the anterior uterine wall and placenta at time of delivery will prompt decisions regarding the need for hysterectomy or other management. A 2013 retrospective case series evaluated 66 pregnancies that ultimately had a placenta increta or percreta identified at time of delivery [92]. Of these, 40 (61%) were identified prior to delivery (via ultrasound during either routine imaging, follow up for a previa, vaginal bleeding, or suspected abnormal placentation) and 26 (39%) were not. Of those identified antenatally, 62% required hysterectomy (versus 50% of the unidentified group), with 12% of the hysterectomies being emergent for severe hemorrhage (versus 69% in the unidentified group, $p = 0.0004$). Those identified in the antepartum period had a significantly lower requirement for massive transfusion, 20% versus 46% ($p = 0.025$).

A retrospective case–control study compared abnormal placentation in 24 women diagnosed in the antepartum period versus 20 diagnosed intrapartum [93]. Estimated blood loss (4500 mL versus 7800 ml, $p = 0.012$) and amount of PRBCs transfused (7 versus 13.5, $p = 0.026$) were noted to be significantly lower in patients with accreta identified in the antepartum period. The length of hospital stay and incidence of surgical complications did not differ between the two groups. Notably, when an antepartum diagnosis was made, it was most often placenta percreta.

Other benefits of early identification of placenta accreta include allowing sufficient time for appropriate planning and referral. Management of placenta accreta by an experienced, multidisciplinary team in a tertiary care center with appropriate resources has been associated with improved outcomes [94]. Pre-operative checklists have been advocated [95] to ensure clear preparations and communication prior to surgery. Antenatal identification of placenta accreta also aids with the decision of delivery timing. Emergent cesarean delivery was required in 44% of women with a placenta accreta when their delivery was planned after 36 weeks [96]. Current recommendations for the gestational age for delivery of a known placenta accreta ranges from 34 to 35 weeks, showing to optimize neonatal and maternal outcomes [97], to the RCOG recommendations of 35–37 weeks

(RCOG). There is evidence that some patients may require earlier delivery, such as those with bleeding or contractions [98], while others may safely be delayed to 36–37 weeks [99]. It has been shown that women with placenta accreta, scheduled to deliver after 36 weeks, will experience emergent delivery 44% of the time [96]. As life-threatening hemorrhage is greatly increased after 36 weeks, and planned delivery from 34 to 35 weeks (with administration of antenatal corticosteroids) has shown decreased blood loss and need for maternal blood transfusion [96, 100] the National Institutes of Health has agreed that delivery timing is best managed between 34 weeks up to 35 completed weeks [101]. The severity of placental invasion, patient history, and patient comoborbidities stress the importance of individualized care.

2. In pregnant patients with morbidly adherent placenta (placenta accreta, increta or percreta) (population), what are potential alternatives to hysterectomy (interventions) to assist with controlling/preventing hemorrhage (outcome)?

Planned hysterectomy at the time of delivery is the definitive management of placenta accreta. In some cases of placenta percreta, when wide excision may cause extreme morbidity, or in women strongly desiring to preserve fertility, conservative management (uterine sparing techniques) may be desirable. In one series of 26 women who chose this option, 21 (80.7%) did not require hysterectomy at the time of delivery, however a majority needed further treatments due to excessive bleeding, including hypogastric artery ligation, UAE, blood transfusion, or curettage [102].

Perhaps the simplest alternative approach to hysterectomy is simply to leave the placenta in situ after delivery, without attempts to forcibly remove it, and allow it to resorb and/or be expelled. Whenever a portion of the placenta is left in-situ, however, there is concern for infection and delayed need for hysterectomy. In a retrospective review of 40 hospitals in France, over a 13-year time span, Senthiles et al. reviewed outcomes when the placenta was left in situ with no attempt at removal versus immediate post-cesarean hysterectomy [103]. Overall, 167 women were treated conservatively, and uterine preservation was successful in 131 patients (78.4%). Of the 36 that required hysterectomies in their series, 18 were performed at time of cesarean and 18 were delayed. Resorption of the placenta was noted in 75% (66.1–82.6%) of cases over an average of 13.5 weeks (range 4–60 weeks).

A single-center retrospective comparison of 26 women diagnosed antenatally with invasive placentation compared scheduled cesarean hysterectomy (n = 16) to planned conservative, in-situ management (n = 10) [104]. Surgical approach was the same for both groups initially, consisting of internal iliac balloon placement preoperatively and a midline vertical skin incision. Those in the conservative management group had the umbilical cord cut and ligated close to the placental insertion and then the hysterotomy was repaired and prophylactic UAE was performed. The internal iliac artery balloons were inflated prior to proceeding with hysterectomy in all women with planned cesarean hysterectomy, but only in those with excessive bleeding in the conservative management group. Of the 10 women desiring conservative management, 4 required hysterectomy due to sepsis, hemorrhage, or coagulopathy. The time from cesarean delivery to hysterectomy for these patients ranged from 10 to 78 days. No statistically significant differences were noted in the mean number of PRBC or FFP transfused, coagulopathy, or bladder/bowel injury. The conservative management group was noted to have a lower estimated blood loss (900 ml) compared to the elective hysterectomy group (3625 ml), $p < 0.05$.

Pre-operative measures such as use of intravascular balloon catheters has recently been adopted. A prospective observational study compared the use of preoperative placement of balloon catheters in the internal iliac arteries with planned cesarean hysterectomy (n = 30) to planned cesarean hysterectomy alone (n = 23) for women with ultrasound identified abnormal placental invasion [105]. The women had various degrees of placental invasion, and hysterectomy alone group had a notably higher estimated blood loss and lower amount of blood products transfused. However, when the accreta/increta patients and the percreta patients were analyzed separately, this data only remained statistically significant for the percreta group: mean estimated blood loss 1507 ml versus 933 ml, $p = 0.0001$ and mean transfused blood products 3.31 units and 0.67 units, $p = 0.0008$ for the planned hysterectomy versus those who received balloon placement prior to planned hysterectomy.

The combination of bilateral uterine artery ligation followed by B-lynch suture was used to control hemorrhage due to uterine atony after cesarean delivery of the fetus in women with known placental invasion [106]. Twenty-six women met inclusion criteria (gestational age at or above 37 weeks, antepartum hemorrhage, PPH, and identified accreta with adherent placenta after delivery). Placental tissue was left in-situ, and the average time to resolution confirmed via ultrasound was 170.7 days +/− 54.7 days. Two of the 26 continued had further bleeding and hypogastric artery ligation was performed; both women experienced disseminated intravascular coagulopathy and died approximately 34 hours later. Of the 24 women who survived, 18 became pregnant after one year.

In one prospective study included 71 patients, specifically with anterior placenta percreta identified antenatally. These women were admitted to the hospital at 32 weeks' gestation and had cesarean delivery scheduled between 37 and 38 weeks; all received antenatal steroids [107]. The goal was then to proceed surgically, in a stepwise fashion, to attempt preservation of the uterus. This included use of a Pfannenstiel incision, transverse hysterotomy avoiding the placenta, uterotonic administration prior to delivery of the fetus, and then no attempt to remove the placenta after cord clamping. The uterus (with placenta in situ) was then exteriorized, rotated anteriorly, and compressed against the pubic symphysis in an attempt to compress the uterine arteries. Thereafter, the anterior division of the internal iliac arteries was ligated bilaterally with injection of pitocin into the myometrial wall to assist with separation of the placental-myometrial interface. The placenta was then removed. Sutures were placed, as needed, for hemostasis and the hysterotomy was then repaired, after identification of the lower uterine segment and internal os digitally, in a running mattress form. Of the 71 patients, 6 (8.5%) required intraoperative hysterectomy, thus the uterus was spared in 91.5% of the patients. This method proved to have an average intraoperative blood loss of 1700 ml (600–2400 ml), postoperative blood loss of 570 ml (400–1300 ml), blood transfusion of 4 U (2–6 U), and operative time of 85 minutes (70–120 minutes); only one patient required delayed postoperative surgery for a vesicouterine fistula.

This technique is also referred to as the "Triple P" procedure, as originally described by Chandraharan et al. [108]. It is important to note that the authors comment, albeit briefly, that this technique may not be suitable for women in whom the placenta invades laterally or into the cervix. Rarely is a single conservative technique used alone. Instead, many authors describe use of a combination of conservative techniques to attain adequate control to optimize treatment [108–111].

The complications associated with conservative management must be anticipated, and the patient adequately counseled prior to attempting such therapy. Such complications include delayed hemorrhage, DIC, endomyometritis, and sepsis [102, 103, 110, 112]. Between 21 and 58% of women managed conservatively may require delayed hysterectomy due to complications [103, 109]. Despite this, in centers with teams experienced in conservative management, successful outcomes have been reported, and with appropriate preparation and counseling, such management may be attractive to select patients.

References

1 Foley, M.R., Strong, T.H., and Garite, T.J. (2010). Postpartum hemorrhage. In: *Obstetric Intensive Care Manual*, 3e, 27–37. The McGraw-Hill Companies Inc.

2 Shakur, H., Elbourne, D., Gulmezoglu, M. et al. (2010). The WOMAN Trial (World Maternal Antifibrinolytic Trial): tranexamic acid for the treatment of postpartum haemorrhage: an international randomized double blind placebo controlled trial. *Trials* **11**: 40.

3 (2010). ACOG practice bulletin no.115: vaginal birth after previous cesarean delivery. *Obstet. Gynecol.* **116** (**2 Pt 1**): 450.

4 O'Brien, D., Babiker, E., O'Sullivan, O. et al. (2010). Prediction of peripartum hysterectomy and end organ dysfunction in major obstetric haemorrhage. *Eur. J. Obstet. Gynecol. Reprod. Biol.* **153** (**2**): 165–169.

5 Creanga, A.A., Berg, C.J., Syverson, C. et al. (2015). Pregnancy-related mortality in the United States, 2006–2010. *Obstet. Gynecol.* **125** (**1**): 5–12. doi: 10.1097/AOG.0000000000000564.

6 The Joint Commission. Preventing Maternal Death. Sentinel Event Alert, Issue 44 January 26, 2010. http://www.jointcommission.org/sentinel_event_alert_issue_44_preventing_maternal_death. accessed 14 July 2018.

7 Duthie, S.J., Ven, D., Yung, G.L. et al. (1991). Discrepancy between laboratory determination and visual estimation of blood loss during normal delivery. *Eur. J. Obstet. Gynecol. Reprod. Biol.* **38**: 119–124.

8 Tall, G., Wise, D., Grove, P., and Wilkinson, C. (2003). The accuracy of external blood loss estimation by ambulance and hospital personnel. *Emerg. Med. (Fremantle).* **15**: 318–321.

9 Beer, H.L., Duvvi, S., Webb, C.J., and Tandon, S. (2005). Blood loss estimation in epistaxis scenarios. *J. Laryngol. Otol.* **119**: 16–18.

10 Glover, P. (2003). Blood loss at delivery: how accurate is your estimation? *Aust. J. Midwifery.* **16**: 21–24.

11 Read, M.D. and Anderton, J.M. (1997). Radioisotope dilution technique for measurement of blood loss associated with lower segment caesarean section. *BJOG* **84**: 859–861.

12 Bose, P., Regan, F., and Paterson-Brown, S. (2006). Improving the accuracy of estimated blood loss at obstetric haemorrhage using clinical reconstructions. *BJOG* **113**: 919–924.

13 Patel, A., Goudar, S.S., Geller, S.E. et al. (2006). Drape estimation vs. visual assessment for estimating postpartum hemorrhage. *Int. J. Gynecol. Obstet.* **93**: 220–224.

14 Zhang, W.H., Deneuz-Tharaux, C., Brocklehurst, P. et al. (2010). Effect of a collector bag for measurement of postpartum blood loss after vaginal delivery: cluster randomized trial in 13 European countries. *BMJ* **c293**: 340.

15 Prendiville, W.J. (1996). The prevention of postpartum haemorrhage: optimizing routine management of the third stage of labour. *Eur. J. Obstet. Gynecol. Reprod. Biol.* **69**: 19–24.

16 Gülmezoglu, A.M., Villar, J., Ngoc, N.T.N. et al. (2001). WHO Collaborative Group to evaluate misoprostol in the management of the third stage of labor. WHO multicenter randomized trial of misoprostol in the management of the third stage of labour. *Lancet* **358**: 689–695.

17 Festin, M.R., Lumbiganon, P., Tolosa, J.E. et al. (2003). International survey on variations in practice of the management of the third stage of labour. *Bull. World Health Organ.* **81** (**4**): 286–291.

18 Gülmezoglu, A.M., Lumbiganon, P., Landoulsi, S. et al. (2012). Active management of the third stage of labour with and without controlled cord traction: a randomised, controlled, non-inferiority trial. *Lancet*, Early Online Publication doi: 10.1016/S0140-6736(12)60206-2.

19 Mitchell, G.G. and Elbourne, D.R. (1993 Aug 13). The Salford Third Stage Trial. Oxytocin plus ergometrine versus oxytocin alone in the active management of the third stage of labor. *Online J. Curr. Clin. Trials.* Do No 83.

20 Wu, L.F., Liu, Y., and Ruan, Y. (2007 Sep). Clinical study on prevention of postpartum hemorrhage of cesarean section using Hemabate in high risk pregnant women. *Zhonghua Fu Chan Ke Za Zhi.* **42** (**9**): 577–581.

21 Zuberi, N.F., Durocher, J., Sikander, R. et al. (2008). Misoprostol in addition to routine treatment of postpartum hemorrhage: a hospital-based randomized-controlled trial in Karachi, Pakistan. *BMC Pregnancy Childbirth* **8**: 40.

22 Prata, N., Mbaruku, G., Campbell, M. et al. (2005). Controlling postpartum hemorrhage after home births in Tanzania. *Int. J. Gynaecol. Obstet.* **90** (**1**): 51–55.

23 Mousa, H.A. and Alfirevic, Z. (2007). Treatment for primary postpartum hemorrhage. *Cochrane Database Syst. Rev.* 1 (Art. No.: CD003249).

24 (2006). ACOG practice bulletin no. 76: postpartum Hemorrhage. *Obstet. Gynecol.* **108**: 1039–1047.

25 Sheehan, S.R., Montgomery, A.A., Carey, M. et al. (2011). Oxytocin bolus versus oytocin bolus and infusion for control of blood loss at elective caesarean section: double blind, placebo controlled, randomised trial. *BMJ* **343**: d4661.

26 Su, L.L., Chong, Y.S., and Samuel, M. (2012). Carbetocin for preventing postpartum haemorrhage. *Cochrane Database Syst. Rev.* 2 (Art. No.: C005457).

27 Zhou, M., Yang, C.Y., Zhao, Y., and Li, P. (2006 Jun). Clinical value of adjuvant therapy with estrogen for postpartum hemorrhage. *Nan Fang Yi Ke Da Zue Zue Bao* **26** (**6**): 865–866.

28 Movafegh, A., Eslamian, L., and Dorabadi, A. (2011). Effect of intravenous tranexamic acid administration on blood loss during and after cesarean delivery. *Int. J. Gynecol. Obstet.* **115**: 224–226.

29 Gai, M.Y., Wu, L.F., Su, Q.F., and Tatsumoto, K. (2004). Clinical observation of blood loss reduced by tranexamic acid during and after caesarian section: a multi-center, randomized trial. *Eur. J. Obstet. Gynecol. Reprod. Biol.* **112** (**2**): 154–157.

30 Gohel, M., Patel, P., Bupta, A., and Desai, P. (2007). Efficacy of tanexamic acid in decreasing blood loss during and after cesarean section: a randomized case controlled prospective study. *J. Obstet. Gynecol. India* **57** (**3**): 227–230.

31 Sekhavat, L., Tabatabaii, A., Dalili, M. et al. (2009). Efficacy of tranexamic acid in reducing blood loss after cesarean section. *J. Matern. Fetal Neonatal Med.* **22** (**1**): 72–75.

32 Gungorduk, K., Yildirm, G., Asicioglu, O. et al. (2011). Efficacy of intravenous tranexamic acid in reducing blood loss after cesarean section: a prospective, randomized, double-blind, placebo-controlled study. *Am. J. Perinatol.* **28** (**3**): 233–240.

33 Kalina, M., Tinkoff, G., and Fulda, G. (2011). Massive postpartum hemorrhage: recombinant factor VIIa use is safe but not effective. *Del. Med. J.* **83** (**4**): 109–113.

34 McMorrow, R.C., Ryan, S.M., Blunnie, W.P. et al. (2008 Apr). Use of recombinant factor VIIa in massive post-partum haemorrhage. *Eur. J. Anaesthesiol.* **24** (**4**): 293–298.

35 Bouma, L.S., Bolte, A.C., and van Geijn, H.P. (2008). Use of recombinant activated factor VII in massive postpartum haemorrhage. *Eur. J. Obstet. Gynecol. Reprod. Biol.* **137** (**2**): 172–177.

36 Sentilhes, L., Gromez, A., Razzouk, K. et al. (2008). B-lynch suture for massive persistent postpartum hemorrhage following stepwise uterine devascularization. *Acta Obstet. Gynecol. Scand.* **87** (**10**): 1020–1026.

37 Rajan, P.V. and Wing, D.A. (2010). Postpartum hemorrhage: evidence-based medical interventions for prevention and treatment. *Clin. Obstet. Gynecol.* **53** (**1**): 165–181.

38 Fenger-Eriksen, C., Lindberg-Larsen, M., Christensen, A.Q. et al. (2008). Fibrinogen concentrate substitution therapy in patients with massive haemorrhage and low plasma fibrinogen concentrations. *Br. J. Anaesth.* **101**: 769–773.

39 Borgman, M.A., Spinella, P.C., Perkins, J.G. et al. (2007). The ratio of blood products transfused affects mortality and patients receiving massive transfusions at a combat support hospital. *J. Trauma.* **63**: 805–813.

40 Dildy, G.A. III, Paine, A.R., George, N.C., and Velasco, C. (2004). Estimating blood loss: can teaching significantly improve visual estimation? *Obstet. Gynecol.* **104**: 601–606.

41 Shields, L.E., Smalarz, K., Reffigee, L. et al. (2011). Comprehensive maternal hemorrhage protocols to improve patient safety and reduce utilization of blood products. *Am. J. Obstet. Gynecol.* **205** (**4**): 368.e1–368.e8.

42 Varatharajan, L., Chandraharan, E., Sutton, J. et al. (2011). Outcomes of the management of massive postpartum hemorrhage using the algorithm "HEMOSTASIS". *Int. J. Gynaecol. Obstet.* **113** (**2**): 152–154.

43 Knight, M. (2007). UKOSS. Peripartum hysterectomy in the UK: management and outcomes of the associated haemorrhage. *BJOG* **114** (**11**): 1380–1387.

44 Heyl, P.S., Stubblefield, P.G., and Phillippe, M. (1984). Recurrent inversion of the puerperal uterus managed with 15(s)-15-methyl prostaglandin F2 alpha and uterine packing. *Obstet. Gynecol.* **63** (**2**): 263, 6607434–264.

45 Loizeaux, L.S. Jr. (1947). Replacement of an inverted uterus with intravaginal packing. *Bull. N. Y. Med. Coll.* **10** (**1**): 53, 18908123–56.

46 Maier, R.C. (1993 Aug). Control of postpartum hemorrhage with uterine packing. *Am. J. Obstet. Gynecol.* **169** (**2 Pt 1**): 317, 8362942–321; . Discussion 321–3.

47 Schmid, B.C., Rezniczek, G.A., Rolf, N. et al. (2013 Sep). Uterine packing with chitosan-covered gauze for control of postpartum hemorrhage. *Am. J. Obstet. Gynecol.* **209** (**3**): 225.e1, 23727525–225.e5. doi: 10.1016/j.ajog.2013.05.055. Epub 2013 May 30.

48 Koyama, S., Maeda, M., Kobayashi, M. et al. (2013). Angiographic findings after vaginal gauze packing: new insight into an old technique. *J. Obstet. Gynaecol. Res.* **39** (**6**): 1212, 23551298–1216. doi: 10.1111/jog.12037. Epub 2013 Apr 3.

49 Bakri, Y.N. (1992). Uterine tamponade-drain for hemorrhage secondary to placenta previa-accreta. *Int. J. Gynaecol. Obstet.* **37** (**4**): 302, 1350550–303.

50 Condous, G.S., Arulkumaran, S., Symonds, I. et al. (2003). The "tamponade test" in the management of massive postpartum hemorrhage. *Obstet. Gynecol.* **101** (**4**): 767, 12681884–772.

51 Johanson, R., Kumar, M., Obhrai, M., and Young, P. (2001). Management of massive postpartum haemorrhage: use of a hydrostatic balloon catheter to avoid laparotomy. *BJOG* **108** (**4**): 420–422.

52 Dildy, G.A., Belfort, M.A., Adair, C.D. et al. (2014). Initial experience with a dual-balloon catheter for the management of postpartum hemorrhage. *Am. J. Obstet. Gynecol.* **210** (**2**): 136.e1, 24055586–136.e6. doi: 10.1016/j.ajog.2013.09.015. Epub 2013 Sep 18.

53 Marasinghe, J.P., Du Plessis, J., Epitawela, D., and Umstad, M.P. (2015). Management of postpartum haemorrhage with uterine balloon tamponade: the way forward. *Aust. N. Z. J. Obstet. Gynaecol.* **55** (**4**): 315, 26130087–317. doi: 10.1111/ajo.12333. . Epub 2015 Jun 30.

54 Tsvetkov, T.S., Kozovski, G., Tsvetkov, K. et al. (2004). Stepwise uterine devascularization in postpartum hemorrhages. *Akush. Ginekol.* **43** (**1**): 9–15.

55 Joshi, V.M., Otiv, S.R., Majumder, R. et al. (2007). Internal iliac artery ligation for arresting postpartum haemorrhage. *BJOG* **114** (**3**): 356–361.

56 Camuzcuoglu, H., Toy, H., Vural, M. et al. (2010). Internal iliac artery ligation for severe postpartum hemorrhage and severe hemorrhage after postpartum hysterectomy. *J. Obstet. Gynaecol. Res.* **36** (**3**): 538–543.

57 Chelli, D., Boudaya, F., Dimassi, K. et al. (2010 Feb). Hypogastric artery ligation for post-partum hemorrhage. *J. Gynecol. Obstet. Biol. Reprod. (Paris).* **39** (**1**): 43–49.

58 Matsubara, S., Yano, H., Ohkuchi, A., Kuwata, T., Usui, R., Suzuki, M. Uterine compression sutures for postpartum hemorrhage: an overview. *Acta Obstet Gynecol Scand.* 2013 Apr;**92** (**4**): 378 –85. doi: 10.1111/aogs.12077. Epub 2013 Feb 9. Review. PubMed PMID: 23330882.

59 Baskett, T.F. (2007). Uterine compression sutures for postpartum hemorrhage: efficacy, morbidity, and subsequent pregnancy. *Obstet. Gynecol.* **110** (**1**): 68–71.

60 Allahdin, S., Aird, C., and Danielian, P. (2006). B-lynch sutures for major primary postpartum haemorrhage at caesarean section. *J. Obstet. Gynaecol.* **26** (**7**): 639–642.

61 Wohlmuth, C.T., Gumbs, J., and Quebral-Ivie, J. (2005). B-lynch suture: a case series. *Int. J. Fertil. Womens Med.* **40** (**4**): 164–173.

62 Ghezzi, F., Cromi, A., Uccella, S. et al. (2007). The Hayman technique: a simple method to treat postpartum haemorrhage. *BJOG* **114**: 362–365.

63 Poujade, O., Grossetti, A., Mougel, L. et al. (2011). Risk of synechiae following uterine compression sutures in the management of major postpartum haemorrhage. *BJOG* **118** (**4**): 433–439.

64 Rathat, G., Do Trinh, P., Mercier, G. et al. (2011 Jan). Synechia after uterine compression sutures. *Fertil. Steril.* **95** (**1**): 405–409.

65 Palacios-Jaraquemada, J.M. (2011 Sep). Efficacy of surgical techniques to control obstetric hemorrhage: analysis of 539 cases. *Acta Obstet. Gynecol. Scand.* **90** (**9**): 1–36, 42.

66 Yong, S.P. and Cheung, K.B. (2006). Management of primary postpartum haemorrhage with arterial embolization in Hong Kong public hospitals. *Hong Kong Med. J.* (**6**): 437–441.

67 Ganguli, S., Stecker, M.S., Pyne, D. et al. (2011). Uterine artery embolization in the treatment of postpartum uterine hemorrhage. *J. Vasc. Interv. Radiol.* **22** (**2**): 169–176.

68 Soncini, E., Pelicelli, A., Larini, P. et al. (2007). Uterine artery embolization in the treatment and prevention of postpartum haemorrhage. *Int. J. Gynaecol. Obstet.* **96** (**3**): 181–185.

69 Maassen, M.S., Lambers, M.D., Tutein Nolthenius, R.P. et al. (2009). Complications and failure of uterine artery embolization for intractable postpartum haemorrhage. *BJOG* **116** (**1**): 55–61.

70 Sidhu, H.K., Prasad, G., Jain, V. et al. (2010). Pelvic artery embolization in the management of obstetric hemorrhage. *Acta Obstet. Gynecol. Scand.* **89** (**8**): 1069–1069.

71 Jung, H.N., Shin, S.W., Choi, S.J. et al. (2011). Uterine artery embolization for emergent management of postpartum hemorrhage associated with placenta accreta. *Acta Radiol.* **52** (**6**): 638–642.

72 Clark, S.L., Belfort, M.A., Dildy, G.A. et al. (2008). Maternal death in the 21st century: causes, prevention and relationship to cesarean delivery. *Am. J. Obstet. Gynecol.* **199**: 36.E1–36.e5.

73 Fargeaudou, Y., Morel, O., Soyer, P. et al. (2010). Persistent postpartum haemorrhage after failed arterial ligation: value of pelvic embolisation. *Eur. Radiol.* **20** (**7**): 1777–1785.

74 Fornet, I., Palacio, F.J., Morillas, P. et al. (2008 Jan). Experience with uterine artery embolization in the treatment of massive postpartum hemorrhage. *Rev. Esp. Anestesiol. Reanim.* **55** (**1**): 21–25.

75 Chauleur, C., Fanget, C., Tourne, G. et al. (2008). Serious primary post-partum hemorrhage, arterial embolization and future fertility: a retrospective study of 46 cases. *Hum. Reprod.* **23** (**7**): 1533–1539.

76 Boulleret, C., Chahid, T., Ballot, D. et al. (2004). Hypogastric arterial selective and superselective embolization for severe postpartum hemorrhage: a retrospective review of 36 cases. *Cardiovasc. Intervent. Radiol.* **27** (**4**): 344–348.

77 Kayem, G., Kurinczuk, J.J., Alfirevic, Z. et al. (2011). Specific second-line therapies for postpartum haemorrhage: a national cohort study. *BJOG* **118** (**7**): 856–864.

78 Silver, R.M., Landon, M.B., Rouse, D.J. et al. (2006). Maternal morbidity associated with multiple repeat cesarean deliveries. *Obstet. Gynecol.* **107**: 1226–1232.

79 Hudon, L., Belfort, M.A., and Broome, D.R. (1998). Diagnosis and management of placenta percreta: a review. *Obstet. Gynecol. Surv.* **53**: 509–517.

80 Belfort, M.A. and Publications Committee, Society for Maternal-Fetal Medicine (2010 Nov). Placenta accreta. *Am. J. Obstet. Gynecol.* **203** (**5**): 430–439. doi: 10.1016/j.ajog.2010.09.013.

81 Wu, S., Kocherginski, M., and Hibbard, J.U. (2005). Abnormal placentation: twenty-year analysis. *Am. J. Obstet. Gynecol.* **192**: 1458–1461.

82 Bailit, J.L., Grobman, W.A., Rice, M.M. et al. (2015). Morbidly adherent placenta treatments and outcomes. *Obstet. Gynecol.* **125** (**3**): 683–689. doi: 10.1097/AOG.0000000000000680.

83 Read, J.A., Cotton, D.B., and Miller, F.C. (1980). Placenta accreta: changing clinical aspects and outcome. *Obstet. Gynecol.* **56**: 31–34.

84 Demirci Oya, T.A.S., Yilmaz, E., Tosun, O. et al. (2011). Emergency peripartum hysterectomy in a tertiary obstetric center: nine years evaluation. *J. Obstet. Gynaecol.* **37** (**8**): 1054–1060.

85 Chou, M.M., Ho, E.S., and Lee, Y.H. (2000). Prenatal diagnosis of placenta previa accreta by transabdominal color Doppler ultrasound. *Ultrasound Obstet. Gynecol.* **15**: 28–35.

86 Finberg, H.J. and Williams, J.W. (1992). Placenta accreta: prospective sonographic diagnosis in patients with placenta previa and prior cesarean section. *J. Ultrasound Med.* **11**: 333–343.

87 Thia, E.W., Lee, S.L., Tan, H.K., and Tan, L.K. (2007). Ultrasounographical features of morbidly-adherent placentas. *Singapore Med. J.* **48**: 799–802.

88 D'Antonio, F., Iacovella, C., and Bhide, A. (2013). Prenatal identification of invasive placentation using ultrasound: systematic review and meta-analysis. *Ultrasound Obstet. Gyecol.* **42**: 509–517.

89 Warshak, C.R., Eskander, R., Hull, A.D. et al. (2006). Accuracy of ultrasonography and magnetic resonance imaging in the diagnosis of placenta accreta. *Obstet. Gynecol.* **108**: 573–581.

90 Comstock, C.H., Love, J.J. Jr., Bronsteen, R.A. et al. (2004). Sonographic detection of placenta accreta in the second and third trimesters of pregnancy. *Am. J. Obstet. Gynecol.* **190**: 1135–1140.

91 Meng, X., Xie, L., and Song, W. (2013). Comparing the diagnostic value of ultrasound and magnetic resonance imaging for placenta accreta: a systematic review and meta-analysis. *Ultrasound Med. Biol.* **39** (**11**): 1958–1965.

92 Chantraine, F., Braun, T., Gonser, M. et al. (2013). Prenatal diagnosis of abnormally invasive placenta reduces maternal peripartum hemorrhage and morbidity. *Acta Obstet Gynecol Scand.* **92** (**4**): 439–444.

93 Tikkanen, M., Paavonen, J., Loukovaara, M., and Stefanovic, V. (2011). Antenatal diagnosis of placenta accreta leads to reduced blood loss. *Acta Obstet. Gynecol. Scand.* **90**: 1140–1146.

94 Shamshirsaz, A.A., Fox, K.A., Salmanian, B. et al. (2015 Feb). Maternal morbidity in patients with morbidly adherent placenta treated with and without a standardized multidisciplinary approach. *Am. J. Obstet. Gynecol.* **212** (**2**): 218.e1–218.e9. doi: 10.1016/j.ajog.2014.08.019. Epub 2014 Aug 27.

95 Hayes, E., Ayida, G., and Crocker, A. (2011). The morbidly adherent placenta: diagnosis and management options. *Curr. Opin. Obstet. Gynecol.* **23**: 448–453.

96 Warshak, C., Ramos, G., Eskander, R. et al. (2010). Effect of predelivery diagnosis in 99 consecutive cases of placenta accreta. *Obstet. Gynecol.* **115**: 65, 20027036–69.

97 Robinson, B. and Grobman, W. (2010). Effectiveness of timing strategies for delivery of individuals with placenta praevia and accreta. *Obstet. Gynaecol.* **116**: 835–842.

98 Bowman, Z.S., Manuck, T.A., Eller, A.G. et al. (2014 Mar). Risk factors for unscheduled delivery in patients with placenta accreta. *Am. J. Obstet. Gynecol.* **210** (**3**): 241, e1–246. doi: 10.1016/j.ajog.2013.09.044. Epub 2013 Oct 2.

99 Rac, M.W., Wells, C.E., Twickler, D.M. et al. (2015 Apr). Placenta accreta and vaginal bleeding according to gestational age at delivery. *Obstet. Gynecol.* **125** (**4**): 808–813. doi: 10.1097/AOG.0000000000000674.

100 O'Brien, J., Barton, J., and Donaldson, E. (1996). The management of placenta percreta: conservative and operative strategies. *Am. J. Obstet. Gynecol.* **175** (**6**): 1632, 8987952–1638.

101 Spong, C.Y., Mercer, B.M., D'Alton, M. et al. (2011). Timing of indicated late-preterm and early-term birth. *Obstet. Gynecol.* **118** (**2 Pt 1**): 323–333. doi: 10.1097/AOG.0b013e3182255999.

102 Bretelle, F., Courbiere, B., Mazouni, C. et al. (2007). Management of placenta accreta: morbidity and outcome. *Eur. J. Obstet. Gynecol. Reprod. Biol.* **133**: 34–39.

103 Sentilhes, L., Ambroselli, C., Kayem, G. et al. (2010). Maternal outcome after conservative treatment of placenta accreta. *Obstet. Gynecol.* **115** (**3**): 526–534.

104 Amsalem, H., Kingdom, J.C.P., Farine, D. et al. (2011). Planned caesarean hysterectomy versus "conserving" caesarean section in patients with placenta accreta. *J. Obstet. Gynaecol. Can.* **33** (**10**): 1005–1010.

105 Cali, G., Forlani, F., Giambanco, L. et al. (2014). Prophylactic use of intravascular balloon catheters in women with placenta accreta, increta, and percreta. *Eur. J. Obstet. Gynecol. Reprod. Biol.* **179**: 36–41.

106 Shahin, A.Y., Farghaly, T.A., Mohamed, S.A. et al. (2010). Bilateral uterine artery ligation plus B-lynch procedure for atonic postpaturm hemorrhage with placenta accreta. *Int. J. Gynecol. Obstet.* **108**: 187–190.

107 Shabana, A., Fawzy, M., and Refaie, W. (2015 May). Conservative management of placenta percreta: a stepwise approach. *Arch. Gynecol. Obstet.* **291** (**5**): 993–998. doi: 10.1007/s00404-014-3496-x. Epub 2014 Oct 7.

108 Chandraharan, E., Rao, S., Belli, A.M., and Arulkumaran, S. (2012). The triple-P procedure as a conservative surgical alternative to peripartum hysterectomy for placenta percreta. *Int. J. Gynaecol. Obstet.* **117** (**2**): 191–194. doi: 10.1016/j.ijgo.2011.12.005. Epub 2012 Feb 11.

109 Clausen, C., Lönn, L., and Langhoff-Roos, J. (2014 Feb). Management of placenta percreta: a review of published cases. *Acta Obstet. Gynecol. Scand.* **93** (**2**): 138–143. doi: 10.1111/aogs.12295. Epub 2013 Nov 25.

110 Legendre, G., Zoulovits, F.J., Kinn, J. et al. (2014 Sep-Oct). Conservative management of placenta accreta: hysteroscopic resection of retained tissues. *J. Minim. Invasive Gynecol.* **21** (**5**): 910–913. doi: 10.1016/j.jmig.2014.04.004. Epub 2014 Apr 24.

111 Lo, T.K., Yung, W.K., Lau, W.L. et al. (2014 Feb). Planned conservative management of placenta accreta – experience of a regional general hospital. *J. Matern. Fetal Neonatal Med.* **27** (**3**): 291–296. doi: 10.3109/14767058.2013.818118. Epub 2013 Jul 24.

112 Kayem, G., Davy, C., Goffinet, F. et al. (2004). Conservative versus extirpative management in cases of placenta accreta. *Obstet. Gynecol.* **104** (**3**): 531–536.

52 CHAPTER 52
Obstetric emergencies

Karin Fox[1,2], Alexandria J. Hill[3,4,5], and Stephanie R. Martin[6]
[1]*Maternal-Fetal Medicine, Baylor College of Medicine, Houston, TX, USA*
[2]*Texas Children's Hospital, Pavilion for Women, Houston, TX, USA*
[3]*High Risk Pregnancy Center, Las Vegas, NV, USA*
[4]*Texas A&M College of Medicine, College Station, TX, USA*
[5]*University of Arizona, Phoenix, AZ, USA*
[6]*Clinical Concepts in Obstetrics, Scottsdale, AZ, USA*

Introduction

This chapter focuses on the role of high-performing team-based care and the use of standardized protocols, particularly in the setting of obstetrical emergencies. There are two clinical scenarios used to illustrate the utility of multidisciplinary team care, one involving the evaluation and management of pulmonary embolism, and the second involving cardiac arrest during pregnancy.

Background

In the last 25 years, there has been a dramatic paradigm shift in medical care. Previously, the physician's role was that as a staunchly independent, all-knowing informational source and leader, with availability at all hours day or night. The pace at which medical knowledge and complexity has advanced makes relying upon one's own resources not only impractical, but also potentially unsafe. According to a discussion paper published by the Institute of Medicine in 2012, entitled, "Core Principles and Values of Effective Team-Based Health Care," the US National Clearinghouse lists over 2700 clinical practice guidelines and more than 25 000 new clinical trials are published annually [1]. No one individual could possibly effectively read, process and apply such a vast amount of information, let alone care for patients with ever more complex chronic and acute disease.

Much like in other industries, such as the commercial aviation or nuclear power industries, in which groups of people must work together in hazardous conditions while maintaining a high level of safety, there has been a push toward development of highly efficient, highly reliable, team-based systems within healthcare. The impetus for this change is in part due to increasing concomitant public demands to improve patient safety and control rising healthcare costs. In 2000, the Institute of Medicine published the report "To Err Is Human," [2] which highlighted the devastating effects of medical error both on patient mortality and national costs, with an estimated 44 000–98 000 deaths per year due to medical errors and estimated adverse health care costs between $17 and $29 billion annually. Since then, national efforts have been led by various medical leadership, education, and credentialing organizations including the Joint Commission [3], the American College of Obstetrics and Gynecology (ACOG) [4], and the American Council for Graduate Medical Education (ACGME) [5], to develop organizational systems that promote a culture in which physicians function as "leaders and participants in team-oriented care." [5]. Standardization in practice may also be leveraged to improve communication and outcomes [4]. The goal of this chapter is to explore the role of high-reliability, team-oriented care specifically in the setting of obstetrical emergencies.

CLINICAL SCENARIO 1

Pulmonary embolism

A 34-year-old G6P1001 Caucasian patient at 32 and 2/7 weeks' gestation, with a body mass index (BMI) of 37, comes to the labor and delivery triage unit having woken up due to chest discomfort. She reports that the pain is worse with inhalation, and her chest feels "heavy." Since she woke up she has the sensation that she needs to cough, but the cough is non-productive. She denies ill contacts or fever. Her heart rate is approximately 130 beats per minute, with a respiratory rate of 30 breaths per minute, and her oxygen saturation is 89% on room

Evidence-Based Obstetrics and Gynecology, First Edition. Edited by Errol R. Norwitz, Carolyn M. Zelop, David A. Miller, and David L. Keefe.

air. She sounds winded when speaking. Upon exam, she has no wheezes or rales. Electrocardiogram shows sinus tachycardia, mild right axis deviation, and no ST changes; an X-ray obtained four hours earlier for cough was without noted abnormalities.

Background

Venous thromboembolism (VTE) remains one of the leading causes of death in industrialized countries [6–8]. Monitoring data from the United Kingdom (UK) indicates that a significant decrease in death due to pulmonary embolism has contributed to the slight decrease in overall maternal deaths between 2006 and 2008. Pulmonary embolism dropped from its former spot as the leading cause of death in the UK for the first time since 1985 [8]. This follows the Royal College's emphasis on prompt recognition and treatment of acute VTEs and recommendations for thromboprophylaxis, initially published in 2001 and updated in 2015 [9, 10]. Similar efforts have been made in the United States, including recommendations from the American College of Obstetricians and Gynecologists [11], the American College of Chest Physicians [12], and the American Thoracic Society and American Society of Radiologists [13, 14].

The aims of this section are to review available evidence regarding diagnosis of pulmonary embolism in pregnancy, to discuss recommendations from the aforementioned medical societies and expert consensus where data is sparse, and to elucidate strategies that may be used to aid healthcare teams in early identification of emergencies such as a VTE. Treatment of venous thrombus embolism is covered in detail in Chapter 34.

Clinical questions

1. Do the normal physiologic and hematologic changes (tests) in the pregnant patient (population) alter the evaluation in working up a patient for pulmonary embolism (outcome)?

2. Are the Wells' criteria of assessment of pretest probability of pulmonary embolism (assessment), useful in pregnancy (population)? Is there another formal assessment that may more accurately determine pretest probability in pregnancy (comparison/outcome)?

3. In pregnant patients admitted to the hospital (population), are the number of deaths from venous thrombotic events reduced (outcome) when using a Modified Early Obstetrical Warning System (MEOWS) (comparison)?

General search strategy

COCHRANE: pulmonary embolism AND pregnancy (yielded 1 Cochrane review, 1 other review, 9 clinical trials, 2 economic evaluations) and PUBMED: pulmonary embolism and pregnancy.

Critical appraisal of the literature

1. Do the normal physiologic and hematologic changes (tests) in the pregnant patient (population) alter the evaluation in working up a patient for pulmonary embolism (outcome)?

Search Strategy

PUBMED: "pregnancy" AND "pulmonary embolism" AND "test" AND (case–control OR cohort OR meta-analysis).

Many of the symptoms of pulmonary embolism such as chest pain and shortness of breath are non-specific, and may lead one to a wide differential diagnosis (Table 52.1). The considerable prevalence of these symptoms during normal pregnancy can either mimic or mask an embolic event (Table 52.2).

Stasis within pelvic vessels increases as the uterus enlarges [11]. The surge in estrogen levels during normal pregnancy increase the levels of prothrombotic coagulation factors to fourfold in normal parturients [17], and the risk of VTE is increased in women with high-risk gene carrier status, such as Factor V Leiden or antithrombin-III deficiency, previous

Table 52.1 Brief list of differential diagnoses based on symptoms of pulmonary embolism

Symptom/signs of VTE	Differential diagnosis
Shortness of breath	Normal pregnancy changes
Tachypnea	Acute asthma exacerbation
Decreased oxygenation	Pulmonary edema (+/− pre-eclampsia)
Cough +/− hemoptysis	Pneumonia
	Congestive heart failure/myocarditis
Mildly elevated temperature/fever	Systemic infection/sepsis
	Chorioamnionitis
Tachycardia	Cardiac tachyarrhythmia
	Thyrotoxicosis/thyroid storm
	Drug toxicity
	Cocaine use
Chest pain (acute)	Myocardial infarction
	Aortic or coronary artery dissection
	Costochondritis/musculoskeletal pain
Calf pain/edema	Normal pregnancy changes
	Muscle spasm
	Pre-eclampsia (although no longer part of diagnostic criteria)
	Congestive heart failure/myocarditis
	Deep venous thrombosis

Table 52.2 Comparison of symptom overlap between physiologic changes in pregnancy and VTE

Physiologic change of normal pregnancy [15]	Symptom of DVT/PE
Shortness of breath (15–75% of patients in 1st and 3rd trimester respectively)	Shortness of breath
Minute ventilation increases 15%	Tachypnea
Physiologic respiratory alkalosis (pH 7.44)	Respiratory alkalosis or acidosis
Functional residual capacity decreases ~20%	Sudden oxygen desideration
Heart rate increases 15–20% (normal range in pregnancy 61–81 bpm)	Tachycardia (mild to >150 bpm)
Lower extremity edema (often bilateral)	Edema of affected limb
Elevation of D-Dimer of 32–39% [16]	Elevated D-Dimer

VTE, or a family history of VTE [12]. Other complications of pregnancy such as infection, premature rupture of membranes or preeclampsia, which can lead to hospitalization and bed rest, may both compound these underlying risks or may lead to signs and symptoms that overlap those associated with VTE such as tachycardia, fever, shortness of breath, and decreased oxygenation [15]. Up to 30% of women have no signs of deep venous thrombosis (DVT) prior development of pulmonary embolus [18], therefore a very high index of suspicion is essential to prompt diagnosis and treatment in a pregnant patient. Diagnostic workup to exclude pulmonary embolism is warranted in any pregnant patient with shortness of breath, and immediate initiation of therapeutic anticoagulation with unfractionated or low-molecular weight heparin (LMWH) is recommended if the pretest probability for pulmonary embolism (PE) is high, until testing can be completed [9–12, 18].

Proposed diagnostic algorithms by expert panels all involve a step-wise assessment involving clinical screening and assessment of risk for VTE using a combination of symptoms and bedside testing such as chest x-ray, electrocardiogram (EKG), pulse oximetry, arterial blood gas evaluation, and initiation of anti-coagulation therapy if clinical suspicion is high. Diagnostic testing follows, however the order varies by specific recommendations and may vary by availability of local resources. The optimal method of imaging during pregnancy remains somewhat contested, especially considering the need to minimize risks of radiation exposure and invasive or repetitive procedures while avoiding a missed diagnosis. These tests include duplex compression sonography of the lower extremities to evaluate for the presence DVT, ventilation-perfusion (V/Q) scanning, computed tomography pulmonary angiogram (CTPA) or V/Q single photon emission computed tomography (SPECT) (Tables 52.2 and 52.3) [11, 12, 14]. Each imaging modality has unique advantages and limitations, and each may require additional testing to confirm a VTE (Table 52.4). For example, the physiologic increase in intravascular volume and cardiac output of 30–50% in pregnancy necessitates alterations to protocols during pregnancy regarding the dose and bolus timing of intravenous contrast to obtain optimal diagnostic accuracy during CTPA evaluation for a pulmonary embolism [16, 19, 20]. Without an increase in contrast concentration, increased venous return from the inferior vena cava creates a small area in which a dilutional effect occurs, causing artifact. Without decreasing the delay between contrast administration and imaging, the pulmonary vasculature contrast may not sufficiently be delineated and the number of non-diagnostic studies increases. This leads to increased exposure of a mother and fetus to either additional doses of radiation, due to repeat or subsequent studies, or to a potential delay in diagnosis and treatment when VTE is present despite low initial clinical suspicion [19, 20]. Regardless of the diagnostic algorithm chosen, more than one test may be required to confirm diagnosis in some pregnant patients, and continued vigilance and treatment are warranted in a patient with an initial high pre-test probability in whom an initial test is non-diagnostic.

2. Are the Wells' criteria of assessment of pretest probability of pulmonary embolism (assessment), useful in pregnancy (population)? Is there another formal assessment that may more accurately determine pretest probability in pregnancy (comparison/outcome)?

Search Strategy

PUBMED: "Wells'" AND "diagnosis of pulmonary embolism in pregnancy".

Several clinical prediction scoring systems have been proposed to estimate pretest probability of a VTE based on patient characteristics, signs, and symptoms (Table 52.5). Scoring systems validated with sufficient numbers of patients include the Modified Geneva Score [20], Wells Criteria [21], and the Pulmonary Embolism Rule-out Criteria (PERC) or Charlotte score [22]. The Wells criteria include factors dependent upon a clinician's implicit judgment about whether a diagnosis other than pulmonary embolism (PE) is less likely than PE, and therefore is not based solely on objective criteria [21]. The PERC score, when initially developed, relied solely on objective variables [22]. It was initially validated in a very low-risk population, and studies in emergency department and internal medicine populations showed that its scoring system alone, or in combination with the revised Geneva score, may not sufficiently exclude patients at risk for pulmonary embolism in high-risk populations without

Table 52.3 Proposed algorithms for evaluation and diagnosis of VTE in pregnancy

Group/ Panel	Diagnostic algorithms/recommendations
ACOG [11]	1) If DVT suspected, obtain compression ultrasonography (CUS) 2) If negative, and no pelvic involvement suspected → surveillance If negative or equivocal and pelvic involvement suspected→further imaging 3) If additional imaging positive, treat, if negative → surveillance 4) If PE suspected, obtain V/Q scan or CTPA. CXR may be used as discriminator to reduce likelihood of non-diagnostic V/Q scan.
RCOG [9, 10]	1) In pregnant women with suspicion of VTE, initiate anticoagulant therapy until testing performed 2) Individual hospitals should have an agreed upon protocol for objective diagnosis of VTE during pregnancy 3) If DVT suspected, CUS should be performed. If negative and low suspicion, anticoagulation may be discontinued 4) When PE suspected, perform CXR. If normal, perform CUS. If both are normal and PE is still suspected, CTPA or V/Q scanning should be performed. 5) Alternate or repeat testing should be performed where V/Q scanning or CTPA are negative, but clinical suspicion is still high. Anticoagulation should be continued until PE definitively ruled out. 6) Women with suspected PE should be counseled that V/Q scanning has a slightly higher risk of childhood cancer compared to CTPA (1/280 000 vs. 1/1 000 000) but carries a slightly lower risk of maternal breast cancer (lifetime risk increased up to 13.6% with CTPA), and when feasible, women should be involved in the decision of which test to undergo, and informed consent given. 7) D-Dimer should not be used in pregnancy
ASR/ATS [14]	1) Do not use D-Dimer in pregnancy to rule out DVT 2) If DVT symptoms, perform compression ultrasonography (CUS) – treat if positive, PERFORM additional testing if negative 3) If pregnant and with PE symptoms, but NO symptoms of DVT, perform studies of pulmonary vasculature rather than CUS 4) Use Chest X-ray (CXR) for initial radiation-producing imaging 5) Pregnant women with PE symptoms and normal CXR, perform lung scintigraphy rather than CTPA as next step 6) PE suspected and a nondiagnostic V/Q scan, further diagnostic testing suggested rather than clinical management alone 7) PE suspected and abnormal CXR, use CTPA as next imaging modality rather than V/Q scan

further testing [23]. Indeed, the most critical value in clinical prediction scoring is in the ability to create an accurate pre-test probability, and no single scoring system without imaging is sufficient to rule out completely VTE.

None of the above-mentioned scoring systems were developed specifically for the pregnant population, nor have they been prospectively validated in pregnancy. The PERC score was derived from logistic regression of 21 independent clinical variables and 3.7% of the 3148 patients from whom clinical variables were analyzed were pregnant [22]. In development of the revised Geneva score, 1% ($n = 10$) of the derivation population were either pregnant or post-partum [20]. Interestingly, although pregnant patients were excluded from the derivation of the Wells criteria [24], only the modified Wells criteria has been validated retrospectively in a single-institution cohort of pregnant patients [25]. In this study, use of the modified Wells score demonstrated a sensitivity of 90% and specificity of 100%, among 125 patients included over a five-year period. Negative CTPA results were considered equivalent to the absence of PE. By using immediate CT results rather than more long-term end-points, such as the lack of diagnosis of PE/DVT or initiation of anticoagulation within a three-month follow-up period, patients with false-negative CT results or who developed a subtle PE within a short time period after imaging might be missed using the scoring system alone. Additionally, 22 patients (18%) were lost to follow-up. The retrospective nature of this study precludes firm conclusions regarding the safety of use of such a scoring when used as the authors intended – to avoid unnecessary imaging, treatment or hospitalization. Nonetheless, the findings in this study suggest that use of a clinical prediction score can aid in developing a reasonable accurate pre-test probability prior to imaging the pregnant or postpartum patients.

3. In pregnant patients admitted to the hospital (population), are the number of venous thrombotic events reduced (outcome) when using a "care bundle" or "Early Obstetrical Warning System" compared to routine care (comparison)?

Search Strategy

PUBMED: pregnancy AND bundles.

PUBMED: "Early Warning Systems" AND "Pregnancy".

PUBMED: "reduction in thromboembolism in pregnancy".

Cochrane Database: "Thromboembolism AND pregnancy".

Hand-searching: references listed in the articles obtained.

One approach to preventing morbidity and mortality from thromboembolism includes utilizing protocols for prophylaxis for patients at risk. Interestingly, in the Cochrane review of Prophylaxis for venous thromboembolic disease in pregnancy and the early postnatal period, reviewers found

Table 52.4 Comparison of imaging modalities used to diagnose VTE in pregnancy

Test	Advantages	Disadvantages
Duplex compression sonography (Doppler)	• No radiation exposure • Treatment similar for PE/DVT	• Cannot detect clots isolated to the pelvic vessels • May not detect thrombi that have already embolized
Computed tomography pulmonary angiogram (CTPA)	• Relatively rapid diagnosis • Lower radiation exposure if single photon emission CT (SPECT) available • Can provide alternative diagnosis (pneumonia, pulmonary edema)	• Some radiation exposure necessary for test • Physiologic changes in pregnancy may result in artifact
Ventilation/perfusion scanning	• Lower radiation exposure to patient and fetus • Reasonably high sensitivity/specificity	• Diagnostic accuracy limited in patients with active or obstructive lung disease due to low specificity (asthma, chronic obstructive pulmonary disease (COPD), pulmonary edema) • Diagnosis less reliable if pre-test probability moderate or low and results indeterminate.

insufficient evidence to guide clinical decision-making [26]. The reviewers attributed this to a lack of reporting of maternal mortality in any of the studies reviewed. Additionally, a majority of studies were relatively small, with only 2592 women included in the 16 trials that were included in the review. The authors' conclusion was that absent evidence from randomized controlled trials that can identify the best means for prophylaxis, practitioners must rely on consensus-derived clinical guidelines, such as those produced or endorsed by the Royal College of Obstetricians and Gynecologists (RCOG) [9, 10], the National Institute for Health and Care Excellence (NICE) [27], the American College of Chest Physicians [12], or other international organizations such as the ACOG [11].

Thromboprophylaxis guidelines were created by the Swedish Society of Obstetrics and Gynecology in 1998, and a prospective study was designed to evaluate the efficacy of the use of LMWH for thromboprophylaxis in women with a prior VTE [28]. Over the five-year study period, 326 women who were prescribed Lovenox for prophylaxis were compared to 1000 controls. With thromboprophylaxis in accordance with the Swedish guidelines, the investigators identified an estimated 88% reduction in the relative risk for recurrent VTE in pregnancy.

These findings are similar to those found in the United Kingdom (UK), whereby thromboprophylaxis guidelines developed in response to the decades old quality and safety initiative "Saving Mothers' Lives: Confidential Enquiry into Maternal Deaths," has led to the sharpest decline in maternal mortality in the UK since 1985 [29]. In a review of nearly 1.5 million pregnancies in one of the largest US hospital systems, pulmonary embolism was the causative factor in 9 (10%) of the 95 deaths identified, and thromboembolism was identified as one of the most accessible targets to effectively aim systematic efforts to reduce maternal mortality [7]. After implementation of a protocol for universal use of sequential compression devices at the time of cesarean delivery, (intervention) and reevaluation of the maternal mortality rate within this same system three years after this intervention, the authors found an 86% reduction in maternal mortality from post-cesarean thromboembolism [30].

The Institute for Healthcare Improvement (IHI) defines the term "bundle" as a way to "describe a collection of processes needed to effectively care for patients undergoing particular treatments with inherent risks." The goal is to "bundle" together several scientifically grounded, essential elements in the care process essential to improving clinical outcomes. Ideally, bundles are relatively straightforward and uncomplicated, and limited to ensure that the bundle can be feasibly carried out [31]. Another critical component of a bundle is the concept that all components work synergistically and must be completed for it to be effective [31]. In other words, bundles work by an all or nothing approach. The Council on Patient Safety in Women's Healthcare is a consortium of organizations across women's healthcare including ACOG, the American Board of Obstetrics and Gynecology (ABOG), the American Academy of Family Physicians, the American College of Nurse Midwives, among others. This consortium uses the term "bundle" to include a collection of materials such as checklists, protocols, educational materials and reporting systems targeted toward a particular morbidity, designed to use a comprehensive treatment approach [32].

The thromboprophylaxis bundle endorsed by the Council on Patient Safety in Women's Healthcare includes development of national and local tools to recognize and prevent VTE in every patient, protocols for every unit, such as utilizing

Table 52.5 Comparison of clinical scoring systems

Scoring system	Finding	Points	Score/probability
Revised Geneva[21]	Age > 65 years	1	0–3 Low Probability 4–10 Intermediate >/= 11 High Probability
	Previous DVT/PE	3	
	Surgery (under general anesthesia) or lower limb fracture within one month	2	
	Active malignancy (within 1 yr)	2	
	Unilateral lower limb pain	3	
	Hemoptysis	2	
	Heart rate 75–94 beats min^{-1}	3	
	HR >/= 95 beats min^{-1}	5	
	Pain on lower limb deep venous palpation and unilateral edema	4	
Modified Well's Criteria[22]	Suspected DVT	3.0	0–2 Low risk 3–6 Moderate risk >6 High risk
	Alternative diagnosis less likely than PE	3.0	
	Heart rate > 100 beats/min	1.5	
	Immobilization/surgery in previous four weeks	1.5	
	Previous DVT/PE	1.5	
	Hemoptysis	1.0	
	Malignancy	1.0	
Pulmonary Embolism Rule-out Criteria (PERC or Charlotte rule)[23]	Age < 50	All criteria must be negative	If negative, likelihood of PE so low that D-Dimer testing not useful (<1.8% likelihood of PE)
	HR < 100		
	SaO_2 > 94%		
	No unilateral leg swelling		
	No recent trauma/surgery		
	No hemoptysis		
	No hormone use		
	No Prior PE/DVT		

standardized recommendations for mechanical and pharmacologic prophylaxis and therapy. Additionally standardized recommendations for timing of use of prophylaxis with neuraxial anesthesia, as well as monitoring process metrics and protocol compliance are recommended [32]. The goal is to encourage use of these bundles throughout the United States by the end of 2016, and long-term data regarding local and regional compliance and outcomes are pending [33]. Some potential limitations to large-scale data collection is the documented need to tailor guidelines to the needs and capabilities of local systems and populations, the potential for variation in compliance amongst individuals and groups and limitations inherent in large-scale data collection [34].

Another approach to reducing adverse outcomes when prophylaxis is contraindicated, otherwise not feasible, or fails, is to facilitate early detection and treatment of thromboembolism. Multiple audits and enquiries into root causes of *preventable* maternal deaths have shown that human failure, specifically failure to recognize the severity of a patient's condition, failure to act, or communication failure, contributed significantly to the outcome [7, 8, 35–37]. Early warning systems, designed to alert care providers to pathologic physiologic parameters that may precede critical illness have been used in fields outside of obstetrics, such as in general medicine [38, 39] and pediatrics wards. A MEOWS was originally proposed in the UK in 2007 as a result of the Confidential Enquiries into Maternal Deaths as a means to systematically improve early identification of women at highest risk for severe morbidity or death [40]. The initially proposed MEOWS allowed any care provider, such as a bedside nurse, to identify abnormal physiologic parameters including: pulse oxygenation, respiratory rate, blood pressure, urine output, level of consciousness, based on color coded values [41]. Values that registered in a "yellow" zone were slightly abnormal, and "red" values were markedly abnormal. To be effective such early warning systems cannot rely upon scoring alone. Instead, mechanisms to encourage appropriate action when abnormal findings are identified must be implemented along with such warning systems. This may include implementing "triggers"; in the above MEOWS example, one "red" or two "yellow" values for any one patient were designed to trigger an action, such as a physician being called to the bedside [41].

In a large, multi-center pilot study conducted in the United States, a Maternal Early Warning Trigger Tool (MEWT) was developed and implemented in 6 of 29 hospitals in a large hospital system [42]. The MEWT was designed to address the four most common causes of maternal morbidity: hemorrhage, preeclampsia, sepsis, and cardiopulmonary dysfunction. During the 13-month study period, the MEWT was used in 93.4% of all patients at the study sites. There were 32 patients who were screened for ICU admission at these sites, and of those, 31 required admission. There was a noted 5.5% increase in ICU admission at participating sites, compared to a 8% decrease in ICU admission at nonparticipating sites, but a significant reduction in Center for Disease Control (CDC)-defined severe maternal morbidity and composite maternal morbidity (18.4% and 13.6% respectively) [42].

CLINICAL SCENARIO 2

Cardiopulmonary arrest

The same 34-year-old G6P1001 Caucasian patient at 32 and 2/7 weeks' gestation in whom pulmonary embolism was suspected underwent appropriate screening and was started on therapeutic Lovenox. Approximately four hours later, a "code" is called, and the responding nurse notifies you that the patient has collapsed, is not breathing, and has no detectable pulse on initial exam.

1. Should pregnant patients past 24 weeks gestation (population) deteriorate rapidly to cardiorespiratory arrest, is maternal survival improved (outcome) if immediate (<5 minutes) versus delayed (>5 minutes) perimortem/resuscitative cesarean section (intervention, comparison) is performed?

Search Strategy

- PUBMED: cardiopulmonary resuscitation AND pregnancy.
- Hand-searching: references listed in the articles obtained.

Perhaps the most alarming event for a clinician is the rapid deterioration of a pregnant patient into cardiopulmonary arrest. Massive pulmonary embolism may either present or progress to cardiopulmonary arrest even when appropriate treatment has been initiated. Cardiac arrest is a rare event, and occurs in approximately 1 : 30 000 pregnancies, of which 29% are due to pulmonary embolism [43]. The fundamentals of resuscitation and advanced cardiac life support are similar in pregnant and non-pregnant patients: the airway must be secured, breathing established, chest compressions promptly and properly performed. Causes must be sought and treatment rendered based on the cardiac rhythm with which the patient presents. Important differences in the pregnant patient, however, particularly in the third trimester include increased airway edema necessitating prompt airway management and aortocaval compression due to the enlarged uterus, which requires placing the patient in a lateral tilt when performing chest compressions [44].

When cardiopulmonary failure occurs, hypoxic injury to the brain begins after approximately five minutes, both in the mother and fetus. To rescue a viable fetus from irreparable brain damage and possible death from an otherwise dying mother, emergent, rescue (perimortem) cesarean section should be performed. Ideally, rescue should be started within four minutes of cardiac arrest in any woman with an estimated gestational age at or beyond 24 weeks [45]; live births have occurred past this time window, however, therefore delivery should be attempted even if more than four minutes have passed since the arrest occurred [46]. Time spent assessing fetal heart tones with Doppler or ultrasound is thought to cause detrimental delay [47]. Additionally, in a recent review, the authors concluded that as up to 90% of cesareans may take longer than one minute, providers should move directly to cesarean once the decision has been made to deliver, rather than waiting for four minutes for the return of a spontaneous pulse, as this, again leads to unnecessary delay [48]. Rose and colleagues have advocated that the terminology should be changed from "perimortem cesarean" to "resuscitative cesarean," and the decision to proceed to cesarean be placed early in standard resuscitation algorithms to prompt early action and thereby optimize neonatal and maternal outcomes [49].

While most of the recommendations for cardiopulmonary resuscitation in the pregnant patient mirror those in other adults, such as establishment of an airway, the depth and rate of compressions, hand placement during compressions and defibrillation when necessary, a few important modifications to cardiopulmonary resuscitation have been identified [44]. Maternal pulmonary functional residual capacity decreases by 10–25%, providing less pulmonary reserve in the unstable pregnant patient, yet oxygen demands increase by 20–30%, and drug metabolism is altered [44]. The need for early 100% oxygen administration and rapid response to an unstable pregnant patient is essential. Especially later in pregnancy, weight gain and tissue edema may result in a "difficult airway," making skilled endotracheal intubation essential, and a smaller endotracheal tube may be required. Continuous capnography is recommended.

Optimal chest compressions have only been studied when the patient is in a supine position, rather than on a tilt, therefore supine positioning is recommended after maternal cardiopulmonary arrest [44]. This may lead to aortocaval compression from the gravid uterus, which impedes blood return to the heart. Therefore, manual left uterine displacement (LUD) is recommended throughout the resuscitative efforts. Delivery must be considered early in the resuscitation, as described previously. Most frequently, this is performed via perimortem (resuscitative) cesarean, however, it is reasonable for a provider experienced in operative vaginal delivery to attempt an assisted vaginal delivery (i.e. with forceps), in a patient who is fully dilated and when the head is sufficiently low.

Finally, planning for personnel and equipment logistics for both maternal and neonatal resuscitation teams is essential. Use of pre-stocked maternal and neonatal carts or equipment bags will allow each team access to essential equipment no matter the location of the cardiac arrest and resuscitation.

2. Do healthcare teams (population) perform better during obstetrical emergencies, such as cardiopulmonary arrest (outcome) if they undergo simulation training (intervention) compared to controls (comparison)?

Search Strategy

PUBMED: cardiopulmonary resuscitation AND simulation AND pregnancy.

PUBMED: simulation AND pregnancy.

Hand searching: references from articles obtained.

Successful resuscitation of any patient with cardiac arrest requires a highly functional team of care providers. Team coordination becomes even more crucial, as the team must prepare to care for two (or potentially more) patients, should resuscitative delivery be required. Cardiac arrest is not likely to occur in pregnant patients only in labor and delivery or an operating suite, but rather may occur anywhere within the hospital, specifically in the emergency department, ICU, or antepartum or postpartum units, underscoring the need to coordinate efforts across units and teams. Simulation training is a means to allow individuals and teams to rehearse and demonstrate medical knowledge, technical and communication skills and evaluate workflows and processes prior to execution of a high-stakes, rare and/or complex event. Perimortem or resuscitative cesarean is indeed a rarely performed procedure. In the 135 years from 1875 to 2010, only approximately 320 cases were reported in the literature [50].

Public demand for provider competency prior to performing procedures on patients, a trend toward non-invasive management whenever possible, and reduced procedure volume due to duty-hour limits have placed demand on training programs. Some providers may not see a rare obstetrical emergency throughout their entire careers. Simulation has been used within several industries, but has proven especially useful in aviation and in the US military since before World War II, and increasingly has been endorsed in obstetrics and gynecology since the turn of the twenty-first century as a means to overcome the challenges mentioned above [51].

In one study of simulation training [52], 12 maternal-fetal medicine faculty and 7 fellows underwent a pre-intervention simulation of a maternal cardiac arrest, then interventional simulation-based training designed to correct identified deficiencies, followed by a post-intervention simulation. Scores of knowledge, confidence and key performance measures in maternal care, critical care and total performance were evaluated before and after the intervention and training, with significant improvements in all measures after simulation training. Specifically, before the training intervention, a majority of providers demonstrated knowledge that cesarean should be initiated within four minutes, but in the pre-intervention exercise, few actually initiated the cesarean within this time. Three participants failed to initiate chest compressions in the initial simulation, yet all participants did so promptly and correctly after the simulation intervention. Interestingly, those participants with more years of experience or who had previously participated in an actual resuscitation appeared to benefit more from the simulation training than did more junior colleagues [52]. This suggests either that simulation provides an opportunity for experienced providers to leverage past experiences or underscores the concept that medical care, especially complex medical care, is subject to an individual learning curve [51].

The return of arterial pulsation during compressions after delivery and successful maternal resuscitation have been well documented [53]. A review of perimortem cesarean deliveries performed before and after emergency skills training demonstrated that of 55 women who had cardiac arrest, 12 underwent perimortem cesarean delivery. Two-thirds of the procedures were performed after skills training. While no cesarean was performed within the recommended five minutes, 67% of women regained cardiac output after delivery, with two maternal and five neonatal survivors [54].

Fortunately, even though cardiac arrest in pregnancy occurs rarely, the survival rate after cardiac arrest during admission for delivery approaches 59% [55], considerably higher than in the average population (18–25%) [56], Still, the rate of maternal mortality and the proportion of maternal deaths attributable to cardiac disease has risen in the last decade [57], which highlights the importance of adequate preparation and training.

Conclusions

Venous thromboembolic events and cardiopulmonary arrest are true obstetrical emergencies that warrant prompt investigation and treatment. Multi-faceted, team-based strategies, such as the use of checklists, bundles, early warning systems and simulation training are designed to reduce variation in practice, reduce medical errors, and improve the overall care given not just by individual providers, but also by the larger care teams.

References

1 Mitchell, P.H. Institute of Medicine (U.S.), Institute of Medicine (U.S.). (2012). *Roundtable on Value & Science-Driven Health Care. Best Practices Innovation Collaborative. Core Principles & Values of Effective Team-Based Health Care*, 30. Washington, DC: Institute of Medicine.

2 Havens, D.H. and Boroughs, L. (2000). "To err is human": a report from the Institute of Medicine. *J. Pediatr. Health Care.* **14** (**2**): 77–80.

3 Chassin, M.R. and Loeb, J.M. (2013). High-reliability health care: getting there from here. *Milbank Q.* **91** (**3**): 459–490.

4 CoPSaQ, I. (2015). Committee opinion no. 629: clinical guidelines and standardization of practice to improve outcomes. *Obstet. Gynecol.* **125** (**4**): 1027–1029.

5 Nasca, T.J., Philibert, I., Brigham, T., and Flynn, T.C. (2012). The next GME accreditation system – rationale and benefits. *N. Engl. J. Med.* **366** (**11**): 1051–1056.

6 Chang, J., Elam-Evans, L.D., Berg, C.J. et al. (2003). Pregnancy-related mortality surveillance--United States, 1991--1999. *MMWR Surveill. Summ.* **52** (**2**): 1–8.

7 Clark, S.L., Belfort, M.A., Dildy, G.A. et al. (2008). Maternal death in the 21st century: causes, prevention, and relationship to cesarean delivery. *Am. J. Obstet. Gynecol.* **199** (**1**): 36.e1, e7–36.e5; discussion 91–2, 11.

8 Cantwell, R., Clutton-Brock, T., Cooper, G. et al. (2011). Saving Mothers' lives: reviewing maternal deaths to make motherhood safer: 2006-2008. The eighth report of the confidential enquiries into maternal deaths in the United Kingdom. *BJOG* **118** Suppl 1: 1–203.

9 Royal College of Obstetricians and Gynecologists (RCOG). *Thrombosis and Embolism during Pregnancy and the Puerperium, Reducing the Risk (Green-Top Guideline No. 37a).* RCOG, London; 2015.

10 Royal College of Obstetricians and Gynecologists (RCOG) (2015). *Thrombosis and Embolism during Pregnancy and the Puerperium, the Acute Management of (Green-Top Guideline No. 37b).* London: RCOG.

11 James, A. (2011). Practice bulletin no. 123: thromboembolism in pregnancy. *Obstet. Gynecol.* **118** (**3**): 718–729.

12 Bates, S.M., Greer, I.A., Middeldorp, S. et al. (2012). VTE, thrombophilia, antithrombotic therapy, and pregnancy: antithrombotic therapy and prevention of thrombosis, 9th ed: American College of Chest Physicians Evidence-Based Clinical Practice Guidelines. *Chest* **141** (**2 Suppl**): e691S–e736S.

13 Leung, A.N., Bull, T.M., Jaeschke, R. et al. (2011). An official American Thoracic Society/Society of Thoracic Radiology clinical practice guideline: evaluation of suspected pulmonary embolism in pregnancy. *Am. J. Respir. Crit. Care Med.* **184** (**10**): 1200–1208.

14 Leung, A.N., Bull, T.M., Jaeschke, R. et al. (2012). American Thoracic Society documents: an official American Thoracic Society/Society of Thoracic Radiology Clinical Practice Guideline--Evaluation of suspected pulmonary embolism in pregnancy. *Radiology* **262** (**2**): 635–646.

15 Monga, M. (2009). *Maternal Cardiovascular, Respiratory and Renal Adaptations to Pregnancy. In: Creasy RK, Editor. Creasy & Resnik's Maternal-Fetal Medicine: Principles and Practice,* 6e, 104–105. Philadelphia, PA: Saunders Elsevier.

16 Kline, J.A., Williams, G.W., and Hernandez-Nino, J. (2005). D-dimer concentrations in normal pregnancy: new diagnostic thresholds are needed. *Clin. Chem.* **51** (**5**): 825–829.

17 Bremme, K.A. (2003). Haemostatic changes in pregnancy. *Best Pract. Res. Clin. Haematol.* **16** (**2**): 153–168.

18 Clark, S.L. and Hankins, G.D. (2012). Preventing maternal death: 10 clinical diamonds. *Obstet. Gynecol.* **119** (**2 Pt 1**): 360–364.

19 Bombeli, T., Raddatz-Mueller, P., and Fehr, J. (2001). Coagulation activation markers do not correlate with the clinical risk of thrombosis in pregnant women. *Am. J. Obstet. Gynecol.* **184** (**3**): 382–389.

20 Le Gal, G., Righini, M., Roy, P.M. et al. (2006). Prediction of pulmonary embolism in the emergency department: the revised Geneva score. *Ann. Intern. Med.* **144** (**3**): 165–171.

21 Wells, P.S., Ginsberg, J.S., Anderson, D.R. et al. (1998). Use of a clinical model for safe management of patients with suspected pulmonary embolism. *Ann. Intern. Med.* **129** (**12**): 997–1005.

22 Kline, J.A., Mitchell, A.M., Kabrhel, C. et al. (2004). Clinical criteria to prevent unnecessary diagnostic testing in emergency department patients with suspected pulmonary embolism. *J. Thromb. Haemost.* **2** (**8**): 1247–1255.

23 Hugli, O., Righini, M., Le Gal, G. et al. (2011). The pulmonary embolism rule-out criteria (PERC) rule does not safely exclude pulmonary embolism. *J. Thromb. Haemost.* **9** (**2**): 300–304.

24 Rac, M.W., Wells, C.E., Twickler, D.M. et al. (2015). Placenta accreta and vaginal bleeding according to gestational age at delivery. *Obstet. Gynecol.* **125** (**4**): 808–813.

25 Aboulafia, Y., Lavie, O., Granovsky-Grisaru, S. et al. (1994). Conservative surgical management of acute abdomen caused by placenta percreta in the second trimester. *Am. J. Obstet. Gynecol.* **170** (**5 Pt 1**): 1388–1389.

26 Bain, E., Wilson, A., Tooher, R. et al. (2014). Prophylaxis for venous thromboembolic disease in pregnancy and the early postnatal period. *Cochrane Database Syst. Rev.* **2**: CD001689. doi: 10.1002/14651858.CD001689.pub3.

27 Hill, J., Treasure, T., and Group, G.D. (2010). Reducing the risk of venous thromboembolism (deep vein thrombosis and pulmonary embolism) in patients admitted to hospital: summary of the NICE guideline. *Heart* **96** (**11**): 879–882.

28 Lindqvist, P.G., Bremme, K., Hellgren, M., and Working Group on Hemostatic Disorders (Hem-ARG) SeSoOaG (2011). Efficacy of obstetric thromboprophylaxis and long-term risk of recurrence of venous thromboembolism. *Acta Obstet. Gynecol. Scand.* **90** (**6**): 648–653.

29 Lewis, G. (2012). Saving Mothers' lives: the continuing benefits for maternal health from the United Kingdom (UK) confidential enquires into maternal deaths. *Semin. Perinatol.* **36** (**1**): 19–26.

30 Clark, S.L., Christmas, J.T., Frye, D.R. et al. (2014). Maternal mortality in the United States: predictability and the impact of protocols on fatal postcesarean pulmonary embolism and hypertension-related intracranial hemorrhage. *Am. J. Obstet. Gynecol.* **211** (**1**): 32.e1–32.e9.

31 Improvement IfH. Bundle Up for Safety http://www.ihi.org/resources/Pages/ImprovementStories/BundleUpforSafety.aspx: Institute for Healthcare Improvement; 2016 accessed 14 July 2018.

32 Council on Patient Safety in Women's Health Care. Patient Safety Bundle: Maternal Venous Thromboembolism Prevention http://www.safehealthcareforeverywoman.org/secure/vte-prevention-patient-safety-bundle.php2015 accessed 15 July 2018.

33 D'Alton, M.E., Main, E.K., Menard, M.K., and Levy, B.S. (2014). The National Partnership for maternal safety. *Obstet. Gynecol.* **123** (**5**): 973–977.

34 Arora, K.S., Shields, L.E., Grobman, W.A. et al. (2016). Triggers, bundles, protocols, and checklists-what every maternal care provider needs to know. *Am. J. Obstet. Gynecol.* **214** (**4**): 444–451.

35 Berg, C.J., Chang, J., Callaghan, W.M., and Whitehead, S.J. (2003). Pregnancy-related mortality in the United States, 1991-1997. *Obstet. Gynecol.* **101** (**2**): 289–296.

36 Geller, S.E., Cox, S.M., and Kilpatrick, S.J. (2006). A descriptive model of preventability in maternal morbidity and mortality. *J. Perinatol.* **26** (**2**): 79–84.

37 Esscher, A., Binder-Finnema, P., Bødker, B. et al. (2014). Suboptimal care and maternal mortality among foreign-born women in Sweden: maternal death audit with application of the 'migration three delays' model. *BMC Pregnancy Childbirth* **14**: 141.

38 Goldhill, D.R., McNarry, A.F., Mandersloot, G., and McGinley, A. (2005). A physiologically-based early warning score for ward patients: the association between score and outcome. *Anaesthesia* **60** (**6**): 547–553.

39 Gao, H., McDonnell, A., Harrison, D.A. et al. (2007). Systematic review and evaluation of physiological track and trigger warning systems for identifying at-risk patients on the ward. *Intensive Care Med.* **33** (**4**): 667–679.

40 Lewis, G. (2007). *Confidential Enquiry into Maternal and Child Health. Saving mothers' Lives : Reviewing Maternal Deaths to Make Motherhood Safer, 2003–2005*. London: CEMACH. xxviii, 267 p.

41 Singh, S., McGlennan, A., England, A., and Simons, R. (2012). A validation study of the CEMACH recommended modified early obstetric warning system (MEOWS). *Anaesthesia* **67** (**1**): 12–18.

42 Shields, L.E., Wiesner, S., Klein, C. et al. (2016). Use of maternal early warning trigger tool reduces maternal morbidity. *Am. J. Obstet. Gynecol.* **214** (**4**): 527. e1–6.

43 Suresh, M.S., LaToya Mason, C., and Munnur, U. (2010). Cardiopulmonary resuscitation and the parturient. *Best Pract. Res. Clin. Obstet. Gynaecol.* **24** (**3**): 383–400.

44 Jeejeebhoy, F.M., Zelop, C.M., Lipman, S. et al. (2015). Cardiac arrest in pregnancy: a scientific statement from the American Heart Association. *Circulation* **132** (**18**): 1747–1773.

45 Katz, V.L., Dotters, D.J., and Droegemueller, W. (1986). Perimortem cesarean delivery. *Obstet. Gynecol.* **68** (**4**): 571–576.

46 Lipman, S.S., Cohen, S., Mhyre, J. et al. (2016). Challenging the 4- to 5-minute rule: from perimortem cesarean to resuscitative hysterotomy. *Am. J. Obstet. Gynecol.* **215** (**1**): 129–131.

47 Katz, V.L. (2012). Perimortem cesarean delivery: its role in maternal mortality. *Semin. Perinatol.* **36** (**1**): 68–72.

48 Benson, M.D., Padovano, A., Bourjeily, G., and Zhou, Y. (2016). Maternal collapse: challenging the four-minute rule. *EBioMedicine* **6**: 253–257.

49 Rose, C.H., Faksh, A., Traynor, K.D. et al. (2015). *Am. J. Obstet. Gynecol.* **213** (**5**): 653–656, 653.e1.

50 Drukker, L., Hants, Y., Sharon, E. et al. (2014). Perimortem cesarean section for maternal and fetal salvage: concise review and protocol. *Acta Obstet. Gynecol. Scand.* **93** (**10**): 965–972.

51 Macedonia, C.R., Gherman, R.B., and Satin, A.J. (2003). Simulation laboratories for training in obstetrics and gynecology. *Obstet. Gynecol.* **102** (**2**): 388–392.

52 Fisher, N., Eisen, L.A., Bayya, J.V. et al. (2011). Improved performance of maternal-fetal medicine staff after maternal cardiac arrest simulation-based training. *Am. J. Obstet. Gynecol.* **205** (**3**): 239.e1–239.e5.

53 Morrison, L.J., Deakin, C.D., Morley, P.T. et al. (2010). Part 8: advanced life support: 2010 international consensus on cardiopulmonary resuscitation and emergency cardiovascular care science with treatment recommendations. *Circulation* **122** (**16 Suppl 2**): S345–S421.

54 Dijkman, A., Huisman, C.M., Smit, M. et al. (2010). Cardiac arrest in pregnancy: increasing use of perimortem caesarean section due to emergency skills training? *BJOG* **117** (**3**): 282–287.

55 Mhyre, J.M., Tsen, L.C., Einav, S. et al. (2014). Cardiac arrest during hospitalization for delivery in the United States, 1998-2011. *Anesthesiology* **120** (**4**): 810–818.

56 Girotra, S., Cram, P., Spertus, J.A. et al. (2014). Hospital variation in survival trends for in-hospital cardiac arrest. *J. Am. Heart Assoc.* **3** (**3**): e000871.

57 Creanga, A.A., Berg, C.J., Syverson, C. et al. (2015). Pregnancy-related mortality in the United States, 2006–2010. *Obstet. Gynecol.* **125** (**1**): 5–12.

53

CHAPTER 53
Methods for spontaneous delivery

Carrie Lynn Johnson
Department of Obstetrics and Gynecology, University of Miami, Miller School of Medicine, Miami, FL, USA

CLINICAL VIGNETTE

A 35-year-old G1P0 at 39 weeks gestation presents with regular uterine contractions every two to three minutes. Cervical exam is three to 4 cm, 100% effaced, −1 station with vertex presentation. Amniotic membranes are intact. Maternal vital signs are reassuring and fetal heart tracing is a Category one.

Background

In 1954–1956 Dr. Emanuel A. Friedman published the sentinel works detailing the normal progress of labor. Friedman pioneered the terms latent phase and active phase of labor as depicted in the eponymous "Friedman's Curve" [1, 2]. Since the 1960s, the demographics and characteristics of our obstetrical patients are older on average (26.8 vs. 24) and with higher Body Mass Index (BMI) (29.1 vs. 26.3) [3]. Obstetrical management has also changed in the ensuing 60 years. For example, in the 1050s and 1960s upwards of 50% of primiparous patients were delivered via forceps with a cesarean delivery rate around 2–3% [1, 3]. Today's obstetrical patient is more likely to receive regional analgesia (80% vs. 4%) and oxytocin in labor (50% vs. 14%) [1–3]. In 2010 the Consortium on Safe Labor (CSL) evaluated data on 228 668 deliveries at 19 US medical centers dating from 2002 to 2008. From this retrospective analysis on spontaneous labor, adjustments and revisions to the previously accepted understandings of active phase and active phase disorders occurred [4].

The CSL also brings to light questions regarding protocols and practices for the second stage of labor. The second stage of labor is the time from complete cervical dilation through delivery of the newborn. Laughon's analysis of the National Collaborative Perinatal Project (CPP) was the first extensive review of the second stage of labor of patients from the 1950s and 1960s. Laughon et al. compared data from the National CPP 39 491 deliveries from 1959 to 1969, with data from the CSL [3]. In spontaneous primiparous deliveries the median time in the second stage was 0.45 hours (CPP) compared to 0.9 hours (CSL) (p value <0.0010) [3]. In operative vaginal deliveries (OVD) of nulliparous women the second stage extended up to 3.1 hours in the CPP group and 4.25 hours in the CSL group (95%, p value <0.001) [3].

American College of Obstetricians and Gynecologists (ACOG) guidelines on the second stage prior to 2014 and the CSL study recommended primiparous patient – 2 hours and multiparous patient – 1 hour. An additional hour was granted if the patient had regional analgesia. The revised guidelines developed by ACOG/SMFM OBSTETRIC CARE CONSENSUS state, "a specific absolute maximum length of time spent in the second stage of labor beyond which all women should undergo operative delivery has not been identified." And the consensus suggests extending the second stage in both primiparous and multiparous by an hour, thus establishing the four-hour mark for primiparous patients and the three-hour mark for multiparous patients. Active and passive activity in the second stage is not elaborated on [5].

The third stage of labor has only become a focus of medical attention over the last few decades. The third stage of labor is defined as beginning after delivery of the newborn through delivery of the placenta and fetal membranes. The majority of maternal blood loss and postpartum hemorrhages (PPHs) occur during the third stage of labor. Active Management of the Third Stage of labor (AMTSL) typically consists of:

- oxytoxic agent administered prior to placental separation
- controlled cord traction
- uterine massage.

AMTSL aims to decrease mean maternal blood loss and PPH. [64]

Evidence-Based Obstetrics and Gynecology, First Edition. Edited by Errol R. Norwitz, Carolyn M. Zelop, David A. Miller, and David L. Keefe.

Clinical questions

First stage of labor

1. When does active labor start?

In Friedman's original articles a specific cervical dilation was not identified as active labor. In his 1978 text *Labor: Clinical evaluation and management* Dr. Emanual Friedman demarcated active labor as the inflection point on the labor curve where the rate of cervical dilation was 1.2 cm hr^{-1} in nulliparous patients and 1.5 cm hr^{-1} in multiparous patients. This inflection point is depicted at 4 cm. Four cm has been accepted as the entry point to active labor until data from the CSL was analyzed. "Nulliparous and multiparous women appeared to progress at a similar pace before six cm. However, after six cm, labor accelerated much faster in multiparous than in nulliparous women." [4]. The inflection point in the CSL labor curves occurred around six cm, moving the start of active labor to 6 cm (Figures 53.1a and b).

2. How long could it take my patient to progress from 4 cm to 6 cm? 6 cm to 10 cm?

According to CSL data, labor may take up to 6.4 hours for a nulliparous women to progress from 4 to 5 cm and an additional 3.2 hours from 5 to 6 cm cervical dilation (95%). The median and 95 percentiles for cervical change before 6 cm for nulliparous and multiparas were close with no significant difference. The nulliparous patient can expect to spend from 2.1 to 8.6 hours in active labor whereas active labor in the multiparous patient lasts 1.5 to 7.5 hours (median to 95 percentiles) [4]. "Historical criteria defining normal labor progress-cervical change of 1.2 cm hr^{-1} for nulliparous women and 1.5 cm hr^{-1} for multiparous women-are no longer valid." [6] (Figures 53.1a and b).

3. How do I diagnosis active-phase arrest?

The traditional diagnosis of arrest of the active-phase was based on several premises:

- Active labor starts at 4 cm.
- Montevideo Units (MVUs) to assess the adequacy of uterine contractions.

The definition was based on the "two hour rule". Lack of cervical change over two hours with adequate contractions, as defined by 200–220 MVU over a 10 minute period, equaled active-phase arrest. In 2001 Rouse et al. challenged the "two hour rule". A standard protocol was implemented to extend the time from two to four hours. A total of 61% of the patients that had arrested at two hours subsequently went on to have a vaginal delivery [7]. Evaluation of the data revealed more cesarean deliveries would have been performed than infections prevented if the "two hour rule" had been followed. For many this study and the follow-up study by Rouse utilizing oxytocin augmentation for four hours prior to diagnosing active labor phase arrest created a point of practice change. [8] The "two hour rule" became the "four hour rule". Additional modifications reflecting the changes noted in the Consortium for Safe Labor are presented in the Table 53.1 below:

4. How does my patient's age affect labor progress?

Most research has focused on maternal and neonatal outcomes related to maternal age. In 2007 Greenberg et al. published a retrospective cohort study to evaluate the length of labor across maternal age groups. The study utilized term nulliparous and multiparous women from 1980 to 2001 at a single California institution, amounting to 31 976 deliveries.

Table 53.1 Diagnosis of active-phase arrest

Cervical change	Uterine activity
No cervical change in 4 h[a]	Adequate uterine contractions (MVU ≥ 200)
No Cervical Change in 6 h[a]	Inadequate uterine contactions (MVU < 200)

[a]Assuming oxytocin augmentation and ruptured membranes.

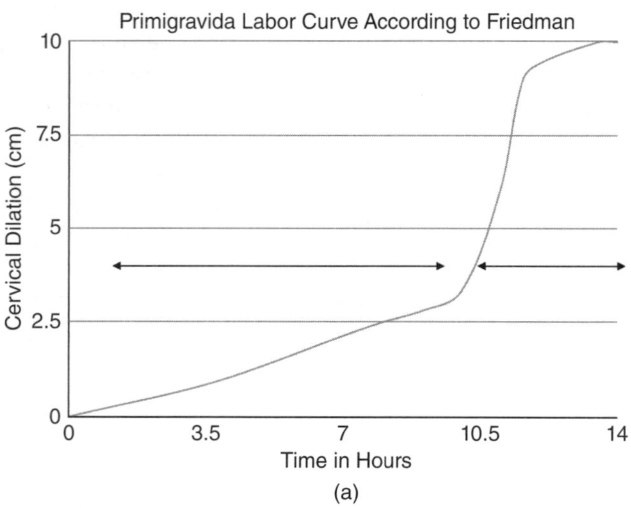

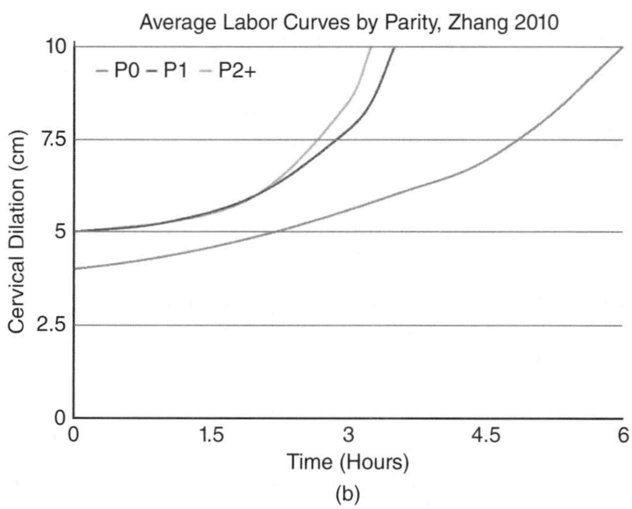

Figure 53.1 (a) Graph. Friedman Labor Curve. (b) Average Labor Curves by parity. (Zhang 2010 [4].)

Table 53.2 Greenberg-maternal age-median length first stage labor

	<20 y/o	35–39 y/o
Total nulliparous women	550 (170–1400)	660 (180–1734)
With epidural ($p < 0.001$)	630 (195–1485)	760 (240–1840)
Without epidural ($p = 0.14$)	435 (127–1300)	470 (125–1365)
Total multiparous women	368 (117–1080)	345 (90–1110)
With epidural ($p < 0.001$)	478 (140–1200)	436 (122–1380)
Without epidural ($p = 0.25$)	308 (100–1005)	290 (75–880)
	Median time reported in minutes (5–95%)	

Table 53.3 Zaki-labor duration from 4–10 cm by maternal age group

	Under 20 y/o	20–29 y/o	30–39 y/o	≥40 y/o
Nulliparous women labor duration 4–10 cm	8.5 (17.2)	7.8 (16.1)	7.4 (15.1)	8.0 (16.9)
Multiparous women labor duration 4–10 cm	8.8 (17.6)	7.5 (15.7)	6.7 (14.5)	6.5 (14.1)

Median time in hours (95%), no significant p values.

Patients were divided into six age groups; under 20, 20–24, 25–29, 30–34, 35–39, and 40 and over. The researchers found that nulliparous women experienced significantly longer labors with increasing age. This effect was intensified if the patient received epidural analgesia. The effect was most pronounced in the 35–39 y/o age group (Table 53.2).

The CSL data was analyzed to answer the same question, with a different result. The CSL data included 120 442 deliveries across 19 institutions from 2002 to 2008. Patients were grouped by parity (nulliparous/multiparous) and by age group (<20, 20–29, 30–39, ≥40). The trend was a shorter first stage of labor with increasing maternal age without reaching statistical significance [9] (Table 53.3).

5. Does obesity affect labor progress?

Four retrospective cohort studies published over the last four years directly answer this question. Labor proceeds more slowly as the BMI increases.

Table 53.4 Impact of body mass index on duration of first stage of labor

	BMI <25.0	BMI 35–39.9	BMI ≥40	p-value
Nulliparous women labor duration 4–10 cm (h)	5.4 (18.2)	6.7 (22.2)	7.7 (25.6)	<0.001
Multiparous women labor dDuration 4–10 cm (h)	4.6 (17.5)	5.0 (19.0)	5.4 (20.6)	<0.001

Median times in hours (95%).

Kominiarek et al. in 2011 analyzed data from the CSL utilizing 118 978 women stratified by BMI (<25, 25–29.9, 30–34.9, 35–39.9 ≥ 40) and parity. The median and 95 percentile duration from 4 to 10 cm were significantly longer in the obese patients for both nulliparous and multiparous women [10]. As shown in Table 53.4.

Hillard et al. and Norman et al. reached similar conclusions of the dose related effect of obesity on the duration of the first stage of labor [11, 12]. Our Swedish colleagues Carlhäll, Källénd, and Blomberg analyzed delivery data gathered through a Swedish regional perinatal database collected from 1995 to 2009 of 63 829 nulliparous women who presented in spontaneous labor. The retrospective cohort study compared women by BMI and duration of labor. Again increasing duration of labor was demonstrated with increasing BMI. The largest difference was noted between BMI <18.5 and BMI >40 with a p value <0.001. Although statistical significance was reached with all classes of obesity in comparison to normal weight parturients [13].

Second stage of labor

1. What is meant by passive or active second stage?

Second stage of labor begins at complete dilation and ends at delivery of the newborn. Passive second stage refers to the absence of maternal expulsive efforts and is often referred to as "laboring down". The intention is to allow the fetus to passively move further down the birth canal via the expulsive forces of the uterus prior to starting the active portion of the second stage. Active second stage indicates the period of time of maternal expulsive efforts.

As part of a 2008–2011 NICHD Maternal-Fetal Medicine Units Network, Yee et al. completed a secondary analysis of the initial 115 502 cohort comparing early with delayed pushing among nulliparous women. 21 034 women were included in the final comparison. Delayed pushing resulted in; a longer second stage with a longer active stage, increased cesarean section rate, increased operative vaginal delivery rate, along with an increased rate of PPH and transfusion [14] (Table 53.5).

A 2015 Cochrane Database review looked at the question of immediate versus delayed pushing. All patients studied had received epidurals. Delaying pushing extended the duration of the second stage by 54 minutes, but decreased the active portion by 22 minutes and increased the rate of vaginal delivery 61.5% versus 56.9% (RR1.09, 95% CI 1.03–1.15). The delayed group had an increased risk of low umbilical artery pH without a difference in neonatal intensive care unit (NICU) admissions. Also evaluated was spontaneous versus directed pushing. There was no significant outcome differences between the two groups in duration, maternal or neonatal complications. In summary delayed versus immediate, spontaneous versus directed show no significant benefit [15].

Table 53.5 Yee maternal and neonatal outcomes with early compared with delayed pushing among nulliparous women

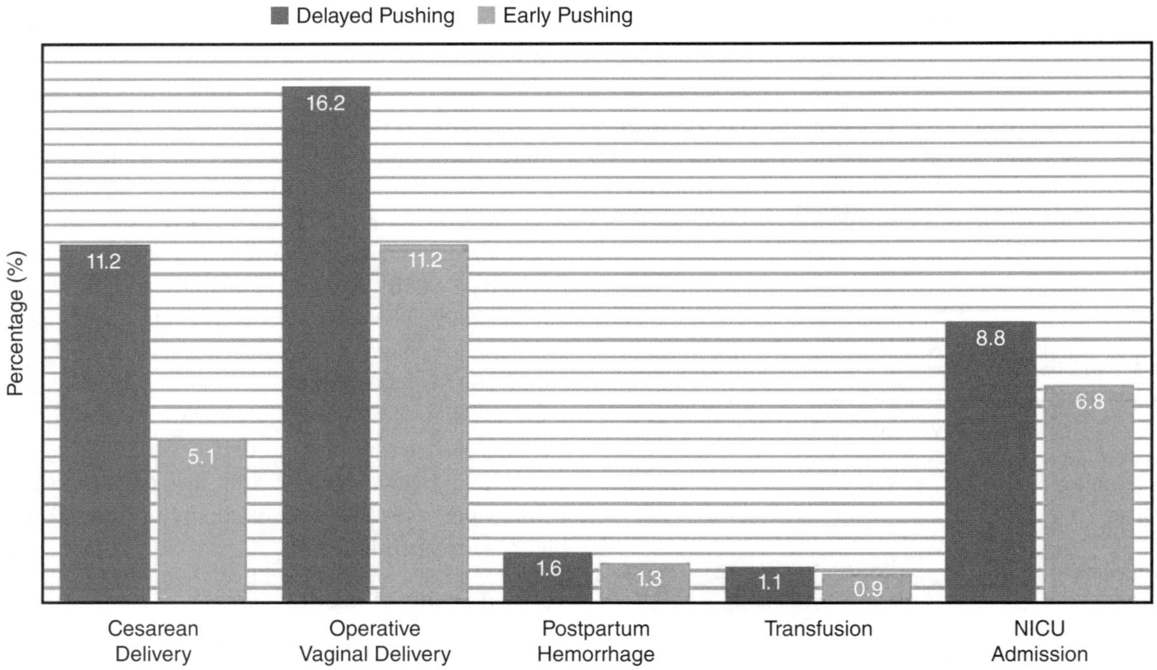

2. Is there a wrong way to push?

The classically propagated maternal expulsive technique involves Valsalva or closed glottis pushing. Across many labor floors you can hear the refrains of one… two… three… and so on as women are coached to hold their breath and bear down to the count of ten. As the standard across the nation and even across the pond there is surprisingly little research to back up the practice. Prins et al. published the best review to date and described the current literature supporting Valsalva pushing as "sparse, and flawed". Furthermore there appears to be no benefit for maternal or neonatal outcome for either Valsalva or physiologic (open glottis) pushing techniques. The researchers final recommendations were for further investigations and for the current time "women should be supported in following the feelings of their bodies and use their own bearing down efforts and urges to push." [16].

3. What effect does maternal position have on the second stage?

A 2012 Cochrane Database Review, "Position in the Second Stage of Labor for Women without Epidural Anesthesia" evaluated 22 studies, 7280 women. The review found most studies were of poor methodological quality with inconsistent clinical interventions. A meta-analysis comparing upright or lateral position versus supine or lithotomy concluded supine position was associated with fewer spontaneous births and more non-reassuring fetal heart rate tracings. The abnormal fetal heart tracings are likely the result of aorto-caval compression. Upright positions were associated with higher rates of blood loss >500 ml (RR 1.65, 95% CI 1.32–2.06) and a shorter but not statistically significant duration of the second stage of labor. [17]. From this review one may infer that the lateral position or supine with lateral uterine displacement maybe advantageous, but until more trials are conducted women should elect the position of their choice.

A similar Cochrane Database Review in 2013 evaluated women with epidural anesthesia. In five randomized controlled trials involving 879 women all with epidural anesthesia identified no statistically significant difference between upright and recumbent positions with regards to operative abdominal or vaginal deliveries. Two trials incorporating 322 women showed no significant difference in duration of second stage of labor. Due to the wide confidence intervals and the insufficient data no conclusions can be made with regards to the effect of maternal position with epidural anesthesia present. [18].

The Italian research team, Gizzo S, Di Gangi S, Novena M, Bacile V, Zambon A, and Battista Nardelli G, of the University of Padua conducted an observational cohort study on nulliparous women divided into two groups. Group A patients spent ≥50% of their labor in the supine or lateral positions whereas Group B patients used alternate positions (sitting, squatting, standing, "on all fours", sitting on the ball). Duration of second stage, analgesia request and presence of persistent occiput posterior were all increased

Table 53.6 Gizzo (2014) [19], comparison of maternal position choice and labor characteristics

	Group A (≥ 50% recumbent)	Group B (alternate positions)	p-value
Mean second stage of labor (min)	84.4 (+/− 57.8)[a]	34.4 (+/− 32.6)[a]	<0.001
Analgesia request (%)	35%	10%	<0.001
Persistent occiput posterior (%)	40%	28%	<0.001

[a]+/− Standard deviation.

with Group A (supine/lateral) with statistical significance (p values <0.001) [19] (Table 53.6).

4. If the second stage extends beyond the ACOG parameters what are the chances for a vaginal delivery versus an operative delivery?

For the nulliparous patient traditional ACOG guidelines recommend a two hour second stage which can be extended to three hours if an epidural is in place. And with a multiparous patient one hour without an epidural and two hours with an epidural. The adoption and implementation of these guidelines extend back to times when the obstetrical population differed and when the operative vaginal delivery rate greatly exceeded both the epidural rate and the cesarean rate [1]. Today's nulliparous patient has an 80% chance of receiving and epidural and at least a 50% of receiving oxytocin during labor [4].

In the last number of years researchers have been exploring the maternal and neonatal risks and benefits to extending the second stage. Data from the CSL showed the 95 percentile for nulliparous patients was 2.8 and 3.6 hours with and epidural. For Multiparous patients the second stage duration 95 percentile was 1 one and two hours with an epidural [4]. Of note the CSL was limited to deliveries with normal neonatal outcomes.

Grobman et al. through the Eunice Kennedy Shriver National Institute of Child Health and Human Development (NICHD) and Maternal-Fetal Medicine Units Networks (MFMU) performed an observational study over 25 hospitals with 53 285 women analyzing active duration of pushing in relation to maternal delivery route (stratified by nulliparous versus multiparous), visualized in the two graphs [20].

With increasing time a patient's risk of operative delivery increases. In nulliparous patients at the three to four hours interval 24.2% cesarean, 35.1% operative vaginal delivery, 40.7% spontaneous vaginal delivery (SVD). [21] (Figures 53.2a and b, Table 53.10)

Bleich analyzed 21 991 nulliparous deliveries that extended beyond three hours and noted a SVD rate of 3% if the second stage ≥4 hours. The majority of OVD occurred in the three to four hour window (Figure 53.3 and Table 53.7).

The contrast between Grobman's data and Bleich's data is the large percentage of OVD performed in the late second stage of labor. In 2009 Rouse et al. studied the second stage beyond five hours. The majority of the vaginal deliveries occurring past the three hour mark were OVD. At three

Table 53.7 Bleich (2012) [24], nulliparous women and route of delivery in relation to length of second stage of labor

	<3 h	3–4 h	≥4 h	p-value
Spontaneous vaginal delivery	93%	29%	3%	p<0.001
Forceps delivery	5%	29%	11%	p<0.001
Cesarean delivery	2%	42%	86%	p<0.001

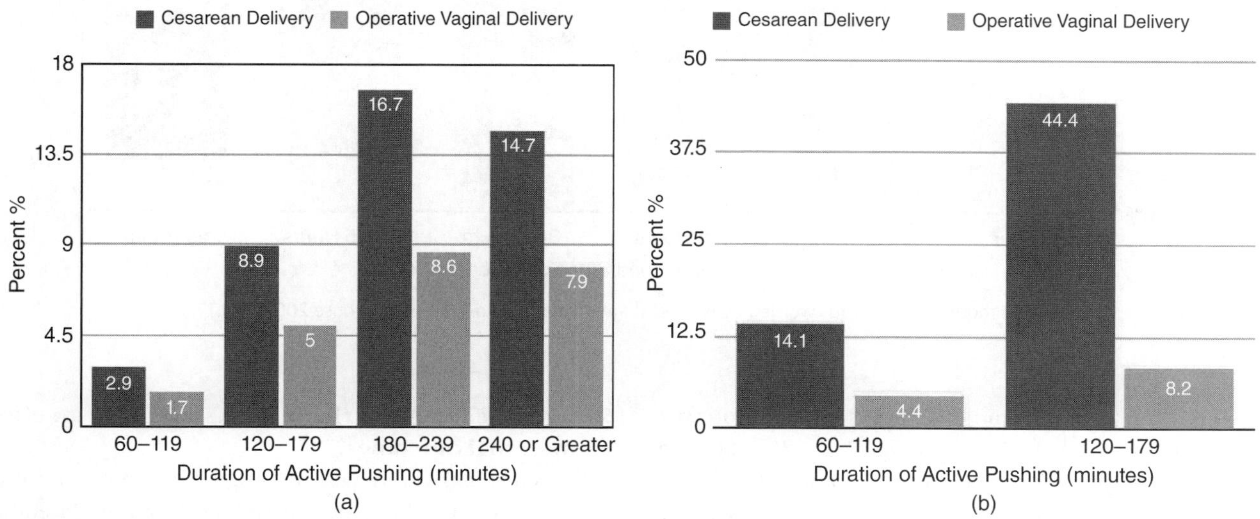

Figure 53.2 (Graph 2a). Duration of active pushing and obstetrical outcomes in nulliparous women. (Graph 2b). Duration of active pushing and obstetrical outcomes in multiparous women.

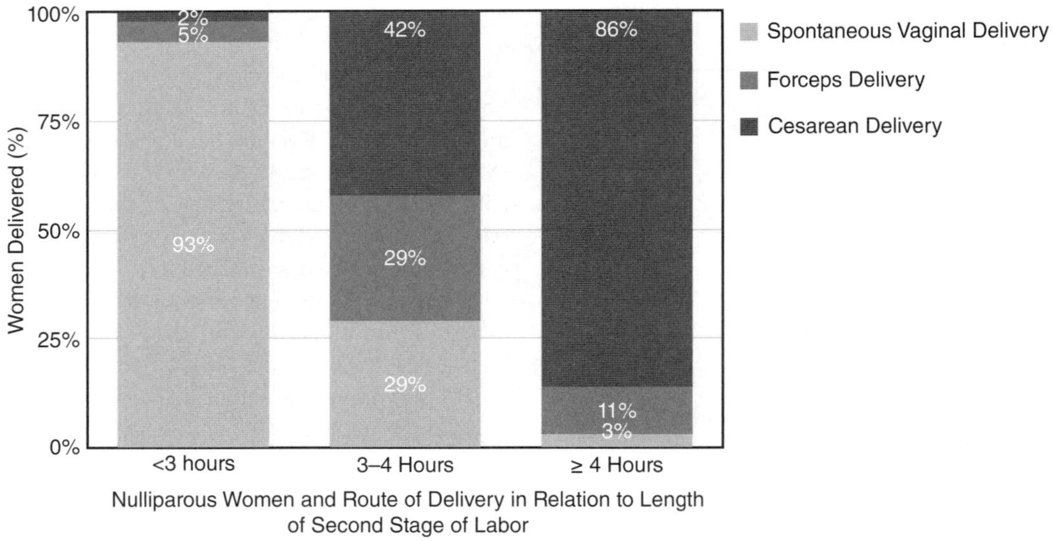

Figure 53.3 Graphic 3. Nulliparous women and route of delivery in relation to length of second stage of labor. (Bleich 2012 [24].)

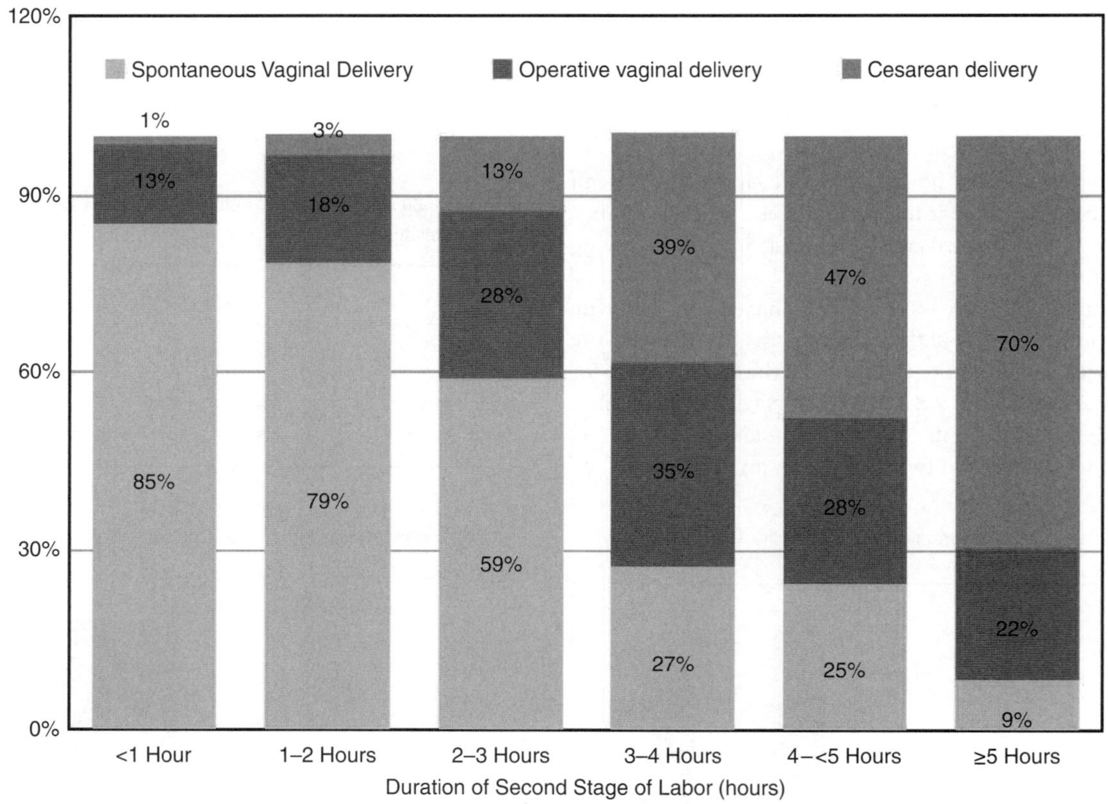

Figure 53.4 Graph 4. Delivery mode in nulliparous women by second stage of labor up to five hours. (Rouse 2009 [20].)

to hours, 34.6% (OVD) and 27.2% SVD. At the four 4 to five5 hours mark OVD 27.8% with SVD 24.7% [20]. The complete table/graph is here (Figure 53.4 and Table 53.8):

The consensus is operative delivery rates increased with longer durations of the second stage. Practitioners skilled at OVD are at an advantage.

5. Does the length of the second stage have an effect on maternal outcomes?

The short answer is yes, although the maternal consequences are related to parity as well as duration. Extending the second stage at what cost to maternal health? The most significant consequences to prolonging the second

Table 53.8 Rouse et al. (2009) [20] delivery mode by duration of second stage of labor

	<1 h	1–2 h	2–3 h	3–4 h	4 to <5 h	≥5 h
Spontaneous vaginal delivery (%)	85	79	59	27	25	9
Operativery vaginal delivery (%)	13	18	28	35	28	22
Cesarean delivery (%)	1	3	13	39	47	70

stage are:

- PPH (>500 ml) (up to 34%) [22, 23]
- Third/fourth degree perineal lacerations (16.3–59%) [20, 22–24]
- Intrapartum fever/chorioamnionitis (12.3–23%) [22, 23]

Uncommon but severe complications from prolonged second stage are:

- Blood transfusions (7%) [24]
- Hysterotomy extensions at time of cesarean delivery (40%) [25]
- Hysterectomy (1%) [24]

Gimovsky and Berghella in 2016 performed a randomized controlled trial of extending the time limit of the second stage by one hour versus the usual guidelines in the nulliparous patient. This extension of the second stage resulted in a primary cesarean section rate of 19.5% while the usual guideline group cesarean section rate was 43.2% (RR 0.45%; CI, 0.22–0.93). No significant differences in neonatal or maternal outcomes were noted. [26]

In Grobman's recent NICHD sponsored observational study PPH (PPH) and third/fourth degree perineal lacerations increased with duration in active pushing for both nulliparous and multiparous patients in a statistically significant fashion, $p < 0.001$ [20] (Table 53.9).

In separate studies Bleich, Le Ray and Cheng confirmed the increased risk for PPH and advanced perineal lacerations but also for intrapartum fever/chorioamnionitis $p < 0.001$ for each study set [22–24] Bleich further noted an increased risk of transfusion and hysterectomy in the ≥4 hours group (7% and 1% respectively, p values <0.001) [24].

A retrospective cohort study by Sung et al. from 2001 to 2004 evaluated pregnant women who underwent primary cesarean sections after failed second stage of labor. The groups were sub-divided into second stage of labor lengths one to three hours and > 4 hours. The study results were significant for an increase in (unintended) hysterotomy extensions in the >4 hours group, with an odds ratio of 2.18 (95% CI 1.13–4.22). Cervical extensions were more commonly seen in the >4 hour group, accounting for 29% of the extensions. Only rarely noted in the one to three hour group where 90% of the extensions were in the lower uterine segment. Oxytocin augmentation also increased the

Table 53.9 Grobman (2016) [21], duration of active pushing with maternal outcomes

	<1 h	1–2 h	2–3 h	3–4 h	≥4h	p-value
Nulliparous postpartum hemorrhage (%)	1.0	1.4	2.5	3.7	3.3	<0.001
Multiparous postpartum hemorrhage (%)	0.6	1.5	3.5			<0.001
Nulliparous third/fourth degree laceration (%)	5.0	8.5	14.0	15.3	16.3	<0.001
Multiparous third/fourth degree laceration (%)	0.9	3.6	5.1			<0.001

Table 53.10 Grobman (2016) [21], duration of active pushing with route of delivery

	<1 h	1–2 h	2–3 h	3–4 h	≥4h
Nulliparous cesarean delivery (%)	3.0	8.2	17.9	24.2	22.4
Nulliparous operative vaginal delivery (%)	7.9	13.3	27.5	35.1	32.8
Nulliparous spontaneous vaginal delivery (%)	89.1	78.5	54.7	40.7	44.8
Multiparous cesarean delivery (%)	0.5	8.5	18.2		
Multiparous operative vaginal delivery (%)	3.2	13.2	18.6		
Multiparous spontaneous vaginal delivery (%)	96.3	78.3	63.2		

risk of an unintended hysterotomy, odds ratio 2.01 (95% CI 1.08–3.75) [25].

6. Does the length of the second stage have on effect on neonatal outcomes?

"A longer duration of pushing is associated with an increased relative risk of neonatal complications." [20]. The Grobman 2016 observational study with 53 285 women is the largest study to date evaluating second stage duration with neonatal outcomes. Newborns of nulliparous women experienced different adverse events in comparison to those born of multiparous women. Nulliparous women were more likely to have:

- Brachial plexus palsy (highest incidence at three to four hours 0.5% p-value 0.009).
- Fracture (non-skull or clavicular) (highest incidence at three to four hour 0.3% p-value <0.001).

While multiparous women were more likely to have newborns with:

- Seizure (0.4% at two to three hours p-value <0.001).
- Hypoxic-ischemic encephalopathy (HIE) (1.1% at two to three hours p-value <0.001) [21].

Bleich's study with nulliparous patients yielded similar data. Brachial plexus injuries in newborns peaked at the three to four hour duration with a rate of 1.4% (p-value

<0.001 compared to <3 hours). Newborn seizures increased significantly with increasing duration of the second stage 0.1% in the <3 hours group compared to 3% in the ≥4 hours group (p value <0.001) [24].

7. Does maternal age affect the length of the second stage?

The two largest studies to date, Greenberg et al. and Zaki et al., are in agreement. The second stage of labor increases in duration with increasing maternal age. Greenberg reviewed 31 976 births from 1980 to 2001 stratified by age, parity and epidural use. The researchers concluded that advancing age was associated with longer second stages regardless of parity or epidural use and with also associated with an increased risk for a prolonged second stage of labor. A 40 y/o nulliparous women had an odds ratio of 3.90 (95% CI 2.70–5.62) compared to a <20 y/o of having a prolonged second stage [27].

Zaki et al. analyzed data from the CS004C with similar results. The length of the second stage of labor with and without epidurals increased directly with age (p value <0.001). The increase in nulliparous as 0.4 hours/ age group and in multiparous the increase was 0.2 hours [9].

8. Does obesity affect the length of the second stage?

Obesity does have an effect on the duration of the second stage of labor. Unlike the first stage obesity shortens the length of the second stage of labor in some cases. Carlhäll et al. utilized a Southern Sweden perinatal database of 63 829 nulliparous women and concluded that the duration of the second stage was significantly shorter in obese women compared to normal weight women (p-value <0.001) [13].

Kominiarek et al., with data from the CSL, arrived at similar conclusions. Once the median traverse times were adjusted for other factors (birthweight) the adjusted times in the nulliparous groups no longer met statistical significance. The multiparous median traverse time was statistically significant before and after adjusted for other factors. (p-value <0.001) [10].

Third stage of labor

The third stage of labor is defined as the time following delivery of the newborn through delivery of the placenta. Hemorrhage is a leading cause of maternal morbidity and mortality in resource poor countries. Excluding hemorrhage from first trimester pregnancy loss the third stage of labor accounts for the majority of pregnancy associated hemorrhage. The average rate of PPH in the US is 3–5%.

Grobman et al. analyzed 115 502 deliveries during the study period 2008–2011 across 25 medical centers for severe maternal morbidity (SMM). For study purposes SMM was defined as:

- maternal transfusion ≥3 units packed red blood cells (PRBC)s
- unanticipated surgical intervention
- ICU admission
- intubation
- organ failure.

SMM occurred in 2.9 per 1000 births with PPH accounting for half of the SMM [28]. Interventions aimed at decreasing or preventing PPH play an important role in obstetrical care.

1. What is the mean duration of the Third Stage? Duration and risk of postpartum hemorrhage

Frolova AI, Stout MJ, Tuuli MG et al. analyzed 7121 women for duration of the placental delivery and risk of PPH. All women delivered vaginally at >37 weeks and received AMTSL. The mean duration of the third stage was 5.46 minutes. Not surprisingly a longer third stage resulted in an increased risk of PPH. What was remarkable was the increased risk started at 20 minutes. Patients with a third stage of 20–24 minutes had a PPH rate of 15.9% (OR 2.04 95% CI 1.03–4.04), 25–29 minutes had a PPH rate of 20% (OR 2.68 95% CI 1.17–6.17) and ≥ 30 minutes 35.1% (OR 5.76 95% CI 3.32–9.99) [29].

2. What is Active Management of the Third Stage of Labor (AMTSL)?

AMTSL is contrasted with physiological management in the table below (Table 53.11).

3. What are the benefits of AMTSL?

In order to best answer this each component on AMTSL needs to be evaluated.

a. Oxytocin

Garabedian et al. performed a single center "before" and "after" study to assess the impact of routine oxytocin use in the third stage of labor.

- Before group (n = 1953, 43% high risk) oxytocin in third stage only for high risk patients.
- After group (n = 1911) oxytocin in third stage for all patients.

High risk was defined as; history of PPH, parity ≥3, estimated fetal weight (EFW) ≥4 kg, uterine over distention, labor ≥12 hours, instrumental delivery, or uterine scar. During the study period oxytocin administration resulted in a reduced risk of moderate hemorrhage (>500 ml) 13.4%

Table 53.11 Comparison of active management versus physiological management of the third stage of labor

	Active management	Physiological management
Uterotonic agent	Prior to delivery of placenta	None or after placental delivery
Controlled cord traction (Brandt-Andrews maneuver)	Applied when uterus has contracted	Deferred
Uterine massage	Variable	Deferred

vs. 9.2% ($p < 0.001$), although no reduction in severe hemorrhage (>100 ml) 2.1% vs. 2.0 ($p = 0.79$) [30].

There are also two significant recent Cochrane Database reviews addressing the issue.

- "Prophylactic oxytocin for third stage of labor to prevent PPH" (2013) [31].
  - * Decreased risk of moderate PPH (>500 ml) RR 0.53 (95% CI, 0.38–7.4) 6 trials 4203 women.
  - * Reduced need for therapeutic uterotonics RR 0.56 (95% CI, 0.36–0.87) 4 trials 3174 women.
- "Active versus expectant management for women in the third stage of labor" (2015) [32].
  - * Decreased risk of severe hemorrhage (>100 ml) RR 0.34 (95% CI, 0.14–0.87) 3 trials 4636 women.
  - * Decreased rate of maternal Hgb < 8 g dl RR 0.50 (95% CI, 0.30–0.83) 2 trials 1522 women.

All of these support the routine use of oxytocin in the third stage of labor.

b. Controlled Cord Traction (CCT)/Brandt-Andrews maneuver

A 2015 Cochrane Database review included three randomized controlled non-blinded studies. No difference in severe hemorrhage (>1000 ml), additional/therapeutic uterotonics, blood transfusions, or SMM were found. The WHO sites utilizing ergotamine had a reduction in manual placental removal, RR 0.69(95% CI, 0.57–0.83). The reviews concluded, "CCT has limited benefits… routine use can be omitted from the "active management" package without increasing risk for severe hemorrhage." [33].

c. Uterine Massage

A 2013 Cochrane Database reviewed studies that addressed the question of the effectiveness of uterine massage. The review included two randomized controlled trials.

One trial compared three groups: oxytocin, uterine massage, or both oxytocin and uterine massage (n = 1964). Uterine massage conferred no additional benefit over oxytocin alone in regards to moderate hemorrhage (500 ml) RR 1.56 (95% C 0.44–5.49) or the need for additional/therapeutic uterotonics RR 102 (95% CI 0.56–1.85).

The second trial simply compared oxytocin with and without uterine massage (n = 200). No significant difference was found for moderate hemorrhage or need for additional/therapeutic uterotonics, although the mean blood loss was found to be significantly less in the uterine massage group, MD −41.60 ml, (95% CI −75.16 to −8.04).

When the two trials were combined and analyzed the average effects using a random effects model revealed no significance between the study and control groups.

The authors concluded, "once an oxytocic has been given, there is limited scope for further reduction in postpartum blood loss." [34].

4. What is the optimum oxytocic medication?

The best way to answer the question is to compare the agents.

- Oxytocin versus ergometrine (Methergine®)

A 2013 Cochrane Database Review evaluated 5 trials with 2226 women comparing oxytocin and ergometrine for AMTSL. Oxytocin was better at preventing moderate PPH (>500 ml) RR 0.76 (95% CI 0.61–0.94). Ergot alkaloids a known to have more side effects including; hypertension, nausea, and vomiting. And are unstable if not refrigerated or exposed to light [31].

- Oxytocin versus misoprostol, prostaglandin E_1, (Cytotec®)

When Misoprostol was compared to oxytocin in AMTSL it was found to be less effective regardless of the route of administration (oral, rectal or sublingual). When given orally misoprostol had an increased risk of severe PPH (>1000 ml) RR 1.33 (95% CI 1.16–1.52), 17 trials n = 29 797. This also held true when administered rectally, RR 1.10 (95% CI 0.69–1.77), 4 trials n = 2221. Although limited data was available for sublingual misoprostol (3 trials n = 270) it did not show any benefit over oxytocin [35]. Misoprostol has dose and route related onset of action and duration of action. See Table 53.12 below: [36].

Misoprostol is also associated with maternal fever. The onset of fever is typically twenty minutes post administration and peaks at one to two hours. [36, 37] The rate of fever is related to the dose:

200–400 mcg – 8%

≥600 mcg – 45% [38]

5. What is the optimum timing of oxytocin administration?

Trials with optimum methodology and power have yet to be performed. The current standard recommendation, (ACOG, WHO, RCOG) is to initiate oxytocin administration after delivery of the anterior shoulder and before the placenta. In recent studies the average time for placental expulsion is 5–6 minutes, with an increased risk of PPH noted if the placenta is not delivered by 17–18 minutes [39, 40]. Initiating oxytocin early in the third stage in theory would allow adequate time for onset on action to enhance uterine contractions and placental separation.

Table 53.12 Misoprostol comparison of route-onset of action and duration of action

Route	Onset of action (min)	Duration of action (h)
Oral[a]	8	~2
Sublingual	11	~3
Vaginal	20	~4
Rectal	100	~4

[a]Due to first pass effect, initial uterine tone is not followed by contractions without repeated doses.

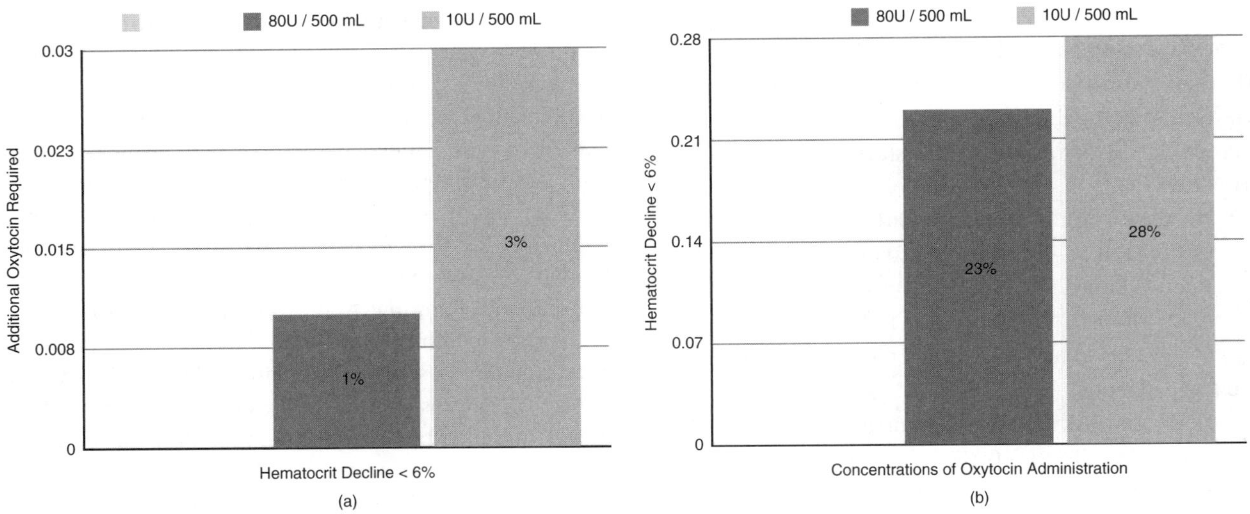

Figure 53.5 (Graph 5a) Effects of higher dose oxytocin on hematocrit. (Graph 5b) Effects of higher dose oxytocin on hematocrit decline. (Tita 2012 [40].)

6. What is the optimum dosage of oxytocin? Route?

Dosage

The largest randomized double blinded trial of three doses of oxytocin (80 U, 40 U, or 10 U) in a 500 ml solution administered over one hour following placental delivery in vaginal delivery patients. Enrollment of the 40 U group was halted due to "futility" while the other study groups continued. 80 U compared to 10 U decreased need for additional/therapeutic uterotonics and decreased the risk of a > 6% decline in hematocrit. Of note the higher concentration of oxytocin were not associated with fluid overload or adverse reactions. A concentrated oxytocin solution administered over the first hour post-delivery shows obvious benefits [35] (Figures 53.5a and b).

Route

Oxytocin may be administered IM, IV solution, or IV bolus. Concern has been expressed over the effect of IV bolus oxytocin may have on maternal vitals. According to a randomized double-blinded double-dummy trial of oxytocin bolus (10 IU IV push) versus oxytocin infusion (10 IU/500 ml at 125 ml hr^{-1}) at delivery of anterior shoulder no significant adverse maternal hemodynamic changes occurred with the IV bolus oxytocin [41].

7. Is there a role for Tranexamic Acid (Lysteda®, Cyklokapron®/Transamin®?

In obstetrics yes! tranexamic acid (TXA) has found a place in the trauma, orthopedic and gynecological operating rooms and can have impact for obstetrics as well. Tranexamic acid is a synthetic derivative of the amino acid lysine. It is a competitive inhibitor of plasminogen, binding to lysine-binding sites and preventing plasminogen activation to plasmin. It is ten times more powerful than aminocaproic acid (Amicar) a similar agent. TXA is not a new drug; data supporting its use dates back 40 years. The WHO recognizes TXA as an essential medicine. TXA is supplied in 1 g/10 ml vials and can be administered as an infusion or slow IV push. In the US a large hospital system cost per vial is ~20$.

The WOMAN trial, evaluated the effect of early tranexamic acid administration on mortality, PPH and hysterectomy. The trial included 20 060 women diagnosed with PPH. Patients were randomized to placebo versus TXA. The TXA group received 1 g slow intravenous push (IVP), with a potential for a second dose. Death due to PPH was greatly reduced in the TXA group; 1.5% vs. 1.9% (RR 0.8, 95% CI 0.65–1.0), especially in women given the treatment within three hours of delivery; TXA group 1.2% vs. 1.7% (RR 0.09, 95% CI 0.52–0.91) A significant deficiency in the study was the decision for study inclusion was often made at the same time as the decision for hysterectomy [42].

A prospective double-blinded randomized controlled trial evaluated the addition of TXA to AMTSL (oxytocin 10 U). The experimental group received a 1 g/10 ml TXA diluted to 50 ml infusion after delivery of the anterior shoulder along with the standard AMTSL. The control group received a 50 ml glucose infusion after the anterior shoulder along with the standard AMTSL. The addition of TXA reduced mean blood loss ($p < 0.001$), reduced the frequency of moderate PPH (>500 ml) ($p < 0.001$), and reduced the need for additional/therapeutic uterotonics ($p = 0.007$). Post-delivery hematocrit and hemoglobin levels with significantly higher in the TXA group ($p < 0.001$). No episodes of thrombosis occurred in the TXA group. The most common side effect in the TXA group was nausea (15%) and vomiting (13.6%) [43].

TXA shows promise in reducing PPH, but with the significant side effect rate it may not be indicated for routine use but rather for select patients.

8. Is AMSTL effective if a patient has received oxytocin during labor?

Sosa et al. analyzed data from 11 323 vaginal deliveries from 24 maternities centers. Exposure to oxytocin through induced or augmented labor compared to unexposed patients did not affect the rate of moderate (>500 ml) or severe (>1000 ml) PPH, or blood transfusion. The researchers concluded that the use of oxytocin for induction or augmentation of labor does not preclude AMSTL with oxytocin [44].

Summary recommendations/considerations

Stage one

- Progress from 4 to 6 cm cervical dilation takes longer than previously thought. Allow more time for a patient to progress from latent to active phase of labor.
- Consider active labor to start at 6 cm cervical dilation.
- Active Phase Arrest is defined as:
  - no cervical change over four hours with adequate uterine contractions (MVU ≥200) with rupture of membranes (ROM);
  - no cervical change over six hours without adequate uterine contractions (MVU <200) with ROM and oxytocin augmentation.
- Age: It is unclear the exact effect age has on the length of labor. Significant data points to increasing maternal age increasing the length of labor.
- Obesity: The length of labor increases with obesity and morbid obesity.

Stage two

- When it comes to the style of maternal pushing maternal choice dominates when consider open versus closed glottis (valsalva) and delayed (laboring down) versus immediate pushing.
- Supine positioning is the least advantageous, causing significant nonreassuring fetal heart rate tracings. While a more upright position is associated with increased blood loss. Consider a lateral or supine with a left uterine displacement. The best option is the one most comfortable for the patient.
- Obese patients will often have shorter second stages.
- Extending the second stage is appropriate:
  - with a reassuring fetal heart rate
  - with providers well versed in operative vaginal delivery
- Maternal complications (third/fourth degree laceration, PPH, fever, difficult delivery) increase when the second stage is extended.
- The risk of adverse neonatal outcomes is most significant in multiparous patients after three hours of pushing.
- For nulliparous patients: ACOG suggests two hours, three hours with an epidural. There is minimal increased maternal or neonatal risk by extending the guidelines by one hour, while still achieving significant AVD rates.
- For multiparous patients: ACOG suggest one hour, two hours with an epidural. Again a one hour extension achieves significant spontaneous vaginal deliveries without significant risk.
- For both nulliparous and multiparous there are diminishing returns with increasing risks with extending the second stage longer than one hour beyond the current ACOG suggestions.

Stage three

- AMTSL decreases PPH.
- The most clinically relevant component of AMSTL is oxytocin.
- A concentrated IV oxytocin solution of IM injection are optimum.
- Oxytocin solutions with higher concentrations are associated with decreased blood loss, with little evidence of adverse maternal side effects. Recommendations are for a minimum concentration of 10 U Oxytocin/500 ml solution up to a concentrations of 80 U Oxytocin/500 ml solution.
- Other uterotonic agents are not as effective and should be reserved for therapeutic treatment of hemorrhage.
- No data supports a specific timing of administration of the oxytocin, but in order to optimize the benefits administration after the anterior shoulder is recommended.
- Tranexamic Acid does not have a role routine AMTSL, but may have a role in AMTSL (in high risk patients).
- Tranexamic Acid is now considered an essential first step in the management of PPH due to its fast onset of action, minimal adverse effects and cost effectiveness. TXA reaches peak plasma levels almost immediately following IV administration in comparison; *sublingual* misoprostol also has a quick onset (5–10 minutes) with peak plasma levels by 30 minutes, methylergonovine maleate reaches peak plasma levels in ~24 minutes, prostaglandin F2-alpha at 15–60 minutes.

References

1 Friedman, E.A. (1955). Primigravid labor; a graphicostatistical analysis. *Obstet. Gynecol.* **6**: 567–589.

2 Friedman, E.A. (1956). Labor in multiparas; a graphicostatistical analy- sis. *Obstet. Gynecol.* **8**: 691–703.

3 Laughon, S.K., Branch, D.W., Beaver, J., and Zhang, J. (2012). Changes in labor patterns over 50 years. *Am. J. Obstet. Gynecol.* **206**: 419.e1.

4 Zhang, J., Landy, H.J., Branch, D.W. et al. (2010). Contemporary patterns of spontaneous labor with normal neonatal outcomes. *Obstet. Gynecol.* **116**: 1281–1287.

5 Caughey, A.B., Cahill, A.G., Guise, J.M., and Rouse, D.J. (2014). Safe prevention of the primary cesarean delivery. *Am. J. Obstet. Gynecol.* (**3**): 179–193.

6 Spong, C.Y., Berghella, V., Wenstrom, K.D. et al. (2012). Preventing the first cesarean delivery: summary of a joint Eunice Kennedy Shriver National Institute of Child Health and Human Development, Society for Maternal-Fetal Medicine, and American College of Obstetricians and Gynecologists Workshop. *Obstet. Gynecol.* **120**: 1181.

7 Rouse, D.J., Owen, J., Savage, K.G. et al. (2001). Active phase labor arrest: revisiting the 2-hour minimum. *Obstet. Gynecol.* **98**: 550–554.

8 Rouse, D.J., Owen, J., and Hauth, J.C. (1999). Active-phase labor arrest: oxytocin augmentation for at least 4 hours. *Obstet. Gynecol.* **93**: 323–328.

9 Zaki, M., Hibbard, J., and Kominiarek, M. (2013). Contemporary patterns and maternal age. *Obstet. Gynecol.* **2013**, **122** (**5**): 1018–1024.

10 Kominiarek, M.A., Zhang, J., Van Veldhuisen, P. et al. (2011). Contemporary labor patterns: the impact of maternal body mass index. *Am. J. Obstet. Gynecol.* **205**: 244.e1–244.e8.

11 Hilliard, A.M., Chauhan, S.P., Zhao, Y., and Rankins, N.C. (2012). Effect of obesity on length of labor in nulliparous women. *Am. J. Perinatol.* **29**: 127–132.

12 Norman, S., Tuuli, M., Odibo, A. et al. (2012). The effects of obesity on the first stage of labor. *Obstet. Gynecol.* **120** (**1**): 130–135.

13 Carhall, S., Kallen, K., and Blomberg, M. (2013). Maternal body mass index and duration of labor. *Eur. J. Obstet. Gynecol. Reprod. Biol.* **171**: 49–53.

14 Yee, L.M., Sandoval, G., Bailit, J. et al. (2016). Maternal and neonatal outcomes with early compared with delayed pushing among nulliparous women. *Obstet. Gynecol.* **2016**, **128**: 1039–1047.

15 Lemos, A., Amorim, M.M., Dornelas de Andrade, A. et al. (2015). Pushing/bearing down methods for the second stage of labour. *Cochrane Database Syst. Rev.*10 (Art. No.:CD009124) doi: 10.1002/14651858.CD009124.pub2.

16 Prins, M., Boxem, J., Lucas, C., and Hutton, E. (2011). Effect of spontaneous pushing versus Valsalva pushing in the second stage of labour on mother and fetus: a systematic review of randomised trials. *BJOG* **118**: 662.

17 Gupta, J.K., Hofmeyr, G.J., and Shehmar, M. (2012). Position in the second stage of labour for women without epidural anaesthesia. *Cochrane Database Syst. Rev.*5 (Art. No.: CD002006) doi: 10.1002/14651858.CD002006.pub3.

18 Kemp, E., Kingswood, C.J., Kibuka, M., and Thornton, J.G. (2013). Position in the second stage of labour for women with epidural anaesthesia. *Cochrane Database Syst. Rev.* 1 (Art. No.: CD008070) doi: 10.1002/14651858.CD008070.pub2.

19 Gizzo, S., Di Gangi, S., Noventa, M. et al. (2014). Women's choice of positions during labour: return to the past or a modern way to give birth? A cohort study in Italy. *BioMed Res. Int.* .

20 Rouse, D.J., Weiner, S.J., Bloom, S.L. et al. (2009). Second-stage labor duration in nulliparous women: relationship to maternal and perinatal outcomes. *Am. J. Obstet. Gynecol.* **201**: 357.e1.

21 Grobman, W.A., Bailit, J., Lai, Y. et al. (2016). Association of the duration of active pushing with obstetric outcomes. *Obstet. Gynecol.* **127**: 667–673.

22 Le Ray, C., Audibert, F., Goffinet, F. et al. (2009). When to stop pushing: effects of duration of second-stage expulsion efforts on maternal and neonatal outcomes in nulliparous women with epidural analgesia. *Am. J. Obstet. Gynecol.* **201**: e361–e367.

23 Cheng, Y.W., Hopkins, L.M., Laros, R.K. et al. (2007). Duration of the second stage of labor in multiparous women: maternal and neonatal outcomes. *Am. J. Obstet. Gynecol.* **196**: e581–e586.

24 Bleich, A., Alexander, J., McIntire, D., and Levano, K. (2012). An analysis of second-stage of labor beyond three hours in nulliparous women. *Am. J. Perinatl.* **29**: 717–722.

25 Sung, J.F., Daniels, K.I., Brodzinsky, L. et al. (2007). Cesarean delivery outcomes after a prolonged second stage of labor. *Am. J. Obstet. Gynecol.* **197**: 306.e301–306.e305.

26 Gimovs.ky, A.C. and Berghella, V. (2016). Randomized controlled trial of prolonged second stage: extending the time limit vs. usual guidelines. *Am. J. Obstet. Gynecol.* **214**: 361.e1–361.e6.

27 Greenberg, M., Cheng, Y., Sullivan, M. et al. (2007). Does length of labor vary by maternal age? *Am. J. Obstet. Gynecol.* **197**: 428.e1–428.e7.

28 Grobman, W., Bailit, J., Rice, M. et al. (2014). Frequency of and factors associated with severe maternal morbidity. *Obstet. Gynecol.* **123** (**4**): 804–810.

29 Frolova, A.I., Stout, M.J., Tuuli, M.G. et al. (2016). Duration of the third stage of labor and risk of postpartum hemorrhage. *Obstet. Gynecol.* **127**: 951–956.

30 Garabedian, C., Simon, M., Closset, E. et al. (2016). Systemic prophylactic oxytocin injection and the incidence of postpartum hemorrhage: a before-and-after study. *J. Gynecol. Obstet. Biol. Reprod. (Paris).* **45**: 147–154.

31 Westhoff, G., Cotter, A.M., and Tolosa, J.E. (2013). Prophylactic oxytocin for the third stage of labour to prevent postpartum haemorrhage. *Cochrane Database Syst. Rev.* 10 (Art. No.: CD001808) doi: 10.1002/14651858.CD001808.pub2.

32 Begley, C.M., Gyte, G.M., Devane, D. et al. (2015). Active versus expectant management for women in the third stage of labour. *Cochrane Database Syst. Rev.* 3 (Art. No.: CD007412) doi: 10.1002/14651858.CD007412.pub3.

33 Hofmeyr, G.J., Mshweshwe, N.T., and Gülmezoglu, A.M. (2015). Controlled cord traction for the third stage of labour. *Cochrane Database Syst. Rev.*1 (Art. No.: CD008020) doi: 10.1002/14651858.CD008020.pub2.

34 Hofmeyr, G.J., Abdel-Aleem, H., and Abdel-Aleem, M.A. (2013; 7 (Art. No.: CD006431)). Uterine massage for preventing postpartum haemorrhage. *Cochrane Database Syst. Rev.* doi: 10.1002/14651858.CD006431.pub3.

35 Tunçalp, Ö., Hofmeyr, G.J., and Gülmezoglu, A.M. (2012). Prostaglandins for preventing postpartum haemorrhage. *Cochrane Database Syst. Rev.* 8 (Art. No.: CD000494) doi: 10.1002/14651858.CD000494.pub4.

36 Durocher, J., Bynum, J., Leon, W. et al. (2010). High fever following postpartum administration of sublingual misoprostol. *BJOG* **117**: 845.

37 Tang, O.S., Gemzell-Danielsson, K., and Ho, P.C. (2007). Misoprostol: pharmacokinetic profile, effects on the uterus and side-effects. *Int. J. Obstet. Gynecol.* **99**: S160–S167.

38 Elati, A., Elmahaishi, M.S., Elmahaishi, M.O. et al. (2011). The effect of misoprostol on postpartum contractions a randomized comparison of three sublingual doses. *BJOG* **118**: 466.

39 Shinar, S., Schwartz, A., Maslovitz, S., and Many, A. (2016). How long is safe? Setting the cut off for uncomplicated third stage length:a retrospective case–control study. *Birth* **43**: 1.

40 Tita, A.T., Szychowski, J.M., Rouse, D.J. et al. (2012). Higher-dose oxytocin and hemorrhage after vaginal delivery: a randomized controlled trial. *Obstet. Gynecol.* **119**: 293.

41 Davies, G.A., Tessier, J.L., Woodman, M.C. et al. (2005). Maternal hemodynamics after oxytocin bolus compared with infusion in the third stage of labor: a randomized controlled trial. *Obstet. Gyneol.* **105** (**2**): 294–299.

42 WOMAN trial collaborators (2017). Effect of early tranexamic acid administration on mortality, hysterectomy, and other morbidities in women with postpartum hemorrhage: an international, randomised, double-blind, placebo-controlled trial. *The Lancet* **389** (**10084**): 2105–2116.

43 Güngördük, K., Asicioglu, O., Celikkol, O. et al. (2010). Use of additional oxytocin to reduce blood loss at elective caesarean section: a randomised control trial. *Aust. N. Z. J. Obstet. Gynaecol.* **50**: 36.

44 Sosa, C., Althabe, F., Belizan, J., and Buekens, P. (2011). Use of oxytocin during early stages of labor and its on active management of third stage of labor. *Am. J. Obstet. Gynecol.* **204** (**3**): 238.e. 238.e5.

54

CHAPTER 54
Operative vaginal delivery

Gary A. Dildy and Steven L. Clark
Department of Obstetrics and Gynecology, Baylor College of Medicine Obstetrics and Gynecology, Service Chief MFM, Texas Children's Hospital, TCH Pavilion for Women, Houston, TX, USA

CLINICAL VIGNETTE

Operative vaginal delivery

A 26-year-old primigravida has progressed in labor to complete dilatation two hours ago, with continued descent of the fetal head to a+2 station. There is mild molding of the fetal cranium and moderate caput succedaneum, rendering determination of the fetal position uncertain. Over the last 30 minutes the fetus has developed tachycardia (165 bpm), minimal beat-to-beat variability and recurrent late decelerations, while maintaining the capacity for evoked accelerations with scalp stimulation. Clinical pelvimetry shows a gynecoid pelvis which is deemed adequate, for an estimated fetal weight of 3500 g.

Your clinical options include all of the following, except:

1. Further expectant management, hoping for vaginal delivery before the fetal acid–base reserve is lost.
2. Proceed with cesarean delivery, which might be avoidable with an attempt at operative vaginal delivery (OVD) if all criteria were fulfilled.
3. Place a vacuum extractor, as precise knowledge of the fetal head position may not be as critical as for a forceps delivery.
4. Perform intrapartum ultrasound to determine the fetal head position and its relationship to the fetal torso, in order to proceed with OVD.
5. Ask a more experienced obstetrician for a second opinion regarding the fetal position and advisability of OVD.

OVD became accepted in obstetric practice with the introduction of obstetric forceps during the eighteenth century and further evolved in the mid-twentieth century with the development of the vacuum extractor [1, 2]. Forceps and vacuum assisted vaginal delivery are important components of contemporary intrapartum care and are accepted as methods to resolve prolonged second stage labor, suspected or potential fetal compromise, and to shorten the second stage of labor for maternal benefit (i.e. maternal cardiac, pulmonary or neurologic medical disorders) [3].

Since the late 1970s when OVD and cesarean delivery each constituted 15% of all births in the United States, there has been a continuing downward trend in rates of OVD accompanied by an increasing trend towards cesarean delivery [4]. As seen in Figure 54.1, by 2014 the cesarean delivery rate was 32.2% and the OVD rate was 3.2%, with the majority (2.6%) of all deliveries being vacuum assisted vaginal delivery and the minority (0.6%) being forceps assisted vaginal delivery. In 1992 the vacuum rate exceeded the forceps rate, and since 1998 both have declined steadily.

The decreasing trend in OVD has contributed to the increasing trend in cesarean delivery, with its attendant immediate risks of immediate complications as well as downstream potentially catastrophic sequelae such as uterine rupture and placental percreta. Appropriate utilization of OVD has been proposed as one strategy to prevent the first cesarean in an effort to safely lower the cesarean rate [6, 7]. While there is no consensus regarding the optimal OVD rate, it is clear that there are valid clinical circumstances where OVD will safely expedite delivery for fetal benefit and avoid cesarean delivery for maternal benefit. In many circumstances, OVD can be performed more safely and quickly than can cesarean delivery.

There are certain clinical scenarios where forceps provides a clear advantage over vacuum, for example, with rotational deliveries or in cases where a vacuum device may be subject to "pop-off", such as mid-station deliveries. With forceps declining to a frequency of <1% of all U.S. births, concerns have arisen that adequate training during residency and maintenance of competency for practitioners will be

Evidence-Based Obstetrics and Gynecology, First Edition. Edited by Errol R. Norwitz, Carolyn M. Zelop, David A. Miller, and David L. Keefe.

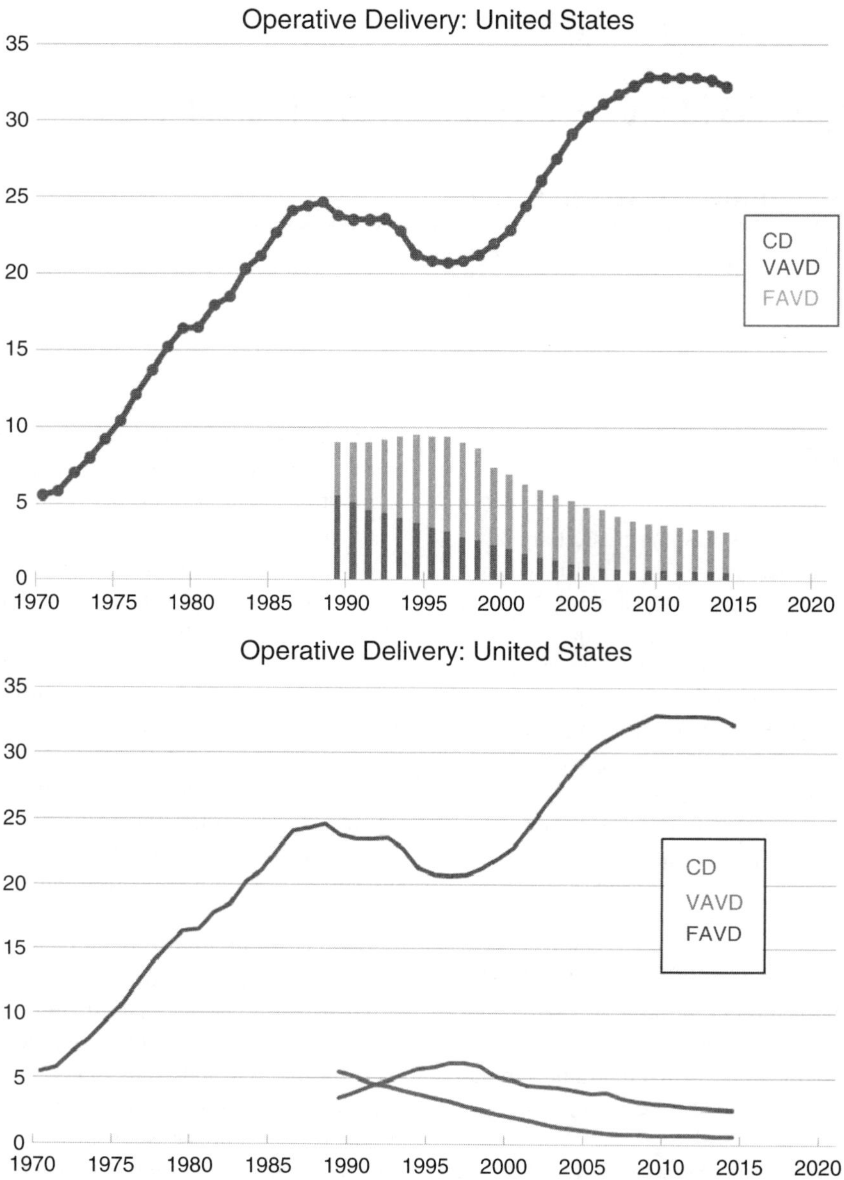

Figure 54.1 Cesarean, forceps, and vacuum delivery rates in the United States (1970–2014) as a percentage of all births. Data for operative vaginal delivery before 1989 were not available. Source: Data were obtained from multiple resources at http://www.cdc.gov/nchs and are specifically cited in reference number [5].

compromised, and that forceps delivery may ultimately face extinction in the near future [5]. These national trends in OVD are also reflected in recent annual Accreditation Council for Graduate Medical Education (ACGME) national residency statistics reports (Figure 54.2), which show declining experience as OVD surgeon for OB/GYN residents; in recent years, OB/GYN residents exit training with a median of only 5 forceps and 16 vacuum deliveries during their four year training program. In 2012 the ACGME recommended a minimum threshold of 15 OVD procedures during OB/GYN residency [8]. For many graduating residents, experience with obstetric forceps and the vacuum extractor is insufficient to develop competency, and even if competent upon completion of residency, limited usage in clinical practice may preclude sufficient maintenance of competency. A decade ago, only one half of U.S. chief residents in OB/GYN programs reported feeling competent to perform forceps deliveries, and things appear to have deteriorated significantly since then [9]. Many graduating OB/GYN residents will likely neither perform forceps in practice, nor pass those skills to the next generation of obstetricians, thus perpetuating the problem.

Our purpose is to address the above concerns and propose evidence-based recommendations towards optimizing

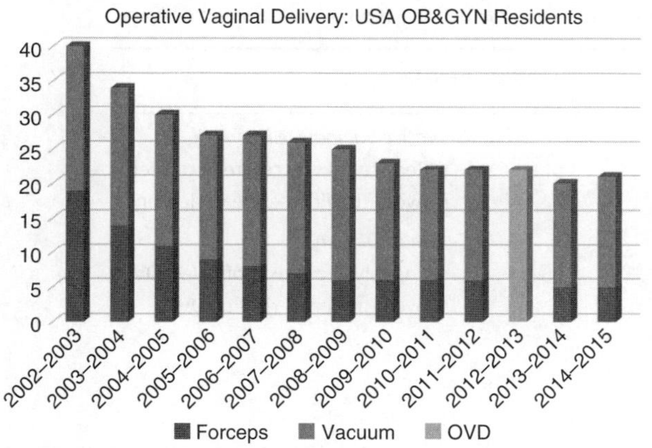

Figure 54.2 Median forceps and vacuum procedures for US Residents completing residency programs between academic years 2002–2003 and 2014–2015, as reported by the ACGME. In 2012–2013 data were reported cumulatively as operative vaginal delivery. Source: Data were obtained from http://www.acgme.org/Data-Collection-Systems/Case-Logs-Statistical-Reports and are specifically cited in reference number [5].

patient safety for women who are candidates for OVD. For technical aspects of OVD, we would refer the reader to the many excellent textbook resources on this subject.

Informed consent

Since there are maternal-fetal benefits and risks to OVD (Table 54.1) with alternatives (i.e. expectant management and cesarean delivery), informed consent is essential to the performance of OVD procedures. Risks, benefits, and alternatives to OVD and contingencies for unsuccessful OVD should be discussed, and when possible, documented before the procedure in the medical record. One retrospective chart review of 100 cases of non-emergent OVD reported that 61% had a general consent for OVD and 22% were given the option for cesarean delivery; maternal and fetal risks of OVD were documented in 3% and 0% of cases, respectively [10]. When delivery is not emergent, ideal informed consent would include a discussion of both maternal risks (e.g. lacerations, bleeding and bladder injury) and fetal injury (e.g. cephalohematoma, retinal hemorrhage), contrasted with the risks of the alternatives – cesarean or continued labor, as circumstances dictate. Such discussions and documentation may improve patient-provider communication, clarify patients' expectations, facilitate decision-making in the setting of an acute intrapartum event, and reduce medical liability for the health care team. In life threatening emergencies, this discussion may be shortened, or in some rare cases (e.g. maternal cardiovascular collapse or cardiac arrest) skipped altogether.

One clinical scenario deserving special mention with regard to OVD informed consent is that in which major shoulder dystocia risk factors are evident. In 1978 Benedetti and Gabbe reported a 23% incidence in shoulder dystocia in the setting of prolonged second stage, mid-pelvic delivery, and birthweight exceeding 4000 g [11]. Bearing in mind differences in clinical definitions (i.e. prolonged second stage, mid-pelvic delivery) used in this study and a low incidence of diabetes in this patient population, it remains evident that the scenario of an OVD in the setting of prolonged second stage and suspected fetal macrosomia should prompt inclusion of shoulder dystocia and its complications in the discussion of alternative management, namely cesarean delivery. A retrospective case–control study of 100 cases of shoulder dystocia at term and 100 controls (singleton term vertex vaginal deliveries without shoulder dystocia) found that the combination of glucose intolerance, birth weight, and OVD were predictive in the occurrence of shoulder dystocia [12]. The major challenge with such models is that birth weight is known only after the fact and the imprecision of estimated fetal weight by any method, whether it be by physical exam, ultrasonography or "ask the parous mother" methods [13]. We do believe that consideration of the estimated fetal weight in conjunction with clinical pelvimetry, maternal diabetes status, and labor progress for risk assessment in the informed consent process for OVD. Thorough medical record documentation cannot be emphasized enough, especially in settings of greater risk, whether contemplating OVD, or managing complications such as shoulder dystocia. In a review of closed medical liability claims, Clark and colleagues showed that poor documentation of shoulder dystocia events with neonatal injuries contributed significantly to liability, underscoring the importance of accurate and detailed documentation [14].

Pre-procedure checklist and clinical documentation

Pre-operative assessment of estimated fetal weight, clinical pelvimetry, adequacy of anesthesia, presence of an empty bladder and fetal station/position serve to reduce the occurrence of an unsuccessful OVD and improvident maternal-fetal complications. Pre-procedure checklists have been shown to be effective in reducing surgical complications and would seem applicable to procedures such as OVD [15]. There may be a tendency to forego checklists in acute emergencies for the sake of critical time, however, a clinical trial using high fidelity simulation of operating room crises such as massive hemorrhage and cardiac arrest showed checklist use to improve performance of critical steps and the potential to improve patient care [16]. Accurate and detailed pre-procedure and post-procedure documentation may benefit patient care, clinical research, peer review, and if needed, medico-legal defense. Proposed elements of an OVD pre-procedure note, pre-operative checklist and post-procedure note are found in Figures 54.3–54.4.

Table 54.1 Reported potential maternal-fetal complications of operative vaginal delivery (OVD) and cesarean delivery

	Risk	Benefit
Maternal	*Operative Vaginal Delivery* • Anal sphincter injury • Pelvic floor injury *Cesarean Delivery* • Increased hemorrhage • Increased infection • Damage to bladder and bowel • Increased venous thromboembolism • Prolonged healing • Increased cost • Increased risk of death • Future risks (placenta previa, invasive placenta, repeat cesareans, uterine rupture)	*Operative Vaginal Delivery* • Reduce risks of cesarean delivery • Avoid the first cesarean delivery *Cesarean Delivery* • Possibly avoid risks of failed OVD • Avoid maternal risks of OVD
Fetal	*Operative Vaginal Delivery* • Cephalohematoma[a] • Retinal hemorrhage[a] • Scalp injuries[a] • Facial injuries[b] • Skull fracture & intracranial bleeding • Shoulder dystocia and brachial plexus palsy • Increased hyperbilirubinemia[a] • Neurodevelopmental complications of above *Cesarean Delivery* • Fetal scalpel laceration • Delay in delivery	*Operative Vaginal Delivery* • Expedite delivery *Cesarean Delivery* • Reduce fetal risks of OVD

[a]More prevalent with vacuum than forceps.
[b]More prevalent with forceps than vacuum.

Guideline considerations

As with any surgical device, the clinician should be familiar with indications, contraindications and operation of devices prior to utilization. This is especially true with vacuum extractors, as the instructions for use (IFU) vary by manufacturer and model, with respect to recommended maximum negative pressure applied, number of pulls, number of pop-offs, traction force, and other considerations. In 1998 the United States Food and Drug Administration (FDA) issued a Public Health Advisory cautioning the use of vacuum assisted delivery devices, with specific emphasis on the importance of familiarity with the manufacturer's IFU [17]. Furthermore, the FDA recommended that the newborn's provider be notified that a vacuum assisted delivery device was used, and that any suspected associated adverse reactions be reported to the FDA as per the Safe Medical Devices Act of 1990. National professional organizations, including the American College of Obstetricians and Gynecologists (ACOG) [3], the Royal College of Obstetricians and Gynecologists (RCOG) [18], the Society of Obstetricians and Gynecologists of Canada (SOGC) [19], and the Royal Australian and New Zealand College of Obstetricians and Gynecologists (RANZCOG) [20], publish clinical management guidelines on OVD.

Evidence-based procedural aspects to performing OVD

Randomized controlled trials focusing upon OVD have generally been small in size and were conducted predominantly in the 1980s. Given the considerable changes in clinical practice over the last several decades (i.e. higher use of intrapartum regional anesthesia, new fetal heart rate monitoring nomenclature, elimination of fetal scalp blood gas analysis, differences in provider experience with OVD, changing maternal demographics, different vacuum extraction devices commercially available, etc.), it would seem that contemporary trials would be in order to study the place of OVD in contemporary practice. Great care must be taken in applying the results of these studies to contemporary practice given the differences in care listed above, as well as changing operator experience.

Operative Vaginal Delivery

Pre-Procedure Note

Indication(s) for operative vaginal delivery

____Prolonged second stage of labor

___ Suspicion of immediate or potential fetal compromise

___ Shortening of the second stage of labor for maternal benefit

Fetal Station_____ Position_____ Caput________ Moulding_________

Adequate pelvis_______________ Estimated fetal weight____________

Fetal heart rate pattern category: I II III Contraction frequency every ______minutes

Informed consent: verbal___ written___

Post-Procedure Note

Anesthesia___________________________

Fetal Station_____ Position_____ at application

Rotation_____degrees Number of vacuum or forceps pulls____ Number of vacuum pop-offs____

Date & time of OVD start:______________________ Date & time of delivery:__________________

Birth weight________________ Apgar@1"_____ Apgar@5"_____ Apgar@10"_____

Umbilical artery pH_______ Umbilical vein pH_______

Estimated blood loss_______mL Episiotomy:________ Perineal lacerations: none, 1°, 2°, 3°, 4°

Forceps instrument used:____

Vacuum instrument used:____

Maternal injury____

Neonatal injury____ Shoulder dydtocia____

Comments____

Figure 54.3 Pre-procedure and Post-procedure delivery notes.

Other safety considerations

Vacuum extraction at cesarean delivery

The use of the vacuum extractor for delivery of the fetal head in order to prevent hysterotomy extension, reduce hysterotomy bleeding, and reduce injury to the fetal head was proposed by Solomons in 1962, soon after introduction of the Malmstrom vacuum extractor [21, 22]. Several subsequent small case series reported satisfactory results and promoted this practice [23, 24]. However, severe complications have been reported with the routine use of the vacuum extractor at cesarean delivery, including cephalohematoma, subgaleal and intracranial hemorrhage [25]. It would seem reasonable to consider vacuum extraction as one option for the difficult delivery of the fetal head during cesarean section, if the only alternative is to effect hysterotomy extension. However it should be noted that none of the reports of routine use of vacuum at cesarean were sufficiently designed to draw any valid conclusions regarding actual safety of this approach. In the absence of data from clinical trials, we believe that routine use of the vacuum extractor at cesarean delivery provides an unfavorable maternal-fetal risk–benefit ratio to the disadvantage of the fetus, as maternal risks of cesarean are combined with the fetal risks of vacuum extraction.

Limitation of pulls and pop-offs (and failed operative vaginal delivery)

There is a reported association between maternal-neonatal complications as the number of forceps/vacuum pulls increase, vacuum pop-offs increase, and also with having to resort to cesarean delivery after unsuccessful attempt at OVD. A study of 393 cases of OVD in the UK found that

Pre-Procedure Checklist

___ Vertex presentation
___ Cervix is fully dilated and retracted
___ Amniotic membranes are ruptured
___ The fetal head is engaged
___ Exact position of the fetal head has been determined
___ Fetal weight estimation has been performed
___ Pelvis is thought to be adequate for vaginal delivery
___ Anesthesia is adequate
___ Maternal bladder has been emptied
___ Patient has agreed after being informed of the risks and benefits of the procedure
___ No suspected fetal demineralization conditions or bleeding disorders
___ Operator has the necessary knowledge, experience and skills
___ Operator is aware of device manufacturer's instructions for use
___ Prepared for potential complications (i.e. shoulder dystocia, postpartum hemorrhage)
___ Neonatal resuscitation team is available or present (if indicated)
___ Determine whether procedure should be performed in labor room or operating room
___ Willingness to abandon trial of OVD and back-up plan in place in case of failure to deliver

Figure 54.4 Pre-operative vaginal delivery checklist.

Rate of OVD
Rate of failed OVD
Rate of sequential instrument use
OVD-related 3rd & 4th degree perineal tears
Composite neonatal trauma (subgaleal hemorrhage, brachial plexus injury, fracture, facial nerve palsy, cerebral hemorrhage, Apgar <7 at 5 minutes, umbilical artery pH <7.1)
Documentation of consent (verbal and/or written) for OVD
Documentation of fetal station and position at OVD
Proper placement of vacuum extractor based upon location of chignon
Accuracy and completeness of hospital OVD record

Figure 54.5 Potential audible standards for operative vaginal delivery (OVD), Modified from RCOG Greentop Guideline No.26 [18].

when compared to OVD requiring 3 or less pulls, those with >3 pulls were associated with a fourfold increase (OR 4.2, 95% CI 1.6–9.5) in neonatal trauma for completed deliveries and a sevenfold increase (OR 7.2, 95% CI 2.1–24.0) in neonatal trauma for failed deliveries [26].

At present ACOG guidelines [3] do not specify a limitation of the number of forceps pulls or vacuum pop-offs before abandoning OVD, but do advise that descent is to be expected with traction, and if no descent is evident, reappraisal of the situation is indicated. One clinical dilemma is when progressive descent of the fetal head occurs with multiple (e.g. 3 or more) pulls but has not resulted in delivery and delivery seems imminent with further reasonable effort; to place an absolute limit of pulls and resort to cesarean delivery may not be in the best interests of the mother and baby, and thus remains a careful clinical decision on a case by case basis. We feel the key is that recognizable descent be achieved with each pull, and the process abandoned if descent has stopped. Using this approach, the number of pulls will be limited but not definitively prescribed.

Of special concern is the attitude observed among some providers, and promulgated by some training programs, that vacuum delivery requires minimal skill and training compared to forceps delivery. Such an attitude has, in a few cases, led to performance of vacuum delivery by individuals with only rudimentary training, with predictably adverse outcomes. While the technical skills associated with vacuum delivery are indeed less complex that those associated with rotational forceps delivery, the often difficult judgment regarding when to attempt OVD, and in particular, when to abandon a trial of OVD remain similar. Patient safety concerns mandate thorough training and ongoing supervision or peer review of any practitioner engaging in any form of OVD. Further, even perfectly justified and performed OVD maneuvers have the potential to cause umbilical cord compression and fetal hypoxia. For this reason, except in emergency situations, we advise against the performance of OVD unless a practitioner with cesarean privileges is immediately available and aware of the patient and the OVD attempt.

Use of sequential instruments

Sequential use of the vacuum then forceps, or vice versa, was once accepted by some obstetric practitioners as a routine method to facilitate delivery. In a survey of ACOG Fellows conducted in the 1990s, free text comments by 4.7% of respondents indicated that they used the vacuum to "gain station in the mid-pelvis" before applying forceps to complete the delivery [27]. Analysis of more recent literature, including a large administrative database study from California [28], a large administrative database study from Washington state [29], and a cohort study from the United Kingdom [26], suggests that there is a significantly increased risk of fetal and maternal injury with sequential use of instruments to effect vaginal delivery, as compared to use of a single instrument.

The retrospective Washington state database study of deliveries between the years 1987–1997 showed statistically significant increases in multiple adverse maternal and fetal outcomes for sequential OVD, compared to forceps or vacuum alone [29]. For some adverse outcomes, the rate was greater for the sequential group, even after combining the forceps and the vacuum group rates together; for the rate (per 1000 infants) of facial nerve injury, the incidence was 0.2 for spontaneous vaginal delivery, 0.3 for vacuum, 2.9 for forceps and 5.1 for sequential instruments. These data do not allow differentiation of planned versus unplanned use of sequential instruments, so it is not possible to determine whether planned sequential use is with less risk. Also, the absolute risk of injury should be considered, as demonstrated in the California study [28], the risk of intracranial hemorrhage with sequential instrument use was 1 in 256 cases.

The ACOG recommends against the *routine* use of sequential instruments at OVD [3]. In clinical practice, when application of the vacuum or forceps is not successful in effecting delivery, the obstetrician should carefully consider the reason (i.e. is there a technical problem primarily with the device, or is there true cephalopelvic disproportion), balance the risks/benefits of using the alternative device with those of cesarean delivery, and document the rationale. Except in life-threatening emergencies, if one device has not worked, cesarean is usually a better option than an attempt with a second instrument.

Training, competency, and simulation

As described in the introduction, with the declining number of OVDs performed nationwide, there has been a parallel drop in resident training experience which threatens to render these techniques extinct in future clinical practice, despite the general belief that OVD remains a superior option to cesarean delivery in a significant subset of patients. Simulation has been shown to improve performance in non-medical fields such as aviation [30, 31]. In the practice of medicine, simulation is becoming integrated into training programs with documented success, showing improved outcomes in communication, teamwork, technical skills and outcomes [32–34]. In other disciplines such as avionics, high-fidelity simulators have been developed and used for training, maintenance and ongoing assessment of pilots' skills and emergency readiness for many years [35]. High fidelity simulation technologies have also been developed for clinical medicine, but have not yet evolved to the same level as aviation simulation. It would seem evident that OVD should be a focus in simulation technology development, given the potential application of OVD in a significant proportion of the roughly four million deliveries in the US per annum, and its potential effect on the national cesarean rate. Such a high-fidelity simulator would need to provide adjustable fetal clinical nuances (i.e. fetal station, fetal position, asynclitism, head deflection), maternal clinical nuances (various bony pelvic architectures, soft tissue interference), maternal-fetal interactions (fetopelvic disproportion), and biofeedback (measurement of traction forces, traction vectors, traction time and fetal descent) experienced in actual clinical practice. Simulation would also be ideal for assessing competency for focused professional practice evaluation, ongoing professional practice evaluation and re-credentialing, given the challenges and limitations in competency assessment from retrospective chart review, especially of low-use providers.

On the horizon

Ultrasound assisted OVD

Furthermore, sound understanding of fetal cranial anatomy, maternal pelvic anatomy and accurate knowledge of the fetal head position and station are prerequisites to safe OVD [3, 18]. Misapplication of either obstetrical forceps or the vacuum extractor can lead to increased risks of maternal-fetal complications and failed OVD resulting in emergency cesarean delivery, with all of its sequelae. Observational studies on intrapartum sonographic assessment of fetal head position have shown a high rate of error in digital examination when compared to ultrasound as a gold standard. In 2001 Kreiser and colleagues showed that digital pelvic exam during the second stage of labor was wrong in 29.6% of cases, with the error being >90° in 9.1%, 90° in 9.1%, and < 90° in 11.4% of 44 cases [36]. Sherer and colleagues found a 65% rate of error in digital pelvic exam (39% if error was defined as >45° difference) in a study of 112 consecutive term singleton cephalic-presenting fetuses [37]. A study from the UK evaluating 496 singleton term pregnancies in labor considered the digital exam to be correct if within 45° of the ultrasound finding; the intrapartum digital exam was indeterminate in one third (n = 166), not in agreement in one third (n = 167), and in agreement in one third (n = 163) of the 496 cases [38]. These data illustrate the difficulty in accurate intrapartum determination of fetal position by digital pelvic examination and the potential utility of ultrasound in correcting such error. At present national guidelines do not recommend intrapartum ultrasound for OVD as prospective studies proving efficacy have not been conducted. Thus use of ultrasound cannot at present be considered mandatory as part of the standard of care. Nevertheless, obstetrical ultrasound is generally available in most high resource settings and this technique would seem easy to learn, thus potentially may in the future prove helpful in optimizing OVD outcomes.

Quality metrics

> Measurement is the first step that leads to control and eventually to improvement. If you can't measure something, you can't understand it. If you can't understand it, you can't control it. If you can't control it, you can't improve it.
>
> H. James Harrington

Payers such as the Centers for Medicare & Medicaid Services (CMS) use quality measures in quality improvement, pay for reporting, and public reporting [39]. At present, pay for reporting and public reporting are not directly relevant to OVD, however quality metrics have been proposed. The ACOG proposed "documentation of station and position at time of forceps or vacuum extractor application" as a performance measure [3]. Suboptimal placement of the vacuum has been reported as a factor in 40% of failed vacuum deliveries [40]. Haikin and Mankuta have proposed assessment of vacuum cup placement as measured by midline and lateral deviation measurements as a quality metric [41]. While OVD may not be a primary reporting metric, the cesarean rate certainly is and will be, thus safe OVD does have an important secondary role considering its potential positive influence on the overall cesarean rate, primary cesarean rate, and nulliparous term singleton vertex (NTSV) cesarean rate [42](Figure 54.5).

Conclusions

Both forceps and vacuum OVD remain valuable tools in the management of second stage labor. The optimal rate of OVD is not well defined, but OVD clearly remains as one option to control the cesarean rate towards an appropriate, balanced level. In the US there has been a steady decline in both forceps and vacuum deliveries over the last two decades, and obstetrical forceps may be on the verge of extinction. We believe that innovative high fidelity simulation, such as used in aviation, is a current critical need in order to both develop and maintain clinical competency in OVD for obstetrical practitioners for future generations of patients [5].

References

1 Sheikh, S., Ganesaratnam, I., and Jan, H. (2013). The birth of forceps. *JRSM Short Rep.* **4**: 1–4.

2 McQuivey, R.W. (2004). Vacuum-assisted delivery: a review. *J. Matern. Fetal Neonatal Med.* **16**: 171–180.

3 Gynecologists ACoOa and Committee on Practice B-O (2015). ACOG practice bulletin no. 154: operative vaginal delivery. *Obstet. Gynecol.* **126**: e56–e65.

4 Notzon, F.C. (1990). International differences in the use of obstetric interventions. *JAMA* **263**: 3286–3291.

5 Dildy, G.A. and Clark, S.L. (2016). Obstetric forceps – a species on the brink of extinction. *Obstet. Gynecol.* **28** (**3**): 436–439.

6 Spong, C.Y., Berghella, V., Wenstrom, K.D. et al. (2012). Preventing the first cesarean delivery: summary of a joint Eunice Kennedy Shriver National Institute of Child Health and Human Development, Society for Maternal-Fetal Medicine, and American College of Obstetricians and Gynecologists Workshop. *Obstet. Gynecol.* **120**: 1181–1193.

7 American College of Obstetrics and Gynecologists (2014). Society for Maternal-Fetal M. Obstetric care consensus no. 1: safe prevention of the primary cesarean delivery. *Obstet. Gynecol.* **123**: 693–711.

8 Minimum Thresholds for Obstetrics and Gynecology Procedures. 2012. (Available at http://www.acgme.org/Portals/0/PFAssets/ProgramResources/220_Ob_Gyn%20Minimum_Numbers_Announcment.pdf.) Accessed 15 July 2018.

9 Powell, J., Gilo, N., Foote, M. et al. (2007). Vacuum and forceps training in residency: experience and self-reported competency. *J. Perinatol.* **27**: 343–346.

10 Nichols, C.M., Pendlebury, L.C., and Jennell, J. (2006). Chart documentation of informed consent for operative vaginal delivery: is it adequate? *South. Med. J.* **99**: 1337–1339.

11 Benedetti, T.J. and Gabbe, S.G. (1978). Shoulder dystocia. A complication of fetal macrosomia and prolonged second stage of labor with midpelvic delivery. *Obstet. Gynecol.* **52**: 526–529.

12 Belfort, M.A., Dildy, G.A., Saade, G.R. et al. (2007). Prediction of shoulder dystocia using multivariate analysis. *Am. J. Perinatol.* **24**: 5–10.

13 Chauhan, S.P., Grobman, W.A., Gherman, R.A. et al. (2005). Suspicion and treatment of the macrosomic fetus: a review. *Am. J. Obstet. Gynecol.* **193**: 332–346.

14 Clark, S.L., Belfort, M.A., Dildy, G.A., and Meyers, J.A. (2008). Reducing obstetric litigation through alterations in practice patterns. *Obstet. Gynecol.* **112**: 1279–1283.

15 Haynes, A.B., Weiser, T.G., Berry, W.R. et al. (2009). A surgical safety checklist to reduce morbidity and mortality in a global population. *N. Engl. J. Med.* **360**: 491–499.

16 Arriaga, A.F., Bader, A.M., Wong, J.M. et al. (2013). Simulation-based trial of surgical-crisis checklists. *N. Engl. J. Med.* **368**: 246–253.

17 FDA Public Health Advisory: Need for CAUTION When Using Vacuum Assisted Delivery Devices. 1998. (Available at http://www.fda.gov/MedicalDevices/Safety/AlertsandNotices/PublicHealthNotifications/ucm062295.htm.) Accessed 15 July 2018.

18 Operative Vaginal Delivery. 2011. (Available at www.rcog.org.uk/globalassets/documents/guidelines/gtg_26.pdf.) Accessed 15 July 2018.

19 Society of O, Gynaecologists of C (2005). Guidelines for operative vaginal birth. Number 148, May 2004. *Int. J. Gynaecol. Obstet.* **88**: 229–236.

20 Instrumental vaginal birth. **2002** (reviewed 2016). (Available at www.ranzcog.edu.au/component/docman/doc_view/950-instrumental-vaginal-birth-c-obs-16.html?Itemid=946.) Accessed 15 July 2018.

21 Malmstrom, T. (1954). Vacuum extractor, an obstetrical instrument. *Acta Obstet. Gynecol. Scand. Suppl.* **33**: 1–31.

22 Solomons, E. (1962). Delivery of the head with the Malmstrom vacuum extractor during cesarean section. *Obstet. Gynecol.* **19**: 201–203.

23 Pelosi, M.A. and Apuzzio, J. (1984). Use of the soft, silicone obstetric vacuum cup for delivery of the fetal head at cesarean section. *J. Reprod. Med.* **29**: 289–292.

24 Arad, I., Linder, N., and Bercovici, B. (1986). Vacuum extraction at cesarean section--neonatal outcome. *J. Perinat. Med.* **14**: 137–140.

25 Clark, S.L., Vines, V.L., and Belfort, M.A. (2008). Fetal injury associated with routine vacuum use during cesarean delivery. *Am. J. Obstet. Gynecol.* **198**: e4.

26 Murphy, D.J., Macleod, M., Bahl, R., and Strachan, B. (2011). A cohort study of maternal and neonatal morbidity in relation to use of sequential instruments at operative vaginal delivery. *Eur. J. Obstet. Gynecol. Reprod. Biol.* **156**: 41–45.

27 Bofill, J.A., Rust, O.A., Perry, K.G. et al. (1996). Operative vaginal delivery: a survey of fellows of ACOG. *Obstet. Gynecol.* **88**: 1007–1010.

28 Towner, D., Castro, M.A., Eby-Wilkens, E., and Gilbert, W.M. (1999). Effect of mode of delivery in nulliparous women on neonatal intracranial injury. *N. Engl. J. Med.* **341**: 1709–1714.

29 Gardella, C., Taylor, M., Benedetti, T. et al. (2001). The effect of sequential use of vacuum and forceps for assisted vaginal delivery on neonatal and maternal outcomes. *Am. J. Obstet. Gynecol.* **185**: 896–902.

30 Lepage, J., Cosson, M., Mayeur, O. et al. (2016). Pedagogical childbirth simulators: utility in obstetrics. *Eur. J. Obstet. Gynecol. Reprod. Biol.* **197**: 41–47.

31 Helmreich, R.L. (2000). On error management: lessons from aviation. *BMJ* **320**: 781–785.

32 Deering, S. and Rowland, J. (2013). Obstetric emergency simulation. *Semin. Perinatol.* **37**: 179–188.

33 Fransen, A.F., van de Ven, J., Merien, A.E. et al. (2012). Effect of obstetric team training on team performance and medical technical skills: a randomised controlled trial. *BJOG* **119**: 1387–1393.

34 Merien, A.E., van de Ven, J., Mol, B.W. et al. (2010). Multidisciplinary team training in a simulation setting for acute obstetric emergencies: a systematic review. *Obstet. Gynecol.* **115**: 1021–1031.

35 F-22 Pilot Training Devices. 2016. (Available at https://www.link.com/military/programs/Pages/F22-pilot-training-devices.aspx.) Accessed 15 July 2018.

36 Kreiser, D., Schiff, E., Lipitz, S. et al. (2001). Determination of fetal occiput position by ultrasound during the second stage of labor. *J. Matern. Fetal Med.* **10**: 283–286.

37 Sherer, D.M., Miodovnik, M., Bradley, K.S., and Langer, O. (2002). Intrapartum fetal head position II: comparison between transvaginal digital examination and transabdominal ultrasound assessment during the second stage of labor. *Ultrasound Obstet. Gynecol.* **19**: 264–268.

38 Akmal, S., Tsoi, E., Kametas, N. et al. (2002). Intrapartum sonography to determine fetal head position. *J. Matern. Fetal Neonatal Med.* **12**: 172–177.

39 Quality Measures. 2016. (Available at https://www.cms.gov/Medicare/Quality-Initiatives-Patient-Assessment-Instruments/QualityMeasures/index.html?redirect=/QualityMeasures/03_ElectronicSpecifications.asp.) Accessed 15 July 2018.

40 Sau, A., Sau, M., Ahmed, H., and Brown, R. (2004). Vacuum extraction: is there any need to improve the current training in the UK? *Acta Obstet. Gynecol. Scand.* **83**: 466–470.

41 Haikin, E.H. and Mankuta, D. (2012). Vacuum cup placement during delivery--a suggested obstetric quality assessment measure. *J. Matern. Fetal Neonatal Med.* **25**: 2135–2137.

42 Specifications Manual for Joint Commission National Quality Measures (v2013A1). 2013. (Available at https://manual.jointcommission.org/releases/TJC2013A/MIF0167.html.) Accessed 15 July 2018.

55

CHAPTER 55

Cesarean delivery in the obese parturient

Diana A. Racusin and Alex C. Vidaeff

Department of Obstetrics and Gynecology, Division of Maternal-Fetal Medicine, Baylor College of Medicine, Texas Children's Hospital Pavilion for Women, Houston, TX, USA

Introduction

The rate of obesity has increased dramatically in the United States, presently with 20.5% of women being obese as they begin pregnancy [1]. Obesity is classified by WHO [2] as:

- Class I (BMI 30.0–34.9)
- Class II (BMI 35.0–39.9)
- Class III (morbid or extreme obesity) (BMI ≥40.0).

An additional category of super-morbid obesity (BMI >50) is sometimes used, especially since the number of women in this category has increased fivefold in the last two decades of the twentieth century [3].

Of all parturients, 4–6% have morbid obesity [1] and it has been estimated that 200 000 morbidly obese women give birth per year in the United States [4]. One of the consequences of prepregnancy obesity has been a greater risk of primary cesarean delivery, both scheduled and unplanned, even after controlling for social and medical risk factors [5]. Given the low rate of vaginal delivery after cesarean, repeat cesareans for these mothers are likely to occur at an increased rate as well. Elevated BMI has been reported to be associated with increased rates of failed trial of labor after cesarean delivery [6] (Hibbard).

Cesarean delivery is the most common major surgical procedure in the United States, but women with BMI >35 have a double risk of cesarean delivery [7] and about 60% of women with BMI >50 undergo cesarean delivery [8]. This trend is present in spite of the physicians' general preference to avoid cesarean delivery in obese women because of the added risk of morbidity with surgery. Obesity alone increases the likelihood of operative wound infections after cesarean delivery by fourfold. Other post-cesarean complications with increased risk of occurrence in obese women, as noted in the Maternal-Fetal Medicine Unit Cesarean Registry, were: wound opening (fivefold increase) and endometritis (26% increased risk) [9]. The rates of surgical site infections and wound disruption increase in parallel with the increase in subcutaneous thickness [10]. Surgical site infections affect not only the mother but also her support system and the healthcare system at large. A wound infection can add over $3000 to the total cost of medical care [11].

Caring for obese patients often requires modification of techniques and practices in order to improve care and safety. The United Kingdom National Collaborating Centre for Women's and Children's Health antenatal guidelines recognize obesity as one of the conditions for which additional care is required [12].

CLINICAL SCENARIO

A 30-year-old G4P3003 at 34 weeks and three days gestation is transferred to your labor and delivery unit for a higher level of care. She is morbidly obese (BMI 70.0), with medical history including chronic hypertension and type II diabetes mellitus. Her obstetrical history is significant for three prior cesarean deliveries, one of which was complicated by incision into the active segment of the uterus. She has just been diagnosed with pre-eclampsia with severe features and pre-term labor. A decision is made for repeat cesarean delivery under magnesium sulfate seizure prophylaxis.

Clinical questions

1. What technical surgical aspects should be considered at cesarean delivery?
2. Are there adjustments necessary in perioperative antibiotic prophylaxis?
3. What particular anesthesia considerations are applicable?
4. What are the post-operative considerations relative to thromboprophylaxis?

Evidence-Based Obstetrics and Gynecology, First Edition. Edited by Errol R. Norwitz, Carolyn M. Zelop, David A. Miller, and David L. Keefe.

1. What technical surgical aspects should be considered at cesarean delivery?

Technical surgical aspects at cesarean delivery

The skin incision type for obese women remains at the latitude of the surgeon, with limited clinical research data to guide the decision-making. In general, the literature contrasts transverse incisions (suprapubic or supraumbilical) with midline vertical incisions (subumbilical, periumbilical, or supraumbilical). The level of evidence is very low, consisting of expert opinions, observational studies, or institutional standards of care. With low transverse incisions, the mainly theoretical concern is placement of the incision under the large panniculus in an area of low oxygen tension and increased microbial flora. On the other hand, a vertical incision is not without wound healing concerns because of longer incisions, higher opposition tension and a deeper subcutaneous layer involved.

Opposing opinions have been expressed in the last century's gynecological literature, with several authors recommending transverse incisions, both in the lower abdomen and above the umbilicus to enter the abdomen in non-pregnant obese women [13, 14], whereas others advocated supraumbilical upper abdominal midline incisions for pelvic surgery in the morbidly obese patients [15]. The literature reports are also inconsistent when recommendations are made specifically for cesarean deliveries. Retrospective data in morbidly obese women undergoing cesarean delivery suggest either no difference in wound outcomes based on the type of skin incision [16], a significantly higher wound complications rate with vertical incisions compared with low transverse incisions [17], or just the opposite, lower wound complications rates with vertical incisions [18].

The operative time and blood loss may be lower with vertical incisions, but, on the other hand, they are more painful, delay the post-operative mobilization and increase pulmonary complications in postpartum [19]. Supraumbilical vertical midline incisions may also require a higher-level of spinal anesthesia and that in turn can cause difficulties with ventilation in an obese patient. A particular aspect related to cesarean delivery in obese women is that high vertical incisions or high transverse incisions are associated with up to an 18-fold increased risk of corporeal, fundal and vertical hysterotomies because the incision often overlies the uterine fundus limiting the access to the lower uterine segment [16, 20–22]. Tixier et al., proponents of transverse incisions, recommend supra- versus subumbilical transverse incisions only in obese women with a voluminous panniculus, in "apron" position [23].

In a recent survey of the American College of Obstetricians and Gynecologists members, for morbidly obese women in nonemergency conditions, 84% of respondents preferred a Pfannenstiel incision and even in emergency conditions, 66% preferred the same type of incision [24]. A common practice when Pfannenstiel incision is employed is to elevate the panniculus using adherent tape. This should be done cautiously to avoid interference with ventilation due to increased intrathoracic pressure. Cephalad retraction of the panniculus can also worsen hypotension. Methods of concomitant cephalad and vertical suspension of the panniculus have been proposed to facilitate ventilation and oxygenation [25]. Two cases of fat necrosis within the abdominal panniculus have been reported following cesarean delivery with suprapubic transverse incisions in morbidly obese patients. The diagnosis was made three to four weeks after delivery and it was postulated that traumatic ischemia during retraction at surgery may have contributed [26].

Taken as a whole, the available data do not allow firm conclusions to be drawn. A randomized clinical trial is underway comparing low transverse and vertical skin incisions for cesarean delivery in morbidly obese women in terms of wound complications (registered at http://clinicaltrials.gov with the ID number NCT 018997376). It will probably be the first randomized trial on this topic. Even if different incisions may have different wound infection risks, the choice of incision should still be individualized because the panniculus is different in different obese patients and the umbilicus may be more or less displaced caudally. The incision choice should focus on adequate exposure for optimal fetal delivery through a low transverse hysterotomy.

Intra-operatively, long instrument trays may be necessary [27], as well as self-retaining retractors, at the discretion of the surgeon. Self-retaining retractors, purported to act as a form of barrier protection while also retracting wound edges, when studied in a randomized controlled trial in 301 obese women, did not decrease the rate of surgical site infection or wound disruption [10].

Regarding *the skin closure method*, a Cochrane review found no difference in wound infection between staple and subcuticular skin closure in the general obstetrical population without separate analysis for obese women [28]. Two randomized controlled trials in obese women undergoing cesarean delivery showed a reduced risk of post-operative wound complications with subcuticular closure, however, when analyzed specifically for wound infection, there was no difference [29, 30]. Using subcutaneous drains has not been shown to be beneficial, whereas closure of the subcutaneous fat layer measuring >2 cm appeared to decrease surgical site infections [31].

Others, in an effort to decrease surgical site infections, have turned their attention to the preoperative skin preparation. A recent study has demonstrated lower rates of surgical site infections when using chlorhexidine – alcohol skin preparation versus iodine-alcohol skin preparation [32]. The reduction in risk was not affected by the presence or absence of obesity.

2. Are there adjustments necessary in perioperative antibiotic prophylaxis?

Antibiotic prophylaxis

Antibiotic prophylaxis is a well-accepted evidence-based practice for all patients undergoing cesarean delivery and is of particular importance in obese women, playing a critical factor in the prevention of surgical site infections. As of 2010, it has been recommended to administer the antibiotics within one hour before the skin incision [33]. Cefazolin is the preferred agent because of its efficacy as a prophylactic agent and excellent safety record in pregnancy [34, 35].

Whether the current antibiotic recommendations are adequate to prevent surgical site infections after cesarean delivery in obese women is unclear. Increased adiposity is accompanied by reduced tissue drug penetration due to decreased vascularity within the tissue. Obesity is also associated with higher glomerular filtration rate for drugs as cefazolin, exclusively cleared by the kidneys. Therefore, BMI increase is associated with lower maternal cefazolin plasma and adipose tissue concentrations. Recent work based on emerging resistance patterns for cefazolin suggests that the old minimal inhibitory concentration (MIC) for Gram-negative organisms of 4 μg cefazolin/g of maternal adipose tissue is insufficient and an MIC of $8\,\mu g\,g^{-1}$ should be observed instead [36]. With the 2 g standard prophylactic cefazolin dose, the majority of obese patients will not achieve above $8\,\mu g\,g^{-1}$ MIC concentrations within the adipose tissue, suggesting that the increased dose of 3 g cefazolin would be advisable [37]. For standard surgical procedures in patients weighing more than 120 kg, the American Society of Health-System Pharmacists also recommends an increased dose of cefazolin (3 g versus the standard 2 g) for preoperative prophylaxis [38]. However, in a retrospective study of 335 obese women, the rate of surgical site infections was not reduced when 3 g cefazolin prophylaxis was used instead of 2 g prophylaxis [39]. In addition to the retrospective design, susceptible to undetected bias, the study may have also been underpowered. Moreover, cefazolin is a concentration-independent antibiotic and factors other than peak concentration may be important for its bactericidal activity, such as the length of time above MIC.

3. What particular anesthesia considerations are applicable?

Anesthesia considerations

According to the 2007 Report on Confidential Enquiries into Maternal Death in the United Kingdom, 67% of deaths directly attributable to anesthesia occurred in obese parturients [40]. Obese pregnant women are at increased risk of failed intubation, aspiration, and nonfunctional epidural anesthesia [41]. In one study, the initial epidural catheter failed, increasing the need for replacement, in 42% of cases of morbid obesity compared to 6% in normal weight women [42]. It also results that obese women have increased odds of requiring general anesthesia, with its additional risks.

The Royal College of Obstetricians and Gynecologists recommends antenatal anesthesiology consultation in cases of morbid obesity [4] and early third trimester may be the ideal time to do that. It is important to point out that, regardless of any potentially existing comorbidities, obesity presents an independent increased risk for mortality and morbidity from both surgery and anesthesia [43].

The obese pregnant women presenting to the labor and delivery unit have to be evaluated by an anesthesiologist early in admission, in order to identify those with difficult airway. Also, the placement of epidural analgesia should be considered early in the labor course, with subsequent low threshold to replace a poorly functioning epidural. Such measures may prevent the need for general anesthesia in an emergency.

In preparation for surgery in morbidly obese patients, longer needles and ultrasound equipment to help with intravenous or arterial catheterization and even neuraxial block placement may prove useful [44]. When general anesthesia is necessary and difficult intubation is anticipated, laryngeal mask airways, fiberoptic bronchoscope and video intubation equipment should be available. It has been found that the risk for difficult intubation at cesarean delivery is increased 16-fold in obese women [45]. Positioning on the table in the ramped-up position (head-up) using a wedge-shaped device or blankets under the patient's upper back and neck improves the laryngoscopic view in extremely obese patients [46].

Most standard operating room tables hold up to 450–500 lb. When the need arises, bariatric tables, which are wider and hold up to 1000 lb, should be obtained. In such extreme cases, specialized equipment for moving the patient may also be necessary, such as bariatric hoist or under-patient air transport system. Appropriate padding must be available to decrease the risk of neural injury and pressure sores and properly sized belts are necessary to minimize intra-operative movement. As one can see, there are logistical delays in transporting the obese patient, positioning the patient in the operating room and obtaining adequate anesthesia. Additional staff are always needed to prepare the patient in the operating room and the so called "30 minute decision-to-incision rule" may prove to be unrealistic at times in morbidly obese women [47]. The skin incision-to-delivery time may also be increased. In women with super-morbid obesity; the average skin incision-to-delivery time was reported to be 16 ± 11 minutes and consequently, in parallel with the BMI increase, a statistically significant raise in the number of cases with umbilical cord blood pH < 7.1–7.2 has been noted [48, 49]. The total operative time at cesarean delivery in morbidly obese women is also increased beyond the delay caused by the prolonged incision-to-delivery interval and independently of the number of prior cesarean deliveries, type of skin incision, or neonatal birth weight [49]. Additionally, obesity poses a risk for increased intra-operative blood loss.

A relationship between increasing BMI and post-operative anemia has been reported [50].

Intra-operatively, standard non-invasive blood pressure monitoring can be challenging due to maternal habitus. Some have suggested the use of invasive monitoring in extremely obese women, especially in those with co-morbid cardiac conditions [51].

Obese pregnant women appear to have a more variable response to intrathecal anesthetic dosing than non-obese women [52]. It has been much published on both the unexpectedly high levels of spinal blockade in morbidly obese women possibly because of decreased cerebrospinal fluid volume [53] and, on the other hand, anesthetic failures in these women even with administration of higher doses of intrathecal anesthetics [52]. In a particular patient, it is impossible to predict if an exaggerated or, on the contrary, an insufficient spinal level will be achieved and general recommendations for reduced or increased spinal doses in obese women cannot be made [4]. Placement of a combined spinal epidural anesthesia (CSE) may allow the anesthesiologist to reduce the spinal dose but also have the option to raise the level of the spinal anesthetic through the epidural catheter if needed or to extend the duration of the anesthesia if surgery is prolonged. CSE, however, is not without risks or failures. Another proposed solution that allows for a lowered-dose spinal anesthetic as well as the ability to extend the block when necessary was the continuous spinal anesthesia (CSA). In this case, an intentional dural puncture is performed. When the patient's BMI is >35, the unintentional dural puncture rate at epidural placement, with the consequent risk of post-dural puncture headache, is double compared to the 2% rate of all placements [42]. With intentional dural puncture at CSA, the rate of post-dural puncture headache is higher than in other types of neuraxial anesthesia and failure is still possible [54]. Although CSA cannot be advocated for routine use, in situations of multiple failed attempts at stand-alone epidural or CSE, or of inadvertent dural puncture, the anesthesiologist may consider intentionally threading an epidural catheter into the intrathecal space [55].

At times, whether for maternal or fetal indication, the use of general anesthesia for cesarean delivery is warranted. Once the patient is successfully intubated, mechanical ventilation may be challenging due to the increased extrathoracic mass weighing on the chest wall. Use of positive end expiratory pressure, pressure control ventilation, and higher FiO_2 may improve ventilation and should be considered [4]. Also, in morbid obesity, the risk of post-operative respiratory failure is higher. In cases of general anesthesia, after extubation, the patient should be maintained on oxygen as needed and longer stays in closely monitored areas may be necessary. Oxygen should be administered continuously until the patient is able to maintain her baseline oxygen saturation on room air. If possible, nonsupine positions in bed are preferred. Obese patients, especially those with obstructive sleep apnea may have an exacerbation of bradypnea, hypoxia and hypercapnia with the use of post-operative opioid analgesics, requiring moderation and increased caution in their use. If patient-controlled systemic opioids are used, continuous background infusions should be used with extreme caution or avoided entirely [55]. Continuous pulse oximetry and capnography may help in monitoring the obese patients. Another option to consider is multimodal analgesia, with the addition of nonsteroidal anti-inflammatory drugs (such as ketorolac) or intravenous acetaminophen if possible.

Compared with systemic analgesia, neuraxial opioids, local anesthetics, or an opioid-anesthetic mixture provide superior analgesia after cesarean delivery, improving the pulmonary status, promoting earlier ambulation and reducing the hospital length of stay [56]. Wound infiltration with local anesthetics at surgery, ilioinguinal nerve block, or ultrasound guided transversus abdominis block [57] may also optimize post-operative analgesia especially in patients who cannot benefit from neuraxial analgesia such as those delivered under general anesthesia [58]. However, some of these nerve block techniques may be challenging in women with a large abdominal panniculus.

4. What are the post-operative considerations relative to thromboprophylaxis?

Thromboprophylaxis

In a large Australian retrospective study, 37.5% of maternal venous thromboembolism cases were related to cesarean delivery and 75% were seen in obese women [59]. However, in current guidelines, obesity alone is considered a minor factor for venous thromboembolism, even in the case of a cesarean delivery. Pneumatic compression devices should be used as recommended for all patients undergoing cesarean delivery [60]. Only if an additional minor risk factor is present (multiple gestation, post-partum hemorrhage, smoking, fetal growth restriction, pre-eclampsia, protein C or S deficiency), the American College of Chest Physicians recommends thromboembolism chemoprophylaxis [61]. This organization has also outlined major risk factors for the development of postpartum thromboembolism and with presence of one such major risk factor they would similarly recommended pharmacologic prophylaxis or mechanical prophylaxis with pneumatic compression devices or elastic stockings in those with contraindications to anticoagulants. Major risk factors are history of venous thromboembolism, pre-eclampsia with fetal growth restriction, high risk thrombophilias, blood transfusion, postpartum infection, or medical comorbidities (sickle cell disease, heart disease, or systemic lupus erythematosus). Chemoprophylaxis may be done with low-molecular weight heparin (LMWH) (such as enoxaparin 40 mg daily) or unfractionated heparin 5000 units every eight hours starting eight hours after delivery. Early ambulation is also encouraged and chemoprophylaxis will be discontinued when the patient ambulates well.

The distribution of LMWH is bodyweight dependent and controversy exists regarding the use of anti-Xa concentrations in thromboembolism chemoprophylaxis monitoring when LMWH is used in obese patients. Anti-Xa concentration is a functional assay that measures the direct inhibition of factor Xa by LMWH. However, anti-Xa concentrations alone do not necessarily correlate with the thrombotic or hemorrhagic risk [62] and the adequate anti-Xa prophylactic range has not been definitely established. Consequently, the American College of Obstetricians and Gynecologists does not recommend routine monitoring of anti-Xa concentrations in women receiving prophylactic anticoagulation [60].

Conclusions

This review has presented the evidence without placing undue emphasis on algorithmic rules. We believe that available evidence must be always individualized for the particular patient because, in the case of the obese surgical patient:

- the abdominal panniculus is not always the same
- additional differences may be generated by gestational age, laboring or non-laboring condition, or the emergency status
- the individual surgeon's experience and preferences should not be neglected.

Given the well-documented risks associated with cesarean delivery in obese women, consideration should be given to developing preventive strategies for reducing the cesarean delivery rate in obese patients. In a French population study, 63% of all primary cesarean deliveries in obese women were either intrapartum deliveries following induction in primiparous women or prelabor deliveries among multiparous women without a scarred uterus [63]. The same findings were reported from Ireland: obesity was associated with an increase in emergency intrapartum cesarean delivery only in primigravidas, particularly post-induction, whereas obese multiparas had an increase in elective cesarean deliveries [64]. Induction of labor is a definite risk factor for cesarean delivery in obese women [63–66]. The empirical observation that inductions tend to be more difficult in obese women is supported by the findings from a secondary analysis of a prostaglandin cervical ripening randomized trial. The investigators reported higher subsequent oxytocin requirements, increased duration of labor and a higher cesarean delivery rate in parallel with BMI increases [67].

Induction in primiparous women and elective cesarean delivery in multiparous women are potentially modifiable practices. It has been reported that primiparous obese women are induced more frequently than normal-weight primiparous women for questionable indications such as nausea, maternal fatigue, previous home delivery, living far away from the hospital [63]. There is no reason why such questionable obstetrical practices could not be changed.

There is little evidence to establish whether elective cesarean delivery is preferable to planned vaginal delivery in morbidly obese women. Older literature seemed to indicate a significantly higher rate of emergency cesarean delivery in morbidly obese women compared to normal weight controls (50% vs 9%) [68]. Anxiety about the need for emergency intrapartum cesarean delivery in technically difficult conditions has undoubtedly contributed to the higher rate of prelabor cesarean deliveries. More recent data, however, indicate that these emergency occurrences are rare, especially in multiparous women, not justifying elective cesarean delivery in obese multiparous women and calling for a change in practice [63]. In a large multicenter cohort study of obese women, it was observed that the majority of obese women attempting vaginal delivery were successful, especially if they had previously delivered vaginally [68].

When deciding on route of delivery in morbidly obese women, the implications of an emergent cesarean delivery in technically difficult conditions and the possibility of neonatal birth injury with attempted vaginal delivery [68] should be considered. Outcome differences between nulliparous and parous women should also be taken into account, with available evidence suggesting that labor induction in obese nulliparous women and elective cesarean delivery in obese multiparous women may not be justified.

References

1 Fisher, S.C., Kim, S.Y., Sharma, A.J. et al. (2013). Is obesity still increasing among pregnant women? Prepregnancy obesity trends in 20 states, 2003-2009. *Prev. Med.* **56**: 372–378.

2 World Health Organization. Obesity and overweight; 2006, http://www.who.int/mediacentre/factsheets/fs311/en/index.html Accessed 15 July 2018.

3 Sturn, R. (2003). Increases in clinically severe obesity in the United States, 1986-2000. *Arch. Intern. Med.* **163**: 2146–2148.

4 Ring, L.E. (2014). The anesthetic approach to operative delivery of the extremely obese parturient. *Semin. Perinatol.* **38**: 341–348.

5 Declercq, E., MacDorman, M., Osterman, M. et al. (2015). Prepregnancy obesity and primary cesareans among otherwise low-risk mothers in 38 U.S. states in 2012. *Birth* **42**: 309–318.

6 Hibbard, J.U., Gilbert, S., Landon, M.B. et al. (2006). Trial of labor or repeat cesarean delivery in women with morbid obesity and previous cesarean delivery. *Obstet. Gynecol.* **108**: 125–133.

7 Poobalan, A.S., Aucott, L.S., Gurung, T. et al. (2009). Obesity as an independent risk factor foe elective and emergency cesarean delivery innulliparous women – systematic review and meta-analysis of cohort studies. *Obes. Rev.* **10**: 28–35.

8 Alanis, M.C., Goodnight, W.H., Hill, E.G. et al. (2010). Maternal superobesity (body mass index ≥ 50) and adverse pregnancy outcomes. *Acta Obstet. Gynecol. Scand.* **89**: 924–930.

9 Smid, M.C., Kearney, M.S., and Stamilio, D.M. (2015). Extreme obesity and postcesarean wound complications in the maternal-fetal medicine unit cesarean registry. *Am. J. Perinatol.* **32**: 1336–1341.

10 Scolari Childress, K.M., Gavard, J.A., Ward, D.G. et al. (2016). A barrier retractor to reduce surgical site infections and wound disruptions in obese patients undergoing cesarean delivery: a randomized controlled trial. *Am. J. Obstet. Gynecol.* **214**: 285.e1–285.e10.

11 Parencevich, E.N., Sands, K.E., Cosgrove, S.E. et al. (2003). Health and economic impact of surgical site infections diagnosed after hospital discharge. *Emerg. Infect. Dis.* **9**: 196–203.

12 Welsh, A. (2008). *Antenatal Care. Routine Care for the Healthy Pregnant Woman*. London: The National Collaborating Centre for Women's and Children's Health.

13 SJ, J.-C. (1978). The place of the abdominal hysterectomy. *Clin. Obstet. Gynaecol.* **5**: 525–543.

14 Krebs, H.B. and Helmkamp, B.F. (1984). Transverse periumbilical incision in the massively obese patient. *Obstet. Gynecol.* **63**: 241–245.

15 Greer, B.E., Cain, J.M., Figge, D.C. et al. (1990). Supraumbilical upper abdominal midline incision for pelvic surgery in the morbidly obese patient. *Obstet. Gynecol.* **76**: 471–473.

16 Alanis, M.V., Villers, M.S., Law, T.L. et al. (2010). Complications of cesarean delivery in the massively obese parturient. *Am. J. Obstet. Gynecol.* **203**: 271.e1–271.e7.

17 Thornburg, L.L., Linder, M.A., Durie, D.E. et al. (2012). Risk factors for wound complications in morbidly obese women undergoing primary cesarean delivery. *J. Matern. Fetal Neonatal Med.* **25**: 1544–1548.

18 Marrs, C.C., Moussa, H.N., and Sibai, B.M. (2014). Skin incision type and wound complications in women with morbid obesity. *Am. J. Obstet. Gynecol.* **210** (**4**): 319.e1.

19 Grantcharov, T.P. and Rosenberg, J. (2001). Vertical compared to transverse incisions in abdominal surgery. *Eur. J. Surg.* **167**: 260–267.

20 Houston, M.C. and Raynor, B.D. (2000). Post-operative morbidity in the morbidly obese parturient woman: supraumbilical and low transverse abdominal approaches. *Am. J. Obstet. Gynecol.* **182**: 1033–1035.

21 Bell, J., Bell, S., Vahratian, A., and Awonuga, A.O. (2011). Abdominal surgical incisions and perioperative morbidity among morbidly obese women undergoing cesarean delivery. *Eur. J. Obstet. Gynecol. Reprod. Biol.* **154**: 16–19.

22 Brocato, B.E., Thorpe, E.M. Jr., Gomez, L.M. et al. (2013). The effect of cesarean delivery skin incision approach in morbidly obese women on the rate of classical hysterotomy. *J. Pregnancy.* **2013**: 890296. doi: 10.1155/2013/890296. Epub 2013 Nov 20.

23 Tixier, H., Thouvenot, S., Coulange, L. et al. (2009). Cesarean section in the morbidly obese woman: supra or subumbilical transverse incision? *Acta Obstet. Gynecol. Scand.* **88**: 1049–1052.

24 Smid, M.C., Smiley, S.G., Schulkin, J. et al. (2016). The problem of the pannus: physician preference survey and a review of the literature on cesarean skin incision in morbidly obese women. *Am. J. Perinatol.* **33**: 463–472.

25 Whitty, R.J., Maxwell, C.V., and Carvalho, J.C. (2007). Complications of neuraxial anesthesia in an extreme morbidly obese patient for cesarean section. *Int. J. Obstet. Anesth.* **16**: 139–144.

26 Chiswick, C., Cooper, E.S., Norman, J.E., and Denison, F.C. (2012). Fat necrosis of the abdominal pannus following caesarean section in patients with morbid obesity. *Eur. J. Obstet. Gynecol. Reprod. Biol.* **160**: 116–119.

27 James, D. and Maher, M. (2009). Caring for the extremely obese woman during pregnancy and birth. *MCN Am. J. Matern. Child Nurs.* **34**: 24–30.

28 Mackeen, A.D., Berghella, V., and Larsen, M.L. (2012). Techniques and materials for skin closure in caesarean section. *Cochrane Database of Syst. Rev.* 11 (Art. No.:CD003577) doi: 10.1002/14651858.CD003577.pub3.

29 Mackeen, A.D., Khalifeh, A., Fleisher, J. et al. (2014). Suture compared with staple skin closure after cesarean delivery: a randomized controlled trial. *Obstet. Gynecol.* **123**: 1169–1175.

30 Figueroa, D., Jauk, V.C., Szychowski, J.M. et al. (2015). Surgical staples compared with subcuticular suture for skin closure after cesarean delivery: a randomized controlled trial. *Obstet. Gynecol.* **121**: 33–38.

31 Dahlke, J.D., Mendez-Figueroa, H., Rouse, D.J. et al. (2013). Evidence-based surgery for cesarean delivery: an updated systematic review. *Am. J. Obstet. Gynecol.* **209**: 294–306.

32 Tuuli, M.G., Liu, J., Stout, M.J. et al. (2016). A randomized trial comparing skin antiseptic agents at cesarean delivery. *N. Engl. J. Med.* **374**: 647–655.

33 American College of Obstetricians and Gynecologists (2010). Committee opinion no. 465: antimicrobial prophylaxis for cesarean delivery: timing of administration. *Obstet. Gynecol.* **116**: 791–792.

34 Tita, A.T., Rouse, D.J., Blackwell, S. et al. (2009). Emerging concepts in antibiotic prophylaxis for cesarean delivery: a systematic review. *Obstet. Gynecol.* **113**: 675–682.

35 Young, O.M., Shaik, I.H., Twedt, R. et al. (2015). Pharmacokinetics of cefazolin prophylaxis in obese gravidae at time of cesarean delivery. *Am. J. Obstet. Gynecol.* **213**: 541:e1–541:e7.

36 Clinical and Laboratory Standards Institute (2010). *Performance Standards for Antimicrobial Susceptibility Testing: Twentieth Informational Supplement*; M100-S20, vol. **30**, No. 1. Wayne (PA): Clinical Laboratory Standards Institute.

37 Swank, M.L., Wing, D.A., Nicolau, D.P. et al. (2015). Increased 3-gram cefazolin dosing for cesarean delivery prophylaxis in obese women. *Am. J. Obstet. Gynecol.* **213**: 415.e1–415.e8.

38 Bratzler, D.W., Dellinger, E.P., Olsen, K.M. et al. (2013). Clinical practice guidelines for antimicrobial prophylaxis in surgery. *Am. J. Health Syst. Pharm.* **70**: 195–283.

39 Ahmadzia, H.K., Patel, E.M., Joshi, D. et al. (2015). Obstetric surgical site infections. *Obstet. Gynecol.* **126**: 708–715.

40 Lewis, G. (2007). *The Confidential Enquiry into Maternal and Child Health (CEMACH). Saving mothers' Lives: Reviewing Maternal Deaths to Make Motherhood Safer – 2003-2005. The Seventh Report on Confidential Enquiries into Maternal Deaths in the United Kingdom.* London: CEMACH.

41 Roofthooft, E. (2009). Anesthesia for the morbidly obese parturient. *Curr. Opin. Anaesthesiol.* **27**: 341–346.

42 Hood, D.D. and Dewan, D.M. (1993). Anesthetic and obstetric outcome in morbidly obese parturients. *Anesthesiology* **79**: 1210–1218.

43 Kramer, C., Zinman, B., and Retnakaran, R. (2013). Are metabolically healthy overweight and obesity benign conditions? A systemic review and meta-analysis. *Ann. Int. Med.* **159**: 758–769.

44 Sahin, T., Balaban, O., Sahin, L. et al. (2014). A randomized controlled trial of preinsertion ultrasound guidance for spinal anaesthesia in pregnancy: outcomes among obese and lean parturients. *J. Anesth.* **28**: 413–419.

45 Rocke, D.A., Murray, W.B., Rout, C.C. et al. (1992). Relative risk analysis of factors associated with difficult intubation in obstetric anesthesia. *Anesthesiology* **77**: 67–73.

46 Collins, J.S., Lemmens, H.J., Brodsky, J.B. et al. (2004). Laryngoscopy and morbid obesity: a comparison of the "sniff" and "ramped" positions. *Obes. Surg.* **14**: 1171–1175.

47 Lucas, D.N. (2010). The 30 minute decision to delivery time is unrealistic in morbidly obese women. *Int. J. Obstet. Anesth.* **19**: 431–435.

48 Conner, S.N., Tuuli, M.G., Longman, R.E. et al. (2013). Impact of obesity on incision-to-delivery interval and neonatal outcomes at cesarean delivery. *Am. J. Obstet. Gynecol.* **209**: 386.e1–386.e6.

49 Girsen, A.I., Osmundson, S.S., Naqvi, M. et al. (2014). Body mass index and operative times at cesarean delivery. *Obstet. Gynecol.* **124**: 684–689.

50 Bodner, L., Siega-Riz, A., and Cogswell, M. (2004). High prepregnancy BMI increases the risk of postpartum anemia. *Obes. Res.* **12**: 941–948.

51 Schwartz, W., Rayburn, W., Turnbull, G., and Christensen, H. (1996). Blood pressure monitoring during pregnancy: accuracy of portable devices designed for obese patients. *J. Reprod. Med.* **41**: 581–585.

52 Carvalho, B., Collins, J., Drover, D.R. et al. (2011). ED(50) and ED(95) of intrathecal bupivacaine in morbidly obese patients undergoing cesarean delivery. *Anesthesiology* **114**: 529–535.

53 Reyes, M. and Pan, P.H. (2004). Very low-dose spinal anesthesia for cesarean section in a morbidly obese preeclamptic patient and its potential implications. *Int. J. Obstet. Anesth.* **13**: 99–102.

54 Gosch, U.W., Hueppe, M., Hallschmid, M. et al. (2005). Post-dural puncture headache in young adults: comparison of two small-gauge spinal catheters with different needle design. *Br. J. Anaesth.* **94**: 657–661.

55 Loubert, C. and Fernando, R. (2011). Cesarean delivery in the obese parturient: anesthetic considerations. *Women's Health* **7**: 163–179.

56 Block, B.M., Liu, S.S., Rowlingson, A.J. et al. (2003). Efficacy of post-operative epidural analgesia: a meta-analysis. *JAMA* **290**: 2455–2463.

57 Belavy, D., Cowlishaw, P.J., Howes, M., and Phillips, F. (2009). Ultrasound-guided transverses abdominis plane block for analgesia after caesarean delivery. *Br. J. Anaest.* **103**: 726–730.

58 Wee, M.Y., Brown, H., and Reynolds, F. (2005). The National Institute of clinical excellence (NICE) guidelines for caesarean section: implications for the anaesthetist. *Int. J. Obstet. Anesth.* **14**: 147–158.

59 Sharma, S. and Monga, D. (2008). Venous thromboembolism during pregnancy and the post-partum period: incidence and risk factors in a large Victorian health service. *Aust. N. Z. J. Obstet. Gynaecol.* **48**: 44–49.

60 American College of Obstetricians and Gynecologists (2011). Thromboembolism in pregnancy. Practice bulletin no. 123. *Obstet. Gynecol.* **118**: 718–729.

61 Bates, S.M., Greer, I.A., Middeldorp, S. et al. (2012). VTE, thrombophilia, antithrombotic therapy, and pregnancy. *Chest* **141**: e691S–e736S.

62 Bergquist, D., Lowe, G., Berstad, A. et al. (1992). Prevention of venous thromboembolism after surgery: a review of enoxaparin. *Br. J. Surg.* **79**: 495–498.

63 Hermann, M., Le Ray, C., Blondel, B. et al. (2015). The risk of prelabor and intrapartum cesarean delivery among overweight and obese women: possible preventive actions. *Am. J. Obstet. Gynecol.* **212**: 241.e1–241.e9.

64 O'Dwyer, V., Farah, N., Fattah, C. et al. (2011). The risk of caesarean section in obese women analysed by parity. *Eur. J. Obstet. Gynecol. Reprod. Biol.* **158**: 28–32.

65 Cnattingius, R., Hoglund, B., and Kieler, H. (2005). Emergency cesarean delivery in induction of labor: an evaluation of risk factors. *Acta Obstet. Gynecol. Scand.* **84**: 456–462.

66 Arrowsmith, S., Wray, S., and Quenby, S. (2011). Maternal obesity and labour complications following induction of labour in prolonged pregnancy. *BJOG* **118**: 578–588.

67 Pevzner, L., Powers, B.L., Rayburn, W.F. et al. (2009). Effects of maternal obesity on duration and outcomes of prostaglandin cervical ripening and labor induction. *Obstet. Gynecol.* **114**: 1315–1321.

68 Clark-Ganheart, C.A., Reddy, U.M., Kominiarek, M.A. et al. (2015). Pregnancy outcomes among obese women and their offspring by attempted mode of delivery. *Obstet. Gynecol.* **126**: 987–993.

Index

Note: Page references in *italics* refer to Figures; those in **bold** refer to Tables and Boxes

Evidence-Based Obstetrics and Gynecology, First Edition. Edited by Errol R. Norwitz, Carolyn M. Zelop, David A. Miller, and David L. Keefe.